FOURTH EDITION

Occupational Therapy
Performance, Participation, and Well-Being

FOURTH EDITION

Occupational Therapy
Performance, Participation, and Well-Being

EDITORS

CHARLES H. CHRISTIANSEN, EdD, OTR, FAOTA

Executive Director
The American Occupational Therapy Foundation
Bethesda, Maryland

CAROLYN M. BAUM, PhD, OTR/L, FAOTA

Elias Michael Director and Professor
Occupational Therapy, Neurology, and Social Work
Washington University School of Medicine
St. Louis, Missouri

JULIE D. BASS, PhD, OTR/L, FAOTA

Professor
Occupational Science and Occupational Therapy
St. Catherine University
St. Paul, Minnesota

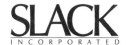

www.healio.com/books

ISBN: 978-1-61711-050-4

Copyright © 2015 by SLACK Incorporated

The procedures and practices described in this publication should be implemented in a manner consistent with the professional standards set for the circumstances that apply in each specific situation. Every effort has been made to confirm the accuracy of the information presented and to correctly relate generally accepted practices. The authors, editors, and publisher cannot accept responsibility for errors or exclusions or for the outcome of the material presented herein. There is no expressed or implied warranty of this book or information imparted by it. Care has been taken to ensure that drug selection and dosages are in accordance with currently accepted/recommended practice. Off-label uses of drugs may be discussed. Due to continuing research, changes in government policy and regulations, and various effects of drug reactions and interactions, it is recommended that the reader carefully review all materials and literature provided for each drug, especially those that are new or not frequently used. Some drugs or devices in this publication have clearance for use in a restricted research setting by the Food and Drug and Administration or FDA. Each professional should determine the FDA status of any drug or device prior to use in their practice.

Any review or mention of specific companies or products is not intended as an endorsement by the author or publisher.

SLACK Incorporated uses a review process to evaluate submitted material. Prior to publication, educators or clinicians provide important feedback on the content that we publish. We welcome feedback on this work.

Published by: SLACK Incorporated
                    6900 Grove Road
                    Thorofare, NJ 08086 USA
                    Telephone: 856-848-1000
                    Fax: 856-848-6091
                    www.Healio.com/books

Contact SLACK Incorporated for more information about other books in this field or about the availability of our books from distributors outside the United States.

Library of Congress Cataloging-in-Publication Data

Occupational therapy (Christiansen)
  Occupational therapy : performance, participation, and well-being / editors, Charles H. Christiansen, Carolyn M. Baum, Julie D. Bass. -- 4th edition.
      p. ; cm.
  Includes bibliographical references and index.
  ISBN 978-1-61711-050-4 (alk. paper)
  I. Christiansen, Charles, editor. II. Baum, Carolyn Manville, editor. III. Bass, Julie D., editor. IV. Title.
  [DNLM: 1. Occupational Therapy. 2. Employment--psychology. WB 555]
  RM735
  615.8'515--dc23
                          2014039446

For permission to reprint material in another publication, contact SLACK Incorporated. Authorization to photocopy items for internal, personal, or academic use is granted by SLACK Incorporated provided that the appropriate fee is paid directly to Copyright Clearance Center. Prior to photocopying items, please contact the Copyright Clearance Center at 222 Rosewood Drive, Danvers, MA 01923 USA; phone: 978-750-8400; website: www.copyright.com; email: info@copyright.com

Printed in the United States of America.

Last digit is print number: 10 9 8 7 6 5 4 3 2 1

DEDICATION

It is with pleasure that I dedicate this edition to my beloved wife, Beth; my esteemed friend and colleague, Kristine Haertl; my children, Carrie, Erik, and Kalle; my friend and colleague, the late Gary Kielhofner; and occupational therapists throughout the world who enact a recognition that participation and quality of life are key outcomes for health care.
Charles H. Christiansen, EdD, OTR, FAOTA

I dedicate this edition to the chapter authors that organized evidence to document the knowledge that occupational therapist can use to address the performance and participation issues faced by people, organizations serving people and populations. My special recognition goes to my daughter, Kirstin Sumner; grandson, Graham; and special friends, Sylvia Rodger, Leeanne Carey, and Helene Polatajko, all who mentor me with their strength and commitment to continued growth.
Carolyn M. Baum, PhD, OTR/L, FAOTA

To family, friends, mentors, colleagues, students, and the people served by occupational therapy—you are my inspiration in all that I do. With gratitude to my daughters, Kathryn and Sarah, and my mother, Lorraine—you are my kindred spirits and your love and support mean the world to me. With special appreciation to Carolyn and Chuck—you welcomed me to be a part of this extraordinary work.
Julie D. Bass, PhD, OTR/L, FAOTA

CONTENTS

Dedication .... *v*

Acknowledgments .... *xi*

About the Editors .... *xiii*

Contributing Authors .... *xv*

Preface .... *xix*

Section I   Occupational Therapy: Promoting Occupational Performance, Participation, and Well-Being and Placing the Focus on Everyday Life 1

Chapter 1   A Welcome to *Occupational Therapy: Performance, Participation, and Well-Being, Fourth Edition* 3
Julie D. Bass, PhD, OTR/L, FAOTA; Carolyn M. Baum, PhD, OTR/L, FAOTA; and Charles H. Christiansen, EdD, OTR, FAOTA

Chapter 2   Health, Occupational Performance, and Occupational Therapy 7
Charles H. Christiansen, EdD, OTR, FAOTA; Carolyn M. Baum, PhD, OTR/L, FAOTA; and Julie D. Bass, PhD, OTR/L, FAOTA

Chapter 3   Theory, Models, Frameworks, and Classifications 23
Carolyn M. Baum, PhD, OTR/L, FAOTA; Julie D. Bass, PhD, OTR/L, FAOTA; and Charles H. Christiansen, EdD, OTR, FAOTA

Chapter 4   The Person-Environment-Occupation-Performance (PEOP) Model 49
Carolyn M. Baum, PhD, OTR/L, FAOTA; Charles H. Christiansen, EdD, OTR, FAOTA; and Julie D. Bass, PhD, OTR/L, FAOTA

Chapter 5   Interventions and Outcomes: The Person-Environment-Occupation-Performance (PEOP) Occupational Therapy Process 57
Julie D. Bass, PhD, OTR/L, FAOTA; Carolyn M. Baum, PhD, OTR/L, FAOTA; and Charles H. Christiansen, EdD, OTR, FAOTA

Chapter 6   Therapeutic Use of Self: A Catalyst in the Client-Therapist Alliance for Change 81
Helene J. Polatajko, PhD, OTReg(Ont), OT(C), FCAOT, FCAHS; Jane A. Davis, MSc, OTReg(Ont), OTR, OT(C); and Sara E. McEwen, PhD, MSc, BSc(PT)

Chapter 7   Using Evidence to Guide Practice 93
Sally Bennett, PhD, BOccThy(Hons)

Section II   Critical Elements of Occupation and Occupational Performance 111

Chapter 8   The Complexity and Patterns of Human Occupations 113
Lena-Karin Erlandsson, PhD, RegOT and Charles H. Christiansen, EdD, OTR, FAOTA

Chapter 9   Occupations of Childhood and Adolescence 129
Sylvia Rodger, BOccThy, MEdSt, PhD; Jenny Ziviani, BAppSc(OT), MOccThy, PhD; and Sok Mui Lim, BOT(Hons), GCert Higher Ed, PhD

Chapter 10   Occupations of Adulthood 157
Kathleen Matuska, PhD, OTR/L, FAOTA and Kate Barrett, OTD, OTR/L

Chapter 11   Occupations of Elderhood 169
Gunilla Eriksson, RegOT, PhD; Margareta Lilja, RegOT, PhD; Hans Jonsson, RegOT, PhD; Ingela Petersson, RegOT, PhD; and Verena C. Tatzer, OT, MSc

Chapter 12   Occupations of Organizations 185
Carol Haertlein Sells, PhD, OTR, FAOTA

Chapter 13   Occupations of Populations 199
Julie D. Bass, PhD, OTR/L, FAOTA

Section III   Person Factors That Support Occupational Performance 215

Chapter 14   Person Factors: Psychological 217
Catana Brown, PhD, OTR/L, FAOTA and Virginia C. Stoffel, PhD, OT, BCMH, FAOTA

Chapter 15   Person Factors: Cognition 233
Adina Maeir, PhD, OT and Shlomit Rotenberg-Shpigelman, MSc, OT

Chapter 16   Person Factors: Sensory 249
Leeanne M. Carey, BAppSc(OT), PhD, FAOTA

Chapter 17   Person Factors: Motor 267
Lisa L. Dutton, PhD, PT and Julie D. Bass, PhD, OTR/L, FAOTA

Chapter 18   Person Factors: Physiological..289
Sandra L. Rogers, PhD, OTR/L

Chapter 19   Person Factors: Meaning, Sensemaking, and Spirituality 313
Aaron M. Eakman, PhD, OTR/L

Section IV   Environment Factors That Support Occupational Performance 333

Chapter 20   Environment Factors: Culture 335
René Padilla, PhD, OTR/L, FAOTA, LMHP

Chapter 21   Environment Factors: Social Determinants of Health, Social Capital, and Social Support..............359
Julie D. Bass, PhD, OTR/L, FAOTA; Carolyn M. Baum, PhD, OTR/L, FAOTA;
Charles H. Christiansen, EdD, OTR, FAOTA; and Kathryn Haugen, REHS/RS

Chapter 22   Environment Factors: Physical and Natural Environment..387
Susan Stark, PhD, OTR/L; Jon Sanford, MArch; and Marian Keglovits, OTD, MSCI

Chapter 23   Environment Factors: Health, Education, Social, and Public Policies........................421
Diane L. Smith, PhD, OTR/L, FAOTA and Stan A. Hudson, MA

Chapter 24   Environment Factors: Technology..441
Jan Miller Polgar, PhD, OTReg(Ont), FCAOT

Section V   Interventions: Principles and Emerging Approaches 465

Chapter 25   Principles Supporting Intervention and Professionalism..467
John D. Fleming, EdD, OTR/L and Penelope A. Moyers Cleveland, EdD, OT/L, FAOTA

Chapter 26   A Person-Centered Strategy: Using Learning Strategies to Enable Performance, Participation, and Well-Being..............485
Timothy J. Wolf, OTD, MSCI, OTR/L and Naomi Josman, PhD, OT(I)

Chapter 27   An Organization-Centered Strategy: Self-Management—An Evolving Approach to Support Performance, Participation, and Well-Being..............499
Joy Hammel, PhD, OTR/L, FAOTA; Marcia Finlayson, PhD, OTReg(Ont), OTR; and
Danbi Lee, OTD, OTR/L

Chapter 28   Educational and Digital Technology Strategies...513
Anita L. Hamilton, BAppSc(OT), MOccThy, Grad Cert(Higher Ed), PhD(Cand) and
Alec I. Hamilton, BEd(Sci), Grad Dip App Child Psych, MAnaly Psych, MCouns(Psych)

Chapter 29   A Population-Centered Strategy: Public and Community Health 527
Gretchen V. M. Stone, PhD, OTR, FAOTA

Section VI   Foundational Knowledge and Resources.. 547

Chapter 30   Enabling Successful Practice Through Application of Business Fundamentals 549
Patricia Nellis, MBA, OTR/L

Chapter 31   Key Occupational Therapy Concepts in the Person-Occupation-Environment-Performance Model: Their Origin and Historical Use in the Occupational Therapy Literature 565
Kathlyn L. Reed, PhD, OTR, FAOTA, MLIS

Financial Disclosures 649
Index 651

ACKNOWLEDGMENTS

We thank the contributors to this edition for their willingness to endure an extended development schedule and to adhere to our requests for specific content and organization. We are grateful to John Bond and Brien Cummings at SLACK Incorporated for believing in this project and having the patience to await its delivery. We also thank April Billick at SLACK Incorporated and students at Washington University in St. Louis and St. Catherine University in St. Paul for "field testing" concepts. Finally, we extend special thanks to Kathryn Haugen for her patient and competent review and editing assistance during the final phases of the project.

ABOUT THE EDITORS

Charles H. Christiansen, EdD, OTR, FAOTA is Executive Director of The American Occupational Therapy Foundation in Bethesda, Maryland, and Clinical Professor, Division of Rehabilitation Sciences, at the University of Texas Medical Branch in Galveston, Texas. Dr. Christiansen is also Principal and Founder, StoryCrafting, Inc, LLC, a private consulting firm for life transitions based in Rochester, Minnesota. As a former senior academic administrator and tenured professor at the University of Minnesota, the University of Texas Medical Branch, and the University of British Columbia, he developed graduate programs and worked on his own research, focusing on patterns of human occupation and their relationship to health, particularly as buffers to create resiliency to stress-related illness and disability. Dr. Christiansen is a Fellow of the American Occupational Therapy Association and a past Vice President and Treasurer of that organization. He is the founding editor of the scientific journal *OTJR: Occupation, Participation and Health*, now well into its fourth decade of publication.

Carolyn M. Baum, PhD, OTR/L, FAOTA is the Elias Michael Director and Professor of Occupational Therapy, Neurology, and Social Work at Washington University School of Medicine in St. Louis, Missouri. Dr. Baum has twice served as President of the American Occupational Therapy Association and was President of the American Occupational Therapy Certification Board (now NBCOT). She currently serves as the Chair of the American Occupational Therapy Foundation's Research Commission and serves on the Executive Board of the Foundation. She has served on the National Center for Medical Rehabilitation Research at the National Institutes of Health and the Institute of Medicine's Committee to Assess Rehabilitation Science and Engineering Needs. In those capacities, she contributed to reports to Congress. Dr. Baum's research is on the relationship of occupation and participation in persons with chronic neurological conditions. She is engaged in research to determine effective interventions and continues her work in the measurement of occupational performance. She consistently contributes her work and the work of her mentees and students to scholarly journals and texts. Dr. Baum was inducted into the AOTF Academy of Research in 2006 for her exemplary and distinguished contributions toward the science of occupational therapy.

Julie D. Bass, PhD, OTR/L, FAOTA is Professor and past Chair, Occupational Science and Occupational Therapy, at St. Catherine University in St. Paul, Minnesota. She was the Founding Director of the Public Health Program at St. Catherine University. Dr. Bass also serves as the Director of Research and Associate Director of the Institute for the Study of Occupation and Health at the American Occupational Therapy Foundation. She is an established and well-published scholar who has been a frequent presenter at national and international conferences and an invited member on several AOTA task force committees. Her areas of expertise include population health and health disparities, program development and evaluation, statistics and research methods, educational methods, and emerging areas of practice for occupational therapy. Dr. Bass is a Fellow of the American Occupational Therapy Association.

CONTRIBUTING AUTHORS

Kate Barrett, OTD, OTR/L (Chapter 10)
OTD Program Director
Occupational Therapy Department
St. Catherine University
St. Paul, Minnesota

Sally Bennett, PhD, BOccThy(Hons) (Chapter 7)
Associate Professor, Occupational Therapy
School of Health and Rehabilitation Sciences
University of Queensland
St. Lucia, Queensland, Australia

Catana Brown, PhD, OTR/L, FAOTA (Chapter 14)
Associate Professor
Midwestern University–Glendale
Glendale, Arizona

Leeanne M. Carey, BAppSc(OT), PhD, FAOTA (Chapter 16)
Professor, Department of Occupational Therapy
School of Allied Health, Faculty of Health Sciences
La Trobe University
Melbourne, Victoria, Australia
Head, Neurorehabilitation and Recovery, Stroke Division
The Florey Institute of Neuroscience and Mental Health
Parkville, Victoria, Australia

Penelope A. Moyers Cleveland, EdD, OT/L, FAOTA (Chapter 25)
Dean of the Henrietta Schmoll School of Health and the
  Graduate College
St. Catherine University
St. Paul, Minnesota

Jane A. Davis, MSc, OTReg(Ont), OTR, OT(C) (Chapter 6)
Lecturer, Department of Occupational Science and
  Occupational Therapy
University of Toronto
Toronto, Ontario, Canada

Lisa L. Dutton, PhD, PT (Chapter 17)
Associate Professor and Director, Doctor of Physical
  Therapy Program
St. Catherine University
St. Paul, Minnesota

Aaron M. Eakman, PhD, OTR/L (Chapter 19)
Assistant Professor
Director of Research, New Start for Student Veterans
Department of Occupational Therapy
College of Health and Human Sciences
Colorado State University
Fort Collins, Colorado

Gunilla Eriksson, RegOT, PhD (Chapter 11)
Researcher, Division of Occupational Therapy
Karolinska Institutet
Stockholm, Sweden
R&D–Neurology Division
University Hospital
Uppsala, Sweden

Lena-Karin Erlandsson, PhD, RegOT (Chapter 8)
Associate Professor, Department of Health Sciences
Lund University
Lund, Sweden

Marcia Finlayson, PhD, OTReg(Ont), OTR (Chapter 27)
Vice Dean (Health Sciences) and Professor and Director
School of Rehabilitation Therapy
Queen's University
Kingston, Ontario, Canada

John D. Fleming, EdD, OTR/L (Chapter 25)
Assistant Professor, Occupational Science and Occupational
  Therapy Department
St. Catherine University
St. Paul, MN

Alec I. Hamilton, BEd(Sci), Grad Dip App Child Psych,
  MAnaly Psych, MCouns(Psych) (Chapter 28)
Psychologist
Matthew Flinders Anglican College
Buderim, Queensland, Australia

Anita L. Hamilton, BAppSc(OT), MOccThy, Grad
  Cert(Higher Ed), PhD(Cand) (Chapter 28)
Lecturer, Occupational Therapy
School of Health & Sport Sciences
Faculty of Science, Health & Education
University of the Sunshine Coast
Maroochydore, Queensland, Australia

Joy Hammel, PhD, OTR/L, FAOTA (Chapter 27)
Professor and Wade Meyer Endowed Chair
Department of Occupational Therapy
Joint Doctoral Program in Disability Studies
University of Illinois at Chicago
Chicago, Illinois

Kathryn Haugen, REHS/RS (Chapter 21)
Preparedness Field Assignee
Centers for Disease Control and Prevention
St. Paul, Minnesota

Stan A. Hudson, MA (Chapter 23)
Associate Director, Center for Health Policy
University of Missouri
Columbia, Missouri

Hans Jonsson, RegOT, PhD (Chapter 11)
Associate Professor, Division of Occupational Therapy
Karolinska Institutet
Stockholm, Sweden

Naomi Josman, PhD, OT(I) (Chapter 26)
Head of PhD Program
Department of Occupational Therapy
Faculty of Social Welfare & Health Sciences
University of Haifa
Haifa, Israel

Marian Keglovits, OTD, MSCI (Chapter 22)
Occupational Therapist
Washington University School of Medicine in St. Louis
St. Louis, Missouri

Danbi Lee, OTD, OTR/L (Chapter 27)
Project Coordinator
University of Illinois at Chicago
Chicago, Illinois

Margareta Lilja, RegOT, PhD (Chapter 11)
Professor, Division of Health and Rehabilitation
Luleå University of Technology
Luleå, Sweden

Sok Mui Lim, BOT(Hons), GCert Higher Ed, PhD (Chaper 9)
Deputy Head of Learning Environment and Assessment
    Development
Assistant Professor
Singapore Institute of Technology
Singapore

Adina Maeir, PhD, OT (Chaper 15)
School Chair and Director of Graduate Studies
School of Occupational Therapy
Faculty of Medicine
Hadassah and Hebrew University
Jerusalem, Israel

Kathleen Matuska, PhD, OTR/L, FAOTA (Chapter 10)
Chair, Occupational Therapy Department
St. Catherine University
St. Paul, Minnesota

Sara E. McEwen, PhD, MSc, BSc(PT) (Chapter 6)
Scientist, Sunnybrook Research Institute, St. John's Rehab
    Program
Assistant Professor, Department of Physical Therapy
University of Toronto
Toronto, Ontario, Canada

Patricia Nellis, MBA, OTR/L (Chapter 30)
Manager of Clinical and Community Services
Program in Occupational Therapy
Washington University School of Medicine in St. Louis
St. Louis, Missouri

René Padilla, PhD, OTR/L, FAOTA, LMHP (Chapter 20)
Associate Dean for Academic and Student Affairs
School of Pharmacy and Health Professions
Executive Director, Office of International Programs
Creighton University
Omaha, Nebraska

Ingela Petersson, RegOT, PhD (Chapter 11)
Deceased

Helene J. Polatajko, PhD, OTReg(Ont), OT(C), FCAOT,
    FCAHS (Chapter 6)
Associate Chair, Graduate Department of Rehabilitation
    Science
Professor, Department of Occupational Science and
    Occupational Therapy
University of Toronto Neuroscience Program
Dalla Lana School of Public Health
University of Toronto
Toronto, Ontario, Canada

Jan Miller Polgar, PhD, OTReg(Ont), FCAOT (Chapter 24)
Professor, School of Occupational Therapy
Western University
London, Ontario, Canada

Kathlyn L. Reed, PhD, OTR, FAOTA, MLIS (Chapter 31)
Associate Professor, Emerita
Texas Woman's University–Houston Center
Houston, Texas

Sylvia Rodger, BOccThy, MEdSt, PhD (Chapter 9)
Division of Occupational Therapy
School of Health and Rehabilitation Sciences
Director of Research and Education
Cooperative Research Centre for Living With Autism
    Spectrum Disorders (Autism CRC)
University of Queensland
St. Lucia, Queensland, Australia

Sandra L. Rogers, PhD, OTR/L (Chapter 18)
Professor, College of Health Professions
School of Occupational Therapy
Pacific University
Hillsboro, Oregon

Shlomit Rotenberg–Shpigelman, MSc, OT (Chapter 15)
Doctoral Student, School of Occupational Therapy
Faculty of Medicine
Hadassah and Hebrew University
Jerusalem, Israel

Jon Sanford, MArch (Chapter 22)
Director, Center for Assistive Technology and
    Environmental Access
Associate Professor, College of Architecture
Georgia Tech
Atlanta, Georgia

Carol Haertlein Sells, PhD, OTR, FAOTA (Chapter 12)
Professor, Department of Occupational Science &
    Technology
University of Wisconsin-Milwaukee
Milwaukee, Wisconsin

Diane L. Smith, PhD, OTR/L, FAOTA (Chapter 23)
Associate Professor, Department of Occupational Therapy
MGH Institute for Health Professions
Boston, Massachusetts

Susan Stark, PhD, OTR/L (Chapter 22)
Assistant Professor of Occupational Therapy, Neurology,
    and Social Work
Washington University School of Medicine in St. Louis
St. Louis, Missouri

Virginia C. Stoffel, PhD, OT, BCMH, FAOTA (Chapter 14)
Associate Professor, Department of Occupational Science
    & Technology
University of Wisconsin–Milwaukee
Milwaukee, Wisconsin

Gretchen V. M. Stone, PhD, OTR, FAOTA (Chapter 29)
Associate Professor Emeritus
Department of Occupational Therapy
School of Health Professions
University of Texas Medical Branch
Galveston, Texas

Verena C. Tatzer, OT, MSc (Chapter 11)
Scientific Staff/Lecturer, Department of Occupational
    Therapy
University of Applied Sciences Wiener Neustadt
Wiener Neustadt, Austria

Timothy J. Wolf, OTD, MSCI, OTR/L (Chapter 26)
Assistant Professor, Program in Occupational Therapy
Department of Neurology
Washington University School of Medicine
St. Louis, Missouri

Jenny Ziviani, BAppSc(OT), MOccThy, PhD (Chapter 9)
Children's Allied Health Research
Children's Health Queensland Health
School of Health and Rehabilitation Sciences
University of Queensland
St. Lucia, Queensland, Australia

PREFACE

The world has changed dramatically since the previous edition of this book was published. As expected, the importance of the global community has become strikingly evident. Occupational therapy has increased in presence, importance, and influence in many countries and is emerging in others—gaining recognition every day. Practice is now driven more than ever by scientific theories and research evidence provided by highly qualified occupational therapy scientists. We expect the trends illustrated by these changes to continue.

The late popular American science writer, Lewis Thomas, is often quoted from an essay about the conditions that lead to progress and result in science:

> What it needs is for the air to be made right. If you want a bee to make honey, you do not issue protocols on solar navigation or carbohydrate chemistry, you put him together with other bees (and you'd better do this quickly, for solitary bees do not stay alive) and you do what you can to arrange the general environment around the hive. If the air is right, the science will come in its own season, like pure honey.[1]

In a similar way, occupational therapy has, for nearly a century, been working to create an environment to "make the air right." That is, it has evolved in a steady manner to identify its place in the family of health care that not only uniquely distinguishes it from other provider groups, but in many ways leads with its awareness that solutions for conditions that significantly interfere with everyday living must be tailored to the individual and planned with particular outcomes in mind. The most important of these outcomes, we assert, enables individuals to engage fully in their lives in a manner that allows them to perform their roles, express their identities, and gain personal satisfaction from this participation. In doing so they flourish and "make the air right" for their own well-being.

One significant and over-arching difference in this edition, as compared with our earlier work, relates to the attention devoted to applying the PEOP Model in practice. We have recognized that while theory is important, it does not always provide a clearly understood road map for those in practice. For this reason, we have devoted a great deal of attention toward explaining how the PEOP Model can be applied in everyday practice. Additionally, we have tried to make clearer the application of the model to systems of care that are provided to groups and populations.

When Adolf Meyer[2] advocated for the mental hygiene movement in the United States during the early 20th century, he recognized that large subsets of the population could benefit from interventions that helped prevent mental illness by addressing problems of living before they resulted in maladaptive behavior and serious illness. The notion that occupational therapy perspectives and interventions can be applied in the service of health promotion and illness prevention is not a new concept; but it has not yet been applied widely among groups and populations. We believe there is great potential in those spheres of care. We hope that this volume contributes to the advancement of efforts in those domains.

We also hope that as this ecological model is applied it will stimulate thought, research, and refinements, so that it can be further evolved as a useful framework for occupational therapists throughout the world.

REFERENCES

1. Thomas L. *The Lives of a Cell. Notes From a Biology Watcher.* New York, NY: Viking Press; 1974:116-117.
2. Christiansen CH. Adolf Meyer revisited: connections between lifestyles, resilience and illness. *Journal of Occupational Science.* 2007;14(2):63-76.

OCCUPATIONAL THERAPY
Promoting Occupational Performance, Participation, and Well-Being and Placing the Focus on Everyday Life

PEOP: Enabling Everyday Living

THE NARRATIVE
The past, current and future perceptions, choices, interests, goals and needs that are unique to the Person, Organization, or Population

PERSON
- Cognition
- Psychological
- Physiological
- Sensory
- Motor
- Spirituality

OCCUPATION
- Activities
- Tasks
- Roles

ENVIRONMENT
- Culture
- Social Determinants
- Social Support and Social Capital
- Education and Policy
- Physical and Natural
- Assistive Technology

Personal Narrative
- Perception and Meaning
- Choices and Responsibilities
- Attitudes and Motivation
- Needs and Goals

Organizational Narrative
- Mission and History
- Focus and Priorities
- Stakeholders and Values
- Needs and Goals

Population Narrative
- Environments and Behaviors
- Demographics and Disparities
- Incidence and Prevalence
- Needs and Goals

OCCUPATION

PERSON

ENVIRONMENT

PARTICIPATION
PERFORMANCE
WELL-BEING

Section I provides the overall framework for our understanding of occupational performance and occupational therapy. Occupational performance is introduced as a central concept that influences health and underpins the profession of occupational therapy. Theories, models and frameworks are used to summarize our knowledge about human occupation and describe the mechanisms by which occupational therapy supports occupational performance, participation, and well-being. The Person-Environment-Occupation-Performance (PEOP) Model and the PEOP Occupational Therapy Process organize and integrate information from occupational science, related disciplines, and occupational therapy professional documentation to support foundational and advanced learning. Therapeutic use of self-based and evidence-based practice are highlighted as core attributes of excellence in occupational therapy practice.

CHAPTER	TITLE	FAQ
1	*A Welcome to* Occupational Therapy: Performance, Participation, and Well-Being, Fourth Edition (Bass, Baum, Christiansen)	• How will this text guide learning about occupational performance, participation, and well-being, as well as the profession of occupational therapy? • What knowledge and skills are needed to be an effective occupational therapy practitioner?
2	*Health, Occupational Performance, and Occupational Therapy* (Christiansen, Baum, Bass)	• What does it mean to be healthy? • How does occupational performance relate to health? • How do specific occupations promote health? • Why is health an important societal issue?
3	*Theory, Models, Frameworks, and Classifications* (Baum, Bass, Christiansen)	• How do theories, models, frameworks, and classifications support problem solving and decision making in occupational therapy practice? • What are some major theories, models, frameworks, and classifications that guide occupational therapy practice?
4	*The Person-Environment-Occupation-Performance Model* (Baum, Christiansen, Bass)	• In the PEOP Model…. ◦ How does the narrative of a person(s), population, or organization influence performance, participation, and well-being? ◦ What are the person factors, environment factors, and occupations that support performance, participation, and well-being?
5	*Interventions and Outcomes: The Person-Environment-Occupation-Performance Occupational Therapy Process* (Bass, Baum, Christiansen)	• In the PEOP Occupational Therapy Process…. ◦ How does a practitioner use narratives and evaluations to guide the occupational therapy process? ◦ What intervention approaches may be used to achieve desired outcomes of occupational therapy? ◦ How is the process similar and different when working with individuals, organizations, and populations?
6	*Therapeutic Use of Self: A Catalyst in the Client-Therapist Alliance for Change* (Polatajko, Davis, McEwen)	• How does an occupational therapy practitioner use self as part of the therapeutic relationship to achieve desired outcomes? • How does therapeutic use of self by occupational therapy practitioners enable their clients' occupational performance, participation, and well-being?
7	*Using Evidence to Guide Practice* (Bennett)	• What is evidence-based practice and how does it support best practice in occupational therapy? • What knowledge and skills are needed in evidence-based practice?

Chapter 1

A WELCOME TO OCCUPATIONAL THERAPY
Performance, Participation, and Well-Being, Fourth Edition

Julie D. Bass, PhD, OTR/L, FAOTA; Carolyn M. Baum, PhD, OTR/L, FAOTA; and Charles H. Christiansen, EdD, OTR, FAOTA

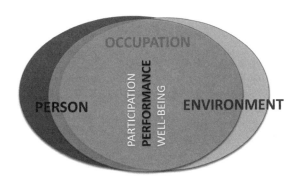

You may be a new student, just beginning your professional education; a faculty member looking for the current evidence in the field; or a practitioner looking for guidance to address problems that your patient, student, client, organization or population is facing. Regardless of your current status, we are all on a journey to acquire the knowledge and skills that support occupational therapy and improve the lives of the people we serve.

If you are a student, it may still be a challenge to explain your chosen profession to others or your rationale for choosing this particular career path. You may know that occupational therapy practitioners "help people" and that the profession is described in terms of both arts and sciences. Your past experiences in occupational therapy may have influenced your current understanding of the profession—maybe you saw a family member have a special relationship with an occupational therapy practitioner or observed a practitioner having fun at their job. You may have realized you weren't quite a fit with related professions—nurses, physical therapists, social workers, teachers, physicians—but couldn't yet define the specific reasons why occupational therapy became the logical choice for a career. You may currently define occupational therapy in terms of a specific intervention or condition that you observed in work or volunteer experiences. You may already have been asked if occupational therapy "helps people find jobs" because a common definition of occupation, of course, relates to vocation. You may have wondered yourself why occupational therapy is called occupational therapy. Stories like these are common among occupational therapy practitioners as they reflect back on their early years of practice—including the authors of this book and some of our most esteemed leaders.

Christiansen CH, Baum CM, Bass JD, eds.
Occupational Therapy: Performance, Participation, and Well-Being, Fourth Edition (pp 3-5).
© 2015 SLACK Incorporated.

If you are a faculty member, you may be looking for an organizing framework for your classes that helps students place the focus on occupations, but also incorporates the critical person and environmental factors that influence performance, participation, and well-being. You may want a core textbook that introduces the essence of current practice, but also provides students with easy access to the evidence that supports practice, prepares students for future opportunities, and positions your program as cutting edge. You also realize that the content in your coursework must be aligned with the *Occupational Therapy Practice Framework,* but you also recognize that our conceptions of practice will change over time and that international perspectives are important to incorporate in your curriculum.

If you are a practitioner, you want your practice to be the best of the best. You have noticed the increasing emphasis on and importance of evidence-based practice, and want to be able to articulate the growing body of knowledge that supports your interventions. You have recognized there are multiple influences on performance, and that environmental influences in particular need more attention in occupational therapy. You realize that there are new opportunities for occupational therapy to support participation and community integration for individuals and groups. You apply Mahatma Gandhi's belief that "you must be the change you wish to see in the world" to your professional development in occupational therapy.

Occupations are central to our engagement in life and the formation of our personal identity. Our occupations may entail work, managing a home, or play. Mary Reilly proposed that the purpose of occupation was to support health—she stated, "Man, through the use of his hands, as they are energized by mind and will, can influence the state of his own health…It falls in the class of one of those great beliefs which has advanced civilization."[1](np)

You are about to learn of the complexity of occupations and how occupational therapy supports performance, participation, and well-being. This learning will help you understand human capacity and environmental supports so you can help people achieve their life goals and overcome the barriers to doing what they want and need to do. Occupational therapy practitioners have a distinct and broad body of knowledge that supports their capacity to help people. This body of knowledge includes human occupation, development, and behavior; environmental supports and barriers; and the biopsychosocial mechanisms that support doing.

We are approaching the 100th anniversary of our profession. In 2017, we will celebrate a century of development. Knowledge has evolved from occupational science, neuroscience, the physical sciences, and environmental science that explains how we as practitioners can use our knowledge and ourselves as tools to help people with developmental disabilities, injuries and illness, mental health problems, and/or chronic health conditions gain the skills to do the ordinary things that are part of everyday living and achieve the profession's Centennial Vision that occupational therapy is a powerful, widely recognized, science-driven, and evidence-based profession with a globally connected and diverse workforce meeting society's occupational needs. In this century, the profession is central to helping society face new populations of children, adults, and older adults whose health is dependent on their engagement in meaningful and challenging physical, cognitive, and social activities. New terms, such as social inclusion and participation, aging in place, primary health care, population health, and self-management, provide occupational therapy practitioners with opportunities to help people gain the skills to manage their health and be active.

Occupational therapy practitioners have many opportunities to exercise their professional roles. You will be called upon to work with children, youth, adults, older adults, families, community residents, organizations, and populations of people. You will find positions in intensive care, acute hospitals, rehabilitation facilities, skilled nursing facilities, home health, hospice, schools, community centers, industry, government, and architectural and engineering firms. All of these roles require occupational therapy practitioners to have a body of knowledge that can be applied across age groups; across practice settings; and with people, organizations, and populations. This body of knowledge is *occupational performance.* Occupational performance requires the practitioner to have knowledge of people's capacity supported by cognitive, psychological, physiological, motor, sensory and spiritual factors, and knowledge of the environment including social support, social capital, culture, the natural, built and physical environment, technology and policy. It also requires the practitioner to view occupations as the activities, tasks, and roles that support development and a meaningful life. This book also introduces the evidence and interventions that that are used in occupational therapy to address the occupational performance issues of people, populations, and organizations.

The following concepts are central to occupational therapy practice and the PEOP Model that serves as the organizing framework for this textbook. These concepts are introduced here and highlighted as important terms that every occupational therapy practitioner will want to integrate into their everyday vocabulary.

- *Occupational performance:* The doing of meaningful activities, tasks, and roles through complex interactions between the person and environment.[2]
- *Occupations:* "The ordinary and familiar things that people do every day."[3](np)

- *Person Factors:* Factors intrinsic to individual(s) that include psychological, cognition, sensory, motor, physiological, and meaning/sense-making/spiritual characteristics that support or limit occupational performance.
- *Environment Factors:* Factors extrinsic to individual(s) that include culture, social, physical and natural, policy, and technology characteristics that support or limit occupational performance.
- *Participation:* Active engagement and involvement in occupations that contribute to well-being.
- *Well-Being:* Satisfaction and quality of life.
- *Narrative:* Important background information from the client in a story format that describes the perception of the current situation and is used to establish goals.
- *Individual:* One person or one small group (eg, a family).
- *Organization:* "Social entities brought into existence and sustained in an ongoing way by humans to serve some purpose, from which it follows that human activities in the entity are normally structured and coordinated towards achieving some purpose or goals."[4(p2),5]
- *Population:* "Body of persons or individuals having a quality or characteristic in common."[6(np),7]

Chapters have been written by national and international authors who have practiced, studied, and compiled the literature to bring you evidence that supports your practice.

We hope you enjoy learning about the many opportunities that occupational therapy has to make a difference in the performance, participation, and well-being for individuals, populations, and organizations.

References

1. Reilly M. Occupational therapy can be one of the great ideas of 20th century medicine. *Am J Occup Ther.* 1962;16:300-308.
2. Baum CM, Christiansen CH, Bass JD. The Person-Environment-Occupation-Performance (PEOP) Model. In: Christiansen CH, Baum CM, Bass JD, eds. *Occupational Therapy: Performance, Participation, and Well-Being.* 4th ed. Thorofare, NJ: SLACK Incorporated; 2015.
3. Christiansen CH, Clark F, Kielhofner G, Rogers J. Position paper: Occupation. *Am J Occup Ther.* 1995;49(10):1015-1017.
4. Rollinson D, Edwards D, Broadfield A. *Organizational Behaviour and Analysis: An Integrated Approach.* New York, NY: Addison Wesley Longman, Inc; 2008.
5. Haertlein Sells C. Occupations of organizations. In: Christiansen CH, Baum CM, Bass JD, eds. *Occupational Therapy: Performance, Participation, and Well-Being.* 4th ed. Thorofare, NJ: SLACK Incorporated; 2015.
6. *Population.* Merriam-Webster Dictionary. http://www.merriam-webster.com/dictionary/population. Updated 2013. Accessed June 6, 2013.
7. Bass JD. Occupations of populations. In: Christiansen CH, Baum CM, Bass JD, eds. *Occupational Therapy: Performance, Participation, and Well-Being.* 4th ed. Thorofare, NJ: SLACK Incorporated; 2015.

Chapter 2

HEALTH, OCCUPATIONAL PERFORMANCE, AND OCCUPATIONAL THERAPY

Charles H. Christiansen, EdD, OTR, FAOTA; Carolyn M. Baum, PhD, OTR/L, FAOTA; and Julie D. Bass, PhD, OTR/L, FAOTA

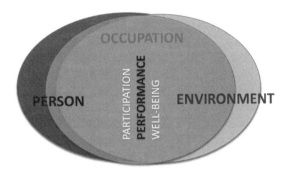

LEARNING OBJECTIVES

- Compare and contrast historical definitions of health.
- Appreciate how differences in the definitions of health influence how health care services are organized and practiced.
- Discuss health status as applied to individuals, organizations, and populations.
- Understand the relationship between health, occupational performance, and quality of life.
- Explain how a focus on occupational performance defines occupational therapy as a service worthy of societal support.
- Appreciate the relationship between services, outcomes, and societal value.

KEY WORDS

- Health
- Health determinants
- Health outcomes
- Occupational performance
- Occupational therapy
- Occupations
- Population health
- Quality of life
- Well-being

INTRODUCTION

In this chapter, we present some basic terms and concepts necessary for understanding the role, purpose, and value of occupational therapy as a client-centered service deserving of societal support. Beginning with an

Christiansen CH, Baum CM, Bass JD, eds.
Occupational Therapy: Performance, Participation, and Well-Being, Fourth Edition (pp 7-21).
© 2015 SLACK Incorporated.

exploration of different definitions of "health," we describe how such definitions evolved and illustrate how they influence societal attitudes, policies, and practices.

We then distinguish among recipients of services, ranging from individuals to organizations to populations. Comprehensive health care requires services that prevent illness and promote and restore health and well-being. Yet, policies and practices differ in the extent to which this scope of services is provided. Moreover, the outcomes that are used to measure the adequacy or quality of health services similarly vary, and these are influenced by definitions that in turn influence policies and laws.

An outcome central to occupational therapy services is *occupational performance,* which we have defined in terms of its connection to everyday living and to broader definitions of participation, health, and well-being. Using this outcome as a lens through which to view occupational therapy services and their overall value to health care, we propose that occupational therapy is a service uniquely capable of bridging the worlds of biomedicine and public health by addressing the everyday life issues that are central to the human condition. Finally, we describe a matrix that illustrates how society's health-related occupational needs can be addressed by different kinds of intervention targeted toward individuals, organizations, and groups. This provides a basis for understanding different occupational therapy models of practice.

DEFINING HEALTH: HOW PERCEPTIONS AND UNDERSTANDINGS OF HEALTH MATTER

The origins of the term *health* derive from words meaning whole, sound, uninjured, and faring well. Within this broad range of concepts related to good fortune or favorable circumstance, one can easily understand how modern definitions of the term *health* vary and may have evolved. In ancient times, ill health was perceived as a state influenced by gods or other supernatural forces. Even today, such divine interpretations of health persist in some cultural and religious practices and traditions.[1]

The ancient Greek physician Hippocrates is credited with influencing a change in definitions of health away from divine explanations to those based in "worldly" conditions. He introduced concepts related to sanitation and nutrition into considerations of health, and proposed that health was related to biological properties requiring a balance of bodily fluids. Clearly, Hippocrates viewed that health involved both the body and its interaction with the surrounding environment.[2]

As medicine evolved, its science was influenced by the views of René Descartes, a 17th century philosopher and mathematician who had a major influence on the scientific revolution. Descartes insisted that knowledge should be guided exclusively by phenomena that can be observed and measured. This "Cartesian" emphasis on observable phenomena had the unfortunate consequence of focusing scientific medicine almost exclusively on the body rather than the mind, with the result that psychological and emotional factors, which we now know are factors that influence the immune system, were disregarded. Science now accepts that health must be seen in a broad, systems-oriented perspective, recognizing that social conditions, attitudes, emotions, habits, and life activities share importance with genetic factors and body functions to determine health status.[3,4]

An additional factor is how people create and derive meaning from their experiences in the world. Both Kielhofner[5] (an occupational therapy practitioner) and Engelhardt[6] (a philosopher and physician) have written about the important role that occupational therapy plays in integrating mind and body phenomena through emphasis on the performance of everyday activities and the meaning of "doing" in the broader life context of the person.

To summarize, as medical science has evolved, it has become clear that personal factors *and* environmental conditions can influence health states. Such changes in understanding have over time influenced health care behaviors and practices at individual, group, and societal (population) levels.

HEALTH FOR INDIVIDUALS, GROUPS, AND POPULATIONS

Scientists have also learned that it is useful to consider health from the standpoint of individuals, groups, and populations. The importance of considering health in these ways has been demonstrated in recent studies that show social networks work to influence health practices and outcomes that affect communities and populations and, of course, the individuals within them. This work has shown that the health of individuals in a social network seems to be influenced both by direct and indirect connections.[7] Thus, obesity, for example, can even be influenced by third-degree relationships (friends of friends that individuals may not have ever met). It is remarkable to consider that a person's lifestyle practices and health habits can have an indirect influence on the health of other members of a larger social group.

Of course, public health professionals have long been concerned with preventing the transmission of infectious disease, and social epidemiologists have studied the social determinants of health, such as attitudes and behaviors. In general, studies have shown that established habits and practices are difficult to change, but they are influenced by social factors, such as societal trends and beliefs. People who believe their behaviors can influence their health may also be more likely to wear seatbelts while driving, avoid smoking and drugs, get regular medical check-ups, and seek immunizations.[8] Different understandings of health by groups can also result in behavioral differences. For example, some religious groups, such as Christian Scientists or Jehovah's Witnesses, oppose traditional medical care and believe that only faith healers should treat illness. Adherents of these religious groups may thus avoid seeking traditional care even during life-threatening emergencies. In other cases, group differences in health behaviors may be influenced by formal policies. For example, employers may differ in how they define and implement sick leave or family leave policies.

Populations may similarly differ in how broadly they define health, and therefore enact social policies that affect the range of services available for preventing or addressing health-related conditions. In the United States, health services provided under Medicaid vary from state to state, based on differences in the policies that govern each state's Medicaid program. Medicaid is a state-federal partnership for providing care for children, adults with low income, pregnant women, impoverished seniors needing long-term care, or persons with disabilities.

Within the enabling legislation[9] (the Social Security Amendments of 1965), Medicaid requires all state programs to meet certain basic requirements. But beyond this, flexibility exists for states regarding the breadth of services they may choose to provide (ie, prosthetic and optometry services), and these may be influenced by budgetary restrictions or the capacity of the state's health and social service infrastructure to provide them. Ultimately, the scope of services provided are also influenced by implicit differences in how health is defined by the policymakers in a given state.

Definitions and understandings of health and illness can also influence societal attitudes toward groups and their individual members. This is readily apparent in the segregation or stigmatization of people with leprosy or other infectious diseases, or how society may assign responsibility for disease states related to behaviors for which there may be moral objections based on social or cultural intolerance (such as sexually transmitted diseases, drug addiction, alcoholism, or obesity).

In an influential paper, medical sociologist Talcott Parsons[10] argued that disease or illness influences everyday social roles by "exempting" persons deemed to be "sick" from fulfillment of their ordinary roles and responsibilities, except for their obligation to seek professional help and to adhere to the treatments prescribed for them. While these social conventions may once have applied to

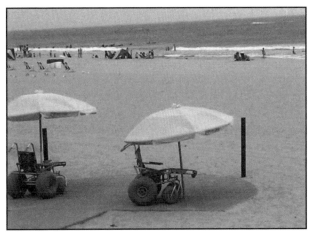

Figure 2-1. Occupational deprivations can also result from public awareness, attitudes and geographical barriers. This accessible park near Virginia Beach, Virginia reflects community awareness that, with accessible accommodations, a day at the beach can be a wonderful leisure experience for everyone, regardless of physical status, thus enabling participation by all. (Reprinted with permission from Edward H.J. Elms, MD.)

acute, transient, and curable illnesses, they become problematic when applied to chronic and disabling conditions; primarily because such conditions are not temporary, but also because the problems that result from them often require self-management rather than medical intervention. Moreover, the consequences of disability are experienced by the persons affected primarily as limitations in their performance of everyday activities and restrictions to their social participation and inclusion. Often, such everyday living consequences can be attributed as much to social policies and environmental characteristics (such as disincentives to work, architectural barriers, or the lack of transportation alternatives) than to ability limitations caused by the condition.

Philosopher/physician H. Tristram Englehardt Jr. expressed the important relationship between health and activity engagement very succinctly when he observed that *"people are healthy or diseased in terms of the activities open to them or denied them."*[11(p672)] His characterization of the experience of illness as framed by participation in everyday activities is consistent with the writing of occupational therapy scientist Gail Whiteford,[12] who makes the distinction between disruptions of everyday occupation that can result from temporary illnesses that restrict social participation and activity engagement (consequences that could result from the flu or travel away from home), and conditions of deprivation that deny an individual the opportunities to participate in valued activities over prolonged periods (Figure 2-1). Whiteford has identified incarceration and refugeeism (voluntary or involuntary) as social conditions that may deprive people of the

Figure 2-2. Differences in how medicine and occupational therapy define order and disorder. (Adapted from Rogers JC. Order and disorder in medicine and occupational therapy. *Am J Occup Ther.* 1982;36[1]:29-35.)

		MEDICINE	
		ORDER= (Health)	**DISORDER=** (Disease)
OCCUPATIONAL THERAPY	**ORDER=** OCCUPATIONAL PERFORMANCE	No intervention from either service or primary prevention and health promotion for well populations.	Medicine needed but occupational therapy not needed. (Example: pneumonia)
	DISORDER= OCCUPATIONAL PERFORMANCE DYSFUNCTION	Occupational therapy needed but medicine unneeded. Example: housing adaptations for normal aging.	Both medicine and occupational therapy are needed. Examples: Arthritis, spinal cord injury, brain injury.

opportunity to participate in necessary or desired everyday activities. Similarly, permanent disabilities, whether involving body or mind, can also lead to deprivation of activity and participation if appropriate social (eg, transportation, financial resources) and rehabilitation services (such as occupational therapy, vocational training, or prosthetic care) are not available or accessible to those so affected.[12]

How concepts are defined can also be useful for explaining how different types of health and social services require different sets of professional skills. Rogers provided a useful illustration of this by comparing medicine with occupational therapy.[3] She described how the ideas of "order" (health) and "disorder" (illness) are defined by medicine and occupational therapy, and how differences in those definitions help explain distinctions in the types of conditions relevant to the two disciplines.

Rogers[13] noted that occupational therapy, with its concern for the everyday living consequences of illness and disease, implicitly sees the desired state (order) in terms of occupational performance, or engagement in life activities important and necessary for the individual. A disordered state is defined by occupational therapy practitioners in terms of occupational performance deficits or the restriction of activity or social participation. In contrast, medicine defines health and illness not by a person's ability to engage in daily activities, but by measures of physiological function.

By making these distinctions between definitions used by medicine and occupational therapy, Rogers was able to illustrate that conditions with physiological and performance consequences require both medicine and occupational therapy, while other circumstances might define conditions where only occupational therapy or medicine

are justified. Figure 2-2 illustrates the manner in which Rogers contrasted medicine and occupational therapy.

ORGANIZATIONAL DEFINITIONS

The manner in which organizations or governments define health is important because such definitions often serve as the starting point for legislative or policy decisions that can affect the type and amount of health services provided within systems.

Typically, policy decisions regarding services that are provided within organizations are influenced by an implicit definition of health that focuses on *preservation of life* rather than *quality of life*. Thus, services for acute care may be given priority over services that support quality of life for chronic, non-urgent, or emergent conditions. Since, as Rogers pointed out, many acute care conditions (such as a bout of pneumonia) represent only temporary disruptions of occupational performance because they are transient, occupational therapy services are not needed. On the other hand, chronic conditions and disabilities are more disruptive and affect quality of life by depriving people of engagement in ordinary daily activities and the inclusive social participation necessary for a meaningful life. Yet, because people can survive with them and may find other ways to cope, occupational therapy services may not be provided because the services are not understood or because of cost concerns.

Ultimately, under current systems of care, it is unlikely that there will ever be sufficient public resources to meet all demands for services that address acute care needs as well as needs important for maintaining a reasonable quality of life. As a result, services will have to be limited (or rationed) in some way. When such policy decisions are made, the principles guiding these decisions are important and they can ultimately be traced back to how policy makers define health and whether or not they see it as an endpoint, or as an enabler for living a life at the highest level of quality possible.

To cite another example, again from the United States, consider the practices of employers who provide health benefits. The system of care in the United States has been dependent for over 60 years on health insurance plans provided by employers as a means for recruiting and retaining employees. Although cost containment efforts have diminished the scope of services covered under such insurance plans and required higher cost sharing by employees, these health insurance plans continue to be offered by employer organizations, who contract with insurance groups to underwrite coverage or manage the plans. As changes in this system have been made over the past 2 decades, more and more choice has been given to employees regarding the kinds of services they are willing to purchase and how much they are willing to pay for the insurance premiums associated with the levels of care they have chosen. Recognizing that overall costs can decline for an employer if employees are healthier, has prompted many employer organizations to encourage healthy behaviors and prevent illness through offering wellness programs and other incentives. These include discounts at health clubs (or the provision of facilities at the worksite) and/or free weight reduction or smoking cessation programs. Employers with more flexible benefit programs may provide options where employees themselves are provided a fixed allocation and decide themselves how to allocate their benefits among many program options. This seems appropriate, as younger workers may want to allocate benefit resources to childcare or maternal and birthing services, while older workers who are caring for aging parents might want to purchase senior care services (such as long-term care or adult daycare). Ultimately, such flexible plans implicitly reflect differences in how organizations define health care benefits.

Naturally, it would be ideal if consensus could be achieved about a single, worldwide or global definition of health. Toward this end, the World Health Organization (WHO), under the aegis of the United Nations, adopted a definition of health in 1948 that serves as the basis for its worldwide health initiatives (Box 2-1). Many governments and organizations—but not all—have embraced the WHO definition of health. It defines health very broadly, as "a complete state of physical, mental, and social well-being, and not merely the absence of disease or infirmity."[14(p100)]

The WHO definition of health has been criticized as too rigid, idealistic, and impractical. For example, critics suggest that use of the word *complete* in the definition

---

BOX 2-1

DEFINING HEALTH: THE WORLD HEALTH ORGANIZATION, THE OTTAWA CHARTER, AND HUMAN RIGHTS

"A state of complete physical, social and mental well-being, and not merely the absence of disease or infirmity."[14(p100)]

In the years since 1948, when the WHO adopted the above definition of health in the preamble to its charter, there has been criticism of the definition as being too vague, impractical, and idealistic. Clearly the definition suggests a broad model of health and wellness that has sociological cultural, psychological, biological, and political elements. The idea, advanced by the WHO, that health is a human right has similarly been criticized, based on specious claims that there is no binding legislation declaring this right or that it is infeasible to ensure that everyone has good health. The Ottawa Charter, adopted by WHO at its first international conference on health promotion in 1986, provided clarity concerning the means to which the right to health should be advanced by member nations, noting that in order to attain optimal health, an individual or group must be able to identify and to realize aspirations, to satisfy needs, and to change or cope with the environment. The charter went on to declare that health is a resource for everyday life, not the objective of living; and that the promotion of health is not just a responsibility for health care providers, but for societies in general. The Ottawa Charter listed the fundamental conditions and resources for health as peace, shelter, education, food, income, a stable ecosystem, sustainable resources, social justice, and equity.[14,15]

---

describes an unachievable state that would be very difficult to attain or maintain. Other critics have observed that "a state of complete physical, mental, and social well-being" seems to correspond more to happiness than to health.

This has led to efforts to propose other definitions that maintain the apparent intent of the WHO definition but add more clarity, flexibility, or practicality to it. For example, Saracci[16] proposed revising the WHO definition as "a condition of well-being, free of disease or infirmity, and a basic and universal human right." In contrast, Bircher's proposed definition is "a dynamic state of well-being characterized by a physical and mental potential, which satisfies the demands of life commensurate with age, culture, and personal responsibility."[17(p337)]

Clearly, definitions of health differ according to their breadth and specificity, and they reflect philosophical differences that are influenced by the practical considerations of health policy. Of course, it is possible for an organization to endorse the ideals behind the WHO definition of health, and yet fail to implement policies or practices that are consistent with that definition. Such lack of alignment or consistency can be the result of insufficient resources or poor implementation strategies.

In this book, a model of occupational therapy practice called the PEOP Model serves as the central organizing framework. The PEOP Model places its emphasis on the person as an individual with unique needs and values, who derives meaning from his or her engagement in the activities, tasks, and roles of everyday life. Personal and environmental factors, and what the person wants and needs to do, influence the individual's occupational performance. When one considers the aims of the model, it is clear that desired outcomes must be considered in terms of a state of well-being that is enabled through occupational performance within an overall context of inclusive social participation. The WHO definition, however idealistic and broad, is therefore consistent with the PEOP Model, which connects the everyday experiences of people with their health and well-being. In the following section, we elaborate on the nature of these relationships.

HEALTH, OCCUPATIONAL PERFORMANCE, AND WELL-BEING

In the early part of the 20th century, a small group of influential and highly committed people recognized that participation in daily occupations both enabled and reflected a person's state of well-being. Nearly a century later, we now know that what people are doing and how they are doing it can often provide many clues about who they are and how they are feeling—both emotionally and physically. What individuals do during a typical day often serves as a window that provides a useful view of their overall well-being.

Activities influence emotions. They may arouse the senses and stimulate attention, motivate people to adapt to challenging or threatening circumstances, impel them to take further action, or stimulate their endocrine systems to release hormones important to their ability to respond. Bruner suggests that the feelings associated with events contribute to the interpretation of experience[18] and help people learn from and remember them. That is, events may

become connected in time with other experiences—and through those connections help people make sense of them. As activities are interpreted in the larger context of personal life stories, they may contribute to identity and provide a sense of continuity or overall coherence.[19,20]

It is clear, then, that our everyday occupations are more complex than they seem. In the following sections we discuss the importance of participation in everyday activities to well-being. We begin with a review of the categories of activity that make up a typical day, and then briefly review the personal and social significance of everyday activities, emphasizing the importance of daily activities to quality of life, personhood, identity, and social roles. Next is a review of how activities influence physiological systems.

DEFINING AND DESCRIBING CATEGORIES OF EVERYDAY ACTIVITIES

Behavioral scientists have tried various approaches to describing or grouping activities according to their characteristics, yet no universal set of categories has been adopted. It is difficult to categorize an activity without knowing more about where it is performed, who it is performed with, when it is performed, and for what purposes.[21] For example, the international game of soccer (known in most countries as football) can be played by professional athletes who earn a living from it or by amateurs as a type of regular recreation. So, is soccer a leisure or play activity, a work activity, or both? The answer depends upon the intended goals of the participants and the context or circumstances of the experience. An activity's context includes the various characteristics of the situation in which it is done.

People don't always do exactly what they want to do, because they have requirements, obligations, and expectations that influence how they use their time. One of the first researchers to develop a classification system proposed that activities be classified according to whether or not they represented endeavors that were necessary (such as sleeping and eating), contracted (such as paid work or school), committed (such as child care, housekeeping, meal preparation, and shopping), or free time (activities chosen during the time remaining after attending to necessary, committed, and contracted activities).[22] Researchers have adopted certain conventions for time-use research that characterize human activity in ways that differ from categories used by occupational therapy practitioners. These categorical differences are influenced by the focus of governments on measuring the economic aspects of time use rather than the social, cultural, and behavioral dimensions of how people spend their time.

EVERYDAY ACTIVITY AS ORGANIZED FROM THE STANDPOINT OF OCCUPATIONAL PERFORMANCE

Occupational therapy practitioners typically divide daily living into several broad categories. These include activities done to earn a living, those related to leisure and recreation, and those related to personal care and self-maintenance, including rest and sleep. The American Occupational Therapy Association (AOTA) groups activities into categories (Table 2-1), including activities of daily living (ADL), instrumental activities of daily living (IADL), rest and sleep, work, education, play, leisure, and social participation.[23(pp631-633)]

Basic and Instrumental Activities of Daily Living

Activities at home and in the community that are designed to enable basic survival and well-being are sometimes referred to as ADLs. These are the duties and chores related to taking care of ourselves, including those related to basic self-care or personal care (such as toileting, bathing, grooming, and dressing), eating, using the telephone, managing medications, and activities related to sexual expression. Sometimes, activities in this category are referred to as personal activities of daily living—and they are fundamental to survival and to living in a social world. This is because they are necessary for good physical and mental health, and also important for group acceptance.

Although not listed in many descriptions of basic activities of daily living (BADL), sleep and its associated routines may also be considered a self-care activity. The revised *Practice Framework* of the AOTA includes rest and sleep as a separate area of human occupation.[23] Sleep constitutes nearly one-third of each day in the lives of typical working adults.[24] In addition to the time it consumes, sleep is also an obligatory occupation that is necessary for health and may have other purposes yet to be fully understood by scientists. Research has shown relationships between activity (including social involvement) and the quality and quantity of sleep.[25]

Instrumental Activities of Daily Living

In 1971, M. Powell Lawton, a gerontologist, recognized that living independently in the community required the ability to accomplish more than personal or basic self-care tasks.[26] These additional and more complex tasks were described by Lawton as IADL. More recently, these have also been referred to as extended activities of daily living, or EADL.[27]

Activities in this category include care of others, care of pets, child rearing, community mobility (getting around in the community), financial management, health management and maintenance, home establishment and management, meal preparation and cleanup, safety and emergency responses, and shopping.

Together, basic self-care tasks and extended self-maintenance activities are viewed as a foundation for survival and for participation in the community. Cross-national research has shown that self-maintenance activities independent of sleep (BADL and IADL together), consume around 20% of the average nondisabled person's waking day.[28] People with disabilities and older persons may require a slightly higher proportion of time to accomplish these self-maintenance activities.[29]

Rest and Sleep

According to the AOTA *Framework*,[23] this category of daily occupations includes activities related to obtaining restorative rest and sleep that support healthy active engagement in other areas of occupation. The particular occupations in this category include rest, sleep, and sleep preparation. Rest includes interruptions in physical or mental activities that promote relaxation and restore energy and interest in resuming active participation. Sleep preparation includes routines related to dressing, grooming, and other practices that prepare the body and its surrounding environment for restorative sleep. Sleep itself includes falling asleep and staying asleep for sufficient duration to enable sleep quality. Sleep quality is a subjective measure, but typically includes feeling a restoration of energy upon awakening.

Because people spend one-third of their lives sleeping, its proportion of human time use is substantial.[30] Despite this, the science underlying sleep remains in its infancy, and scientists are still not in agreement about all of the functions of sleep. Measurement of electrical activity in the brain has consistently shown that restorative sleep involves defined stages, leading to progressively deeper sleep and culminating in REM or rapid eye movement sleep.[31] During REM sleep the individual is dreaming, and it is widely believed that this stage of deep sleep is important for physical and mental restoration.

Research has shown that sleep deficits are related to the incidence of impaired cognition and safety issues, as well as chronic disease and life expectancy.[31-33] In addition to the mental and physical causes, disturbed sleep can be caused by lifestyle factors related to time use, including jet lag, shift work, and other factors leading to disturbances in a person's regular routine. Depression, shift work, conditions that obstruct breathing, noisy environments, stress, and other circumstances can lead to sleep disturbances that, if left untreated, can lead to diminished immune function

Table 2-1.   Areas of Occupation and Specific Activities Within the Areas Found in the American Occupational Therapy Association Practice Framework: Domain and Scope

Activities of Daily Living	Instrumental Activities of Daily Living	Rest and Sleep	Education	Work	Play	Leisure	Social Participation
• Bathing and showering • Toileting and toilet hygiene • Dressing • Swallowing/eating • Feeding • Functional mobility • Personal device care • Personal hygiene and grooming • Sexual activity	• Care of others, (including selecting and supervising caregivers) • Care of pets • Child rearing • Communication management • Driving and community mobility • Financial management • Health management and maintenance • Home establishment and management • Meal preparation and clean up • Religious and spiritual activities and expression • Safety and emergency maintenance • Shopping	• Rest • Sleep preparation • Sleep participation	• Formal educational participation • Informal personal educational needs or interests exploration (beyond formal education) • Informal personal education participation	• Employment interests and pursuits • Employment seeking and acquisition • Job performance • Retirement preparation and adjustment • Volunteer exploration • Volunteer participation	• Play exploration • Play participation	• Leisure exploration • Leisure participation	• Community participation • Family participation • Peer-friend participation

Adapted from American Occupational Therapy Association. Occupational therapy practice framework: domain and process, 3rd edition. *Am J Occup Ther.* 2014;68(Suppl 1):S1-S48.

and other health consequences.[34] The relationship between daily routines and sleep duration and quality is not fully understood, but there does appear to be useful guidance for sleep hygiene, or practices, that contribute to falling and staying asleep in a consistent manner.[35]

Work

Work includes activities needed for engaging in paid employment or volunteer activities.[23] This category includes employment and related activities (such as job seeking and acquisition), job performance, retirement-related activities, and exploration and participation in volunteerism. Time-use scientists recognize that work occurs both in the home and at workplaces outside the home. When scientists want to distinguish between the work of maintaining households and that of earning a living, they refer to the latter category as paid work. With increases in flexibility for where work is performed as well as increases in part-time employment arrangements, the nature of paid work is changing. However, traditional work sites and work groups provide more than income for the people employed there. Even in manufacturing jobs where wages are paid based on piecework (or per each item manufactured or completed), there develops over time a set of relationships among those sharing work time that helps meet human needs for socialization and esteem. Regular work schedules also impose a temporal order on lives, so that the structure of the day and week become important parts of a person's habit patterns, routines, and lifestyle.[36] It is a small wonder that unwanted changes in work routines affect health. For example, there is substantial evidence that unemployment impairs mental health.[37]

Volunteerism consists of contributing one's time and talent toward an area of interest that benefits society or a specific group. Although it is generally accepted that public volunteerism fosters goodwill and trust in groups and in societies by promoting social capital, it also is said to offer the benefit of participation to greater numbers of people, and in so doing provides opportunities for learning and relationship building.[38] Volunteerism enables an individual to contribute knowledge and skills for the benefit of others without obligation and with minimal social expectation beyond altruism and earnest effort. Recent studies have shown a relationship between volunteerism and health and longevity.[39-41]

Education

Education includes activities needed for participating in a learning environment. This classification of activity includes participation in both formal and informal educational pursuits and involves sensory and cognitive processing as well as motor, physiological, and emotional systems.

Although education of both a formal and informal nature occurs throughout life, formal education constitutes a significant portion of time use during a typical week for children and adolescents.[42]

Play

Any spontaneous or organized activity that provides enjoyment, entertainment, amusement, or diversion can be considered play.[43(p252)] According to Sutton-Smith,[44] play is almost impossible to define because it is so ambiguous. He notes that many categories of play that have been named in the scientific literature, including celebrations, rituals, contests, risky play, vicarious or audience play, mind play, solitary play, and informal social play; with each category having multiple examples of activity within it.[44] Huizinga, a highly regarded play scholar, contends that play is fundamental to culture and that it is contained within definite space and time, and pursued voluntarily.[45] Sociologist Caillois,[46] building on Huizinga's work, identified character play, including role playing, competition, chance, and sensation seeking. Societal changes in the 21st century are increasingly mixing features of work and play, presumably thus making the category less distinct as an area of occupation. Professional (paid) sports and gaming businesses are examples of this increasing ambiguity. Moreover, cultural trends toward reshaping workplaces that encourage play, relaxation, innovation, and creativity by workers will contribute to a modification of existing delineations between work and play.[47]

Leisure

Nonobligatory activity that is intrinsically motivated and engaged in during discretionary time is described as leisure.[43] Similar to play, leisure is freely chosen, seems to have an attitudinal component, and is culturally defined.[48] Stebbins identified 2 broad categories of leisure, which he termed *serious leisure* (including hobbies, volunteerism, and self-development efforts), and *casual leisure* (consisting of those activities requiring little effort that are pleasurable, of short duration, and intrinsically rewarding).[49]

Some theories have posited that leisure fulfills needs for agency, novelty, belongingness, service, sensual enjoyment, cognitive stimulation, self-expression, creativity, competition, vicarious competition, and relaxation.[50] A study of unemployed persons conducted by Waters and Moore[51] sought to determine the validity of the needs-based leisure hypothesis. Groups of employed and unemployed subjects were asked to report on their unmet needs, moods, and participation in leisure activities. Unemployed participants engaged in social leisure activities less and solitary activities more, and showed higher levels of depression, lower self-esteem, and greater unmet needs. The results suggested that participation in leisure activities that are meaningful might represent a constructive and readily achievable coping response during unemployment.

In a manner similar to the championing of play in the workplace that is now being introduced in some companies, leisure too has become more ambiguous as societal practices have changed. Digital wireless devices have enabled people to participate in work and social networking anytime and nearly anywhere, while globalization and entrepreneurship have made mixing work and leisure more common. This raises the question of whether or not leisure may soon become an outmoded concept.[52-54]

Social Participation

Social participation constitutes the final area of occupation identified in the contemporary occupational therapy literature. Social participation includes activities that result in successful interaction at the community level, as well as activities that help fulfill required or desired familial or friendship roles. This category also includes activities at different levels for intimacy, including engaging in desired sexual activity.

Christiansen[20] and Bruner[18] assert that an individual's social identity is achieved mainly through activities, and that many activities are pursued as a manifestation of self. This expression of selfhood occurs through the choice of activity, with whom the activity is shared, and even where or how well the activity is conducted.[55]

STUDIES OF PARTICIPATION AND WELL-BEING

The importance of engagement and full participation to well-being and a high quality of life has been demonstrated in recent research involving people with and without functional performance deficits that could limit participation in activities. Many of the studies involving people with disabilities illustrate that functional ability is often not a significant determinant of either participation or well-being.[56] For example, studies of persons with spinal cord injury have found that life satisfaction is most influenced by role performance and the extent of participation in everyday activities, and is not significantly influenced by degree of impairment or disability.[57,58] A study of survivors of traumatic brain injury (TBI) similarly concluded that factors associated with engagement in valued activities in the community predicted life satisfaction.[59]

Studies of able-bodied people have also shown that engagement in valued activities is related to higher levels of perceived well-being (happiness) and life satisfaction. For example, Menec[60] reported a study of elderly persons

in Canada that found happiness was related to activity level. Engagement in social and productive activities predicted greater happiness, increased functional ability, and longer lifespan; whereas participation in more solitary activities (such as hobbies requiring careful handwork) predicted happiness, but not functional ability or longevity. The study suggested that social and productive activities may be more active and therefore result in greater physical benefit as related to function and longer life; whereas solitary activities (such as reading) might provide important psychological benefits that promote well-being. Everard[61] found that activities engaged in for social purposes predicted better well-being than activities pursued simply to pass time.

IMPORTANT BIOLOGICAL CONNECTIONS BETWEEN ACTIVITIES AND HEALTH

Activities also influence physical health, fitness, and cognition. Because technology and lifestyle have created sedentary behavioral patterns that are problematic for maintaining fitness and weight, most people are familiar with admonitions to participate in active exercise to promote cardiovascular fitness or weight maintenance. Abundant evidence supports the value of regular physical regimens for physical and mental health.[62] Literature has also demonstrated that regular physical activity confers cognitive benefits for children and adults.[63-65] However, relationships between activity participation and less obvious influences on physiological states of the body are also important, such as stress and its effects on the immune system (psychoneuroimmunology) and through the role of activity in regulating the body's internal clocks (chronobiology). We explain each of these influences in the sections to follow.

Activity and Stress

Activities influence feelings, inviting reactions that we commonly call emotions. Emotions are increasingly being studied using a construct known as core affect.[66] The concept of core affect is intended to create an understandable structure to explain the very broad area of human emotion.[67]

The idea behind *core affect* is that people have a central disposition, or feeling state. Core affect is based upon 2 dimensions or continua: activation and pleasure. People experience activation along a continuum from fatigue or listlessness to states of high alertness or excitement. Feelings at points along the activation continuum explain the level of energy with which people engage in activity. A tandem continuum is one of pleasure and displeasure. People feel happy, pleased, or positive—or they may feel sad or depressed. This dual continuum of core affect helps to explain why people with depression often feel lethargic or disinclined to act. On the other hand, it also provides a framework for understanding observed associations between energy and positive feelings.

Beyond their core affect, people may also exhibit changes in emotion based on particular events or situations. These shorter duration feelings have been described as prototypical emotional episodes and most closely resemble how activity-related emotions are described and understood by people in everyday life. These episodes have been labeled with commonly understood terms such as surprise, fear, anger, sadness, and happiness. According to current theory, however, they are labels that are more fully explained by examining how underlying levels of activation and pleasure interact with situations to produce the short-term emotional states they represent.

Regardless of the theoretical structures explaining affect, as emotional states change, the human endocrine system releases different hormones designed to ready the body for action. Through the vascular system, the body channels cells carrying nutrients or repair mechanisms to where they will be needed. In stressful circumstances, this system acts as a useful defense. If overused, this process can damage the body's immune system, much as a fireman would get fatigued following too many false alarms. The degree of wear and tear on the human immune system is now calculated through a measurement called allostatic load.[68] The entire process, from emotion to physiological changes, including the consequences of these changes over time, defines an important area of study called psychoneuroimmunology.[69] The term and the process are easy to remember if the term is broken down into its component parts. Psychoneuroimmunology describes how thoughts and feelings work through the neuroendocrine system to influence the body's immune system.

Although it is important to understand how stressful circumstances can influence the immune system through the feelings or emotion-based reactions that accompany them, it is also important to recognize that a person's ability to cope with stressful circumstances involves multiple factors—many of which pertain to activities.[70] Aaron Antonovsky,[19] who developed a widely respected theory of adaptation to stress called *salutogenesis,* identified the creation of meaning as an important component of resilience to the harmful affects of stress. His theory emphasizes the importance of being competent in the performance of tasks, an aspect of coping he called manageability, as another central feature. Manageability of life's roles requires social competence, self-confidence, and other activity-related dimensions of life.

Viewed altogether, this section emphasizes that activity-related dimensions seem to play a central role in helping people manage stress, reduce allostatic load, and thus prevent the chronic diseases that have been found to be associated with the body's physiological reactions to stress.[71]

Activities and Internal Clocks

Another important relationship between activity and health concerns chronobiology, or the science concerning biological rhythms or internal clocks. These clocks influence the rest-activity cycle that influences when people have the energy to pursue greater levels of activity or, conversely, are inclined to be less active. The regularity of habits and routines is greatly influenced by the consistency of these cycles, which seem to be "set" in tune with the environment through a person's performance of activities, tasks, and roles at regular or predicable times. When internal clocks are not "in tune" with the environment, people feel fatigued and "out of sorts." Experienced after intercontinental travel, many people experience know this disruptive state by its common name of *jet lag.*

Regular activities such as social interaction, routine chores such as walking the dog or the timing of meals, and when a person goes to bed help to keep the body's clocks properly set. Research has shown that life events, such as the birth of a baby, death, or even unemployment, can disrupt ordinary rhythms and have a harmful effect on lifestyle and relationships, decrease immune function, and have been associated with depression and anxiety.[72-75]

As the relationship between biological clocks and activity has become better understood, this understanding has led to interventions such as the use of melatonin supplements, regular exposure to light, and practicing consistent routines. This latter approach is strikingly reminiscent of habit-training programs for persons with mental illness that were used as an intervention during the era of Adolf Meyer's theory of psychobiology.[76-79] Further discussion of chronobiology in the context of its influence on patterns of occupation is contained in Chapter 8.

OCCUPATIONAL PERFORMANCE AND THE HEALTH OF POPULATIONS

As an emerging focus of attention, population health is concerned with both the definition and measurement of health outcomes, as well as the roles of health determinants.[80] Population health highlights the influential role of social and economic forces in combination with biological and environmental factors that shape the health of entire populations. Wilcock[81] proposed that participation in valued activities is an important social determinant of the health of populations. This idea led to the concept of occupational justice, an argument that when opportunities for occupational engagement are denied or restricted within a population because of social disadvantage, the individuals so affected are at least indirectly subjected to conditions leading to diminished health.[82] A large body of research documents the associations among various social conditions that limit participation (such as economic disadvantage, discrimination, isolation, unemployment, and inadequate transportation systems) with diminished health outcomes.[83-85]

Illness and Disability as Participation Restrictions

People expect to pursue their goals and participate in the world through their actions and activities. They seldom anticipate that these pursuits will be interrupted by unforeseen events, as they can people are isolated from opportunity, or restricted from participation by environmental circumstances, or worse yet, by illness and disability. For example, in a study of persons 1 year after suffering stroke and receiving acute rehabilitation, Hartman-Maier and colleagues[86] found that dissatisfaction with life was associated with activity limitation and restricted participation. These findings have been confirmed in numerous quantitative and qualitative studies, underscoring the important need for services that go beyond addressing symptoms to enabling the performance of activities that afford full participation in life.[87-89]

Attitudinal Barriers to Participation

Persons with conditions that limit their participation in society, rehabilitation professionals, and social activists have banded together to influence legislation and language in an attempt to change prejudicial attitudes and influence social policy. Recognizing that language influences thought and attitudes, they have worked hard to introduce new terminology that does not perpetuate outdated views, as reflected in outmoded terms such as handicap and disability. The word *disablement* portrays a view that an individual's ability to participate in society is based on a combination of factors, not just the ability of the body to move, sense, or comprehend. These factors include (in addition to body structure and function) people's attitudes; social policies; and physical structures in the built environment, such as buildings, vehicles, and streets. The evolution of this more inclusive perspective on function can lead to a global perspective that reduces stigma and prejudice; encourages inclusive attitudes and policies; and fosters cohesive, healthier communities.[90]

Systems, Services, and Quality of Care

At one level, the extent to which health systems reflect definitions of health and national and political priorities can be examined through comparative statistics. The WHO gathers and reports data on national expenditures and population measures of health, using outcomes such as the percent of gross domestic product (GDP) spent on health services, per capita expenditures on health, how funds are expended, and outcomes such as life expectancy and infant mortality.[91]

Most developed, industrialized countries currently have systems of care that are national in scope and publicly administered (from the standpoint of financing), recognizing that the health of populations requires a coordinated approach if it is to be affordable, accessible, comprehensive, and universal. The United States is a notable exception, in that it does not have a system that provides universal care, even though services funded by states and the federal government account for the vast majority of health care expenditures in the country.[92]

Fineberg[93] points out that despite spending more in total and per capita than any other country, the United States compares poorly to other countries on objective measures of health outcome, including life expectancy and infant mortality (Figure 2-3).[94,95] More problematic is the manner in which health care resources are spent. The amount spent on prevention and community-based management of chronic illness, or on mental health services, is a small fraction of expenditures on acute care services, the majority of which are rendered during the last months of life.[93]

In the United States, the reasons for this have been expressed in many reports of the Institute of Medicine, the medical arm of the National Academies of Science in the United States. These reports consistently point to the lack of coordination of services, provider errors, and a patchwork of policies and regulations among the states and federal government that lead to waste, fraud, and poor alignment of service capabilities with health needs.[96,97] As new systems of care are implemented that decrease hospital use (and thus costs), the focus of occupational therapy at the person, community, and organization level will engage occupational therapy practitioners to demonstrate leadership in building coordinated, client-centered, evidence-based services and community health initiatives that improve health and function.

SUMMARY

In this chapter, we have reviewed definitions of health to illustrate how they have changed to include social and lifestyle factors that influence health, including how people spend their time. We have described how limited definitions of health can influence the provision of services, and we have identified many of the mechanisms that help explain how occupation influences health and how restrictions on participation can diminish the well-being of

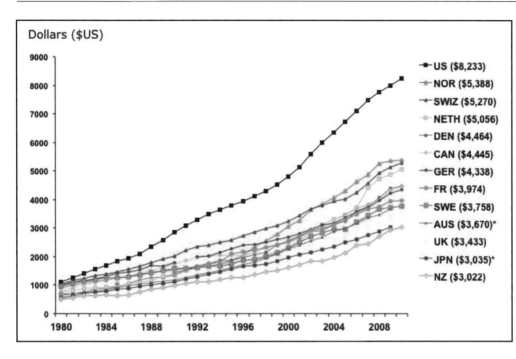

Figure 2-3. Average health care spending per capita, 1980-2010 (adjusted for differences in cost of living). (Adapted from *The US Health System in Perspective: A Comparison of Twelve Industrialized Nations*, [June 2011], published with permission from The Commonwealth Fund, New York, New York.)

persons, groups and populations. We have argued that because meaningful occupational engagement is such an essential element of promoting and maintain health, occupational therapy must be viewed as an essential component of comprehensive health care, including in primary care roles that have previously been seen as less traditional. This underscores the important reality that health outcomes for well populations, as well as those who have disabilities or chronic illnesses, can be influenced by the degree of alignment between services provided and the important person, environment, and performance factors that affect health.

REFERENCES

1. Spector RE. *Cultural Diversity in Health and Illness*. Norwalk, CT: Appleton-Century-Crofts; 1985.
2. Leder D. Medicine and paradigms of embodiment. *J Med Phil.* 1984;9(1):29-44.
3. Engel GL. The need for a new medical model: a challenge for biomedicine. *Science.* 1977;196(4286):129-136.
4. Sullivan M. In what sense is contemporary medicine dualistic? *Cult Med Psych.* 1986;10(4):331-350.
5. Kielhofner G. Motives, patterns, and performance of occupation: basic concepts. In: Kielhofner G. *A Model of Human Occupation: Theory and Application.* 3rd ed. Baltimore, MD: Lippincott Williams & Wilkins; 2002:13-27.
6. Engelhardt H. Occupational therapists as technologists and custodians of meaning. In: Kielhofner G. *Health Through Occupation*. Philadelphia, PA: FA Davis Co; 1983:139-144.
7. Christakis NA, Fowler JH. The spread of obesity in a large social network over 32 years. *N Eng J Med.* 2007;357(4):370-379.
8. Wallston KA. The validity of the multidimensional health locus of control scales. *J Health Psychol.* 2005;10(5):623-631.
9. The Social Security Amendments of 1965. 42. Sect. 226, 89-97 July 30, 1965.
10. Parsons T. The sick role and the role of the physician reconsidered. *The Milbank Memorial Fund Quarterly: Health and Society.* 1975;53(3):257-278.
11. Engelhardt HT Jr. Defining occupational therapy: the meaning of therapy and the virtues of occupation. *Am J Occup Ther.* 1977;31(10):666-672.
12. Whiteford G. Occupational deprivation: global challenge in the new millennium. *Br J Occup Ther.* 2000;63(5):200-204.
13. Rogers JC. Order and disorder in medicine and occupational therapy. *Am J Occup Ther.* 1982;36(1):29-35.
14. Preamble to the Constitution of the World Health Organization as adopted by the International Health Conference, New York, 19-22 June, 1946; signed on 22 July 1946 by the representatives of 61 States (Official Records of the World Health Organization, no. 2, p. 100) and entered into force on 7 April 1948.
15. World Health Organization, Health and Welfare Canada, Canadian Public Health Association. *Ottawa Charter for Health Promotion.* Ottawa, Canada: World Health Organization; 1986.
16. Saracci R. The World Health Organization needs to reconsider its definition of health. *BMJ.* 1997;314(7091):1409-1410.
17. Bircher J. Towards a dynamic definition of health and disease. *Med Health Care Philos.* 2005;8(3):335-341.
18. Bruner JS. *Acts of Meaning.* Boston, MA: Harvard University Press; 1990.
19. Antonovsky A. *Unraveling the Mystery of Health: How People Manage Stress and Stay Well.* San Francisco, CA: Josey-Bass; 1987.
20. Christiansen CH. Defining lives: occupation as identity: an essay on competence, coherence, and the creation of meaning. *Am J Occup Ther.* 1999; 53(6):547-558.
21. Christiansen CH, Townsend EA. *Introduction to Occupation: The Art and Science of Living: New Multidisciplinary Perspectives for Understanding Human Occupation as a Central Feature of Individual Experience and Social Organization.* Upper Saddle River, NJ: Pearson; 2010.

22. Aas D. Designs for large scale time use studies of the 24 hour day. In: Staikov Z, ed. *It's About Time: International Research Group on Time Budgets and Social Activities*. Sofia, Bulgaria: Institute of Sociology at the Bulgarian Academy of Sciences; 1982.

23. American Occupational Therapy Association. Occupational therapy practice framework: domain & process, 3rd edition. *Am J Occup Ther*. 2014;68(Suppl 1):S1-S48.

24. Basner M, Fomberstein KM, Razavi FM, et al. American time use survey: sleep time and its relationship to waking activities. *Sleep*. 2007;30(9):1085-1095.

25. Carney CE, Edinger JD, Meyer B, Lindman L, Istre T. Daily activities and sleep quality in college students. *Chronobiol Int*. 2006;23(3):623-637.

26. Lawton MP. The functional assessment of elderly people. *J Am Ger Soc*. 1971;19(6):465-481.

27. Christiansen C, Rogers S, Haertl K. Functional evaluation and management of self care and other activities of daily living. In: Frontera WR, DeLisa J, Gans B, et al, eds. *DeLisa's Physical Medicine & Rehabilitation*. 5th ed. Philadelphia, PA: Lippincott Williams & Wilkins; 2010:243-288.

28. Fraire M. Multiway data analysis for comparing time use in different countries-application to time-budgets at different stages of life in six European countries. *International Journal of Time Use Research*. 2006;3(1):88-109.

29. McKinnon AL. Time use for self care, productivity, and leisure among elderly Canadians. *Can J Occup Ther*. 1992;59(2):102-110.

30. Roehrs T, Roth T. Sleep disorders: an overview. *Clin Cornerstone*. 2004;6(1):S6-S16.

31. Dew MA, Hoch CC, Buysse DJ, et al. Healthy older adults' sleep predicts all-cause mortality at 4 to 19 years of follow-up. *Psychosom Med*. 2003;65(1):63-73.

32. Chaput JP, Després JP, Bouchard C, Tremblay A. Short sleep duration is associated with reduced leptin levels and increased adiposity: results from the Quebec family study. *Obesity*. 2007;15(1):253-261.

33. Landis CA, Frey CA, Lentz MJ, Rothermel J, Buchwald D, Shaver JL. Self-reported sleep quality and fatigue correlates with actigraphy in midlife women with fibromyalgia. *Nurs Res*. 2003;52(3):140-147.

34. Murphy K, Delanty N. Sleep deprivation: a clinical perspective. *Sleep and Biological Rhythms*. 2007;5(1):2-14.

35. Atkinson G, Davenne D. Relationships between sleep, physical activity, and human health. *Physiol Behav*. 2007;90(2):229-235.

36. Zerubavel E. *Hidden Rhythms: Schedules and Calendars in Social Life*. Berkeley/Los Angeles, CA: University of California Press; 1985.

37. Paul KI, Moser K. Unemployment impairs mental health: meta-analyses. *J Vocat Behav*. 2009;74(3):264-282.

38. Brudner J, Kellough K. Volunteers in state government: involvement, management and benefits. *Nonprofit and Voluntary Sector Quarterly*. 2000;29(1):111-130.

39. Harris AH, Thoresen CE. Volunteering is associated with delayed mortality in older people: analysis of the longitudinal study of aging. *J Health Psychol*. 2005;10(6):739-752.

40. Ayalon L. Volunteering as a predictor of all-cause mortality: what aspects of volunteering really matter? *Int Psychogeriatr*. 2008;20(5):1000-1013.

41. Yaffe K, Fiocco A, Lindquist K, et al. Predictors of maintaining cognitive function in older adults: the Health ABC Study. *Neurology*. 2009;72(23):2029-2035.

42. Hofferth SL, Sandberg JF. How American children spend their time. *J Marriage Fam*. 2001;63(2):295-308.

43. Parham LD, Fazio LS. *Play in Occupational Therapy for Children*. 2nd ed. St. Louis, MO: Mosby/Elsevier Health; 2008.

44. Sutton-Smith B. *The Ambiguity of Play*. Cambridge, MA: Harvard University Press; 2009.

45. Huizinga J. *HomoLudens*. Boston, MA: Beacon Press; 2011.

46. Caillois R. *Man, Play, and Games*. Chicago, IL: University of Illinois Press; 2001.

47. Hirst G, Van Knippenberg D, Zhou J. A cross-level perspective on employee creativity: goal orientation, team learning behavior, and individual creativity. *Acad Manage J*. 2009;52(2):280-293.

48. Thibodaux L, Bundy A. Leisure. In: Jones D, Blair SE, Hartery T, Jones RK, eds. *Sociology and Occupational Therapy: An Integrated Approach*. Philadelphia, PA: Churchill Livingstone; 1998:157-169.

49. Stebbins RA. Casual leisure: a conceptual statement. *Leisure Studies*. 1997;16(1):17-25.

50. Tinsley HE, Eldredge BD. Psychological benefits of leisure participation: a taxonomy of leisure activities based on their need-gratifying properties. *J Couns Psych*. 1995;42(2):123-132.

51. Waters LE, Moore KA. Reducing latent deprivation during unemployment: the role of meaningful leisure activity. *J Occup Organizat Psychol*. 2002;75(1):15-32.

52. Rojek C. *Decentring Leisure: Rethinking Leisure Theory*. London, UK: Sage Publications Limited; 1995.

53. Blackshaw T. *Leisure*. New York, NY: L Routledge; 2010.

54. Rojek C, ed. *Key Issues for the 21st Century: Leisure Studies*. London, UK: Sage Publications Limited; 2010.

55. McAdams DP. *The Stories We Live By: Personal Myths and the Making of the Self*. New York, NY: The Guilford Press; 1993.

56. Dijkers MP. Correlates of life satisfaction among persons with spinal cord injury. *Arch Phys Med Rehab*. 1999;80(8):867-876.

57. Boschen KA, Tonack M, Gargaro J. Long-term adjustment and community reintegration following spinal cord injury. *Int J Rehabil Res*. 2003;26(3):157-164.

58. LoBello SG, Underhil AT, Valentine PV, Stroud TP, Bartolucci AA, Fine PR. Social integration and life and family satisfaction in survivors of injury at 5 years post-injury. *J Rehabil Res Dev*. 2003;40(4):293-300.

59. Corrigan JD, Bogner JA, Mysiw WJ, Clinchot D, Fugate L. Life satisfaction after traumatic brain injury. *J Head Trauma Rehabil*. 2001;16(6):543-555.

60. Menec VH. The relation between everyday activities and successful aging: a 6-year longitudinal study. *The Journals of Gerontology Series B: Psychological Sciences and Social Sciences*. 2003;58(2):S74-S82.

61. Everard KM. The relationship between reasons for activity and older adult well-being. *J Appl Gerontol*. 1999;18(3):325-340.

62. Penedo FJ, Dahn JR. Exercise and well-being: a review of mental and physical health benefits associated with physical activity. *Curr Opin Psychiatry*. 2005;18(2):189-193.

63. Ratey JJ, Loehr JE. The positive impact of physical activity on cognition during adulthood: a review of underlying mechanisms, evidence and recommendations. *Rev Neurosci*. 2011;22(2):171-185.

64. Sibley BA, Etnier JL. The relationship between physical activity and cognition in children: a meta-analysis. *Pediatr Exerc Science*. 2003;15(3):243-256.

65. Hillman CH, Erickson KI, Kramer AF. Be smart, exercise your heart: exercise effects on brain and cognition. *Nature Reviews Neuroscience*. 2008;9(1):58-65.

66. Russell JA. Core affect and the psychological construction of emotion. *Psychol Rev*. 2003;110(1):145-172.

67. Russell JA, Barrett LF. Core affect, prototypical emotional episodes, and other things called emotion: dissecting the elephant. *J Pers Soc Psychol*. 1999;76(5):805-819.

68. Goodkin K, Visser A, Song C, Leonard B. Psychoneuro-immunology: stress, mental disorders, and health. *Psychosomatic Medicine*. 2002;64:847-849.

69. McEwen BS. Central effects of stress hormones in health and disease: understanding the protective and damaging effects of stress and stress mediators. *Eur J Pharmacol*. 2008;583(2):174-185.

70. McEwen BS, Wingfield JC. What's in a name? Integrating homeostasis, allostasis and stress. *Horm Behav*. 2010;57(2):105-111.

71. Ganzel BL, Morris PA, Wethington E. Allostasis and the human brain: integrating models of stress from the social and life sciences. *Psychol Rev*. 2010;117(1):134-174.

72. Monk TH, Reynolds CF, Kupfer DJ, Hoch CC, Carrier J, Houck PR. Differences over the life span in daily life-style regularity. *Chronobiol Int*. 1997;14(3):295-306.

73. Grandin LD, Alloy LB, Abramson LY. The social zeitgeber theory, circadian rhythms, and mood disorders: review and evaluation. *Clin Psychol Rev*. 2006;26(6):679-694.

74. Shen GH, Alloy LB, Abramson LY, Sylvia LG. Social rhythm regularity and the onset of affective episodes in bipolar spectrum individuals. *Bipolar Disord*. 2008;10(4):520-529.

75. Lieverse R, de Vries R, Hoogendoorn AW, Smit JH, Hoogendijk WJ. Social support and social rhythm regularity in elderly patients with major depressive disorder. *Am J Geriatr Psychiatry*. 2013;21(11):1144-1153.

76. Slagle EC. Training aides for mental patients. *Am J Phys Med Rehabil*. 1922;1(1):11-18.

77. Meyer A. *Psychobiology: A Science of Man*. Oxford, UK: Charles C. Thomas; 1957.

78. Meyer A. The philosophy of occupation therapy. *Am J Occup Ther*. 1977;31(10):639-649.

79. Rutter M. Meyerian psychobiology, personality development, and the role of life experiences. *Am J Psychiatry*. 1986;143(9):1077-1087.

80. Kindig D, Stoddart G. What is population health? *Am J Public Health*. 2003;93(3):380-383.

81. Wilcock AA. *An Occupational Perspective of Health*. 2nd ed. Thorofare, NJ: SLACK Incorporated; 2006.

82. Stadnyk R, Townsend EA, Wilcock A. Occupational justice. In: Christiansen C, Townsend E, eds. *Introduction to Occupation: The Art and Science of Living*. Upper Saddle River, NJ: Pearson; 2010:329-358.

83. Wilkinson RG, Marmot MG. *Social Determinants of Health: the Solid Facts*. Geneva, Switzerland: World Health Organization; 2003.

84. Dixon J. Social determinants of health. *Health Promot Int*. 2000;15(1):87-89.

85. Pickett KE, Pearl M. Multilevel analyses of neighborhood socioeconomic context and health outcomes: a critical review. *J Epidemiol Community Health*. 2001;55(2):111-122.

86. Hartman-Maeir A, Soroker N, Ring H, Avni N, Katz N. Activities, participation, and satisfaction one-year post stroke. *Disabil Rehabil*. 2007;29(7):559-566.

87. James BD, Boyle PA, Buchman AS, Bennett DA. Relation of late-life social activity with incident disability among community-dwelling older adults. *Journals of Gerontology Series A: Biological Sciences and Medical Sciences*. 2011;66(4):467-473.

88. Young FW, Glasgow N. Voluntary social participation and health. *Res Aging*. 1998;20(3):339-362.

89. Depp CA, Jeste DV. Definitions and predictors of successful aging: a comprehensive review of larger quantitative studies. *Am J Geriatric Psych*. 2006;14(1):6-20.

90. Breslow L. From disease prevention to health promotion. *JAMA*. 1999;281(11):1030-1033.

91. World Health Organization. *World Health Statistics 2012*. Geneva, Switzerland: World Health Organization; 2012.

92. Martin AB, Lassman D, Washington B, Catlin A, National Health Expenditure Accounts Team. Growth in US health spending remained slow in 2010; health share of gross domestic product was unchanged from 2009. *Health Aff*. 2012;31(1):208-219.

93. Fineberg HV. A successful and sustainable health system—how to get there from here. *N Engl J Med*. 2012;366(11):1020-1027.

94. Organisation for Economic Co-Operation and Development. *Health: Health Indicators: Health Expenditure and Financing: Main Indicators*. OECD StatExtrats. http://stats.oecd.org/. Published 2012. Accessed February 23, 2014.

95. Murray CJ, Frenk J. Ranking 37th—measuring the performance of the US health care system. *N Engl J Med*. 2010;362(2):98-99.

96. Kohn LT, Corrigan JM, Donaldson MS, eds. *To Err is Human: Building a Safer Health System*. Washington, DC: National Academies Press; 2000.

97. Institute of Medicine, National Academies of Science. *Crossing the Quality Chasm: A New Health System for the 21st Century*. Washington, DC: National Academies Press; 2001.

Chapter 3

THEORY, MODELS, FRAMEWORKS, AND CLASSIFICATIONS

Carolyn M. Baum, PhD, OTR/L, FAOTA; Julie D. Bass, PhD, OTR/L, FAOTA; and Charles H. Christiansen, EdD, OTR, FAOTA

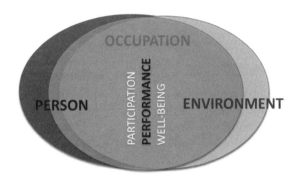

LEARNING OBJECTIVES

- Describe the relationship of theories, models, frameworks, and classifications; and how they work together to support the practitioner's clinical reasoning and ongoing professional growth.
- Highlight major theories and how they support our understanding of the person, environment, and occupational factors, what needs to be assessed and principles underlying interventions that contribute to occupational performance in the people, populations, and organizations that we serve.
- Summarize 4 contemporary models (The Model of Human Occupation [MOHO], The Kawa [River] Model, the Canadian Model of Occupational Performance-Enabling [CMOP-E], and PEOP Model) that can guide the practice of occupational therapy.
- Describe 3 major frameworks that support occupational therapy practice: The AOTA *Practice Framework: Domain and Process*, 3rd Edition; *The Biomechanical Framework for Occupational Therapy*; and *A Cognitive Behavioral Framework*.
- Summarize the International Classification of Functioning, Disability and Health (ICF) from the World Health Organization (WHO) as a classification system.

KEY WORDS

- Classification
- Framework or frame of reference
- Model
- Theory

Christiansen CH, Baum CM, Bass JD, eds.
Occupational Therapy: Performance, Participation, and Well-Being, Fourth Edition (pp 23-47).
© 2015 SLACK Incorporated.

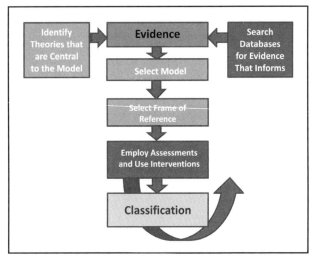

Figure 3-1. The Relationship of Theory, Models, Frames of Reference, and Classifications in the Practice of Occupational Therapy.[1]

INTRODUCTION

Students often ask why we need to study theories and models, and just what are the differences between models and frameworks? Theories, models, frameworks, and classifications are tools that help you, the practitioner, gather and organize information that will allow you to make your unique contribution to health care, education, management, science, or policy. You are entering a profession. As an occupational therapy practitioner, you will make a unique contribution to improving society. Each profession has the obligation to serve a need of society. Occupational therapy's unique contribution to society is the knowledge and skills to support occupational performance. Every profession has its uniqueness. For example, physical therapy's uniqueness is movement, and speech language pathology's is communication, and occupational therapy's is occupational performance (doing). The people that occupational therapy serves may be limited in doing what they want or need to do because of developmental problems, chronic disease, or disability. Or, their conditions or circumstances may put them at risk of being unable to pursue necessary or desired activities, tasks, or roles. They need your services to help them recover and/or develop compensatory strategies or use environmental supports to manage their daily lives, which in addition to caring for themselves may involve caring for others, working, and community participation.

This chapter will introduce the relationship of theories, models, frameworks, and classifications. Each serves a specific purpose in your learning, your practice, and your lifelong learning. Actually, once you understand the role

each plays, you will have resources that will help you organize your approach to your practice and support you as you dialogue with your clients and their families, your colleagues, policy makers in the systems in which you work, payers, the public, and elected officials.

Figure 3-1 describes the relationships of theories, models, frameworks, and classifications. Each element of the figure will be described, and examples of theories, models, frameworks, and classifications will be presented. The work we have elected to describe is not exhaustive, but provides examples for how information is integrated to support your practice. This book is organized around the Person-Environment-Occupational-Performance (PEOP) Model. However, 3 other contemporary occupational performance models are introduced to help you to know how to integrate information to fit the model that will best serve your practice.

At the core of the decision-making process for intervention are 2 things: goals and evidence to inform strategies. *What the client wants from your services is the basis for your goals.* This client may be a person, an organization, or a population with occupational performance needs. The second important element is *evidence.* There is an excellent chapter (Chapter 7) that introduces the process and the knowledge and skills for evidence-based practice. It also describes the process of knowledge translation and how evidence supports clinical reasoning and reflectivity, which are essential to support you in serving those who need your services. We recommend that you read Chapter 7 as a way of understanding how the models presented in this chapter can guide the decision-making process.

THEORIES SUPPORTING WHAT PEOPLE DO

This chapter will put occupation in a developmental context. Primeau and Ferguson support viewing occupation from a developmental perspective, and offer the following assumptions that underpin the value of occupation to persons of all ages[2]:

- Humans have a drive to engage in occupation
- Occupation is complex and multidimensional
- Occupation must be considered within an environmental context
- Occupation is experienced within the context of time
- Occupation holds meaning for the person
- Occupation influences health and well-being

It is important as you read this chapter to focus on occupation as both the product and process of development, the activity as the process used to support

---

BOX 3-1

THEORIES THAT SUPPORT OUR UNDERSTANDING OF PERSON FACTORS

- Motor Behavior Models and Theories[3-7]
- Well-Being[8-27]
- Social Learning Theory and Self-Efficacy[28]

BOX 3-2

THEORIES THAT SUPPORT OUR UNDERSTANDING OF ENVIRONMENT

- Environmental Press[29-31]
- Brofenbrenner's Ecological Systems Theory[32]

---

intervention that will enhance the person's capacity, and the environment as the support for the accomplishment of activities that are central to daily life.

Theories provide knowledge that informs our understanding of major concepts, mechanisms, or constructs that explain the human behavior of performing occupations. Theories are the highest order of knowledge, as they have been tested and their principles are accepted. There are many theories that guide the measurement and interventions aimed at improving occupational performance. For this chapter we have chosen to introduce theories to serve as examples that guide our understanding of occupation—the person factors and the environmental factors (Boxes 3-1 and 3-2)—all of which are central to the occupational therapy practitioner's understanding of occupational performance.

PIAGET'S THEORY OF COGNITIVE DEVELOPMENT

Piaget's theory explains the nature and development of human intelligence. It is a developmental stage theory that addresses the nature of knowledge and how humans acquire, construct, and use knowledge. Many occupational therapy clients have cognitive impairments that require us to understand the processes involved in acquiring, constructing, and using knowledge to support everyday life.

Basic to Piaget's theory are 2 conditions that are present in a dynamic system of continuous change. These dynamic systems are *transformations* and *states*.[33] Transformations refer to the change that humans undergo; states refer to the conditions in which things or persons can be found between transformations (eg, change in shape, change in age, change in the color of objects, or placement of objects). Piaget's position was that human intelligence must be adaptive, as it must represent both the transformation and state aspect of daily life. He proposed that *operative intelligence* manipulates information to follow, recover, or anticipate the transformation of objects or

people. *Figurative intelligence* is the state aspect of intelligence that involves perception, imitation, imagery, and language to retain forms, shapes, and location. These 2 types of intelligence cannot exist independently. Piaget believed that the figurative aspects of intelligence are supportive to the operative and dynamic aspects of operative intelligence that is associated with understanding.[33] Piaget focused on 2 concepts that have become central for occupational therapy practitioners to employ in their interventions: *accommodation* and *assimilation*.[34] Assimilation is how humans perceive and adapt to new information from new learning and from one's environment. Assimilation occurs when humans are faced with new or unfamiliar information and they refer to previously learned information to make sense of it. Accommodation is the process of taking new information and altering previous understanding to fit in the new information. Piaget believed that it is through assimilation that accommodation is derived.[34] Accommodation is essential, as it is through accommodation that people will continue to interpret new information and concepts that support daily life. Other scholars have worked to extend Piaget's theories with newer concepts in learning and cognition as neuroscience research has evolved. One thing that has not changed is the theory supporting assimilation and accommodation, these concepts are central to his theory and rehabilitation approaches.

VYGOTSKY'S SOCIAL DEVELOPMENT THEORY

The work of Lev Vygotsky is a foundation for research and theory development in cognition in both education and rehabilitation. Vygotsky stressed the fundamental role of social interaction in the development of cognition.[35,36] Unlike Piaget's notion that development must proceed learning, Vygotsky perceived that "learning is a necessary and universal aspect of the process of developing culturally organized, specifically human psychological

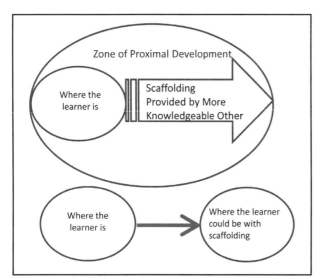

Figure 3-2. The Zone of Proximal Development.[35,37,39]

function."[36(p90)] Vygotsky developed his theories in the 1920s and 1930s, at the same time as Piaget, but he died at an early age; his theories were translated from Russian well into the 1980s. Vygotsky placed more emphasis on culture and social factors as they shaped cognitive development. Both Piaget and Vygotsky claimed that infants are born with the basic abilities for intellectual development; Piaget focused on motor reflexes and sensory abilities, while Vygotsky saw attention, sensation, perception, and memory as essential mental functions.[35]

There are 2 main principles of Vygotsky's work that add a dimension to rehabilitation approaches. The first, the *More Knowledgeable Other* (MKO), and the second, the *Zone of Proximal Development* (ZPD). The MKO refers to someone who has a better understanding or higher ability than the learner with respect to the task, process, or concept. This can be a parent, friend, therapist, teacher, peer, or non-human factor like technology and electronic tools that can assist the learning process.[35] The ZPD relates to the difference between what a child can achieve independently and what a child can achieve with guidance. Wertsch and Tulviste stressed that the instructor or occupational therapy practitioner working with someone inside of the zone of proximal development must be a highly skilled individual who can take into account the teacher-student (occupational therapy practitioner-client) learning process.[37] They proposed that it matters how we are taught, how we practice and refine skills, and who guides us from dependence to independence.

Vygotsky's work is still perceived as very contemporary, as evident in the educational and rehabilitative methods of scaffolding and apprenticeship or mentoring. *Scaffolding* is a strategy in cognitive rehabilitation and the ZPD is a central concept in addressing *excess disabilities,* the gap

between a person's capacity and their performance.[38] Business principles used in rehabilitation have also adopted ZPD; group members with different levels of abilities and advanced peers help others operate within their zone of proximal development. Later in this chapter you will see how Lawton and Nemahow use the term *zone of maximum performance potential* as a concept central to the interaction of capacity and environment to support their aging theory. Figure 3-2 depicts the ZPD and where a learner could be with appropriate scaffolding.[39]

BALTES SELECTIVE OPTIMIZATION WITH COMPENSATION THEORY

The Selective Optimization With Compensation Theory states that older adults maximize their positive and minimize their negative experiences and activities by selection, optimization, and compensation.[40] Older adults choose the most rewarding activities, and select fewer and more meaningful goals and activities as they age, to optimize their experiences through practice and use of new technologies. They also compensate for their losses by finding other ways to accomplish tasks and activities. The occupational therapy practitioner may be helpful in helping the older adult select, optimize, and compensate. This can be done on an individual or population level.

Ontogeny is a scientific term used to describe human development, or the study of development. Ontogeny, or ontogenesis, is defined as "the origin and development of the individual."[41(np)] Baltes proposed the following general principles of lifespan human development[42,43]:

- Growth, stability, and change in behavior occurs throughout life
- There is a continuous interplay between growth (gains) and decline (losses) in ontogeny
- Selection, optimization, and compensation constitute fundamental elements of development
- There is age associated change in adaptive potential (plasticity). These principals are central to occupational therapy's understanding of occupation and the reason for delivering client-centered care

According to Baltes and his colleagues, development is embedded in biological, historical, and cultural contexts. The Selective Optimization With Compensation Theory stresses the interplay among biological, historical, and cultural contexts over time. The influence of different components depends on the particular developmental stage of the individual and the demands of the environment. Development is a lifelong process that is both multidirectional and multidimensional.[43] In early life, the gains outnumber the losses, but the balance shifts as the individual grows older. Multidirectionality creates a

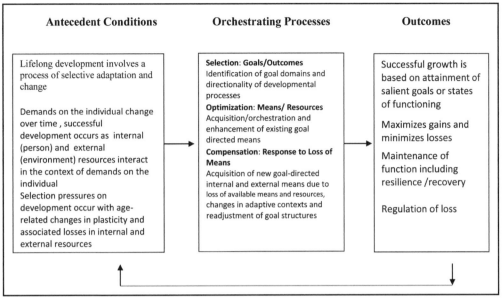

Antecedent Conditions	Orchestrating Processes	Outcomes
Lifelong development involves a process of selective adaptation and change Demands on the individual change over time , successful development occurs as internal (person) and external (environment) resources interact in the context of demands on the individual Selection pressures on development occur with age-related changes in plasticity and associated losses in internal and external resources	**Selection: Goals/Outcomes** Identification of goal domains and directionality of developmental processes **Optimization: Means/ Resources** Acquisition/orchestration and enhancement of existing goal directed means **Compensation: Response to Loss of Means** Acquisition of new goal-directed internal and external means due to loss of available means and resources, changes in adaptive contexts and readjustment of goal structures	Successful growth is based on attainment of salient goals or states of functioning Maximizes gains and minimizes losses Maintenance of function including resilience /recovery Regulation of loss

Figure 3-3. The Lifespan Model of Selective Optimization With Compensation. (Reproduced with permission from Baltes PB, Staudinger UM, Lindenberger U. Lifespan psychology: theory and application to intellectual functioning. *Annual Review of Psychology.* 1999;50[1]:471-507. ©1999 Annual Reviews.)

balance between growth and decline. As some behaviors and capacities are lost, new skills, abilities, and attitudes emerge.[44] In later life, physical capacities often decline but wisdom, emotional, and creative energy are believed to increase; it is possible to achieve the same goal by the use of different mechanisms. Older adults and persons with disabilities may maintain important roles by guiding the actions of others rather than by physically performing the specific tasks. For example, a grandmother may share her recipes for holiday foods with her granddaughter rather than prepare the meal herself, or a person with a disability may hire a personal attendant to perform tasks that are difficult or require time they want to use for something else. Neither diminishes their contributions because they don't do the task themselves.

Multidimensionality also insures that the individual has a variety of resources available to support engagement in roles and responsibilities at each stage of life. The relative allocation of physical, cognitive, and emotional resources shifts across the lifespan. In early life, growth functions are prominent, maintenance functions characterize mid-life, and regulation and accommodation of loss occurs when maintenance and recovery are no longer possible (Figure 3-3).

MOTOR BEHAVIOR MODELS AND THEORIES

Human movement is beautiful, complex, and challenging to explain. How does a musician learn to master the coordinated movements of 2 hands to play a guitar or violin? How is it possible that a toddler develops skill in walking over such a short period of time? Why do movement patterns sometimes change after an injury or illness?

Our understandings and explanations of movement have evolved significantly over the last century. Many disciplines have contributed to models and theories of human movement (Table 3-1), including physics, engineering, statistics, behavioral science, cognitive science, human factors, physiology, medicine, and allied fields. Each discipline has areas of inquiry that has advanced the science and provided important questions for research. However, the disciplinary nature of movement science has also led to variations in the use of terminology and inconsistency in the naming and framing of theories and models. Thus, this chapter represents one explanation of concepts, models, and theories of movement.

Motor behavior has sometimes been used as an overarching term for all of the areas of study related to human movement.[3,4] Motor learning, motor control, and motor development are commonly used concepts used to organize the major theories and models of motor behavior (Table 3-2). The models and theories of motor behavior that are used to guide occupational therapy intervention approaches have evolved from 3 disciplinary traditions: physiology (neurophysiology), neuroscience, and behavioral science (psychology). In recent years, researchers from these 3 traditions have collaborated to propose more comprehensive understandings of movement and motor behavior. In this chapter, an overview of recent motor behavior theories and models will be provided, with an emphasis on ideas that are congruent with the PEOP Model.

The systems model of motor behavior has been proposed as an overarching model for recent theories of

Table 3-1.   *Contributions of Disciplines to Models and Theories of Movement*

Discipline	Main Contributions
Physics	Identification of factors that enable and limit performance
Engineering	Role of feedback in motor control
Statistics	Variability in movement
Behavioral science	Prediction and control of observable behaviors
Cognitive science	Internal processes that contribute to movement
Human factors	Application of science to practical problems involving movement
Physiology	Biomechanical and neuroscience factors contributing to movement
Medicine	Diagnosis of conditions resulting in motor behavior problems
Allied health professions	Treatment of conditions resulting in motor behavior problems

Table 3-2.   *Definitions of Motor Concepts*

Concept	Definition
Motor behavior	An area of study stressing primarily the principles of human skilled movement generated at a behavioral level of analysis.[3(p455)]
Motor learning	The changes in performance that occur as a direct result of practice; a set of internal processes associated with practice or experience leading to a relatively permanent change in the capability for skilled behavior; (does not include) changes in behavior that are due to maturation or growth, or momentary fluctuations in performance attributable to temporary factors[3(p320)]; changes, associated with practice or experience, in internal processes that determine a person's capability for producing a motor skills.[4(p11)]
Motor control	An area of study dealing with the understanding of neural, physical, and behavioral aspects of movement.[3(p455)]
Motor development	A field of study concerning the changes in motor behavior occurring as a result of growth, maturation, and experience.[3(p466)]
Motor performance	The observable production of a voluntary action, or a motor skill; susceptible to fluctuations in temporary factors such as motivation, arousal, fatigue, and physical condition.[4(p11)]
Motor skill	A skill for which the primary determinant of success is the quality of the movement that the performer produces.[4(p4)]

motor control, motor development, and motor learning. It is consistent with the explanation of occupational performance in the PEOP Model, and includes assumptions that have been introduced in recent theories of motor learning, motor control, motor skills, and motor development, including the following[5(p188)]:

- Personal and environmental systems interact to achieve functional goals

- Movement emerges from the interaction of many systems
- Systems are dynamical, self-organizing, and heterarchical
- Movement used for a task is the preferred means for achieving a functional goal
- Changes in one or more systems can alter behavior.

There are many similarities in the motor behavior theories that have been proposed in the physiology

Table 3-3.   Systems Models and Theories of Motor Behavior

Theory	Description	Resources
Dynamical Systems Theory of Motor Control[6]	• Coordinated movement, as observed in effective performance, is possible because the many parts of the body are constrained to work together as a unit or coordinative structure to achieve a functional goal. • The complexity of the motor system (ie, degrees of freedom) is controlled by the development of coordinative structures that act as a functional unit. • Stable and preferred movement patterns (ie, attractors) are self-organizing and developed for specific tasks, but also allow for flexibility in movement.	*Theorists:* Nikolai Bernstein Karl Newell Michael Turvey *Disciplines:* Neuroscience Physiology Kinesiology
Ecological Approach to Perception and Action[7]	• There is a close link between perception and action. • Perception and action is influenced by functional goals and environmental factors. • Affordances, or the perceived functional utility of an object, as identified by an individual influences the relationship between perception and action.	*Theorists:* James Gibson *Disciplines:* Ecological psychology Human factors Kinesiology Cognitive neuroscience
Dynamic Systems Theory of Motor Development[6]	• Temporal: Engagement in movement at one point in time sets the stage for changes in future movement. • Nonlinear, softly assembled systems: Movements are shaped by the interaction of many systems and are flexible and variable. • Embodiment: Perception, action, and cognition are embodied in an integrated system. • Individuality: Individuals develop individual solutions for individual problems.	*Theorists:* Esther Thelen *Disciplines:* Human development Kinesiology
Motor Learning[4,6]	• Stages of Learning: The stages of learning a task (cognitive, associative, automatic) influence the nature of observed movement and the level of cognitive effort required. • Types of Tasks: The nature of motor learning is influenced by the type of task (discrete, continuous, serial) and the predictability of the environment (open, closed). • Practice: Different types of practice (eg, massed, distributed, blocked, random, whole, parts) result in different outcomes for motor learning. • Feedback: Different types of feedback (intrinsic/implicit, extrinsic/explicit, concurrent, immediate, terminal, delayed, knowledge of results [KR], knowledge of performance [KP]) for motor performance influence outcomes for motor learning.	*Theorists:* Paul Fitts and Michael Posner Richard Schmidt Antoinette Gentile Anne Shumway-Cook *Disciplines:* Kinesiology Exercise science Neuroscience

(neurophysiology), neuroscience, and behavioral science (psychology) traditions (Table 3-3). The Dynamical Systems Theory of Motor Control, Ecological Approach to Perception and Action, Dynamic Systems Theory of Motor Development, and Recent Motor Learning Theories have emphasized the importance of studying movement within a task; both person and environment factors as influencing movement, cognitive contributions to movement, and the aspects of movement that are unique to the person.

A brief summary of these 4 theories are provided here. The Dynamical Systems Theory of Motor Control provides an explanation for how coordinated, stable movements are possible in performing a complex task (eg, writing your signature), despite the many body structures and functions that contribute to the motor behavior; body parts are constrained to work together to achieve a performance goal.[6] The Ecological Approach to Perception and Action emphasizes the links among person factors (perception), environmental factors, and performance (action); each individual develops a perception of an object in terms of its functional use (eg, affordance) which in term influences motor behavior.[7] The Dynamic Systems Theory of Motor Development describes the influence of many person and environmental systems on movement and how integration and interaction of these systems shape the individuality and flexibility of motor behavior over time.[6] Recent motor learning theories identify how stages of learning, types of tasks, practice experiences, and feedback on performance are important in understanding changes in movement.[4,6]

WELL-BEING: AN OUTCOME RELATED TO HEALTH AND OCCUPATION

In seeking to clarify people's ideas about the relationships between health, well-being, and occupation, it is important to state that the ideas held and practices associated with health have been dominated by medical science. This is not suggesting the medical science approach is necessarily incorrect, but our understanding can be informed by other knowledge bases. Additionally and, in part because of acceptance of a medical science view, current social and political thinking does not fully acknowledge people's need for a range of meaningful occupations as important for health; rather, occupations are seen principally as an economic requirement. The WHO's holistic view of health and well-being includes an appreciation of the association between positive health and what people do.[8] It is possible to state, quite categorically, that people have occupational needs that are related to health. The doing of something is used to overcome physiological, psychological, or social discomfort and maintain the well-being of the organism. Well-being may be defined as "a subjective assessment of health which is less concerned with biological function than with feelings such as self-esteem and a sense of belonging through social integration;"[9(p126)] and a "sense of contentment and order"[10(pp312-313)] that contributes to meaning, acceptance, and belonging in one's life.

Well-being has been linked with income, employment, social supports, community adhesion, perceived status and marital state, education, religious attitudes, beliefs and activities, the quality of the environment, and quality of life in general.[11-19] In some instances it is used interchangeably with wellness. The term *wellness* has become increasingly popular and is used to represent a range of notions about what are deemed to be healthy behaviors such as physical fitness; not smoking; not overeating or drinking excessively; adequate and regular sleep and meals; meaningful and productive work; and loving, caring relationships.[20] Thus, well-being is firmly linked with holistic notions of health.

Physical, mental, and social well-being appears to call for a variety of prerequisite skills and abilities.[21] Physical well-being is the aspect of health that has received the most attention and is the easiest to understand. When people experience physical well-being, they are able to carry out occupations they need or wish to do without undue consideration of body functioning. Mental well-being encompasses ideas about the development of emotional, intellectual, and spiritual capacities, which, in combination, enables people to interact effectively with others, be reflective, problem solve, make decisions, cope with stress, clarify values and beliefs, be flexible, and find meaning in their lives.[22] Social well-being is dependent on satisfying interpersonal relationships within "just" cultural and social parameters that permit or encourage people to develop ideas deemed of benefit to society or to challenge injustice. What constitutes well-being varies for different people, not only because of the uniqueness of human beings, but because of the potential for variation in the physical, mental, and social dimensions frequently used to describe well-being, and also because individuals may assign different levels of significance and meaning to those dimensions.

Nutbeam viewed well-being within the broad context of a social model of health,[9] and Doyal and Gough went so far as to suggest that "to be denied the capacity for potentially successful social participation is to be denied one's humanity."[23(p184)] If social participation is a precondition of basic needs, then community well-being must consider a community's cultural and spiritual philosophies, socially dominant views, and type of economy. One challenge in post-industrial societies is individualistic and material values, as sustained by market forces that often take precedence over community well-being. Individuals in large urban communities may be particularly at risk of having a paucity of social contacts, and as a result may be susceptible to stress and illness. That is perhaps particularly true for people with disabilities, who may have occupational deprivation and, thus, fewer personal contacts. Blaxter found that "those who had the fewest family, friendship, working, and community roles had the lowest psychosocial well-being, and—for all age/gender groups except the young men—it is obvious that low income and lack of social support are each associated with high illness." She found that "not only socioeconomic circumstances and the external environment, but also the individual's psychosocial environment, carry rather more weight as determinants of health than healthy or unhealthy behaviors."[24(pp105-109,223,233)]

A Holistic View of Health, Well-Being, and What People Do

The Ottawa Charter for Health Promotion is a central document in world health policy which resulted from the combined wisdom of 212 delegates representing 38 countries at the first WHO Health Promotion Conference in 1986.[8] The document stresses that the favored roles of health professionals should be those of advocate, enabler, and mediator. The charter states "to reach a state of complete physical, mental and social well-being, an individual or group must be able to identify and to realize aspirations, to satisfy needs and to change or cope with the environment."[8(p2)]

Wilcock challenged occupational therapy to recognize and build services to support people in realizing their aspirations, satisfying their needs, and coping with their environments.[25] People in general may not adequately understand the central place of occupation in health and well-being in their lives, and such understanding is of primary and general importance. As health practitioners adopt a health promotion direction they must[25]:

- Give stronger attention to occupation for health research and make changes in professional education and training to help enable all people to better understand occupation for health
- Work toward changing attitudes and the organization of health services to increase an understanding and inclusion of occupation for health concepts
- Refocus on the needs of individuals as whole persons including their occupational personae

Well-being from an occupation and health perspective needs to embrace the notions of happiness, personal potential, community action, and client-centeredness. It requires facilitation and utilization of a range of physical, social, and emotional experiences as people go about meeting their basic needs. Engagement in occupation provides physical exercise, motivation, socialization, opportunities to develop self-esteem, meaning, and purpose, as well as intellectual challenge.[26,27]

SOCIAL LEARNING THEORY AND SELF-EFFICACY

Learning would be exceedingly laborious, not to mention hazardous, if people had to rely solely on the effects of their own actions to inform them what to do. Fortunately, most human behavior is learned observationally through modeling; from observing others one forms an idea of how new behaviors are performance, and on later occasions this coded information serves as a guide for action.[28(p22)]

Bandura introduced a social element to learning theory in the early 1970s. His theory states that people can learn both information and behaviors by watching other people. This concept has become central to rehabilitation; however, practitioners do not often discuss the theory nor make it explicit. His work has become known as Social Learning Theory. There are 3 key concepts imbedded in Social Learning Theory[28]:

1. People can learn through observation
2. Internal mental states are necessary to support the learning
3. Learning does not necessarily result in changed behavior

Observational Learning

There are 3 basic elements of observational learning, all of which are important in a client-occupational therapy practitioner interaction. First, the individual or the client demonstrates or acts out the behavior that the occupational therapy practitioner is enabling the person to learn. Second, the practitioner and the client describe and explain the behavior. Third, a symbolic model with either real or fictional characters displays the target behavior in books, films, TV, or other electronic media. It is important to remember new behaviors can be learned by observation, but people can learn new information without demonstrating behavioral change.[28]

The Importance of Mental States

Although external or environmental reinforcement can influence behavior, Bandura believed intrinsic reinforcement or rewards like pride, satisfaction, and a sense of accomplishment were also essential. By relating internal thoughts to cognition, his theory incorporates memory, performance, and judgment (among other things).[28]

Learning Does Not Necessarily Lead to a Change in Behavior

There are important approaches that must be used by the occupational therapy practitioner and the client to enable social learning to be successful. Learning requires *attention to the model.* Anything that detracts attention is going to have a negative effect on observational learning. The material must be interesting or novel in order to dedicate full attention to learning. The ability to *store information* is important to the learning process; linking a prior experience to the current experience will help with retention. Later, access of the information and reproduction are also necessary to change behavior. After the person has paid attention to the model and retained the information, practicing the learned behavior will lead to improvement and skill advancement.[28]

In social learning theory, the individual has to be motivated to imitate the behavior that has been modeled and regulate or control behavior. People can perform *self-observation* by reviewing their behavior. People also can *compare their performance with standards* such as rules. They also can *set a goal, make a resolution, or set up a competition* with others or even with themselves. At the center of this theory, individuals' actions and reactions are influenced by the actions observed in others. Social learning theory can provide a theoretical context for occupational therapy approaches, as learning through observation is central in helping people manage disabling and chronic health conditions.[28]

Self-efficacy is also a key component in Bandura's social cognitive theory. Self-efficacy is one's belief in one's ability to perform specific actions; self-efficacy develops from the person's perception of others.[28] Self-efficacy does affect human behavior; people generally avoid activities where self-efficacy is low. Self-efficacy that is beyond a person's actual ability leads to overestimation of abilities; self-efficacy that is significantly lower than ability discourages growth and skill development. The optimum level of self-efficacy is slightly above ability, and when this is the situation a person attempts tasks and gains experience.[45] People with high self-efficacy are more likely to make efforts to complete a task, persist longer, and are more active in their efforts.[28] People with low self-efficacy believe tasks to be harder than they are, and those with high self-efficacy are stimulated to greater efforts. Self-efficacy also influences how people set their health goals.[46]

People with high self-efficacy generally believe that they are in control of their own lives. Bandura identifies 4 factors that affect self-efficacy[28]:

1. Success raises self-efficacy, failure lowers it.
2. Modeling success increases self-efficacy.
3. Social persuasion or encouragement is helpful in increasing self-efficacy.
4. Physiological responses of distress, fatigue, and fear may be interpreted by someone with low self-efficacy as inability.

These factors must be understood to create a better learning and therapeutic environment.

THEORIES AT THE ENVIRONMENT LEVEL

Historically, occupational therapy literature has recognized the importance of creating opportunities for meaningful interactions with the environment as the basis for promoting health through occupation.[47,48] Although these visionaries challenged the profession to address the environment, it was not until the 1970s and 1980s that occupational therapy practitioners began to talk about the environment as central to the experience of occupation. Two theorists, Lawton and Brofenbrenner, influenced occupational therapy's understanding of the environment and will be discussed in this section.

Environmental Press Theory

Powell Lawton, an environmental psychologist, described the "good life" as composed of 4 elements that are central to an occupational therapy practitioners approach to measurement and intervention.[29] The elements are behavioral competence (person factors), psychological well-being, perceived quality of life, and the objective environment (environmental factors). He was explicit in stating that each of these elements implies individual and social goals that are defensible, without regard to how much the effect of change in one is reflected in change in another. Thus, all are important and involve the engagement in occupations with others.[29] He and his colleague, Lucille Nahemow, proposed a model (the Environmental Press Model) describing that stress and adaptation depend on the fit between environmental demands and an individual's competence to meet them. Their initial work led to the Ecological Theory of Adaptation and Aging,[30] and proposed that the theory can be used to understand how the person and environment interact regardless of age. A number of occupational therapy practitioners continue to use this theory to pose questions to guide their research and clinical practices. We think it is an important theory that highlights the importance of the person-environment interactions that are central to occupational performance.[30]

The Ecological Theory of Adaptation and Aging considers the person as an individual whose collective abilities, identified as biological, cognitive, motor, and sensory/perceptual capacities, are defined as competence. Competence is influenced by environmental press, or the forces present in the environment and their demand characteristics. In occupational therapy, these environmental factors would be social support, social capital, determinants of health, culture, policy, the physical environment and technology (adaptive and mobility equipment), and the natural environment (terrain and weather). All of these factors will be introduced in the PEOP Model and reported in chapters in this book. Press can be negative and positive or even neutral. Their theory is expressed as the "environmental docility hypothesis." This hypothesis states that the more competent the organism, in terms of health, intelligence, ego strength, social role performance, or cultural evolution, the less will be the proportion of variance in behavior attributable to physical objects or conditions around him or her. With high degrees of competence, a person may rise above his or her environment; however, a reduction in competence heightens the person's behavioral dependence on external conditions.[31]

The theory is represented graphically in Figure 3-4. It shows that individual competence and environmental press as represented by the adaptation level of the competence interacting with the environment. In rehabilitation we want to create the opportunity for the individual to be in the zone of maximum performance potential to foster improvement. When the environmental press increases slightly, the problems the client/patient faces increase—but remain within the individual's capacity. This can be equated to the term *activity analysis* used by occupational therapy practitioners to support recovery and progress toward the client's goal. The principles of the theory are in Table 3-4. This theory posits that the individual is operating at his best when the environmental press is moderately challenging. If the environment offers little challenge, the individual adapts by functioning below his or her capacity. If the environment is too challenging or stressful the individual may adapt by disengaging from the activity. It is the responsibility of the occupational therapy practitioner to provide the just right challenge.[30]

Ecological Systems Theory

Brofenbrenner's Ecological Systems Theory emanated from his roots in developmental psychology and his perception of the inadequacies and limitations of the understanding of the interdependencies of people and their social settings, as it related to their development.[32] In his theory, the person is viewed as a social agent who interacts with multiple levels of the environment in order to develop and bring understanding and meaning into his or her life. The environment is described in terms of the social and cultural milieu of the individual. It is depicted as a series of nested circles that radiate from the individual to include personal groups, informal social structures, and societal institutions. Figure 3-5 depicts the specific levels included in the theory.[32]

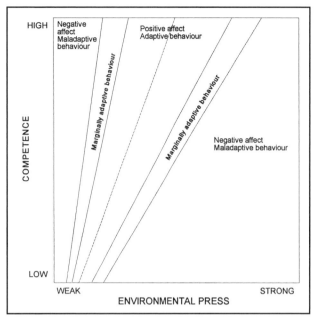

Figure 3-4. Ecological Theory of Adaptation and Aging: Environmental Press and Competence.[30]

Brofenbrenner's work is of importance to occupational therapy practitioners, as it places the emphasis on the social nature of the individual and helping clients understand and use resources in their social environment that create a person, environment, and occupational interaction. The theory was developed to describe human development and it can be used by occupational therapy practitioners to understand life span changes within the context of social systems. The interaction between the person and environment is critical for child development, but also for the learning and development that must occur when a disability or chronic health condition affects a person at any stage in their development.[32]

MODELS AND THEIR USE

A model is an image of an object, system, or process.[49] It also describes the general functional relationship among components of a system.[50] Of particular importance to the occupational therapy practitioner, it allows the practitioner to formulate a problem in a written description and visual representation of predicted relationships between entities and the stressors to which they may be exposed.[51] By understanding the components of models, the practitioner knows the information that must be collected and uses it to frame the problems the client may have that may benefit by occupational therapy services.

In this section we have chosen to introduce 4 of the evolving occupational therapy models.[1] Having models is

Table 3-4.   *Principles Central to the Lawton and Nahemow Theory[30]*

Principles

- Individual competence is the ability that enables an individual to function (person factors).
- Environmental press is the concept that is attributable to Murray in 1938. The aspects of the environment that act in concert with a personal need (occupations) to evoke behavior by the person.
- Adaptive behavior is the externally observable behavior of the individual based on the assumption that fulfillment of one's own potential pleasure to others and performances of complex tasks are equally important and can be achieved. The goal is to have an adaptive behavior that fits between the zone of maximum comfort and the zone of maximum performance potential.
- Affective response is the self-evaluated quality of the experience.
- Adaptation level is being able to screen out awareness of our visual, auditory, thermal, and other environments in order to concentrate attention and effort on the tasks that are central to living.
- Optimization function is the behavior that will be optimized if it fits within the zone of maximum comfort and the zone of maximum performance potential. As stimuli proceed further toward either higher or lower levels in intensity, the person may begin to evoke a negative response (bored, acting out).

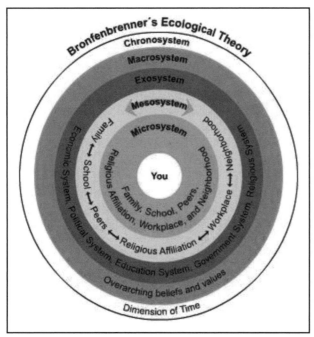

Figure 3-5. Brofenbrenner's Ecological Theory and its definitions.[32]

relatively new to our profession, as they have evolved in the last 30 years from new knowledge emerging from theory and evidence. Students often ask, "Why don't all of you that are developing models get together and come up with one model?" The answer is that models serve different purposes and have different degrees to which the constructs are explicated. Our hope in presenting 4 key

---

BOX 3-3

EXAMPLES OF MODELS USED IN OCCUPATIONAL THERAPY

- The Model of Human Occupation (MOHO)[52-56]
- The Kawa River Model (KAWA)[57,58]
- The Canadian Model of Occupational Performance-Enabling (CMOP-E)[59-61]
- The Person-Environment-Occupation-Performance Model (PEOP)[62-68]

models is to teach you how to recognize and use them to organize the information that will be central to your practice. It is our intent to introduce you to these models and suggest resources you can use to obtain an in-depth understanding of the ones that will best serve in your practice.

All 4 models (Box 3-3) have some common characteristics. For example:

1. All are client-centered and have the person, environment, and occupation as key elements that support the occupational therapy practitioner in understanding the client's occupational needs
2. All are ecological models that recognize the importance of stages of development as they influence motivation, skills, and roles
3. All emphasize the complex interactions of biological, psychological, and social phenomena

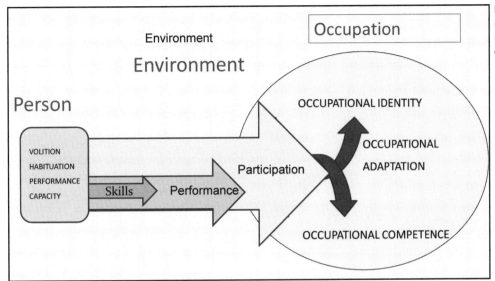

Figure 3-6. Model of Human Occupation (MOHO): Person, Environment, Occupation.[55,56]

4. All recognize the importance of the match between person, task, and situation for performance to be supported

You will note some differences in language or terminology and, as previously stated, they will have differences in how the constructs are explicated.

THE MODEL OF HUMAN OCCUPATION: A PERSON-CENTERED MODEL OF OCCUPATIONAL PERFORMANCE

The MOHO emerged in the late 1970s when Gary Kielhofner and Janice Burke were graduate students of Mary Reilly at the University of Southern California.[52-56] MOHO was first published in 1980. It first emerged with the expressed purpose of organizing concepts to guide occupational therapy practice.[69-71] The first fully explicated model was published in 1985, with revisions in 1995, 2002, and 2008.[52-56] The 2008 edition is the most current in the understanding and application of MOHO.[56] The concepts are displayed in the Modified MOHO, where all the original concepts are used but are now labeled as Person, Environment, and Occupation. Core concepts of the model that the practitioner must address are the motivation for occupation, the individual's routines that support performance, the skills the individual employs to perform their daily occupations, and the influence of the environment of occupation.[72] The model will be explained by the Person, Environment, and Occupation sections of the model (Figure 3-6).

The Person Components of MOHO

MOHO conceptualizes how people choose and create patterns and perform the occupations that are meaningful to them (ie, participation). The process of participation is supported by volition, habituation, and performance capacity. *Volition* is the process that motivates choices and actions. It proposes that humans have a desire to engage in occupations that is shaped by ongoing experience.[72] Kielhofner asserts that volition is concerned with personal causation, values, and interests.

Personal causation reflects our awareness of our present and potential abilities, and our capacity to do what we need or want to do.[73,74] Evolving concepts of cognitive awareness and self-efficacy also fit into the concept of personal causation.[75] *Values* are central to our choice of occupations. Values, such as fairness, friendliness, honor, kindness, loyalty, reliability, resourcefulness, self-reliance, service to others, tolerance, truth, and many others, help us define right from wrong and good from bad. This in turn helps select how to use our time and effort. If we cannot live up to our values it is not possible to feel adequate[76]; we do things that are of *interest* or are pleasurable. We are likely to enjoy things that are within our skills and capacities, yet illness and/or disability interferes with doing what is interesting.[72] Choosing a meaningful activity is a function of volition. The satisfaction of doing activities that are meaningful enables people to exercise reasonable control.[72]

Habituation involves habits and roles. *Habits* are the learned ways of doing occupations that unfold automatically in our daily lives. They are environmentally dependent, and when faced with doing a task in an unfamiliar environment or after a health condition or disability, the task becomes novel. *Roles* define how people see themselves. Much of what we do is done to fulfill a role. Our roles serve as a framework for viewing responsibilities and for what we choose to do in our daily occupations. Acquiring a disability or an illness will likely impact the ability to engage in the occupations that support roles. *Performance capacity* is the client's capacity for performance that relates to his/her musculoskeletal, neurological, and cardiopulmonary (and other body systems) capabilities. MOHO does not explicitly address performance capacity, as Kielhofner felt that other frameworks (eg, Trombly, Ayres, and others) contributed to our understanding for addressing performance capacity.[72] MOHO does however offer a complementary way of thinking about performance capacity as it builds on clients' subjective experiences and how they feel about their performance. The occupational therapy practitioner pays attention to how the person performs, and the role that pain, fatigue, confusion or other subjective aspects can influence performance.

The Environment in MOHO

The environment offers opportunities, resources, demands, and constraints. Because each individual is unique, each environment will provide different levels of support to doing. The environment can be physical, either natural-made or human-made spaces or tools, that are used in everyday life. The environment can also be social, including groups of people that create a sense of belonging. All settings in which an activity or task is performed is made up of spaces and objects. Such settings can be an enabler or a barrier for people with a physical and or mental impairment.[72]

Occupational Performance in MOHO: Doing

Doing is examined at different levels—skills, occupational performance, occupational participation, occupational identity, competence, and occupational adaptation. Each will be briefly introduced. MOHO describes skills as purposeful actions. *Skills*, in contrast to performance capacity (eg, underlying abilities of motor, cognition, strength, etc), refers to the discrete actions seen within the performance. Kielhofner described 3 types of skills: motor skills, process skills, and communication and interaction skills.[55,56,72] These skills support the actions of the person as they perform tasks that are meaningful and necessary in their daily lives. These skills can be influenced by personal and environmental factors. *Occupational performance* is the completion of an occupational form or task. Occupational performance involves daily tasks such as walking a pet,

mowing the lawn, teaching, care of self, care of others, etc. These tasks/occupational forms are what we do. Occupational *participation* refers to engagement in work, play, or ADL that are part of one's own sociocultural context.[56]

Occupational Identity and Occupational Competence

Kielhofner relates participation to identity.[56] It is through participation that identities are created and maintained. He defines occupational identity as having a sense of who one is and who one wishes to become as an occupational being; this is generated from one's history of participation. Occupational identity is formed by one's sense of capacity and effectiveness for doing and includes interests, roles, relationships, and habits. *Occupational competence* comes from sustaining a pattern of occupational participation that reflects identity and that is "putting your identity into action."[72(p58)] Occupational competence is achieved when an individual can fulfill the expectation of his or her roles and values; performs and maintains a routine that supports responsibilities; and participates in the occupations that provide a sense of ability, control, and satisfaction and fulfillment.[72] This all leads to *occupational adaptation*, which occurs when the person has constructed a positive occupational identity and achieved occupational competence over time in the environments that support their meaningful and necessary activities.[56]

The primary reference for the MOHO Model is the book *A Model of Human Occupation: Theory and Application*, 4th edition, by Kielhofner.[56]

THE KAWA (RIVER) MODEL: A PERSON-CENTERED MODEL OF OCCUPATIONAL PERFORMANCE

The Kawa Model (Figure 3-7) was developed in response to a growing need to provide occupational therapy in a relevant and responsive way to an increasingly global population. The meaning of human occupation is uniquely tied to sociocultural contexts, which make a universal interpretation of the construct of occupation impossible. Iwama asks what happens when cultural norms and imperatives of autonomy, personal causation, and self-determinism are foisted onto clients who come from a culture of shared learning and experience and whose values include dependency, group harmony, and collective determinism.[57] The Kawa Model emerged from a group of Japanese occupational therapy practitioners who were grappling with this question. They needed an approach that would bring their occupational therapy practice more

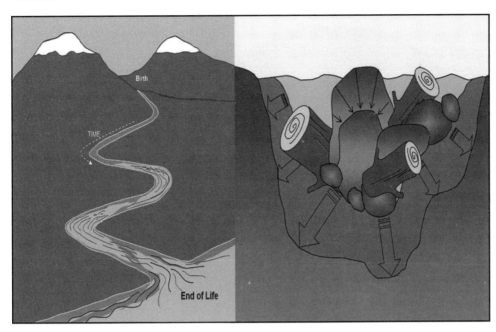

Figure 3-7. The Kawa (River) Model.[58] (Reprinted with permission from Michael K. Iwama, PhD, OT[C].)

in line with the day-to-day realities and experiences of the clients they were serving in an Eastern culture.[58] The approach they took identified the overlooked issue of culture in the design of models that would serve them as they sought to value each client's unique narrative and the richness of the client's experiences and explanations of their day-to-day realities.[58] The Kawa Model includes 4 basic concepts that are elements of a river; the river serving as a metaphor for a life journey. The river flows through time and space, and a state of well-being can be portrayed by the image of a strong, deep, river unimpeded in its flow. Life circumstances are like certain structures in a river (eg, rocks, driftwood, and river beds) that provide an understanding of the assets and problems that the client faces in daily life. The occupational therapy practitioner's role is to enable and support the person to enhance their life flow. An unrestricted flow represents personal health and well-being.[58]

The first component of the Kawa Model is *water*. Water represents the individual's life energy or life flow. The water provides a spirit, cleansing, and renewing process. The volume and rate of the flow can reflect the state of one's health. The water is a fluid and its form comes from its container, in this case the river sides and bed. People in collective-oriented societies often interpret their social world as the container, and as such the river bed can serve to shape the individual self. The second components are the *river sides and bed*, which metaphorically represent the individual's physical and social environment. Structures or factors in the physical environment can enable and constrain human action. The social environment is the most important determinant of a person's life flow in a

collectivist social context because of the affordances the environment provides for the meaning and experience of personal action. It is comprised mainly of others who share a direct relationship with the person.[58] The third components are the *rocks* that represent discrete circumstances that the person considers are limiting or impeding his or her life or life flow. The rocks are considered by the client to be problems and matters that are difficult to manage, that interrupt the flow. Rocks can be bodily impairments that can become disabling without the supportive environment. The fourth component is *driftwood*, which represents the person's attributes. The can include values (honesty, rightness), character (optimism, insightful), personality (introvert, extrovert), skills (cooking, woodworking, fishing), and immaterial (friends and family) and material things (wealth, home, transportation). These assets can positively or negatively influence the person's circumstances. The driftwood can get stuck between the rocks and river walls, resulting in a larger impedance to flow. The driftwood can also be transient and can be used to clear the rocks from the river.[57]

The final element of the Kawa Model is the obstructions or the *space* created in the area between the rocks, driftwood, river sides, and river bed.[58] This is the area where the occupational therapy practitioner works with the client to self-identify goals and make plans and strategies to assist the client in reestablishing the flow of the river, thus their life flow translates into health and well-being.

The full description of the Kawa Model can be studied in detail in the book *The Kawa Model: Culturally Relevant Occupational Therapy* by Iwama.[58]

Figure 3-8. The CMOP-E Model.[61] (Reprinted with permission from Townsend EA, Polatajko HJ. *Enabling Occupation II: Advancing an Occupational Therapy Vision for Health, Well-Being & Justice Through Occupation.* Ottawa, ON: CAOT ACE; 2007.)

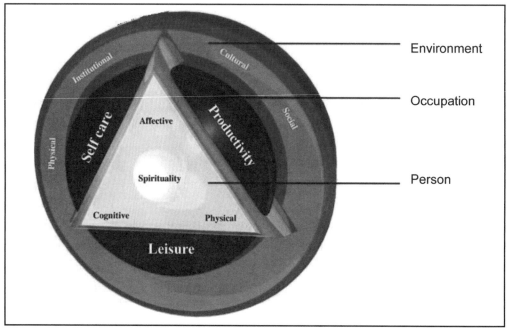

THE CANADIAN MODEL ENABLING OCCUPATION: A PERSON-CENTERED MODEL OF OCCUPATIONAL PERFORMANCE

The first step in building the Canadian model started with funding from the Canadian Association of Occupational Therapy (CAOT) and the Department of National Health and Welfare of Canada back in the 1980s. The (Canadian) Model of Occupational Performance, based on the work of Reed and Sanderson,[66] was an outcome of this effort. In 1997, the Canadian Model of Occupational Performance (CMOP) introduced a social model that put the person in a social environmental context.[60] In 2007, the Canadian Association released Enabling Occupation II (CMOP-E), which is the model presented in the following description (Figure 3-8).[61]

In the CMOP-E, occupational performance is the result of the interaction and interdependence between the person, the environment, and the person's occupations.[61] Occupation is at the center of the CMOP-E model representing the doing (physical), feeling (affective), and thinking (cognitive) components of the person. The points of the interaction extend beyond the person to interact with the environment, depicting the interaction with the person and environment components. Self-care, productivity, and leisure are the main components of occupation; the central sphere now focuses on the person, including their spiritual, affective, cognitive, and physical elements. The environ-

ments in the outer sphere are physical, institutional, cultural, and social.[60]

The Components of the Canadian Association's Enabling Occupation II

There are 3 components of occupation: *self-care*, the occupations for looking after the self; *productivity*, the occupations that make a social or economic contribution or provide for economic sustenance; and *leisure*, the occupations for enjoyment.[60(p37)] There are also 4 components for performance. *Performance* reflects the interaction of affective, physical, cognitive, and spiritual components. *Affective* relates to feeling, the domain that comprises all social and emotional functions that include interpersonal and intrapersonal factors.[60(p44)] *Physical* relates to doing and comprises all sensory, motor, and sensorimotor functions. *Cognitive* or thinking is the domain that addresses all mental functions, both cognitive and intellectual, and includes concepts like perception, concentration memory, comprehension, judgment, and reasoning. Spiritual is defined as residing in the person and gives meaning to occupation.[60]

Environment includes cultural, physical, and social components, as well as legal and political components in institutional environments. The legal and political environments in institutions were added in the 2007 edition. The *physical environment* can be a support or barrier. It includes issues such as physical accessibility and proximity to family or services like food and entertainment. The

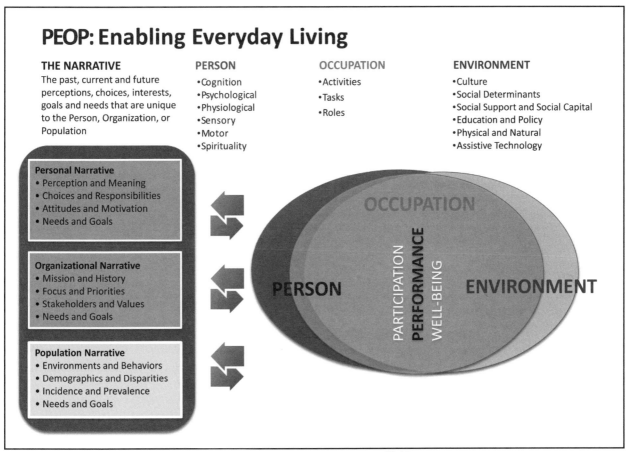

Figure 3-9. The Person-Environment-Occupation-Performance (PEOP) Model.[62-66]

social environment is composed of social groups (family, co-workers, and friends) and the activities in which people engage with others, like playing cards, bicycling, going out to dinner, or to a place of worship. The *institutional environment* includes legal, policy, and political environments where issues such as accessible transportation and building access are of particular concern.

The 2007 enhancement of the CMOP-E added the concept of engagement, which brings depth to the CMOP Model[60] in that the occupational therapy practitioner's area of "concern is what is related to human occupation and its connection with the occupational person and the occupational influences of the environment."[61(p24)]

The full description of the CMOP-E Model can be studied in detail in the book *Enabling Occupation II: Advancing an Occupational Therapy Vision for Health, Well-Being and Justice Through Occupation* by Townsend and Polatajko.[61]

THE PERSON-ENVIRONMENT-OCCUPATION-PERFORMANCE MODEL: A PERSON, POPULATION, AND COMMUNITY MODEL OF OCCUPATIONAL PERFORMANCE

The final model highlighted in this chapter is the PEOP Model (Figure 3-9). This chapter will give a brief overview, as this model is central to this text and will be fully discussed in Chapter 4 along with the process that supports it in Chapter 5.

The PEOP Model was first published in 1991 and has now had 3 additional iterations.[62-66] It was conceived to organize the growing body of knowledge generated by occupational science, neuroscience, physiology, psychology, and environmental science that could identify, clarify, and emphasize the unique contributions of occupational

---

BOX 3-4

EXAMPLES OF FRAMES OF REFERENCE COMMONLY USED IN OCCUPATIONAL THERAPY

- The *AOTA Practice Framework*[77]
- The Biomechanical Framework[56,58,64,77,78]
- The Cognitive Behavioral Framework[79-84]

---

therapy practitioners to the health, participation, and well-being of individuals, groups, and populations. The goal was to have a model of occupational performance that would be relevant regardless of the setting or level of care in which occupational therapy practitioners worked; the type of client they served; and the age, life stage, or diagnosis of the client. The model was designed to encourage a balanced approach to care that would encourage occupational therapy practitioners to use a client-centered approach with a focus on the life situations of the clients. Such an approach would require that practitioners consider the person-related and environment-related resources and barriers to enable their clients to perform or accomplish the occupations necessary to live satisfying lives.[67]

The PEOP Model was designed to make explicit the occupational therapy practitioner's contribution to client-centered care; as such it is designed to facilitate collaboration in the medical system and the community. Occupational therapy's unique contribution is the interaction of person, environment, and occupation factors, and by involving those 3 factors it enables occupational performance.

The concept of occupational performance is common to all occupational therapy models. Occupational performance serves to connect the individual to a role and the sociocultural environment.[67(p23)] The PEOP Model's definition of occupational performance is the doing of meaningful activities, tasks, and roles through complex interactions between the person and environment.[66]

The PEOP is a systems model, recognizing that the interaction of person, environment, occupation, and performance is dynamic and reciprocal and the client (whether person, family, organization of community) must be central to planning care. Only the client can determine what outcomes are most important and necessary. Figure 3-9 is a graphic depiction of the model's 4 parts: the narrative, the person factors, the occupational factors, and the environmental factors. These factors are explicitly described on the figure and will not be repeated here. All of the 4 key elements are essential to understanding occupational perfor-

mance and building an intervention plan of care for a person, an organization, or a population. The occupational therapy practitioner must have current knowledge of these elements depending on the population being served and the level of care that must be delivered. The PEOP Model can provide the structure for knowledge that enables the performance of occupation (doing), for participation (engagement in everyday life), and well-being (health and quality of life). These are the outcomes of occupational therapy.[66]

The PEOP processes for person-centered, population-centered, and organization-centered practice are described in Chapter 5. Because the knowledge of occupational performance is at the person, environment, and occupation level, it works well in both the medical system of care and the sociocultural system of care. In fact occupational therapy is the bridge between the medical system where the person receives diagnosis-based care and the sociocultural level of care where the person receives intervention relevant to everyday living.

Three common frameworks will be used for illustration purposes (Box 3-4). As a clinician you will need to apply these Frameworks using knowledge of theory and having organized your knowledge in a practice model that will serve as a lens for viewing and interpreting your observations.[66]

Framework Definition and Purpose

A framework or frame of reference is "a structure of concepts, values, customs, views, with which an individual or group perceives or evaluates data, communicates ideas, and regulates behavior."[68(np)] Frameworks use knowledge from theories and may be organized within the model that you have chosen for your practice. Information from the AOTA *Practice Framework* will clarify why theory, models, and classifications (taxonomys) are necessary in order to apply a practice framework.

> The *Framework* was originally developed to articulate occupational therapy's distinct perspective and contribution to promoting the health and participation of persons…and populations through engagement in occupation. The *Framework* does not serve as a taxonomy, theory, or model of occupational therapy…. By design, the *Framework* must be used to guide occupational therapy practice in conjunction with the knowledge and evidence relevant to occupation and occupational therapy….[77(pS2-S3)]

The AOTA *Practice Framework* is in its 3rd edition.[77] It was developed by the Commission on Practice and approved by the Representative Assembly of the AOTA. It is a document that reflects the profession's core beliefs, defines the profession's language, and describes the occupational therapy domain and process occupational therapy practitioners should use in their practice. The AOTA *Practice Framework* is a document that articulates occupational therapy's

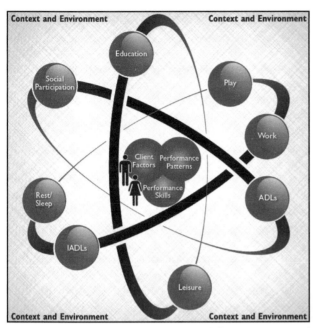

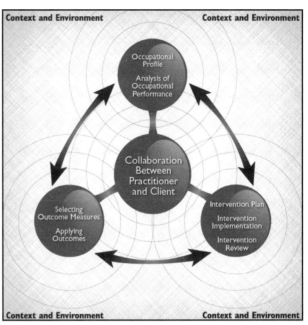

Figure 3-10. The domain of occupational therapy. (Reprinted with permission from American Occupational Therapy Association. Occupational therapy practice framework: domain and process [3rd ed]. *Am J Occup Ther.* 2014;68[Suppl 1]:S1-S48. © 2014 AOTA.)

Figure 3-11. Occupational Therapy Process. (Reprinted with permission from American Occupational Therapy Association. Occupational therapy practice framework: domain and process [3rd ed]. *Am J Occup Ther.* 2014;68[Suppl 1]:S1-S48. © 2014 AOTA.)

contribution to promoting the health and participation of people, organizations, and populations. It is meant to be used by occupational therapy practitioners to organize their practice and by people external to the profession to describe occupational therapy's contribution to health.[77]

The domain identifies the profession's purview and areas with a body of knowledge that contribute to expertise in practice. The occupational therapy practitioner has and integrates knowledge of *occupations, client factors, performance skills, performance patterns,* and *contexts and environments.*[77] Each will be introduced here.

The *occupations* include activities of daily living (ADLs), instrumental activities of daily living (IADLs), rest and sleep, education, work, play, leisure, and social participation. For *client factors,* the therapy practitioner addresses values, beliefs, and spirituality in addition to the person's body functions and structures (based on the ICF).[85] *Performance skills* are observable, concrete, goal-directed actions that clients use to engage in daily life. Performance skills are interrelated and include motor skills, process skills, and social interaction skills. *Performance patterns* "are the habits, routines, roles, and rituals used in the process of engaging in occupations or activities that can support or hinder occupational performance."[77(pS8)] *Habits* are automatic behaviors, and routines are sequences of occupations that provide structure to daily lives.[77] *Roles* are behaviors that people use to construct their occupations to fulfill their perceived roles and identity. *Rituals* are actions with

cultural, spiritual, and social meaning—rituals contribute to the client's identities. Again, the information to inform this area of concern comes from research and practice.[77]

The *contexts and environments* include cultural, personal, physical, social, temporal, and virtual and are the interrelated conditions that influence performance.[77] The *cultural aspects* include customs, beliefs, activities, behavioral standards, and expectations from the society of choice. *Personal* context includes factors such as age, gender, education, and socioeconomic status. *Temporal* is the location of occupations in time. This includes the stages of life, time of day, rhythm of activity, or history.[77] *Virtual* is the environment where communication is supported by technology in the absence of physical contact. *Physical* is the natural and built environment and the tools that provide support or create barriers to performance. The *social* environment is constructed by relationships at the family, community, or system level at which the client is a member. The knowledge the practitioner uses in the *Practice Framework* comes from knowledge of theory and models, and he or she will use that knowledge in practice in the clinical reasoning process. The occupational therapy domains are listed in Figure 3-10, and the *Practice Framework* explicitly states all aspects of the domain.[77]

The process of occupational therapy (Figure 3-11) includes evaluation (occupational profile, analysis of occupational performance), intervention (plan, implementation, review), and outcomes. Service delivery models, therapeutic

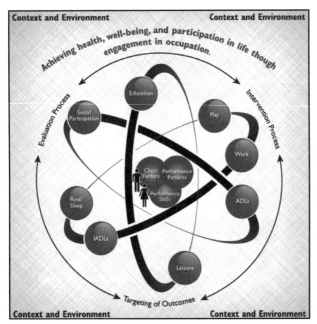

Figure 3-12. The relationship of the occupational therapy domain and process. (Reprinted with permission from American Occupational Therapy Association. Occupational therapy practice framework: domain and process [3rd ed]. *Am J Occup Ther*. 2014;68[Suppl 1]:S1-S48. © 2014 AOTA.)

use of self, activity analysis, and clinical reasoning must be considered within the occupational therapy process. Figure 3-12 depicts the relationship between the occupational therapy domains and process in the *Framework*.[77]

THE BIOMECHANICAL FRAME OF REFERENCE USED IN OCCUPATIONAL THERAPY

Many people experience injuries that limit their capacity to move, limit their strength and endurance, create problems of immobilization, have peripheral nerve impairment or damage, and experience pain. All of these conditions limit the person's daily life function, including their ability to care for themselves (self-care and instrumental tasks), care for others (family roles), work (may have a condition that temporarily limits work or may require a vocational change), and be limited in their leisure and community activities. The occupational therapy practitioner is a member of a medical team that is expected to contribute to the acute management of a condition to restore movement, prevent secondary problems, and provide compensatory strategies that will address the factors that limit the person's occupational performance.

The term *biomechanics* means life mechanics, and the study of biomechanics addresses the structure and func-

tion of biological systems by means of mechanics. The concept of biomechanics became the focus of health care in the 1970s when medical systems and biological mechanisms addressed the payment systems request to report progress in biomechanical terms like strength, range, and endurance, all terms that relate to how a person moves. Occupational therapy practitioners are in a unique position to understand movement, as well as the psychological, cognitive, sensory, and spiritual issues of the person as they interact in their environment.[56,58,64,77] Thus, occupational therapy practitioners are in a good position to address the movement and performance problems of people with conditions like arthritis, amputations, burns, soft-tissue damage, fractures, back strain, overuse syndrome, and chronic pain using both the biomechanical approach and an occupational performance approach.

Because occupational therapy practitioners have a unique perspective on the biomechanical approach, they have the knowledge to understand both the physiology and mechanics of movement (see Chapter 18). Occupational therapy practitioners are not only a valuable resource for programs that address biomechanical problems, but also have the skills to understand and address the occupational needs of the person who may have a temporary or long-term disability. Any of the models addressed in this chapter (MOHO, Kawa, CMOP-E, and PEOP) will provide structure to the biomechanical approach to care, employing an occupational performance perspective.

There are limits to the biomechanical frame of reference, as the person must have the ability to initiate and coordinate skilled movements and have the cognitive ability to follow through with strategies that will promote recovery. If the person has damage to the central nervous system and resulting cognition or emotional problems, the biomechanical frame of reference would have to be reconsidered; as the knowledge of motor learning would be central to support the individual's recovery (see Chapter 17). The biomechanical frame of reference actually relates very well to the person-centered factors addressed in the PEOP, if the recovery is not to be immediate, as secondary emotional, cognitive, and physiological problems often occur with these conditions.[78]

THE COGNITIVE-BEHAVIORAL FRAMEWORK

Occupational therapy services can be thought of as a learning activity. In order to teach activities as effectively as possible, occupational therapy practitioners must choose an appropriate instructional method that is compatible with the client's cognitive skills/abilities, and then structure the learning environment appropriately.[79] An intervention approach that can help therapy practitioners achieve this is the Cognitive-Behavioral Intervention Framework.

As the name implies, the Cognitive-Behavioral Intervention Framework is the combination of 2 theories of learning: behavioral and cognitive. A psychologist named John B. Watson is credited with forming the school of thought called *behaviorism*. According to Watson, the behaviorist view is purely objective; the goal of which is to predict and control behavior, and only observable behaviors are worthy of being studied.[80] He believed that all behavior was the result of learned responses and that any person could be conditioned to react to a given situation in a certain way, without regard for understanding the cognitive processes involved in achieving the behavior. Two of the most prominent concepts associated with behavioral learning are *classical conditioning* and *operant conditioning*. Classical conditioning is a behavior modification technique in which a subject produces a desired behavior in response to a previously neutral stimulus that has been repeatedly paired with an unconditioned stimulus to elicit the behavior.[81] Operant conditioning states that a specific behavior is increased or decreased through positive or negative reinforcement each time the behavior is exhibited, as the subject will associate pleasure or displeasure with the behavior in response to the reinforcement.[82] The basic premise of behavioral training is still very much reflective of the work of Watson, Pavlov, and Skinner; behavior can be trained through stimulus-response pairings that are positively or negatively reinforced in accordance with the desired behavior regardless of cognitive ability. *Cognitive* learning theory does not attribute all learning to observable behavior, but rather states that learning also includes unobservable cognitive processes (eg, attention, memory, metacognition/awareness, executive function) that are used to acquire and use information to adapt to environmental demands.[83,84] In essence, cognitive learning theory focuses on the mental acquisition and organization of knowledge that is deployed to learn and perform behaviors. Cognitive-behavioral learning theory is based on the notion that these 2 theories do not exist in isolation; that using cognitive processes can change behavior. Therefore, according to this theory, while behavior can be trained using methods rooted in behavioral modification (ie, stimulus-response pairing, reinforcement), it can be supported by training thinking patterns.[86]

While a lot of health care professionals use the cognitive-behavioral framework in some form, occupational therapy practitioners are uniquely positioned for an application with a focus on the person, environment, and occupation. At the person level, we understand the cognitive capacities of the client to know if he or she is capable of cognitive learning and the combination of behavioral techniques and cognitive capacity that will be necessary to achieve skill acquisition. At the environment level, we understand the context in which the person will be required to perform the occupation so we can structure the learning environment to promote generalization and transfer as appropriate. Finally, at the occupation level, we understand the activities we are helping our clients learn, which informs the behavioral techniques used and helps guide clients to develop their own strategies to achieve their optimal performance.

Classification Definition and Purposes

The *Oxford Dictionary* defines classification as the action or process of classifying something, for example, the classification of disease according to symptoms. In biology, classification is defined as the arrangement of animals and plants in taxonomic groups according to their observed similarities (including at least kingdom and phylum in animals; division in plants; and class, order, family, genus, and species). The WHO's International Classification of Functioning, Disability and Health (ICF) provides a standard language and framework for the description of health and health-related states.[85] It is a multipurpose classification intended for a wide range of uses in different sectors. It is a classification of health and health-related domains—domains that help us to describe changes in body function and structure, what a person with a health condition can do in a standard environment (their level of capacity), as well as what they actually do in their usual environment (their level of performance). These domains are classified from body, individual, and societal perspectives by means of 2 lists: a list of body functions and structures and a list of domains of activity and participation. In the ICF, the term *functioning* refers to all body functions, activities, and participation, while *disability* is similarly an umbrella term for impairments, activity limitations, and participation restrictions. ICF also lists environmental factors that interact with all these components.[85]

Definitions Used in the International Classification of Functioning, Disability and Health

Body functions are physiological functions of body systems (including psychological functions). Body structures are anatomical parts of the body such as organs, limbs, and their components. Impairments are problems in body function or structure such as a significant deviation or loss. Activity is the execution of a task or action by an individual. Activity limitations are difficulties an individual may have in executing activities. Participation is involvement in a life situation. Participation restrictions are problems an individual may experience in involvement in life situations. Environmental factors make up the

---

BOX 3-5

THE CHAPTERS OF THE INTERNATIONAL CLASSIFICATION OF FUNCTIONING, DISABILITY AND HEALTH[85]

Body Function	*Body Structure*
• Mental Functions	• Structure of the Nervous System
• Sensory Functions and Pain	• The Eye, Ear, and Related Structures
• Voice and Speech Functions	• Structures Involved in Voice and Speech
• Functions of the Cardiovascular, Hematological, Immunological, and Respiratory Systems	• Structure of the Cardiovascular, Immunological, and Respiratory Systems
• Functions of the Digestive, Metabolic, Endocrine Systems	• Structures Related to the Digestive, Metabolic, and Endocrine Systems
• Genitourinary and Reproductive Functions	• Structure Related to Genitourinary and Reproductive Systems
• Neuromusculoskeletal and Movement-Related Functions	• Structure Related to Movement
• Functions of the Skin and Related Structures	• Skin and Related Structures
Activities and Participation	*Environmental Factors*
• Learning and Applying Knowledge	• Products and Technology
• General Tasks and Demands	• Natural Environment and Human-Made Changes to Environment
• Communication	• Support and Relationships
• Mobility	• Attitudes
• Self-Care	• Services, Systems, and Policies
• Domestic Life	
• Interpersonal Interactions and Relationships	
• Major Life Areas	
• Community, Social, and Civic Life	

---

physical, social, and attitudinal environment in which people live and conduct their lives.[85]

Underlying Principles From the International Classification of Functioning, Disability and Health

There are general principles that underlay the conception of ICF as a health classification of functioning and disability. They are closely linked to the biopsychosocial model of disability that bridges from the biomedical model, which is focused on treatment and the sociocultural model that provides services and resources that supports people in their everyday lives. There are 4 principles:

1. The ICF is designed to be universal, it is applicable to all people irrespective of health condition. It concerns everyone's functioning and it should not become a tool for labeling persons with disabilities as a separate group.[85]

2. The ICF does not make a distinction between different health conditions such as "mental" and "physical" that affects the structure of content of a classification of functioning and disability.[85]

3. The domain names are worded in neutral language so that the classification can express both positive and negative aspects of each aspect of functioning and disability.

4. The ICF includes contextual factors in which environmental factors range from physical factors such as climate and terrain, to social attitudes, institutions, and laws. Interaction with environmental factors is an essential aspect of the scientific understanding of the phenomena included under the umbrella terms *functioning* and *disability*.

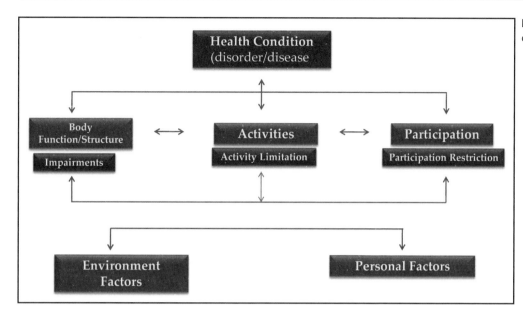

Figure 3-13. The ICF classification system.[85]

Box 3-5 lists the chapters in the ICF; these chapters are the essential elements of the classification. Of particular interest to the occupational therapy practitioner are the activity and participation elements, as they are the focus of our interventions.[85]

How Will the International Classification of Functioning, Disability and Health Be Used?

The classification offered by the ICF is the basis for the standardization of data concerning all aspects of human functioning and disability around the world.[85] It offers a language to be used by persons with disabilities and professionals alike to evaluate health care settings across a continuum of care such as rehabilitation centers, nursing homes, psychiatric institutions, and community services. It can be useful for persons with disabilities to identify their health care and rehabilitative needs, as well as the effect of the physical and social environment on the situation that they experience in their lives. The ICF serves a policy function, as it will help monitor and explain health care and other disability costs and quantify the productivity loss and its impact on the lives of the people in society. In some of the developed countries, ICF has been introduced into legislation and social policy. And it is expected that ICF will become the world standard for disability data and social policy modeling and be introduced in the legislation of many more countries around the globe.[85]

In summary, the ICF is the WHO's taxonomy for health and disability. It is the conceptual basis for the definition, measurement, and policy formulations for health and dis-ability. It is a universal classification of disability *and* health for use in health and health-related sectors.

SUMMARY

This chapter has introduced the knowledge and language that will serve you well in your understanding of theory, models, frameworks, and classifications. Many people do not use these terms correctly, and some go directly to frameworks—bypassing theories and models that are central to the clinical reasoning process. You should now have a level of understanding of the relationship of these concepts and should be able to identify why they are critical for supporting your clinical reasoning and communication with client's, their families, your peers, administrators, and policy makers. To recap, the relationships are described in the following diagram (Figure 3-13). In Chapters 4 and 5 you will receive specific information on how to apply the knowledge you have learned from this diagram to people, organizations, and populations.

REFERENCES

1. Duncan EAS. An introduction to frames of reference and conceptual models of practice. In: Duncan EAS, ed. *Foundations for Practice in Occupational Therapy.* 5th ed. Edinburgh, United Kingdom: Elsevier/Churchill Livingstone; 2011.

2. Primeau LA, Ferguson JM. Occupational frame of reference. In: Kramer P, Hinojosa J, eds. *Frame of Reference for Pediatric Occupational Therapy.* Philadelphia, PA: Lippincott Williams & Wilkins; 1999:469-516.

3. Schmidt RA, Lee TD. *Motor Control and Learning: A Behavioral Emphasis.* 4th ed. Champaign, IL: Human Kinetics; 2005.

4. Schmidt RA, Wrisberg CA. *Motor Learning and Performance.* 3rd ed. Champaign, IL: Human Kinetics; 2004.

5. Mathiowetz V, Bass Haugen J. Assessing abilities and capabilities: motor behavior. In: Radomski MV, Trombly Latham CA, eds. *Occupational Therapy for Physical Dysfunction.* 6th ed. Baltimore, MD: Lippincott Williams & Wilkins, Wolters Kluwer; 2008.

6. Thelen E. Motor development: a new synthesis. *Am Psychol.* 1995;50(2):79-95.

7. Turvey MT, Kugler PN. An ecological approach to perception and action. In: Whiting HTA, ed. *Human Motor Actions: Bernstein Reassessed.* Philadelphia, PA: Elsevier Science; 1984:373-412.

8. World Health Organization, Health and Welfare Canada, Canadian Public Health Association. *Ottawa Charter for Health Promotion.* Ottawa, Canada: World Health Organization: 1986.

9. Nutbeam D. Health promotion glossary. *Health Promot.* 1986;1(1):113-127.

10. Depoy E, Kolodner EL. Psychological performance factors. In: Christiansen C, Baum C, eds. *Occupational Therapy: Overcoming Human Performance Deficits.* Thorofare, NJ: SLACK Incorporated; 1991.

11. Argyle M. *The Psychology of Happiness.* New York, NY: Methuen & Co; 1987.

12. Cohen P, Struening EL, Genevie LE, Kaplan SR, Muhlin GL, Peck HB. Community stressors, mediating conditions, and well-being in urban neighborhoods. *J Community Psychol.* 1982;10:377-390.

13. Warr P. The measurement of well-being and other aspects of mental health. *J Occup Psych.* 1990;63(4):193-210.

14. Ullah P. The association between income, financial strain, and psychological well-being among unemployed youths. *The British Psychological Society.* 1990;63(4):317-330.

15. Burckardt C, Woods S, Schultz A, Ziebarth D. Quality of life of adults with chronic illness: a psychometric study. *Res Nurs Health.* 1989;12:347-354.

16. Homel R, Burns A. Environmental quality and the well-being of children. *Soc Indic Res.* 1989;21:133-158.

17. Koeing H, Kvale J, Ferrel C. Religion and well-being in later life. *Gerontol.* 1988;28(1):19-27.

18. McConatha JT, McConatha D. An instrument to measure self-responsibility for wellness in older adults. *Educational Gerontol.* 1985;11:295-308.

19. Isaksson K. A longitudinal study of the relationship between frequent job change and psychological well-being. *J Occup Psych.* 1990;63:297-308.

20. Gross SJ. The holistic health movement. *Pers Guid J.* 1980;59(2):96-100.

21. Kanner AD, Coyne JC, Schaefer C, Lazarus RS. Comparison of two modes of stress management: daily hassles and uplifts versus life events. *J Behav Med.* 1981;4:1-39.

22. Payne WA, Hahn DB. *Understanding Your Health.* 4th ed. St. Louis, MO: Mosby; 1995.

23. Doyal L, Gough I. *A Theory of Human Need.* New York, NY: Palgrave Macmillan; 1991.

24. Blaxter M. *Health and Lifestyles.* New York, NY: Tavistock/Routledge; 1990.

25. Wilcock AA. Biological and sociocultural aspects of occupation, health, and health promotion. *Br J Occup Ther.* 1993; 56(6):200-203.

26. Lilley J, Jackson L. The value of activities: establishing a foundation for cost effectiveness: a review of the literature. *Activ Adapt Aging.* 1990;14(4):12-13.

27. Foster P. Activities: a necessity for total health care of the long-term care resident. *Activ Adapt Aging.* 1983;3(3):17-23.

28. Bandura A. Self-efficacy: toward a unifying theory of behavioral change. *Psychol Rev.* 1977;84(2):191-215.

29. Lawton MP. The varieties of well-being. *Exp Aging Res.* 1983;9(2):65-72.

30. Lawton MP, Nahemow L. Ecology and the aging process. In: Eisdorfer C, Lawton MP, eds. *Psychology of Adult Development and Aging.* Washington, DC: American Psychological Association; 1973:619-674.

31. Lawton MP, Simon B. The ecology of social relationships in housing for the elderly. *Gerontol.* 1988;8:108-115.

32. Brofenbrenner U. *The Ecology of Human Development: Experiments in Nature and Design.* Cambridge, MA: Harvard University Press; 1979.

33. Sutherland P. *Cognitive Development Today: Piaget and His Critics.* London, UK: Sage Publications; 1992.

34. Block J. Assimilation, accommodation, and the dynamic of personality development. *Child Dev.* 1982;53(2):281-295.

35. McLeod SA. *Vygotsky—social development theory.* Simply Psychology. http://www.simplypsychology.org/vygotsky.html. Published 2007. Updated 2013. Accessed December 2, 2013.

36. Vygotsky LS. *Mind in Society: The Development of Higher Psychological Processes.* Cambridge, MA: Harvard University Press; 1978.

37. Wertsch JV, Tulviste PLS. Vygotsky and contemporary developmental psychology. *Dev Psychol.* 1992;28:548-557.

38. Brody EM, Kleban MH, Lawton MP, Silverman HA. Excess disabilities of mentally impaired aged: impact of individualized treatment. *Gerontol.* 1971;11(2):124-133.

39. Kail RV. *Children and Their Development.* 5th ed. Upper Saddle River, NJ: Pearson Education Inc; 2010.

40. Baltes MM, Baltes PB, eds. *The Psychology of Control and Aging.* Hillsdale, NJ: Erlbaum; 1986.

41. Burchfield R. Ontogeny. In: Burchfield R, ed. *The Compact Edition of the Oxford English Dictionary: Volume III.* New York, NY: Oxford University Press; 1987.

42. Baltes PB. On the incomplete architecture of human ontogeny: selection, optimization, and compensation as foundation of developmental theory. *Am Psychol.* 1997;52:366-380.

43. Baltes PB, Smith J. Multilevel and systemic analyses of old age: theoretical and empirical evidence for a fourth age. In: Bengtson VL, Schaie KW, eds. *Handbook of Theories of Aging.* New York, NY: Springer; 1999:153-173.

44. Datan N, Rodelheaver D, Hughes F. Adult development and aging. In: Rosenzweig M, Porter L, eds. *Ann Rev Psychol.* Vol 38. Palo Alto, CA: Annual Review Inc; 1987:153-180.

45. Csikszentmihalyi M. *Finding Flow: The Psychology of Engagement with Everyday Life.* New York, NY: BasicBooks; 1997.

46. Luszczynska A, Schwarzer R. Social cognitive theory. In: Conner M, Norman P, eds. *Predicting Health Behaviour.* 2nd ed. Buckingham, UK: Open University Press; 2005:127-169.

47. Meyer A. The philosophy of occupation therapy. *Arch Occup Ther.* 1922;1:1-10.

48. Reilly M. Occupational therapy can be one of the great ideas of 20th century medicine. *Am J Occup Ther.* 1962;16:1-9.

49. University of Oklahoma. *An abbreviated glossary of system terminology.* OU Earth Science Education. http://www.esse.ou.edu/glossary_st.html. Updated August 19, 2001. Accessed December 4, 2013.

50. Meteorology glossary. American Meteorological Society glossary of meteorology. http://glossary.ametsoc.org/wiki/Main_Page. Updated August 30, 2013. Accessed December 4, 2013.

51. US Environmental Protection Agency. *Water home.* EPA: US Environmental Protection Agency. http://water.epa.gov/index.cfm. Updated December 4, 2013. Accessed December 4, 2013.

52. Kielhofner G, ed. *A Model of Human Occupation: Theory and Application.* Baltimore, MD: Williams & Wilkins; 1985.

53. Kielhofner G. *A Model of Human Occupation: Theory and Application.* 2nd ed. Baltimore, MD: Williams & Wilkins; 1995.

54. Kielhofner G. Habituation. In: Kielhofner G, ed. *A Model of Human Occupation: Theory and Application.* 2nd ed. Baltimore, MD: Lippincott Williams & Wilkins; 1995:63-82.

55. Kielhofner G. *A Model of Human Occupation: Theory and Application.* 3rd ed. Baltimore, MD: Williams & Wilkins; 2002.

56. Kielhofner G. *A Model of Human Occupation: Theory and Application.* 4th ed. Baltimore, MD: Williams & Wilkins; 2008.

57. Lim H, Iwama MK. Emerging models—an Asian perspective: the Kawa (River) Model. In: Duncan EAS, ed. *Foundations for Practice in Occupational Therapy.* 5th ed. London, UK: Elsevier Limited; 2011.

58. Iwama M. *The Kawa Model: Culturally Relevant Occupational Therapy.* Edinburgh, UK: Churchill Livingstone-Elsevier Press; 2006.

59. Reed KL, Sanderson SR. *Concepts of Occupational Therapy.* 2nd ed. Baltimore, MD: Williams & Wilkins; 1983.

60. Canadian Association of Occupational Therapists. *Enabling Occupation: An Occupational Therapy Perspective.* Ottawa, ON: CAOT Publications ACE; 1997.

61. Townsend EA, Polatajko HJ. *Enabling Occupation II: Advancing an Occupational Therapy Vision for Health, Well-Being & Justice Through Occupation.* Ottawa, ON: CAOT ACE; 2007.

62. Christiansen C, Baum CM. *Occupational Therapy: Overcoming Human Performance Deficits.* Thorofare, NJ: SLACK Incorporated; 1991.

63. Christiansen C, Baum CM. *Occupational Therapy: Enabling Function and Well-Being.* 2nd ed. Thorofare, NJ: SLACK Incorporated; 1997.

64. Christiansen C, Baum CM, Bass Haugen J. *Occupational Therapy: Performance, Participation, and Well-Being.* 3rd ed. Thorofare, NJ: SLACK Incorporated; 2005.

65. Baum CM, Bass Haugen J, Christiansen CH. Person-environment-occupation-performance: a model for planning interventions for individuals and organizations. In: Christiansen CH, Baum CM, Bass Haugen J, eds. *Occupational Therapy: Performance, Participation, and Well-Being.* 3rd ed. Thorofare, NJ: SLACK Incorporated; 2005:372-392.

66. Baum CM, Christiansen CH, Bass JD. The Person-Environment-Occupation-Performance (PEOP) Model. In: Christiansen CH, Baum CM, Bass JD, eds. *Occupational Therapy: Performance, Participation, and Well-Being.* 4th ed. Thorofare, NJ: SLACK Incorporated; 2015.

67. Reed KL, Sanderson SN. *Concepts of Occupational Therapy.* Baltimore, MD: Wolters Kluwer Health, Lippincott Williams & Wilkins; 1999.

68. *Frame of reference.* Dictionary.com. http://dictionary.reference.com/browse/frame%20of%20reference?&o=100074&s=t. Updated 2013. Accessed December 4, 2013.

69. Kielhofner G. A model of human occupation, part three: benign and vicious cycles. *Am J Occup Ther.* 1980;34:731-737.

70. Kielhofner G. A model of human occupation, part two: ontogenesis from the perspective of temporal adaptation. *Am J Occup Ther.* 1980;34:657-663.

71. Kielhofner G, Burke J. A model of human occupation, part one: conceptual framework and content. *Am J Occup Ther.* 1980;34:572-581.

72. Forsyth K, Kielhofner G. The model of human occupation: integrating theory into practice and practice into theory. In: Duncan EAS, ed. *Foundations for Practice in Occupational Therapy.* 5th ed. London, UK: Elsevier Churchill Livingstone; 2011.

73. Harter S. Developmental perspectives on the self-system. *Handbook of Child Psychology.* 1983;4:275-385.

74. Rotter JB. Some implications of a social learning theory for the prediction of goal directed behavior from testing procedures. *Psychol Rev.* 1960;67(5):301-316.

75. Bandura A. Self-efficacy mechanism in human agency. *Am Psychol.* 1982;37:122-147.

76. Bruner JS. *Acts of Meaning.* Cambridge, MA: Harvard University Press; 1990.

77. American Occupational Therapy Association. Occupational therapy practice framework: domain and process (3rd ed). *Am J Occup Ther.* 2014;68(Suppl 1):S1-S48.

78. Bailey R, Kaskutas V, Fox I, Baum CM, Mackinnon SE. Effect of upper extremity nerve damage on activity participation, pain, depression, and quality of life. *J Hand Surg.* 2009;34(9):1682-1688.

79. Richardson P. Teaching activities in occupational therapy. In: Pendleton HM, Schultz-Krohn W, eds. *Pedretti's Occupational Therapy: Practice Skills for Physical Dysfunction.* 6th ed. St. Louis, MO: Mosby Elsevier; 2006:102-108.

80. Watson JB. Psychology as the behaviorist views it. *Psychol Rev.* 1913;20(2):158-177.

81. Gray P. *Psychology.* 4th ed. New York, NY: Worth Publishers; 2002.

82. Nye RD. *The Legacy of BF Skinner: Concepts and Perspectives, Controversies and Misunderstandings.* New York, NY: Brooks/Cole Publishing Company; 1992.

83. Haywood HC, Lidz C. *Dynamic Assessment in Practice: Clinical and Educational Applications.* New York, NY: Cambridge University Press; 2007.

84. Lidz CS. Cognitive deficiencies revisited. In: Lidz CS, ed. *Dynamic Assessment: Evaluating Learning Potential.* New York, NY: Guilford Press; 1987:444-478.

85. World Health Organization. *Classifications: International Classification of Functioning, Disability, and Health.* World Health Organization. http://www.who.int/icidh. Published May 22, 2001. Updated 2013. Accessed December 2, 2013.

86. Meichenbaum DH, Goodman J. Training impulsive children to talk to themselves: a means of developing self-control. *J Abnorm Psychol.* 1971;77(2):115-126.

THE PERSON-ENVIRONMENT-OCCUPATION-PERFORMANCE (PEOP) MODEL

Carolyn M. Baum, PhD, OTR/L, FAOTA; Charles H. Christiansen, EdD, OTR, FAOTA; and Julie D. Bass, PhD, OTR/L, FAOTA

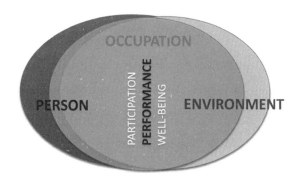

LEARNING OBJECTIVES

- Describe the characteristics of the PEOP Model.
- Discuss how person, environment, and occupation contribute to performance, participation, and well-being.

KEY WORDS

- Environment
- Narrative
- Occupation
- Occupational performance
- Participation
- Performance
- Person
- Well-being

INTRODUCTION

The PEOP Model is a model for practice. It was first conceived during the 1980s in the United States. During that time, a number of scholars around the world were creating conceptual models to help organize the expanding knowledge base of occupational therapy. These frameworks were designed to guide the development of measures and interventions that could be used by occupational therapy practitioners to improve the lives of those they served. (Some of these models are discussed in Chapter 3 of this text.) The PEOP Model was originally published in 1991,[1] and was previously updated in 1997[2] and 2005.[3] These updates were developed to keep pace with the evolution of knowledge in occupational therapy practice.

As a guide to occupational therapy intervention, the PEOP Model can be considered an ecological-transactional systems model.[4] This means the model focuses on the characteristics of the person and his or her living environment. Within the support of the environment, the

Christiansen CH, Baum CM, Bass JD, eds.
Occupational Therapy: Performance, Participation, and Well-Being, Fourth Edition (pp 49-55).
© 2015 SLACK Incorporated.

person performs the activities, tasks, and roles of everyday life. Understanding how the characteristics of the person and environment interact to influence the performance of everyday occupations is fundamental to occupational therapy practice and constitutes the framework of the PEOP Model. The model can be applied to individuals, groups (or organizations), and populations.

The PEOP Model bridges biomedical and sociocultural models in that it identifies 3 relevant domains of knowledge for occupational therapy practice:

1. *Person factors,* which if used alone describe capacities and help identify impairments
2. *Environment factors,* which include physical, social, cultural, policy, and technological influences by enabling or creating barriers of what and how people do what they do
3. *Occupations* (activities, tasks, and roles) that individuals want and need to do as they pursue their lives

The doing of these activities, tasks, and roles are supported by person and environmental factors and constitute occupational performance. The PEOP Model is transactional, in that it views everyday occupations as being affected by and affecting both the person factors and the environments that characterize a client's home, work/school, and community life.

The PEOP Model has several characteristics that are aligned with current and emerging areas of practice. The PEOP Model supports client-centered practice, in that it values and requires the input of individuals to define the context, identify resources, and formulate important goals. The narrative provides the foundation for synthesizing and interpreting data provided by clients to describe their perceptions, choices, interests, and goals. The model also reinforces a "top-down" approach to problem identification and decision-making, as it emphasizes the highest-order factors (the performance, participation, and well-being of individuals, organizations, and populations in context) and their interaction with specific factors (person and environmental capabilities/enablers and constraints/barriers). Besides helping to organize knowledge, the purpose of the PEOP Model is to provide a tool that offers practitioners a useful, logical, systematic, and comprehensive means to plan interventions that can be used in all practice settings with all age ranges, life stages, or occupational performance problems. The PEOP Model focuses on applying knowledge relevant to the occupational performance needs of clients whether they are individuals, an organization, or a population. The PEOP Model makes the person, environment, and occupational factors explicit in the PEOP Occupational Therapy Process (presented in Chapter 5) and supports practitioners in their practice at the person, organization, and/or population levels.

ORIGINS AND AIMS OF THE PERSON-ENVIRONMENT-OCCUPATION-PERFORMANCE MODEL

When work began on this model in 1985, there was a growing awareness that the developing knowledge being used by occupational therapy practitioners required an organizing structure to identify, clarify, and emphasize the field's unique contribution to the health and well-being of individuals, groups, and populations. We knew that occupational therapy could provide practical and relevant interventions that enabled people to preserve or improve the quality of their lives. Yet, at that time, the most influential textbooks in the field were continuing to organize their content using a biomedical approach that resembled the diagnosis and pathology-focused approach of allopathic medicine. Influenced by writers from medicine who were calling for more health-oriented approaches,[5,6] as well as writers from occupational therapy who openly lamented the field's apparent divergence from ideas central to its founding (Box 4-1),[14,16,17] we undertook the challenge to reframe the organizing structure for knowledge relevant to occupational therapy theory and practice. We intended to propose a model that would provide practitioners with an intuitive and organized way to understand the areas relevant to supporting people's ability to perform or do the activities, tasks, and roles necessary for everyday living. Through creating such a framework, we aimed to facilitate thinking in ways that would guide assessment, planning, and the delivery of interventions. We also felt that creating such a model would enable a more practical, logical, and balanced approach that would encourage occupational therapy practitioners to plan interventions with a focus on the life situations of their clients. This focus, we surmised, would require that practitioners consider the person-related and environment-related resources and barriers relevant to a full understanding of how to enable their clients to perform or accomplish the particular occupations necessary to live satisfying and meaningful lives.

This text introduces the 4th generation of the PEOP Model. Since its inception, the knowledge generated from occupational science, neuroscience, environmental science, and other biological and social sciences has permitted us to extend our original ideas and to provide a more solid scientific basis for the factors that we believe are central to understanding (and thus, facilitating) the occupational performance of humans. Throughout this process of elaboration, we have been influenced by many emerging ideas and innovations in health care, disability studies, social policy, technology, rehabilitation science, and public health. Although some terminology has changed, definitions have been revised, and new concepts have been added; the basic philosophical orientations of the model and its central

---

BOX 4-1

OCCUPATION BASED MODELS VERSUS BIOMEDICAL-BASED MODELS

In his seminal work on how ideas evolve in science, the sociologist Thomas Kuhn wrote that new paradigms tend to emerge when existing models are seen as inadequate or unable to address the problem-solving needs of the time.[7] During the first 60 years of occupational therapy's history, very little research was conducted,[8] and practice was based largely on experience and tradition.[9] Although it was clear that the founders agreed that human occupation was the central and organizing concept underlying practice,[10] there were no established "conceptual models" and just a handful of books and articles that shared experiences and beliefs about the importance of occupation and its potential value in helping people recover from mental and physical diseases.[11]

Yet even then, there was concern about how to understand and explain the value of occupation-based interventions. For example, in 1923, Norman Burnette, a Canadian author, wrote:

> We make specious claims for the therapy of occupation when advocating work among the insane. There remains the task of proving this by quantitative or even qualitative measurement. The difficulties of this field of research should not deter us from entering it. Until we do so, we will never be sure of holding ground over which we have advanced because we are armed with nothing more than speculative theories.[9(p182)]

Yet, it would be many years before serious efforts at supporting theory would bear fruit.

Historians have observed that for several decades occupational therapy practitioners working outside of mental health, in hospitals and medical rehabilitation facilities, were influenced by biomedical models.[12] It is likely that advances in medical science accounted for this tendency, relegating occupation to an incidental role in interventions designed to strengthen muscles or normalize neuromotor function.

During the late 1970s, however, a movement occurred in the United States that led to a resurrection of the original and founding concepts about the importance of occupation as a central organizing concept in the practice of occupational therapy. This movement has been labeled the "occupational behavior" era,[13] which gradually led to the development of conceptual frameworks where occupation assumed a more central focus. These included the MOHO,[14] the CMOP,[15] and, of course, the PEOP Model.[1] Some key differences between the biomedical models and the occupation-based models include:

- Biomedical models tend to start with the diagnosis and be less concerned about the system as a whole. These models are sometimes described as "bottom-up" approaches.

- Biomedical approaches are more likely to view the therapeutic process as one where the occupational therapy practitioner is an expert and the client or patient becomes a passive recipient of care, rather than being actively involved in the process.

- Biomedical models are less likely to devote concern to how the patient views the intervention and how the dysfunction has an influence on the client's everyday life experiences. This happens because the goals of intervention are often measured by physiologic or system specific outcomes, such as muscle strength, coordination, or range of motion.

---

features have remained consistent. This, we believe, indicates that we were successful in developing a model that was not only conceptually sound and parsimonious, but also robust in its ability to organize evidence-based knowledge useful for education, practice, research, and policy.

The Person-Environment-Occupation-Performance Model Values Collaboration

Because occupational therapy is based on a cooperative approach toward care,[18] the PEOP Model was designed to facilitate the development of a collaborative intervention plan with the client—who must be central to the plan of care and the intervention process because only the client is able to determine what outcomes are most valued and necessary. Additionally, care is planned with other professionals. Use of the term *client* is meant to apply whether the intervention is provided directly with a patient, a child, an adult, or a family or done in consultation with a physician, a social worker, a student, an architect, an employee, an organization, or an entire community. All these "clients" seek the knowledge and skills of an occupational therapy practitioner to address issues that could enhance their ability (or the ability of those they serve) to participate fully in their lives. Occupational therapy practitioners use their knowledge and skills to bridge the world of the client with the systems of care provided in health and medical care, whether at a hospital, a school, a clinic, or community-based program.[19] A core assumption of occupational therapy is that in order to be considered healthy, one must be able to engage in daily occupations that are desired, meaningful, and satisfying.

The Person-Environment-Occupation-Performance Model Is Focused on Occupational Performance

The concept of occupational performance has become a mainstay in the development of most models of occupational therapy. It operates as a means of connecting the individual to roles and the sociocultural environment.[19] We previously defined occupational performance as "the complex interactions between the persons' capacities and their environments that involve the activities, tasks, and roles that are meaningful or required of them."[13] In this edition, we expand upon this idea to emphasize the active nature of *occupational performance* and define it as *the doing of meaningful activities, tasks, and roles through complex interactions between the person and environment.* We believe occupational performance supports *participation* (active engagement and involvement that contributes to the well-being of individuals and communities) and *well-being* (satisfaction and quality of life). Implicit with any conceptual model is a purpose of guiding the application of knowledge to make informed decisions. So it is with the PEOP Model, conceived to organize evidence-based knowledge to guide the practitioner's clinical reasoning necessary to address the occupational performance needs of clients being served.

The Person-Environment-Occupation-Performance Model Emphasizes a Systems Perspective

The PEOP Model is a systems model,[4,20] proposing that the factors involved in occupational performance involve characteristics of the activity, task, or role; features of the environment (cultural, social support, social determinants and social capital, physical and natural environments, health education and public policy, assistive technology); and characteristics of the person (physiological, psychological, motor, sensory/perceptual, cognitive, or spiritual). Systems models assert the principle that each component has the potential to impact other components and the function of the system as a whole.[21] When people

perform occupations, they interact with their environments in ways that have reciprocal consequences. This reciprocal person-environment interaction, or more properly transaction, can be considered the throughput of the model. Goals and intentions influence actions (occupational performance) that result in outcomes (finishing a chore, enjoying an activity, taking care of one's health). The person, through the occupation, changes some aspect of the environment (whether through a conversation, written idea, or task performed) and at the same time changes herself (or himself) in some way (physically, cognitively, psychologically, spiritually, or emotionally). Viewed in this way, any change in individuals' capabilities, their occupational choices, or the environmental features of their situations, could potentially influence the results—the outcomes of a given occupational situation. These human "doings" result in a variety of outcomes, ranging from the mundane to the magnificent. But only clients themselves (whether a person, family, organization, or community) are able to determine the outcomes that are important to them. Viewing the PEOP Model as a system where factors or components work together to influence an occupational outcome provides a useful framework that supports the systematic analysis and reasoning necessary to guide decision making for intervention.

The Person-Environment-Occupation-Performance Model Supports Client-Centered Practice

In the PEOP Model, a partnership between the client and practitioner is necessary because the client must actively set goals and participate in determining a beneficial approach that supports performance, participation, and well-being. A client-practitioner partnership, important to the PEOP Model, serves as a bridge between the scientific, biological, and technological world of biomedicine to the practical, social, cultural, and spiritual world of everyday living.[19] This bridge includes a full panorama of person and environmental factors that positively or negatively influence occupational performance, participation, and well-being. The context of individuals' life circumstances is where they live, how they live their lives, and what they need to do; and it is how all of those factors, when considered together, combine to support or limit activities and participation (and ultimately, well-being). Performance and participation problems, then, are redefined so that factors that facilitate or support occupational performance are considered alongside those that limit or restrict performance of what individuals need and want to do. Individuals' stories, or narratives about their lives, provide important information for considering the enabling and disabling characteristics of a situation in context. In occupational therapy, then, interventions are aimed at enabling individuals to perform the activities and tasks that are central to their lives, whether these pertain to management of self and others, work/school, or community engagement. It is important to recognize that a central theme of the PEOP Model is that the client's context and preferences shape the goals for performance, participation, and well-being.

The PEOP Model can be used as a guide for forming a complete occupational profile of an individual. This profile includes information about individuals' perceptions of their performance history, abilities, and problems and their roles, interests, responsibilities, and values. For individuals, this profile includes a personal narrative that includes perceptions and meaning, choices and responsibilities, attitudes and motivation, and needs and goals. For organizations, the narrative can include the mission and history of the organization, its culture and priorities, the organization's stakeholders, and the organization's needs and goals. For communities or populations, the narrative provides a description of the social, cultural, geographic, and political features of the environment, including the incidence and prevalence of health problems; a description of the community; and the needs and goals of the population.

The PEOP Model is also grounded in evidence. When there are problems that limit occupational performance and participation, knowledge of person and environmental factors and the partnership of a practitioner and client may foster occupational performance (doing) and enable participation (engagement in everyday life), all of which contribute to a sense of well-being (satisfaction). Loche and Latham[22] have provided useful reasons for having individuals establish their own goals (Box 4-2).

DESCRIPTION OF THE MODEL

It is often said that a picture is worth a thousand words. Figure 4-1 provides a graphic representation of the PEOP Model. This representation is intended to convey that occupational performance is determined not only by the nature of the activity, task, or role to be performed, but also by the characteristics of the person and the environment that supports the person's occupations. To paraphrase an often observed systems theory adage, *environments, people, and occupations are perfectly aligned to result in the performance that occurs.* In other words, occupational performance successfully leads to participation and well-being when there is a person-environment fit that optimally supports the client and his or her valued occupations.

It should be noted that for a given situation, the applicability or importance of the person and environmental factors will vary. The PEOP Model assumes that consideration of each of the relevant factors that bear upon the

---

BOX 4-2

COLLABORATIVE GOAL-SETTING PRINCIPLES[23]

- Goals that are established by individuals themselves focus attention and direct efforts
- Establishing challenging, but realistic, goals leads an individual to greater effort and persistence
- Encouraging goals that are challenging leads to higher performance than goals that simply ask for best performance
- A goal-setting process helps individuals apply or develop skills to achieve the goal
- Ongoing feedback that recognizes progress toward a goal is important for goal achievement.

---

performance, since some will offer challenges and others will provide the support that will make doing possible. Accordingly, the PEOP Model visually depicts the factors that must come together to support performance, participation, and well-being. Application of the PEOP Model in practice requires (a) forming a collaborative relationship with the client and eliciting the client's narrative by asking the right questions, and (b) being able to use that information to better understand the issues and options presented by the client's needs and goals. The PEOP Model identifies targeted factors to address the personal performance capabilities/constraints and the environmental performance enabler/barriers that are central to the occupational performance.

Person Factors

In the previous sections, we identified how the PEOP Model begins with an understanding of the roles, activities, and goals of a client, which provide the motivation to address occupational performance problems. Motivation is one of several psychological factors that can influence performance. Others include self-concept, self-esteem, sense of identity, self-efficacy, metacognition, and self-awareness. Another important psychological factor is emotional state. This includes core affect and situational-based feelings (Chapter 14). Other important psychological factors include the client's life story, or narrative. This story provides the context for a person's perceived meaning and sense of coherence—how they understand and interpret the world. Spiritual or transcendental beliefs are often important to this overall understanding (Chapter 19). Other person factors in the PEOP Model that are central

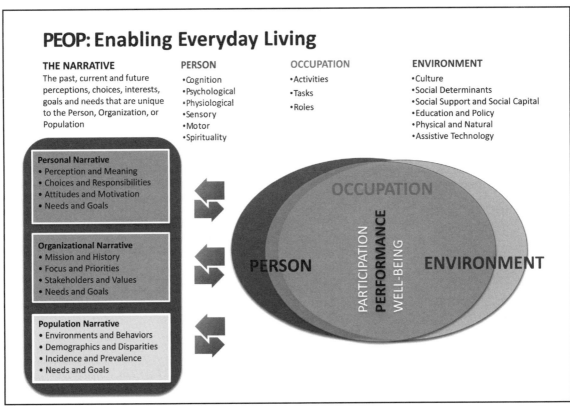

Figure 4-1. PEOP Model. Occupational performance (doing) enables participation (engagement) in everyday life that contributes to well-being (health and quality of life).

to occupational performance include the person's physiological status, including strength, endurance, flexibility, inactivity, and stress; as well as their sleep habits, nutrition, and general health (Chapter 18). Of great importance are the factors associated with cognitive processing, including memory, thought organization, attention, awareness, and the key reasoning, decision making, and goal achievement skills provided by executive function (Chapter 15). Other person factors important to task performance involve the neurobehavioral subsystems, which include sensing and perceiving the self and environment through the somatosensory, olfactory, gustatory, visual, auditory, proprioceptive, and tactile senses; and moving within the environment through use of movement-related subsystems, including motor control, motor planning (praxis), and postural control (Chapters 16 and 17).

Environment Factors

Environment factors in the PEOP Model that are central to occupational performance include social support, practical or instrumental support, and informational support; all based on relationships, networks, and group affiliations. Social groups have characteristics that can influence performance and participation (including social attitudes such as stigmas), or more formal laws and policies (Chapter 21). The cultural environment includes values, beliefs, customs, rituals, and time use, all of which can influence performance (Chapter 20). The policy environment governs access to and the availability of societal resources (Chapter 23). The physical features of an environment are both obvious and subtle. These factors include the built environment and its accessibility and usability features, as well as the natural environment, including geography, terrain, climate, air quality (Chapter 22), and tools and assistive technologies (Chapter 24). All of these factors impact occupational performance either as a barrier or enabler, and must be considered within a comprehensive environmental scan.

To incorporate key elements of planning, the occupational therapy practitioner uses an analytic or process approach. This analysis (process approach) seeks information from the client by interview and by employing assessments that give the practitioner a clear understanding of the environment-related and person-related enablers or constraints that may enhance or limit the person's activity and participation. While the practitioner will gain key information by considering person-related, environment-related, and occupation-related factors individually, the most important insights will come by examining the factors in combination—that is, how these features interact to support or impede the performance of valued activities, tasks, and roles.

Using the Person-Environment-Occupation-Performance Model to Plan Occupational Therapy Services

The PEOP Model provides occupational therapy practitioners with foundational knowledge of concepts and relationships that inform understanding of occupational performance at the person, organization, and population levels. The core principles of the model, including client-centeredness, collaboration between practitioner and client, and the identification of valued outcomes (leading to increased participation and well-being), combine with an understanding of the key components of persons, environments, and occupations, as these interact to support occupational performance and provide the framework for systematic analysis. This analytic approach becomes a guide for assessment and, later, decision making for intervention.

We refer to this analytic approach as the occupational therapy process, and it is the heart of occupational therapy practice. It is also of high ethical importance, because according to the principle of beneficence, the occupational therapy practitioner is obligated to select the interventions that are likely to result in the *best* possible outcome for the client.[24] This can only be done through use of a conceptual framework that systematically guides the practitioner through a process of data gathering, assessment, collaborative decision making, and intervention.

Thus, in this fourth edition of the PEOP Model we introduce the PEOP Occupational Therapy Process, designed to guide the practitioner through all of the steps necessary for implementing the PEOP Model in traditional and emerging areas of practice—whether with individual clients, groups and organizations, or populations. The PEOP Model identifies the factors that must come together to support both the practitioner and the client in developing a realistic and sequenced plan of care. Success in this process depends on the practitioner's skills in forming a relationship and eliciting the client's motivation by asking the right questions, as well as being able to access that knowledge to understand the issues and options presented by the client's needs and goals. In Chapter 5 we describe the PEOP Occupational Therapy Process and further define and discuss its essential elements: the narrative, assessment/evaluation, intervention, and outcome.

REFERENCES

1. Christiansen C, Baum C. *Occupational Therapy: Overcoming Human Performance Deficits.* Thorofare, NJ: SLACK Incorporated; 1991.
2. Baum CM, Christiansen C, eds. *Occupational Therapy: Enabling Function and Well-Being.* Thorofare, NJ: SLACK Incorporated; 1997.
3. Christiansen C, Baum CM, Bass Haugen J, eds. *Occupational Therapy: Performance, Participation, and Well-Being.* Thorofare, NJ: SLACK Incorporated; 2005.
4. Von Bertalanffy L. General system theory. *Gen Syst.* 1956;1:1-10.
5. Engel GL. The need for a new medical model: a challenge for biomedicine. *Science.* 1977;196(4286):129-136.
6. Kleinman A, Eisenberg L, Good B. Culture, illness, and care: clinical lessons from anthropologic and cross-cultural research. *Ann Intern Med.* 1978;88(2):251-258.
7. Kuhn TS. *The Structure of Scientific Revolutions.* Chicago, IL: University of Chicago Press; 2012.
8. Quiroga VAM. *Occupational Therapy: The First 30 Years 1900 to 1930.* Bethesda, MD: AOTA; 1995.
9. Burnette NL. The status of occupational therapy in Canada. *Am J Phys Med Rehab.* 1923;2(3);179-182.
10. Christiansen C, Haertl K. A contextual history of occupational therapy. In: Schell B, Gillen G, Scaffa M, Cohn ES, eds. *Willard and Spackman's Occupational Therapy.* 12th ed. Philadelphia: Lippincott Williams & Wilkins; 2014:9-34.
11. Hall HJ. Work-cure: a report of five years' experience at an institution devoted to the therapeutic application of manual work. *JAMA.* 1910;54(1):12-14.
12. Friedland J. Occupational therapy and rehabilitation: an awkward alliance. *Am J Occup Ther.* 1998;52(5):373-380.
13. Reed KL, Sanderson SN. *Concepts of Occupational Therapy.* Baltimore, MD: Wolters Kluwer Health; 1999.
14. Kielhofner G, Burke JP. A model of human occupation, part 1: conceptual framework and content. *Am J Occup Ther.* 1980;34(9):572-581.
15. Canadian Association of Occupational Therapists. *Enabling Occupation: An Occupational Therapy Perspective.* Ottawa, Ontario: CAOT Publications ACE; 1997.
16. Shannon PD. The derailment of occupational therapy. *Am J Occup Ther.* 1977;31(3):229-234.
17. Kielhofner G, Burke J. Occupational therapy after 60 years: an account of changing identity and knowledge. *Am J Occup Ther.* 1976;31(10):675-689.
18. Meyer A. The philosophy of occupation therapy. *Arch Occup Ther.* 1922;1(1):1-10.
19. Engelhardt Jr HT. Defining occupational therapy: the meaning of therapy and the virtues of occupation. *Am J Occup Ther.* 1977;31(10):666.
20. Kielhofner G. General systems theory: implications for theory and action in occupational therapy. *Am J Occup Ther.* 1978;32(10):637-645.
21. Boulding KE. General systems theory—the skeleton of science. *Management Science.* 1956;2(3):197-208.
22. Locke EA, Latham GP. Building a practically useful theory of goal setting and task motivation: a 35-year odyssey. *Am Psychol.* 2002;57(9):705-717.
23. Loche RA, Latham GP. Building a practical useful theory of goal setting and task motivation. *Am Psychol.* 2002;57(9):705-717.
24. Rogers JC. Eleanor Clarke Slagle Lectureship—1983; clinical reasoning: the ethics, science, and art. *Am J Occup Ther.* 1983;37(9):601-616.

INTERVENTIONS AND OUTCOMES
The Person-Environment-Occupation-Performance (PEOP) Occupational Therapy Process

Julie D. Bass, PhD, OTR/L, FAOTA; Carolyn M. Baum, PhD, OTR/L, FAOTA;
and Charles H. Christiansen, EdD, OTR, FAOTA

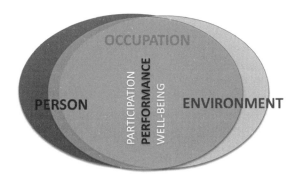

LEARNING OBJECTIVES

- Describe the components of the PEOP Occupational Therapy Process for individuals, populations, and organizations.
- Discuss why the terms occupation-based, client-centered, and evidence-based are essential components in the PEOP Occupational Therapy Process.
- Use the PEOP Occupational Therapy Process to develop an intervention plan for individuals, populations, and organizations.
- Describe occupational therapy intervention approaches and principles that should be applied in the PEOP Occupational Therapy Process.

- Identify and define terminology that has been used to document occupational therapy outcomes.
- Discuss historical influences on the PEOP Occupational Therapy Process.

KEY WORDS

- Assessment/evaluation
- Intervention
- Narrative
- Outcomes

Christiansen CH, Baum CM, Bass JD, eds.
Occupational Therapy: Performance, Participation, and Well-Being, Fourth Edition (pp 57-79).
© 2015 SLACK Incorporated.

INTRODUCTION

The phrase *occupational therapy process* is often used to describe the components and process of clinical reasoning that an occupational therapy practitioner uses when working with a client. The AOTA states the occupational therapy process involves "the delivery of services and includes evaluating, intervening, and targeting outcomes"[1(pS73)] with an occupation and client-centered focus. The PEOP Model provides the basis for an occupational therapy process that practitioners may use in addressing problems that limit occupational performance. This chapter will explain how the PEOP Model can serve as part of a process, the PEOP Occupational Therapy Process, to organize knowledge for practice with an individual, a population or community, and/or an organization. The PEOP Model is designed to support practitioners as they build collaborative plans with clients (ie, the patient, the child, the family, the physician, the social worker, the student, the architect, the employee, the organization, the employer, or the community); this plan incorporates the knowledge and skills of an occupational therapy practitioner to address issues that impact occupational performance.

Mattingly and Fleming[2] in their seminal work on clinical reasoning in occupational therapy made a statement that captures the essence of the occupational therapy process. They said that what occupational therapy practitioners do appears so simple; but it is so complex. Occupational therapy practitioners are problem solvers and consultants. Meyer said, "We provide opportunities, not prescriptions."[3(p7)] The problems of clients have to be solved in the context of the client's life, characteristics of the community, or the organization's culture. The client's internal and external resources must be mobilized to address the problems, and the resolution has to capture the client's motivation and also occur in the client's time frame. The practitioner is an agent of change, bringing to the situation knowledge of interventions that can enable clients to meet their goals.

Before we start planning treatment for someone else, let's think about occupational performance from your perspective. Imagine—you were riding your bike in the park (occupation: activity). You came up over a hill going at a pretty fast clip and someone had left a tricycle in the path (environment: physical and natural). You fall off your bike and the next thing you know you are in the hospital in a great deal of pain (person: psychological, physiological, and sensory). You learn that you have broken your shoulder and pelvis (person: physiological), and have a mild head injury (person: physiological and cognitive). If that is not enough, you touch the bandages on your face and find that you have some serious abrasions on your face that will require plastic surgery (person: physiological and psycho-

logical). You don't have time for this, you have to study for your finals (occupation: task), you are in a friend's wedding in 3 weeks (occupation: activity and role), and your family lives over 1000 miles away (environmental: social support).

As you begin to comprehend what has happened, you think, "I can't do what I did before, but I need to get back to my life as soon as possible." You want to go home, but you wonder how is it going to work; you live on a 3rd floor with no elevator (environment: physical) and you live alone and all of your good friends are at universities and jobs all over the country (environment: social support). You realize you are weak (person: physiological), your vision is not clear (person: physiological and sensory), you can't remember your new phone number (person: cognitive), and you are concerned over who is going to pay for this (environment: social determinants)... "What am I going to do?" To provide the most appropriate care for you, your providers need to know who you are and what you need. What do you want people to know about you and your previous activities and roles? Do you want them to know what you need and want to do? How would it be to turn control over to someone else—or should you? In walks your occupational therapy practitioner. The story is really just beginning and you can use your imagination regarding the scenarios that follow.

In your role as an occupational therapy practitioner, people won't always choose to be your client—a series of events has created the occupational performance issue that requires your service. Clients come to you because you have the knowledge and skills to help them build and execute a plan to accomplish what they want and need to do for themselves. It becomes your task to identify how impairments or problems have limited their activities and how barriers are limiting their participation, and to do this in a client-centered context.

OVERVIEW OF THE PERSON-ENVIRONMENT-OCCUPATION-PERFORMANCE OCCUPATIONAL THERAPY PROCESS

The PEOP Occupational Therapy Process builds upon capabilities and environmental resources that can support the client in the occupations they want and need to do. The Process may appear somewhat complex, but you have (or will have at the end of your educational program) the knowledge to promote occupational performance using this PEOP Model. In the PEOP Occupational Therapy Process, all of the knowledge you have acquired in your occupational therapy program, prerequisite courses, and related experiences comes together. Many sources of knowledge will contribute to your understanding of person

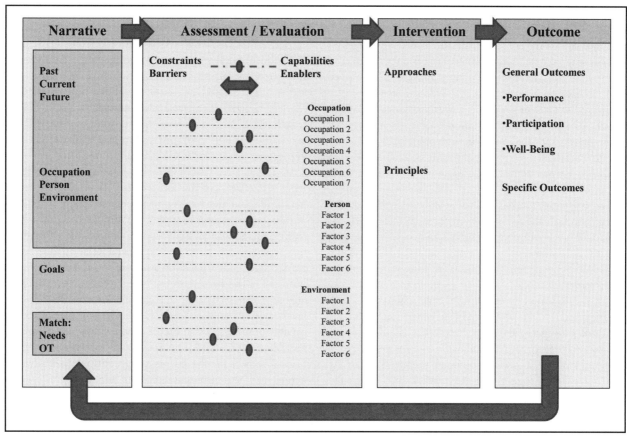

Figure 5-1. Introduction to the PEOP Occupational Therapy Process.

factors (eg, anatomy, physiology, neuroscience, medical lectures, psychology, ethics, and religion), environmental factors (eg, sociology, anthropology, political science, geography, engineering, and public health), and occupations (eg, occupational science, occupational therapy theory, psychology, education, industry, family, and consumer science). Fieldwork and case studies will provide you with opportunities to integrate concepts as you interact with real people and real situations. This knowledge, applied to the occupational performance needs of your client, defines your professional role as an occupational therapy practitioner and differentiates you from other professionals. You will employ client-centered and occupation-based strategies that engage individual(s) to develop or use resources that enable successful occupational performance.

The PEOP Occupational Therapy Process has 4 primary components that occur concurrently throughout the time you are with a client or clients: narrative, assessment and evaluation, intervention, and outcomes. This process may be applied to individuals, populations, and organizations. It is challenging to visually represent the dynamic nature of the PEOP Occupational Therapy Process, as it involves humans engaged in solving real problems (Figure 5-1). The Process includes a number of constructs that

must come together to support both the practitioner and the client in developing a realistic and sequenced plan. These constructs and the dynamic nature of the PEOP Occupational Therapy Process will be introduced in this chapter. The PEOP Occupational Therapy Process also depends on the practitioner's skills in forming a relationship with the client(s), asking the right questions, and being able to access knowledge to understand the issues and options presented by the client's occupational issues and goals. The Process requires the skills of a professional. An individual who lacks the conceptual ability, knowledge, or access to resources cannot perform it.

The Person-Environment-Occupation-Performance Occupational Therapy Process: Occupation-Based

Many health, social service, and education professionals use a process that includes assessment/evaluation, interventions, and outcomes as the basis for providing services. What, then, is the unique contribution of occupational therapy in our different practice settings? Occupations and occupational performance serve as threads that connect the different components of the PEOP Occupational Therapy Process and give occupational therapy a scope of practice that is different from all other health professions.

An occupation-based framework is the foundation for the PEOP Occupational Therapy Process. Occupations and occupational performance provide the lens for understanding the client's narrative, summarizing the results from assessment and evaluation, selecting intervention approaches, and analyzing the outcomes of occupational therapy services. Occupational therapy scholars and leaders have emphasized the importance of occupations in promoting health and framing the role of occupational therapy as a profession. In 1962, Reilly hypothesized that "man, through the use of his hands, as they are energized by mind and will, can influence the state of his own health"[4(p87)] and that occupational therapy's calling was to apply this knowledge to promote performance, participation, and well-being.

It is important to point out that when the PEOP Occupational Therapy Process is used with an individual, it is not pathogenic-based or diagnostic-based. It is based on the occupational performance problems presented by the individual. As an occupational therapy practitioner, you have knowledge about the relationships of impairments to a diagnosis; and while this information will give you clues about problems that the person might be experiencing, relying only on what one expects to find based on an impairment or diagnosis does not give credit to the client's ability to share his or her experiences concerning the problem nor to your knowledge about occupational performance. To further explain the point, a person is not seen as having a hand injury, a stroke, autism, or a mental illness. The person is presented to you as an individual who is limited in his or her capacity to do that which he or she wants or needs to do. In the process of developing a plan, you will use a variety of strategies to help the person address the problems that are limiting his or her occupational performance. This is the defining characteristic of an occupational therapy practitioner.

The Person-Environment-Occupation-Performance Occupational Therapy Process: Client-Centered

A client-centered approach is central to the occupational therapy process and requires 1) the practitioner to engage the client in problem solving and goal achievement, and 2) the client to fully participate as a collaborator in occupational therapy.[5] It also requires the occupational therapy practitioner to adopt the role of collaborator with the client instead of decision maker. Asking clients to be partners in their own care requires the occupational therapy practitioner to explore the extent to which the client

understands his or her circumstances, and whether or not he or she feels that their objectives can be accomplished.

Self-efficacy, or believing that a task or activity can be accomplished, allows one to feel competent. This, in turn, contributes to improved occupational performance and well-being.[6] Self-efficacy is at the core of client-centered care. By viewing clients as individuals with unique characteristics and roles and focusing the plan on the client's needs, the person can gain motivation from their own perceptions and emotional efforts.

A model of care can only be described as client-centered when the client explains the problems, and defines his or her needs and experiences in an environment of understanding, trust, and acceptance.[7] It also requires the client and occupational therapy practitioner to work together to define the nature of the occupational performance problems, the focus and need for intervention, and the preferred outcome of therapy supported by evidence. Clients must be encouraged to participate in planning their care at their own levels, depending on their capabilities; but all people are capable of making some choices about how their treatment should be approached. The practitioner must have a fundamental respect for the clients' values and for their style of coping with the current situation.

A recent definition of client-centered occupational therapy highlights the many elements of this approach that are important in practice, eg, partnership, empowerment, occupational roles, active participation, negotiation, listening, respect, and informed decision-making.[8] There are additional concepts related to client-centered practice that also deserve consideration as we strive to implement client-centered principles. Family-centered care recognizes the important role of the family in occupational therapy services; relationship-centered care acknowledges the variations in client engagement that are associated with limitations and the external and environmental influences that influence the nature of decision making that occurs within the relationship.[9] The PEOP Occupational Therapy Process considers the client central to the planning process and implementation of the occupational therapy program.

The Person-Environment-Occupation-Performance Occupational Therapy Process: Evidence-Based

Evidence underpins the practitioner's decisions of what measures to include, interventions to employ, and outcomes to use. All professionals are being held to a standard—that of competent practice using best-practice methods that have been determined to be effective. Thus, evidence becomes the filter through which clinical decisions about the type of evaluation or assessment and the interventions that will support the client in achieving goals. Traditionally, intervention decisions were made based primarily on experience and training. Students looked to their teachers and fieldwork supervisors, and new practitioners looked to more experienced colleagues to guide their approach to both assessment and intervention. Evidence-based practice takes into account the practitioner's experience and the unique perspectives of the client and adds to this evidence from relevant publications as decisions are made about interventions that will be effective.[10] You will note in this book that many chapters end with a table of evidence that supports the content of the chapter. This was done to integrate evidence into the basic learning process. It then becomes available for planning interventions that will be effective given the problems as presented by the client.

NARRATIVE

The PEOP Occupational Therapy Process begins with the narrative (personal story) from your client(s); conversations and observations are used to understand issues and to have a clear picture of what is needed and wanted. The client's narrative includes perspectives on person, occupation, and environment in the past, present, and future, as well as consideration of long-term and short-term goals. The client and the practitioner then decide together whether there is a match between the client's goals and the interventions that occupational therapy can provide.

There has been renewed interest in using narrative in medicine and health care.[11] Narrative provides a means to fully understand the client's problems and their meaning within the broader context of a person's life. Narrative is one aspect of a holistic approach to health care, because it uncovers unique perspectives and addresses the innermost emotions that emerge as a result of problems. The hypothetical example of having an injury as an occupational therapy student at the beginning of this chapter highlighted the personal feelings and concerns that might be shared in the PEOP Occupational Therapy Process. Narratives are unique to the person, but examples of clients' perspectives and experiences can be explored through published qualitative research and websites like Health Talk Online (http://www.healthtalkonline.org/).

ASSESSMENT AND EVALUATION

The assessment and evaluation phase of the PEOP Occupational Therapy Process is grounded in evidence. Formal assessments that have strong measurement characteristics and established reliability and validity will contribute to baseline information on the person, environment, and occupations and the overall evaluation that is the basis for intervention planning. Assessments may give the practitio-

ner a clear understanding of the constraints and barriers that are limiting activities and participation. As well, the practitioner will gain insight into capabilities and enablers that will support engagement in meaningful occupations.

The outcome of the evaluation is a summary of the client's current status on multiple occupation, person, and environment factors along a continuum scale of constraints and barriers to capabilities and enablers. Capturing an overall profile of a client's status is a challenging, but important, part of the evaluation process. In the representation of the PEOP Occupational Therapy Process, a graphic organizer[12] of a continuum scale is used to represent the complex connections across different factors and summarize the client's overall current status. A marker on each continuum scale represents the practitioner's evaluation of the client's current status on a specific factor along the continuum. A marker closer to the constraints and barriers end of the scale indicates a potential problem area, while a marker closer to capabilities and enablers suggests a strength that may be used.

Let's consider a couple of simple examples of continuum scales; a graphic organizer is used to summarize the case study at the beginning of the chapter. Recall that you, as the hypothetical occupational therapy student who was involved in a bike accident, have a great deal of pain, blurry vision, a broken shoulder and pelvis, a mild head injury with thinking and memory difficulties, and facial abrasions. You live on the 3rd floor, have friends who live far away, and don't have much money. Although we don't have the results from actual assessments, let's imagine the findings in several areas at the initial assessment. Where would you put your markers on the constraints and barriers to capabilities and enablers continuum scale? Would it look something like Box 5-1?

Now imagine that it is 2 weeks later. You had a fabulous team of health professionals in the hospital (including occupational therapy of course!) that addressed the many constraints and barriers that occurred as a result of the accident. Your occupational therapy practitioner provided you some equipment and taught you some dressing techniques you can use while your shoulder and pelvis are healing. You worked with the health care team and your university to obtain a temporary living situation in one of the accessible dorms and are able to postpone taking your final exams a few weeks and take an incomplete in your courses. Although you don't feel ready to take the exams, you are at least able to concentrate better after getting some ideas on how to organize your day. Two of your classmates who live on campus have generously agreed to help you get around campus. Your brother brought you a wheelchair that your grandmother had used. We still don't have the results from actual assessments, but we can imagine the changes in the findings. Where would you put your markers on the constraints and barriers to capabilities and

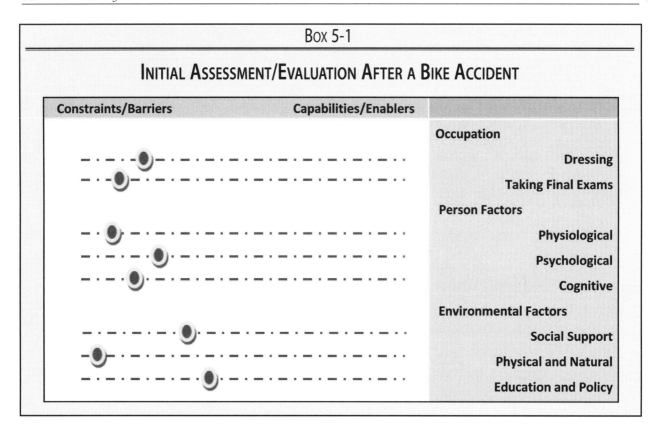

enablers continuum scale given this update 2 weeks later? Would it look something like Box 5-2?

The assessment and evaluation process provides direction for the intervention phase. The clients should enter into the intervention phase with a clear understanding of the potential outcomes that will result with the effort exerted by both the practitioner and the client. Assessment, evaluation, and intervention occur concurrently throughout the time you are with a client or clients.

INTERVENTIONS

Intervention planning is based on the information gathered from the narrative and assessment and evaluation. In collaboration with the client, the occupational therapy practitioner selects intervention approaches that will help the client reach short-term and long-term goals and produce desired outcomes. A variety of intervention approaches may be used in working with each client (Table 5-1). A description of common approaches will include create-promote, establish-restore, maintain-habilitate, modify-compensate, prevent, educate, consult, and advocate. Throughout the PEOP Occupational Therapy Process, the occupational therapy practitioner considers whether the approaches selected are occupation-based, client-centered, and evidence-based. Categories and prin-

ciples of interventions[13] were discussed in the previous edition of this text, and provide the foundation for the approaches and principles adopted in the PEOP Occupational Therapy Process.

Occupational therapy practitioners also operate from principles in planning and implementing interventions. Principles serve as parameters and guideposts that are important across different intervention approaches. You are already familiar with 2 of these principles: client-centered and evidence-based. The PEOP Occupational Therapy Process incorporates additional principles related to ethics and advocacy, communication, culture, professional lifelong development, business fundamentals, and therapeutic use of self (Table 5-2). There may be additional principles that guide your practice for specific intervention approaches and settings.

OUTCOMES

In order for a profession to earn the respect of the people it serves, it must offer a service of demonstrable value. This means that the public must perceive that there is measurable benefit, result, or consequence for the services delivered. A profession must deliver what it says it will. Medicine has earned public support through, among other things, the provision of medical and surgical

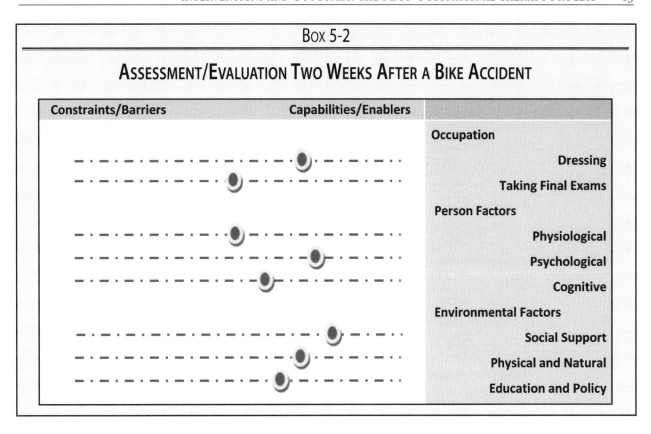

techniques that increase life expectancy, save lives, and reduce pain and suffering. Public health has acquired respect by its leadership in vaccinations, infectious disease control, and health education programs that improve the health of populations. Education has developed a strong reputation for providing early childhood programs that result in better academic outcomes for at-risk children. These are outcomes, or results, that the public values and expects in exchange for its considerable support of professional programs and services. Outcomes are the deliverables or benefits that a profession brings to society.

All professions achieve their status by providing a service to society. Society will either accept or support that contribution with payment for services, or will limit what the professions can do by denying payment and the privileges to practice. In more recent times, accountability for results has increased. Regulatory bodies and financial authorities in the business, education, and health sector and in local as well as national government are seeking to know the potential impact on interventions employed in the health, education, and social services. This interest has encouraged the use of outcomes focused on quality of life, and other measures to assist in resource allocation and assessing the impact of policy decisions.[16]

Many of the outcomes of concern to our profession have not changed since occupational therapy was founded. The field remains dedicated to help people achieve health,

well-being, and a high quality of life (QOL). However, in directing their efforts toward these ultimate outcomes, therapy personnel may often set interim goals that may also be viewed as outcomes. Because of its broad scope of concerns about humans as occupational beings, occupational therapy personnel deliver services that range from helping children acquire the functional skills necessary for everyday living to helping older adults identify ways in which they can maintain their health and continue living in the community. With this range of concerns, the number of potential outcomes of interest is large. However, this broad scope does not reduce the importance of thinking carefully about how outcomes are identified, defined, measured, and demonstrated. Additional discussion on outcomes will be provided at the end of this chapter.

Using the Person-Environment-Occupation-Performance Occupational Therapy Process to Plan Person-Centered Interventions

A person-centered PEOP Occupational Therapy Process (Figure 5-2) may be used to address the occupational needs and goals of an individual, family, or formal/informal caregivers. In the following description of the person-centered PEOP Occupational Therapy Process, an

Table 5-1.   *Occupational Therapy Interventions: Approaches*

Approach	Key Characteristic
Create-promote	• Focus on enhancing well-being or quality of life • Enhance opportunities for engagement in occupation, give meaning to participation in daily life, and promote a balanced lifestyle
Establish-restore	• Focus on physiological, neurobehavioral, cognitive, or psychological skills • Enhance personal performance capabilities and/or diminishing constraints • Restore: Recovering a skill that was lost • Establish: Attainment of a new skill • Activities are selected to meet the current skill level of the individual or population and then are graded to increase ability level • Devices or technology may be used
Maintain-habilitate	• Focus on maintaining current levels of performance and participation • Important in situations that pose a risk of declining personal capabilities or increased barriers in the environment • An important part of an overall intervention plan to ensure successful outcomes from other intervention approaches • For example, self-management programs for individuals with chronic conditions, home and school routines for children with developmental disabilities
Modify-compensate	• Focus on diminishing personal constraints or eliminating environmental barriers • Compensate: Use of environmental supports to avert occupational performance problems associated with a personal performance constraint (eg, assistive technology) • Modify: Reduce environmental barriers in the physical environment, social support systems, societal policies and attitudes, cultural norms and values (eg, educational programs to reduce social stigma)
Prevent	• Focus on limiting impact of anticipated problem • Primary: Problem is prevented by avoiding risk factors and threats • Secondary: Problem is interrupted before it becomes significant • Tertiary: Problem is evident, but consequences/complications are limited
Educate	• Focus on providing knowledge and skills • Transfer specific knowledge related to client's needs and priorities
Consult	• Focus on providing knowledge and skills • Collaborate with client to mutually define problems, identify solutions, and develop strategies; enable client to solve own problems
Advocate	• Focus on changes needed to promote performance, participation, and well-being • Collaborate with client to promote changes in policies, procedures, and practices

Adapted from Youngstrom MJ. Categories and principles of interventions. In: Christiansen C, Baum C, Bass Haugen J, eds. *Occupational Therapy: Performance, Participation, and Well-Being*. Thorofare, NJ: SLACK Incorporated; 2005:396-419.

individual is used to describe the process. What are some examples of individuals who have occupational needs and goals?

• A child who needs to engage in play activities that are important for learning and development.

Table 5-2.   *Principles to Apply in Occupational Therapy Interventions*

Principle	Key Characteristic
Client-centered	Incorporates clients' goals, perspectives and values in addressing their occupational needs[13,14]
Evidence-based	Uses a systematic process to find, evaluate, and applies evidence from research into practice[13,14]
Ethics and advocacy	Employs ethical and socially responsible practices; advocates for access and equitable policies for people served[14]
Communication	Adopts effective communication strategies and resources to support interprofessional teamwork and ensures understanding by lay audiences[14]
Culture	Demonstrates cultural sensitivity to the health beliefs and practices of clients[14]
Professional lifelong development	Recognizes that knowledge evolves; demonstrates currency in practice[14]
Business fundamentals	Develops innovative and evidence-based programs that fit with the mission and business plans of the organization or agency where services are delivered[14]
Therapeutic use of self	Strives for "intentional, planned use of personal behaviors, insight, perception, judgment, skill, and knowledge to optimize our working alliance with our clients and enable change"[15]

Adapted from Youngstrom MJ. Categories and principles of interventions. In: Christiansen C, Baum C, Bass Haugen J, eds. Occupational Therapy: Performance, Participation, and Well-Being. Thorofare, NJ: SLACK Incorporated; 2005:396-419.
Baum C, Barrows C, Bass Haugen J, et al. Blueprint for entry-level education. *Am J Occup Ther.* 2009;64:186-203.
Polatajko HJ, Davis, JA, McEwen SE. Therapeutic use of self: a catalyst in the client-therapist alliance for change. In: Christiansen CH, Baum CM, Bass JD, eds. *Occupational Therapy: Performance, Participation, and Well-Being.* 4th ed. Thorofare, NJ: SLACK Incorporated; 2015.

- A young adult who wants to better manage medications and household responsibilities that have been disrupted by mental health issues.
- An adult who wants to resume work roles after a traumatic brain injury.
- An older adult who wants to maintain involvement in volunteering and community activities.

It is important to note that a person-centered PEOP Occupational Therapy Process may also be used to address the occupational needs and goals of families and formal/informal caregivers. What are some examples of families and caregivers who may need occupational therapy services?

- The teachers of a special needs student who want to develop a classroom routine that supports learning.
- The parents of a young adult with mental health issues who need respite activities that promote wellness.
- The spouse or partner of an adult with a traumatic brain injury who needs to assume new responsibilities in the home.

- The children of an older adult who have been assisting with transportation because they are concerned about their parent driving to volunteering and community activities.

The Person-Centered Narrative

Except in an emergency situation, a physician does not begin to make decisions about a medical plan without a medical history. The occupational therapy practitioner should find it impossible to build a client-centered, occupation-based plan without an occupational history and profile. It is during the process of obtaining a history that the practitioner learns what the person has done previously and how values impact his or her priorities and everyday life. An occupational history should include a description of leisure interests and social activities and should provide a clear understanding of the responsibilities the client has for work, self, and home management tasks. Such a history can be accomplished with an interview or an instrument like the *Activity Card Sort*[17] or the

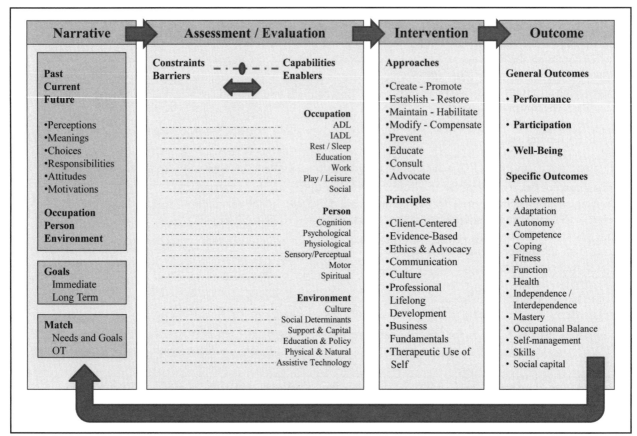

Figure 5-2. Person-Centered PEOP Occupational Therapy Process.

Interest Checklist.[18] Another key element is the person's perception of the situation. Every person has different levels of knowledge and awareness regarding his or her person and environmental factors, along with occupational issues of concern. So it is important to know how the person describes his or her past and current life in terms of person, environment, and occupations. It is also important to form an occupational profile that includes the client's hopes for the future. The *Role Checklist*[19] is a valuable resource to the practitioner to determine the past, current, and future roles of the client. It is especially important to understand the client's roles and responsibilities that must be maintained during the time he or she is receiving occupational therapy services. The profile should include a description of lifestyle issues and routines that enable daily occupation.

The narrative also provides an understanding of the client's goals. Often, the client will be more clear on his or her long-term goals (eg, I want to take my final exams this semester, I want to participate in my friend's wedding), than the immediate goals that are essential to address in working toward long-term goals (eg, I need to be able to

write to take my exams and get dressed to go to a wedding). Determining the long-term goals is useful in structuring a discussion around the immediate goals. The practitioner can help the client plan the steps to accomplish long-term goals. By knowing the person's interests, skills, roles, cultural beliefs, and values, it is possible to help formulate immediate goals that will not only be achievable, but will also be meaningful. The Canadian Occupational Performance Measure[20] is an excellent tool to use in planning goals; it also detects change in a client's self-perception of occupational performance over time.

The final step in the narrative of the PEOP Occupational Therapy Process is to determine the match between the person's goals and the occupational therapy approach. If there is not a match, the occupational therapy practitioner should make an appropriate referral to another professional or to other resources to address the client's goals. When there is a match, the practitioner should begin the second step of the PEOP Occupational Therapy Process to determine the person's capabilities and enablers and identify constraints and barriers that will need to be overcome.

Person-Centered Assessment and Evaluation

After obtaining the narrative, assessments are used to evaluate person factors, environmental factors, and occupations. The findings from assessments enable the occupational therapy practitioner to understand and document the constraints/barriers and capabilities/enablers along a continuum scale. The occupation areas include ADLs, IADLs, rest/sleep, education, work, play/leisure, and social. The person factors include cognition, psychological, physiological, sensory/perceptual, motor, and spiritual. The environmental factors include culture, social support, social determinants and capital, education and policy, physical and natural, and assistive technology. The occupational therapy practitioner carefully selects assessments that effectively and efficiently examine the occupations, person factors, and environmental factors that emerged as important from the client's narrative and other information.

Person-Centered Interventions

A person-centered intervention plan is constructed from the client's narrative and the results of assessment and evaluation. The practitioner uses his or her skill and expertise to help the client understand the issues that must be addressed in order to achieve immediate and long-term goals. The client has the right to question and the practitioner has the responsibility to identify the evidence that the interventions will enable goal attainment. Person-centered occupational therapy interventions may generally be classified as create-promote, establish-restore, maintain, modify-compensate, prevent, and educate-consult. Often, a combination of approaches will be used to meet the needs and goals of an individual. The selection of specific approaches are guided by intervention principles (client-centered, evidence-based, ethics/advocacy, communication, culture, professional lifelong development, and business fundamentals) that influence the integrity of therapy services. A general description of intervention approaches and principles will be provided later in this chapter.

Person-Centered Outcomes

The implementation of the intervention plan hopefully enables the client to achieve his or her immediate and long-term goals. Outcomes should be measured, not only to demonstrate the progress to the client, but also to demonstrate the effectiveness of the occupational therapy interventions to the referral source, to the payer, and to the public. The effectiveness of occupational therapy must be public to shape policies of institutions and payment sources. The entire PEOP Occupational Therapy Process leads to achieving the goals identified by the client and helping him or her to engage in life and meet roles, responsibilities, and interests. Because many individuals have lifelong occupational issues that require self-management strategies, part of the outcome should include planning for other periodic services from a practitioner if occupational performance issues emerge in the future.

USING THE PERSON-ENVIRONMENT-OCCUPATION-PERFORMANCE OCCUPATIONAL THERAPY PROCESS TO PLAN POPULATION-CENTERED INTERVENTIONS

The process described previously fits well when the occupational therapy practitioner is working with individuals or small groups of people (ie, families). However, an emerging area of practice for occupational therapy addresses the occupational issues of populations and communities. Population-based care may theoretically range from as large as all of the people in the world who fit some characteristic (eg, people with AIDS, children who are homeless) or may reflect a small group of people or a community with issues of concern (eg, mid-life women with family issues that affect their work for a company, or seniors who have become isolated in a neighborhood because of transportation issues). Sometimes, these issues are identified within a more obvious or defined organizational structure, such as within a community group, business, or a group of people within a designated government category (eg, people over 65 within a designated political or geographic jurisdiction). One might guess that the PEOP Occupational Therapy Process conducted will look different in these different situations. A population-centered PEOP Occupational Therapy Process may serve as the starting point for occupational therapy practitioners who are interested in improving the health of populations or communities in general or working within specific organizations.

Consider that you are an occupational therapy practitioner who has worked with older people in long-term care settings for several years and you wish to continue to work with older people, but would like to work with well elders to enable them to remain at home and improve their quality of life. How do you begin? Do you already have the background and knowledge that will enable success in this new practice arena? Are you ready to jump in and promote your services to organizations that work with this population or in these communities? Perhaps, but not likely.

In this situation, a population-centered PEOP Occupational Therapy Process may better prepare you to

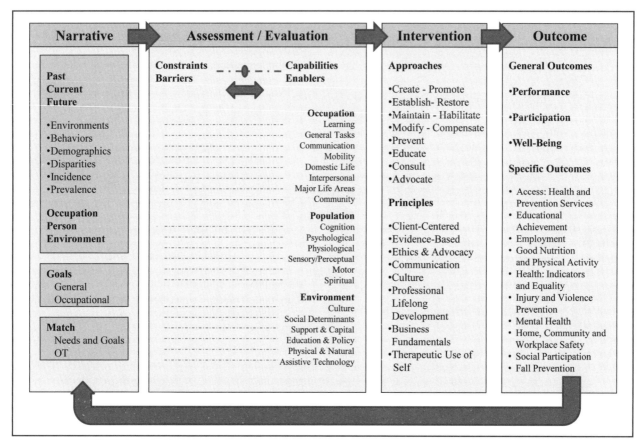

Figure 5-3. Population-Centered PEOP Occupational Therapy Process.

understand the general characteristics and issues of the older population, the community in which they live, and most importantly, to plan interventions that will meet the needs and goals of specific organizations. Let's follow this example through a population-centered PEOP Occupational Therapy Process. Although you have worked with elders who have health conditions and diminished abilities in the long-term care setting, you do not have a clear understanding of well elders. So you begin this process by acquiring general information and a narrative of population issues. What things would you look at (Figure 5-3)?

The Population-Centered Narrative

The population-centered narrative will help you define the population or community (eg, age, gender, income, education, employment, religion, and geographic area), obtain statistics of interest (eg, risk factors), and identify characteristics that are associated with people who are part of this population (eg, knowledge, attitudes, beliefs, habits, preferences, and sensitivities). This narrative may support some of your assumptions and/or dispel myths that are commonly held. Identification of areas of concern for this population requires you to look outside of occupational therapy to gain a broader understanding of the array of critical issues (eg, environments, behaviors, demographics, disparities, incidence, and prevalence). You will often find areas of concern identified by local, national, and international agencies and organizations; census information; public health; school districts; and even in the popular press. In a sense, you are conducting an environmental or informational scan to learn more about the priorities for a population, the incidence and prevalence of the issues, and the major stakeholders. For example, transportation has been identified as a major issue for older adults living in communities. Some of these population issues may not have occupational performance implications, while others will. An important step in the narrative is to explore the occupational therapy literature, use your knowledge of factors that support occupational performance, and employ strong critical thinking skills to help you make links between general population issues (eg, transportation for older adults) and related occupations (eg, shopping, financial transactions, and socialization).

Table 5-3.   Occupations of Populations: International Classification of Functioning, Disability and Health Areas

ICF General Areas: Activities and Participation Areas	ICF Specific Areas: Most Relevant to Occupational Therapy
Learning and applying knowledge	Basic learning Applying knowledge
General tasks and demands	Carrying out a daily routine Handling stress and other psychological demands
Communication	Conversation and use of communication devices and techniques
Mobility	Carrying, moving and handling objectives Walking and moving Moving around using transportation
Self-care	Activities of daily living Looking after one's health
Domestic life	Acquiring a place to live Acquisition of goods and services Household tasks Caring for household objects and assisting others
Interpersonal interactions/relationships	General interpersonal interactions
Major life areas	Education Work and employment Economic life; transactions and self-sufficiency
Community, social, and civic life	Community life Recreation and leisure Religion and spirituality Human rights—self-determination, autonomy, dignity Political life and citizenship

Adapted from World Health Organization. International Classification of Functioning, Disability, and Health (ICF). World Health Organization. http://www.who.int/classifications/icf/en/. Published 2001. Updated 2013. Accessed June 6, 2013.

Population-Centered Assessment and Evaluation

The occupational therapy practitioner selects appropriate assessments to understand person and environment factors that are enabling as well as constraining the occupations of the population. The person and environment factors include the same areas as the person-centered assessment and evaluation, but are analyzed at the population rather than the individual level. Occupation factors in populations are generally more focused on occupations that are important in public and community health and represented at the participation level in the ICF[21] (eg, learning, general tasks, communication, mobility, domestic life, interpersonal, major life, and community) (Table 5-3). Some assessment findings may be obtained from published evidence on a population. For example, it has been documented that over 60% of older adults over the age of 70 have a hearing loss.[22] This finding would be important information in planning interventions that address isolation and the need for social occupations by older adults. At the population level, many of the constraints and barriers will be environmental (eg, the lack of an accessible playground for children, inadequate public transportation to support older adult's participation in the community, and poor or confusing signage at the health clinic). Environmental factors may in turn affect the person factors (eg, poor air quality affects respiratory status). As with a person-centered assessment and evaluation, the evaluation of a population results in a summary of occupational performance, person factors, and environmental factors along a continuum scale. This summary provides the foundation for intervention planning.

Population-Centered and Community-Centered Interventions

Evidence is considered in understanding the intervention approaches that have already been tried to address occupational goals in the population. Examination of the evidence is important to select strategies that work for this population, discard ideas that do not have evidence to support them, and identify intervention approaches that have not yet been evaluated. If an untried strategy will be used, it is important for the client (ie, the population) to understand the principles on which you will base the intervention and agree to its use. If your work entails population initiatives (eg, public health, labor, and legislation), you may collaborate with others to implement intervention strategies. If your work involves developing partnerships with organizations and agencies, you may also need to complete an organization-centered PEOP Occupational Therapy Process to address the priorities of a specific organization. The intervention approaches and principles of the population-centered PEOP Occupational Therapy Process are similar to the person-centered Process, although some intervention aspects may be emphasized more than others.

Population-Centered Outcomes

The implementation of the intervention plan should result in improved outcomes for the population. Outcomes should be measured, not only to demonstrate the achievement of population goals, but also to document the effectiveness of the occupational therapy interventions to the referral source, to the funding sources, and to the public. The effectiveness of occupational therapy must be public in order to shape policies of institutions and payment sources. The entire process leads to achieving the goals identified by the population related to occupational performance, participation, and well-being of individuals in their communities. Achievement of goals related to performance, participation, and well-being will in turn contribute to the health of the population and community. Since many communities are facing new problems with an emerging population of older adults and many persons living with chronic diseases and disabling conditions, infrastructure is needed to enable full participation of all members of the community. One outcome may include the possibility of additional occupational therapy services if occupational performance issues emerge in the future that could benefit from an occupational therapy practitioner's expertise.

USING THE PERSON-ENVIRONMENT-OCCUPATION-PERFORMANCE OCCUPATIONAL THERAPY PROCESS TO PLAN ORGANIZATION-CENTERED INTERVENTIONS

The organization-centered PEOP Occupational Therapy Process begins with a population-centered Process related to the types of clients served by the organization. This step in the process enables the occupational therapy practitioner to approach the organization with a level of credibility that will open doors of opportunity. After developing expertise with regard to a specific population, an occupational therapy practitioner may not need to do this step in an explicit manner. Rather, the knowledge base of the professional includes this foundational information. Entry-level practitioners, however, will likely need to begin with a population-centered process as a preliminary step prior to any discussions with a specific organization. Although the organization-centered PEOP Occupational Therapy Process also includes a narrative, assessment and evaluation, interventions, and outcomes; it also requires consideration of the unique priorities of the organization (Figure 5-4).

Organization-Centered Narrative

The narrative of the organization includes not only the people served by the organization, but also its mission, history, focus, values, activities, funding, and stakeholders. Some of this information may be obtained in publications about the organization. Other information may be acquired through initial conversations with a contact person in the organization. The narrative helps the occupational therapy practitioner to identify the organization's needs and the potential for providing occupational therapy services. As part of the conversation with the organization's stakeholders, the occupational therapy practitioner explores areas of concern and unmet needs for the clients served. Many of these concerns may be expressed in terms of general issues. For example, a community agency might be concerned about the adaptation of recent immigrants to the expectations of the larger culture. A school district may be concerned about the social and emotional health of some student groups. A corporation may be concerned about retention of workers who are mothers or caregivers. In this step, the occupational therapy practitioner also uses critical reasoning skills to identify and communicate the occupational issues that may be influencing the general areas of concern for the organization. For example, recent immigrants may have vocational backgrounds that are different from the work opportunities currently available. Some

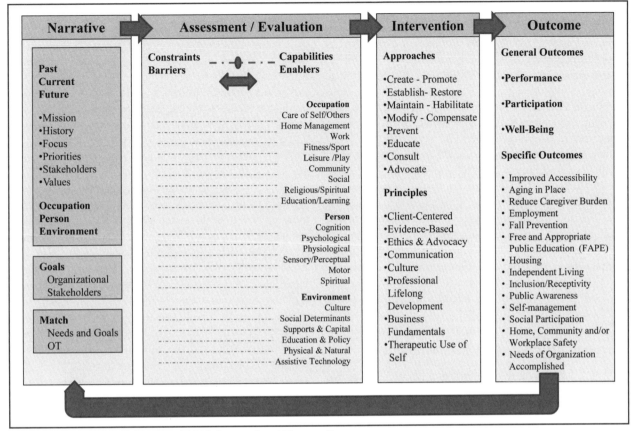

Figure 5-4. Organization-Centered PEOP Occupational Therapy Process.

adolescents may only have access to extracurricular activities that are sports-related. Workers may not have sufficient support systems to solve parenting or caregiving problems as they arise.

The goals of the organization and its stakeholders are considered next in the process. The occupational therapy practitioner inquires about the organization's immediate and long-term goals as they relate to general and occupational areas of concern. The practitioner also asks for information that will help determine the organization's commitment and ability to achieve these goals. The final part of the narrative step is to evaluate the match between the organization's goals and the occupational therapy services you can provide. You will use your population-centered PEOP Occupational Therapy Process, all the information you have gathered about the organization, and your discussions with people in the organization to decide whether to continue the process. At this point, your personal investment in the organization has been limited. However, if you continue the process, you and the organization may make a considerable commitment of personnel and resources to conduct assessment and evaluation and provide interventions.

Organization-Centered Assessment and Evaluation

The occupational therapy practitioner selects assessments to evaluate the person and environment factors that are enabling as well as constraining the occupations of the clients served by the organization. Clinical reasoning supports the occupational therapy practitioner in applying knowledge of the person, environment, and occupations to the programs and initiatives of the organization. At the organization level, many factors affecting occupational performance will be environmental (eg, lack of teacher training that fosters full participation of children in a mainstreamed classroom or managers who need ideas on how to make accommodations for workers who wish to return to work after an accident or injury). There may also be specific organizational problems that affect the person; for example, some work demands may foster poor posture or repetitive motion injuries.

Organization-Centered Interventions

With the organization's narrative and the results of the assessment and evaluation, an intervention plan may be constructed. The organization has the right and the practitioner has the responsibility to discuss the level of available evidence regarding interventions that target general and occupational goals. You are now ready to develop an organization-centered intervention plan. You will want to consider your initial population-centered plan, variations of this plan that are appropriate for this organization, and the current evidence that is available. It may also be important to pilot any interventions, especially if this represents a new area of occupational therapy practice. Pilot studies are a way to establish relationships with organizational clients, as initial outcomes can pave the way for additional work and funding. The organization may use the time to evaluate your capacity to help them achieve their goals. Implementation of your intervention plan may include any of the approaches and principles identified in the person-centered or population-centered plan. However, promote/prevent and educate/consult approaches are probably more common and effective when the target of the intervention is an organization and its clientele.

Organization-Centered Outcomes

Your success with this organization can only be verified and documented if you conduct an evaluation of your interventions for their effectiveness in achieving goals. This step is important in helping you solidify your relationship with the organization and preparing you to work with other related organizations. Disseminating the outcomes of your interventions to the broader occupational therapy community is also essential for expanding practice into new areas.

OUTCOMES OF THE PERSON-ENVIRONMENT-OCCUPATION-PERFORMANCE OCCUPATIONAL THERAPY PROCESS

Goals and Outcomes of Occupational Therapy

The types of goals toward which occupational therapy personnel provide their expertise are as varied as the occupations of life. For a child, the goals may be to be able to engage in sports, to learn in a classroom, to be able to play with siblings or to acquire the skills to be able to work when they are older. For an adult, the goals may be to return to work, to live safely in a community environment, to be able to care for a child, or to have the skills to support an important relationship. Older adults may want to be able to continue to work, to remain in their own homes, to be able to read to their grandchildren, or to go to a place of worship. Despite their variety, these goals have something in common. Each goal reflects an individual's desire to participate fully in society. Thus, it can be said that an important, perhaps universal, outcome of occupational therapy services is to enable people to participate in society through engaging in the occupations that are meaningful and important to them.

An organization may want to reduce its absenteeism due to injury, help an employee return to work after an injury, or provide knowledge to employees on how to manage their aging parents. Communities may want to provide more services to enable older adults to remain in their own homes, design a new playground that will accommodate all children with and without disabilities, or plan new street signs that older adults will be able to use to navigate safely. Each of these goals can be supported by an occupational therapy practitioner using an occupational performance approach. In each case, the expected outcome is one of increased participation, brought about by increases in capacities or skills and the elimination of environmental barriers (Table 5-4).

Efficacy and Effectiveness

The words *efficacy* and *effectiveness* are often used as synonyms to describe the results of intervention demonstrated through research. Although they have slightly different meanings, they each refer to studies of outcomes. Professions demonstrate the efficacy of their services through highly controlled clinical trials, research, and the general effectiveness of their services through other types of outcome studies done under less controlled and more natural conditions. The idea in both instances is to objectively demonstrate whether or not an expected goal or result of intervention was achieved. Typically, the degree of confidence that one has in a given procedure or technique increases as the evidence accumulates in support of its effectiveness.

The public is interested in evidence that a procedure, treatment, or program of intervention provides the results or outcomes that were intended. The term *evidence-based practice* aptly describes the expectation that services delivered have been shown to result in expected outcomes.[28] The randomized clinical trial, or RCT, is the "gold standard" for demonstrating efficacy. However, because of the difficulty and expense associated with conducting clinical trials, as well as ethical problems associated with denying potentially beneficial treatment to a control or comparison group, other types of evidence-related studies are often conducted. These effectiveness studies often have less stringent controls and, as a result, the confidence that one may have in their findings is limited.

Table 5-4.   *Description of Outcomes That Reflect Performance, Participation, and Well-Being*

Description	Source
Occupation is the vehicle to acquire, maintain, or redevelop skills necessary to fulfill occupational roles and provide satisfaction.	Fidler & Fidler[23]
Occupation can contribute to a person's sense of well-being and state of health.	Reed[24]
Occupation can be used to help a person learn to organize his or her life and use resources to reduce the impact of disability.	Reed[24]
The lack of occupation leads to a breakdown in habits and physiological deterioration—this leads to loss of ability and competency to support daily life.	Kielhofner[25]
Individuals with cognitive loss who remain engaged in occupations retain higher levels of functional status and demonstrate fewer disturbing behaviors.	Baum[26]
Engagement in individually motivating and ongoing occupations supplies sustenance for survival and safety and enhanced health.	Wilcock[27]
Meaningful occupations provide individuals with exercise to maintain homeostasis; to keep body parts, neuronal physiology, and mental capacities functioning at peak efficiency; and enable maintenance and development of satisfying and stimulating social relationships.	Wilcock[27]

When several studies of this type, showing the same or similar results, have been completed, this adds to the level of confidence that one can have in the effectiveness of an intervention. The aggregate results of these types of studies (as well as RCTs), can be summarized in a systematic review or estimated using a technique called meta-analysis. A meta-analysis considers various characteristics of many studies by using statistical techniques to estimate the overall benefit of a particular type of intervention.[29]

Placing Outcomes in a Historical Context

As occupational therapy personnel consider the expected outcomes of their interventions, it is reassuring to find that many of the desired outcomes popular today in health care (such as participation, well-being, QOL, life satisfaction, and prevention) have been central to occupational therapy since its inception as an organized profession in the United States in 1917. The earliest work of occupational therapy practitioners was focused primarily with individuals with mental illness.[30] The interventions used in occupational therapy were designed to establish and reinforce personal habits and provide structure in the daily routines of individuals who were placed in institutions. Occupational therapy practitioners provided opportunities for experiences and practice in activities and tasks to build skills (this occurred at a time when drugs were not available to control behavior). Here, the expected outcomes were improvements in the client's daily habits and time use.

Eleanor Clarke Slagle, a distinguished practitioner of the period, emphasized the need for a balance between work and restorative activities. She also emphasized the need for graded activity and the use of the environment to support habits and occupations.[31] Other pioneers of the occupational therapy movement applied techniques to elicit natural interests and childhood occupations (such as care of self) to foster healthy development.[32,33] The expected outcomes in these cases were well-being and the ability to care for oneself. The practical approach of using natural interests and opportunities for learning in these treatment programs was consistent with the emerging philosophy of pragmatism being advanced at the time by the American philosopher and educator John Dewey.[34]

The expectation that occupational therapy would lead to improved mental status and habits persisted well into the 1940s. For example, Dutton[35] wrote of the importance of providing the patient with the activities to allow him or her to control attention and focus on productive thoughts. Stanley[36] placed emphasis on establishing habits that would make individuals more aware of their environment and show interest in achievement. Here, the expected outcomes were improved attention and motivation.

Habits and mental function were not the only concerns of the occupational therapy workshops of the 1940s. With the emergence of physical therapy and physical medicine, there was a concurrent interest in how occupations could be used to improve a client's physical function. Licht and Reilly[37] viewed occupational therapy as a treatment process to improve physical or functional performance. It

Table 5-5. *Relationship of Contemporary and Historical Outcomes*

Contemporary Outcome	Historical Outcome	Source
Health and participation	"Our conception of man is that of an organism that maintains and balances itself in the world of reality and actuality be being in active life and active use...It is the use that we make of ourselves that gives the ultimate stamp to our every organ"	Meyer[3(p5)]
Satisfaction and achievement	"A pleasure in achievement, a real pleasure in the use and activity of one's hands and muscles and a happy appreciation of time began to be used as incentives in the management of our patients"	Meyer[3(p3)]
Demonstration of initiative and participation	Occupational therapy through the use of light manual occupations arouses interest and develops the initiative of men and women with handicapping or serious medical conditions	Hall[40]
Health, work, and participation	Occupational therapy uses objects to arouse interest, courage, and confidence to exercise mind and body in healthy activity to overcome disability and to re-establish capacity for industrial and social usefulness	AOTA[41]

should be noted that the outcomes for these clients during the early decades of occupational therapy were documented by observation of the patient's behavior. At the time, the availability of objective measures for these outcomes was limited.

Later, Ayres[38] called attention to the importance of the treatment of physical disabilities through occupation. Purposeful function was used to achieve maximal rehabilitation. Ayres was convinced that since the human motor system evolved to permit purposeful motion, it was logical that purposeful activity would elicit the highest level of recovery of function for this system. Ayres was one of the first occupational therapy practitioners to engage in a program of research to demonstrate links between neuromotor components viewed as central to development and learning behaviors in children. This led to the emergence of sensory integration theory and a battery of tests that were used to identify deficits and measure function. Through her dedicated work, Ayres had identified maximum performance as a desired outcome of occupational therapy.

In 1968, Ainsley and colleagues[39] reported a program of occupational therapy services aimed at assisting older adults, persons with mental retardation, criminals, and culturally deprived individuals with social adjustment. Their program focused on developing the skills to adjust to community life, and their desired outcome was community participation.

More recently, researchers at USC completed a study of occupational therapy with well elderly persons living in the community. This study demonstrated that community based services aimed at engaging clients in learning new occupations and lifestyle habits can improve health status and well-being. Table 5-5 highlights key statements that identify the importance of occupation—these can be directly translated into outcomes that practitioners can address today as they plan client-centered care for individuals, for communities, and for organizations.

Occupational Therapy Outcomes

A number of central occupational therapy outcomes have been proposed in the literature, including participation, occupational role performance, identity and realization of self, life satisfaction, happiness and well-being, quality of life, and creation of meaning. Some outcomes are adopted to provide direct evidence for occupational therapy services (eg, participation, occupational role performance, QOL, and well-being). Other outcomes contribute to changes in the narrative of the person, population, or organization (eg, identity and realization of self, life satisfaction, happiness, and creation of meaning).

Participation

Being able to go where you want to go and do what you want to do is central to personal freedom. Participation describes the extent to which a person is engaged in life situations in a societal context. The ICF[21] asks health professionals to measure participation across 9 domains:

1. Learning and applying knowledge
2. General tasks and demands
3. Communication
4. Mobility
5. Self-care

6. Domestic life
7. Interpersonal interactions and relationships
8. Major life areas
9. Community, social, and civic life

While the concept of participation is not new to occupational therapy practitioners, the concept of participation as central to health care delivery has taken hold only in the last decade. In its report to the US Congress, the National Medical Rehabilitation Research Center at the National Institutes of Health introduced the possibility that it is social limitation due to societal policy, attitudes, and actions (or lack of) that creates physical, social, or financial barriers to access of health care, housing, and vocational/avocational opportunities.[42]

In 1997, the Institute of Medicine developed the report *Enabling America*.[43] This report introduced the Enabling-Disabling Process to describe the outcome of rehabilitation as both restoring the individual's function and employing environmental strategies to remove barriers that limit performance and participation. More recently the WHO (ICIDH-2) released the ICF.[21] This model shifts the view of the indicators of health from one based on mortality rates of the populations, to one focused on how people live with health conditions and how the individual can achieve a productive, fulfilling life. It introduces and defines the concept of *participation* as an individual's involvement in life situations or occupations. Such things reflect the individual's desire to participate fully in society, performing the occupations that are meaningful and personally important. Participation enables other high level outcomes, such as the creation of meaning, satisfactory role performance, life satisfaction, well-being (happiness), and the creation of meaning. Each of these outcomes is discussed briefly in the sections to follow.

Occupational Role Performance

Reilly[4] first introduced the concept of occupational role to occupational therapy when she proposed a framework of occupational behavior. She emphasized that occupational therapy should help people achieve satisfaction in their occupational roles. This focus on occupational roles is related to the concept that to be competent in daily life, the occupational therapy practitioner has to understand what daily activities are related to an individual's roles.

In the first description of the MOHO, Kielhofner and Burke[44] emphasized that social roles help organize daily life. Such roles are positions that individuals hold, including worker, spouse, parent, friend, member, student, and scientist. Each social role carries obligations and expectations that influence actions and, therefore, help structure the daily lives of the people who occupy them. People with illness or injury and whose role performance is compromised are clients in occupational therapy. Because per-

forming their valued roles is important to them, satisfaction with role performance is often an important goal or outcome for occupational therapy intervention. Sadly, it is often overlooked, despite attention to it in the literature and the availability of role performance measures,[45] some of which are specifically designed for use by occupational therapy practitioners.[46,47]

Identity and Realization of Self

The areas of participation and role performance are critical elements in the creation and realization of selfhood. Existential philosophy proposes that throughout life, humans seek to answer questions about their existence, such as:

- Who am I?
- What is the purpose of existence?
- Why am I here?
- What is the nature of reality?
- How shall I live my life?

Kaufman,[48] Christiansen,[49] and McAdams[50] have proposed that the realization of both meaning and identity come largely through self-construction, or shaping the self through engagement in occupations. These writers suggest that humans get their sense of selfhood from agency, or the reactions and changes they engender through participation in occupations that lead to creation, personal expression, and influencing others, particularly as these take place within an understandable life story.

Life Satisfaction

The concept of life satisfaction is very subjective, since what is satisfying to one person is not necessarily satisfying to another. The concept reminds the occupational therapy practitioner of the importance of implementing a client-centered plan—helping the person do what he or she wants and needs to do. The concepts central to life satisfaction are pursuing valued interests, meaningful experiences, relationships, and a sense of comfort with one's life plan.[51] Branholm and her colleagues have studied occupational roles and activity preferences as antecedents of life satisfaction.[52,53] She proposed that satisfaction is based on the person's contentment in daily life, and the extent to which a person achieves his or her goals under different circumstances throughout life depends upon the person's abilities to adapt or to cope.[53] Branholm identified 8 life satisfaction domains that extend the concept of satisfaction to daily activities and are represented in the Life Satisfaction Checklist[53]:

1. Ability to manage self-care
2. Leisure situations
3. Vocational situation
4. Financial situation

5. Sexual life

6. Partnership relations

7. Family life

8. Contacts with friend and acquaintances

Each of these domains may be affected by an injury or chronic condition and addressed as part of a client-centered plan to enable the client to do what he or she wants and needs to do.

Well-Being and Happiness

A concept closely related to life satisfaction is subjective well-being (SWB), or happiness. Much research has shown that subjective well-being is explained by 3 factors: life satisfaction, negative affect or feelings, and positive affect or feelings.[54] Diener has developed a measure of happiness called the Satisfaction with Life Scale (SWLS). The SWLS was developed to assess satisfaction with people's lives as a whole, and does not assess satisfaction with life domains such as health or finances, but allows subjects to integrate and weigh these domains in whatever way they choose. Research has consistently shown that economics and material goods do not predict happiness or subjective well-being. Christiansen et al[55] have studied the relationship between goal-directed occupations (called personal projects) and well-being. This research has shown that certain characteristics of a person's projects, such as their progress, structure, stressfulness, outcomes, importance, and time adequacy, help explain differences in well-being.

Another view holds that well-being includes the concepts of physical and mental health as well as the person's perception of confidence and self-esteem.[27,56] Wilcock asserted that relationships including social friends, family, partnerships, neighbors, and strangers and the availability of surroundings including home, school, place of worship, peace, terrain, and weather contribute to a person's perception of well-being.

Quality of Life

Well-being is also one of the concepts that contributes to an individual's perception of QOL. The WHO defines QOL as an individual's perception of his or her position in life in the context of the culture and value systems in which he or she lives, and in relation to his or her goals, expectations, standards, and concerns. "It is a broad-ranging concept, incorporating in a complex way the person's physical health, psychological state, level of independence, social relationships, and their relationship to salient features of their environment."[57(p43)]

There are many measures of QOL described in the literature. Some focus on outcomes associated with specific disease states, and these instruments are often described as measuring Health-Related Quality of Life

(HRQOL). The WHO has also developed a measure of quality of life that includes 6 domains and 24 facets or concepts.[58]

Creation of Meaning

Victor Frankl, a psychologist who proposed the theory of *logotherapy*, suggested that all humans have a need to find meaning in existence, and that this is an elementary driving force in who we become.[59] Frankl observed that people can lead 3 types of meaningful lives: the active life, which affords the opportunity to realize values in creative work; the passive life of enjoyment, which allows the experience of beauty, art, and nature; and the life of moral excellence, which may impart meaning through suffering, as in the ascetic existence of some religious orders. It is easy to see the relationship between occupations and meeting the essential drive for meaning that Frankl described in his important psychological theory.

Another psychologist, Aaron Antonovsky, proposed a theory attempting to explain why some people adapt better to life's challenges and difficult circumstances than others. Antonovsky's salutogenic theory proposes that people are best able to adapt when they perceive that their world of existence is comprehensible, manageable, and meaningful.[60] Collectively, these 3 factors, which Antonovsky described as "the Sense of Coherence," are defined by what people do, how effectively they can do it, and what meanings they derive from their daily endeavors. The Sense of Coherence scale, which measures these factors, has consistently predicted well-being and other indicators of health in numerous studies.[61]

A related measure of personal meaning reported in the literature is the Life Regard Index (LRI).[62] This 28-item scale measures personal meaning from the standpoint of life structure (goals and purposes) and fulfillment. The scale has demonstrated impressive psychometric properties, and research has shown that it has evidence of conceptual validity.[63] For example, it correlates significantly with measures of well-being, intimacy, commitment, happiness, and self-esteem.[64] The scale has also been used as an outcome measure following psychological interventions, but there are no reports of its use following occupational therapy.

Another measure of personal meaning, the Personal Meaning Profile (PMP), has been reported by Wong.[65] This instrument hypothesizes the existence of 8 domains that contribute to a meaningful life, including achievement, relationship, religion, self-transcendence (making a difference in the world), fulfillment, self-acceptance, intimacy, and fair treatment. The PMP, while still in its developmental stages, is designed for use in counseling and seems highly consistent with goal-setting and activity-related intervention strategies. The scale has satisfactory psychometric properties, and has correlated with measures of physical and psychological well-being.[66] No examples of its use as a measure of occupational therapy outcome have been reported in the literature.

Tristram Englehardt, a medical historian and philosopher, once observed the uniqueness of occupational therapy as a bridge between a patient's world of meaning and the scientific, technologically dominated world of medicine.[67] He described occupational therapy practitioners as custodians of meaning precisely because the field enables participation in the occupations of life through which people derive meaning. Clearly, life meaning is an important outcome of therapy, and one that should continue to be studied and documented by practitioners and occupational scientists.

Defining Expectations for Evidence-Based Practice Outcomes

All health care professionals are expected to inform their clients about what results or outcomes they can expect from different intervention approaches; whether such approaches involve strategies to support recovery, remove barriers, educate consumers, or employ assistive technologies. This requires that the expected outcomes are made explicit to the client so that he or she can collaborate in the selection of approaches that are most likely to lead to the achievement of goals. Occupational therapy intervention should always be aimed at achieving improved occupational performance in occupations and tasks that the individual wants and needs to do.

When an occupational therapy practitioner interacts with a client, the client has the right to know about the interventions that will be employed to help them meet their goals, and the probability that the outcome will be achieved. This approach is becoming known as using an evidence-based approach to care. Evidence-based practice is about asking questions and "finding, appraising, and using contemporaneous research findings as the basis for clinical decisions."[68(p2233)]

Selecting Suitable Outcome Measures

In the earlier section on occupational therapy goals and outcomes, several outcome instruments were identified and described. However, the instruments listed were provided as examples. Any measure that can reliably and validly document change as a result of planned intervention can be a suitable measure of therapeutic outcome. Once occupational performance needs or issues have been identified, an appropriate assessment approach or instrument should be selected. Criteria for selection include theoretical consistency, clinical utility (which includes factors such as cost, time required for administration, training required for administration and interpretation), and the reliability

and validity of a measure. A reliable measure will yield consistent results over time and across practitioners, while also being sensitive to change in the performance of a client. A valid measure has face or content validity and yields findings that are intuitively sound, logical, and consistent with theory. Practitioners are encouraged to consult test manuals and published reviews of measures to determine their suitability for use in measuring the attainment of specified client or program goals.

SUMMARY

This chapter introduced the PEOP Occupational Therapy Process as an organizing framework for providing interventions for individuals, populations, and organizations. Occupation-based, client-centered, and evidence-based are foundational concepts for using the process in practice. Three versions of the PEOP Occupational Therapy Process introduce narrative, assessment and evaluation, interventions, and outcomes components for planning services for individuals, populations, and organizations. Occupational therapy outcomes were discussed as central to evaluating the effectiveness of the PEOP Occupational Therapy Process.

REFERENCES

1. AOTA. Scope of practice. *Am J Occup Ther.* 2010;64:S70-S77.
2. Mattingly C, Fleming MH. *Clinical Reasoning: Forms of Inquiry in a Therapeutic Practice.* Philadelphia, PA: FA Davis Co; 1994.
3. Meyer A. The philosophy of occupational therapy. *Arch Occup Ther.* 1922;1(1):1-10.
4. Reilly M. Occupational therapy can be one of the great ideas of 20th century medicine. *Am J Occup Ther.* 1962;16:1-9.
5. Maitra K, Erway F. Perception of client-centered practice in occupational therapists and their clients. *Am J Occup Ther.* 2006;60(3):298-310.
6. Gage M, Polatajko H. Enhancing occupational performance through an understanding of perceived self-efficacy. *Am J Occup Ther.* 1994;48(5):452-462.
7. Gerteis M, Edgman-Levitan S, Walker JD, Stoke DM, Cleary PD, Delbanco TL. What patients really want. *Health Manage Q.* 1993;15(3):2-6.
8. Sumsion T. A revised OT definition of client-centred practice. *Br J Occup Ther.* 2000;63(7):304-309.
9. Kyler PPL. Client-centered and family-centered care: refinement of the concepts. *Occupational Therapy in Mental Health.* 2008;24(2):100-120.
10. Law M, Baum C. Evidence-based occupational therapy. *Can J Occup Ther.* 1998;65(3):131-135.
11. Greenhalgh T, Hurwitz B. Narrative-based medicine: why study narrative? *BMJ.* 1999;318(7175):48-50.
12. Kools M, van de Wiel MWJ, Ruiter RAC, Cruts A, Kok G. The effect of graphic organizers on subjective and objective comprehension of a health education text. *Health Education and Behavior.* 2006;33(6):760-772.

13. Youngstrom MJ. Categories and principles of interventions. In: Christiansen C, Baum C, Bass Haugen J, eds. *Occupational Therapy: Performance, Participation, and Well-Being.* Thorofare, NJ: SLACK Incorporated; 2005:396-419.

14. Baum C, Barrows C, Bass Haugen J, et al. Blueprint for entry-level education. *Am J Occup Ther.* 2009;64:186-203.

15. Polatajko HJ, Davis, JA, McEwen SE. Therapeutic use of self: a catalyst in the client-therapist alliance for change. In: Christiansen CH, Baum CM, Bass JD, eds. *Occupational Therapy: Performance, Participation, and Well-Being.* 4th ed. Thorofare, NJ: SLACK Incorporated; 2015.

16. Rogerson R. Environmental and health-related quality of life: conceptual and methodological similarities. *Soc Sci Med.* 1995;41:1373-1382.

17. Baum CM, Edwards DF. *The Activity Card Sort.* 2nd ed. Bethesda, MD: AOTA Press; 2008.

18. Matsutsuyu JS. The interest check list. *Am J Occup Ther.* 1969;23(4):323-328.

19. Oakley F, Kielhofner G, Barris R, Richler RK. The role checklist: development and empirical assessment of reliability. *Occup Ther J Res.* 1986;6:157-169.

20. Law M, Baptiste S, Carswell A, McColl MA, Polatajko H, Pollock N. *Canadian Occupational Performance Measure.* Ottawa, ON: Canadian Association of Occupational Therapists; 2005.

21. World Health Organization. International Classification of Functioning, Disability, and Health (ICF). World Health Organization. http://www.who.int/classifications/icf/en/. Published 2001. Updated 2013. Accessed June 6, 2013.

22. Lin FR, Thorpe R, Gordon-Salant S, Ferrucci L. Hearing loss prevalence and risk factors among older adults in the United States. *The Journals of Gerontology Series A: Biological Sciences and Medical Sciences.* 2011;66(5):582-590.

23. Fidler GS, Fidler JW. *Occupational Therapy: A Communication Process in Psychiatry.* New York, NY: MacMillan; 1963.

24. Reed KS. *Concepts of Occupational Therapy.* Philadelphia, PA: Lippincott Williams & Wilkins; 1999.

25. Kielhofner GW. *A Model of Human Occupation: Theory and Application.* Baltimore, MD: Williams & Wilkins; 1995.

26. Baum M. The contribution of occupation to function in persons with Alzheimer's disease. *J Occup Sci: Australia.* 1995;2(2):59-67.

27. Wilcock AA. A theory of the human need for occupation. *J Occup Sci: Australia.* 1993;1(1):17-24.

28. Law M, Baum C. Evidence-based occupational therapy. *Can J Occup Ther.* 1998;65(5):131-135.

29. Naylor CD. Meta-analysis and the meta-epidemiology of clinical research. *BMJ.* 1997;315:617-619.

30. Bing RK. Occupational therapy revisited: a paraphrastic journey. *Am J Occup Ther.* 1981;35:499-518.

31. Slagle EC. Training aids for mental patients. *Arch Occup Ther.* 1922;1:11-17.

32. Whitter I. The modern hospital. *Occupational Therapy for Children.* 1923;21:330-334.

33. Sellew G. Occupational therapy for children. *Occup Ther Rehabil.* 1932;11:379-381.

34. Dewey J. Human Nature and Conduct. New York, NY: Henry Holt; 1922.

35. Dutton WR. The mechanisms of recovery by occupation. *Can J Occup Ther.* 1941;8:42-46.

36. Stanley J. Habit training. *Occup Ther Rehabil.* 1942;21:82-85.

37. Licht S, Reilly M. The correlation of physical and occupational therapy. *Occup Ther Rehabil.* 1943;22:171-175.

38. Ayres A. Basic concepts of clinical practice in physical disabilities. *Am J Occup Ther.* 1958;12(6):300-302,311.

39. Ainsley J, Barnes SS, Grove EA, Johnson T, Kooiman CA, Stephens F. On change. *Am J Occup Ther.* 1968;22(3):186-189.

40. Hall HJ. *OT: A New Profession.* Concord, MA: Rumford Press; 1923.

41. AOTA. *Principles of Occupational Therapy.* Bulletin No. 4. New York, NY: AOTA; 1923.

42. NCMRR. *Research Plan for the National Center for Medical Rehabilitation Research: (NIH publication no. 93-3509).* Washington, DC: National Institutes of Health: US Government Printing Office; 1993.

43. Brandt EN, Pope AM. Executive summary. In: Brandt EN, Pope AM, eds. *Enabling America: Assessing the Role of Rehabilitation Science and Engineering.* Washington DC: National Academy Press; 1977:1-23.

44. Kielhofner G, Burke JP. A model of human occupation: part 1: conceptual framework and content. *Am J Occup Ther.* 1980;34:572-581.

45. Goodman SH. Assessing levels of adaptive functioning: the Role Functioning Scale. *Community Ment Health J.* 1993;29(2):119-131.

46. Good-Ellis MF, Spencer JH. Developing a role activity performance scale. *Am J Occup Ther.* 1985;41(4):232-241.

47. Jackoway I, Rogers J, Snow T. Role change assessment. *Occup Ther Mental Health.* 1987;7(1):17-37.

48. Kaufmann W. *Existentialism: From Dostoevsky to Sartre.* New York, NY: Penguin; 1989.

49. Christiansen CH. Defining lives: occupation as identity: an essay on competence, coherence and the creation of meaning. *Am J Occup Ther.* 1999;53(6):547-558.

50. McAdams D. Unity and purpose in human lives: the emergence of identity as a life story. In: Zuker RA, ed. *Personality Structure in the Life Course.* New York, NY: Springer; 1992:323-376.

51. Neugarten BL, Havighurst RJ, Tobin SS. The measurement of life satisfaction. *J Gerontol.* 1961;16(2):134-143.

52. Lundmark PBI. Relationship between occupation and life satisfaction in people with multiple sclerosis. *Disabil Rehabil.* 1996;18(9):449-453.

53. Branholm IB. Occupational role preferences and life satisfaction. *Occupational Therapy Journal of Research.* 1992;12(3):159-171.

54. Diener E, Suh E, Lucas RE, Smith HL. Subjective well-being: three decades of progress. *Psychol Bull.* 1999;125(2):276-302.

55. Christiansen C, Backman C, Little BR, Nguyen A. Occupations and subjective well-being: a study of personal projects. *Am J Occup Ther.* 1999;53(1):91-100.

56. Wilcock AA. *An Occupational Perspective of Health.* Thorofare, NJ: SLACK Incorporated; 1998.

57. Group TW. The development of the World Health Organization Quality of Life Assessment Instrument (the WHOQoL). In: Orley WKJ, ed. *Quality of Life Assessment: International Perspectives.* Heidelberg, Germany: Springer-Verlag; 1994.

58. World Health Organization. *WHO Quality of Life-BREF (WHOQOL-BREF).* World Health Organization. http://www.who.int/substance_abuse/research_tools/whoqolbref/en/. Published 1993. Updated 2013. Accessed June 10, 2013.

59. Frankl V. *Man's Search for Meaning.* New York, NY: Washington Square Press; 1984.

60. Antonovsky A. *Health, Stress, and Coping: New Perspectives on Mental and Physical Well-Being.* San Francisco, CA: Jossey-Bass; 1979.

61. Antonovsky A. The structure and properties of the Sense of Coherence Scale. *Soc Sci Med.* 1993;36:725-733.

62. Debats D. Measurement of personal meaning: the psychometric properties of the Life Regard Index. In: Wong P, ed. *The Human Quest for Meaning.* Mahwah, NJ: Lawrence Erlbaum; 1998:237-259.

63. Debats D. Meaning in life: clinical relevance and predictive power. *Br J Clin Psychol*. 1996;35:503-516.

64. Debats D, Wezeman FR. On the psychometric properties of the Life Regard Index: a measure of meaningful life. *Pers Individ Dif*. 1993;14:337-345.

65. Wong T. Implicit theories of meaningful life and the development of the personal meaning profile. In: Wong P, ed. *The Human Quest for Meaning*. Mahwah, NJ: Lawrence Erlbaum; 1998:111-140.

66. Wong P. Personal meaning and successful aging. *Canadian Psychology*. 1989;30:516-525.

67. Englehardt HT. Defining occupational therapy: the meaning of therapy and the virtues of occupation. *Am J Occup Ther*. 1977;31(10):666-672.

68. Rosenberg W, Donald A. Evidence-based medicine: an approach to clinical problem-solving. *BMJ*. 1995;310:1122-1126.

THERAPEUTIC USE OF SELF
A Catalyst in the Client-Therapist Alliance for Change

Helene J. Polatajko, PhD, OTReg(Ont), OT(C), FCAOT, FCAHS;
Jane A. Davis, MSc, OTReg(Ont), OTR, OT(C); and Sara E. McEwen, PhD, MSc, BSc(PT)

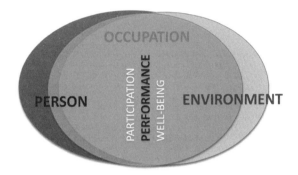

LEARNING OBJECTIVES

- Identify the occupational imperatives for our work.
- Name theories of change relevant to the occupational imperatives.
- Relate therapeutic use to "core occupational therapy outcomes."
- Define therapeutic use of self.
- Place the therapeutic use in context of the working alliance.
- Discuss the dimensions of the self, in alliance.
- Relate the dimensions of self to client needs, therapy goals, tasks, and bond.
- Understand and use tools for reflection on the self in a working alliance.

KEY WORDS

- Learning
- Occupational imperatives
- Reflexive
- Responsible collaborator
- Therapeutic relationship
- Therapeutic use of self
- Working (therapeutic) alliance

INTRODUCTION

Every artist dips his brush in his own soul, and paints his own nature into his pictures.

—Henry Ward Beecher[1](np)

Christiansen CH, Baum CM, Bass JD, eds.
*Occupational Therapy: Performance, Participation,
and Well-Being, Fourth Edition (pp 81-92).*
© 2015 SLACK Incorporated.

Our profession is described by 2 terms: *occupation* and *therapy*. The former names our domain of concern; the latter names the nature of our work.[2] By calling our work therapy, we profess a particular kind of work.

The AOTA defines our work as "the therapeutic use of everyday life activities (occupations)."[3(p199)] This definition indicates that the therapy in our work emanates from the use of activity/occupation. In contrast, the current guidelines of the CAOT define occupational therapy as "the art and science of enabling engagement in everyday living, through occupation."[4(p2)] This definition implicitly gives prominence to the role of the occupational therapy practitioner in our work; that is, it names the work as enablement, which requires the action of a person. Further, by defining occupational therapy as an *"art,"* it indicates the importance of the specific occupational therapy practitioner carrying out the work. To paraphrase Henry Ward Beecher: *every occupational therapy practitioner paints her own nature into her practice.* This is the essence of therapeutic use of self.[1]

Taken together, these definitions point to the 2 primary active ingredients in occupational therapy: the occupation and the occupational therapy practitioner. The former is dealt with extensively throughout this text; the latter is the focus of this chapter. In particular, in this chapter, we will focus on the occupational therapy practitioner as the therapeutic agent—on the *therapeutic use of self.*

As will be seen in this chapter, *therapeutic use of self* is a broad construct. Emerging initially from psychotherapeutic traditions, the concept is now discussed from multiple perspectives, in multiple knowledge traditions, amid numerous controversies. It is not the intent to discuss these in this chapter. Rather, we have chosen to present only those aspects that are most widely discussed, seem to enjoy consensus, and have particular relevance for occupational therapy. We have taken this approach to all aspects of the material presented in this chapter, including the definition of therapeutic use of self itself. Accordingly, the definition we use in this chapter is an amalgam of various definitions. We define the therapeutic use of self as *the intentional, planned use of personal behaviors, insight, perception, judgment, skill, and knowledge to optimize our working alliance with our clients and enable change.*

Notwithstanding the focus on therapeutic use of self, it must be acknowledged that the form and function of therapeutic use is affected by the domain of concern of the therapy. After all, enabling clients to engage in occupation is inherently different from, say, maintaining joint mobility through passive range of motion exercises. Accordingly, in this chapter we will position therapeutic use of self within the context of occupation.

Overview

This chapter starts with an overview of the essential aspects of human occupation and their imperatives for our work. As human occupation is covered extensively throughout this text, in this chapter we will only discuss those points that have particular relevance to therapeutic use of self. Accordingly, we will focus on the nature of human occupation and occupational change and identify the imperatives those hold for the therapeutic use of self. Arguing that occupational therapy practitioners essentially must be client-centered enablers of client-enacted occupational change, we then turn to the discussion of therapeutic use of self. We consider its use in our profession and note that therapeutic use of self is positioned within the relationship, or more specifically, the alliance we form with our clients. We then present a discussion of the key elements of the self and its use as a therapeutic agent in alliance, and the essential components of the working alliance, and for each we provide reflexive tools for the practitioner. The chapter ends with a reflexive exercise that enables you to initiate the development of your therapeutic use of self in alliance.

HUMAN OCCUPATION AS OUR CONTEXT

Bonnie Sherr Klein, an accomplished filmmaker, author, and disability activist who has written and spoken extensively about her process of recovery from a debilitating brain stem stroke and her experience of being a disabled person in a world that is not really ready for them, offered this observation:

> The occupational therapist worked with humiliating seriousness. We played shuffleboard, and ping-pong, but no one explained that they were to practice our balance and I was too out of it to understand. Everything seemed random and irrelevant.[5(pviii)]

Just as the work of the artist is affected by the subject matter he intends to capture, so too, the work of the occupational therapy practitioner is affected by his/her subject matter, or domain of concern. In occupational therapy, that is human occupation.

As described throughout this text, the role of the occupational therapy practitioner is to enable clients to meet their occupational goals by enhancing occupational performance through building personal capabilities, modifying occupations or environments, and/or reconsidering occupational processes and goals. To be effective in enacting change in occupation, it is important to understand the aspects of human occupation and occupational change.

Essential Aspects of Human Occupation

Human occupation is a complex phenomenon. Loosely speaking, occupation refers to everything that people do. However, for the purposes of this chapter, we determined that a more formal definition is appropriate. From among the many definitions available, we have chosen to use that of the CAOT, as it provides important directions for the nature of our work and the therapeutic use of self.

Occupation refers to groups of activities and tasks of everyday life, named, organized, and given value and meaning by individuals and a culture. Occupation is everything people do to occupy themselves, including looking after themselves (self-care), enjoying life (leisure), and contributing to the social and economic fabric of their communities (productivity).[5(p34)]

This definition identifies 3 essential aspects of occupation that are germane to our work as occupational therapy practitioners. First, *people do* occupations. In other words, occupations are not passive; we, as practitioners, cannot do occupations unto our clients as you might with passive range of motion. Rather, *our clients have to actively engage in occupation themselves*. For the practitioner's therapy to be enacted, Bonnie Sherr Klein, herself, had to engage in shuffleboard and ping-pong. Second, *occupations have value and meaning ascribed by the individual*. Had the occupational therapy practitioner working with Bonnie incorporated this aspect of the definition into her work, she might have chosen to make explicit the purpose of the occupations she was requiring of her client, thereby enabling Bonnie to ascribe value and meaning to them rather than leaving her to consider them as *"random and irrelevant."*[5(pviii)] Third, *human occupation is idiosyncratic*. That is, everyone has a different constellation of occupations in which they engage and to which they ascribe their personal value and meaning.[6] Had Bonnie's practitioner recognized the idiosyncratic nature of human occupation, she might have chosen to engage Bonnie in occupations that Bonnie valued or considered meaningful and thereby enhance her engagement and, in turn, the therapeutic potency of the occupations chosen.

The potential of occupations to have therapeutic potency has been a basic tenet of occupational therapy since its inception. As was first voiced by Dunton in his Credo of 1919, "Sick minds, sick bodies, and sick souls may be healed thru [sic] occupation."[7(p10)] The AOTA definition, cited previously, reaffirms the centrality of therapeutic activity to our practice.[3] However, therapeutic potency is not an essential characteristic of occupation Bonnie did not find shuffleboard therapeutic. *Occupations have the potential to be therapeutic, but are not necessarily therapeutic*. It is part of our work to determine which occu-pations have therapeutic potency, for which clients, and under which circumstances. It is also part of our work to recognize that an important component of the therapeutic potency of an activity or occupation is the occupational therapy practitioner herself, as excruciatingly pointed out by Bonnie: "The occupational therapist worked with humiliating seriousness."[5(pviii)] Had Bonnie's practitioner understood this, she might have used her interpersonal skills to note Bonnie's reactions to the occupations being offered and to explain their purpose to Bonnie, thereby engaging her more fully and mitigating against the experi-ence of the session as *"random and irrelevant."*[5(pviii)]

While Dunton's Credo is often cited with respect to the therapeutic potency of occupation, the far more important offering of the Credo is that "occupation is as necessary to life as food and drink."[7(p10)] The realization that *occupation is a basic human need* has tremendous impli-cations for our work; it makes us concerned with occupa-tion in the broadest sense, not simply as a means to health but as an end in and of itself. This realization suggests that the nature of our work with our clients must go beyond practicing balance through activities, such as shuffleboard and ping-pong, to enabling meaningful occupation.

The aspects of occupation discussed previously indicate that in our work we must *actively engage our clients in doing* and that we must *know our clients occupationally*, be they individuals, groups, organizations, or populations. That is, we must *form a relationship with our clients* that allows us to know the occupations they want to, need to, and are expected to perform, to understand the value and meaning they ascribe to those occupations, and to know the occu-pational change that needs to occur in their lives. We must be able to uncover their occupational issues and enable them to enact solutions. Occupational therapy can neither be done passively, nor unilaterally; it can be done only with the active cooperation and engagement of the client in the therapy.[8] Accordingly, as occupational therapy practitio-ners, we must *work in partnership* with our clients and our practice must be client-centered.

"Client-centred practice in occupational therapy embraces a philosophy of respect for, and partnership with, the people who are engaging in occupational therapy services."[5(p49)] Taken together, this discussion of the essential features of occupation indicates that to be thera-peutic in the context of occupation therapy we must *form a relationship with our clients, actively engage them in doing, know our clients occupationally, and work in respectful part-nership*.

The Nature of (Occupational) Change

Our clients come to us at a time when they need occu-pational change. Frequently, it is because life circumstanc-es have brought them to a point of occupational disequilibrium; occasionally, because they have chosen to make an occupational change in their lives. In either case, the goal of occupational therapy is to enable our clients to affect the occupational change they want to, need to, and are expected to make in their lives.

While change can be affected in many ways, occupational change, because of the nature of occupation, requires the active involvement of the client. Given the breadth of human occupation, the nature of the change we need to enable our clients to affect is broad; it can range from using a padded spoon temporarily, to (re)learning to ride a bike, to renovating an entire house, to reconstructing their occupational lives. The AOTA *Blueprint for Entry-Level Education*[3] captures this breadth under 4 major outcomes: adaptation/coping, competence/mastery, independence/autonomy, and occupational performance/function. Each of these outcomes, although enabled by the occupational therapy practitioner, must be enacted by the client.

As evidence of the importance of the client in enacting occupational change, we need only consider the extensive literature on the patterns of utilization of occupational therapy practitioner-prescribed assistive devices. A summary of findings from a systematic review suggests abandonment rates are as high as 65% (with reported usage patterns ranging from 35% to 86.5%).[9] Through in-depth interviews, Lund and Nygård uncovered that the perceptions and attitudes of the users toward their device determined whether or not they ultimately used it.[10] In a similar vein, Krantz recently proposed that the pattern of assistive device utilization is reflective of the personal meaning that an individual associates with the device, as well as needs, motivation, and perceived value.[11]

Gage provides a real world example of how a client's perceptions affects device use.[12] She describes her interactions with Fred, a 50-year-old antique car enthusiast, who experienced severe pain with most movements, resulting in difficulty with even the simplest of tasks. As a solution, Gage suggested the use of a motorized wheelchair, which she saw as *adapting* the occupational requirements to match her client's capacity, enabling her client's *mastery*, and supporting his *independence/autonomy*. The client adamantly rejected her suggestion, as he saw the chair as a vivid reminder of his level of disability, as stigmatizing, and as cumbersome. Had he shared Gage's perspective (which he came to do a year later), he would have seen the chair as liberating, as an aid to independence and mastery, and he would have used it (as he did a year later). Gage's case description demonstrates that for occupational change to occur, the client has to be an active partner in enacting the change; thus, enabling occupational change is essentially a process of *enabling our clients to enact occupational change.*

Theories of Occupational Change: How Change Happens

Since occupational performance is the complex interaction among person, occupation, and environment, and change in occupational performance can result from change in the person, occupation, environment, or some combination thereof, numerous theories of change have relevance for occupational therapy. However, as has been argued previously, the nature of occupation is such that ultimately, the client must enact the occupational change. The role of the occupational therapy practitioner is to use her skills and talents to enable the client to enact that change. Accordingly, in this chapter we will limit our discussion of change theories to those that discuss client action.

Numerous models and theories of change exist that focus on encouraging of motivating an individual, community, or society toward the intention to change and ultimately enacting actual change. Among the most relevant theories to occupational change and therapeutic use of self and the most frequently cited within the occupational therapy literature is that of Kielhofner in relation to occupational adaptation. In the Model of Human Occupation (MOHO), Kielhofner identifies 3 essential components to selecting, organizing, and undertaking occupations: volition (one's thoughts and feelings related to personal causation, values, and interests), habituation (one's habits and internalized roles), and performance capacity (one's objective capacity to do as well as one's subjective experiences of doing).[8(p12)]

Kielhofner's construct of volition, especially in relation to ideas of personal causation, invokes the idea of attribution which is at the center of what is perhaps the most long-standing theory of personal change.[8] *Attribution theory*, derived from the ideas of Fritz Heider, refers to various ideas that speak to the attributions an individual (or group) makes with respect to his, or another's, behavior or performance and the resultant possible actions due to this attribution.[13,14] Locus of causation, whether a challenge or issue is perceived to be the result of internal or external factors, is a central element of attribution theory. This theory proposes that the best predictor of a behavior or action is intention or perceived readiness to act, and that intention is immediately followed by the behavior.

The Theory of Reasoned Action and Planned Behavior focuses on understanding the elements that predict intention to change and actual change.[15-19] It defines 3 predictive dimensions: (1) attitudes, (2) subjective norms, and (3) perceived behavioral control. *Attitudes* result from the weighting of all beliefs related to the nature of a particular behavior. *Subjective norms* convey the weighted perceived importance of the beliefs and opinions of the people who inhabit an individual's social environment on his or her behavioral intentions. *Perceived behavioral control* is defined as an individual's perceived control over the opportunities, resources, and skills required to perform the desired behavior (or occupation). Thus, the outcome of behavioral intention is viewed as a function of an individual's attitudes toward a behavior, in association with the subjective norms an individual encounters toward that behavior, and an individual's perceived behavioral control influences whether the intention to act will result in action.[20]

The dimension of *perceived behavioral control* emanated from the concept of self-efficacy proposed by Bandura in 1977 in his Social Cognitive Theory.[21,22] *Self-efficacy* is defined as the conviction that one can successfully execute the behavior required to produce the outcomes. Bandura argues that self-efficacy is the most important precondition for behavioral change, since it determines the initiation of coping behavior.[23] Expectations such as motivation, performance, and feelings of frustration associated with repeated failures determine effect and behavioral reactions.

With respect to occupation, these theoretical ideas point to the importance of understanding people's perceptions of the occupations they are performing or are being asked to perform with respect to value and interest, perceived locus of causation, and expectations of their performance. Uncovering this information helps to discern their motivation and intention for affecting change in their own performance to achieve their desired occupational outcomes.

Although it is commonly understood in occupational therapy that environmental conditions and sociocultural contexts can be barriers to (or enablers of) occupational change, our client's attitudes, values, aspirations, and self-efficacy are presented here as crucial in affecting occupational change.[24] Applying these theories to practice, therapy would be required to take the form of supporting the development of clients' intentions to perform and enabling that performance to be actualized by encouraging shifts in clients' beliefs and attitudes, and possibly those around him (ie, sociocultural context), while advocating for the creation of a supportive environment. Thus, occupational therapy practitioners would need to learn to use their self therapeutically.

THERAPEUTIC USE OF SELF

There are no therapeutic interventions delivered from a position of neutrality or transcendent objectivity; rather all interventions reflect the person of the analyst [therapist] ... it is precisely the personal

elements contained in the intervention that are most responsible for its therapeutic impact.[25(p93)]

Our therapy takes many forms. We can be seen engaging a client in therapeutic macramé to increase range of motion at the shoulder, (re)teaching a client a skill so he can dress independently, working with builders to remodel a home to make it accessible, consulting with a community to design a center that meets the needs of a variety of users, or enabling a client to reframe his occupational self after a catastrophic event. Regardless of the form our therapy takes, it is the practitioner who delivers the therapy and imprints her own nature in it. The therapeutic ingredients in our work are more than just the techniques we use. The practitioner herself is an active therapeutic ingredient in occupational therapy.

Therapeutic Use of Self: A Matter of Alliance

Mosey, a major proponent of the importance of the occupational therapy practitioner *self* to the therapeutic process, conceptualizes the therapeutic use of self, or as she refers to it, the *conscious* use of self, in interaction with the client.[26] The conscious use of self, she writes:

... involves a planned interaction with another person in order to alleviate fear or anxiety, provide reassurance, obtain necessary information, provide information, give advice, and assist the other individual to gain more appreciation of, more expression of, and more functional use of his or her latent inner resources.[26(p199)]

Current definitions also place therapeutic use of self within the context of the relationship between client and occupational therapy practitioner. As Taylor, Lee, and Kielhofner point out in their summary of the literature, therapeutic use of self is "therapists' conscious efforts to optimize the therapeutic relationship."[27(p6)] Practicing occupational therapy practitioners also subscribe to this idea. Further, they view the relationship as the most critical determinant of treatment outcomes.[28-30]

The interaction between client and occupational therapy practitioner is referred to in a number of ways: *helping alliance*,[31] *helping encounter*,[32] *intentional relationship*,[33] *interactive encounter*,[34] *therapeutic alliance*,[35] *therapeutic relationship*,[26,36,37] and *working alliance*.[38] Among these, one of the most commonly appearing terms and one that has been the focus of a considerable body of empirical research is *working alliance* and, thus, it is the term we use throughout the rest of the chapter.

Working alliance, as a construct, has had a long and influential history. Despite controversy as to the precise nature of the construct,[39] a theory of working alliance put forward by Bordin,[38,40] one of the earliest and most widely used, has been deemed robust.[41] Bordin describes the working alliance as the degree to which the therapy dyad, that is the client and practitioner, is engaged in *collaborative, purposeful work*.[38] According to Bordin's theory, working alliance has 3 core features:

1. Goals: Practitioner-client agreement as to the client's problems and possible solutions
2. Tasks: Practitioner-client agreement on what will be done to achieve the goals
3. Bond: Practitioner-client trust and attachment[38]

The working alliance is developed and maintained through active negotiation at the initiation of the therapeutic relationship and continually renegotiated thereafter, although the manner in which these negotiations are operationalized varies with different therapeutic techniques.[41] The alliance is not a therapeutic technique in itself, but rather an overarching entity that permeates all aspects of therapy. In the following section we elaborate on both the science and the art of the construct as a means of enhancing therapeutic use of self.

Therapeutic Use of Self in Alliance: The Science

Very good evidence from occupational therapy and other health professions acknowledges the importance of the working alliance to outcomes. In clinical psychology, for example, the quality of the therapeutic relationship has been shown to account for 30% of the therapeutic effect of therapy, regardless of the therapeutic techniques being used or the severity of the client's presenting problems and motivation.[42] In psychotherapy, a meta-analysis of 68 studies reported that alliance has a moderate association with overall outcomes, including mood and anxiety.[31] A similar finding emerged from a systematic review of the literature conducted by Hall and colleagues on the impact of the practitioner-client alliance (they used the term *therapeutic alliance*) in physical rehabilitation settings.[35] They concluded that a working alliance is positively associated with treatment adherence in clients with brain injury and multiple pathologies, reduction in depressive symptoms in clients with cardiac conditions and brain injury, better treatment satisfaction in clients with musculoskeletal conditions, and improved physical function in older clients and those with low back pain.

Gunnarson and Eklund examined therapeutic alliance specifically between occupational therapy practitioners and 35 adults seen in an outpatient clinic for personality disorders, affective syndromes, anxiety/obsession syndromes, or eating disorders.[43] Higher therapeutic alliance ratings by both practitioners and clients were associated with larger changes in occupational performance and self-mastery, and higher overall client satisfaction.

Although working alliance, as a construct, originated in psychotherapy, an important observation to be made from this empirical work is that the impact of the alliance is not restricted to the psychotherapeutic relationship; rather it applies to all manner of enabling change. Indeed, as Davidson summarized in a recent paper,

> The quality of the relationship between client and therapist is foundational to successful outcomes at every level: attainment of therapeutic goals (Cole & McLean, 2003), follow through on self-care plans (DiMatteo, Reiter, & Gambone, 1994; Stewart, Bhagwanjee, Mbakaza, & Binase, 2000), clients' sense of satisfaction (Corring & Cook, 1999; Darragh, Sample, & Krieger, 2001), and practitioners' sense of professional competence and enjoyment (Rosa & Hasselkus, 1996; Taylor, Wook Lee, Kielhofner, & Ketkar, 2009).[44(p87-88)]

Therapeutic Use of Self in Alliance: The Art

Every therapist dips her brush in her own soul, and paints her own nature into her practice.[1]

As we have discussed throughout this chapter, occupational therapy is unique with respect to the nature of its therapy, because its outcomes of concern require the active involvement of the client; that is, the client (individual, community, group, or population) enacts the occupational change. *Thus, the therapeutic use of self is the intentional, planned use of personal behaviors, insight, perception, judgment, skill, and knowledge to optimize the working alliance with clients and enable change.* As part of our education and continued development as professionals, we learn to have the insights, perception, judgment, skills, and knowledge that are germane to our practice. However, as the definition implies, how we enact these is necessarily modified by the personal behaviors. Then, intentional use of personal behaviors first requires an understanding of those personal behaviors; in other words, an understanding of the self and then matching that self to the client's needs.

The Self

"First, know thyself."[45] Personal behaviors emanate from the self. The self is a complex and dynamic entity comprised of diverse affective and cognitive elements and interacting with a number of sociocultural contexts. As our *person* develops, our *self* organizes our thoughts and feelings, related to our experiences within the external context, into coherent over-arching structures—our sense of self. Our sense of self is comprised of our self: values, social and cultural beliefs, spiritual nature, and the meaning and purpose behind our behaviors and actions. Based on our sense of self, we enact personal behaviors that are complex and fluid.[46,47]

The self is frequently discussed as having 2 key interrelated aspects: personal/private and social/public, each continually influencing the other.[48] This distinction has relevance for a discussion of the therapeutic use of self because our personal experiences and behaviors influence our interactions with others; in the working alliance, the "others" are our clients. In our interactions with our clients we must make a conscious choice about which aspects of our self to use at what time to enable our clients to enact occupational change.

The personal self is composed of one's self-concept that develops through cognitive processes pertaining to one's personality traits and temperament, actualized as personal behaviors.[47,48] Attitudes, beliefs, intentions, norms, roles, and values are key elements of the personal self as constructed through our interactions with society.[48] Although the personal self is proposed as being shaped early on by the social context, it is viewed as "an alternate means of being in the world,"[49(p63)] alternate to the public self.

The public self is contextually dependent and shaped to varying extents by local, societal, global, structural, and temporal contexts. It is viewed as a socially-constructed identity that is fluid, shaped by other individuals, groups, cultures, and aspects of society; thus it is essentially "coauthored" and continually evolves over time.[46] The public self is constructed through reflexivity of our position in the world, that is, the generalized views held by "others" toward our self. As occupational therapy practitioners, our public self (in other words, our professional self) is constructed within the context of enabling our clients' occupation.

The Self in Alliance

An occupational therapy practitioner's capacity to develop, modify, and transform her public self to suit the requirements of the client-therapist relationship is an important professional skill. There are 5 key elements of the self within the client-therapist relationship to consider:

1. Authenticity
2. Empathy
3. Reflexivity
4. Responsible collaboration
5. Enablement

Table 6-1 outlines the goals of each of these key elements and provides examples of actions that are compatible and incompatible with each. The first 3, authenticity ("one's relationship to oneself"),[46(p124)] empathy (knowing and conveying an appreciation of another person's experiences), and reflexivity (awareness of the self as an "other" who has the capacity to adapt)[54] are requisite elements brought to the client-therapist relationship to allow for responsible collaboration and enablement to occur.

Responsible collaboration is defined as a therapeutic interaction for which the occupational therapy practitioner takes on the responsibility for the development of a working alliance with her client that supports mutual, respectful, and transparent collaboration, as well as for the outcomes of the therapy. Responsible collaboration requires that occupational therapy practitioners ensure that clients understand the "intent" of their partnership, and the roles and responsibilities of each partner (in other words, the nature of their working alliance).

Enablement is "the core competency of occupational therapy—what occupational therapists actually do."[55(p367)] Through experience and reflexivity, an occupational therapy practitioner develops awareness of how the practitioner's *self* can both enable and hinder occupational change in her clients. Townsend, Polatajko, Craik, and Davis identified 10 specific enablement skills: adapt, advocate, coach, collaborate, consult, coordinate, design and build, educate, engage, and specialize.[56]

Tools for Understanding the Self and the Self in Alliance

Coming to know the *self* is a reflexive process. Here we highlight 3 tools: an occupational therapy practitioner-specific reflexive tool developed for this chapter based on the work of Taylor; a formal, widely-used personality typing instrument; and a published inventory to estimate the strength of the working alliance.

Taylor identified a number of characteristics that are important to the client-therapist relationship.[33] We have created a chart (Figure 6-1) that uses those characteristics as a source of critical self-reflexivity. Consider each characteristic and reflect upon whether it is a lot like you, somewhat like you, or not at all like you. Then, consider the needs of a particular client, and whether or not the characteristics you have identified in yourself are a good match for those needs.

A widely-used personality typing tool is the Myers-Briggs Type Indicator.[57] This instrument was developed by Myers and Briggs, based on the work of Carl Jung, and distinguishes 16 different personality types based on 4 pairs of personality characteristics:

1. Introversion-extraversion
2. Intuition-sensing
3. Thinking-feeling
4. Perceiving-judging

The test can be taken from a licensed administrator or online at The Center for Applications of Psychological

Table 6-1.   *Key Elements of the Occupational Therapy Practitioner Self to Support the Development of a Strong Working Alliance*

Key Element	Goal	Actions Supporting the Goal	Actions Incompatible With the Goal
Authenticity	• To act in practice following one's self-values. Self-values are desired conceptualizations that "serve as standards or criteria for self-judgment.[50(p18)]	• Bring forward into practice one's self-values. Commit to the role-identity of *occupational therapy practitioner* and the collective values captured by the occupational therapy profession. • Reconcile one's self-values with the values of the profession and commit to action following these values within therapeutic situations.	• Actions that stem from conflicting values will weaken the therapeutic relationship.
Empathy	• To encourage dialogical interactions by constructing a mutual and reciprocal empathic understanding.[51]	• Take on role of learner by encouraging client to tell story in own words.[52] • Listen/attune for understandings of sociopolitical contexts that underlie personal meaning.[53] • Use techniques of restating and incorporating client's actual words to privilege his experiences.[51]	• Rephrasing and reframing techniques may lead to possible misinterpretation or marginalization of client's true meaning.[51]
Reflexivity	• To understand how one's *self* can greatly influence the occupational outcomes of clients. • To consciously adapt the *self* to needs of the "other," fostering an equal, supportive, and just alliance.[54]	• Be conscious of the *self* in action. • Critically examine one's actions within/reactions to all interactions and alter behavior to enable a strong alliance. • Reflect on one's personality and modify greetings and interactions based on the reactions, needs, and personality of the client • Reflexively manage conflicts/inconsistencies with authentic nature and demands of context.	• Actions based on the broad assumptions about clients will lead to weaker alliances. • Lack of reflexivity in practice will create stagnation of potential and could perpetuate situations in which the clients face occupational marginalization.
Responsible collaboration	• To make intent of relationship understood and take on responsibility of working in alliance with client as mutual agent of change.	• Clearly communicate reasons for and goals of therapy. • Negotiate role responsibilities of all parties. • Outline parameters of client-practitioner relationship. • Be transparent with all actions. • Listen to client's successes and concerns. • Encourage client participation in process.	• Making all decisions for therapy for client will not enable the development of a strong working alliance and will diminish occupational engagement outcomes.

(continued)

Table 6-1 (continued).   *Key Elements of the Occupational Therapy Practitioner Self to Support the Development of a Strong Working Alliance*

Key Elements	Goal	Actions Supporting the Goal	Actions Incompatible With the Goal
Enablement	• To support and facilitate clients in making meaningful occupational changes in their lives.	• *Encourage* ◦ Recognize capacities and strengths ◦ Support client decisions ◦ Reward successes, both small and large • *Engage* ◦ Bring clients into working alliance. ◦ Help clients realize their key role in the collaboration. ◦ Listen to client's occupational life stories. • *Exemplify or leading by example* ◦ Advocate for resources and supports ◦ Convey positive, compelling, and consistent messages pertaining to client's occupational challenges.	• Being closed to possibilities for enablement leading to missed enablement, or creating situations of ineffective enablement will lead to client disengagement and discouragement.[2]

Type (http://www.capt.org/take-mbti-assessment/mbti.htm).[57]

In some cases, it may be useful to estimate the strength of the working alliance. While a number of tools exist, the Working Alliance and Theory of Change Inventory (WATOCI) has been modified for use with people receiving physical rehabilitation.[35]

REFLEXIVE EXERCISES

Derived from our discussion of occupational change and elements of self, the following is a reflexive exercise to initiate the development of your therapeutic use of self (see Figure 6-1). Starting with 2 client-therapist situation examples, the exercise provides a series of questions you can use to begin to appreciate your self and how aspects of your personal self may influence your occupational therapy practitioner self.

Occupational therapy practitioners gain an appreciation of their clients' *self* through 3 key sources: communication (written and verbal) with other health professionals or stakeholders, clinical observations and assessments, and communication (questioning and listening) with the client. Practitioners need to ensure that communication with other health professionals or stakeholders does not bias their initial views of their clients; however, having some information about your client before meeting them can help to set the stage to a stronger working alliance by allowing the practitioner to be aware of possible reactions from the client. To enable clients to realize occupational change, practitioners need to understand their client's habits and routines, attitudes and beliefs, and perception of social norms and self-efficacy (Figure 6-2).

To effectively use the self therapeutically, occupational therapy practitioners must be reflexive of their actions and attitudes and gain a thorough appreciation of clients' behaviors, routines, and motivation and intent to enact occupational change. Ultimately, building a strong client-therapist working alliance requires that occupational therapy practitioners ask, listen, observe, and assess.

Client-Occupational Therapy Practitioner Situation (use these examples, or please substitute situations from your own practice):

- A man who sustained a skydiving injury leaving him with complete paralysis asks you to enable him to go skydiving.
- A woman admitted to hospital because of her long-term issues with addiction, who is pregnant with her third child and is in threat of having the child taken from her, asks you to help her learn the skills she needs to care for her soon-to-be born child.

ASK YOURSELF:

PERSONAL AND PROFESSIONAL VALUES AND BELIEFS

- What are my essential personal values—those that guide my decisions and come out in all my actions? (Are these values your authentic characteristics?)
- How do my essential personal values fit with the values of the profession?
- How do my essential values fit with the values held by the practice context and culture?
- How do my values influence my responses to these clinical situations and client actions?
- Why do I believe what I believe?
- What will I do if my beliefs differ from those of the client?
- Will my decision lead to successful occupational change for the client?

PERSONALITY TRAITS, TEMPERAMENT, and PERSONAL BEHAVIORS: HABITS, MOODS, AND ROUTINES

- What are my dominant characteristics? (Refer to Table 6-1.)
- How will my personality traits fit with those of my client and his current mood and situation?
- What strategies have I learned that help me to manage aspects of my personality that might be viewed as undesirable in certain situations?
- How are my habits, moods, and routines affecting my client's success in reaching his goals?

SELF-EFFICACY

- Do I think that I have the capacity to help this client?

ENABLEMENT

- Do I adapt, advocate, coach, collaborate, consult, coordinate, design/build, educate, engage, specialize? (These are the 10 enabling skills that comprise the Canadian Model of Client-Centered Enablement[2].)
- Which enabling skills do I use least frequently? Why?
- Are there enabling skills I could use more frequently?
- How will my use of enablement skills affect my client's success?

Figure 6-1. Reflexive exercise for developing therapeutic use of self.

CLIENT'S HABITS AND ROUTINES

- What are my client's habits and occupational routines that will shape our interventions?

CLIENT'S ATTITUDES, BELIEFS, AND PERCEIVED SOCIAL NORMS

- What is my client's attitude toward the occupation he is to perform or performing?
- How much weight does my client place on each of his beliefs about that occupation?
- What does my client perceive to be the subjective social norms pertaining to the occupation or activities in which he is participating or will participate?

CLIENT'S PERCEPTIONS OF OWN CAPACITY

- How does my client perceive his capacity to engage in therapy, perform his desired occupation(s), and enact occupational change?

Figure 6-2. Reflexive exercise for developing an understanding of your client and his or her potential for occupational change.

REFERENCES

1. Beecher HW. Every artist dips his brush. *BrainyQuote*. http://www.brainyquote.com/quotes/quotes/h/henrywardb100771.html. Updated 2013. Accessed December 2, 2013.

2. Townsend EA, Beagan B, Kumas-Tan Z, et al. Enabling: occupational therapy's core competency. In: Townsend EA, Polatajko HJ. *Enabling Occupation II: Advancing an Occupational Therapy Vision for Health, Well-Being, and Justice through Occupation.* 2nd ed. Ottawa, ON: CAOT Publications ACE; 2013:87-133.

3. AOTA. Blueprint for entry-level education. *American Journal of Occupational Therapy.* 2010;64:186-203.

4. Townsend EA, Polatajko HJ. Introduction. In: Townsend EA, Polatajko HJ. *Enabling Occupation II: Advancing an Occupational Therapy Vision for Health, Well-Being, and Justice through Occupation.* 2nd ed. Ottawa, ON: CAOT Publications ACE; 2013:1-8.

5. Canadian Association of Occupational Therapists. *Enabling Occupation: An Occupational Therapy Perspective.* Ottawa, ON: CAOT Publications ACE; 1997.

6. Polatajko HJ, Davis J, Stewart D, et al. Specifying the domain of concern: occupation as core. In: Townsend EA, Polatajko HJ. *Enabling Occupation II: Advancing an Occupational Therapy Vision for Health, Well-Being, and Justice through Occupation.* 2nd ed. Ottawa, ON: CAOT Publications ACE; 2013:13-36.

7. Dunton WR. *Reconstruction Therapy.* Philadelphia, PA: WB Saunders; 1919.

8. Kielhofner G. Introduction to the model of human occupation. In: Kielhofner G, ed. *Model of Human Occupation: Theory and Application.* 4th ed. Baltimore, MD: Lippincott Williams & Wilkins; 2008:1-7.

9. Steel DM, Gray MA. Baby boomers' use and perception of recommended assistive technology: a systematic review. *Disability and Rehabilitation: Assistive Technology.* 2009;4:129-136.

10. Lund ML, Nygård L. Incorporating or resisting assistive devices: different approaches to achieving a desired occupation self-image. *OTJR: Occupation, Participation and Health.* 2003;23:67-75.

11. Krantz O. Assistive devices utilisation in activities of everyday life—a proposed framework of understanding a user perspective. *Disability and Rehabilitation: Assistive Technology.* 2012;7:189-198.

12. Gage M. Sense of doing—the impact of occupational restoration in the home. *Occupational Therapy Now.* 2003;5(5):35-37. http://www.caot.ca/default.asp?pageid=695. Updated 2013. Accessed December 2, 2013.

13. Heider F. Social perception and phenomenal causality. *Psychological Review.* 1944;51:358-374.

14. Lewis FM, Daltroy LH. How causal explanations influence health behavior: attribution theory. In: Glanz K, Lewis FM, Rimer BK, eds. *Health Education and Health Behavior: Theory, Research, and Practice.* San Francisco, CA: Jossey-Bass; 1990:92-114.

15. Ajzen I. From intentions to actions: a theory of planned behavior. In: Kuhl J, Beckmann J, eds. *Action Control: From Cognition to Behavior.* Heidelberg, Germany: Springer; 1985:11-39.

16. Ajzen I. The theory of planned behavior. *Organizational Behavior and Human Decision Processes.* 1991;50:179-211.

17. Ajzen I. Perceived behavioral control, self-efficacy, locus of control, and the theory of planned behavior. *Journal of Applied Social Psychology.* 2002;32:665-683.

18. Ajzen I, Fishbein M. *Understanding Attitudes and Predicting Social Behavior.* Englewood Cliffs, NJ: Prentice Hall; 1980.

19. Fishbein M, Ajzen I. *Belief, Attitude, Intention, and Behavior: An Introduction to Theory and Research.* Reading, MA: Addison-Wesley; 1975.

20. Miller K. *Communications Theories: Perspectives, Processes, and Contexts.* New York, NY: McGraw-Hill; 2005.

21. Fishbein M, Cappella JN. The role of theory in developing effective health communications. *Journal of Communication.* 2006;56(S1):S1-S17.

22. Bandura A. Self-efficacy: toward a unifying theory of behavioral change. *Psychological Review.* 1977;84:191-215.

23. Bandura A. *Social Foundations of Thought and Action: A Social Cognitive Theory.* Englewood Cliffs, NJ: Prentice Hall; 1986.

24. Knott D, Muers S, Aldridge S. *Achieving Culture Change: A Policy Framework.* London, UK: Strategy Unit, Government of UK; 2008.

25. Aron L. *A Meeting of Minds: Mutuality in Psychoanalysis.* Hillsdale, NJ: Analytic Press; 1996.

26. Mosey A. *Psychosocial Components of Occupational Therapy: New Psychosocial Components of Occupational Therapy.* New York, NY: Raven Press; 1986.

27. Taylor RR, Lee SW, Kielhofner G. Practitioners' use of interpersonal modes within the therapeutic relationship: results from a nationwide study. *OTJR: Occupation, Participation and Health.* 2011;31:6-14.

28. Ayres-Rosa S, Hasselkus BR. Connecting with patients: the personal experience of professional helping. *Occupational Therapy Journal of Research.* 1996;16:245-260.

29. Cole B, McLean V. Therapeutic relationships redefined. *Occupational Therapy in Mental Health.* 2003;19(2):33-56.

30. Taylor RR, Lee SW, Kielhofner G, Ketkar M. Therapeutic use of self: a nationwide survey of practitioner's attitudes and experiences. *American Journal of Occupational Therapy.* 2009;63:198-207.

31. Martin DJ, Garske JP, Davis MK. Relation of the therapeutic alliance with outcome and other variables: a meta-analytic review. *Journal of Consulting and Clinical Psychology.* 2000;68;438-450.

32. Norrby E, Bellner AL. The helping encounter—occupational therapists' perception of therapeutic relationships. *Scandinavian Journal of Caring Science.* 1995;9(1):41-46.

33. Taylor RR. *The Intentional Relationship: Occupational Therapy and Use of Self.* Philadelphia, PA: FA Davis; 2008.

34. Burke JP. What's going on here? Deconstructing the interactive encounter (Eleanor Clarke Slagle Lecture). *American Journal of Occupational Therapy.* 2010;64:855-868.

35. Hall AM, Ferreira PH, Maher CG, Latimer J, Ferreira ML. The influence of the therapist-patient relationship on treatment outcome in physical rehabilitation: a systematic review. *Physical Therapy.* 2010;90:1099-1110.

36. Punwar AJ. Defining occupational therapy. In: Punwar AJ, Peloquin SM, eds. *Occupational Therapy: Principles and Practice.* 3rd ed. Philadelphia, PA: Lippincott Williams & Wilkins; 2000:3-6.

37. Wright KM. Therapeutic relationship: developing a new understanding for nurses and care workers within an eating disorder unit. *International Journal of Mental Health Nursing.* 2010;19(3):154-161.

38. Bordin ES. The generalizability of the psychoanalytic concept of the working alliance. *Psychotherapy: Theory, Research.* 1979;16:252-260.

39. Samstag LW. The working alliance in psychotherapy: an overview of the invited papers in the special section. *Psychotherapy: Theory, Research, Practice, Training.* 2006;43:300-307.

40. Bordin ES. Theory and research on the therapeutic working alliance: new directions. In: Horvath AO, Greenberg LS, eds. *The Working Alliance: Theory, Research, and Practice.* New York, NY: Wiley; 1994:13-37.

41. Hatcher RL, Barends AW. How a return to theory could help alliance research. *Psychotherapy: Theory, Research, Practice, Training.* 2006;43:292-299.

42. Lambert MJ. Psychotherapy outcome research: implications of integrative and eclectic therapists. In: Norcross JC, Goldfried MR, eds. *Handbook of Psychotherapy Integration.* New York, NY: Basic Books; 1992:94-129.

43. Gunnarsson AB, Eklund M. The Tree Theme Method as an intervention in psychosocial occupational therapy: client acceptability and outcomes. *Australian Occupational Therapy Journal.* 2009;56:167-176.

44. Davidson DA. Therapeutic use of self in academic education: a mixed-methods study. *Occupational Therapy in Mental Health.* 2011;27(1):87-102.

45. Know thyself. Wikipedia: The Free Encyclopedia. http://en.wikipedia.org/wiki/Know_thyself. Updated November 28, 2013. Accessed December 5, 2013.

46. Hewitt JP, Shulman D. *Self and Society: A Symbolic Interactionist Social Psychology.* Boston, MA: Allyn & Bacon; 2011.

47. Nowak A, Vallcher RR, Tesser A, Borkowski W. Society of self: the emergence of collective properties in self-structure. *Psychological Review.* 2000;107(1):39-61.

48. Triandis HC. The self and social behavior in differing cultural contexts. *Psychological Review.* 1989;96:506-520.

49. Modell AH. *The Private Self.* Cambridge, MA: Harvard University Press; 1993.

50. Rosenberg M. *Conceiving the Self.* Malabar, FL: RE Krieger; 1986.

51. Clark J. *Beyond Empathy: An Ethnographic Approach to Cross-Cultural Social Work Practice.* Toronto, ON: University of Toronto; 2000. http://www.mun.ca/cassw-ar/papers2/clark.pdf. Published 2000. Accessed December 2, 2013.

52. Sells SP, Smith TE, Newfield N. Teaching ethnographic research methods in social work: a course model. *Journal of Social Work Education.* 1997;33(19):167-184.

53. Green JW. *Cultural Awareness in the Human Services.* 2nd ed. Toronto, ON: Allyn & Bacon; 1995.

54. Bennett-Levy J, Thwaites R. Self and self-reflection in the therapeutic relationship: a conceptual map and practical strategies for the training, supervision, and self-supervision of interpersonal skills. In: Gilber P, Leahy R, eds. *The Therapeutic Relationship in the Cognitive Behavioural Therapies.* London, UK: Routledge; 2007:255-281.

55. Townsend EA, Polatajko HJ. Glossary. In: Townsend EA, Polatajko HJ. *Enabling Occupation II: Advancing an Occupational Therapy Vision for Health, Well-Being, and Justice through Occupation.* 2nd ed. Ottawa, ON: CAOT Publications ACE; 2013:364-374.

56. Townsend EA, Polatajko HJ, Craik J, Davis J. Canadian Model of Client-Centred Enablement. In: Townsend EA, Polatajko HJ. *Enabling Occupation II: Advancing an Occupational Therapy Vision for Health, Well-Being, and Justice through Occupation.* 2nd ed. Ottawa, ON: CAOT Publications ACE; 2013:110.

57. Myers and Briggs Foundation. *MTBI Basics.* The Myers & Briggs Foundation. http://www.myersbriggs.org/my-mbti-personality-type/mbti-basics/. Accessed December 2, 2013.

Chapter 7

USING EVIDENCE TO GUIDE PRACTICE

Sally Bennett, PhD, BOccThy(Hons)

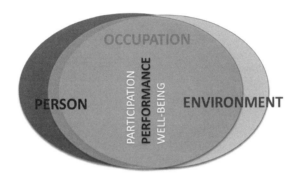

LEARNING OBJECTIVES

- Summarize the key components of evidence-based practice.
- Describe the process, knowledge, and skills for evidence-based practice.
- Compare and contrast individual, organization, and population perspectives of evidence-based practice.
- Describe the process of knowledge translation.
- Understand the role of meta-cognitive processes of reasoning, reflexivity, and critical thinking in becoming a wise practitioner.

KEY WORDS

- Decision making
- Evidence-based practice

INTRODUCTION

Decision making is central to occupational therapy practice, and shapes the way in which we support clients to achieve their goals. Occupational therapy practitioners make many decisions each day about which assessments to utilize, which interventions to use (if any), or how to modify an intervention depending on the context. As health professionals, we draw on many different types of knowledge and pool information from many different sources to direct the encounters we have with clients. Clinical (or professional) decision making is a complex process. It is dynamic and fluid, involves gathering data from multiple sources, interpreting and reasoning about the information, collaborating with both the client and other professionals, choosing a course of action, and evaluating the outcomes of that choice.[1] Further, decision making is highly contextualized and influenced by personal, professional, and societal values.

Christiansen CH, Baum CM, Bass JD, eds.
*Occupational Therapy: Performance, Participation,
and Well-Being, Fourth Edition (pp 93-109).*
© 2015 SLACK Incorporated.

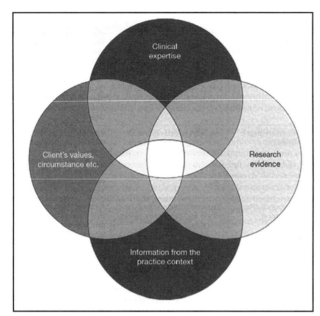

Figure 7-1. Integration of research, clinical, practice, and client. Evidence-based practice involves the integration of research evidence with our clinical expertise, our client's unique values and circumstances, and information from the practice context. (Reprinted with permission from Hoffmann T, Bennett S, Del Mar C. Introduction to evidence-based practice. In: Hoffmann T, Bennett S, Del Mar C, eds. *Evidence-Based Practice Across the Health Professions.* Sydney, Australia: Churchill Livingstone; 2010:1-16.)

We have seen in earlier chapters that the PEOP Occupational Therapy Process provides a framework for organizing information that has been gathered from the client's narrative, helps guide selection of assessments that aims to understand the factors that are intrinsic and extrinsic to the client, and helps to choose interventions with the client that enables the client to achieve their goals and desired outcomes. Thus, decisions require reasoning about different types of information from a range of sources in order to develop and evaluate intervention plans. Ideally, these decisions will be client-centered, draw on clinical expertise, take the context into account, and also consider evidence from research. Taken together, the integration of these information sources in practice is known as evidence-based practice.

This chapter provides an introduction to evidence-based practice, considers each of these sources of information and how they might be integrated, and also addresses the challenge of knowledge translation.

EVIDENCE-BASED PRACTICE

Evidence-based practice is a paradigm that proposes an approach to decision making that has been described as "the integration of the best research with our clinical expertise and our client's unique values and circumstances."[2,3] More recently the influence of information from the context in which we practice has been recognized and specifically incorporated into this definition.[4-6] A diagrammatic representation of evidence-based practice can be seen in Figure 7-1.[6]

Evidence-based practice adds to our understanding of decision making by explicitly inviting health professionals to consider research as a source of information in the decision making mix. We are reasonably proficient at gathering information from client narratives; have typically sought to refine our knowledge of assessments and interventions through practice evidence—observing and evaluating what works and what does not; developed clinical experience though practice, reflection, attending continuing education, and observing our colleagues; but have not, until more recently, been particularly aware of how we might use research information to inform our decisions. Understanding the nature, strengths, and limitations of each of these sources of information is critical to understanding evidence-based practice as an integrated decision-making concept, and each will be discussed in more detail later in this chapter.

Origins of Evidence-Based Practice

A complex interplay of social, political, and economic factors stimulated the adoption of evidence-based practice. Against a backdrop of an escalating volume of research information and technologies, the 1980s and 1990s also saw an increased demand for efficient use of resources and simultaneous improvements in the quality of health care.[7] This placed pressure on health care professionals to ensure that clinical practice was based on sound research evidence or "doing the right things right."[8] At the same time, the introduction of the Internet allowed rapid sharing of research information across the globe, and significantly opened the doors for consumers to access similar information as their health providers. By the late 1980s in the United Kingdom and Canada,[2] initiatives were underway that have had a momentous impact on the use of research within health care. The potential for systematic reviews as a means of synthesizing the results of RCTs was progressed considerably with the development of the first Cochrane Centre in Oxford, and later the development of the Cochrane Collaboration in 1993.[9] In Canada, the teaching of clinical epidemiology using a problem-based learning approach at McMaster University Medical School placed fresh emphasis on the integration of research and practice. The term *evidence-based medicine* was introduced in the literature in 1991 to describe a process that focused on "the conscientious, explicit, and judicious use of current best evidence in making decisions about the care of individual patients."[10] Briefly, the Working Group proposed a set of skills for lifelong learning that clinicians could use to identify their information needs, locate relevant research literature that may address these needs, and evaluate and apply it in practice.

The Process of Evidence-Based Practice

Specifically, the Evidence-Based Medicine Working Group proposed a series of 5 steps that could be used to facilitate the use of research evidence in practice.[11] These included the following:

1. Forming clinical questions reflecting the information needed
2. Searching for the best research evidence most appropriate for answering the clinical question
3. Critically appraising research evidence for its validity or rigor, impact (size of effect), and applicability (usefulness)
4. Integrating the research evidence with clinical experience, client's values and circumstances (and information from the practice context)
5. Evaluating the effectiveness and efficiency with which the previous steps were carried out and how it might be improved in future

These steps are briefly illustrated in the example in Box 7-1.

However, as evidence-based practice evolved it has been recognized that it is not always practical to work through each of these steps each time one has a new need for information that might be informed by research, because of the amount of time required to do so.[16] Depending on the situation, some health professionals may continue to work through each of these steps, whereas others may seek out research evidence that has already been appraised and therefore skip appraising the validity of research for instance.[3] These steps have been described in detail in many texts on evidence-based practice and therefore will not be the focus of this chapter. However, a number of pertinent observations will be made later in this chapter concerning the nature of research evidence, the availability of research evidence that might guide practice decisions, and how different types of information might be integrated.

The Context of Evidence-Based Practice

Evidence-based practice may be thought of differently depending on the context and level of "system" in which it is being used. Most often, evidence-based practice is applied at the microsystems level of the individual client; however, it can also be considered at the mesosystem level of large organizations, such as hospitals or nationwide health care providers, and has often been used to inform policies at the macrosystem level (eg, in government policies). As a relatively new paradigm, evidence-based practice has therefore had a substantial impact not just in the clinical domain, but also in the province of health management, policy, and purchasing.[8] Its influence can be seen in many of the major health systems and government health strategies and policies around the world. For example, the integration of research in practice has been central to the strategic plan of the National Health and Medical Research Council of Australia,[17] the policies of the Agency for Health Research and Quality in the United States,[18] and the Department of Health in the United Kingdom.[19]

The original stated aim of evidence-based practice was to improve clinical care. This important goal, and many other factors, continue to foster its use across all areas of health care and beyond. One of the drivers of evidence-based practice is the exponential increase in the quantity of research that continues as new advances, technologies, and approaches to health care are introduced. This makes it simply impossible for students (and occupational therapy practitioners for that matter) to keep up to date with everything they need to know. The explosion of information that has occurred over the last century has also meant that there is often a time lag of many years between when important research findings have been published and when they are actually translated into practice.[20] The process of evidence-based practice provides a self-directed means for organizing our thinking about the types of information that are needed to address particular issues or questions as they arise. This targeted "judicious" approach to finding and selecting research information therefore increases the likelihood that health professionals may stay up to date with research relevant to their practice.

The availability of the Internet, allowing clients' rapid access to health care information, has reinforced the growing trend toward consumer-driven health care. During the last few decades, clients have become more autonomous and assertive in interactions with health professionals, actively searching for information to bring to their healthcare provider and enquiring about evidence that might demonstrate the effectiveness of interventions offered. Accordingly, expectations for accessible health care, quality of services, and the accountability of health care providers have also increased.[8]

The need for both professional and economic accountability has afforded evidence-based practice a strong role in the occupational therapy profession. In many countries occupational therapy practitioners are guided by competency standards that indicate the need to be accountable for the safety and effectiveness of the services we provide.[21] Occupational therapy practitioners are

---

BOX 7-1

THEORIES THAT SUPPORT OUR UNDERSTANDING OF PERSON FACTORS

Assume for a moment that you are a new occupational therapy practitioner and that you are working with people with arthritis. You know that for people with arthritis, joint protection approaches can help to reduce hand deformities[12] and that activity pacing can reduce the impact of fatigue.[13] However, you don't know whether occupational therapy is effective for enabling people with arthritis to remain at work. So the question you have in mind might be: *Does occupational therapy enable people with rheumatoid arthritis to remain at work for longer than those who have not received occupational therapy?*

While the possible answer to this might be thought through based on theories or might have been observed by practitioners with extensive experience in this area, research information can provide data that is helpful for communicating effectiveness of interventions; not just to purchasers and managers, but also to clients. To find research addressing this question one needs to know about the type of question that it is that is being asked. This is because different types of research are more appropriate than others for providing information depending on the question at hand. This will be considered in more detail later in this chapter. For now however, you want to find research about an intervention and therefore look initially for systematic reviews of intervention studies or individual randomized controlled trials. By searching the freely accessible PubMed database (www.ncbi.nlm.nih.gov/sites/entrez) or OTseeker (www.otseeker.com)—a database of systematic reviews and RCTs relevant to occupational therapy,[14] you locate the following article citation and obtain a copy of it to read in detail: Macedo AM, Oakley SP, Panayi GS, Kirkham BW. Functional and work outcomes improve in patients with rheumatoid arthritis who receive targeted, comprehensive occupational therapy. *Arthritis Rheum.* 2009;61(11):1522-30.[15] This study compared the effects of 6 to 8 sessions of comprehensive occupational therapy spread over 6 months, as well as usual rheumatology care, or with rheumatology usual care alone (ie, these participants did not routinely receive occupational therapy). Participants in this study were people who had rheumatoid arthritis, were currently employed, and had medium or high work disability risk. Assessments were conducted at baseline and 6 months using the Canadian Occupational Performance Measure (COPM); the disability index (DI) of the Health Assessment

Questionnaire (HAQ); Disease Activity Score in 28 joints (DAS28); RA Work Instability Scale (RIS); EuroQol Index; visual analog scales (VAS) for pain, work satisfaction, and work performance; and days missed per month.

One of the tenets of evidence-based practice is that we cannot assume that all published research is methodologically sound, and that it is possible for bias in the design of a research study to influence the reported results. The idea of critical appraisal (Step 3 in the process outlined earlier) is that we need to read articles with a critical eye, to consider how rigorous the methods were, or how serious the risk of bias might be. The study we are interested in was an RCT: a study design that requires attention to particular features when it is carried out to reduce the risk of bias. The OTseeker database considers these features of internal validity for thousands of trials relevant to occupational therapy. By looking this study up quickly in OTseeker we can see that the authors have attempted to reduce the risk of bias when carrying out this trial. However, they were not able to blind participants or occupational therapy practitioners to which groups participants had been randomly assigned (a common problem in non-pharmacological interventions) and many outcomes were provided by self-report. Therefore, the possibility of expectation bias inflating the results needs to be considered. The discussion of risk of bias and rigor in different study designs is a substantial topic that cannot be adequately addressed here. Many textbooks are available on evidence-based practice that provide detailed explanations and worked examples of the various issues to consider for critical appraisal. Suffice to say that the risk of bias in the study by Macedo et al[15] is moderate.

So what did they find? Using the RA Work Instability Scale (RIS), which has a scale range of 0 to 23 with higher scores indicating greater work instability, participants had an average RIS of approximately 15.29 at the commencement of the study (when considering average baseline means of the 2 groups). At 6 months following the intervention period, those in the occupational therapy group had a reduction in work instability of 5.33 points on the RIS and those in usual care had a reduction of 2.53 on the RIS. Therefore, the difference in reduction of work instability scores between the 2 groups was 2.8, in favor of those who had received the comprehensive occupational therapy program—which is a statistically significant result. If

(continued)

BOX 7-1 (CONTINUED)

THEORIES THAT SUPPORT OUR UNDERSTANDING OF PERSON FACTORS

we then compare that difference of 2.8 (reduction of work instability) with the original baseline scores average of the 2 groups of 15.29, this may well represent a clinically significant change also. However we need to remember of course that this is an average, and therefore some will have had better scores and some will not have done as well. To consider the applicability of these results to the population you are interested in, you might then compare the people who were eligible for participating in this research study with those you are interested in working with to see how similar or otherwise they might be.

Moving on to Step 4 of this evidence-based practice process, you would need to have a conversation with the people for whom you were considering this research information. If this is an individual client, is this amount of change (for the effort required) worth their time and effort to participate? For some it will be

and for some it may not be, depending on their values and circumstances. The context of the practice you work in will also influence the subsequent decision to commence this intervention or not. If you have looked at this research with the view to using it with clients on a routine basis, then it will be important to discuss this with your colleagues and manager to determine if it is possible to provide this service routinely in your local setting. From the perspective of purchasers and policy makers though, it is fair to say this study provides good initial evidence for the effectiveness of occupational therapy for people with rheumatoid arthritis in reducing work instability. Importantly, this study measured many other outcomes and also found improvements in work performance and satisfaction, reduced the number of work days missed, reduction in pain, improved quality of life, and found significant results on the COPM.

---

encouraged to participate in continuing professional development (CPD) activities, engage in evidence-based practice, and evaluate their clinical practices in order to meet professional standards.[22]

The issue of economic accountability is more challenging. The cost of providing health care is increasing. Organizations purchasing health care services, whether they are part of the private or public sector, are concerned with achieving maximum value and with being accountable for how health care dollars are spent.[8] As Gray puts it, we need to not just be concerned with *"doing the right things,"* but also *"doing the right things right."*[8] Thus the parameters for health care purchasing have shifted over time from ensuring clinical effectiveness to ensuring the best value for health care. This has driven demand for evidence about the effectiveness and cost-effectiveness of service provided by those responsible for providing services and the need to demonstrate value for money.

The implication for occupational therapy is substantial. As a profession we are being asked to provide research evidence to demonstrate the effectiveness and value of our services. This is a challenge for occupational therapy as a research-emergent profession.[23] Although rigorous research testing the effects of occupational therapy is rapidly increasing,[24] it is simply not possible to have sufficient research to support all that health providers do. Unfortunately, some governments and health funds have increasingly adopted the position of allocating health resources depending on research demonstrating effective-

ness.[25] Given the difficulty providing definitive statements about the effectiveness (or otherwise) of many interventions, and the fact that many interventions simply do not require evidence from research to demonstrate their necessity (which shall be discussed later), this stance is untenable. Nevertheless, where this model of health care purchasing does exists, we need to be able to clearly articulate our concerns. Under these circumstances, one principle that needs greater understanding by all is that "absence of evidence" is not "evidence of absence,"[26] and that when there is no clear research evidence available this is not justification for rejection of innovation[27] or associated funding. We therefore need to be skilled communicators, to understand the different interests of policy makers and purchasers, and to engage them in dialogue about the nature of the services provided by occupational therapy practitioners.

A closely related issue is one of distributive justice. The goals of evidence-based practice at the level of the person are to improve or maintain the health of the individual. In contrast, the goal of evidence-based public health is the health of populations. These goals may at times be complementary and at others times conflict, most obviously concerning resource allocation. The agenda of social justice frameworks that emphasize health as a moral right for all may at times clash with the agenda of distributive justice frameworks that require some "leveling" of health care service provision to enable at least a minimal level of benefit to all.[28] Different stakeholders in health care value different types of outcomes and, thus, funding based on demonstrating one type of outcome will not represent the interests of all.[29] Unfortunately the complexity of health care is such that there is no easy solution. Evidence-based practice at the level of the individual, organization, and population requires understanding of the values of different stakeholders and, further, this necessitates that we learn more about managing value conflicts.[25]

Evidence-Based Practice Is Not Just About the Evidence

We have emphasized that evidence-based practice is a decision-making paradigm, one which integrates information from research, from clients, and is informed by clinical experience and practice contexts. A common misrepresentation that occurs in the literature is that evidence-based practice is synonymous with research. The way in which language is used is pivotal to our mutual understanding—to discourses and conversations about particular issues. Too often the terms *evidence* and *evidence-based practice* are used interchangeably when they are not one and the same. Research evidence is only one aspect of evidence-based practice, as the original authors who coined the phrase "evidence-based medicine" were at pains to point out.[27] In order to understand the full meaning of evidence-based practice, we shall look in more detail at information from research, from clinical experience, from the client, and from the practice context before considering how we integrate this information.

RESEARCH EVIDENCE

The original definitions of evidence-based medicine specifically spoke of evidence as meaning evidence from systematic research.[11,27] During the last decade it has been contended that the term *evidence* should also include evidence from sources other than research. This is because the term *evidence* is commonly used in everyday language when speaking about all sorts of information that health professionals gather to inform their decisions.[30] The importance of these other sources of information and other ways of knowing is not contested in evidence-based practice. However, the use of the term *evidence* to denote "evidence from research" in this framework serves a particular purpose. This term was specifically chosen to emphasize research as a source of information that, at the time, received little attention in clinical decision making. In this chapter then, when the term *evidence* is used, it is taken to mean evidence from research.

It is not surprising that there have been many attempts to find a phrase other than evidence-based practice (for example *research-based practice* or *research-informed prac-*

tice), to avoid the contentiousness about what evidence is and what it is not within this paradigm. Nevertheless, the phrase evidence-based practice has persisted and now permeates most areas of health care. Given how embedded this phrase has become, equating the term *evidence* with "research" may be accepted as long as the phrase *evidence-based practice* is also understood as an integration of information from multiple sources: clients, clinical experience, practice context, and research (evidence).

What Sort of Research?

Research within the evidence-based practice paradigm emphasizes the use of clinically relevant research. "By best available external clinical evidence we mean clinically relevant research, often from the basic sciences of medicine, but especially from patient-centred clinical research."[2(p71)]

Given that evidence-based practice derived from evidence-based medicine, the majority of examples of research evidence initially described in the literature have demonstrated how quantitative research could inform practice. However, one of the first articles about evidence-based medicine from The Evidence-Based Medicine Working Group at McMaster University also recognized the value of research techniques from behavioral sciences.[27] "The new paradigm (evidence-based medicine) would call for using the techniques of behavioral science to determine what patients are really looking for from their physicians and how physician and patient behavior affects the outcome of care."[27(p2422)]

In its broad application, behavioral sciences might be taken to include qualitative research, with explicit recognition of the value of qualitative research within the evidence-based practice paradigm occurring at least as early as 1997.[31] Thus, both quantitative and qualitative methods were embraced, despite concerns to the contrary expressed in subsequent critiques of evidence-based practice.

One of the tenets of evidence-based practice is the use of "best" available evidence from systematic research. The use of the term *best* here indicates selection of information from the most **appropriate** type of research to address the type of issue/question being considered and the most **rigorous** research available.

Appropriateness of Research

Let's consider appropriateness of research first. This is about the fit or potential of research designs to answer different type of information needs we might have. There are two questions we can ask ourselves to clarify what sort of research information to look for. The first is a screening question which may appear obvious, but is worth explaining here.

- *Can research help us to address this particular information need/question that we have, or are other sources of information/knowledge more appropriate for this particular issue?*

Quite clearly, many different sources of information other than research information are important for addressing the many questions we might have in occupational therapy. We have, however, gradually become accustomed to the importance of research evidence for addressing questions about the effectiveness of interventions. There are exceptions to this "rule." Not *all* interventions that we offer as occupational therapy practitioners need to be tested by research to demonstrate their effectiveness (or value for that matter). Where interventions have a direct and/or significant benefit[32,33] (as some assistive technologies and many home modifications do for instance), such interventions may not require research to demonstrate their effects. A satirical example of this principle is the use of parachutes to prevent death amongst skydivers[34]—a technique never tested with research! We may, however, seek research to understand the acceptability, comfort, perceived usefulness, usage, and so on, for these types of interventions—which are different questions to that of effectiveness.

The second question then becomes:

- *If the issue can be informed by research, what type of research would be best suited (appropriate) for addressing what I want to know?*

Some of the questions we commonly ask are:

- How common is this problem?
- What are the concerns and experiences of people with a particular condition or disability?
- What are the long-term outcomes likely to be?
- Which assessment might be best to use?
- What interventions might help?
- Why do some interventions not seem to work?

Different types of research methods have specific design features that are better able to inform us about different types of questions.[31,35] For example, qualitative research is much more useful than any quantitative research methods for providing us with information about why things occur (or don't), how they occur, and what clients' experiences might be. Within qualitative research there are also many different approaches to be aware of (eg, phenomenology, ethnography, discourse analysis) that are suited to addressing different types of issues. *Quantitative research* on the other hand provides information about likelihoods, probabilities, patterns, and associations between variables—with some quantitative methods being particularly suited to information about long-term outcomes (eg, cohort or longitudinal studies), and others

being suited to helping us consider the effects of interventions (eg, experimental designs).[31]

This brings us to the concept of hierarchies of evidence. Hierarchies of evidence are frameworks that present different study designs in hierarchies according to a) their ability to address different types of questions and b) to control for bias (with those toward the top being more suited to the type of question and having more potential to control for bias).[36] One persistent misunderstanding in the occupational therapy literature (and elsewhere) is that there is only one hierarchy of evidence that promotes systematic reviews of RCTs and, following that, individual RCTs are the "best" type of evidence.[37] What is not commonly known is that this well-known hierarchy of evidence was only ever meant for research about the effects of interventions and, further, that *different hierarchies of evidence have existed for different types of clinical issues* since the 1990s. A current example of multiple hierarchies of evidence from the Oxford Centre for Evidence-Based Medicine[38] can be found at www.cebm.net/index.aspx?o=5513. Hence, hierarchies of evidence match study designs to different types of questions in a type of matrix. Applying one type of research hierarchy with little regard for the type of question at hand is a misuse of this concept that has permeated many dialogues in health care. It is not surprising then that there is great concern regarding the overemphasis on RCTs, when they are often not the most appropriate research design for the question and are simply not appropriate for many concerns of occupational therapy.

Hierarchies of evidence also take potential for bias into account. Bias occurs when there is a systematic error in the way in which participants are selected for a study, how outcomes might be measured, or how data is analyzed and, if present, may lead to either overestimation or underestimation of the study results.[39] Thus studies toward the top (or beginning) of any one hierarchy have more potential to control for bias. It is important to note here that hierarchies of evidence are intended as guidelines or heuristics for thinking about different types of study designs and were not designed to be treated rigidly as rules.[38] For example, a hierarchy of evidence can provide guidelines for efficient search strategies for guiding a health professional to initially consider research from a particular research design before moving on to others.

Rigorous Research

The second consideration regarding the idea of "best" available evidence is that using the most *rigorous* research available helps to increase our confidence in the results or findings from the research, whether this is from quantitative or qualitative research. Regardless of the study design used, not all studies are able to be undertaken utilizing all the design principles recommended. Each study type has a range of different techniques that may be used to control for risk of bias (quantitative research) or improve rigor and credibility (qualitative research) within the research project. For instance, in a cohort study considering long-term outcomes post-TBI it is important that the group of participants are recruited at as similar and early time point as possible following brain injury, to minimize selection bias.[40] In an RCT testing the effect of home modifications for reducing risk of falls, it is ideal that trial participants are blind to (unaware of) whether they were allocated to the experimental or control condition, so that their expectations about the trial do not influence their behavior during the trial or the assessment or reporting of outcomes. In qualitative research the data representation and analysis should be congruent with the research methodology chosen, and clearly reported.[41] While many of these design principles are possible, some are simply not able to be achieved due to the nature of occupational therapy and due to practical issues. In these cases the size of resulting estimates (quantitative research) or credibility (qualitative) may be affected. Therefore appraising the potential for bias (quantitative research) and rigor (qualitative research) in individual studies is an important aspect to identifying "best" research evidence. Critical appraisal checklists provide a series of key questions that can help health professionals establish the internal validity and clinical usefulness of an article's results. Checklists for critical appraisal of both quantitative and qualitative studies exist, and many of these can be accessed through the Internet.

And so, we are encouraged to use the best research evidence available. This implies that **all** types of research should be understood and valued for what information they can provide and their strengths and limitations taken into account as we seek to make decisions.

Problems and Opportunities in Occupational Therapy Research

Research is a difficult undertaking. The nature of a discipline, pragmatic constraints, and ethical issues determine how research is undertaken. In occupational therapy much has been written about the difficulty undertaking RCTs due to the highly individualized nature of occupational therapy interventions.[42] Many questions concerning the effectiveness of occupational therapy treatments are therefore more suited to quasi-experimental or single-case experimental designs.[43,44]

Having said this, there are increasing numbers of RCTs relevant to occupational therapy that either directly involve occupational therapy or may inform occupational therapy practice. At time of writing this chapter, the OTseeker database[45] (www.otseeker.com) provided citations and

critical appraisals of RCTs of over 8250 RCTs relevant to occupational therapy. Just a few examples of evidence from RCTs support the benefits of occupational therapy for the following:

- People with dementia[46,47]
- People with rheumatoid arthritis[48,49]
- People at risk of falling[50,51]
- People who have had a hip fracture[52,53]
- People who have had a stroke[54-57]
- People with multiple sclerosis[58,59]
- People with psychotic conditions living in the community[60]
- Children's handwriting development[61-63]
- Wellness in healthy older people[64,65]

But what of study designs addressing issues other than effect of interventions? There are increasing numbers of research studies determining the utility and properties of a wide range of assessments used in occupational therapy (eg, the COPM,[66] the Assessment of Motor and Process Skills,[67] the Executive Function Performance Test,[68] Occupational Therapy Adult Perceptual Screening Test,[69] and so on). There are also many studies providing predictive information from longitudinal studies investigating, for example, the relationship between pre-discharge occupational therapy home assessment and prevalence of post-discharge falls,[70] or identifying predictors of social and functional outcomes for individuals sustaining pediatric TBI.[71]

The breadth and depth of evidence from qualitative research in occupational therapy is impressive. Qualitative research can tell us about what matters most to consumers, what their experiences are, why approaches to health care may or may not work, help describe and characterize contextual issues, and can sensitize health professionals and governments to the diversity of concerns needing to be addressed. For example qualitative research has informed us about the following:

- Parent perspectives of therapy services for their children with physical disabilities[72]
- Goal setting in neurological rehabilitation—patients' perspectives[73]
- The experience of loss of the driving role following TBI[74]
- Perceptions of persons with multiple sclerosis on cognitive changes and their impact on daily life[75]
- Consumer-identified barriers and strategies for optimizing technology use in the workplace[76]
- The bodily experience of apraxia in everyday activities[77]
- Hopes and aspirations of teenagers with cerebral palsy[78]

• Clinicians' experience with occupation-based practice[79]

The difficulties with the production, relevance, and availability of research evidence are real. Concerns are frequently raised about how research is influenced by pragmatic factors, such as ease of measurement, availability of participants, and funding opportunities, and may not readily be able to address issues of real clinical and professional concern.[29] It is acknowledged that many aspects of clinical practice cannot, or will not, ever be adequately tested through research,[27] particularly given the complexity and changing nature of practice. Nonetheless, the research we **do** have available in occupational therapy, regardless of whether it is quantitative or qualitative in nature and regardless of the types of issues it might address, is an *opportunity*, not just for guiding individual clinical decisions, but for informing the wider health care agenda.

CLINICAL AND PROFESSIONAL EXPERTISE

Concern has been raised in the literature that the construction of hierarchies of evidence devalues experiential knowledge.[80] Initial versions of the hierarchy of evidence that dated from the late 1970s[81] regarding the effect of interventions, placed expert knowledge at the bottom of the hierarchy of evidence. However, including it as a category of "evidence" created confusion,[82] given that expert knowledge is essential to making decisions about many different aspects of health care and it has thus been removed from many published versions of hierarchies about intervention effects.

However, there are limits to clinical experience, just as there are limits to scientific understanding that we need to be aware of. At times, clinical experience is subject to flaws of thinking. For example, we may overemphasize some information and experiences and may underestimate others. Further, while information from colleagues who are older and more experienced may certainly be valuable and accurate, at times the information may be out of date or based on tradition rather than careful observations, as we would hope. However the Evidence-Based Medicine Working Group[27] argues that recognizing the limitations of experience should not be misinterpreted as rejecting these routes to knowledge. As more research is undertaken about judgment and decision making, the nature and importance of experiential knowledge has been increasingly understood. Clinical experience and the wider concept of professional expertise is so important to evidence-based practice that it is a key feature of its definition:

The practice of evidence-based medicine means integrating individual clinical expertise with the best available external clinical evidence from systematic research. By individual clinical expertise we mean the proficiency and judgment that individual clinicians acquire through clinical experiences and clinical practice. Increased expertise is reflected in many ways, but especially in more effective and efficient diagnosis and in the more thoughtful identification and compassionate use of individual patients' predicaments, rights, and preferences in making clinical decisions about their care.[2(p7)]

Thus, knowledge and expertise developed through practice is essential for selecting and using assessments and interventions, and for communicating with clients. Clinical experience is generated from observation and reflection of practical experiences, and requires thoughtfulness and compassion as well as knowledge about the practices and activities specific to a discipline.[6] It is developed over time, through observing more experienced colleagues, trialing interventions and observing what works and what does not, listening carefully to the experiences of clients, systematically collecting data from practice, attending conferences and workshops, reading research, discussing cases and experiences with colleagues, and (perhaps most importantly) being a reflective practitioner.[5,83,84] Deliberate reflective practice is used to process experiences and information and involves critical analysis of thoughts, feelings, and knowledge to develop new perspectives, which in turn influence decision making.[5] Clinical experience develops as different types of knowledge are assimilated: knowledge of theory and of science, professional craft knowledge (knowing the practical "what," "when," and "how" of practice), and personal knowledge (reflection on personal experiences, which forms a frame of reference for interpreting the world).[85]

The lines between practice knowledge founded on clinical experiences and research evidence blur as health professionals seek to systematically observe and measure their practice. "When optimal care is taken to both record observations reproducibly and avoid bias, clinical and institutional experience evolves into the systematic search for knowledge that forms the core of evidence-based medicine."[27(p2423)]

In a study involving focus groups with 9 occupational therapy practitioners with between 5 to 24 years clinical experience, Copley and Allen[84] noted that participants used the phrase *practice evidence* to describe an ongoing process of testing what they had learned from training and research into the evaluation of their clinical experiences. The authors conclude that practice-generated evidence can be useful when professionals seek to systematically plan, conduct, evaluate, and report their practices in a consistent manner.[84]

It is therefore not surprising that many studies have found occupational therapy practitioners rely more on clinical experience than on other information when making clinical decisions.[86-88] It is both a source of information itself, and influences how research information is integrated in practice.[89] To quote Sackett, Richardson, Rosenberg, and Haynes, "without clinical expertise, practice risks becoming tyrannized by external evidence, for even excellent external evidence may be inapplicable to or inappropriate for an individual patient."[11(p5)]

CLIENTS' PREFERENCES, VALUES, AND CIRCUMSTANCES

Central to evidence-based decision making is the consideration of clients' preferences, values, and circumstances. Clients come to the health care context with unique beliefs, values, and experiences: the lens through which they filter information relevant to their health. Similarly, health care professionals enter the interaction with a client with their own personal and professional beliefs, values, and experiences. Because health professionals and clients think differently from each other about health care issues, and have very different personal and contextual perspectives, their values and preferences with respect to health outcomes also differ. Therefore, explicitly enquiring about a client's preferences and values with respect to decisions about their health is essential. Understanding clients' preferences and values necessitates that the research evidence that does exist is communicated to clients clearly, that uncertainties are acknowledged, and that clients are able to express their preferences and goals.

Understanding a client's circumstances also directly affects the shape of therapy. For example, if clients need to travel long distances or arrange child care in order to receive therapy, this may make them less inclined to attend. Similarly, the financial and social supports they have available to them can facilitate or limit a client's ability (and sometimes motivation) to maintain involvement in therapy. While some of these circumstances may become evident during occupational therapy assessment, specifically enquiring about a client's available supports and possible constraints to participation in therapy is important.

Using the process of evidence-based practice, health professionals (where appropriate) provide clients with information from research, share their experience and reasoning with clients, and seek to identify the clients' values and preferences for therapy. In the PEOP Model, clients are similarly invited to be actively involved in selecting goals for their therapy. This active involvement of clients in decision making can also be understood as shared decision making. *Shared decision making* requires a partnership between the client and health professional, with clients being invited to be actively involved in determining goals, weighing up intervention options, and evaluating outcomes.[90] The extent of involvement the client may wish to have in decision making varies greatly, with many clients wanting information but still wanting to rely on the health professional to make the decisions.[91] It is therefore important for occupational therapy practitioners to determine to what extent a client might want to be involved in decision making.

This consideration of a client's values, preferences, and circumstances in the evidence-based practice paradigm is congruent with client-centered practice.[92] A practitioner's consideration of a client's contexts and what he or she values is also described in the PEOP Model, as found earlier in this text. At the person level, this model proposes the use of a narrative perspective to understand more about the client's perceptions, meanings, motivations, attitudes, needs, and goals. This narrative, or story, then provides the backdrop against which occupational therapy practitioners seek to understand the person and environment factors influencing occupational performance, and to establish goals for therapy in conjunction with the client. At the organizational level, this narrative enquiry pays attention to the mission and history of an organization, its focus, priorities, and values in order to establish an organization-centered intervention to achieve the organization's goals. At the population level, the narrative provides the practitioner with an understanding of the environments, behaviors, demographics, incidence, and prevalence about the population and helps them to identify needs and goals of the population that might be met through occupational therapy. Much more remains to be said about the type of information we gather from clients that informs our decisions and how this information might be gathered, and is addressed within other chapters of this text.

THE PRACTICE AND CLINICAL CONTEXT

Decision making is highly contextualized, and this can be seen most clearly by the influence of practice contexts on the decisions that might be made. Smith, Higgs, and Ellis[93] note that social, professional, organizational, physical, and environmental aspects of the practice setting influence decisions and that these factors assume different importance according to the particular circumstances at any point in time. As our understanding of evidence-based practice has evolved, an increasing number of authors note the importance of taking the practice context into account when making decisions.[4,35-41]

One of the most direct ways we can observe the influence of contexts on decision making is how the availability of resources influences decisions.[4] The resources of a particular practice setting do not just include the funding available, but also the space, time available, staffing levels, and availability of equipment.[83] For example, even though there might be rigorous research evidence that a particular intervention is effective, the intervention can only be provided if the required equipment is available. Similarly, what practitioners do is greatly influenced by the time they have available for carrying out assessments or interventions. In turn, resource availability is determined by a number of factors, such as where a service is based (eg, metropolitan versus rural settings), the model of care being provided (eg, acute care versus community-based care), or the financial structures and policies of an organization.

It is impossible to separate individual practitioners' decision making from the influences of the system within which one works; whether that be microsystems (clinic or hospital ward), mesosystems (organizations), or macrosystems (governments and their associated healthcare policies).[94] At the microsystem level, for instance, physicians or specialists may determine that all their clients are to receive care based on a clinical pathway and/or specific protocol. This in turn directly influences the individual occupational therapy practitioner's decision making. At the mesosystem level, the organization's policies and structures, for example, determine the amount of time practitioners have available, the equipment available to use, and scope of practice that is supported. These, each in turn, influence individual practitioners' decisions. At the macrosystem level of government, policies are shaped by ideological, social, legal, and economic issues,[95] which then filter through to influence the way in which health care service delivery is structured, and ultimately to what individual occupational therapy practitioners are able or not able to do.

Less tangible is the influence of social contexts on decision making. The more complex a decision is and the greater the uncertainty, the more likely it is that health care professionals will consult others. A number of surveys have found that occupational therapy practitioners commonly rely on their colleagues when making clinical decisions.[86,96] This is also true of other health professions. In-depth interviews with hundreds of nurses revealed many different reasons why they relied on "human" sources of information when making decisions.[97] Just some of these were that a person can directly answer a question that has been asked (and is therefore a more efficient means of finding an answer), they may be seen as experienced and trustworthy, they seem to provide a balanced picture (although this may not be the case), they may provide a range of different types of knowledge, provide information that is unlikely to be challenging and likely to be supportive, and do not require the additional skills of critical appraisal.[97] An extension of this reliance on others is the concept of *communities of practice*. Communities of practice can be thought of as groups of people held together by a common interest in a body of knowledge, common concerns, and passions,[98] and as such are powerful influences on knowledge acquisition, knowledge management, ways of thinking, and decision making. While such communities of practice occur within individual practice settings, the *professional* community of practice of occupational therapy sets standards and ethical expectations for practice that also guide what we do and how we do it.

INTEGRATING SOURCES OF INFORMATION

We have seen that evidence-based practice is a decision-making paradigm, one which integrates information from research, from clients, and is informed by clinical experience and practice contexts. We have also seen that there are different types of knowledge we might draw on. Just how do we integrate all this information? *Professional (clinical) reasoning*, the over-arching thinking processes associated with practice,[99] is used to determine what information is needed, to interpret that information, and then weigh up information from each of these sources. The aim of this reasoning is to guide the health professional to make wise choices, particularly in the face of uncertainty.

Clinical reasoning is the higher-order thinking that we use when discerning the relevance and import (or not) of research evidence, theoretical, and practice knowledge for a particular client within a particular context. What should be clear by now is that evidence-based practice is not **just** about using research, but requires considerable reasoning skills to integrate information from many different sources. Our reasoning skills can be improved by *reflective practice* and by *critical thinking*. Whereas reflective practice is a deliberate processing of experiences and information,[5] critical thinking is a process of mindful monitoring and self-correction of thought processes. Critical thinkers examine their thinking. They consider whether they are asking the right question, think about what the underlying assumptions of an idea might be, think about the consequences of their decisions prior to them being made, think about alternative viewpoints, and embrace different ways of knowing. Critical thinking is a lifelong process aimed at improving the quality of one's thinking.[100] Used with integrity and fairness, it underpins wise practice.

Kemmis observed that expert practitioners:

...have highly developed capacities to search for saliences that allow them to respond wisely and prudently to each situation, taking into account the likely consequences of their actions in relation to the many, often competing or conflicting aims, understandings, values, and self-interests they bring to the situation and that others bring to it, and that reveal themselves in and through action and interaction—practice—in the situation as it unfolds.[101(p392-393)]

And so, a balanced view of evidence-based practice that values all ways of knowing and that uses research evidence judiciously "without overinflating its practical significance"[80] is warranted.

USING KNOWLEDGE IN PRACTICE (KNOWLEDGE TRANSLATION)

Much has been written about the complexities involved in using evidence-based practice on a day-to-day basis. Embracing evidence-based practice requires changes in attitudes, values, skills, knowledge, and work practices.[102] Numerous factors influence the ease with which evidence-based practice skills and processes might be used. For instance, lack of time and access to research information in the workplace limits the ease with which relevant information can be located,[86,103] whereas positive leadership at the level of the organization enables evidence-based practice activities to be valued and become part of the organization culture.[94] Discussion of methods for overcoming barriers to evidence-based practice is beyond the scope of this chapter and has been discussed in detail elsewhere.[104,105] However, in part, these challenges have increased interest in understanding factors influencing how research knowledge is translated into practice.

Translation of research into practice has been described as occurring in 2 phases. The first phase (T1), also known as *translational research*, is the translation of research from basic biomedical sciences into clinical applications. The second phase (T2) refers to translation of research knowledge into practice and improved health care.[106] It is this second phase that is often referred to simply as *knowledge translation*. Knowledge translation has been defined by the Canadian Institutes of Health Research as "a dynamic and iterative process that includes the synthesis, dissemination, exchange, and ethically sound application of knowledge to improve health, provide more effective health services and products, and strengthen the health care system."[107(np)]

The purpose of knowledge translation is to try to improve health care by reducing the gap between research knowledge and practice.[108] Numerous terms related to knowledge translation have been in use in the literature for some time, with different terms being used in different countries or between organizations. Some of the most commonly used terms are *knowledge transfer* or *exchange, implementation, research utilization, diffusion of innovations,* and *knowledge uptake.*[108]

The reasons why clinically important research is often published but not routinely implemented can be seen diagrammatically in the "research-to-practice pipeline," which identifies points at which "leaks" in knowledge translation might occur.[109] As can be seen in Figure 7-2, in order for evidence to be put into practice, the health professional or organization needs to be aware of the research evidence, accept what the research might indicate, recognize which clients it might apply to, be able to carry out the assessment or intervention, and actually act on the evidence. The last 2 points require the client's involvement in agreeing to the assessment or intervention and adhering to the intervention. Where any of these do not occur, there is "leakage" in the evidence-to-practice pipeline.[109] This model is helpful for considering where we may need to focus efforts for improve the use of research in practice.

A number of theories or models exist that can be used to guide the planned use of rigorous research evidence more systematically in practice. The "knowledge to action" (KTA) process conceptualizes knowledge translation as including a knowledge creation phase and an "action cycle." The action cycle (similar to the idea of T2 knowledge translation) is based on a review of commonly identified steps of existing planned-action models and frameworks, and outlines the following phases in the cycle[108]:

- Identify a problem that needs addressing
- Identify, review, and select the knowledge or research relevant to the problem (eg, practice guidelines or research findings)
- Adapt the identified knowledge or research to the local context
- Assess barriers to using the knowledge
- Select, tailor, and implement interventions to promote the use of knowledge (ie, implement the change)
- Monitor knowledge use
- Evaluate the outcomes of using the knowledge
- Sustain ongoing knowledge use

The first 2 phases enable knowledge-practice gaps to be identified; either by identifying a problem or issue that needs attention and locating knowledge and/or research that might address it that is not currently being used, or by health providers being aware of knowledge from rigorous sources (such as systematic reviews) and determining if it is being implemented. The appropriateness and value of this knowledge/research to the local setting is then

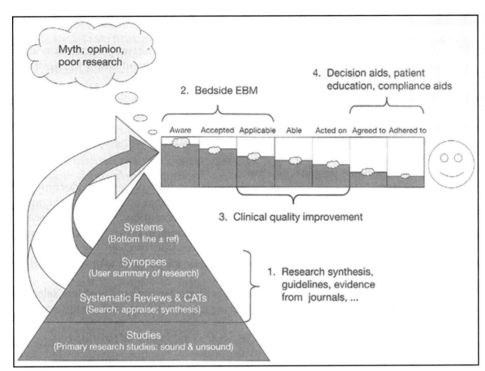

Figure 7-2. The research-to-practice pipeline. (Reprinted with permission from Glasziou P, Haynes B. The paths from research to improved health outcomes. *ACP Journal Club.* 2005;142[2]:A8-A10.)

considered by relevant stakeholders and may be tailored to the local context.[108]

Identifying the types of barriers that might limit the use of this knowledge by those who will be involved in its use is then critical. Barriers to its use might be due to a lack of knowledge or skills, attitudinal issues, or lack of resources, for instance.

A particularly useful framework for understanding the range of barriers (and enablers) to behavior change required for knowledge translation is the Theoretical Domains Framework.[110] It is a framework developed from 33 behavior change theories, and its validated version[111] describes 14 domains of theoretical constructs thought to influence or mediate behavioral change. These domains include knowledge, skills, social/professional role and identity, beliefs about capabilities, optimism, beliefs about consequences, reinforcement, intentions, goals, memory, attention and decision processes, environmental context and resources, social influences, emotions, and behavioral regulation.

The use of surveys and interviews are particularly useful for identifying where key barriers might occur. Once these barriers are identified, interventions relevant to the stakeholders involved can be selected to address them.[108] A substantial amount of research has been undertaken to develop and test specific approaches for bringing about behavior change. The simple provision of information or one-off educational sessions appear to be insufficient on their own to change what we do as health professionals, but approaches that are more active show promise.[112,113]

For instance, a systematic review of guideline dissemination and implementation strategies indicated that it is possible to bring about a small degree of behavior change using strategies such as reminders, dissemination of educational material, audit, feedback, and educational outreach.[114]

In order to track the use of the knowledge or research that is being targeted, it is necessary to measure its use. This next phase of the action cycle is to monitor use of this knowledge, measuring not just if it is used, but how, by whom, what additional barriers might be evident, and so on. Of course it is also important to determine the impact that this process has had on knowledge use. While it is possible to just measure knowledge usage, it is also important to measure the impact of that knowledge use on health outcomes. At a minimum, this involves measuring relevant variables before and after the process undertaken or the use of more sophisticated research designs to determine impact. Finally, sustaining systematic use of the targeted knowledge or research may involve the use of similar strategies all over again; hence, a feedback loop is created and explains the term *action cycle*.[108]

Strategies used for knowledge translation may need to differ between different types of stakeholders (that is, clinicians, academics, and managers).[115] They need to take into account the actual innovation, local barriers, different types of stakeholders, and the setting, as well as the social and economic contexts.[113,115] Grimshaw and Eccles[114] suggest that better understanding of behavior change at both the level of the individual and the organization is necessary, and that this may be enhanced by appreciating how differing theoretical models for behavior change, such as behavioral, educational, economic, social, and organizational learning theories, may apply in health care settings.

SUMMARY

In this chapter, we have discussed evidence-based practice as a clinical (or professional) decision-making approach that requires the integration of information from research evidence; clinical experience; clients' values, preferences, and circumstances; and information from the practice context. We have briefly considered the nature of these different sources of information before highlighting the importance of clinical reasoning for integrating this knowledge. The importance of knowledge translation to close the gaps between what we know and what we do was then discussed. It is hoped that the thoughts expressed in this chapter will clarify some of the complexities about evidence-based practice, although much remains to be understood, discussed, and debated. Finally, and most importantly, it is important to have a balanced view of evidence-based practice that values all ways of knowing and that uses research evidence as one source of knowledge wisely.

REFERENCES

1. Smith M, Higgs J, Ellis E. Characteristics and processes of physiotherapy clinical decision making: a study of acute care cardiorespiratory physiotherapy. *Phys Res Int.* 2008;13(4):209-222.
2. Sackett DL, Rosenberg WM, Gray JA, Haynes RB, Richardson WS. Evidence-based medicine: what it is and what it isn't. *BMJ.* 1996;312(7023):71-72.
3. Straus SE, Richardson WS, Glasziou P, Haynes RB. *Evidence-Based Medicine: How to Practice and Teach EBM.* 3rd ed. Edinburgh, Scotland: Elsevier/Churchill Livingstone; 2005.
4. Rycroft-Malone J, Seers K, Titchen A, Harvey G, Kitson A, McCormack B. What counts as evidence in evidence-based practice? *J Adv Nurs.* 2004;47(1):81-90.
5. Bannigan K, Moores A. A model of professional thinking: integrating reflective practice and evidence-based practice. *Can J Occup Ther.* 2009;5(76):342-350.
6. Hoffmann T, Bennett S, Del Mar C. Introduction to evidence-based practice. In: Hoffmann T, Bennett S, Del Mar C, eds. *Evidence-Based Practice Across the Health Professions.* Sydney, Australia: Churchill Livingstone; 2010:1-16.
7. Trinder L. Introduction: the context of evidence-based practice. In: Reynolds S, Trinder L, eds. *Evidence-Based Practice: A Critical Appraisal.* Oxford, UK: Blackwell Science; 2000:1-16.
8. Gray M. *Evidence-Based Healthcare.* 2nd ed. Edinburgh, Scotland: Churchill Livingston; 2001.
9. Chalmers I. The Cochrane collaboration: preparing, maintaining, and disseminating systematic reviews of the effects of health care. *Ann N Y Acad Sci.*1993;703:156-163.
10. Guyatt G. Evidence-based medicine. *ACP J Club.* 1991;A-16:114.
11. Sackett DL, Richardson WS, Rosenberg WM, Haynes RB. *Evidence-Based Medicine: How to Practice and Teach EBM.* New York, NY: Churchill Livingstone; 1997.
12. Hammond A, Freeman K. The long-term outcomes from a randomized controlled trial of an educational-behavioural joint protection programme for people with rheumatoid arthritis. *Clin Rehab.* 2004;18(5):520-528.
13. Murphy SL, Lyden AK, Clary M, et al. Activity pacing for osteoarthritis symptom management: study design and methodology of a randomized trial testing a tailored clinical approach using accelerometers for veterans and non-veterans. *BMC Musc Dis.* 2011;12:177.
14. Bennett S, Hoffmann T, McCluskey A, McKenna K, Strong J, Tooth L. Introducing OTseeker (Occupational Therapy Systematic Evaluation of Evidence): a new evidence database for occupational therapists. *Am J Occup Ther.* 2003;57(6):635-638.
15. Macedo AM, Oakley SP, Panayi GS, Kirkham BW. Functional and work outcomes improve in patients with rheumatoid arthritis who receive targeted, comprehensive occupational therapy. *Arthritis Rheum.* 2009;61(11):1522-1530.
16. Guyatt G, Meade M, Jaeschke R, Cook D, Haynes R. Practitioners of evidence-based care: not all clinicians need to appraise evidence from scratch but all need some skills. *BMJ.* 2000;320(7240):954-955.
17. Council NHaMR. *NHMRC Strategic Plan 2010-2012.* Canberra, Australia: NHMRC; 2010.
18. US Department of Health and Human Services: Agency for Healthcare Research and Quality. AHRQ at a Glance. US Department of Health and Human Services: Agency for Healthcare Research and Quality (AHRQ). http://www.ahrq.gov/about/mission/glance/index.html. Updated September 2012. Accessed October 7, 2013.
19. UK Department of Health. *Department of Health Annual Report and Accounts 2010-11.* London, UK: The Stationary Office Limited; 2011. https://www.gov.uk/government/publications/department-of-health-annual-report-and-accounts-2010-11. Published September 5, 2011. Accessed October 7, 2013.
20. Contopoulos-Ioannidis D, Alexiou G, Gouvias T, Ioannidis J. Life cycle of translational research for medical interventions. *Implement Sci.* 2008;328:1298-1299.
21. AOTA. Guidelines for supervision, roles, and responsibilities during the delivery of occupational therapy services. *Am J Occup Ther.* 2009;63:173-179.
22. Rappolt S, Mitra AL, Murphy E. Professional accountability in restructured contexts of occupational therapy practice. *Can J Occup Ther.* 2002;69(5):293-302.
23. Ilott I. Challenges and strategic solutions for a research emergent profession. *Am J Occup Ther.* 2004;58:347-352.
24. Bennett S, Hoffmann T. Evidence about effects of interventions. In: Hoffmann T, Bennett S, Del Mar C, eds. *Evidence-Based Practice Across the Health Professions.* Sydney, Australia: Churchill Livingstone; 2010:59-96.
25. Kerridge I, Lowe M, Henry D. Ethics and evidence-based medicine. *BMJ.* 1998;316(7138):1151-1153.
26. Altman DG, Bland JM. Absence of evidence is not evidence of absence. *BMJ.* 1995;311(7003):485.
27. Evidence-Based Medicine Working Group. Evidence-based medicine: a new approach to teaching the practice of medicine. *JAMA.* 1992;268(17):2420-2425.
28. de Chesnay M, Anderson B. *Caring for the Vulnerable: Perspectives in Nursing Theory, Practice, and Research.* 3rd ed. Sudbury, MA: Jones & Bartlett; 2012.

29. Turpin M, Higgs J. Clinical reasoning and evidence-based practice. In: Hoffmann T, Bennett S, Del Mar C, eds. *Evidence-Based Practice Across the Health Professions*. Sydney, Australia: Churchill Livingstone; 2010:300-317.

30. Haynes R. What kind of evidence is it that evidence-based medicine advocates want health care providers and consumers to pay attention to? *BMC Health Services Research*. 2002;2(1):3.

31. Sackett DL, Wennberg JE. Choosing the best research design for each question. *BMJ*. 1997;315(7123):1636.

32. Glazsiou P, Chalmers I, Rawlins M, McCulloch P. When are randomised trials unnecessary? Picking signal from noise. *BMJ*. 2007;334(7589):349-351.

33. Howick J, Glasziou P, Aronson JK. The evolution of evidence hierarchies: what can Bradford Hill's 'guidelines for causation' contribute? *J R Soc Med*. 2009;102(5):186-194.

34. Smith P, Pell J. Parachute use to prevent death and major trauma related to gravitational challenge: systematic review of randomised controlled trials. *BMJ*. 2003;327:1459-1461.

35. Bennett S, Bennett JW. The process of evidence-based practice in occupational therapy: informing clinical decisions. *Aust Occup Ther J*. 2000;47(4):171-180.

36. Council NHaMR. *NHMRC Levels of Evidence and Grades for Recommendations for Developers of Guidelines*. Canberra, Australia: National Health and Medical Research Council; 2009.

37. Tomlin G, Borgetto B. Research pyramid: a new evidence-based practice model for occupational therapy. *Am J Occup Ther*. 2011;65(2):189-196.

38. Howick J, Chalmers I, Glasziou P, et al. *The 2011 Oxford CEBM Levels of Evidence (introductory document)*. University of Oxford: Centre for Evidence-Based Medicine (CEBM). http://www.cebm.net/index.aspx?o=5653. Published 2011. Updated September 16, 2013. Accessed October 7, 2013.

39. Del Mar C, Hoffmann T. Information needs, asking questions and some basics of research studies. In: Hoffmann T, Bennett S, Del Mar C, eds. *Evidence-Based Practice Across the Health Professions*. Sydney, Australia: Churchill Livingstone; 2010:16-37.

40. Elkins M. Evidence about prognosis. In: Hoffmann T, Bennett S, Del Mar C, eds. *Evidence-Based Practice Across the Health Professions*. Sydney, Australia: Churchill Livingstone; 2010:166-185.

41. Pearson A. Evidence about clients' experiences and concerns. In: Hoffmann T, Bennett S, Del Mar C, eds. *Evidence-Based Practice Across the Health Professions*. Sydney, Australia: Churchill Livingstone; 2010:206-222.

42. Ottenbacher KJ. Clinically relevant designs for rehabilitation research: the idiographic model. *Am J Phys Med*. 1990;69(6):286-292.

43. Johnston MV, Ottenbacher KJ, Reichardt CS. Strong quasi-experimental designs for research on the effectiveness of rehabilitation. *Am J Phys Med*. 1995;74(5):383-392.

44. Backman CL, Harris SR. Case studies, single-subject research, and N of 1 randomized trials: comparisons and contrasts. *Am J Phys Med*. 1999;78(2):170-176.

45. Bennett S, McCluskey A, Hoffmann T, Tooth L. Resources to help occupational therapists access and appraise research evidence: progress from Australia. *WFOT Bull*. 2011;64:18-23.

46. Graff MJ, Vernooij-Dassen MJ, Thijssen M, Dekker J, Hoefnagels WH, Rikkert MG. Community-based occupational therapy for patients with dementia and their care givers: randomised controlled trial. *BMJ*. 2006;333(7580):1196.

47. Gitlin LN, Winter L, Dennis MP, Hodgson N, Hauck WW. Targeting and managing behavioral symptoms in individuals with dementia: a randomized trial of a nonpharmacological intervention. *J Am Geriatr Soc*. 2010;58(8):1465-1474.

48. Niedermann K, de Bie RA, Kubli R, et al. Effectiveness of individual resource-oriented joint protection education in people with rheumatoid arthritis: a randomized controlled trial. *Patient Educ Couns*. 2011;82(1):42-48.

49. Macedo AM, Oakley SP, Panayi GS, Kirkham BW. Functional and work outcomes improve in patients with rheumatoid arthritis who receive targeted, comprehensive occupational therapy. *Arthritis Rheum*. 2009;61:1522-1530.

50. Pighills AC, Torgerson DJ, Sheldon TA, Drummond AE, Bland JM. Environmental assessment and modification to prevent falls in older people. *J Am Geriatr Soc*. 2011;59(1):26-33.

51. Clemson L, Cumming RG, Kendig H, Swann M, Heard R, Taylor K. The effectiveness of a community-based program for reducing the incidence of falls in the elderly: a randomized trial. *J Am Geriatr Soc*. 2004;52:1487-1494.

52. Hagsten B, Svensson O, Gardulf A. Early individualized postoperative occupational therapy training in 100 patients improves ADL after hip fracture: a randomized trial. *Acta Orthop Scand*. 2004;75:177-183.

53. Hagsten B, Svensson O, Gardulf A. Health-related quality of life and self-reported ability concerning ADL and IADL after hip fracture: a randomized trial. *Acta Orthop*. 2006;77:114-119.

54. Logan PA, Gladman JRF, Avery A, Walker MF, Dyas J, Groom L. Randomised controlled trial of an occupational therapy intervention to increase outdoor mobility after stroke. *BMJ*. 2004;329:1372-1375.

55. Walker M, Gladman J, Lincoln N, Siemonsma P, Whitely T. Occupational therapy for stroke patients not admitted to hospital: a randomised controlled trial. *The Lancet*. 1999;354:278-280.

56. Sackley C, Wade D, Mant D, et al. Cluster randomized pilot controlled trial of an occupational therapy intervention for residents with stroke in UK care homes. *Stroke*. 2006;37:2336-2341.

57. Jing ZW, Han QY, Wang Z, et al. Effect of early occupational therapy on the activities of daily life in stroke patients. *Chin J of Clin Rehab*. 2006;10:54-56.

58. Vanage SM, Gilbertson KK, Mathiowetz V. Effects of an energy conservation course on fatigue impact for persons with progressive multiple sclerosis. *Am J Occup Ther*. 2003;57:315-323.

59. Mathiowetz VG, Finlayson ML, Matuska KM, Chen HY, Luo P. Randomized controlled trial of an energy conservation course for persons with multiple sclerosis. *Mult Scler*. 2005;11:592-601.

60. Cook S, Chambers E, Coleman JH. Occupational therapy for people with psychotic conditions in community settings: a pilot randomized controlled trial. *Clin Rehab*. 2009;23:40-52.

61. Peterson CQ, Nelson DL. Effect of an occupational intervention on printing in children with economic disadvantages. *Am J Occup Ther*. 2003;57:152-160.

62. Ratzon N, Efraim D, Bart O. A short-term graphomotor program for improving writing readiness skills of first-grade students. *Am J Occup Ther*. 2007;61:399-405.

63. McGarrigle J, Nelson A. Evaluating a school skills programme for Australian Indigenous children: a pilot study. *Occ Ther Int*. 2006;13:1-20.

64. Yamada T, Kawamata H, Kobayashi N, Kielhofner G, Taylor RR. A randomised clinical trial of a wellness programme for healthy older people. *Br J Occup Ther*. 2010;73:540-548.

65. Clark F, Azen S, Zemke R, et al. Occupational therapy for independent-living older adults: a randomized controlled trial. *JAMA*. 1997;278:1321-1326.

66. Law M, Baptiste S, McColl M, Opzoomer A, Polatajko H, Pollock N. The Canadian occupational performance measure: an outcome measure for occupational therapy. *Can J Occup Ther.* 1990;57(2):82-87.

67. Fisher AG, Bray Jones K. *Assessment of Motor and Process Skills. Vol. 1: Development, Standardization, and Administration Manual.* Fort Collins, CO: Three Star Press, Inc; 2010.

68. Baum CM, Connor LT, Morrison T, Hahn M, Dromerick AW, Edwards DF. Reliability, validity, and clinical utility of the Executive Function Performance test: a measure of executive function in a sample of people with stroke. *Am J Occup Ther.* 2008;62(4):446-455.

69. Cooke DM, McKenna K, Fleming J, Darnell R. Construct and ecological validity of the Occupational Therapy Adult Perceptual Screening Test (OT-APST). *Scand J Occup Ther.* 2006;13(1):49-61.

70. Johnston K, Barras S, Grimmer-Somers K. Relationship between pre-discharge occupational therapy home assessment and prevalence of post-discharge falls. *J Eval Clin Prac.* 2010;16(6):1333-1339.

71. Wells R, Minnes P, Phillips M. Predicting social and functional outcomes for individuals sustaining paediatric traumatic brain injury. *Dev Neurorehabil.* 2009;12(1):12-23.

72. Egilson S. Parent perspectives of therapy services for their children with physical disabilities. *Scand J Caring Sci.* 2011;25(2):277-284.

73. Holliday RC, Ballinger C, Playford ED. Goal setting in neurological rehabilitation: patients' perspectives. *Disabil Rehab.* 2007;29(5):389-394.

74. Liddle J, Fleming J, McKenna K, Turpin M, Whitelaw P, Allen S. Adjustment to loss of the driving role following traumatic brain injury: a qualitative exploration with key stakeholders. *Aust Occup Ther J.* 2012;59(1):79-88.

75. Shevil E, Finlayson M. Perceptions of persons with multiple sclerosis on cognitive changes and their impact on daily life. *Disabil Rehab.* 2006;28(12):779-788.

76. De Jonge DM, Rodger SA. Consumer-identified barriers and strategies for optimizing technology use in the workplace. *Disabil Rehab Assist Tech.* 2006;1(1-2):79-88.

77. Arntzen C, Elstad I. The bodily experience of apraxia in everyday activities: a phenomenological study. *Disabil Rehab.* 2013;35(1):63-72.

78. Cussen A, Howie L, C. I. Looking to the future: adolescents with cerebral palsy talk about their aspirations—a narrative study. *Disabil Rehab.* 2012;34(24):2103-2110.

79. Aiken FE, Fourt AM, Cheng IK, Polatajko HJ. The meaning gap in occupational therapy: finding meaning in our own occupation. *Can J Occup Ther.* 2011;78(5):294-302.

80. Kinsella EA, Whiteford GE. Knowledge generation and utilisation in occupational therapy: towards epistemic reflexivity. *Aust Occup Ther J.* 2009;56(4):249-258.

81. Fletcher S, Spitzer W. Approach of the Canadian Task Force to the Periodic Health Examination. *Ann Intern Med.* 1980;92(1):253-254.

82. Guyatt GH, Oxman AD, Vist GE, et al. GRADE: an emerging consensus on rating quality of evidence and strength of recommendations. *BMJ.* 2008;336(7650):924-926.

83. Copely J, Bennett S, Turpin M. Clinical reasoning, evidence, and practice with children. In: Rodger S, ed. *Occupation Centred Practice for Children: A Practical Guide for Occupational Therapists.* West Sussex, UK: Wiley-Blackwell; 2010:320-338.

84. Copley J, Allen S. Using all the available evidence: perceptions of paediatric occupational therapists about how to increase evidence-based practice. *Int J Evid Based Healthc.* 2009;7(3):193-200.

85. Higgs J, Titchen A. Knowledge and reasoning. In: Higgs J, Jones M, eds. *Clinical Reasoning In The Health Professions.* 2nd ed. Oxford, UK: Butterworth Heinemann; 2000: 23-32.

86. Bennett S, Tooth L, McKenna K, et al. Perceptions of evidence-based practice: a survey of Australian occupational therapists. *Aust Occup Ther J.* 2003;50(1):13-22.

87. Dubouloz CJ, Egan M, Vallerand J, von Zweck C. Occupational therapists' perceptions of evidence-based practice. *Am J Occup Ther.* 1999;53:445-453.

88. Dysart AM, Tomlin GS. Factors related to evidence-based practice among US occupational therapy clinicians. *Am J Occup Ther.* 2002;56:275-284.

89. Craik J, Rappolt S. Theory of research utilization enhancement: a model for occupational therapy. *Can J Occup Ther.* 2003;70:266-275.

90. Entwistle V, Watt I. Patient involvement in treatment decision-making: the case for a broader conceptual framework. *Patient Educ Couns.* 2006;63:268-278.

91. Levinson W, Kao A, Kuby A, Thisted RA. Not all patients want to participate in decision making: a national study of public preferences. *J Gen Intern Med.* 2005;20(6):531-535.

92. Law MC, Baum CM, Dunn W, eds. *Measuring Occupational Performance: Supporting Best Practice in Occupational Therapy.* Thorofare, NJ: SLACK Incorporated; 2001.

93. Smith M, Higgs J, Ellis E. Factors influencing clinical decision making. In: Higgs J, Jones M, Loftus S, Christensen N, eds. *Clinical Reasoning in the Health Professions.* Sydney, Australia: Elsevier/Butterworth Heinemann; 2008:89-100.

94. Stetler CB, Ritchie JA, Rycroft-Malone J, Schultz AA, Charns MP. Institutionalizing evidence-based practice: an organizational case study using a model of strategic change. *Implement Sci.* 2009;4(78):1-13.

95. Dobrow MJ, Goel V, Upshur RE. Evidence-based health policy: context and utilisation. *Soc Sci Med.* 2004;58(1):207-217.

96. Dubouloz CJ, Egan M, Vallerand J, von Zweck C. Occupational therapists' perceptions of evidence-based practice. *Am J Occup Ther.* 1999;53(5):445-453.

97. Thompson C, Cullum N, McCaughan D, Sheldon T, Raynor P. Nurses, information use, and clinical decision making—the real world potential for evidence-based decisions in nursing. *Evid Based Nurs.* 2004;7(3):68-72.

98. Boateng W. Communities of practice as conduit for knowledge management: a sociological analysis of the macro level health care decision-making in Canada. *Int J Human and Soc Sci.* 2011;14(1):29-36.

99. Higgs J, Jones M. Clinical reasoning in the health professions. In: Higgs J, Jones M, eds. *Clinical Reasoning In The Health Professions.* 2nd ed. Oxford, UK: Butterworth Heinemann; 2000:3-14.

100. Scriven M, Paul R. *Critical Thinking as Defined by the National Council for Excellence in Critical Thinking.* The Critical Thinking Community. http://www.criticalthinking.org/pages/about-critical-thinking/FULLRULpages/defining-critical-thinking/766. Published 1987. Accessed March 10, 2012.

101. Kemmis S. Knowing practice: searching for saliences. *Pedagogy, Culture, and Society.* 2005;13:391-426.

102. McCluskey A, Cusick A. Strategies for introducing evidence-based practice and changing clinician behaviour: a manager's toolbox. *Aust Occup Ther J.* 2002;49:63-70.

103. Gosling AS, Westbrook JI. Allied health professionals' use of online evidence: a survey of 790 staff working in the Australian public hospital system. *Int J Med Inform.* 2004;73:391-401.

104. Lin SH, Murphy SL, Robinson JC. Facilitating evidence-based practice: process, strategies, and resources. *Am J Occup Ther.* 2010;64(1):164-171.

105. Solomons NM, Spross JA. Evidence-based practice barriers and facilitators from a continuous quality improvement perspective: an integrative review. *J Nurs Manag.* 2011;19(1):109-120.

106. Grimshaw JM, Eccles MP, Lavis JN, Hill SJ, Squires JE. Knowledge translation of research findings. *Implement Sci.* 2012;7(1):50-67.

107. Canadian Institutes of Health Research. *About Knowledge Translation and Commercialization.* Canadian Institutes of Health Research. http://www.cihr-irsc.gc.ca/e/29418.html. Updated May 15, 2013. Accessed October 7, 2013.

108. Graham ID, Logan J, Harrison MB, et al. Lost in knowledge translation: time for a map? *J Contin Educ Health Prof.* 2006;26(1):13-24.

109. Glasziou P, Haynes B. The paths from research to improved health outcomes. *ACP Journal Club.* 2005;142(2):A8-10.

110. Michie S, Johnston M, Abraham C, Lawton R, Parker D, Walker A, on behalf of the Psychological Theory Group. Making psychological theory useful for implementing evidence based practice: a consensus approach. *Qual Saf Health Care.* 2005;14:26-33.

111. Cane J, O'Connor D, Michie S. Validation of the theoretical domains framework for use in behaviour change and implementation research. *Implementation Science.* 2012;7:37.

112. Davis D, Evans M, Jadad A, et al. The case for knowledge translation: shortening the journey from evidence to effect. *BMJ.* 2003;327:33-35.

113. Sanson-Fisher RW, Grimshaw JM, Eccles MP. The science of changing providers' behaviour: the missing link in evidence-based practice. *Med J Aust.* 2004;180:205-206.

114. Grimshaw JM, Eccles MP. Is evidence-based implementation of evidence-based care possible? *Med J Aust.* 2004;180(6 Suppl):S50-51.

115. Grol R. Beliefs and evidence in changing practice. *BMJ.* 1997;315:418-421.

CRITICAL ELEMENTS OF OCCUPATION AND OCCUPATIONAL PERFORMANCE

PEOP: Enabling Everyday Living

THE NARRATIVE
The past, current and future perceptions, choices, interests, goals and needs that are unique to the Person, Organization, or Population

PERSON
•Cognition
•Psychological
•Physiological
•Sensory
•Motor
•Spirituality

OCCUPATION
•Activities
•Tasks
•Roles

ENVIRONMENT
•Culture
•Social Determinants
•Social Support and Social Capital
•Education and Policy
•Physical and Natural
•Assistive Technology

Personal Narrative
• Perception and Meaning
• Choices and Responsibilities
• Attitudes and Motivation
• Needs and Goals

Organizational Narrative
• Mission and History
• Focus and Priorities
• Stakeholders and Values
• Needs and Goals

Population Narrative
• Environments and Behaviors
• Demographics and Disparities
• Incidence and Prevalence
• Needs and Goals

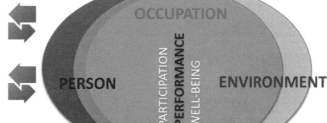

OCCUPATION

PERSON

PARTICIPATION
PERFORMANCE
WELL-BEING

ENVIRONMENT

Section II introduces foundational concepts of occupation and occupational performance and explores the occupations of individuals across the lifespan and of organizations and populations.

Foundational knowledge is essential in every discipline and profession. For example, anatomy and kinesiology are critical elements for athletic trainers and exercise scientists. Similarly, calculus and physics are critical elements for engineers. Occupation and occupational performance are critical elements for occupational therapy practitioners.

Developing a comprehensive understanding of occupations for individuals, organizations, and populations is a necessary prerequisite for obtaining narratives, completing evaluations, providing interventions, and measuring outcomes of occupational therapy.

Upon completion of this section, you will have a new appreciation that occupations are both beautiful in their simplicity and amazing in their complexity. The authors have also provided an abundance of resources to help you further your learning.

CHAPTER	TITLE	FAQ
8	*The Complexity and Patterns of Human Occupations* (Erlandsson, Christiansen)	• What are human occupations and how are they studied? • What other words and ideas are used to explore the complexity of human occupation? • What factors influence the habits, routines, and rituals of human occupation?
9	*Occupations of Childhood and Adolescence* (Rodger, Ziviani, Lim)	• What is typical development and occupations for children and youth and important periods of transition? • How do developmental theories inform the understanding of childhood occupations? • How do individuals, communities, and environmental factors support occupational performance of children and youth?
10	*Occupations of Adulthood* (Matuska, Barrett)	• What are the important occupations and stages of adulthood? • What are the typical challenges in and barriers to healthy adult development? • How do essential skills and environmental factors support competence in occupational performance during adulthood?
11	*Occupations of Elderhood* (Eriksson, Lilja, Jonsson, Petersson, Tatzer)	• How do demographic characteristics, health status, and other aspects of aging contribute to variation in older adults' occupations? • How does the environment support or limit occupational performance for older adults? • How does active living support healthy aging?
12	*Occupations of Organizations* (Haertlein Sells)	• What are the roles of organizations in society? • What are the occupations of organizations and how can they be analyzed? • What are examples of occupation-centered needs in organizations?
13	*Occupations of Populations* (Bass)	• How are the occupations of populations identified and described in population health and public health? • What are some current occupational issues of concern in populations? • What are examples of opportunities for occupational therapy to address the occupations of populations?

Chapter 8

THE COMPLEXITY AND PATTERNS OF HUMAN OCCUPATIONS

Lena-Karin Erlandsson, PhD, RegOT and Charles H. Christiansen, EdD, OTR, FAOTA

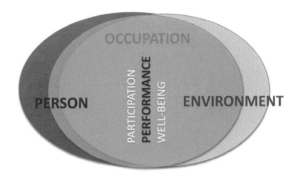

LEARNING OBJECTIVES

- Summarize key components of daily human occupation and how they are related to the PEOP Model.
- Differentiate between occupation, project, and activity and give examples.
- Describe how patterns of daily occupations are characterized and developed through time and life stages.
- Describe how occupation and complexity in patterns of daily occupations impact on humans' health and well-being.
- Give examples of methods for collecting data and analyzing daily occupations.

KEY WORDS

- Activity
- Chronobiology
- Cultural factors
- Environment
- Habit
- Hidden occupations
- Life balance
- Lifestyle
- Main occupation
- Occupation
- Occupational disruption
- Occupational performance
- Pattern of daily occupations
- Ritual
- Routines
- Stages of life
- Time budget
- Time geography
- Time use
- Unexpected occupations
- Zeitgebers

Christiansen CH, Baum CM, Bass JD, eds.
Occupational Therapy: Performance, Participation, and Well-Being, Fourth Edition (pp 113-127).
© 2015 SLACK Incorporated.

INTRODUCTION

In this chapter we will discuss what those interested in human occupation need to know about the patterns of occupations and why studying and understanding these patterns may be important.[1-3] When Swedish occupational therapy students in their first year defined occupation they expressed it in contextual terms, as something that depends on who is performing the occupation and where the occupation is performed; influenced by temporal rhythms and imprinted by social cultural influences that create a unique context.[1-4]

Thus, occupation refers to something that is done at a particular time and in a particular place. That is, occupations are the ordinary and familiar things that people do everyday. Furthermore, a person (or more than one person) may be performing the occupation.

These multiple dimensions of occupations and their performance create complexity that challenges scientists and other observers. For example, depending on the time and place, the leisure occupation known as floor ball may be practiced by a boy or a girl, together with his or her team, on Wednesday evenings. (Floor ball is an indoor team sport similar to hockey but not played on ice.) However, the occupation changes considerably the coming Saturday when the team goes away to a nearby town and meets another team in a local competition. The occupation is the same, the team members are the same, but the time and place differ; thereby presumably the experiences and challenges related to the occupation are different. In other words, the multiple factors that describe and influence occupations are complex and make it challenging to devise taxonomies to organize and systematically study human occupation.

Since occupations are fundamental to the profession of occupational therapy, are used "both as means and ends,"[5(p127)] and are unique to each individual and situation; finding a way to untangle the complexity in ways that are useful for guiding occupational therapy is a worthwhile goal. In a larger sense, understanding patterns of daily occupations and their influence on health can be useful for planning and implementing programs of health promotion and disease prevention.

THE WHEN, WHAT, AND WHERE OF HUMAN OCCUPATIONS

Individual Level

People seldom stop to think about how they actually spend their time. Most people can tell you something about what they did during the day, and they may recall some of their specific occupations during the past week. If they are goal-oriented and structure their time use through careful planning, they may be better informed. Some individuals may develop routines that vary little unless they experience a significant life change, such as relocation, becoming a parent, starting a new job, getting married or divorced, experiencing a significant illness or injury, or the death of someone close to them. Thus, unless an occupation is notable for some reason or changes from the usual routine, it will fade from memory rather quickly. As a result, most people have only a vague idea about how they allocate their occupations over time. Yet, for occupational therapy practitioners who treat individuals with problems related to their daily occupations, it is useful to get a more accurate picture of the patterns of human occupation than what may be gleaned from personal accounts of daily time use.

Group Level

There are practical benefits to understanding how people use time. Because time allocations for different occupations influence the consumption of goods and services, people who manufacture and sell products are interested in time use data to determine the potential for marketing their products. People who provide services are interested in tailoring their businesses to the lifestyles of their customers. Because there is often a close association between how time is used and a person's location, city planners and architects may have an interest in this information. Economists are interested in the production of goods and services to measure the wealth of regions and nations and to understand trends in economic development. Public health officials are also interested in time use statistics to determine potential exposure to hazardous substances or pathogens. Psychologists, anthropologists, sociologists, and occupational scientists are interested in time use data as everyday measures of typical behavior, cultural patterns and trends, and lifestyles. How people use time also indicates their underlying beliefs, values, interests, needs, and personality dispositions.[6]

The Complexity of Human Occupation

We know that occupational performance (or what, when, where, and how daily activities are performed) is influenced by the characteristics of the performer, the environment and the nature of the occupation. In this section we will explore in more detail the structure of daily occupation; and how human occupation can be viewed as consisting of smaller units (or time segments) and how these segments, when combined to form larger units, create larger patterns that can be observed and described on a daily basis as well as from a life perspective.

There are several examples in the literature describing the structure of occupations[7-9]; they are all theoretically seeking to provide a systematic approach to observing and analyzing how occupations are performed. Haglund and Henriksson[7] developed a hierarchical terminology for illuminating the complexity related to the performance of single occupations. The smallest parts in their hierarchy are actions, and a number of consecutively performed actions make up action sequences, which in turn become fulfilled occupations. Furthermore, several occupations are performed to reach higher goals. Nelson,[8] introduced the concept of levels of occupation and incorporated the aspect of time. There are several levels of occupation. The base level concerns the most immediate performance of an act (eg, painting a wall), whereas higher-level occupations by their nature are seldom completed in one session (eg, building a garage).

Persson, Erlandsson, Eklund, and Iwarsson[9] introduced a structure of 3 interacting perspectives in dynamic interplay, from which occupations can be viewed and analyzed. The perspectives reflect occupation in a lifelong panorama, as well as the momentary experience a person gets from performing an occupation. From a *meso* perspective, daily occupations make up larger units in time when viewed over a day or a week's time. These units, in turn, build up the individual's life repertoire of occupations, which the authors describe as the *macro* perspective. Analyzing occupations from the macro perspective implies considering an individual's past occupations as well as that person's future occupations. Thus, a young boy's occupations on an everyday basis are different from what he will be doing as a teenager, and his occupations will continue to change and adapt as he grows into early, middle, and late adulthood.

Just as chains of occupations on the meso level build a life course repertoire that forms a broader macro level, each of the single occupations in the meso perspective can be viewed from a narrower *micro* perspective, where the occupation is regarded as built up of small segments, called actions, that are in turn composed of operations.

DEFINING PATTERNS OF DAILY OCCUPATIONS

Activities and Tasks: Sequences Building Up Occupations

An occupation is made up of smaller units of actions or tasks with identifiable start and end points.[10] Occupations are culturally imprinted, and thereby the characteristics defining the start and end points are to some extent predictable. For every occupation in a certain sociocultural context there is a pre-designed norm, an idea of how the specific occupation is to be performed.[8,11] However, an occupation is almost never performed fully in accordance with the norm. The sequence of actions is, to a high extent, dependent on the occupational circumstances[8] (ie, the person and the specific physical and psychosocial context in which the occupation is performed). For example, the act of eating breakfast is often a routine, and it may be easy to assume that it is performed in nearly the same way every day.

A typical Swedish breakfast may consist of having a cup of coffee, juice, and a sandwich while reading the morning paper. However, if you look more closely there are likely daily, yearly, and seasonal variations. The ingredients may differ, for example, which changes the way one makes the breakfast. The social context has an impact—family members participating (or not participating) in the occupation affect the experience and the way it's performed. Finally, and maybe most importantly in this example, there may be different amounts of time available to perform the occupation. Therefore, there is likely daily variation in the common occupational experience of having breakfast. For example, the breakfast routine when one is traveling may be very different from what is typical at home.

Each specific sequence of actions in an occupation is always unique; even if the same person performs the same occupation again, he or she will have a new and slightly different way of performing it. This also means that the experience of performing every occupation is more or less unique.[9] The uniqueness of the unrepeatable performance of an occupation is described by Pierce, as "a subjective event in perceived temporal, spatial, and sociocultural conditions that are unique to that one-time occurrence."[12(p139)]

The variation in actions and tasks that can occur in the same occupation was highlighted in the case study of Anne, a Swedish woman who worked full time from home and lived with her husband, 3 children, and several domestic animals.[13] Anne was observed on 2 Wednesdays performing the occupation of cooking dinner. In other words, the person, context, day of week, physical location, and occupation were the same. In Figure 8-1, the pattern of actions within this occupation is shown in detail from the first day of observation.

The actions were understood as having different purposes, and together they made up a complex pattern and formed the unique occupation. Included in the occupation of cooking as performed by Anne was, on this occasion, also caring for her dogs, looking for a sock in the laundry, and cleaning the dinner table. Further, since her daughter was helping that day, she performed actions that were related to coaching and helping her. The grey area in

Figure 8-1. The sequences of actions building up the occupation cooking one afternoon in Anne's every day. (Adapted with permission from Erlandsson L-K, Eklund M. Describing patterns of daily occupations—a methodological study comparing data from four different methods. *Scand J Occup Ther.* 2001;8[1]:31-39.)

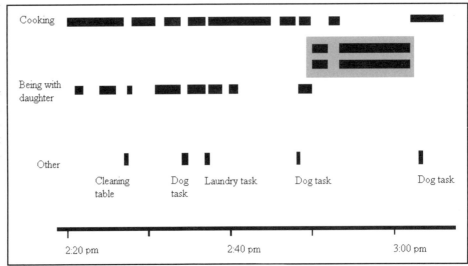

Figure 8-2. The sequences of actions building up the occupation cooking one other afternoon in Anne's every day. (Adapted with permission from Erlandsson L-K, Eklund M. Describing patterns of daily occupations—a methodological study comparing data from four different methods. *Scand J Occup Ther.* 2001;8[1]:31-39.)

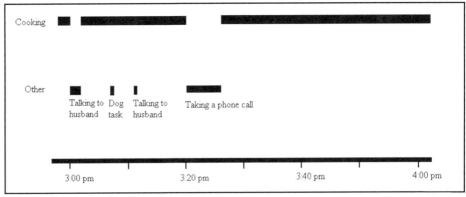

Figure 8-1 illustrates a sequence where Anne and her daughter are both doing actions related to the same occupation: making spaghetti in a pasta machine. Anne is holding the dough while it's going through the machine and her daughter grinds the handle. Occupations are often shared, as illustrated in this example, and those that implicitly involve 2 or more individuals can be termed *co-occupations*.[14] Co-occupation has been described by Pierce as a dance between 2 individuals that sequentially shapes the singular occupations of both people.[15]

In Figure 8-2, Anne performs the same occupation in her kitchen, but 1 week later. The main difference between the 2 sets of actions is in the sequence of actions. In the latter example, Anne is alone and interrupted less often, and is thereby able to perform consecutive actions specifically related to cooking. The 2 figures illustrate how the same occupation (eg, cooking dinner) could on different occasions be built of different action sequences.

In conclusion, the case study of Anne illuminates how patterns of daily occupations are made of building blocks that consist of a blend of actions performed in integrated or separated sequences. Together, these blocks of actions

create occupations. Thus, using a detailed level of analysis, the process of doing an occupation can be analyzed to reveal a complex weave of several actions that become integrated, creating a recognizable pattern that usually leads to completion of a goal.

Occupations Building Patterns of Daily Occupations

The sum of all occupations, with the individual's personal use and organization of time, is reflected in a unique pattern of occupations for each individual.[16] Occupations are performed during a course of time, forming a pattern of occupations that is unique for each individual throughout his or her life.[9,17] The patterns consist of a variety of different occupations. Some are performed in order to maintain the daily routine and fulfill prerequisites for survival.[18] Others are labeled work occupations and are product-generating or service-generating. By performing them, the individual supports himself or herself either directly (eg, by getting a salary) or indirectly (eg, by taking care of household and children, making it possible for a partner to be employed and have an income).[9] In contrast to work and maintenance occupations, which can bear the stamp of obligation, the patterns of occupations also include play, recreation, and sleep. Participation in these occupations is generally undertaken for purposes of enjoyment and rest or rejuvenation.

In addition to the time perspectives presented by Persson et al,[9] the patterns of occupations on a meso level and daily basis can be described as "a pattern built up of building blocks in the shape of all occupations (and sleep) performed by one individual during one day and one night, in a 24-hour cycle."[19] The blocks of time used for different purposes are related, and more or less organized into certain temporal orders. Some occupations are located in time and have to be performed before (or after) others. For example, having dinner usually means having to prepare food (in one way or another) before the dinner can be served. After the dinner it is a good idea to clean the table and the dishes. Some occupations are performed in segments integrated with other occupations, such as making a phone call to change an appointment at the dentist while at work. The occupations have a peer relationship that impacts on the complexity and flexibility in the pattern.

If we consider the order in which blocks of time are used in a person's daily occupations, the patterns are dominated in time and awareness by a few *main occupations*.[13] These are the occupations that we most often refer to if we are asked, for example, what we did the day before. The main occupations vary with age, interests, and context. For example, since children's days are often dominated by play and school, their main occupations reflect these contexts. Playing with a friend or taking an exam would be examples of such occupations. In contrast, most working-age adults' patterns are influenced by job-related occupations. Main occupations for this group could be something that engaged them in the work setting, such as participating in an important conference or meeting with a prospective client. For older adults, a decline in their ability to easily or quickly perform daily routines related to self-care may take up a considerable part of their daily pattern of occupations, and thus the main occupations that would occupy the time and awareness for some older adults might be related to self-care and recreation.

Intertwined with the main occupations in the daily patterns are the so-called *hidden occupations*.[13] Hidden occupations are important as they belong to, and are necessary for, the rhythm of the daily pattern, but are performed in between the dominating main occupations and with less attention from the performer. The hidden occupations are the activities people do in support of their main occupations. Examples of hidden occupations may be taking a shower in the morning, dropping off recycling on the way to the grocery store, driving to work, having a cup of coffee in between meetings, or going through the not-yet-read morning paper before starting to cook dinner in the evening. Even if these occupations are performed in between the more interesting and attention-demanding daily chores, hidden occupations should be recognized for their importance. When a person experiences functional limitations in any way, it is often the hidden occupations that are hindered. Thus, actions we once performed automatically suddenly demand more attention and time; there is a risk that the hidden occupations will become main occupations in disproportion to the occupations that they want and need to do at home, at work, and during free time.

Patterns of daily occupations also include a third category, *unexpected occupations*.[13] Such occupations occur unexpectedly in one's regular pattern of daily occupations and may interrupt the ongoing rhythm of main and hidden occupations being performed. The unexpected occupations are sometimes generated from positive events and can bring joy and happiness. For example, a good friend shows up unexpectedly or a child experiences delight because school is closed due to heavy snow. However, there are a significant number of unexpected events that may interrupt and disturb a daily pattern and these may be experienced as negative. Examples might include a bike or car that has a flat tire in the morning when a person is on the way to school, a computer malfunctions at work, or a power outage occurs as dinner is being prepared. Unexpected situations like these force the individual to change the anticipated or expected plan for the day and engage in the occupations that are necessary to cope with the situation at hand.

The fourth building block in this terminology to describe patterns of daily occupations is *sleep*. Sleep is a prerequisite for the ability to participate in occupations during the waking hours. This is especially evident in young children's patterns of daily occupations, since they tend to fall asleep even in the middle of an occupation in order to gain new energy (Figure 8-3).

The amount of time spent in sleep is dependent on the time spent in other occupations and the physical locations in which these take place. For example, if main occupations related to work or leisure take place during the night, it is likely that the time for sleep occurs during the day. The quality of sleep may differ if the context is suitable for sleep or not; it is easier to sleep in a bed in a bedroom than, for example, on a bench at an airport or on a plane. Sleep during night may also be interrupted by hidden or unexpected occupations, such as a need to care for a sick child or waking up due to back pain. Having broken sleep periods in the long-term constitutes a risk for developing ill health.[20]

Integrated Patterns of Daily Occupations

An individual's pattern of daily occupations is also influenced by the patterns of other people in his or her life.

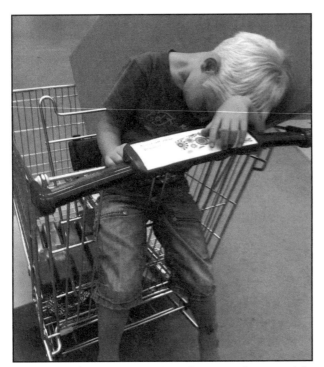

Figure 8-3. Sleep is a prerequisite for occupation, especially evident among children. This boy has fallen asleep while shopping with his mother. (Reprinted with permission from Virginia Christensson.)

People coordinate and synchronize their occupations for a variety of reasons. For example, workplaces often require coordination and teamwork, and these requirements influence the occupational patterns of everyone in a workgroup, whether during one day or over an extended period for longer-term projects. Similarly, members of the same family will influence the occupational patterns of each other. Because their actions and routines are linked together, their different schedules must be taken into account; competing time requirements must be coordinated or synchronized. For example, if the family has only one car, members must coordinate their schedules in order to commute together to daycare, school, or work. Thus, family members may share time together as well as divide available time between each other.[21] In Figure 8-4, we present 2 integrated patterns of daily occupations, one of a mother and one of a father with mutual children living together. The time and place for different occupations by these subjects during a 24-hour period are illustrated in graphs. This data are from a weekday, and both parents are attending paid work outside the home. Therefore, the subjects' patterns are integrated in the morning and evening and separate but parallel during working hours.

These examples depict how the available family time at home is divided. The father is going to fitness training while the mother is cooking dinner, and later the father is cleaning the kitchen and in parallel the mother is putting the children to bed. Such social coordination of daily occupations is defined by Larson and Zemke[21] as complex, requiring consideration of individuals' routines and competing desires and needs in daily life. When applied to family units, complexity with integrated patterns means that a change in one individual's pattern affects other members as well. Likewise, an individual change in everyday routines at work may prove more difficult to implement due to the people with whom it is integrated. For occupational therapy practitioners, understanding the social coordination of patterns of daily occupations forms an important consideration in planning intervention. For example, knowing a family's typical patterns may be helpful in recommending changes related to avoiding disruptive situations in caring for a child with autism.

PATTERNS OF DAILY OCCUPATIONS AND HEALTH

Conceptualizations of Balance

The idea that some patterns of occupations may reflect characteristics that are better suited to health and adaptation has been a concept of interest in the literature of occupational therapy and occupational science.[22-24] This concept has been widely termed *occupational balance* in the occupational therapy literature. To balance can mean to make adjustments or changes in conditions within a system seeking equilibrium, such as balancing on a seesaw. This idea is implicit in public understanding of the term *work-life balance*, where it is believed that too much time in the workplace spills over onto personal or family time and creates difficulties with roles and relationships. Balancing may also mean providing a complete pattern, and therefore being able to participate in a variety of occupations. An example of this type of balance is shown in a study of adults with cerebral palsy, which demonstrated the benefit of engagement in leisure occupations, along with already-established routines involving daily occupations of self-care and productivity.[25] Participation in leisure activities was hypothesized as improving the balance of the subjects' patterns of daily occupations, which in turn increased well-being.

Another study of balance assessed the efficacy and clinical utility of an occupational time-use intervention for community-dwelling people with serious mental illness. Edgelow[26] and colleagues demonstrated that treatment group participants increased their occupational balance by spending an average of 47 minutes more per day in activity than the control group. In this study, by participating in

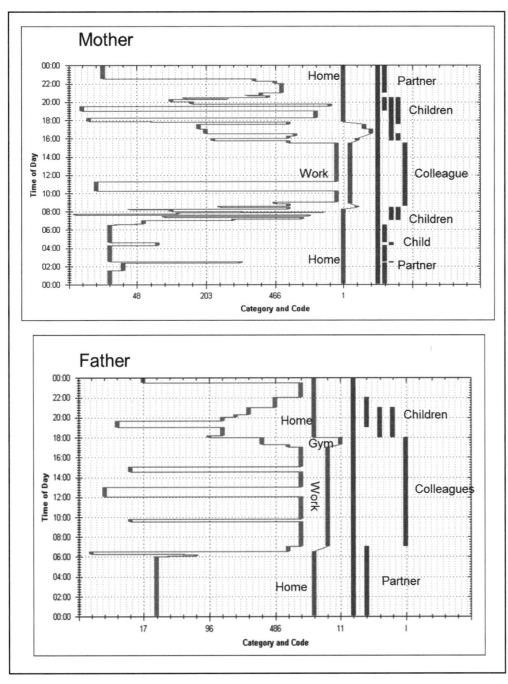

Figure 8-4. The patterns of daily occupations of one mother and one father in the same family. (Reprinted with permission from Kristina Orban, PhD, RegOT, MSc.)

more occupations, the treatment group achieved an increased balance based on the improved variety within their overall pattern of occupations, as well as through a change in the ratio of the amount of time spent in periods of activity and no activity.

An additional concept of balance relates to maintaining a pattern where occupations shown to be related to overall health and well-being are regularly included. Within this conceptualization, the absence of occupations seen as necessary for health within an individual's ongoing pattern

would be considered unhealthful. Based on a synthesis of current research, Matuska and Christiansen[27] proposed a model of *life balance* (a term they chose in place of occupational balance) comprising 5 need-based occupational dimensions viewed as important for health and well-being. Their model defines balance as a perceived congruence between desired and actual patterns of occupation, as well as a state where an individual's pattern reflects participation in occupations that address needs seen as important to health. The model includes an ability related need associated with developing the skill necessary to plan and manage occupational patterns in order for the identified needs to be met.

Balance can also mean considering how an individual's patterns of occupation are aligned with typical patterns of time use within a culture or larger social group. Such larger patterns may influence when stores are open or services are available. Thus, individual patterns that are not aligned with an overall social pattern may create difficulties and challenges. An example would be people whose shiftwork requires atypical patterns, such as working at night and sleeping during the day. A study involving a group of people in Slovenia illustrates this concept. The participants interviewed during the study described increased difficulties in performing desired occupations when being out of synch with the clock time, and as a consequence they experienced discomfort.[28]

Based on studies of working-age women, some of whom had children living at home, and some who did not, Erlandsson and Håkansson[29] described how occupational patterns are influenced by environmental conditions. The authors concluded that both physical factors (eg, weather conditions, non-working tools, or changed schedules) and social factors (eg, family members, colleagues, and customers) may create conditions that result in patterns of occupation that are challenging or stressful. For example, family members and colleagues may create occupational demands that challenge the person, and if he or she fails to adapt to these challenges it is likely that increased stress will result. Thus, research suggests that there are several conditions affecting patterns of daily occupations that can be addressed if a person is to maintain a healthful, satisfactory balance in everyday life.

Complexity in Patterns of Occupation

Patterns of daily occupations have different levels of complexity. These patterns can differ temporally (ie, daily, monthly, and yearly) as well as individually through changing task or role demands. One way to measure this level of complexity can be to recognize the transitions between the 3 categories of main, hidden, and unexpected occupations, as well as sleep with respect to frequency of change, frequency of unexpected occupations, and whether these shifts are concentrated in limited parts of the day (eg, the mornings). In a study exploring the patterns of daily occupations and health among 100 Swedish working mothers, participants were grouped according to complexity in their everyday patterns. In the "low-complexity" patterns, the daily time span was dominated by a few main occupations, which were seldom or never interrupted by unexpected or hidden occupations. Women with "medium-complexity" patterns of daily occupations were dis-

turbed during sleeping hours, and their daily patterns all contained unexpected occupations. The women in the "high-complexity" category had patterns that contained many interruptions of both main and hidden occupations. Moreover, both hidden and unexpected occupations interrupted ongoing main occupations.[30] It was assumed that individuals having patterns of daily occupations characterized as typically "low-complexity" (ie, fewer shifts between the categories and few unexpected occupations during sleep) would rate their health and well-being higher than women with typically medium and high complexity patterns.[31] The results indicated that among the women studied, an increased level of complexity was correlated with lower self-rated health.

Perhaps the level of complexity in a pattern of daily occupations could be the result of whether the individual's use of time is primarily continuity and cyclic or discontinuity and linear.[32] Linear and discontinuing time use, according to Karen Davies,[32] means performing the daily occupations one after another, allowing for pauses between them. To have a cyclic and continuing time use means that occupations are integrated; performed in parallel and recurring in the pattern (as in multitasking). In this view, high-complex patterns are seen as reflecting a more cyclical time use (ie, having parallel occupations and not finishing occupations before starting new ones). In such continuing time use the risk for occasions of being interrupted by the social environment or by ideas and impulses from the performer herself increases.

Lack of Occupations: Low Complexity

The opposite of high complexity in patterns of daily occupations is low complexity; having few or a lack of occupations to fill the daily time span. Lack of occupations may occur for several reasons. Functional limitation and disease may be one reason. For example, studies of persons with schizophrenia have shown the diagnosis affecting the extent to which the person can coordinate and engage in everyday occupations.[33] Bejerholm[34] assessed whether subjects with schizophrenia were under-occupied, over-occupied, or occupationally balanced; meaning that there was a balance between the capability of the individual, the circumstances in the environment, and the challenges in their occupations. Among the 72 participants aged 20 to 55 years, no more than 5 participants were assessed as being over-occupied, and a majority were assessed as under-occupied. According to Bejerholm, people with schizophrenia "are not exposed to an overload of occupational opportunities and a too stimulating environment on a daily basis."[34(p11)] Eklund and colleagues[35] concluded in a literature review that occupations among people with psychiatric disabilities are often restricted to sleeping, eating, caring for oneself, and performing quiet activities. Such use of time and occupational patterns influence their experience of occupational balance and well-being.

There are several other situations where individuals may experience lack of occupations. For example, retirement or unemployment may be situations that result in involuntary occupation reductions. In an Australian study, Scanlan et al[36] compared the time use among people aged 18 to 25 who were unemployed, unemployed but pursuing education, working part-time, or employed full-time. The study illustrated how patterns of daily occupations resulting from unemployment led to large amounts of time occupied by non-directed occupations, such as watching television or occupations expressed as "doing nothing."

Thus, patterns of daily occupations with low complexity may result from several factors, including functional limitations of disease or illness, social policies, or organization-related circumstances (such as layoffs). For people in these circumstances, strategies to increase the number of occupations in their daily lives may lead to more complex patterns of daily occupations and increased health and well-being.

Occupational Patterns and Resilience

There are several areas of research that study occupational patterns in order to identify characteristics that may be related to health and well-being or, conversely, to identify conditions that may pose threats to those states. Epidemiologists concerned with lifestyle issues have traditionally focused on characteristics of human occupation that are unsafe or unhealthy, such as wearing seatbelts and helmets, or avoiding practices that lead to physiological consequences (eg, smoking, drug use, unhealthy diets).

More recently, however, epidemiologists and others have become aware of the less obvious but equally harmful consequences of prolonged stress. A growing body of research has now shown conclusively that exposure to stress is related to nearly every chronic illness and disease that threaten human populations, ranging from heart disease and diabetes to substance abuse and cancer. The physiological mechanisms explaining the connection between stress and illness constitute the focus for an emerging specialty known as *psychoneuroimmunology*. The title of this specialty reveals the mechanisms involved in the process, which include the emotional response to life experiences, the resulting neurological responses to that emotional response (which include the release of stress hormones such as cortisol), and the harmful effects that high levels of these hormones have on the immune system over time.[37]

For many years, social epidemiologists and others have been interested in the characteristics and lifestyle factors that seem to protect or buffer some people from the con-

sequences of stress; and thus, occupational scientists have also been interested in how occupational patterns might also provide resilience to stress. This interest lies at the heart of attempts to construct models of life balance.

A few studies have been completed that have investigated the relationship between occupational patterns and measures of stress. However, because studies of occupational patterns differ in the characteristics under investigation (whether the factors being measured involve levels of complexity, the number of unexpected occupations, conflicts with external factors, or regular participation in need-based occupations, for example) no definitive conclusions can yet be drawn about how occupational patterns relate to stress. A study underway by Rogers and Christiansen is measuring whether or not regular participation in valued activities reduces levels of cortisol and other measures of allostasis in students during stressful events. Results of this study have not yet been published.

Temporal Dimensions: Relationships Between Time and Occupation

Despite the uniqueness of every individual's pattern of daily occupations, certain groups and sub-groups in society share similar characteristics in their patterns of daily occupations. The sociologist Zerubavel[38] introduced the term *temporal pattern*. As mentioned before, occupations cannot be performed simultaneously and they are therefore segregated from one another; some are to be performed before and some after the others. Sometimes the order in which the occupations are performed may be purely random, but very often they are, according to Zerubavel, regulated by different temporal influences. In this section, we review the literature on how time is used, depending on different regulators and in different cultures and subgroups, thus resulting in a variation of lifestyles.

INTRINSIC FACTORS IMPACTING ON OCCUPATION IN TIME

The Experience of Time

The experience of time is, according to Zemke and Clark,[14] shaped by occupations. Despite the standardization of time-keeping, people differ in the manner in which time is perceived. That is, different occupations can provide different experiences of time. For example, a boring lecture may seem endless, while an engaging conversation may seem to make the time pass quickly. On the other hand, the same occupation can result in different perceptions of time depending on the context in which it is done. Consider committee meetings, for example. The agenda or purpose, the people present, the time of day, and even the comfort of the meeting room may influence how time is perceived during the meeting.

Explaining how people experience the passage of time has been a topic of interest to both philosophers and scientists for centuries. Individual differences appear to be based on age, personality, cultural experiences, and attitudes. Psychophysical and physiological variables, such as the temperature of the body, the state of arousal, and the effect of drugs,[39] can also affect time perception. The extent to which accurate perception of the passage of time influences the performance of everyday occupations can be shown among musicians, dancers, and skilled athletes. The skilled performance of music, dance, and sport depends on the precise timing of human movements.

Scientists believe they have now identified areas in the brain that are responsible for time perception. The basal ganglia located deep within the base of the brain and the parietal lobes located on the surface of the right side of the brain are critical areas for this time-keeping system.[40]

Physiological factors, such as lower body temperatures, high levels of arousal, and concentrations of dopamine, are thought to influence the perception of time through the body's internal biological clocks.[41] Experiments have shown that as people age, their estimates of the amount of time that has passed, particularly while doing an activity, are higher than people at younger ages. This suggests that as people mature, they perceive that time is moving faster than it actually is, which may explain why there is the nearly universal perception that years get shorter as we get older.

Physiological Influences on Patterns of Occupation

The term *chronobiology* is derived from the Greek words chronos (time), bios (life), and logos (reason). There are several biological systems (eg, blood pressure, body temperature, and rest activity cycle) that are influenced by internal time keepers or physiological systems of temporal regulation.[38] These internal clocks are dependent on external, environmental phenomena to synchronize them according to social and physical environmental factors.

Such external phenomena are called "zeitgebers" (time-keepers). They include light, darkness, and ambient temperature, as well as social influences related to human occupation such as meals, social interaction, and regular habits and routines performed at consistent times (eg, walking the dog).[42] These timekeepers in turn influence the rest activity cycle of the body, making us alert, energized, and active during some periods and drowsy and less energized at other times. As might be expected, the human's daily rhythm of occupations is highly influenced

by these biotemporal patterns, and the need for certain activities (eg, eating and sleep) does not entirely depend on the individual's impulses or motivation, but also on recurrent biological needs and pace.

Chronobiology explains why, during any one day, a person goes through periods of higher and lower arousal or activity. This is known as the rest/activity cycle, and has a profound impact on occupational engagement. Environmental changes can disrupt that cycle and can cause physiological disturbances. Scientists are now aware that biological rhythms provide optimal times for human function and can significantly influence the value of medical or therapeutic interventions. This knowledge is the basis for an emerging focus in medicine called *chronotherapeutics*.[43]

Most people know about jet lag, which occurs when travelers cross many time zones. The disruption that sometimes occurs following such travel is called circadian *desynchronosis*. This disruption of internal biological clocks can also occur as a result of shift work and can be of limited duration or longer term. Common symptoms of desynchronosis include sleep loss, fatigue, diminished performance, loss of appetite, nervous tension, and a feeling of malaise or ill health. Scientists have shown that the physiological consequences of long distance travel can influence sleep and alertness for as long as 1 month following the completion of long distance travels. Similarly, people who experience erratic schedules because of shift work, or experience changes that disrupt normal routines (such as unemployment or loss of a partner or spouse), can similarly experience desynchronosis.

Scientists at the University of Pittsburgh have examined the relationship between social factors and patterns of occupation that demonstrate greater or lesser degrees of consistency. Using a measure called the Social Rhythm Metric, they have demonstrated that significant social changes can disrupt the body's timekeeping systems, resulting in significant consequences with health implications.[44] Their work has demonstrated an important link between health (especially bipolar mood disorders) and the consistency of daily activity rhythms, as these may be influenced by habits and routines.[44,45]

Habits and Routines

Some behaviors are repeated so often that they become habitual, performed on an automatic, preconscious level. In the extreme, recurring behavior may meet a strong physiological and psychological need, which is described as an addiction. Habits influence behavior in a semiautomatic way without need for conscious, deliberate action. They are established through prior repetition of a series of acts and serve to enable higher occupations. Habits are more likely to occur in familiar environments and conserve energy needed for attention and decision making while enabling us to do things we must do regularly without requiring high levels of motivation or energy.

Routines are occupations with established sequences, such as the morning ritual surrounding showering and dressing for the day. Routines provide an orderly structure for daily living, as suggested in this description by Bond and Feathers,[3] who write that "a routine has a stability about it that extends over time and pertains to a particular set of activities within a defined situation."[3(p328)]

Studies have supported the idea that certain activities naturally take place at certain times of the day. For example, a study of the daily lives of older adults in Germany[46] observed that work and self-maintenance activities tended to predominate in the morning and early afternoon, whereas leisure and restful activities were associated with late afternoon and evening periods. Similar activity rhythms have been found in studies of higher-order group living animals, such as mountain gorillas.[47]

Studies of biological rhythms tend to support the idea that routines are highly influenced by internal clocks. Routines are also provided structure by social and environmental factors that provide behavioral expectations; for example, working for an employer imposes a workday routine, while business hours at a favorite store may dictate shopping routines, just as religious services influence the times when spiritual occupations occur on days of worship.

Viewed over extended periods, habits and routines comprise important dimensions of lifestyles, components of which have been shown to influence health and well-being. For example, regular exercise, rest, and appropriate dietary habits (ie, lifestyle behaviors) can be influenced by daily routines. Additionally, adherence to therapeutic regimens, such as eating or taking medications at prescribed times, can also be influenced by habits and routines. Unfortunately, the extent to which habits and regular routines contribute to healthful consequences (independent of specific practices) is not yet well understood.

EXTRINSIC FACTORS IMPACTING ON OCCUPATION IN TIME

Society and Cultural Structures

The sociotemporal patterns of a society reflect the structure of its social life. Western society is to a great extent scheduled, and many occupations take place during certain hours, days, and seasons. Thereby, concepts such as cleaning days, lunchtime, and weekends become commonly understood blocks of time in this society. By analyzing statistics from the Canadian adult population's time use, Zuzanek and Smale[48] confirmed that what people do with their time differs significantly between weekdays and weekends, particularly regarding the occupational category of work. In a more recent study, factors impacting on time use by a sample of United States citizens was explored. The study found that the most important factors[49] influencing what and when people do occupations included the season of the year, whether they occupations were performed on weekdays or weekends, and whether the occupations were classified as work or non-work.

Gender impacts on patterns of occupations in all life stages—at least in western societies. For example, in comparing United States teenagers aged 12 to 17, the main differences found were that girls spent 1 hour more per week in household work than did boys, and took care of siblings or babysat 1.5 hours more per week than boys. Moreover, the girls spent much more time on shopping and grooming, while the boys spent more time on sports and education.[50] The oldest age group showed the same patterns; ie, women aged 65 years and above spent more time on household work and shopping, while men in the corresponding age group used more time for sports and watching television.[50] In comparing these findings with current figures from people aged 20 to 64 years in the Swedish population, it is clear that such gender differences are sustained. Swedish men spend more time on paid work than women do. Women do more household work and have less leisure time than men do.[51] However, since 1990 the average Swedish woman has reduced her time spent with housework by more than 1 hour a day, and 14 minutes less on unpaid housework per day in 2010 compared to 2000. Instead Swedish women spend more time in gainful employment, or 21 minutes more a day. For men the time spent in paid work has decreased by 14 minutes, and they have somewhat increased time with daily household tasks.

Besides gender, there are other aspects that impact on time use. Patterns of daily occupations differ with one's life stage. In later life stages, patterns of time use change. Elderly people spend less time in paid work and household tasks and more time in self-care and leisure.[52,53] In examining data from the Canadian population, Singleton and Harvey[54] found that persons with children at home spent more time on household chores than those who had no children. Furthermore, the study showed that adults who lived in traditional families with children and a spouse tended to spend more time in different occupations (ie, had a different variation of occupations, as compared to those who were unmarried and/or had no children). The same pattern is found in more recent research. When comparing nationally representative time-use data from more than 5000 individuals living in Australia, Italy, France, and Denmark, Craig and Mullan[55] found that parents in all countries have higher, less gender-equal workloads than non-parents.

To work outside the home is another variable that clearly impacts time use and pattern of daily occupations. Time use studies indicate that for adults in the United States (on average) approximately 30% of a typical 24-hour day is spent sleeping; 10% is allocated to personal care activities (including eating); and another 10% is allocated to household work such as cooking, laundry, and cleaning. For those who are employed, approximately 25% of one's daily time is spent on actual paid work (excluding breaks). Thus, nearly 60% of the waking day is devoted to obligatory or required activities, including employment, for a typically employed adult. This proportion of obligatory activity has also been found for adolescents, though related to school occupations instead of paid work.[56]

Daily occupations work as regulators for patterns, and there is international consistency in time allocation. Percentages reported for the United States are similar to data collected in other countries, showing remarkably consistent patterns both for obligatory and discretionary categories of occupation, as well as in more specific areas of occupation such as self-care and household maintenance.[46,57,58] Furthermore, the latest time use exploration in Sweden comparing time use in the general population between year 2000 and 2010[51] may be interpreted as illustrating that time use in populations are fairly consistent, since the average changes in time use in 10 years regarding different categories of occupation were less than 60 minutes.

Strategies for Observing and Measuring Daily Occupations at the Person, Organization, and Population Level

We have now presented several aspects of the complexity of patterns of human occupation. What remains to be illuminated is how to document and analyze the time and place for occupation. In this section we will present 2 main perspectives: one regarding methods for documenting the time used for occupations in minutes and hours, and another focusing on the ability to explore the temporal rhythm in patterns of daily occupations (eg, how single occupations, such as driving to work, are related in time to other occupations in daily life, eg, filling up gas, picking up children at daycare, and visiting the gym). Furthermore, if an individual is facing a need for change and to reorganize his or her daily pattern of daily occupations, it might be important to understand in what order the occupations are performed and whether or not this order is restricted or constrained by circumstances.

Time Budget Methods

In the literature, a pattern of occupations commonly refers to trends or similarities in measures of how much time people spend on different occupations. The main sources for such knowledge are time-use or time-budget studies. The measure is quantitative and time use is recorded based on the type of occupation noted in diaries, so that the reported time spent on different occupations can be totaled and analyzed on a group level. A large number of time-use studies conducted with large populations in several different countries across the globe have provided important information on what people do and to what extent. Much of the current information on time use comes from consumer research, although governmental agencies and scientists studying gerontology and leisure have also made useful contributions to the general understanding of how people "spend" their time. However, certain types of time-use studies attempt to link the use of time to perceived experiences and health-related factors. The research on patterns of occupations within the area of occupational therapy has contributed to this body of knowledge.

Several studies have applied a time-budget perspective with an occupation/health standpoint,[59-61] studying how time is used by persons with varying types of health conditions. Peachey-Hill and Law[62] examined the impact of the condition of environmental sensitivity on the lifestyles of persons with this disorder by collecting and analyzing their 24-hour diaries. They found that such persons experienced a decline in their ability to devote time for engagement in the tasks and roles that were valued and necessary for their well-being.

Time Geographic Method

Time geography methodology[63,64] complements the study of patterns of human occupation previously discussed in this chapter. The geographic method studies human occupation with respect to their relationships to place and time. Originally this method was developed to support different aspects of community planning (eg, studies of work processes or energy use in communities), but has also been used for describing and comparing how different groups in the society use their time. More recently, time geography-inspired methodology has increasingly been applied in studies of daily life.[64] For example, time geographic visualizations of family members' time diaries have been used to describe the diversity of everyday life of households and when, where, and what energy-related activities occurred in the home.[65]

More recently, the time geography method has been applied in occupational therapy and occupational science research. For example, the method has been used to describe the everyday life of adolescents with low vision,[66,67] parents' shared patterns of daily occupations,[68] and the habits of elderly people.[69]

In Sweden, the approach has been used to study ways for helping people to change their daily occupations in order to lower their energy use.[65] There are examples of occupational therapy practitioners applying the method in interventions,[70] since transforming time use diaries into graphs has been shown to enable individuals to gain insight into their own patterns of daily occupations.[71]

Essentially, time geography is based on the representation of individuals as paths in a 3-dimensional coordinate system, where 2 dimensions represent geographic space, (ie, room and action) and the third represents time.[63] Time geography implies presenting the everyday life in a linear context of moments in time and space.[72] From an occupational therapy and occupational science perspective, the method thereby is suitable for illustrating individual's *doing* in time and place. The basis for the method is used for exploring individuals' doing in diary notes covering a 24-hour day. Such a diary may be collected by interview or be self-reported continuously during a day. The notes about when, what, and where are then basically transformed as coordinates in a 2-dimensional (or 3-dimensional) coordinate system. The coordinates are connected and graphs are drawn. More recently, digital technology has provided the means for graphs to be drawn by computers, with variations in the graphic presentation dependent on the software being used.

In Figure 8-4, 2 pictures were presented illustrating a mother's and a father's occupations in time. Far to the left in each picture, the trajectory of the individual's occupations in time is illustrated from bottom to the top. Here it becomes evident how the father is spending longer periods in the same occupations as compared to the mother, who changes occupations more often. In addition, to the right in each picture there are lines describing where the person is doing the occupation, as well as whether or not others are involved. Thus, the second line from left shows how the mother is at home, goes to the daycare, and to her work. On her way home she does some errands before coming home again.

New Technologies

An increasing selection of technology can be applied to measuring occupational behavior and allowing scientists to study and describe the patterns of occupational performance or engagement. Computers have now been used for several years to analyze and describe patterns of daily occupations; applying different perspectives for analysis. However, emerging technologies are opening up new possibilities to record and measure what people do. In Sweden, the time geographers of today have developed advanced computer programs for the categorization and description of what people do in relation to time and space, eg, Daily Life[73] and the VISUAL-TimePAcTS.[65]

Wood[74] developed the program Activity in Context and Time (ACT), a computer-assisted observational tool designed to record environmental correlates of the time use of people with dementia. Video has been used in studies of the occupations of family members during a normal day.[75] However, even if technology development is tempting to use for documenting human occupations, there are other methods that may be just as important to apply and develop. This is especially important if human occupation is regarded as a worldwide, cultural-dependent phenomenon. To explore and record what is being done may not be possible if the doing is not understood by the spectator. In this perspective, qualitative approaches (such as ethnographic field studies and participant analysis) may also be relevant. Time use research may therefore be useful for the application of mixed methods research designs, where scientists can derive both qualitative and quantitative approaches that yield insights with both individual and group relevance.

SUMMARY

In this chapter, we have described how human occupation can be described and measured based on patterns of engagement as they change in time and place. Such patterns may recur (as occurs with habits, routines, and rituals), and the nature of the patterns may have a certain regularity, predictability, or consistency.

We have noted that patterns are influenced by both intrinsic and extrinsic factors, which include biological, social, cultural, and environmental phenomena, and that these factors can influence the complexity of the patterns observed. Some people have greater complexity in the variety of occupations undertaken within a given interval (ie, day, week, month, or year), whereas others exhibit less complexity. Because of the multiple factors that may influence occupational patterns, each individual can be viewed as having a unique occupational pattern within a specified interval. Because of the relationship between internal or biological clocks and the regulation of hormones within the endocrine system, there are physiological influences on occupational patterns; disruption of these physiological influences can have health consequences. Because of the relationship between the endocrine system and physiological stress responses, it is logical to assume that there is a relationship between occupational patterns and resilience to stress. Occupational scientists and others are studying whether certain patterns of occupational engagement over time may contribute to health and longevity.

When describing daily occupations with respect to category, a person's day typically includes engagement in main or primary occupations, occupations that are hidden between or within main occupations (such as having a cup of coffee), and unexpected occupations that people undertake to deal with events and situations that are unusual or unexpected.

A variety of approaches to measuring occupational patterns were reviewed, including time budget approaches (such as time diaries), time geographic methods that record patterns of movement, changes between occupations and the places where occupations are performed, and videography and newer digital technologies that can combine multiple methods for recording and analysis. Despite the impressive progress in conceptualizing and studying occupational patterns, it can be said that the science of measuring, describing, analyzing, and understanding the occupational patterns of humans, though promising, is still in its infancy.

REFERENCES

1. Elliott DS. *Health Enhancing and Health Compromising Lifestyles.* New York, NY: Oxford University Press; 1993.
2. Reed K, Sanderson S. *Concepts of Occupational Therapy.* 4th ed. Philadelphia, PA: Lippincott Williams and Wilkins; 1999.
3. Bond MJ, Feathers MT. Some correlates of structure and purpose in the use of time. *J Pers Soc Psychol.* 1988;55(2):321-329.
4. Mullersdorf M, Ivarsson AB. Occupation as described by novice occupational therapy students in Sweden: the first step in a theory generative process grounded in empirical data. *Scand J Occup Ther.* 2008;15(1):34-42.
5. Hasselkus B. Reaching consensus. *Am J Occup Ther.* 2000;54(2):127-128.
6. Little B, Lecci L, Watkinson B. Personality and personal projects: linking big five and PAC units of analysis. *J Pers.* 1992;6(20):501-525.
7. Haglund L, Henriksson C. Activity—from action to activity. *Scand J Caring Sci.* 1995; 9:227-234.
8. Nelson D. Occupation: form and performance. *Am J Occup Ther.* 1988;42:633-641.
9. Persson D, Erlandsson L-K, Eklund M, et al. Value dimensions, meaning, and complexity in human occupation—a tentative structure for analysis. *Scand J Occup Ther.* 2001;8(1):7-18.
10. Clark F. Actions for activity and occupation: WFOT core theme. Paper presented at: 13th WFOT Conference; Stockholm, Sweden; June 23-28, 2002.
11. Nelson DL. Therapeutic occupation: a definition. *Am J Occup Ther.* 1996;50(10):775-782.
12. Pierce D. Untangling occupation and activity. *Am J Occup Ther.* 2001;55:138-146.
13. Erlandsson L-K, Eklund M. Describing patterns of daily occupations—a methodological study comparing data from four different methods. *Scand J Occup Ther.* 2001;8(1):31-39.
14. Zemke R, Clark F. *Occupational Science: An Involving Discipline.* Philadelphia, PA: FA Davis; 1996.
15. Pierce D. Co-occupation: the challenges of defining concepts original to occupational science. *J Occup Sci.* 2009;16(3):203-207.
16. Kielhofner G. *A Model of Human Activity: Theory and Application.* 3rd ed. Baltimore, MD: Williams & Wilkins; 2002.
17. Polatajko HJ. The study of occupation. In: Christiansen CH, Townsend E, eds. *Introduction to Occupation. The Art and Science of Living.* Upper Saddle River, NJ: Pearson Education Inc; 2004:29-61.
18. Wilcock A. *An Occupational Perspective of Health.* 2nd ed. Thorofare, NJ: SLACK Incorporated; 2006.
19. Erlandsson L-K. 101 Women's pattern of daily occupations: characteristics and relationships to health and well-being. In: *Dept of Clinical Neuroscience, Div. of Occupational Therapy.* Lund, Sweden: Lund University; 2003:157.
20. Maume DJ, Sebastian RA, Bardo AR. Gender, work-family responsibilities, and sleep. *Gend Soc.* 2010;24:746-768.
21. Larson EA, Zemke R. Shaping the temporal patterns of our lives: the social coordination of occupation. *J Occup Sci.* 2003;10(2):80-89.
22. Meyer A. The philosophy of occupation therapy. *Arch Occup Ther.* 1922;1:1-10.
23. Wilcock AA, Chelin M, Hall M, et al. The relationship between occupational balance and health: a pilot study. *Occup Ther Int.* 1997;4(1):17- 30.
24. Christiansen CH, Matuska K. Lifestyle balance: a review of concepts and research. *J Occup Sci.* 2006;(13):63-73.
25. Specht J, King G, Brown E, et al. The importance of leisure in the lives of persons with congenital physical disabilities. *Am J Occup Ther.* 2002;56(4):436-445.
26. Edgelow M, Krupa T. Randomized controlled pilot study of an occupational time-use intervention for people with serious mental illness. *Am J Occup Ther.* 2011;65(3):267-276.
27. Matuska KM, Christiansen CH. A proposed model of lifestyle balance. *J Occup Sci.* 2008;15(1):9-19.
28. Piskur B, Kinebanian A, Josephsson S. Occupation and well-being: a study of some Slovenian people's experiences of engagement in occupation in relation to well-being. *Scand J Occup Ther.* 2002;9(2):63-70.
29. Erlandsson L-K, Håkansson C. Aspects of daily occupations that promotes life balance. In: Matuska K, Christiansen CH, eds. *Life Balance: Multidisciplinary Theories and Research.* Thorofare, NJ: SLACK Incorporated and AOTA Press; 2009:115-131.
30. Erlandsson L-K, Rögnvaldsson T, Eklund M. Recognition of similarities (ROS): a methodological approach to analysing and characterising patterns of daily occupations. *J Occup Sci.* 2004;11(1):3-13.
31. Erlandsson L-K, Eklund M. Levels of complexity in patterns of daily occupations in relation to women's well-being. *J Occup Sci.* 2006;13(1):27-36.
32. Davies K. *Women, Time and the Weaving of the Strands of Everyday Life.* Aldershot, UK: Avebury; 1990.
33. Bejerholm U, Eklund M. Engagement in occupations among men and women with schizophrenia. *Occup Ther Int.* 2006;13(2):100-121.
34. Bejerholm U. Occupational balance in people with schizophrenia. *Occup Ther Ment Health.* 2010;26(1):1-17.
35. Eklund M, Leufstadius C, Bejerholm U. Time use among people with psychiatric disabilities: implications for practice. *Psychiatr Rehabil J.* 2009;32(3):177-191.
36. Scanlan JN, Bundy AC, Matthews LR. Promoting well-being in young unemployed adults: the importance of identifying meaningful patterns of time use. *Aust Occup Ther J.* 2011;58(2):111-119.
37. Sapolsky RM. *Why Zebras Don't Get Ulcers: The Acclaimed Guide To Stress, Stress-Related Diseases, and Coping.* New York, NY: Henry Holt and Company, LLC; 2004.
38. Zerubavel E. *Hidden Rhythms; Schedules and Calendars in Social Life.* Chicago, IL: The University of Chicago Press; 1981.
39. Eisler AD, Eisler H. Subjective time scaling: influence of age, gender and Type A and Type B behavior. *Chronobiologia.* 1994;(21):185-200.

40. Rao SM, Mayer AR, Harrington DL. The evolution of brain activation during temporal processing. *Nat Neurosci.* 2001;4:317-323.

41. Schleidt MK, Kien J. Segmentation in behavior and why it can tell us about brain function. *Hum Nat.* 1997;8:77-111.

42. Moore-Ede M, Sulzman F, Fuller C. *The Clocks That Time Us: Psychology of Circadian Timing System.* Cambridge, UK: Harvard University Press; 1982.

43. Decousus H. Chronobiology in hemostatis. In: Touitou HE, ed. *Biologic Rhythms in Clinical and Laboratory Medicine.* New York, NY: Springer-Verlag; 1994:555-565.

44. Monk TH, Flahert, JF, Frank E, et al. The Social Rhythm Metric: an instrument to quantify the daily rhythms of life. *J Nerv Ment Dis.* 1990;178(2):120-126.

45. Frank E, Kupfer DJ, Thase ME, et al. Two-year outcomes for interpersonal and social rhythm therapy in individuals with bipolar I disorder. *Arch Gen Psychiatry.* 2005;62:996-1004.

46. Baltes MM, Wahl HW, Schmid-Furstoss U. The daily life of elderly Germans: activity patterns, personal control, and functional health. *J Gerontol.* 1990;45(4):173-179.

47. Harcourt AH. Social relationships among adult female mountain gorillas. *Anim Behav.* 1979;27(1):251-264.

48. Zuzanek J, Smale B. Life-cycle variations in across-the-week allocation of time to selected daily activities. *Soc Leis.* 1992;15:559-586.

49. Mccurdy T, Graham SE. Using human activity data in exposure models: analysis of discriminating factors. *J Expo Anal Environ Epidemiol.* 2003;13:294–317.

50. Robinson J, Godbey G. *Time for Life: The Surprising Ways Americans Use Their Time.* University Park, PA: Penn State Press; 1997.

51. Statisitics Sweden. *Swedish Time Use Survey 2010.* Örebro, Sweden: Statistical Agency and Producer; 2010.

52. McKenna K, Broome K, Liddle J. What older people do: time use and exploring the link between role participation and life satisfaction in people aged 65 years and over. *Aust Occup Ther J.* 2007;54(4):273-284.

53. Chilvers R, Corr S, Singlehurst H. Investigation into the occupational lives of healthy older people through their use of time. *Aust Occup Ther J.* 2010;57(1):24-33.

54. Singleton J, Harvey A. Stage of life cycle and time spent in activities. *J Occup Sci.* 1995;(20):522-672.

55. Craig L, Mullan K. Parenthood, gender and work-family time in the United States, Australia, Italy, France, and Denmark. *J Marriage Fam.* 2010;72:1344-1361.

56. Csikszentmihalyi M. *Flow—The Psychology of Optimal Experience.* New York, NY: Harper and Row; 1990.

57. Castles I. *How Australians Use Their Time.* Canberra, Australia: Australian Bureau of Statistics; 1994.

58. Sjöberg LM. Action and emotion in everyday life. *Scand J Psychol.* 1990;(31):9-27.

59. Larson KB. Activity patterns and life changes in people with depression. *Am J Occup Ther.* 1990;44(10):902-906.

60. Fricke J, Unsworth C. Time use and importance of instrumental activities of daily living. *Aust Occup Ther J.* 2001;(48):118-131.

61. Liedberg G, Hesselstrand M, Henriksson C. Time use and activity patterns in women with long-term pain. *Scand J Occup Ther.* 2004;(11):26-35.

62. Peachey-Hill C, Law M. Impact of environmental sensitivity on occupational performance. *Can J Occup Ther.* 2000;(67):304-313.

63. Hägerstrand T. Survival and arena: on the life-history of individuals in relation to their geographical environment. In: Carlstein T, Parkes D, Thrift NJ, eds. *Human Activity and Time Geography: Timing Space and Spacing Time.* 2nd ed. New York, NY: Wiley; 1978:122-143.

64. Ellegård K. A time-geographical approach to the study of everyday life of individuals—a challenge of complexity. *Geo J.* 1999;(48):167-175.

65. Palm J, Ellegård K. Visualizing energy consumption activities as a tool for developing effective policy. *Int J Consum Stud.* 2011;35(2):171-179.

66. Kroksmark U, Nordell K. Adolescence: the age of opportunities and obstacles for students with low vision in Sweden. *J Vis Impair Blind.* 2001;95:213-220.

67. Kellegrew DH, Kroksmark U. Examining school routines using time-geography methodology. *Phys Occup Ther Pediatr.* 1999;19(2):79-91.

68. Orban K, Ellegård K, Thorngren-Jerneck K, Erlandsson L-K. Shared patterns of daily occupations among parents of children Aged 4-6 years old with obesity. *J Occup Sci.* 2012;19(3):241-257.

69. Rowles GD. Habituation and being in place. *Occup Ther J Res.* 2000;20:526-676.

70. Erlandsson L-K. The Redesigning Daily Occupations (ReDO)-programme: supporting women with stress-related disorders to return to work - knowledge base, structure, and content. *Occup Ther Ment Health.* 2013;29(1):85-101.

71. Orban K, Edberg A-K, Erlandsson L-K. Using a time-geographical diary method in order to facilitate reflections on changes in patterns of daily occupations. *Scand J Occup Ther.* 2011;19(3):249-259.

72. Ellegård K, Cooper M. Complexity in daily life—a 3-D visualization showing activity patterns in their contexts. *Int J Time Use Research.* 2004;1(1):37-59.

73. Ellegård K, Nordell K. *Daily Life: Version 2008.* Linköping, Sweden: Linköping University; 2008.

74. Wood W, Womack J, Hooper B. Dying of boredom: an exploratory case study of time use, apparent affect, and routine activity situations on two Alzheimer's special care units. *Am J Occup Ther.* 2009;63(3):337-350.

75. Rönkä A, Korvela P. Everyday family life: dimensions, approaches, and current challenges. *J Family Theory Rev.* 2009;1(2):87-102.

Chapter 9

OCCUPATIONS OF CHILDHOOD AND ADOLESCENCE

Sylvia Rodger, BOccThy, MEdSt, PhD; Jenny Ziviani, BAppSc(OT), MOccThy, PhD; and Sok Mui Lim, BOT(Hons), GCert Higher Ed, PhD

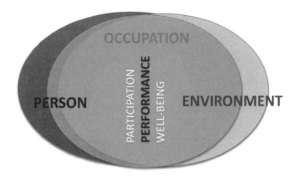

LEARNING OBJECTIVES

- Describe typical development at various ages and occupations engaged in by children and youth, highlighting the interaction between development and these occupations. Identify potential barriers and enablers that impact occupations of children and youth (eg, personal factors [such as health conditions] and environmental factors [such as family, culture, and socioeconomic circumstances]).

- Identify key developmental theories that underpin the development of children's occupations and the relationship between independence and interdependence (eg, social learning theory, socioecological theory, attachment theory, and cognitive theories).

- Identify the skills and environmental supports required for educational transitions from early childhood settings to school, primary to high school, and post-school.

- Identify some key measures of occupations for children and youth (eg, play, school, self-maintenance).

- Identify key roles of families, peers, and communities in enabling daily occupations of children and youth.

KEY WORDS

- Attachments
- Flow
- Learning style
- Motivation
- Play
- Resilience
- Roles
- Self-efficacy
- Temperament
- Transitions
- Volition

Christiansen CH, Baum CM, Bass JD, eds.
Occupational Therapy: Performance, Participation, and Well-Being, Fourth Edition (pp 129-155).
© 2015 SLACK Incorporated.

INTRODUCTION

Occupation has been defined as a "goal-directed pursuit that typically extends over time, has meaning to the performer, and involves multiple tasks."[1(p548)] Depending on their age, children and youth engage in a range of daily occupations, including looking after themselves (self-care), play, recreation (leisure), productivity (such as education, school work), and contributing to their social and economic community (such as volunteering and doing household chores), as well as rest and relaxation. Occupational performance refers to the act of "doing" an occupation.[2] Children engage in different occupational roles, including those of player, self-carer, and school student,[3] as well as social roles such as friend, sibling, and grandchild. Roles have been defined as "position(s) in society having expected responsibilities and privileges."[2(p56)]

In this chapter, the roles, occupations, and occupational performance of children and youth will be described. This chapter addresses 4 stages that encompass specific age groups:

1. Infancy and toddlerhood (up to 2 years old)
2. Early childhood (2 to 6 years old)
3. Middle childhood (7 to 12 years old)
4. Adolescence (12 to 18 years old)

The terms *youth* and *young people* will be used interchangeably to describe individuals during the stage of adolescence.

This chapter focuses on normal development and the relevant occupations engaged in during childhood and adolescence. Developmental theories that support these life stages are discussed alongside the occupations in which children and youth are engaged. We will broadly address some illustrative health conditions, personal, and environmental factors that impact on occupational performance and present measures of occupational performance that can be used by occupational therapy practitioners.

A large amount of learning through exposure to new experiences occurs during infancy and early childhood. Hence, it is a period of great developmental significance. Similar to building a house, typical brain development or neuromaturation occurs sequentially. This developmental blueprint supports an individual's expression of his or her genetic potential. Just as a lack of the right materials can result in changes to housing blueprints, a lack of appropriate experiences can lead to alterations in genetic plans.[4] Although the brain retains the capacity to adapt and change throughout life (known as plasticity), this capacity decreases with age.[5-7] More recent neuroscience research indicates that the brain continues to be plastic throughout life, even in the face of specific neurological damage. It is far more effective to support healthy development from the outset compared to building more advanced motor, cognitive, social, and emotional skills on weak neurological foundations. Hence, providing children with appropriate, stimulating environmental opportunities and experiences alongside responsive and nurturing social relationships is of utmost importance.

While the course of typical development enables the child to engage in age-appropriate occupations in a recurring process, engagement in these occupations also enhances healthy development and the attainment of developmental milestones and acquisition of skills. This occurs through a dynamic and reciprocal process whereby the individual interacts with his or her environment and, through these experiences/interactions, his or her development and neurological maturation are enhanced. For example, children in middle childhood often play games such as hide and seek that require motor skills (eg, running, agility, speed), problem-solving and reasoning related to where to hide, perceptive taking (to understand the view of the person who is "up" or "it" and is searching for the other children), and interpersonal relationships with other players.

Middle childhood and adolescence remain periods of considerable psychological, physiological, perceptual, cognitive, and sensory/motor development. These are elements of the person as described in the PEOP Model that is central to this book. During middle childhood, children gain refinement in their motor abilities and cognitive development continues, especially in memory and language. Adolescence is a time of adjustment to bodily changes, increased awareness of sexuality, and changing status within family and society. Accompanying these changes, occupational roles are further refined. Physically, young people undergo puberty. Cognitively, they develop more abstract thinking and advanced reasoning skills. Socioemotionally, they search for personal identity and develop a more mature sense of morality alongside exerting greater autonomy and independence from parents and family. Each of these stages will now be addressed in more detail in the following sections.

TYPICAL DEVELOPMENT AND OCCUPATIONS

Infancy and Toddlerhood

The first 12 months of life is a period of significant development. In no other developmental period does so much change occur during such a short time frame. Physically, an infant's weight is expected to double between birth and 5 months, and increases 3 times by the age of 1 year. Babies are born with reflexes that help them survive. For example, the rooting reflex enables an infant to orient in response to his or her cheek being stroked and begin to make sucking motions followed by swallowing, thereby enabling the child to perform the occupation of feeding. Most infant reflexes disappear as the infant develops (eg, rooting, sucking), although some reflexes, such as the pain reflex (withdrawal from painful stimulus) and reactions (allowing the body to maintain alignment and right or protect itself when placed off balance), are adaptive and remain throughout life.[8]

Within the first 12 months of life, infants are dependent on their caregivers for all of their needs. In fact, the main occupations of infants in the first 3 months of life are limited to sleeping, crying, feeding, and developing attachment relationships with primary caregivers.[9] Crying enables infants to communicate their needs (eg, pain, hunger, and relational). In response to stressors such as pain, fatigue, fearful events, and separation from attachment figures, infants use specific behaviors such as crying to gain proximity to caregivers and to experience reassurance and security.[10] Around 6 months of age, the infant develops some mobility; now being able to roll, sit, reach out or move towards toys. Such abilities enable the child to engage in more occupations such as exploratory play (eg, grasping and mouthing rattles, body parts, and moving about the environment). Bathing is another occupation that is enjoyed by many infants, particularly during this period when they are dependent on adults to ensure their safety and cleanliness. Around 9 months, the child's socialization with caregivers increases through games like peek-a-boo and pat-a-cake. The child becomes more mobile and may be crawling, pulling to stand, or cruising around low furniture.[8(p156)] This enhanced mobility allows further exploration of the environment, which brings with it issues of safety as well as socioemotional challenges, such as caregivers being out of sight. An important theory to understand alongside the development of infant's occupations is *Attachment Theory*.[11]

According to Attachment Theory, human biology guarantees that all infants become attached to at least one caregiver.[12] However, the quality of attachment differs depending on various factors, such as caregiver's or parent's sensitivity to the infant's signals. Attachment Theory originated with the seminal work of John Bowlby[13] in the 1950s. According to Bowlby,[10(p11)] the attachment system is developed through ongoing social and care-giving interactions between the child's developing cognitive capacities and the caregivers' responses within the environment. Early attachment styles have been found to organize emotions and behavior throughout life, contributing to the development of intimate relationships in adulthood.[14]

It is generally believed that the first 12 months of life represents the most important stage for the human infant to become securely attached to an adult caregiver/parent. After this it becomes ever more difficult for the child to form his or her first attachment relationship.[10(p11)] Attachment promotes survival in 3 main ways[10(p11-12,131)]:

1. *Through safety:* Attachment keeps the primary caregiver and child close to each other. Separation results in feelings of anxiety for both mother and child.

2. *Through providing a safe base for exploration:* The child is happy to explore the physical environment away from his or her parent, which is important to facilitate his or her cognitive and motor development. While exploring, the attached child knows that he or she can return to an attachment figure or safe place near the attachment figure when threats arise or he or she feels insecure. This also aids in the development of independence in later life.

3. *Through providing a means for forming an internal working model:* Attachment allows the child to form a schema that provides him or her with a sense of what relationships are all about. This schema is used in future years when the child forms other social relationships, particularly intimate ones.

The quality of attachment provides a foundation that continues to impact on the child's development.[12(p47)] If a child feels secure, he or she will actively explore his or her physical and social environment. The child with a secure attachment relationship will also later be more confident in problem solving independently.[12(p48)] Conceptually, Rubin and Krasnor[15] suggested that children who believe that their parents are available and responsive to their needs will feel secure, confident, and self-assured when they are introduced to novel settings such as kindergarten. In turn, when children confidently explore their social environment, this leads to positive experiences of peer play and the development of healthy peer relationships through the refinement of social skills in their early childhood years. Conversely, attachment insecurity has been associated with maladaptive personal and social characteristics such as difficulties with emotional regulation, less adaptive social behaviors, and lower self-efficacy, all of which are long-lasting.[14(p286)]

Piaget's Stages of Cognitive Development informs our understanding of an individual's learning, problem solving, play, and later academic abilities. The first stage is known as the *Sensory Motor Stage*, which occurs in children from birth to approximately 2 years. During this stage, infants and toddlers gain knowledge about objects and the ways that they can be manipulated.[16] Through the acquisition of information about self and the world and the people in it, infants and toddlers begin to understand concepts like cause and effect (eg, shaking a rattle leads to an entertaining noise, pressing a button on a toy car leads to a noise, such as a siren) and begin to develop simple ideas about time and space. This stage is also consistent with their simultaneous engagement in exploratory play. They are interested in toys that make noise, containers that can be stacked and knocked down, and other cause and effect toys. During this stage, a child around 8 to 12 months learns to look for objects or people when they move out of sight, commonly known as "object permanence."[17] This is also when infants begin to play social games, such as peek-a-boo.

Children enter toddlerhood either when they start walking (typically around 12 months) or when they pass their first birthday. Toddlers are typically busy as they can walk and soon learn to run and climb allowing them to more fully explore their physical environment. Toddlers require less sleep, having fewer daytime naps and spending their time watching and imitating adults and other children around them. Toddlers begin to form their first words, and by the end of the toddler period put 2 word sentences together.[17] They have little regard of danger and are interested in all household items, including fans, drawers, and electric sockets. This is a time where it is very important that adults "baby proof" the house and provide a safe environment for the child to explore. At this stage they play in parallel with other toddlers (eg, 2 children may sit in a sandpit and play with sand or dig but not play interactively).[18] As toddlers grow and pass their second birthday, they enter early childhood.

Early Childhood

Early childhood is the period from approximately 2 to 5 years of age in which young children are growing rapidly, losing their baby features, slimming down, and becoming taller, as well as developing further motor, language, cognitive, and social emotional skills.[19] As they move away from infancy and toddlerhood, they are able to do more for themselves. In fact, by the time most children go to school (around age 5 years) they can usually undress and dress (except for difficult fastenings or shoelaces), get themselves a drink or simple snack, manage their lunch box at school, toilet themselves independently (may need help with wiping), and seek help from an adult when required. These are all important skills necessary for managing a day at school on their own. They remain active in exploring the world and developing peer relationships and engage in a range of occupations such as play and self-care, and kindergarten activities such as art, craft, story time, and show-and-tell.

Young children gain independence and develop self-care abilities. They are involved in self-feeding and eating as they gain better control in use of tools such as a spoon and fork. They develop manual dexterity and calibration, enabling them to drink from a cup without spilling. Calibration refers to the judgment of force, speed, and

directional control to successfully manage a desired task.[19(p180)] With the guidance of caregivers, young children learn to undress and dress themselves, and take on a more active role during bath time and with basic grooming activities. Mastering toileting is an important developmental task and occupation of early childhood, as this can influence the child's ability to enter regular formal schooling.

According to Piaget's Stages of Cognitive Development, at 2 to 7 years of age, children enter the *Pre-Operational Stage*.[20] They start being able to categorize objects according to function not just appearance, and distinguish between animate and inanimate objects. At the same time, young children begin to use mental representations to think about things that are absent (eg, what they did yesterday at kindergarten). Pre-operational children are considered "egocentric." This means that they are only able to consider things from their own point of view, and imagine that everyone shares this view. As they grow older, a certain amount of "decentering" occurs, where the child stops believing that they are the center of the world, and they are more able to imagine that something or someone else could be the center of attention. At this stage they also begin to be able to entertain the thoughts of others, which is known as perspective taking.[20(p32)]

Young children's stage of cognitive development also influences their development of play skills. Between 2 and 3 years of age, typical children engage in parallel play, where they play beside each other with minimal interaction, drawing from a common pool of toys. There is minimal sharing and turn-taking, as children at this age cannot consider anyone else's point of view. As they continue to grow and develop, children begin to accept other's views, enabling them to delay gratification and to share and take turns, hence permitting more interactive play—known as associative and then cooperative play.[19(p192)]

With regard to productive roles, young children may attend playgroups, daycare, or kindergarten, gradually learning the student or learner role. In early childhood environments, they participate in a variety of occupations, such as sports, writing, and craft activities (cutting, pasting). In their learner role they develop *learning-related skills*,[21] such as paying attention to the teacher, sitting in a group for stories, and taking turns. At the same time, they take on roles as friends or playmates and develop early friendships. This early socioemotional development can be understood in terms of Bandura's Social Learning Theory.[20(p35)]

Bandura's Social Learning Theory focuses on the importance of observing and modeling the behaviors, attitudes, and emotional reactions of others.[20(p35)] It explains human behavior in terms of the interaction between cognitive and behavioral aspects of the child and his or her environmental influences. For children to be able to learn effectively from adult or peer modeling there are 4 necessary conditions.[22] First, they need to attend to what is shown. Second, they need to remember what they attend to. Next, they need to perform the behavior observed. Fourth, it is necessary for them to have the motivation to imitate. Reinforcement (especially social reinforcement) plays an important role in the development of such behaviors. For example, social conventions or school rules are learned—after watching how a child is praised for raising his hand during a circle time at kindergarten, another child will learn to raise his hand too in order to ask a question.

While socioemotional development is important for play and learning, language development is also crucial. Around 3 years of age, children's vocabularies have about 900 to 1000 words, and nearly 90% of what they say should be intelligible.[17(p173)] They are able to use pronouns, such as "I," "you," "me," as well as some plurals and past tenses. At 4 years of age, they are able to use verbs more than nouns and can form sentences of between 4 to 5 words. By 5 years, children can use some compound and complex sentences and are able to follow 3 commands given without interruptions.[17(p183)] With the development of more complex language, children gain the ability to regulate their behavior and emotions as they are able to express their thoughts, negotiate with others, and explain their actions. The ability to express themselves and understand instructions allows children to be prepared to enter formal schooling, which marks the beginning of middle childhood.

Transitions

A *transition* is defined as the passing from one condition, place or activity to another, and often involves a psychological response to change.[23] The transition from early to middle childhood is typically heralded by entering school. Times of transition are known to be challenging for children and their families, as they need to become accustomed to new environments—both in terms of locale, physical spaces, and the people who occupy these environments. It is important that both children and their families are prepared well for transitions so that they become positive learning experiences. Points of transition are likely to become more challenging when children experience occupational performance issues as a result of health or developmental conditions, which makes these times focal points for intervention (eg, school readiness preparation).

Middle Childhood

The ages of 7 to 12 are commonly referred to as the middle childhood stage of development. Children are typically enrolled in school during this period and spend a large portion of the day interacting with peers and teachers. Physically, their growth is slower but consistent, with an average gain of 6 to 7 cm in height and 3 kg in weight yearly.[24] They increase in their strength capabilities and coordination, speed, and balance. For example, they can throw and catch a tennis ball at about 6 years of age, learn to skip and play hopscotch, and balance well enough to ride a bicycle, skate, rollerblade, etc. Children improve in their anticipatory postural control, which means they are able to make some adjustments to their movements in anticipation of the task (eg, running to catch a ball on a basketball court, anticipating where a football will be passed or kicked). With such gross motor development, children are able to participate in team sports and physical education classes and gain proficiency at a range of ball games. During middle childhood, their fine motor skills become more refined and they have a well-established hand preference and become skilled in handwriting and arts and craft activities.[24(p207)] As their attention span and memory improves they are able to sit longer in class, pay closer attention to lessons, and have increased memory capacity (eg, for spelling, times tables, facts, and school rules).

According to Piaget's Stages of Cognitive Development, children between ages 7 and 12 go through the *Concrete Operational Stage.*[25] This stage is characterized by:

1. *Conservation:* The ability to recognize that 2 equal quantities of matter remain equal, even though they may appear different in shape or size.
2. *Seriation:* The understanding of relationships, indicated by the ability to arrange objects by size and length in sequence.
3. *Classification:* The ability to classify objects on more than one dimension, such as color and size.
4. *Decentering:* The ability to take into account multiple aspects of a problem to solve it.

For example, instead of believing that someone taller must be older, they understand many features need to be considered when age is being determined. This provides children with an ability to understand mathematics and science concepts, and helps them learn more about the world. Children at this stage enjoy playing games with rules and games that challenge them cognitively, requiring them to problem solve[24(p209)] (eg, board games and computer games).

During middle childhood, children demonstrate basic safety awareness in familiar situations. They are able to function independently in a variety of familiar community settings without assistance. This increased independence impacts the types of occupations they can perform. Not only do they become independent in self-care, they are able to get themselves ready for school and can prepare a simple snack, such as making themselves toast.[24(pp208-209)]

In addition, they are able to help out with chores at home (eg, taking out the trash, and feeding or walking the dog) and at school (eg, running an errand or taking orders to the school cafeteria).

With regard to social development, egocentric thought tends to decline during middle childhood. Children are able to work with others to solve problems in ordinary situations and are capable of performing in teams.[25(p335)] The peer group is central to children's personality development, and they often turn to friends and siblings for social support. They continue to do so during adolescence and may be subjected to increased pressure to conform in a variety of ways, such as the way they dress or talk. New roles and occupations during this period may include that of a team member (eg, playing in sports teams, scouting, music/gymnastics or ballet student) or member of chess or drama club. These occupations take the child away from immediate family members, positions them more independently in school and community contexts away from home, and situates them with peers who provide support as they experience new challenges as team or club members together. Inter-school or club sports and other competitions (debating or chess) provide avenues for group cohesion, team spirit, and the interdependence of team members.

Transitions

The transition to adolescence is recognized as a time of change for children and is often marked by the change from primary to secondary or high school, during which children frequently change school locations, have to cope with a larger peer group, a larger number of teachers, bigger size of schools, new curricula, and new modes of transport to and from school. It is common for the transition to secondary school to evoke anxiety, uneasiness, and worry in students prior to leaving primary school.[26,27] Some students transition from primary to secondary school smoothly, while others have difficulty maintaining support from friends when existing friendship networks are compromised by school change. This often leads to a shift in reliance upon family support during this transition period. Children with fewer social support resources initially may have difficulty expanding their support base in adolescence. Individual coping strategies adopted by the students are also recognized as a potential influence in the successful transition from primary to secondary school.[28(p80)]

When children experience conditions such as cerebral palsy (CP), this transition has the potential to be more difficult as the physical, communication, and perceptual challenges of this condition can make it more difficult to master larger physical spaces, use public transportation, carry books and materials over greater distances and between classes, and manage physical education and other aspects of the curriculum such as home economics and science experiments, etc, since these may require significant fine motor control. Adaptations to the curriculum and accommodations made within the school environment become necessary to enhance educational participation.[29]

Adolescence

Adolescence is described as a period of developmental transition from childhood to adulthood. It begins with puberty, and the "end of adolescence" is usually defined more by social and emotional choices and economic independence than by age.[30] Adolescence is a period of rapid physical and social emotional development and change. It is a time of adjustment to sexuality, bodily changes, role changes, and changing status within family and society. Physically, individuals undergo puberty, which includes an adolescent growth spurt, maturation of reproductive organs, and development of secondary sexual characteristics (eg, growth of pubic and underarm hair, development of breasts for girls, and voice changes and facial hair growth for boys). With these physical developments, adolescents become more aware of their appearance at the same time that their bodies begin changing dramatically.[30(p219)] This can make physical changes difficult to deal with emotionally. Beside basic self-care occupations, new grooming occupations develop during puberty in response to increasing awareness of appearance. For example, adolescents engage in self-care activities such as applying make-up, shaving, styling hair, using female hygiene products, and contraception.

In addition, adolescent youth also participate in a range of instrumental self-care occupations. As they increase in independence, they are involved in a range of new occupations, related to participation in their own health care, taking care of finances, using transport in the community, participating in home maintenance (eg, tidying bedroom, yard work), and preparing food. With more autonomy, they may be involved in a range of structured and unstructured leisure occupations.[30(p231)] Structured leisure occupations include team sports, youth groups, art, and classes. Examples of unstructured leisure occupations are hanging out with friends at the beach, watching television, window shopping, and reading a magazine. The productivity occupations that adolescents engage in include pursuing education and training, full time or part time work, and volunteering.

According to Piaget's Stages of Cognitive Development, adolescents are in the *Formal Operations Stage*, from the age of around 11 to 16 and onwards. They develop more logical thought processes and the ability to think about things hypothetically. This facilitates their development in faith, trust, beliefs, and spirituality.[31] Youth are able to think creatively and critically. They also develop enhanced *meta-cognition*, which is the ability to monitor and be aware of one's own mental processes and strategies. This allows individuals to think about and reflect on how they feel and what they are thinking. However, youth may also appear indecisive because their thinking becomes multidimensional rather than linear.

In terms of *social emotional development*, adolescent youth are establishing a sense of identity. They begin to integrate the opinions of influential others (eg, parents, other adults such as teachers, friends, etc) into their own views, influencing their likes and dislikes. They gain the ability to take on another's perspective and show empathy, the ability to understand the other's emotional responses. Young people become more altruistic, which is the conscious or unconscious effort to consider others with equal or greater concern than one's own self. At the same time, they feel more strongly about guilt and shame, which are negative feelings associated with the activation of the conscience. With these developments, they join in groups or align themselves with peers who share interests or beliefs; for example, an animal rights group or an environmental group. Adolescence is also the stage where they learn more about intimacy and sexuality. Intimacy is usually first learned within the context of same-sex friendships, and then further develops in romantic relationships. How teens are informed about their bodily changes and developing sexuality will largely determine whether or not they develop a healthy sexual identity.[30(p219)] Young people learn to become interdependent, in that they start to become more emotionally and economically self-reliant, while at the same time being responsible to their family, peers, and wider communities; learning that they need others' support to varying extents with particular tasks while they can be quite independent at others.

Assessing the Occupations and Performance of Children and Youth

As the individual develops through childhood into adolescence, he or she becomes more independent in many tasks, such as doing school work, self-care, choosing friends, and engaging in play/leisure activities. There are a number of measures that occupational therapy practitioners can use to assess occupational performance in children and young people depending on their age and the occupational focus required. Table 9-1 lists assessments that focus on play and leisure occupations, Table 9-2 presents measures of school participation, and Table 9-3 presents measures of self-care performance. A new assessment that does not fit into the categorization of the 3 tables but is worth noting is the Participation and Environment Measure for Children and Youth (PEM-CY).[53] It is a parent-report instrument that examines participation frequency, extent of involvement, and desire for change in

sets of activities typical for the home, school, or community. This measure has demonstrated moderate-to-good reliability and ability to detect differences between groups of children and young people with and without disabilities.[53(p1034)]

Families have a significant role in shaping the development of childrens' well-being during their early years. As children grow older, peers take on a more important role in shaping their personalities and belief systems. Their communities either afford opportunities for engagement or provide barriers to the growing child's and young person's engagement in different occupations. For example, within a safe community or neighborhood that has child friendly spaces, traffic-calmed streets, and a neighborhood child safety watch program, it is more likely that children will be allowed to walk to school, play in the local park or on the sidewalk, or have access to the local shops. The next section of this chapter will discuss factors that impact on occupational performance of children and youth.

FACTORS IMPACTING OCCUPATIONAL PERFORMANCE

Health and Developmental Conditions

Health conditions caused by disease processes such as juvenile arthritis or leukemia can influence a child's occupational performance. Developmental conditions, on the other hand, are not related to diseases per se, but refer to cognitive, physical, and/or neurological difficulties that usually occur in the early years of life. As listed in Table 9-4, many of these developmental conditions result in significantly reduced capacity to engage in major life activities, such as play learning, community mobility, and self-care. Early detection of and early intervention for children with developmental conditions are both critical to the well-being of children and their families.[65] While congenital conditions are present at birth (eg, Down syndrome), acquired conditions refer to those that develop during childhood, such as head injury or childhood cancer. Accidents are a major cause of many acquired conditions, such as brain injury and fractures. Some of the conditions listed in Table 9-5 may result in short-term or long-term hospitalization, causing children to lose opportunities to perform their typical daily occupations.

A number of mental health conditions can be acquired and are listed in Table 9-6. These more often declare themselves during middle childhood and adolescence although their antecedents may have been obvious earlier. Depending on the severity of the developmental, acquired and/or mental health conditions, some have short-term or transient effects on the child's occupational performance.

Table 9-1. *Measures of Play/Leisure Occupations*

Assessment	Construct or Factor Assessed	Description and Reference	Where It Can Be Obtained
Revised Knox Pre-school Play Scales (PPS-R)	Play behavior	A rated observation tool for children between 0 to 6 years old. Knox S. The Revised Knox Preschool Play scale. In: Parham LD, Fazio LS, eds. *Play in Occupational Therapy for Children*. 2nd ed. St. Louis, MO: Mosby Elsevier; 2008:55-70.[32]	Can be found in the book titled *Play in Occupational Therapy for Children* (2nd ed), as referenced.[32] http://www.assessment-toolshop.com/category.php3?category=Ass%20Play
Test of Playfulness	Playfulness during free play	A rated observation tool for children between 6 months to 18 years. Bundy A. *Test of Playfulness*. Lidcombe, NSW: University of Sydney; 2003.[33]	Can be found in the book titled *Play in Occupational Therapy for Children* (2nd ed), as referenced.[34] http://www.assessment-toolshop.com/category.php3?category=Ass%20Play
Symbolic Play Test	Symbolic play	A rated observation tool with a set of standardized toys, for children between 1 to 3 years old; takes 10 to 15 minutes to complete. Lowe M, Costello AJ. *Symbolic Play Test*. London, England: NFER-Nelson; 1989.[35]	http://www.gl-assessment.co.uk/products/symbolic-play-test
The Symbolic and Imaginative Play Developmental Checklist (SIPDC)	Pretend play	A tool that can be scored via interview or observation; suitable for 18 months to 5 years. Stagnitti K. *Learn to Play: A Practical Program to Develop a Child's Imaginative Play Skills*. West Brunswick, Victoria: Co-Ordinates Publications; 1998.[36]	Can be found in the book titled *Learn to Play: A Practical Program to Develop a Child's Imaginative Play Skills,* as referenced.[36] http://www.therapy-bookshop.com/category.php3?category=Play
Child-Initiated Pretend Play Assessment (ChiPPA)	Pretend play	A rated observation tool with a set of standardized toys, for ages 3 to 7; takes 30 minutes to administer and score. Stagnitti K. *The Child-Initiated Pretend Play Assessment. Manual and Kit*. Melbourne: Co-Ordinates Publications; 2007.[37]	http://www.assessment-toolshop.com/category.php3?category=Ass%20Play
Play History	Play experiences and opportunity	An interview to find out about play experiences and opportunities; suitable from infancy to adolescence. Bryze K. Narrative contributions to the play history. In: Parham LD, Fazio LS, eds. *Play in Occupational Therapy for Children*. 2nd ed. St Louis, MO: Mosby Elsevier; 2008:43-54.[38]	Can be found in the book titled *Play in Occupational Therapy for Children* (2nd ed) as referenced.[38] http://www.assessment-toolshop.com/category.php3?category=Ass%20Play

(continued)

Table 9-1 (continued).   *Measures of Play/Leisure Occupations*

Assessment	Construct or Factor Assessed	Description and Reference	Where It Can Be Obtained
Pediatric Interest Profiles (PIP)	Play and use of leisure time	A self-report tool to assess level of participation in play and leisure for children and youth 6 to 21 years old. Henry AD. *Pediatric Interest Profiles*. San Antonio, TX: Harcourt Assessment; 2000.[39]	http://www.cade.uic.edu/ moho/productDetails. aspx?aid=43
Paediatric Activity Card Sort (PACS)	Engagement in a range of activities (including play)	A self-report tool that allows children to identify activities they are currently doing as well as they want to, need to, or are expected to do; suitable for children and youth 5 to 14 years old; takes 20 to 25 minutes to complete. Mandich A, Polatajko H, Miller L, Baum C. *Paediatric Activity Card Sort*. Ottawa, ON: CAOT Publication ACE; 2004.[40]	http://www.ot.utoronto.ca/ faculty/documents/pacs.pdf
Children's Assessment of Participation and Enjoyment/ Preferences for Activities of Children (CAPE/PAC)	Participation in, enjoyment of, and preferences for activities	A self-administered or interviewer-assisted tool for assessing day-to-day participation in activities outside of the school curriculum; suitable for children and youth 6 to 21 years old. King G, Law M, King S, Hurley P, Hanna S, Kertory M. *Children's Assessment of Participation and Enjoyment/ Preferences for Activities of Children*. San Antonio, TX: Harcourt Assessment; 2004.[41]	The CAPE and PAC are packaged together and are available through Harcourt Assessment, Inc. http://www.pearson-assessments.com/ HAIWEB/Cultures/en-us/ Productdetail.htm?Pid=076-1606-432&Mode=summary

Other mental health conditions may result in disabilities that lead to a long-term impact on children's ability to perform various different occupations and engage in appropriate occupational roles.

Table 9-7 provides a summary of several occupation-centered interventions for children with CP and Developmental Coordination Disorder (DCD), both of which impact on children's motor skill acquisition. Some of the evidence underpinning these interventions is summarized in Tables 9-8 and 9-9.

Environmental Influences

Contemporary development theories accept that both a child's biology and his or her environment play a role in shaping developmental change and growth. **Bronfenbrenner's Bioecological or Ecological Systems Theory**[89] describes influences on behavior as a series of layers, or

onion rings, where each ring has an influence on the next. The innermost level represents the individual, which is then surrounded by differing levels of environmental influences known as the microsystems, mesosystems, exosystems, macrosystems, and chronosystems. The microsystem refers to a setting in which a child interacts with others on a daily basis.[89] The family is the most important influence on a young child, because that is where the child spends the most time and these relationships have the most emotional influence on the child. Other important environments may include the child's extended family, early care and education programs, health care settings, and other community learning sites (eg, schools, neighborhoods, libraries and playgrounds). The child's and adolescent's social environment of family, friends, and workplace (microsystem) are embedded within the physical environment and characterized by a geographic location and presence or absence of community facilities (mesosystem),

Table 9-2.   *Measures of School Work Occupations*

Assessment	Construct or Factor Assessed	Description and Reference	Where It Can Be Obtained
School Version of the Assessment of Motor and Process Skills (School AMPS)	Motor and process skills, as reflected in performance of school-related activities	A naturalistic, observation-based assessment conducted in the context of a student's natural classroom setting during his or her typical routine, while the student performs schoolwork tasks assigned by the teacher; suitable for children 3 to 12 years old. Fisher AG, Bryze K, Hume V, Griswold LA. *School AMPS: School Version of the Assessment of Motor and Process Skills.* 2nd ed. Fort Collins, CO: Three Star Press; 2005.[42]	http://www.ampsintl.com/SchoolAMPS/
School Function Assessment	Functional performance in school	A teacher-report assessment tool to assess a student's performance of functional tasks and activities in school; suitable for children 5 to 12 years old or kindergarten through grade 6. Coster W, Deeney T, Haltiwanger J, Haley S. *School Function Assessment.* San Antonio, TX: Psychological Corporation; 1998.[43]	http://www.pearsonassessments.com/HAIWEB/Cultures/en-us/Productdetail.htm?Pid=076-1615-709&Mode=summary
School Setting Interview (SSI)	Student-environment fit	A semi-structured interview designed to assess student-environment fit and identify the need for accommodations for students with disabilities in the school setting; suitable for children and youth 10 years old and above. Hemmingsson H, Egilson S, Hoffman O, Kielhofner G. *A User's Manual for the School Setting Interview, Version 3.0.* Chicago, Il: MOHO Clearinghouse; 2005.[44]	http://www.cade.uic.edu/moho/productDetails.aspx?aid=10 http://www.fsa.akademikerhuset.se/Global/Om_forbundet/Other%20languages/English/schoolsettinginterview.pdf
School Outcomes Measure	Functional performance in school	A rated observation tool to assess functional performance in school; suitable for children and youth 3 to 21 years old; can be completed in approximately 10 minutes. McEwen IR, Arnold SH, Hansen LH, Johnson D. Interrater reliability and content validity of a minimal data set to measure outcomes of students receiving school-based occupational therapy and physical therapy. *Physical and Occupational Therapy in Pediatrics.* 2003;23(2):77-95.[45]	http://www.ah.ouhsc.edu/somresearch/adminGuide.pdf

Table 9-3.   Measures of Self-Maintenance and Self-Care Occupations

Assessment	Construct or Factor Assessed	Description and Reference	Where It Can Be Obtained
Pediatric Evaluation of Disability Inventory (PEDI)	Self-care, mobility and social function	An assessment tool that can be scored via observation, interview, or caregiver report to determine the functional levels of children age 6 months to 7 years old; takes 45 to 60 minutes to complete. Haley SM, Coster WJ, Ludlow L, Haltiwanger J, Andrellos P. *Administration Manual for the Pediatric Evaluation of Disability Inventory.* San Antonio, TX: Psychological Corporation; 1992.[46]	http://www.pearsonassessments.com/HAIWEB/Cultures/en-us/Productdetail.htm?Pid=076-1617-647&Mode=summary
Functional Independence Measure for Children (WeeFIM)	Self-care, mobility, and cognition	This assessment can be completed via clinician observation or interview with caregiver; suitable for children between 6 months and 7 years old. Uniform Data System for Medical Rehabilitation. *WEEFIM II System Clinical Guide.* Ver.sion 6.0. Amherst, NY: Uniform Data System for Medical Rehabilitation; 2006.[47]	http://www.weefim.org/WebModules/WeeFIM/Wee_About.aspx
Activities Scales for Kids (ASK)	Basic and IADL	A child or parent report assessment tool to assess the physical functioning of children and youth between 5 and 15 years old. Young NL. *The Activities Scale for Kids Manual.* Toronto, ON: The Hospital for Sick Children; 1996.[48]	http://www.activitiesscaleforkids.com/
Assessment of Motor and Process Skills (AMPS)	Motor and process skills in ADL	An observation-based assessment conducted while the person is doing chosen, familiar, and life-relevant ADL tasks; suitable for children 2 years old and above. Fisher AG. *The Assessment of Motor and Process Skills.* 3rd ed. Fort Collins, CO: Three Star Press; 1999.[49]	http://www.amps-intl.com/AMPS/
Vineland Adaptive Behavior Scales, Second Ed. (Vineland-II)	Daily living skills, communication, socialization, motor skills	A semi-structured interview or rating scale for caregiver and teacher to report the daily living skills of a child; suitable for individuals between birth to age 90; takes 20 to 60 minutes to complete. Sparrow SS, Cicchetti DV, Bella DA. The Vineland *Adaptive Behavior Scales.* 2nd ed. Circle Pines, MN: AGS Publishing; 2005.[50]	https://www.pearsonclinical.com.au/products/view/244
Adaptive Behavior Assessment System, Second Ed. (ABAS-II)	Adaptive skills including self-care, communication, community use	An assessment that can be completed by observation, interview or parent and teacher report; suitable from birth to 89 years old; takes 15 to 20 minutes to complete. Harrison P, Oakland T. *Adaptive Behavior Assessment System Manual.* 2nd ed. San Antonio, TX: Psychological Corporation; 2003.[51]	http://www.pearsonpsychcorp.com.au/productdetails/21
Children Helping Out: Responsibilities, Expectations and Supports (CHORES)	Household task performance	It is a tool that measures school-age children's participation in household tasks (including self-care and family-care activities); suitable for children between 6 to 11 years old; based on parent/caregiver report. Dunn L. Validation of the CHORES: A measure of school-aged children's participation in household tasks. *Scandinavian Journal of Occupational Therapy.* 2004;11:179-190.[52]	Contact author to enquire about assessment tool.

Table 9-4.   *Examples of Common Developmental Conditions*

Common Developmental Conditions	Brief Description of Condition
Autism spectrum disorder (ASD)	ASDs are a group of developmental disabilities that can cause significant social, communication, and behavioral challenges that include autistic disorder, asperger syndrome, and pervasive development disorder-not otherwise Specified (PDD-NOS).[54]
Attention deficit hyperactivity disorder (ADHD)	ADHD is diagnosed in children who display developmentally inappropriate levels of inattention or hyperactivity with impairments in adaptive functioning at home, at school, and/or in social situations.[55]
Cerebral palsy (CP)	CP is a disorder of movement and posture that is caused by a nonprogressive abnormality of the immature brain.[56]
Down syndrome	Down syndrome is a chromosomal abnormality associated with mental retardation. Affected individuals have similar facial features. Children with Down syndrome have an increased risk of medical problems such as congenital heart disease, sensory impairments, and epilepsy.[57]
Developmental coordination disorder (DCD)	DCD is a condition where, despite average intelligence and the absence of identifiable medical or neurological conditions, children have marked impairment in the development of motor coordination that significantly affects their daily activities at school and home.[58]
Language impairment	Language impairment is diagnosed based on language abilities that are below age expectations in one or more language domains. It affects the acquisition and use of spoken language, as well as written language.
Fragile X syndrome	Fragile X syndrome is the most common inherited cause of mental retardation. It is an X-linked disorder, in which most affected boys present with a characteristic pattern of physical, cognitive, and behavior impairments, whereas a fraction of carrier girls manifest less severe symptoms.[59]
Fetal alcohol syndrome (FAS)	FAS is a condition resulting from alcohol abuse during pregnancy. Children experience neurobehavioral abnormalities, including developmental delay, growth problems, and other physical effects.[60]
Specific learning disabilities (SLD) or dyslexia	SLD is a disorder in which a healthy child with average intelligence fails to learn adequately in one or more school subjects.[61] Children with SLD appear to have impairment in some language and/or visual perceptual development that interferes with learning. A specific learning difficulty in the area of literacy (reading/spelling) is also referred to as dyslexia, where as specific learning difficulties with numerical information and arithmetic is referred to as dyscalculia.
Mental retardation (intellectual disability)	A person with mental retardation has significantly below average intellectual functioning and impairment in adaptive abilities.[62]
Prader-Willi syndrome	Prader-Willi syndrome is a chromosomal abnormality characterized by short stature, failure to thrive during infancy, hyperphagia (increased appetite), and small hands and feet. Associated complications include mental retardation, behavioral problems, obstructive sleep apnea, and neonatal temperature instability.[63]
Tourette syndrome	Tourette syndrome is a severe tic disorder, and the criteria for diagnosis include motor tics in combination of vocal tics and symptoms that persist for more than 1 year. Tics are involuntary movements during wakefulness. Motor tics may include head shaking, eye blinking, and shoulder shrugging. Examples of vocal tics include coughing, humming, sniffing, and repetitive grunting.[64]

Table 9-5.   *Examples of Common Acquired Childhood Health Conditions*

Common Childhood Health Conditions	Brief Description of Condition
Asthma	Asthma is a common childhood condition with widespread narrowing of the bronchial airways that changes in severity over short periods of time, leading to cough, wheezing, and difficulty in breathing. The onset of asthma is usually early in life and may be accompanied by other manifestations of hypersensitivity, such as hay fever and dermatitis.[66]
Juvenile rheumatoid arthritis	Juvenile rheumatoid arthritis is an autoimmune disease that can cause inflammation of synovium (synovial cells), increased joint fluid, and arthritic changes in childhood.[67]
Leukemia and other childhood cancers	Leukemia is a cancer of the bone marrow and blood. It is the most common type of childhood cancer. The most common types in children are acute lymphocytic leukemia (ALL) and acute myelogenous leukemia (AML). Leukemia may cause bone and joint pain, weakness, bleeding, fever, weight loss, and other symptoms. Other common types of childhood cancer include brain and other nervous system tumors and bone cancer.[68]
Meningitis	Meningitis is a disease caused by the inflammation of the protective membranes covering the brain and spinal cord, known as the meninges. It can be caused by bacteria, viruses, physical injury, or certain drugs. The inflammation is usually caused by an infection of the fluid surrounding the brain and spinal cord.[69]
Musculoskeletal injuries	Musculoskeletal injuries in childhood are common, due largely to patterns of childhood play and behavior. Common injuries include limb fractures and joint injuries.[70]
Traumatic brain injury (TBI)	Head trauma is a common childhood event with a broad spectrum of consequences. Depending on the severity, type, and location of the injury, outcome may range from complete recovery to severe functional disability. Persistent motor, communication, cognitive, behavior, and sensory impairments may result from TBI.[71]

which is in turn embedded within the institutional or policy environment of different levels of government (exo-system).

One example of the policy environment is the interest/concern shown by politicians, health economists, and those involved with the health and well-being of children with physical inactivity in children and consequent growing levels of obesity. Socioenvironmental considerations contribute to this health issue.[90] With the expanding influence of digital technologies such as televisions, computers, the Internet, and hand-held games, children are spending more and more time in sedentary occupations. Researchers are exploring sustainable approaches to ensuring children engage in adequate amounts of physical activity. For example, children's involvement in incidental physical activity such as active travel that includes walking or riding a bicycle to or from local destinations (eg, school or a park)[91] has become a recent focus. Factors influencing engagement in such activities include physical, economic,

and political-cultural considerations. Occupational therapy practitioners are also taking on a more active role in advocating for promotion of a more engaging urban design to support physical activity, as well as community occupation-based approaches targeted at increasing activity participation.[90(p9),92]

Environments clearly have an impact on the healthy development of young people. Young people living in unsafe neighborhoods are more vulnerable to risky behaviors such as substance and alcohol abuse. When they are exposed to failure at school or family financial problems, they may inadequately manage stress and develop poor coping mechanisms, such as alcohol and illicit drug use. Accidents are the most common cause of injury and death for adolescents, the most common cause being motor vehicle accidents.[31(p400)] Political-social-cultural efforts can be made to reduce adolescents' engagement in risky activities. For example, education and health promotion efforts have focused on advising against substance abuse

Table 9-6.   *Examples of Common Mental Health Conditions in Children and Youth*

Mental Health Conditions	Brief Description of Condition
Separation anxiety disorder	Children with separation anxiety disorder experience excessive anxiety and often panic whenever they are separated from home or a parent. They may be extremely anxious being in school or away from home.[72]
Oppositional defiant disorder	Children with this condition argue repeatedly with adults, lose their temper, and feel great anger and resentment. They frequently defy rules and requests, annoy others, and blame others for their own mistakes and problems.[72]
Conduct disorder	Conduct disorder can be considered a more severe pattern of oppositional defiant disorder. Children may go further in repeatedly violating the rights of others. They are often aggressive and may be physically cruel to persons or animals, deliberately destroy others' property, lie and cheat, skip school, or run away from home.[72]
Mood disorders	Depression and mania are 2 extreme dominating emotions in mood disorder. Depression is a low, sad state in which life seems bleak and its challenges seem overwhelming. Sufferers from depression lose interest in daily activities such as play and school.[72] Sufferers from mania experience excessive cheerfulness, are bursting with energy, and may have an exaggerated belief that the world is theirs for the taking.[72] People who undergo periods of mania that alternate with periods of depression are diagnosed as having bipolar disorder.
Elimination disorders	Enuresis refers to repeated involuntary (or in some case intentional) bed wetting or wetting's of one's clothes, which can happen at night or during the day.[72] Encopresis is the repeated defecating in inappropriate places.[72]
Eating disorders	Eating disorders refer to an obsession with thinness. With anorexia nervosa, one relentlessly pursues thinness and loses so much weight that he or she may starve himself or herself to death.[72] Sufferers of bulimia nervosa go on frequent eating binges during which they uncontrollably consume large quantities of food, then force themselves to vomit or take other strong steps to prevent gaining weight.[72]
Schizophrenia	Sufferers from schizophrenia may hear voices other people do not hear or have a false belief that others are plotting to harm them. It is understood as a developmental brain disorder that leads to hallucination and delusion.[73]
Suicide	Suicides refer to a self-inflicted death in which a person acts intentionally, directly or consciously. Teenage suicides have been linked with clinical depression, low self-esteem, and feeling of hopelessness, and can be caused by long-term pressures, such as social isolation, inadequate peer relationships, and family conflict.[72]
Post-traumatic stress disorder (PTSD)	PTSD is considered an anxiety disorder that some people develop after seeing or living through an event that caused or threatened serious harm or death. Symptoms of PTSD include strong and unwanted memories of the trauma, bad dreams, emotional numbness, intense guilt, or worry.[74]

and setting up youth information networks to assist youth and their families in identifying affordable, and interest-linked activities and accessible recreation options within the local community.[93]

Personal Factors

Apart from environmental factors, there are personal factors that influence the occupational performance of an individual. According to the International Classification of Functioning, Disability and Health ICF,[94] personal

Table 9-7. Interventions Supporting Children's Skill Acquisition for Children With Developmental Coordination Disorder and Cerebral Palsy as Illustrations of Developmentally Appropriate and Occupation-Centered Interventions

Construct, Mechanism/Factor, Intervention Goal	Intervention and Reference	How It Relates to PEOP
Examples for Developmental Coordination Disorder		
Acquisition of child-chosen occupational goals for children with DCD (eg, dressing, bike riding, hair brushing/styling, basketball, shoelace tying).	Cognitive Orientation for Daily Occupational Performance (CO-OP) uses a global problem-solving strategy and domain-specific strategies to support skill acquisition using therapist-guided child discovery of strategies.[75]	Focuses on the child's occupations of choice through child chosen goals, and enhancing their occupational performance through promoting and enhancing skill acquisition.
Improvement of academic skills in classroom of children with DCD (eg, handwriting, other motor-based school and learning skills).	MATCH Strategy (Modify task, Alter expectations, Teach the task, Change the environment, Help by understanding) is used by occupational therapists working with teachers to help them enhance children's performance at school.[76,77]	Focuses on changing the task (occupation), the environment, and/or improving the child's abilities; hence enhancing occupational performance.
Children's and parents' goals related to their children/parenting (eg, children with DCD handwriting, homework, bike riding, morning routine).	Occupational Performance Coaching (OPC)—occupational therapists work with parents to coach them to assist their children to develop skills needed for goal achievement at home, school, or in the community.[78]	Focuses on coaching parents to help their children or improve the parents' occupational performance. Focuses on environmental changes, improving child's abilities/skills, and also altering the task/occupations over which parents have control.
Examples for Cerebral Palsy		
Enhancing uni-manual ability to support the development of self-identified skills necessary for the performance of occupational goals for children with congenital hemiplegia.	Constraint-induced movement therapy (CIMT) involves constraint, by means of glove, splints, or other device, to the non-hemiplegic hand; coupled with engaging the child in activities (either intensively delivered or distributed over time) requiring the use of the child's hemiplegic hand/limb.[79]	CIMT is child-focused, as it imposes a constraint on a child's upper limb on the assumption that forced use will enhance upper limb abilities in the child's hemiplegic arm. It is delivered through engagement in meaningful daily activities (either in the child's environment or in a group setting) that are related to the child's occupational goals and are developmentally appropriate.
Enhancing bimanual abilities to support the development of self-identified skills necessary for the performance of occupational goals.	Hand Arm Bimanual Intensive Training (HABIT) provides intensive training of bimanual coordination.[80]	HABIT is occupational goal-focused and involves practice of self-identified activities alongside engaging developmentally appropriate activities, which rely on bimanual performance. Engagement in these activities is subjected to practice.

(continued)

Table 9-7 (continued).   *Interventions Supporting Children's Skill Acquisition for Children With Developmental Coordination Disorder and Cerebral Palsy as Illustrations of Developmentally Appropriate and Occupation-Centered Interventions*

Construct, Mechanism/Factor, Intervention Goal	Intervention and Reference	How It Relates to PEOP
Enabling the performance of child- and family-identified functional goals.	Task/Context-Focused Approach focuses on achievement of child-identified and family-identified functional goals through a range of solution options, not necessarily requiring a change in the way the child performs the activity. Some key tenets are optimizing motivation for engagement by selection of age-appropriate tasks, identifying and modifying constraints to achieving these, and providing opportunity for practice.[81]	The primary focus of this intervention is identification and planning strategies which address constraints/enablers in the task and/or environment for the child. Any involvement of measures addressing the way the child performs a task is time-limited and only at the level of activity/participation.
Enhancing functional performance in seating.	Adaptive seating interventions for children with CP aim to improve postural control, activity performance, and participation in everyday activities by enhancing postural stability and optimizing volitional arm and hand function by modifying abnormal tonal patterns.[82]	Environment is the primary means of intervention. Modifications to seating are individualized to optimize an individual's comfort and function.

factors include gender, age, coping styles, social background, education, past and current experience, overall behavior pattern, character, and other factors that influence how a health condition is experienced by the individual. Personal factors affect an individual's ability to function and participate in the society. In this section, the following *personal factors* will be discussed in more details: gender and culture, temperament, resilience, learning style, and motivation.

Gender and Culture

Gender and culture interact in society to influence the occupations and activities engaged in by children and young people. There are particular behavioral expectations and ceremonial activities that are expected rites of passage for boys and girls from various religious and cultural groups. For example, Jewish boys at approximately 13 years of age prepare for their Bar Mitzvah to recognize their coming of age and ability to be responsible for their own actions allowing them to become fully engaged in Jewish rituals, traditions, and all areas of Jewish community life. The equivalent ritual and ceremony for girls at age 12 years is the Bat Mitzvah.

In Islamic society, girls are required to conform to particular dress codes and their societal roles, and opportunities are governed by Islamic law and beliefs; the extent of which varies in different communities. These traditions may restrict opportunities for Muslim girls to fully participate in the same activities and occupations of their non-Muslim friends when living in Western societies. These differences in roles and expectations need to be understood and are either accepted or rejected by young people as they develop the capacity to make independent decisions and become more self-determined. Particular roles determined by cultural and religious beliefs will impact on the occupations engaged in by children and young people and the environments in which they perform these occupations.

Table 9-8.   Evidence Table for Selected Interventions for Developmental Coordination Disorder

Study/Reference	Aim of Study	Methods	Participants	Results and Outcome(s)	Conclusion(s) and Implications	Level/Type of Evidence	Statistical Probability or Effect Size
Pilot RCT of CO-OP[83]	This study aimed to determine whether CO-OP was more effective than standard occupational therapy intervention for children 7 to 12 years with DCD.	RCT with 2 arms: (1) CO-OP and (2) standard occupational therapy treatment	20 children age 7 to 12 with motor difficulties <15% on motor test; normal intelligence	Improvement in CO-OP group greater than CTA group on COPM scores, VABS, and PQRS, but not on BOTMP.	Needs replication with larger numbers plus control group. At follow up, CO-OP group had maintenance of motor skills and acquired strategies.	Single RCT	Not provided.
Partnering for Change (P4C)[77]	The goals of P4C are to facilitate earlier identification, build capacity of educators and parents to manage DCD, and improve children's participation in school and at home.	Descriptive study about outcomes using questionnaires and interviews; 8 practitioners worked in schools during 2009-2010. Their mandate was to build capacity through collaboration and coaching, the school became the "client," rather than any individual student.	Over 2600 students and 160 teachers in 11 elementary schools received services during the project	Results from questionnaires and individual interviews indicated that this model was highly successful in increasing teachers' knowledge and capacity.	P4C intervention holds promise for transforming service delivery in schools. Still needs testing with control schools who receive standard occupational therapy school-based services aimed at child vs classroom.	Phase 2 Feasibility Study Mixed Methods.	Not provided.
OPC Study[84]	This study examined the effectiveness of occupational performance coaching in improving children's and mothers' occupational performance and mothers' parenting self-competence.	A one-group time series design was used to evaluate changes in children's (n = 29) and mothers' (n = 28) occupational performance at: (1) pre-waitlist, (2) pre-intervention, (3) post-intervention, and (4) 6 weeks follow-up	Twenty-nine mothers of children aged 5 to 12 years who had concerns with their children's occupational performance	Significant improvements in occupational performance occurred post-intervention for children $P<.001$, and mothers $P<.001$, which were maintained 6 weeks following intervention. Mothers' self-competence in parenting also improved $P<.001$.	Findings provide preliminary evidence supporting the effectiveness of OPC to improve children's and mothers' occupational performance and mothers' parenting self-competence. Improvements sustained at 2 months follow up. Replication needed with other therapists and control group.	One-group time series design	$P<.001$

Table 9-9.   Evidence Table for Selected Interventions for Cerebral Palsy

Study and Reference	Aim of Study	Methods	Participants	Results and Outcome(s)	Conclusion(s) and Implications	Level or Type of Evidence	Statistical Probability or Effect Size
Sakzewski, Ziviani, Abbott, MacDonell, Jackson, and Boyd (2011)[85]	To determine if CIMT is more effective than bimanual training (BIM) in improving upper limb activity outcomes for children with congenital hemiplegia	Matched-pairs randomized trial. Children allocated to either CIMT or BIM group day camps (60 hours over 10 days)	63 children (mean age, 10.2 ± 2.7 years; 33 males, 30 females; 16 in Manual Ability Classification Level I, 47 level II, all cognitively and behaviorally capable of group participation	CIMT had superior outcomes compared to BIM for uni-manual capacity at 26 weeks (estimated mean difference, 4.4; 95% confidence interval, 2.2 to 6.7; P <.001 on the Melbourne Assessment of Unilateral Upper Limb Function (MUUL). There was no other significant difference between groups post-intervention. Both demonstrated significant improvements in bimanual performance at 3 weeks, with gains maintained by BIM at 26 weeks.	Only small differences between CIMT and BIM with both delivering significant gains in activity performance. CIMT resulted in greater changes to uni-manual capacity of hemiplegic upper limb compared to BIM highlighting the impact of specificity of practice. Both interventions support improvement in bimanual upper limb activity performance (NB lack of no/standard care intervention comparison group.)	RCT (Level II evidence)	P <.001 in favor of CIMT on MUUL at 26 weeks; no other statistical difference between groups

(continued)

Table 9-9 (continued).   Evidence Table for Selected Interventions for Cerebral Palsy

Study and Reference	Aim of Study	Methods	Participants	Results and Outcome(s)	Conclusion(s) and Implications	Level or Type of Evidence	Statistical Probability or Effect Size
Wallen, Ziviani, Naylor, Evans, Novak, and Herbert (2011)[86]	To determine if modified constraint-induced therapy (mCIT) confers significant benefits over intensive occupational therapy on self-identified occupational goals and upper limb outcomes for children with hemiplegic CP	Assessor-blinded pragmatic RCT. Children allocated to either mCIT or occupational therapy delivered in the family environment (dose goal was 2 hours/day × 6 days per week for 8 weeks).	50 children (27 males, 23 females; age range 19 months to 7 years 10 months) with hemiplegic CP (Manual Ability Classification System Levels I, $n = 2$; II, $n = 37$; III, $n = 8$; IV, $n = 1$).	No clinically or statistically significant difference between groups on COPM performance or satisfaction. Within group differences supported a mean increase in performance of 3.3 ± 1.9 and satisfaction of 3.5 ± 2.5.	Children in both intervention arms demonstrated clinically significant improvement on goal performance and satisfaction (COPM). No added advantage was conferred by mCIT on achieving occupational goals. (NB lack of no/standard care intervention comparison group.)	RCT (Level II evidence)	Group difference was not significant on primary outcome measure (COPM)
Law, Darrah, Pollock, Wilson, Russell, Walter, Rosenbaum, and Galuppi (2011)[87]	To evaluate the efficacy of a child-focused versus context-focused intervention in improving performance of functional tasks and mobility in young children with CP	Randomized controlled cluster designed trial	128 children (49 females, 79 males, Mean age 3 years 6 months ± 1 year 5 months; Gross Motor Classification System I–V). Therapists from 19 children's rehabilitation centers were block randomized to a treatment arm.	There were no significant differences on the primary outcome measure (Pediatric Evaluation of Disability Inventory) between intervention arms. The mean scores changed significantly for both groups on Functional Skills Scales ($P < .001$) and Caregiver Assistance Scales ($P < .02$).	Child or context focused approaches are equally effective and frequency of intervention maybe a critical component of successful intervention. (NB lack of no/standard care intervention comparison group.)	RCT (Level II evidence)	Group difference was not significant on primary outcome measure (PEDI)

(continued)

Table 9-9 (continued).   *Evidence Table for Selected Interventions for Cerebral Palsy*

Study and Reference	Aim of Study	Methods	Participants	Results and Outcome(s)	Conclusion(s) and Implications	Level or Type of Evidence	Statistical Probability or Effect Size
Ryan (2012)[88]	To review systematic reviews of adaptive seating interventions for children with cerebral palsy	Synthesis of systematic reviews of children and young people to the age of 20 with cerebral palsy.	Cochrane Database of systematic reviews, Ovid MEDLINE, Ovid HealthStar and PsychINFO data bases from 1990 to 2010 for search terms inclusive of children and young people to 20 years with CP and terms related to seating.	Search yielded 5 reviews of adaptive seating interventions that reported generally positive, but inconclusive evidence of effectiveness for postural control, seating posture, upper extremity function, and overall clinical outcomes.	Review authors consistently reported an inability to combine data from original studies, lack of appropriate outcome indicators, and lack of clarity around participant characteristics and intervention specificity. Recommendations were made for higher quality research evidence.	Systematic review of range of study designs.	Not appropriate on basis of data.

Temperament and Resilience

Rothbart and Bates[95] defined temperament as constitutionally-based individual differences in reactivity and regulation, with reactivity referring to the child's responsiveness to changes in the external and internal environment and regulation referring to ability to sustain focused attention and control impulses. By the term *constitutional*, they referred to the biological bases of temperament influenced over time by heredity, maturation, and experience. They distinguished among 3 dimensions of temperament during early childhood. The first is where the child falls in the range from shy to extroverted. The second refers to how readily a child shows negative emotions (eg, fearful, sad, anxious, anger). It is worth noting that temperament describes tendencies that are not continually expressed, but require eliciting conditions. For example, fearful children are not continually distressed, but under conditions of sudden change they may be more prone to a fearful reaction. The third is how well a child can sustain focused attention and inhibit certain actions.[96] Other terms that have been used to describe the dimension of self-regulation in various literatures include *inhibition*[97] and *effortful control*.[98]

Temperament plays a role in how children learn to regulate and express who they are.[97(p106)] Temperament has been found to support children in their attempts to play well and make friends. In a study with 135 preschool and kindergarten children, Fabes et al[98(p439)] found that children who were more self-regulated were observed to respond in more socially competent ways than those with low self-regulation. Apart from social participation, temperament also affects how children learn. Children who are able to sustain focused attention are able to participate better in their roles as students and engage better in learning.

Resilience has been defined as "the manifestation of positive adaptation despite life adversity."[99(pxxix)] The study of resilience involves identifying risk and protective factors. Risk factors increase a child's chances of developing psychological, emotional, and behavioral problems, and as a result possibly not functioning well in occupational performance. Examples of risk factors include parental unemployment, poverty, maternal depression, and residential instability. Protective factors range from intrapersonal (eg, intellectual ability, temperament, outlook on life), to familial (eg, supportive family), to educational (eg, school connectedness), and beyond.[100] The greater the number of protective factors, the more likely children will be resilient in the face of adverse circumstances.

Volition, Motivation, and Flow

Volition, the drive for occupation (or the decision to undertake an activity), is influenced by 3 factors. The first factor, personal causation, is a person's sense of personal effectiveness while performing a task.[101] The second factor is a child's values. Values are shaped by culture and context, and they define what is meaningful and important for a person who belongs to a certain family, community, society, or culture. The third factor that influences volition is interest. This refers to the enjoyment and satisfaction that a person gets from engaging in an activity.[101(p42)] Occupational performance is enhanced when the child feels that he or she is competent in doing the task, that it is meaningful, and he or she enjoys doing it.[102] For example, a child may not do well in skipping or moving lightly from one foot to another if he or she does not feel that he or she is good at skipping or has parents who perceive skipping as a waste of time compared to academic tasks or do not provide opportunities or materials for developing such physical skills, such as a rope or space to skip. Similarly, a child may not develop the skill if he or she does not enjoy skipping.

Along with volition, intrinsic motivation refers to engaging in authentic, self-authored, and personally endorsed activities.[103] When children are intrinsically motivated, they have high levels of spontaneous interest, excitement, confidence, persistence, and creativity. They want to do more of an occupation and persist to do better in it. This leads to enhanced performance, self-esteem, and general well-being.[103(p84)] The highest level of intrinsically motivated activity engagement is described by Cszentmihalyi as being the state of flow.[103(p84)] Flow is characterized by fulfilling personal enjoyment associated with engaging in an activity that is perceived as providing a "just-right" challenge for an individual's skills or capacities.[104] This occurs when there is an optimal match between the individual, the occupation, and the environment, hence ongoing activity engagement is facilitated. When flow occurs, an individual feels intense concentration or focusing on the task at hand. Loss of self-consciousness, self-control, and concept of time occur because he or she is enjoying intensely. In summary, occupational performance is enhanced when a child or young person feels that he or she has choice in what is being done, has a sense of competence in the performance of the task or activity, and undertakes the activity in the context of others who value and understand him or her and the importance of the activity. Ultimately, addressing these aspects enhances the individual's motivation and supports his or her self-efficacy[105] or a child's personal belief in his or her ability to make things happen.

Learning Styles

It is well-recognized that individuals have preferred learning styles and techniques. Learning styles group common ways that people learn. Learning styles have also been defined as those educational conditions under which a student is most likely to learn.[106] Everyone has a mix of learning styles; however, some individuals have a dominant style of learning with far less use of other styles. Others may find that they use different styles in different circumstances. To enhance occupational performance during daily activities, it is important to identify the child's learning style and help the child learn to use different ways. There are many different categorizations of the various learning styles. One common categorization is Fleming's VAK model,[107] which categorizes learning styles as follows:

- *Visual:* A preference to use pictures, images, and spatial understanding.
- *Auditory:* Learning better through listening to information by using sound and music.
- *Kinesthetic:* A preference to learn using body, hand, and sense of touch.

As children are developing and gaining independence, they are constantly learning. It is important to apply insights gained by understanding their learning styles during formalized classroom learning, as well as when they are learning other skills, such as sports, self-care, and games. For example, when teaching a game, instead of verbally describing the instructions, some children may require adults to show them how to do it and allow them to experience through doing and using trial and error.

SUMMARY

In this chapter we have briefly summarized the key occupations engaged in by children and youth throughout the stages of infancy and toddlerhood, early childhood, middle childhood, and adolescence. In describing the key developmental stages, we have referenced relevant theories that provide insights for practitioners working with children and youth, specifically Piaget's cognitive theories, Bronfenbrenner's ecological theory, and Bowlby's attachment theory. We have also provided a brief list of assessments that can be used to measure occupational performance during childhood and adolescence in relation to key occupations of self-care, school work, and productivity. Common developmental, health, and mental conditions have been described that may be experienced by children and adolescents and have the potential to impact on their occupational performance and participation. Table 9-10 lists organizations that support children and adolescents in the United States, and Table 9-11 lists relevant journals for these age groups. It is hoped that this brief introduction to these important life stages will provide a basis for undertaking further study and work in providing effective interventions for children and adolescents.

Table 9-10.   *Organizations That Serve Children and Adolescents*

Organization	Description	Website
American Academy of Child and Adolescent Psychiatry	Contains depression resource center with useful information resources for professionals on a range of mental health conditions affecting children and adolescents	http://www.aacap.org/AACAP/Families_and_Youth/Resource_Centers/Depression_Resource_Center/Home.aspx
Autism Speaks	Funds research and promotes public awareness of autism spectrum disorders; provides information on latest research	http://www.autismspeaks.org
BrainlineKids	Special website section of brainline.org with information on pediatric brain injury and resources	http://www.brainline.org/landing_pages/features/blkids.html
Center for Parent Information and Resources	US Department of Education–sponsored central information resource center for parent service organizations focusing on evidence and best practices for the education of children and adolescents with special needs	http://www.parentcenterhub.org
MyChild	Provides resources, support, and encouragement to persons affected by cerebral palsy and other neurological conditions.	http://cerebralpalsy.org
Federation for Children with Special Needs	Serves parents and professionals with information, training programs, and transition planning guidance	http://fcsn.org
Kids Get Arthritis Too	Provides information and other resources under the auspices of the Arthritis Foundation	http://www.kidsgetarthritistoo.org
National Organization for Rare Diseases (NORD)	Provides assistance, advocacy, and information for patients with rare diseases, their families, and other professionals	https://www.rarediseases.org
Rehabilitation Research and Training Center on Developmental Disabilities and Health	Conducts research and serves as an information resources for professionals and families serving persons with intellectual and developmental disabilities	http://www.rrtcadd.org
Early Childhood Technical Assistance Center	Provides extensive information for parents of infants and toddlers with disabilities regarding services available under federal legislation in the United States	http://ectacenter.org

Table 9-11. *Key Journals Relevant to Childhood and Adolescence*

Journal	Description	Website
Developmental Medicine and Child Neurology (DMCM)	A leading interdisciplinary journal in pediatrics. *DMCN* publishes a range of articles relevant to children with disabilities and their families; also of interest to professionals concerned with children with neurological conditions.	http://www.blackwellpublishing.com/journal.asp?ref=0012-1622&site=1
Child Indicators Research	*Child Indicators Research* is an international, peer-reviewed quarterly that focuses on measurements and indicators of children's well-being, and their usage within multiple domains and in diverse cultures. It explores how child indicators can be used to improve the development and well-being of children.	http://www.springer.com/social+sciences/well-being/journal/12187
Child: Care, Health and Development	A multidisciplinary journal that publishes research findings relevant to children's and young people's health care and development. It also addresses global health issues.	http://www.blackwell-publishing.com/journal.asp?ref=0305-1862
Journal of Adolescent Health	A multidisciplinary scientific journal publishing research findings in the field of adolescent medicine and health, ranging from the basic biological and behavioral sciences to public health and policy.	http://jahonline.org/aims
Journal of Developmental and Physical Disabilities	An interdisciplinary research journal featuring theory and research on the problems and strengths of persons with developmental and physical disabilities.	http://www.springer.com/psychology/child+%26+school+psychology/journal/10882
Journal of Learning Disabilities	An interdisciplinary journal with a broad range of articles on theory, research, intervention, and policy.	http://intl-ldx.sagepub.com/
The Journal of Special Education	Provides research articles and scholarly reviews on special education for individuals with mild to severe disabilities. Publishes traditional, ethnographic, and single-subject research; intervention studies, integrative reviews on timely issues, and critical commentaries; and special thematic issues.	http://sed.sagepub.com/
Physical & Occupational Therapy in Pediatrics	Publishes a wide range of research and editorial commentary relevant to practitioners working with children.	http://informahealth-care.com/pop
American Journal of Play	Includes material that describes major themes of play scholarship; including research about play and play theory, play and human development, public policy related to play, and cultural history through the world of play.	http://www.journalofplay.org/
Topics in Early Childhood Special Education	A practical journal for improving service delivery systems for preschool children with special needs.	http://tec.sagepub.com/

REFERENCES

1. Christiansen C, Baum MC, Bass-Haugen J, eds. *Occupational Therapy: Performance, Participation, and Well-Being*. Thorofare, NJ: SLACK Incorporated; 2005.

2. Christiansen C, Baum C. Person-environment-occupational performance: a conceptual model for practice. In: Christiansen C, Baum C, eds. *Occupational Therapy: Enabling Function and Well-Being*. 2nd ed. Thorofare, NJ: SLACK Incorporated; 1997:47-70.

3. Rodger S, Ziviani J. Children, their environments, roles and occupations in contemporary society. In: Rodger S, Ziviani J, eds. *Occupational Therapy with Children: Understanding Children's Occupations and Enabling Participation*. Oxford, England: Blackwell Publishing; 2006:3-21.

4. National Scientific Council on the Developing Child. *The Timing and Quality of Early Experiences Combine to Shape Brain Architecture*. Boston, MA: Center on the Developing Child at Harvard University; 2007.

5. Keuroghlian AS, Knudsen EI. Adaptive auditory plasticity in developing and adult animals. *Progress in Neurobiology*. 2007;82:109-121.

6. Buonomano DV, Merzenich MM. Cortical plasticity: from synapses to maps. *Annual Review of Neuroscience*. 1998;21:149-186.

7. Karmarkar UR, Dan Y. Experience-dependent plasticity in adult visual cortex. *Neuron*. 2006;52:577-585.

8. Mandich M. Infancy. In: Cronin A, Mandich M, eds. *Human Development and Performance: Throughout the Lifespan*. Clifton Park, NY: Thomson Delmar Learning; 2005:139-163.

9. Koontz-Lowman D. Family and disabilities issues in infancy. In: Cronin A, Mandich M, eds. *Human Development and Performance: Throughout the Lifespan*. Clifton Park, NY: Thomson Delmar Learning; 2005:164-175.

10. Bowlby J. *A Secure Base*. New York, NY: Basic Books; 1988.

11. Ainsworth M. Attachment retrospect and prospect. In: Parkes CM, Stevenson-Hind M, eds. *The Place of Attachment in Human Behavior*. New York, NY: Basic Books; 1982.

12. Sroufe L. Infant-caregiver attachment and patterns of adaptation in preschool: roots of maladaptation and competence. In: Perlmutter M, ed. *Development and Policy Concerning Children with Special Needs*. Vol. 16. The Minnesota Symposia on Child Psychology. Hillsdale, NJ: Erlbaum; 1983:41-83.

13. Bowlby J. The nature of the child's tie to his mother. *International Journal of Psychoanalysis*. 1958;39:350-371.

14. Meredith P. Introducing attachment theory to occupational therapy. *Australian Occupational Therapy Journal*. 2009;56:285-292.

15. Rubin KH, Krasnor L. Interpersonal problem solving and social competence in children. In: VanHassett VB, Hersen M, eds. *Handbook of Social Development*. New York, NY: Plenum; 1992:283-323.

16. Mandich M. Theoretical framework for human performance. In: Cronin A, Mandich M, eds. *Human Development and Performance: Throughout the Lifespan*. Clifton Park, NY: Thomson Delmar Learning; 2005:139-163.

17. Papalia DE, Olds SW, Feldman RD. Cognitive development during the first three years. In: Papalia DE, Olds SW, Feldman RD, eds. *Human Development International Edition*. 9th ed. New York, NY: McGraw Hill; 2004:147 -184.

18. Parten MB. Social participation among pre-school children. *Journal of Abnormal Social Psychology*. 1932;27(3):243-269.

19. Cronin A. Development in the preschool years. In: Cronin A, Mandich M, eds. *Human Development and Performance: Throughout the Lifespan*. Clifton Park, NY: Thomson Delmar Learning; 2005:176-197.

20. Papalia DE, Olds SW, Feldman RD. Theory and research. In: Papalia DE, Olds SW, Feldman RD, eds. *Human Development International Edition*. 9th ed. New York, NY: McGraw Hill; 2004:25-57.

21. Lim SM, Rodger S, Brown T. Assessments of learning-related skills and interpersonal skills constructs within early childhood environments in Singapore. *Infant and Child Development*. 2010;19(4):366-384.

22. Bandura A. *Social Learning Theory*. New York, NY: General Learning Press; 1977.

23. Turner SL. Introduction to special issue: transitional issues for K-16 students. *ASCA: Professional School Counseling*. 2007;10(3):224-226.

24. Cronin A. Middle childhood and school. In: Cronin A, Mandich M, eds. *Human Development and Performance: Throughout the Lifespan*. Clifton Park, NY: Thomson Delmar Learning; 2005:198-214.

25. Papalia DE, Olds SW, Feldman RD. Physical and cognitive development in middle childhood. In: Papalia DE, Olds SW, Feldman RD, eds. *Human Development International Edition*. 9th ed. New York, NY: McGraw Hill; 2004:307-347.

26. Sweetser GK. *Transition From Primary School to Secondary School: The Beginning of a Journey*. New Zealand Association for Research in Education and Australian Association for Research in Education (NZARE & AARE) Conference. Auckland, New Zealand: University of Queensland, Australia; 2003.

27. Carter EW, Clark NM, Cushing LS, Kennedy CH. Moving from elementary to middle school: supporting a smooth transition for students with severe disabilities. *Teaching Exceptional Children*. 2005;37(3):8-14.

28. Qualter P, Whiteley HE, Hutchinson JM, Pope DJ. Supporting the development of emotional intelligence competencies to ease the transition from primary to high school. *Educational Psychology in Practice*. 2007;23(1):79-95.

29. Jones F. *Experiences Informing Decisions Around the Transition from Primary to Secondary School for Adolescents with Cerebral Palsy*. Brisbane, Australia: The University of Queensland; 2011.

30. Simons DF. Adolescence development. In: Cronin A, Mandich M, eds. *Human Development and Performance: Throughout the Lifespan*. Clifton Park, NY: Thomson Delmar Learning; 2005:215-245.

31. Papalia DE, Olds SW, Feldman RD. Physical and cognitive development in adolescence. In: Papalia DE, Olds SW, Feldman RD, eds. *Human Development International Edition*. 9th ed. New York, NY: McGraw Hill; 2004:385-421.

32. Knox S. The Revised Knox Preschool Play scale. In: Parham LD, Fazio LS, eds. *Play in Occupational Therapy for Children*. St. Louis, MO: Mosby Elsevier; 2008:55-70.

33. Bundy A. *Test of Playfulness*. Lidcombe, NSW: University of Sydney; 2003.

34. Parham LD, Fazio LS, eds. *Play in Occupational Therapy for Children*. St. Louis, MO: Mosby Elsevier; 2008:55-70.

35. Lowe M, Costello AJ. *Symbolic Play Test*. London, England: NFER-Nelson; 1989.

36. Stagnitti K. *Learn to Play: A Practical Program to Develop a Child's Imaginative Play Skills*. West Brunswick, Victoria: Co-Ordinates Publications; 1998.

37. Stagnitti K. *The Child-Initiated Pretend Play Assessment: Manual and Kit*. Melbourne, Australia: Co-Ordinates Publications; 2007.

38. Bryze K. Narrative contributions to the play history. In: Parham LD, Fazio LS, eds. *Play in Occupational Therapy for Children.* St Louis, MO: Mosby Elsevier; 2008:43-54.

39. Henry AD. *Pediatric Interest Profiles.* San Antonio, TX: Hardcourt Assessment; 2000.

40. Mandich A, Polatajko H, Miller L, Baum C. *Pediatric Activity Card Sort.* Ottawa, ON: CAOT Publication ACE; 2004.

41. King G, Law M, King S, Hurley P, Hanna S, Kertory M. *Children's Assessment of Participation and Enjoyment/Preferences for Activities of Children.* San Antonio, TX: Harcourt Assessment; 2004.

42. Fisher AG, Bryze K, Hume V, Griswold LA. *School AMPS: School Version of the Assessment of Motor and Process Skills.* 2nd ed. Fort Collins, CO: Three Star Press; 2005.

43. Coster W, Deeney T, Haltiwanger J, Haley S. *School Function Assessment.* San Antonio, TX: Psychological Corporation; 1998.

44. Hemmingsson H, Egilson S, Hoffman O, Kielhofner G. *A User's Manual for the School Setting Interview Version 3.0.* Chicago, IL: MOHO Clearinghouse; 2005.

45. McEwen IR, Arnold SH, Hansen LH, Johnson D. Interrater reliability and content validity of a minimal data set to measure outcomes of students receiving school-based occupational therapy and physical therapy. *Physical and Occupational Therapy in Pediatrics.* 2003;23(2):77-95.

46. Haley SM, Coster WJ, Ludlow L, Haltiwanger J, Andrellos P. *Adminstration Manual for the Pediatric Evaluation of Disability Inventory.* San Antonio, TX: Psychological Corporation; 1992.

47. Uniform Data System for Medical Rehabilitation. *WEEFIM II System Clinical Guide. Version 6.0.* Amherst, NY: Uniform Data System for Medical Rehabilitation; 2006.

48. Young NL. *The Activities Scale for Kids Manual.* Toronto, ON: The Hospital for Sick Children; 1996.

49. Fisher AG. *The Assessment of Motor and Process Skills.* 3rd ed. Fort Collins, CO: Three Star Press; 1999.

50. Sparrow SS, Cicchetti DV, Bella DA. *The Vineland Adaptive Behavior Scales.* 2nd ed. Circle Pines, MN: AGS Publishing; 2005.

51. Harrison P, Oakland T. *Adaptive Behavior Assessment System— Second Edition Manual.* San Antonio, TX: Psychological Corporation; 2003.

52. Dunn L. Validation of the CHORES: a measure of school-aged children's participation in household tasks. *Scandinavian Journal of Occupational Therapy.* 2004;11:179-190.

53. Coster W, Bedell G, Law M, et al. Psychometric evaluation of the Participation and Environment Measure for Children and Youth. *Developmental Medicine and Child Neurology.* 2011;53(11):1030-1037. doi: 10.1111/j.1469-8749.2011.04094.x.

54. Centers for Disease Control and Prevention. *Autism Spectrum Disorders: Data and Statistics.* Centers for Disease Control and Prevention. http://www.cdc.gov/ncbddd/autism/data.html. Accessed November 29, 2011.

55. Stein MA, Efron LA, Schiff WB, Glanzman M. Attention deficit and hyperactivity. In: Batshaw ML, ed. *Children with Disabilities.* 5th ed. Baltimore, MD: Paul H. Brookes Publishing Co; 2002:389-416.

56. Pellegrino L. Cerebral palsy. In: Batshaw ML, ed. *Children with Disabilities.* 5th ed. Baltimore, MD: Paul H. Brookes Publishing Co; 2002:443-466.

57. Roizen NJ. Down syndrome. In: Batshaw ML, ed. *Children with Disabilities.* 5th ed. Baltimore, MD: Paul H. Brookes Publishing Co; 2002:307-320.

58. Rodger S, Liu S. Cognitive orientation to (daily) occupational performance: changes in strategy and session time use over the course of intervention. *OTJR: Occupation, Participation & Health.* 2008;28(4):168-179.

59. Meyer GA, Batshaw ML. Fragile X Syndrome. In: Batshaw ML, ed. *Children with Disabilities.* 5th ed. Baltimore, MD: Paul H. Brookes Publishing Co; 2002:321-331.

60. Wunsch MJ, Conlon CJ, Scheidt PC. Substance abuse: a preventable threat to development. In: Batshaw ML, ed. *Children with Disabilities.* 5th ed. Baltimore, MD: Paul H. Brookes Publishing Co; 2002:107-122.

61. Shapiro B, Church RP, Lewis MEB. Specific learning disabilities. In: Batshaw ML, ed. *Children with Disabilities.* 5th ed. Baltimore, MD: Paul H. Brookes Publishing Co; 2002:417-442.

62. Batshaw ML, Shapiro B. Mental retardation. In: Batshaw ML, ed. *Children with Disabilities.* 5th ed. Baltimore, MD: Paul H. Brookes Publishing Co; 2002:287-305.

63. Scacheri C. Syndromes and inborn errors of metabolism. In: Batshaw ML, ed. *Children with Disabilities.* 5th ed. Baltimore, MD: Paul H. Brookes Publishing Co; 2002:749-773.

64. Weinstein S. Epilepsy. In: Batshaw ML, ed. *Children with Disabilities.* 5th ed. Baltimore, MD: Paul H. Brookes Publishing Co; 2002:493-523.

65. Council on Children With Disabilities. Identifying infants and young children with developmental disorders in the medical home: an algorithm for developmental surveillance and screening. *Pediatrics.* 2006;118(1):405-420.

66. Martin EA. *Oxford Concise Medical Dictionary.* Oxford, United Kingdom: Oxford University Press; 1998.

67. Leet AI, Dormans JP, Tosi LL. Muscles, bones and nerves: the body's framework. In: Batshaw ML, ed. *Children with Disabilities.* 5th ed. Baltimore, MD: Paul H. Brookes Publishing Co; 2002:493-523.

68. American Cancer Society. *Learn About Cancer.* American Cancer Society. http://www.cancer.org/Cancer/CancerinChildren/DetailedGuide/cancer-in-children-types-of-childhood-cancers. Accessed November 29, 2011.

69. Centers for Disease Control and Prevention. *Meningitis.* Centers for Disease Control and Prevention. http://www.cdc.gov/meningitis/index.html. Accessed November 29, 2011.

70. The Royal Children's Melbourne Hospital. *114 Musculoskeletal Injury.* The Royal Children's Melbourne Hospital. http://www.rch.org.au/paed_trauma/manual.cfm?doc_id=12602. Accessed November 29, 2011.

71. Michaud LJ, Semel-Concepcion J, Duhaime A-C, Lazar MF. Traumatic brain injury. In: Batshaw ML, ed. *Children with Disabilities.* 5th ed. Baltimore, MD: Paul H. Brookes Publishing Co; 2002:287-305.

72. Comer RJ. *Abnormal Psychology.* 3rd ed. New York: W.H. Freeman and Company; 1998.

73. National Institutes of Health. *Schizophrenia.* National Institutes of Health: research portfolio online reporting tools (rePORT). Available at: http://report.nih.gov/NIHfactsheets/ViewFactSheet.aspx?csid=67&key=S#S. Accessed December 9, 2011.

74. National Institude of Health. *Post-Traumatic Stress Disorder.* National Institutes of Health: research portfolio online reporting tools (rePORT). http://report.nih.gov/NIHfactsheets/ViewFactSheet.aspx?csid=58&key=P#P. Accessed December 9, 2011.

75. Polatajko H, Mandich A. *Cognitive Orientation for Daily Occupational Performance (CO-OP).* Ottawa, ON: CAOT; 2004.

76. Missiuna C, Rivard L, Pollock N. They're bright but they can't write: DCD in school-aged children. *TEACHING Exceptional Children Plus.* 2004;1(1):3.

77. Missiuna C, Pollock N, Levac D, et al. Partnering for change: An innovative school-based occupational therapy service delivery model for children with developmental coordination disorder. *Can J Occup Ther.* 2012;79(1): 41-50.

78. Graham F, Rodger S. Occupational performance coaching: enabling parents' and children's occupational performance. In Rodger S, ed. *Occupation Centered Practice for Children: A Practical Guide for Occupational Therapists.* Oxford, United Kingdom: Wiley Blackwell; 2010:203-226.

79. Eliasson AC, Krumlinde-Sundholm L, Shaw K, Wang C. Effects of constraint-induced movement therapy in young children with hemiplegic cerebral palsy: an adapted model. *Developmental Medicine and Child Neurology.* 2005;47:266-275.

80. Gordon AM, Scheider JA, Chinnan A, Charles JR. Efficacy of a hand-arm bimanual intensive therapy (HABIT) in children with hemiplegic cerebral palsy: a randomized control. *Developmental Medicine and Child Neurology.* 2007;49:830-838.

81. Law M, Darrah J, Pollock N, et al. Focus on function—a randomized trial comparing two rehabilitation interventions for young children with cerebral palsy. *BMC Pediatrics.* 2007;7:31.

82. Cook AM, Polgar J. *Cook and Hussey's Assistive Technologies: Principles and Practice.* 3rd ed. St. Louis, MO: Elsevier; 2007.

83. Miller L, Polatajko H, Missiuna C, Mandich A, Mcnab JJ. A pilot trial of a cognitive treatment for children with developmental coordination disorder. *Human Movement Science.* 2001;20(1):183-200.

84. Graham F, Rodger S, Ziviani J. Effectiveness of occupational performance coaching in improving children's and mothers' performance and mothers' self-competence. *Am J Occup Ther.* 2013;76(1):10-18.

85. Sakzewski L, Ziviani J, Abbott DF, MacDonell RA, Jackson GD, Boyd RN. Randomized trial of constraint-induced movement therapy and bimanual training on activity outcomes for children with congenital hemiplegia. *Developmental Medicine and Child Neurology.* 2011;53:313-320.

86. Wallen M, Ziviani J, Naylor O, Evans R, Novack I, Herbert,RD. Modified constraint-induced therapy for children with hemiplegic cerebral palsy: a randomized trial. *Developmental Medicine and Child Neurology.* 2011;53:1091-1099.

87. Law MC, Darrah J, Pollock N, et al. Focus on function: a cluster, randomized controlled trial comparing child- versus context-focused intervention for young children with cerebral palsy. *Developmental Medicine and Child Neurology.* 2011;53:621-629.

88. Ryan SE. An overview of systematic reviews of adaptive seating interventions for children with cerebral palsy: where do we go from here? *Disability and Rehabilitation: Assistive Technology.* 2012;7(2):104-111.

89. Bronfenbrenner U. *The Ecology of Human Development: Experiments by Nature and Design.* Cambridge, MA: Harvard University Press; 1979.

90. Ziviani J, Wadley D, Ward H, Macdonald D, Jenkins D, Rodger S. A place to play: socioeconomic and spatial factors in children's physical activity. *Australian Occupational Therapy Journal.* 2008;55(1):2-11.

91. Pont K, Ziviani J, Wadley D, Abbott R. The Model of Children's Active Travel (M-CAT): a conceptual framework for examining factors influencing children's active travel. *Australian Occupational Therapy Journal.* 2011;58:138-144.

92. Ziviani J, Poulsen A, Hansen C. Movement skills proficiency and physical activity: a case for Engaging and Coaching for Health (EACH)–Child. *Australian Occupational Therapy Journal.* 2009;56:259-265.

93. Poulsen A. Children with attention deficit hyperactivity disorder, developmental coordination disorder and learning disabilities. In: Bazyk S, ed. *Mental Health Promotion, Prevention, and Intervention with Children and Youth.* Bethesda, MD: AOTA Press; 2011:231-265.

94. World Health Organization. *International Classification of Functioning, Disability and Health (ICF).* Geneva, Switzerland: WHO; 2001.

95. Rothbart MK, Bates JE. Temperament. In: Damon W, Lerner RM, eds. *Handbook of Child Psychology: Vol. 3. Social, Emotional, and Personality Development.* 6th ed. Hoboken, NJ: John Wiley & Sons; 2006:99-166.

96. Rothbart MK, Bates JE. Temperament. In: Damon W, ed. *Handbook of Child Psychology: Vol. 3. Social, Emotional, and Personality Development.* 5th ed. New York, NY: John Wiley & Sons; 1998:105-176.

97. Shonkoff JP, Phillips DA. *From Neurons to Neighborhoods: The Science of Early Childhood Development.* Washington, DC: National Academy Press; 2000.

98. Fabes RA, Eisenberg N, Jones S, et al. Regulation, emotionality, and preschoolers' socially competent peer interactions. *Child Development.* 1999;70(2):432-442.

99. Luthar SS, ed. *Resilience and Vulnerability: Adaptation in the Context of Childhood Adversities.* Cambridge, England: Cambridge University Press; 2003.

100. Petrenchik TM, King GA, Batorowicz B. Children and youth with disabilities: enhancing mental health through positive experiences of doing and belonging. In: Bazyk S, ed. *Mental Health Promotion, Prevention, and Intervention with Children and Youth.* Bethesda, MD: AOTA Press; 2011:189-205.

101. Kielhofner G, ed. *Model of Human Occupation: Theory and Application.* 4th ed. Baltimore, MD: Williams & Wilkins; 2008.

102. Lim SM, Rodger S. An occupational perspective on the assessment of social competence in children. *British Journal of Occupational Therapy.* 2008;71(11):469-481.

103. Poulsen A, Rodger S, Ziviani J. Understanding children's motivation from a self-determination theoretical perspective: implications for practice. *Australian Occupational Therapy Journal.* 2006;53:78-86.

104. Csikszentmihalyi M. *Flow: The Psychology of Optimal Experience.* New York, NY: Harper & Row; 1990.

105. Ziviani J, Poulsen A, Cuskelly M. *Motivation: Engaging Children in Therapy.* London, England: Jessica Kingsley Publishers; in press.

106. Stewart KL, Felicetti LA. Learning styles of marketing majors. *Educational Research Quarterly.* 1992;15(2):15-23.

107. Leite WL, Svinicki M, Shi Y. Attempted validation of the scores of the VARK: Learning Styles Inventory with multi-trait–multi-method confirmatory factor analysis models. *Educational and Psychological Measurement.* 2010;70(2):323-339.

Chapter 10

OCCUPATIONS OF ADULTHOOD

Kathleen Matuska, PhD, OTR/L, FAOTA and Kate Barrett, OTD, OTR/L

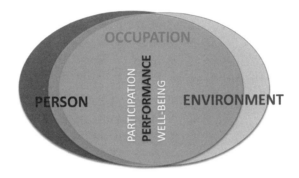

LEARNING OBJECTIVES

- Describe the role that occupations play in normal adult development.
- Identify challenges and barriers to healthy adult development.
- Discuss essential skills needed to progress into healthy aging.
- Identify the contextual factors that influence adult development.
- Define occupational competence and relate its components to the characteristics of stages of adulthood.

KEY WORDS

- Adult stage theories
- Affordances
- Burnout

- Capacity
- Effectivities
- Family Leave Act
- Life balance
- Life coaching
- Life imbalance
- Maturation
- Middle age
- Occupational competence
- Sandwich generation
- Self-efficacy
- Workaholism

INTRODUCTION

In this chapter, we consider adult development from the standpoint of occupational performance. Through this lens, we identify key concepts from the PEOP Model and

Christiansen CH, Baum CM, Bass JD, eds.
Occupational Therapy: Performance, Participation, and Well-Being, Fourth Edition (pp 157-168).
© 2015 SLACK Incorporated.

BOX 10-1

CASE EXAMPLE

Karen is 47 years old; married; and has 3 children, ages 17, 15, and 10. She works 32 hours a week as an administrative assistant in the high school her children attend. Although she enjoys her work, she is taking classes to become an accountant because she wants a more meaningful career. Her mother died about 4 years ago and her father is living alone in the old family home about 8 miles away. Karen's 2 siblings live in other states. Lately, Karen feels like she can't keep up with all the demands on her time and attention. Her oldest daughter is acting out and hangs out with a group who drink and smoke and she does not help with chores or driving. Her middle son is very active in soccer and basketball and has a practice or game almost every evening. Karen's husband helps with the driving when he can, but he often works in the evening. Her accounting classes also meet in the evening, so she often has to problem-solve ways to manage everyone's schedule. Finally, her father recently had a knee replacement surgery; he is not fully weight-bearing and is having difficulty making his meals and doing the housework. On weekends, Karen brings groceries and meals to her father and spends a few hours cleaning and laundering for him. Karen feels stressed and cranky and worries about the deteriorating relationships in her busy life. Occupational therapy practitioners would use a preventive approach to working with adults like Karen. For example, the occupational therapy practitioner may help Karen examine each of her habits and routines, and discuss time use and priorities—with the goal of balancing her roles and responsibilities to prevent illness from accumulated stress.

note how personal and environmental factors influence the conditions under which adults progress through the stages of adulthood by facilitating or constraining an individual's ability to competently perform role requirements. Drawing from theories of adult stage development, we identify key roles and their competencies. We then identify factors that can limit role performance, using the concepts of life balance and balance as one way to consider how occupational and role performance engender states of health and well-being, including life satisfaction. We begin with the case study of a middle-aged adult woman (Box 10-1).

Karen's life, summarized in Box 10-1, may seem very familiar for many adults. Adulthood, especially with work and caregiving responsibilities, is a very demanding period

in life and requires a different set of occupational performance skills and patterns than in other periods of life. It is a very important and busy time in the human lifespan, yet the period seems less visible compared to other developmental periods, such as childhood, adolescence, and old age. It includes the period of life when people complete their formal education, work to develop financial independence and security, develop significant relationships, reproduce and form families, and make contributions through their vocations to broader society. During this period of life, people also develop, maintain, and may transition through multiple roles (eg, adult child, parent, caregiver, citizen, worker, community member, volunteer). In the last half of adulthood, many people begin to experience the effects of aging and health conditions that influence activity and participation. The occupational performance demands for adulthood are arguably the most challenging, and this chapter will explore the population requirements.

The characteristics of current and future adult populations are important to note. In the United States, there have been gradual and multiple changes in the demographic profiles of some individuals in this age group (eg, higher educational levels, longer hours at work), their families (eg, delayed reproduction, non-traditional families, increased geographic distances among members, two-worker families), and their communities (eg, diversity in race, culture, language, disability, aging work force, increased disparities, global influences, labor opportunities). All of these changes in turn influence changes in occupational performance.

Public policy initiatives in the United States will influence many aspects of life for the adult population of the future. Social security benefits may be lower, or recipients may be required to wait longer to receive them. People will live longer and healthier lives because of advances in and access to medical technology. The make-up of the workforce will include an increased mix of cultures, ages, genders, and races. Industry will continue moving from mass-production occupations to office-worker, service-provider occupations. Increased global competition, due in part to advances in communication, will continue to increase the demand for new technologies.[1]

STAGES OF ADULTHOOD

Stages of adulthood are often defined by developmental tasks and characteristic roles and activities, rather than by specific ages. Young adults are often involved in education and career training, decisions about life roles, and establishing social and intimate relationships. In the United States and Canada, there is some blurring of the transition from late adolescence and young adulthood. This blurring occurs for that segment of the population undertaking professional or graduate education, as extended years of education and training delay entry into the workforce.

Major shifts in the economy and dramatic changes in the roles of women have had a significant impact on the norms and expectations for young adults in Western industrialized nations. For example, even in the recent past, women were expected to forego careers and assume homemaking and child-rearing responsibilities. Today, the shift toward dual-career families, the growing acceptance of same-sex unions, and the loosening of gender-based roles represent some of the significant social and cultural changes influencing young adults. These changes will influence the characteristic occupations of middle age and later life for young adults born during the past 3 decades of the 20th century. Recent census data in the United States and other developing nations suggest that decisions about marriage and life partners, childbearing, and work are being deferred until later in the stage of young adulthood than was typical even a few decades ago.[2,3]

Often, middle age is a time during which adjustments are made based on past experiences to make positive changes while there is still time. This redefinition of values and lifestyles that sometimes occurs often associates middle adulthood with the term *mid-life crisis,* but in fact, some research suggests that few people experience stress at a level that warrants the term *crisis* and such redefinition may not be a universal "marker" event of this stage after all.[4] During middle adulthood, parental responsibilities for children may be decreasing, while responsibilities for one's adult parents may be increasing. Career responsibilities may change, and achievement of significant life goals may become realized. There may be more time and recognition for contributions to community and social activities. Middle adulthood is also marked by a growing awareness of the physical and emotional changes experienced in later life.

Developmental theorists have identified stages of growth that occur through adulthood. Erikson proposed that young adults must develop intimate relationships and mid-life adults must contribute to society or risk isolation and self-absorption.[5,6] Levinson, drawing on a concept of life structures influenced by the patterns of a person's life, theorized that early adulthood demands development of mature behaviors in both family and career, middle adulthood involves reassessing the meaning, direction, and value of life, with attention to the neglected parts of the self (eg, talents, desires, aspirations).[7,8] Middle adulthood is also when choices and commitments are made, a new life structure is formed, and one transitions into later adulthood where attention is directed to leaving a legacy. A key feature of Levinson's work was his emphasis on the importance of transitions from one stage to the next. According to Levinson, the primary tasks of every transition period are to reappraise the existing life structure, to explore possibilities for change, and to make crucial choices that will enable stable life structures in the ensuing stage.

OCCUPATIONAL COMPETENCE IN ADULTHOOD

Occupational therapy practitioners assert that adults progress through stages of development by engagement in occupations as they fulfill role demands and develop personal skills. People have an innate need to develop competence in their roles and seek out activities and challenges to meet their need for role fulfillment. This helps to explain why a person with a poorly defined role is uncomfortable; and why people feel sad, frightened, and angry when they lose their ability to fulfill their roles as a consequence of injury or illness.

Occupational competence is tied to individual roles and varies as the demands of the roles vary, usually in a gradual developmental progression. As the individual matures and ages, various roles are undertaken, each composed of numerous demands that pose varying levels and types of challenge to the person. For example, the transition from adolescence to adulthood is accompanied by societal role expectations to become a productive, self-supporting member of the social group. Acquisition of this worker role often involves training or study along a chosen vocational or professional career track, followed by entry into the workforce as an apprentice or beginning worker.

Similarly, the transition from worker to retiree requires a successful shift in daily routine that often affects the types of activities in which an individual participates, whether these are mostly leisure, such as travel and hobbies, or involved volunteer pursuits. Jonsson, Josephsson, and Kielhofner completed a longitudinal study of the transition to retirement and found that many people replaced their work roles with very engaging occupations that required vast amounts of their free time.[9]

These role expectations vary from culture to culture, and may be impeded by either personal or environmental limitations or barriers, such as illness or social conditions (eg, high unemployment). As digital technologies and social media create more cross-cultural awareness, it is likely that attitudes and expectations about role transitions may change. However, it is important to recognize that group expectations are powerful influences on behavior, and that perceptions of competence, both by the individual or the group, are influenced by role demands.

To the degree that the individual is able to meet the role demands, he or she becomes occupationally competent.[10] Occupational development occurs in the individual's quest to establish and maintain occupational competence in systematic patterns of behavioral response to culturally determined role-based challenges that typically are referred to as "growth and development" in the early years and as "aging" in the later years.[10]

Adults choose careers, housing, partners, etc, that reflect their values, aspirations, and goals with a belief that they are the best opportunities to develop and maintain competence as an adult in society. The drive for competence is a hallmark of adult life and is highly influenced by the interaction of personal attributes, roles, and opportunities or barriers in the environment. One's *capacity* to develop competence in roles refers to the physiological, psychological, and sociocultural attributes available to an individual. These capacities are unique to each individual and may change over time with development and age. To develop competence, individuals must also have the necessary *effectivities;* the sub-set of attributes and abilities that are relevant to role demands.[11] For example, the individual in the student role develops effectivities for that role that are not pertinent to some of the student's other roles of sister, aunt, or daughter. After graduation, if the role that replaces the student role does not require these "student" effectivities, they continue to exist as abilities, but because they are not necessary to meet a role challenge (to maintain occupational competence as a student) they lie fallow or may degrade.[10] Fulfillment of roles also requires affordances, which are features within an environment or situation that are perceived as pertinent to the role challenge and can facilitate role competence.[12-14] For example, in a student role, access to computers, books, and a quiet place to study will support occupational competence. Developing occupational competence is also guided by *self-efficacy* beliefs; the perception of personal abilities that guides how people behave, their level of motivation, thought processes and emotional reaction to challenging circumstances.[15] Self-efficacy affects the degree to which the individual perceives that he or she has the effectivities and affordances to successfully address a challenge. Self-efficacy beliefs make it more likely that the individual will attempt to overcome a particular task or role challenge and will increase perseverance in the face of initial performance failure, so that competence can be achieved. In addition, self-efficacy beliefs facilitate exploration in new areas of task role performance. In this way, task competence becomes generalized to the role. Occupational competence is role-directed and develops in adults because they need to look for and accept challenges that are part of their social roles. It is sustained when the adult roles are meaningful and the individual perceives he or she has adequate abilities and environmental support.

Although individuals are unique, in Western societies there are some common occupations in adulthood, such as paid work, caregiving, and leisure activities. The following sections will discuss typical occupations of adulthood, including some of the rewards and challenges that accompany them.

WORK

Work is one of the primary occupations of early and middle adulthood. Paid employment patterns have changed over the past few decades, with people much more likely to change jobs or hold multiple jobs. In the United States, adults between the ages of 18 to 44 have a mean of 11 different jobs and 26.2% work part-time.[16] For full-time employees, the typical work week is 42.2 hours.[17]

In the United States, the rate of women entering the workforce has stabilized from the significant increase in the past decades of the 20th century. Women continue to be employed primarily in education, health care, and service occupations. Globally, the participation of women in the paid workforce varies greatly among different regions and is related to such factors as literacy and fertility rates within countries.[18] However, women experience unfavorable disparities in compensation and representation in positions of power and influence in all regions. In the United States, men continue to hold the majority of jobs in architecture, engineering, protective service, and construction occupations.[19,20] Two-income families are common, with 52% of families with small children having both parents employed. Adults who are single parents are more likely to be employed with 67% of single mothers and 76% of single fathers working.[21]

Many adults experience *occupational deprivation, employment disparities,* or *occupational imbalance* related to paid employment. When people are willing and able to work but cannot find adequate or sustainable employment, they may be experiencing *occupational deprivation.*[22] *Employment disparities* are conditions where work participation is different among groups because of racial, ethnic, gender, disability status, or other differences. Combinations of these differences, such as being an immigrant woman with a disability, creates even greater barriers to participation in the workforce.[23] When people find that the demands of work impinge on their enjoyment of other parts of life, such as family time and recreation, they may be experiencing *occupational imbalance.*[24]

Unemployment and Underemployment

The most obvious form of occupational deprivation is when someone is unemployed and unable to find work. Unemployment rates reflect the state of the general economy, but certain demographic groups are at more risk. For example, unemployment rates are higher for people with low levels of education. In 2010, the unemployment rate for those with less than a high school diploma was 14.9% and only 4.7% for those with a bachelor's degree or higher.[25] Unemployment is more likely for single adults than for married adults, and almost twice as high for Blacks (16%) than for Whites (8.7%).[25] People with mental health problems also have higher rates of unemployment.[26]

Underemployment means people may be working, but at jobs that are below their capability, at lower rates of pay, or involuntarily less than full time. Both unemployment and underemployment can be detrimental to health and well-being.[27] Underemployment brings loss of a previous standard of living, insecurity of income, stigma, loss of self-esteem, and loss of social contacts, all with negative impact on mental health.[26] A recent Gallup poll found that the longer people were unemployed, the poorer their physical health (more pain, lower energy level, and less rest), especially for the 18- to 29-year-old age group.[28]

Workaholism

The concept of *workaholism* has been used for many years, with most common understandings about an over-extension at work, usually related to an individual's own drive to work. This over-extension is believed to impinge on other areas of life, such as time with family, leisure, and rest, representing an occupational imbalance.[24] Although there is still no agreement on the definition or characteristics of workaholism, some scientists have defined a profile whereby workaholics have high work involvement, high drive to work, and low work enjoyment.[29] People who displayed this profile delegated responsibility less, were more perfectionist and stressed, and had more health complaints than people without the profile.[29] People who exhibited all the 3 characteristics also had lower life satisfaction and higher work–life imbalance than people who had only 1 or 2 of the characteristics.[30]

Workaholism must also be viewed within the broader sociocultural and economic environments that influence it, such as competitive job markets, stagnant wages and salaries, and higher costs of living. People bemoan the blending of work and non-work, and blame technological advances for the ease of doing work tasks at home or on vacation.[31] For example, the Internet and mobile digital devices have made it easier than ever to perform work functions away from the office and at all hours of the day and night. Other factors that lead to work and non-work blending may stem from the employer, such as increased productivity demands, incentive systems for higher productivity, and a culture that values job loyalty.[32] The global market, economic insecurity, and cultural value of consumerism may also influence perceived job insecurity, creating a sense of urgency in work and fueling the beginning stages of over-work.

Burnout

Burnout is a result of perceived imbalance in work or in other major responsibilities. It is commonly described as a state of mental weariness with 3 major components: exhaustion, cynicism, and inefficiency.[33] The exhaustion component refers to feelings of being overextended and depleted of one's emotional and physical resources, and is the strongest predictor of negative health outcomes.[34] The cynicism component refers to a negative, callous, or excessively detached response to various aspects of the job. The component of inefficacy refers to feelings of incompetence and a lack of achievement and productivity.[35,36] Burnout is seen often in high-stakes and high-stress jobs, such as critical health care and disaster relief, where there is an intense emotional component.[37,38] People who are experiencing burnout may not find opportunities for renewal and experience-reduced productivity, thus diminishing their self-esteem and overall affect. For example, significantly more self-reported depression, anxiety, sleep disturbance, memory impairment, and neck and back pain was reported by Swedish health care workers who were burned-out than workers who were not.[37] On the other hand, getting adequate sleep seems to be a buffer against the risk for long-term burnout.[39]

Working adults in the United States who are struggling to manage major family crisis may benefit from the Family and Medical Leave Act (FMLA), which entitles eligible employees to take unpaid, job-protected leave for specified family and medical reasons with continuation of group health insurance coverage.[40] Many employers are discovering that by offering flextime, compressed workweeks, shift flexibility, job sharing, and sabbaticals it is proving to be cost-effective morale boosters that benefit company bottom-lines.[41] Many worksites offer employee wellness programs, such as incentives for exercise and healthy habits, because the outcome is a more productive and contented worker. Wellness programs also lower their overall health costs and are supported by the *Healthy People 2020*, naming increased employee wellness programs as one of its objectives.[42] Occupational therapy practitioners can be useful in helping workers manage their stress by balancing their habits, routines, and roles.

CAREGIVING

Most people at one time in their adult life find themselves assuming some kind of caregiving role. Typically these include caring for children or aging parents. Most of the caregiving is informal or unpaid, and carried out because of an emotional bond and sense of obligation and love. The cost of informal caregiving is staggering when the hours of service and lost hours at work are considered.

Women in the United States take an average of 11.5 years out of the paid labor force because of caregiving responsibilities (including that of elder care and raising children) and men average 1.3 years.[43] The cost of caregiving includes the actual hours of direct and indirect care, and the cost to businesses in lost productivity time and replacement costs when employees leave to do caregiving.[44]

Parenting

Parenting is a common role for adults, but many adults may find themselves as parents with little experience or knowledge about how to fulfill the role. Even in the best situations, parenthood can be demanding and challenging. One parent summed it up this way,

> I had a pretty good idea of the kind of parent I would like to be and the kinds of things I should do for my children. I just didn't know I'd be so tired while trying to do it! (T. O'Neill, personal communication, September 1989).

Parents learn by doing and by using whatever resources are available to them, including relying on past memories of their own experiences as children. By age 44, 85.1% of women and 78% of men have become parents.[45] Women have on average 2.27 children and the average age of having a first child is 25.[46] The more educated a woman is, the fewer children she is likely to have, and women living at or below the poverty level are likely to have more children.[47]

There is increasing support for mothers working, with 70% of fathers and 82% of mothers agreeing that working mothers can establish just as warm and secure a relationship with her children as a mother who does not work.[46] The perception of the fatherhood role has also strengthened with the majority of mothers and fathers (over 70%) believing that it is more important for a man to spend a lot of time with his family than to be successful at his career.[46] The great majority (over 95%) of mothers and fathers agree that the rewards of being a parent are worth it, despite the cost and the work it takes.[46]

Caregiving of Elderly Parents

More than half of the adults 85 years and older require the assistance of another person to perform ADL. Family members are the primary source of such assistance, and the majority of them are women. In 2009, almost 30% of United States households had a member that had served as an unpaid caregiver to an adult in the past year. Spouses provide the most care (38%), followed by daughters (19%) and others.[48] Only 9% of those needing assistance use paid providers.[49]

Many adults want to help their aging parents, but there may be a geographic barrier. The distance caregiving demographic trends are noteworthy. Of the estimated 44.4 million Americans who provide informal care, 15% (or approximately 6.7 million individuals) live at least 1 hour from the care recipient. The reasons for this distance include career or education, children, military deployment, divorce, or simply choice.[50] Fifteen percent of all family caregivers travel an average of 450 miles (up to 8 driving hours) to provide care for elderly, disabled, or chronically ill family members. With distance an important factor in the intensity of caregiving dynamics, experts say emotional strain and financial sacrifice are the chief dilemmas.[43]

Caregiving has an enormous impact on the work life of the caregiver and the work environment. Employers report an increase in the number of requests for time off to care for aging parents. Eighty percent of these men and women work full time and nearly one quarter are the only or the primary caregiver.[44] A total of 5% of the men and 7% of the women reported that they left the workplace as a result of caregiving. Men were just as likely as women to report they retired early as a result of caregiving responsibilities.[44] An additional 10% of the employed caregivers reduced their hours from full to part time. More than 6 in 10 had to rearrange their work schedules in order to take care of their caregiving responsibilities, with more than a third (36%) reporting missing days of work and 12% taking a leave of absence.[44]

Some adults provide care to both their children and aging parents, commonly referred to as being in the *sandwich generation*. This has become more prevalent as people live longer, as they delay marriage, as more adult children are choosing (or find it necessary) to live at home during their early adult years, and as increased numbers of adult children are returning home after divorce.[51]

Caregiving responsibilities may contribute to a risk of occupational interruption and occupational imbalance for the sandwich generation population. Caregiving can interrupt performance of all other occupations and result in imbalance in some occupations, notably work and leisure. The challenges have a tremendous impact on the overall lifestyle of middle-aged adults, including personal time, career development, and financial stability.[51] The effects of providing elder care increase with time spent. For example, half of those spending more than 8 hours per month (high-intensity caregivers) had to change their social activities, and over a third had to change their work schedule.[52]

Typically, middle-aged adults are at the peak of their careers and face extensive demands in the workplace. Thirty (30%) percent of caregivers report a moderate or high degree of financial hardship. Seventy percent (70%) of caregivers have had to make changes at work, such as leaving early, going in late, changing to part time, or taking time off during the day to accommodate caregiving. Nine percent (9%) of workers providing care report having to give up work entirely as a result of care giving responsibilities.[48]

Sandwiched workers were more likely to feel generally stressed—about 70% compared with about 61% of workers with no child-care or elder-care responsibilities. However, almost all (95%) felt satisfied with life in general—about the same percentage as those with fewer caregiving responsibilities.[52] Women who are sandwiched and had attitudes and behaviors that valued caregiving reported the fewest burdens and had greater awareness of community resources including elder care programs.[51] Over half of those working and caring for an older person while still having children at home felt that caring for a senior was simply giving back what they had received and that the relationship was strengthened.[53]

LEISURE

Activities that are classified as leisure typically occur in discretionary time, involve choice, and are intrinsically satisfying.[54] In the occupational therapy literature, the term *play* is typically used when referring to children and *leisure* is most often used when referring to adults. In general, perhaps because of its strong history of providing early education and school-based services, the occupational therapy literature has devoted more attention and research to childhood play occupations than to adult leisure occupations.

According to the US Department of Labor, over 95% of people engage in some form of leisure per day.[55] Although most people spend more time on leisure during weekends and holidays, the typical person also spends a significant amount of time (over 4.5 hours) engaging in leisure activities on weekdays as well. People are also more likely to engage in leisure activities for longer periods of time on weekends. People spend more leisure time watching television (an average of 2.73 hours per day) than other activities, such as socializing or participating in sports. Almost 80% of people watch television on an average day.

Women are more likely to engage in household activities, most notably housework and food preparation and clean up. In addition, women also spend more time caring for and helping household members. Men spend more time working and doing work-related activities outside of the home, and also dedicate more time to leisure and sports. These statistics remain consistent across racial/ethnic lines, even when taking into account only people who have engaged in the activity that day (for example, out of men and women that do housework on an average day, women spend almost 30 minutes more on the task).[55]

Hispanic people are more likely to spend time caring for and helping household members than other groups, and Blacks are more likely to engage in organizational, civic, and religious activities. Of all of the groups surveyed, Hispanic women spend the least amount of time on leisure and sports.

Work and leisure are not mutually exclusive, but more often than not, work influences how people spend their leisure time. The type of work and when it is done influences when and how much time one is available for leisure. When people are highly satisfied with their work and feel a certain level of autonomy and creativity, work may spill over into leisure pursuits.[54] On the other hand, when work is dominated by routine, leisure is often used to compensate for that work and the leisure choices are radically different from work. In all models explaining the work-leisure relationship, feelings about work is what dominated the leisure choice.

How people experience a balance of leisure and employment seems to be a predictor of their health. Hakansson and Ahlborg found that for women, the strongest predictor of health was low stress outside of the workplace.[56] Women value having energy left for both leisure and domestic work after completing their paid work. For men, the strongest predictor of health was having low stress at work. In this study, both men and women felt healthier when able to participate in rigorous exercise. The results of this study may demonstrate that for women to experience health, they need to handle stress both within and outside of the workplace, whereas men may be more singularly focused on stress within the workplace.[56]

While occupational therapy practitioners value leisure as a significant area of occupation, most practitioners do not formally assess leisure. In occupational therapy, leisure is most often assessed through informal assessment and, although leisure assessments have been developed in other disciplines, there is a need for valid and reliable assessment tools specific to leisure developed from an occupational therapy perspective.[57,58]

LIFE IMBALANCE

One challenge for adults is to find ways to balance the multiple role demands in work, caregiving, and leisure and manage their own health needs at the same time. Within the general population, lifestyle imbalance is often experienced as a difficulty in meeting the demands of modern life because of perceived or actual time constraints. These constraints limit peoples' ability to meet important personal or social needs in a satisfactory or meaningful manner and lead to stress.[58-60] People often adapt to these time-stress demands by seeking new strategies, such as attending time management seminars, learning to multi-task, taking working vacations, or making more drastic changes in lifestyle by downsizing living environments, changing jobs, or moving to the country (or even other countries). Time-coping strategies are also facilitated by digital technologies such as laptop computers; smart phones; or use of the Internet for banking, shopping, social networking, or correspondence.[61]

A life coaching approach may be useful for adults who are otherwise healthy, but feeling imbalanced or dissatisfied with how their lives are going. People seem to readily recognize when they are feeling imbalanced, but often have difficulty achieving or maintaining more satisfactory patterns of living. Occupational therapy practitioners can use strategies developed by professional coaches when helping people regain life balance or achieve their goals. For example, coaches do not make recommendations or provide solutions. Instead, they work with a client in a conversation and question-based process to foster the client's self-awareness and clarifying what is important to them.[62] Occupational therapy practitioners understand how performance patterns can impact health and well-being, and would have excellent background knowledge to serve as a coach using a preventative approach.

Insomnia and Sleep Disorders

The literature on sleep disorders shows that sleep quality is related to what people do during the day, their experiences of stress, and the manner in which they cope with stressful circumstances.[63,64] Sleep is an important and obligatory daily human occupation, and on average normal healthy adults spend nearly one-third of their lives sleeping.[65] Recent research has shown that it is vital for health, and that sleep deficits are related to the emergence of many chronic diseases, as well as life expectancy.[66,67] Many adults have difficulty sleeping at various times in their lives. When work schedules or sleeping problems require adults to disregard their natural biological rhythms, they are at risk of disentrainment and negative health consequences. For example, airline workers, emergency personnel, and a host of other shift workers may be at greater risk for performance decrements and diminished safety, as well as insomnia, immune dysfunction, and increased risk for cancer and cardiac conditions, among others.[68-71] Occupational therapy practitioners can evaluate sleep performance and work with adults to develop helpful routines and patterns that promote sleep quality.

Obesity and Inactivity

Approximately 60% of American adults are obese, and sedentary lifestyles have been directly linked to an increased risk of obesity.[72,73] However, environmental factors also contribute to the obesity epidemic in the United States. Environmental factors are largely ignored in the medical systems, where the focus is only on personal lifestyle change. The production and marketing of food that is more fully prepared, readily available, and promoted through competitive business strategies contributes to diets that have higher fat and caloric content.[74] Poor food options driven by environmental and economic factors may partially explain why socioeconomically disadvantaged populations have a greater prevalence of obesity, as compared to economically advantaged populations.[75] Occupational therapy practitioners can help people examine their habits and routines that lead to obesity and advocate for healthier food and activity options in their communities.[76]

Poverty

Poverty can also negatively impact life balance for adults. People living in poverty experience higher levels of stress about finances and employment. This stress may cause sleep disturbance, leading to exhaustion and increased stress levels. People living in poverty often experience underemployment or unemployment, which also impacts one's ability to achieve balance.[59,60] While people who are unemployed may have more discretionary time, they may experience limited choices about how to spend that time due to financial constraints.

SUMMARY

Adulthood is an important developmental period that requires personal and environmental supports to navigate successfully. Occupational performance in adulthood requires the ability to meet the demands of employment and family, while growing and developing new personal skills and attributes. This period is often wrought with competing demands for time and attention and can result in stress and poor health. Occupational therapy practitioners provide a useful perspective of examining the roles, routines, and habits that make up the occupational profile of adults. When adults experience employment disparities, occupational disruptions or deprivations, or imbalance, they are at risk for negative health consequences and may benefit from wellness programs, coaching, or advocacy by occupational therapy. Tables 10-1 and 10-2 provide information about additional resources and assessments for many of the issues of adulthood.

TABLE 10-1. ASSESSMENTS FOR WORKAHOLISM, LIFE BALANCE, PARENTING HASSLES, AND SLEEP

ASSESSMENT	CONSTRUCT OR FACTOR ASSESSED	DESCRIPTION AND REFERENCE	WHERE IT CAN BE OBTAINED
The Work Addiction Risk Test (WART)	Specifies 5 risk factors for workaholism: compulsive tendencies, control, impaired communications/self-absorption, inability to delegate, and self-worth.	Self-rating on 30 items related to work habits. Four response choices from "never true" to "always true." Scores are summed and divided into 3 ranges indicating highly workaholic, mildly workaholic, and not workaholic.[77]	http://www.thecounseling team.com/interactive/ tests/Work-Addiction%20 Risk%20Test.pdf
The Life Balance Inventory (LBI)	Assesses perceived congruence between how people want to spend their time in various activity categories and how they actually spend their time in those categories. It is used for both research and as a personal assessment of life balance for making meaningful changes.	Self-rating on 53 items taken online. Total life balance score is given and sub-scores in 4 areas: relationships, health, challenge, and identity.[60]	http://minerva.stkate.edu/ LBI.nsf
Parenting Daily Hassles (PDH)	Assesses the frequency and intensity/impact of 20 experiences that can be a "hassle" to parents. Each of the 20 hassles is rated for frequency and intensity.	Parent/caregiver fills out the survey. It takes about 10 minutes to complete. It is used as a basis for discussion.[78]	http://www.excellence forchildandyouth.ca/ sites/default/files/ meas_attach/ Parenting_Daily_Hassles_ Scale_%28PDH%29.pdf.pdf
Pittsburgh Sleep Quality Index (PSQI)	Measures sleep quality and disturbance over a 1-month period.	Self-rating on 19 items yields a global sleep score and 7 sub-scores for subjective sleep quality, sleep latency, sleep duration, habitual sleep efficiency, sleep disturbance, use of sleep medication, and daytime dysfunction.[79]	http://www.sleep.pitt.edu/ content.asp?id=1484& subid=2316

TABLE 10-2. RESOURCES TABLE

ORGANIZATION	DESCRIPTION OF WHO THEY SERVE	WEB ADDRESS
Medicare—Support for Caregivers	All caregivers of aging, seriously ill, or disabled family members or friends	http://www.medicare.gov/campaigns/caregiver/caregiver.html
AgingCare.com	Connect people caring for elderly parents	http://www.agingcare.com/Caregiver-Support
VA Caregiver Support Services	For caregivers of United States veterans	http://www.caregiver.va.gov/support_landing.asp
SleepCenters.org	Compiled and published by the American Academy of Sleep Medicine (AASM) as a reference source of professional information on AASM accredited center and laboratory members.	http://www.sleepcenters.org/
American Academy of Sleep Medicine	For clinicians, students, and research professionals specializing in sleep medicine.	http://www.aasmnet.org/
Mayo Clinic: Insomnia	A resource for people who have trouble getting to sleep or poor sleep quality.	http://www.mayoclinic.com/health/insomnia/DS00187
Centers for Disease Control and Prevention Obesity Resource Center	Provides a wide variety of resources covering obesity and weight loss: medical problems, exercise and diet, Q&A with medical professionals, weight-loss surgery, forums, information, and education.	http://www.cdc.gov/nccdphp/dch/programs/CommunitiesPutting PreventiontoWork/resources/obesity.htm
SandwichGeneration.org	Provides resources to address the many challenges of caring for older parents and children.	http://sandwichgeneration.org/index.html
Working America AFL CIO: Unemployment Lifeline	Providing people who are unemployed the opportunity to talk to others and share support and lessons learned.	http://www.unemploymentlifeline.com/
US Department of Labor: Unemployment Insurance	Provides information about who is eligible for unemployment benefits and how to file a claim.	http://www.dol.gov/dol/topic/unemployment-insurance/

REFERENCES

1. US Department of Labor: Bureau of Labor Statistics. *TED: The Editor's Desk: Employment Characteristics of Families—2010.* US Department of Labor: Bureau of Labor Statistics. http://www.bls.gov/opub/ted/2011/ted_20110328.htm. Published March 28, 2011. Accessed September 22, 2013.
2. United Nations Statistics Division. *Statistics and indicators on women and men.* United Nations. http://unstats.un.org/unsd/demographic/products/indwm/indwm2.htm. Published April 22, 2005. Updated 2006. Accessed September 22, 2013.
3. US Census Bureau. *Marriage and Divorce: Current Population Survey Data on Marriage and Divorce.* US Census Bureau. http://www.census.gov/hhes/socdemo/marriage/data/cps/index.html. Updated August 15, 2012. Accessed September 22, 2013.
4. Kruger A. The mid-life transition: crisis or chimera? *Psychological Reports.* 1994;75:1299-1305.
5. Erickson E. *Identity, Youth and Crisis.* New York, NY: WW Norton; 1968.
6. Erickson E. *Identity and the Life Cycle.* New York, NY: WW Norton; 1994.
7. Levinson D, Darrow CN, Klein EB, Levinson MH, McKee B. *The Seasons of a Man's Life.* New York, NY: Alfred A. Knopf; 1978.
8. Levinson D. *The Seasons of a Woman's Life.* Toronto, ON: Random House of Canada; 1996.
9. Jonsson H, Josephsson S, Kielhofner G. Narratives and experience in an occupational transition: a longitudinal study of the retirement process. *American Journal of Occupational Therapy.* 2001;55(4):424-432.

10. Matheson LN, Bohr PC. Occupational competence across the life span. In: Christiansen C, Baum C, eds. *Occupational Therapy: Enabling Function and Well-Being.* Thorofare, NJ: SLACK Incorporated; 1997:429-457.

11. Kadar E, Shaw RE. Toward an ecological field theory of perceptual control of locomotion. *Ecological Psychology.* 2000;12:141-180.

12. Chemero A. What we perceive when we perceive affordances. *Ecological Psychology.* 2001;13:111-116.

13. Gibson JJ. *The Senses Considered as Perceptual Systems.* Boston, MA: Houghton Mifflin; 1966.

14. Gibson JJ. *The Ecological Approach to Visual Perception.* Boston, MA: Houghton Mifflin; 1979.

15. Bandura A. Self-efficacy: toward a unifying theory of behavioral change. *Psychological Review.* 1977;84:191-215.

16. US Department of Labor: Bureau of Labor Statistics. *Number of Jobs Held by Individuals From Age 18 to Age 44 in 1978 to 2008 by Educational Attainment, Sex, Race, and Hispanic or Latino Ethnicity.* US Department of Labor: Bureau of Labor Statistics. http://www.bls.gov/nls/nlsy79r23jobsbyedu.pdf. Published 2011. Accessed Sept 22, 2013.

17. US Department of Labor: Bureau of Labor Statistics. *Persons at Work in Agriculture and Related and in Nonagricultural Industries by Hours of Work.* US Department of Labor: Bureau of Labor Statistics. http://www.bls.gov/cps/cpsaat19.pdf. Published 2011. Accessed September 22, 2013.

18. United Nations Department of Economic and Social Affairs. *The World's Women 2010: Trends and Statistics.* New York, NY: United Nations; 2010.

19. US Department of Labor: Bureau of Labor Statistics. *Employed Persons by Detailed Occupation, Sex, Race, and Hispanic or Latino Ethnicity.* US Department of Labor: Bureau of Labor Statistics. http://www.bls.gov/cps/cpsaat11.pdf. Published 2011. Accessed September 22, 2013.

20. US Department of Labor: Bureau of Labor Statistics. *Employment Status of the Civilian Noninstitutional Population 25 Years and Over by Educational Attainment, Sex, Race, and Hispanic or Latino Ethnicity.* US Department of Labor: Bureau of Labor Statistics. http://www.bls.gov/cps/cpsaat7.pdf. Published 2011. Accessed September 22, 2013.

21. US Department of Labor: Bureau of Labor Statistics. *Multiple Jobholders by Selected Demographic and Economic Characteristics.* US Department of Labor: Bureau of Labor Statistics. http://www.bls.gov/cps/cpsaat36.pdf. Published 2011. Accessed September 22, 2013.

22. Whiteford G. Occupational deprivation: global challenge in the new millennium. *British Journal of Occupational Therapy.* 2000;63(5):200-204.

23. Smith DL, Alston R. Employment disparities for minority women with disabilities. *University of Minnesota, Institute on Community Integration: Impact: Feature Issue on Employment and Women With Disabilities.* 2008:21(1):16-18.

24. Matuska K. Workaholism, life balance, and well-being: a comparative analysis. *Journal of Occupational Science.* 2009;17(2):104-111.

25. US Department of Labor: Bureau of Labor Statistics. *Unemployed Persons by Marital Status, Race, Hispanic or Latino Ethnicity, Age, and Sex [Data File].* US Department of Labor: Bureau of Labor Statistics. http://www.bls.gov/cps/cpsaat24.pdf. Published 2011. Accessed September 22, 2013.

26. Institute for Work and Health. *Unemployment and mental health.* Institute for Work and Health. http://www.iwh.on.ca/briefings/unemployment-and-mental-health. Published 2009. Accessed February 7, 2012.

27. Rosenthal L, Carroll-Scott A, Earnshaw VA, Santilli A, Ickovics JR. The importance of full-time work for urban adults' mental and physical health. *Social Science and Medicine.* 2012;75(9):1692-1696.

28. Marlar J. *Young, Longer Term Unemployed Experience Health Decline: Also Experience Greater Rates of Physical Pain and Lower Rates of Rest and Energy.* Gallup Wellbeing. http://www.gallup.com/poll/141206/young-longer-term-unemployed-experience-health-decline.aspx. Published July 9, 2010. Updated 2013. Accessed September 22, 2013.

29. Spence J, Robbins A. Workaholism: definition, measurement, and preliminary results. *Journal of Personality Assessment.* 1992;58:160-178.

30. Aziz S, Zicker MJ. A cluster analysis investigation of workaholism as a syndrome. *Journal of Occupational Health Psychology.* 2006;11:52-62.

31. Erase-Blunt M. The busman's holiday. *HR Magazine.* 2001;46:76-80.

32. Piotrowski C, Vodanovich SJ. The workaholism syndrome: an emerging issue in the psychological literature. *Journal of Instructional Psychology.* 2008;35(1):103.

33. Maslach C. Burnout: a multidimensional perspective. In: Schaufeli WB, Maslach C, Marek T, eds. *Professional Burnout: Recent Developments in Theory and Research.* Washington, DC: Taylor & Francis; 1993:19-32.

34. Schaufeli WB, Taris TW, van Rhenen W. Workaholism, burnout, and work engagement: three of a kind or three different kinds of employee burnout? *Applied Psychology: An International Review.* 2008;57(2):173-203.

35. Breso E, Salanova M, Schaufeli WB. Search of the "third dimension" of burnout: efficacy or inefficacy? *Applied Psychology.* 2007;56(3):460-478.

36. Maslach C, Leiter MP. Early predictors of job burnout and engagement. *Journal of Applied Psychology.* 2008;93(3):498-512.

37. Peterson U, Demerouti E, Bergström G, Samuelsson M, Asberg M, Nygren A. Burnout and physical and mental health among Swedish healthcare workers. *Journal of Advanced Nursing.* 2008;62(1):84-95.

38. Figley C. *Treating Compassion Fatigue.* New York, NY: Brunner-Routledge; 2002.

39. Sonnenschein M, Sorbi MJ, Verbraak MJ, Schaufeli WB, Maas CJ, Van Doornen LJ. Influence of sleep on symptom improvement and return to work in clinical burnout. *Scandinavian Journal of Work, Environment & Health.* 2008;34(1):23-32.

40. US Department of Labor. *Wage and Hour Division (WHD): Family and Medical Leave Act.* US Department of Labor. http://www.dol.gov/whd/fmla. Accessed September 22, 2013.

41. HR Focus. Employers embracing programs as morale booster, business strategy. *HR Focus.* 2011;88(9):1-4.

42. US Department of Health and Human Services. *Educational and Community Based Programs.* Healthypeople.gov. http://www.healthypeople.gov/2020/topicsobjectives2020/objectiveslist.aspx?topicId=11. Updated August 28, 2013. Accessed September 22, 2013.

43. Smith C. Engaging the emotional, financial, and physical ramifications of long-distance caregiving. *Home Health Care Management & Practice.* 2006;18(6):463-466. doi:10.1177/1084822306290347.

44. MetLife Mature Market Institute: National Alliance for Caregiving. *The Metlife Caregiving Cost Study: Productivity Losses to US Business.* National Alliance for Caregiving. http://www.caregiving.org/data/Caregiver%20Cost%20Study.pdf. Published July 2006. Accessed September 22, 2013.

45. US Department of Health and Human Services. Fertility, contraception, and fatherhood: data on men and women from cycle 6 (2002) of the National Survey of Family Growth. *Vital and Health Statistics.* 2006;23(26):32.

46. US Department of Health and Human Services. Fertility, contraception, and fatherhood: data on men and women from cycle 6 (2002) of the National Survey of Family Growth. *Vital and Health Statistics.* 2006;23(26):110-119.

47. US Department of Health and Human Services. Fertility, family planning, and reproductive health of US women: data from the 2002 national survey of family growth. *Vital and Health Statistics.* 2005;23(25):42.

48. National Alliance for Caregiving. *The National Alliance for Caregiving.* NAC: National Alliance for Caregiving: advancing family caregiving through research, innovation, and advocacy. http://www.caregiving.org/. Updated 2013. Accessed September 22, 2013.

49. US Department of Labor: Bureau of Labor Statistics. *American Time Use Survey—2012 Results.* US Department of Labor: Bureau of Labor Statistics. http://www.bls.gov/news.release/pdf/atus.pdf. Published June 20, 2013. Accessed September 22, 2013.

50. Bevan JL, Sparks L. Communication in the context of long-distance family caregiving: an integrated review and practical applications. *Patient Education and Counseling.* 2011;85(1):26-30.

51. Riley LD, Bowen C. The sandwich generation: challenges and coping strategies of multigenerational families. *The Family Journal.* 2005;13(1):52-58.

52. Williams C. The sandwich generation. *Perspectives: Statistics Canada.* 2004;75001-XIE:1-8. http://www.statcan.gc.ca/pub/75-001-x/10904/4212007-eng.pdf. Published September 2004. Accessed September 22, 2013.

53. Williams C. The sandwich generation. *Canadian Social Trends.* 2005;77:16-21.

54. Lobo F. Social transformation and the changing work-leisure relationship in the late 1990s. *Journal of Occupational Science.* 1998;5(30):147-154.

55. US Department of Labor: Bureau of Labor Statistics. *American Time Use Survey.* US Department of Labor: Bureau of Labor Statistics. http://www.bls.gov/news.release/atus.nro.htm. Published 2011. Accessed September 22, 2013.

56. Hakansson C, Alhborg G. Perceptions of employment, domestic work, and leisure as predictors of health among women and men. *Journal of Occupational Science.* 2010;17(3):150-157.

57. Turner H, Chapman S, McSherry A, Krishnagiri S, Watts J. Leisure assessment in occupational therapy: an exploratory study. *Occupational Therapy in Health Care.* 2000;12(2/3):73-85.

58. Bundy A. Assessment of play and leisure: delineation of the problem. *American Journal of Occupational Therapy.* 1993;47(3):217-222.

59. Matuska K. Validity evidence for a model and measure of life balance. *OTJR: Occupation, Participation and Health.* 2012;32(1):229-237.

60. Matuska K. Development of the Life Balance Inventory. *OTJR: Occupation, Participation and Health.* 2012;32(1):220-228.

61. Matuska K, Christiansen C. A theoretical model of life balance and imbalance. In: Matuska K, Christiansen C, eds. *Life Balance: Multidisciplinary Theories and Research.* Thorofare, NJ: SLACK Incorporated; 2009:149-163.

62. Heinz A, Pentland W. Professional coaching for life balance. In: Matuska K, Christiansen C, eds. *Life Balance: Multidisciplinary Theories and Research.* Thorofare, NJ: SLACK Incorporated; 2009:241-254.

63. Atkinson G, Davenne D. Relationships between sleep, physical activity and human health. *Physiology and Behavior.* 2007;90(2-3):229-35.

64. Landis CA, Frey CA, Lentz MJ, Rothermel J, Buchwald D, Shaver JL. Self-reported sleep quality and fatigue correlates with actigraphy in midlife women with fibromyalgia. *Nursing Research.* 2003;52(3):140-147.

65. Roehrs T, Roth T. Sleep disorders: an overview. *Clinical Cornerstone.* 2004;6(1):S6-S16.

66. Chaput JP, Després JP, Bouchard C, Tremblay A. Short sleep duration is associated with reduced leptin levels and increased adiposity: results from the Quebec family study. *Obesity.* 2007;15(1):253-261.

67. Dew MA, Hoch CC, Buysse DJ, et al. Healthy older adults' sleep predicts all-cause mortality at 4 to 19 years of follow-up. *Psychosomatic Medicine.* 2003;65(1):63-73.

68. Boivin DB, Tremblay GM, James FO. Working on atypical schedules. *Sleep Medicine.* 2007;8(6):578-589.

69. Boggild H, Knuttson A. Shift work, risk factors and cardiovascular disease. *Scandinavian Journal of Work, Environment and Health.* 1999;2:85-99.

70. Costa G, Sartori S, Akerstedt T. Influence of flexibility and variability of working hours on health and well-being. *Chronobiology International.* 2006;23(6):1125-1137.

71. Haus E, Smolensky M. Biological clocks and shift work: circadian dysregulation and potential long-term effects. *Cancer Causes and Control.* 2006;17(4):489-500.

72. Ogden CL, Carroll MD, McDowell MA, Flegal KM. *Obesity Among Adults in the United States: No Change Since 2003-2004.* NCNS Data Brief No. 1. Hyattsville, MD: National Center for Health Statistics; 2007.

73. Jebb S, Moore M. Contribution of a sedentary lifestyle and inactivity to the etiology of overweight and obesity: current evidence and research issues: roundtable Consensus statement. *Medicine & Science in Sports & Exercise.* 1999;31(11):S534-S531.

74. Tillotson J. America's obesity: conflicting public policies, industrial economic development, and unintended consequences. *Annual Reviews of Nutrition.* 2004;24:617-643.

75. Ford PB, Dzewaltowski DA. Disparities in obesity prevalence due to variation in the retail food environment: three testable hypotheses. *Nutrition Reviews.* 2008;66(4):216-228.

76. Forhan M, Law M, Taylor V, Vrkljan B. Factors associated with the satisfaction of participation in daily activities for adults with class III obesity. *OTJR: Occupation, Participation and Health.* 2012;32(2):70-78.

77. Robinson BE. *Chained to the Desk: A Guidebook for Their Partners and Children and the Clinicians Who Treat Them.* New York, NY: University Press; 1998.

78. Crnic KA, Greenberg MT. Minor parenting stresses with young children. *Child Development.* 1990;61(5):1628-1637.

79. Buysse DJ, Reynolds CF, Monk TH, Berman SR, Kupfer DJ. The Pittsburgh Sleep Quality Index (PSQI): a new instrument for psychiatric research and practice. *Psychiatry Research.* 1989;28(2):193-213.

Chapter 11

OCCUPATIONS OF ELDERHOOD

Gunilla Eriksson, RegOT, PhD; Margareta Lilja, RegOT, PhD; Hans Jonsson, RegOT, PhD;
Ingela Petersson, RegOT, PhD; and Verena C. Tatzer, OT, MSc

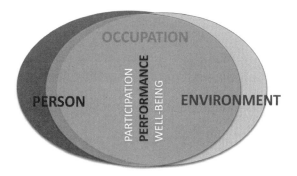

LEARNING OBJECTIVES

- Understand demographic and epidemiologic aspects related to older adults.
- Understand how culture/context affects older adults and occupation at the individual, organization, and population/community level.
- Describe different faces of aging and how environment influences older adults' occupational performance.
- Compare and contrast assessment and interventions regarding older adults and occupational therapy practice.
- Describe different settings for occupational practice.
- Understand the importance of promoting active living strategies and healthy aging.

KEY WORDS

- Age coding
- Ageism
- Continuity theory
- Disengagement theory
- Elder
- Elderhood
- Engaging occupations
- Fourth age
- Gerontology
- Healthy life years (HLY)
- Narratives
- Third age

Christiansen CH, Baum CM, Bass JD, eds.
*Occupational Therapy: Performance, Participation,
and Well-Being, Fourth Edition* (pp 169-183).
© 2015 SLACK Incorporated.

INTRODUCTION

This chapter focuses on the occupations of *elderhood*, or advanced age. In introducing the topic, a few important points must be made. The first concerns a perspective that regards older adults as a group of quite special people who have certain characteristics that differentiates them from other people. In the gerontological literature, this view has sometimes been critiqued as a form of "ageism"[1] that can lead to a number of consequences that potentially discriminate against older adults in society. Although this chapter focuses on older adults, it is important to note that "older adults" represent a large and diverse group whose ages span over more than 30 years, if one considers that the age of 65 is typically the criterion for being called an older adult.[2] Thus, there is great variability within this larger group and it is therefore understandable that subgroups within it have emerged. Included among these is the category *the oldest old*, which has been introduced to describe older adults over the age of 85. As the focus of this chapter is on occupation, a second important distinction concerns a concept known as *age coding*.[3] This type of stereotyping based on chronological age can be misleading and discriminatory, and in an occupational sense may include views that some occupations are not appropriate for people of a certain age. For example, a view that backpacking is not appropriate for a woman aged 75 could be seen as age coding. These views may also be internalized by individuals themselves, who may view that occupations such as backpacking are not appropriate for them, thus influencing their attitude toward participation despite the fact that they may be interested and physically capable of engaging in that occupation. To "age code" occupations is thus to engage in a particular form of ageism.

Despite these caveats, one must acknowledge that age and older age do influence lifestyle, behavior, and socialization. In this chapter you will read Hertha's story. She expresses awareness that she is old; yet she does not feel old. How Hertha's story relates to occupation will provide information pertinent to the concepts in this chapter. From Hertha's individual perspective, the chapter will move toward a discussion about the aging society, about activity patterns and about retirement as an important occupational transition. An occupational view on aging will be discussed in relation to gerontological theories such as Disengagement Theory, Continuity Theory, and the Theory About the Third and Fourth Age. Occupational engagement as predictor of survival in old age will also be discussed. From this general view on aging and older adults we will turn to occupation-based interventions for older adults. Beginning with descriptions of community-based interventions to help prevent physical and mental decline for well elderly persons, the chapter will progress

to descriptions of occupational therapy interventions in 4 countries.

In the third and final part of the chapter, *occupational dysfunction* will be the focus. Reduced performance capacities in older adults are discussed in relation to barriers and inaccessibility in the environment. This section will also give an overview of assessments and how they are used to evaluate individual performance, environmental conditions and/or both in combination.

NARRATIVE: AN OCCUPATIONAL PERSPECTIVE ON GROWING OLD

Hertha's Story: The Maid of Orleans

(The Maid of Orleans refers to a play by Friedrich Schiller that is based on Jean d'arc. It is a metaphor that resulted from the narrative analysis.)

In the following section, the life story of Hertha is described. Hertha was 81 years old when the interview was done and was living in her apartment in Vienna, Austria. She was a very active and energetic person, despite her chronic illness requiring her to use oxygen for cardiopulmonary weakness. Her cardiopulmonary condition was limiting her activities. Hertha's story was documented as part of a narrative research project on life stories and is described in more detail elsewhere.[4] The participants in the study were 4 older women with different occupational experiences who were living in Vienna, Austria. The main finding of this qualitative study was that the participants each described occupational engagement as crucially related to helping them maintain their true identities and to enable them to experience aging without "feeling old."

Part One: Hertha, The Maid of Orleans

Hertha starts her story at her birth in 1927 in Vienna. She continues with the first major change in her life,

"I was 12 when the war started and 18 when it was over."[4](pp138-149)

Her grandfather was of Jewish denomination and she therefore suffered under the Nazi regime in Austria. Theater and writing were her early passions; she wanted to become a journalist. When she was forced to work in an ammunition factory, she learned the play "Maid of Orleans" by heart. After the war, she started her studies of art history and drama. When she got to know her husband she got pregnant, then married and passed her final exams when her first son was 6 weeks old. She took care of her child, but wrote for different student newspapers. After the war she started working for "Rot-weiß-Rot," the first radio broadcasting station in Austria supported by the Americans. After a marriage of 4 years and the birth of her second son, she divorced her husband and since then has supported herself and her family on her own, also financially.

"I had no money, no job, no apartment and nobody who helped me."[4](pp138-149)

She had to overcome all these difficulties at a time when divorce was not accepted in society and pursuing a higher professional career was rare among women. She started taking whatever jobs could support her financially, and finally became the chief executive of a public design institution. In all those years, she enjoyed the work and managed to raise her children alone.

"That I raised my children was never valued, it surely was exhausting, because I never had leisure time in 25 years, never had a Sunday off... I never avoided work, not even doing stupid things if necessary in order to make money."[4](pp138-149)

She also judges her life as something "atypical."

"most of the women, if they have a profession, they stick with it or give it up for their children. They are married. And good wives. Or divorced... I mean, this is... not the usual." "you get used to making your own decisions."[4](pp138-149)

This period of her life was shaped by challenges and survival, in both her private and professional lives.

"There was something different every day. One was always challenged. And that is important to me."[4](p138-149)

Part Two: Second Career, A New Start

Hertha did not wish to retire.

"The idea to stop working never really occurred to me."[4](pp138-149)

When the political pressure was rising, she was forced to leave work at the age of 58. She overcame difficulties finding a new job.

"In the meantime, for a few months, I worked as a secretary in an enterprise selling... [laughs]... cattle testicles, well you really can do business with that kind of thing..."[4](pp138-149) *"I was forced to retire. And at the age of 58. And have made up. Another thing. But I have to admit that it was what I really wanted. To be a journalist."*[4](pp138-149)

She started her second career as a teacher of art history and worked as a journalist, something she has wanted to do all her life but couldn't because of her responsibility for her family and the challenge involved in being a single parent.

Part Three: Theater, An Experiment of Survival and Challenge—"Not a Princess and the Pea"

At the time of the interview, Hertha was 81 years old and contending with the physical limitations linked to a chronic disease that forced her to use a portable oxygen

tank to assist in sustaining her limited physical activities. Her mobility outside her apartment was limited to short distances—she compensated by using her car even for short distances. Even while sitting and talking, she was using her oxygen tank for support.

"My doctor always tells me I was expected to die 5 years ago and that I have broken all the records with my disease." "More and more people from my... time, my youth or even older years have died. I like to remember. I am not sentimental... But I cannot say that this has changed my life, my daily life a lot. This is surely related to the fact, that I have never been dependent on anybody my whole life."[4](pp138-149)

She tells a story that seems to characterize her attitude toward aging and the physical restraints related to aging as follows:

"I really wanted to go to the theatre... And I used to go without having a ticket in advance. And then I had this idea. The Volkstheater. They presented the "Präsidentinnen." I called, but it was all sold out. I said to myself. Well, I can park there. Because I have this parking ticket for people with disability... And I went there. And certainly, I got a ticket! And I did it partly to prove to myself that I can still do it... This is my way. That is what I am used to...This: More than ever! If one says: this was difficult. Then I roll up my sleeves and then: more than ever... This is what I did for years."[4](pp138-149)

Hertha gave up teaching when she realized that it required too much energy and money. She judges this step as:

"rather stopping when one's still loved."[4](pp138-149)

She has a very rational, intellectual, and ironic attitude toward aging. As an example, she relates a story about the limitation of activities she can do due to her disease and aging process. In former times, "only" going to the pharmacy was not acceptable for her as a main activity of the day. Now, there are days for her where going to the pharmacy and the doctor consumes most of her energy.

"Today, I did something disagreeable... And then I went to the pharmacy. That was always the embodiment. I have always said, if I come to the point where I go to the pharmacy and say, this is what I have done the whole day—that is terrible. Well, that's how it is now."[4](pp138-149)

Hertha wants to delay reaching the state when she is no longer able to do anything, but feels that this day might come soon. She knows that she is able to withstand difficult times. The meaning of activities has changed significantly as Hertha discusses dressing herself.

"What do I wear. This is always a big problem. In former times, it should be suitable for the occasion or if I wanted to please someone or not... But I had a lot of fun doing it; I also liked to wear something crazy... And now it is...well, what you wear, for it is neither too cold nor too hot."[4](pp138-149)

Hertha must contend with a chronic disease that hinders her from many physical activities. She feels healthy in spite of it and keeps up with her habits.

"It is some sort of exercise. If one over a longer period had to overcome obstacles, it's certainly easier. I imagine. If I had been a 'princess and a pea' all my life. And then I have a problem... That's maybe some sort of adjustment."[4(pp138-149)]

The main changes of occupation are dealing with physical issues and the restraint of her body for example when travelling.

"I can only experience Venice while browsing through books or watching films. And what goes with it, the smelling and the feeling... the... experience... that is not possible anymore."[4(pp138-149)]

She is still writing and this is also when she experiences some sort of flow.

"I have to say that the moments when I feel most comfortable are while sitting at the table working on something or driving a car."[4(pp138-149)]

A Woman Full of Stories

Hertha's life narrative is full of minor stories that have all influenced her life in different ways. Her personal narrative is an important starting point for understanding her as a person, but to get a fuller understanding her life narrative must be understood within the context of when it was lived and is now recalled. World War II, the sociocultural circumstances to be a working single mother in Austria during the decades after the war, labor regulations about retirement, possibilities to have societal support when facing functional limitations, and other contextual factors are important subtexts for understanding Hertha's story. These social and cultural realities provide an important context that is sometimes apparent in the narrative account but also sometimes invisible, much as the air we breathe. The metaphor of the "Maid of Orleans"—a story of a strong heroine, who retains her reputation and identity despite enduring unfair and difficult life situations—strongly expresses her situation and attitude.

For Hertha, occupations have changed over her lifetime, as some have faded out and others faded in. Energy levels might decrease for an old person due to natural aging processes or to the presence of impairments; Hertha faces both challenges. Yet, she manages well in her aging process. She performs valued occupations and even has maintained connections to old passions and made them bloom again after retirement. She successfully overcomes challenges due to physical limitations, not allowing them to take over her life. She has lost valued occupations, but this seems acceptable for her as she still has valued occupations in her life. However, she worries that she might soon reach a point where she cannot fight her physical limitations and constraints anymore. For Hertha, it means that she not only will *be* quite old but also *feel* very old.[4]

Hertha's story serves to illustrate some points that are useful in understanding elderhood:

- An elderly person is a person full of stories.
- The personal story is a good starting point for understanding the individual, but is not sufficient.
- The organizational and community features of a narrative are important if one is to fully understand a person's story, since the story is told in this context (and sometimes taken for granted).
- Occupations come and go; for elderly persons the amount of energy available for activities and participation might decrease due to the natural aging process or due to the presence of impairments.
- The aging process, as well as the activity limitations that might come from impairments, is important as one aspect for understanding occupational performance.
- Loss of some occupations can be acceptable if other valued occupations and/or social community participation are present in a person's life.
- As the aging process progresses, limitations may lead to a point where the person begins to fear not only that others perceive them as old, but that they perceive themselves as very old because they cannot do what they value and need to do.

Hertha's dynamic life narrative is one story among an increasing population of older adults. We will keep this individual story in mind as we examine the characteristics of older adults in general—all persons situated in what has been called "the aging society."

AGING IN RELATION TO AN OCCUPATIONAL PERSPECTIVE

The Aging Society: Burden, Resource, or Both? (Demographic Aspects)

It is well known that the number of older persons as a proportion of the entire population is increasing in most Western countries, and that this growth will continue and lead to significant societal affects. Social security systems will be challenged, and requirements for health care, as well as long-term care, will increase. Further, there will be a need for more gerontological knowledge among health workers and more openness to secure older people's rights and opportunities in society-at-large.[5] Older adults are typically defined as those 60 years or older.[6] People 80 years or older were earlier called the *oldest old*, but the WHO has changed this term to *very old*.[5] Owing to a substantial decline in the age-specific mortality of the very old (80+ years) within the last 50 years, this group has become the fastest growing age segment in most western countries.[7]

According to WHO, 2 billion people will be aged 60 and older by 2050.[5] In 2008, there were an estimated 39 million people age 65 and over in the United States, accounting for just over 13% of the total population. In 2010, there were 1.9 million people aged 90 and older; the majority were women. The older population in 2030 is expected to be nearly 20% of the total United States population.[8] In Europe in 2010 there was a slightly higher proportion of the population (17%) that was 65 years or older,[9] and older persons will continue to account for an increasing share of the total population so that by 2060 those aged 65 years or over will account for about 30% of the population.[9] Moreover, the share of those aged 85 years or older is projected to almost triple by 2060 (12%).

Life Expectancy and Disability-Free Life Expectancy

Life expectancy and disability-free life expectancy are 2 different summary measures of population health. Life expectancy is the expected number of years of life remaining at a given age. Disability-free life expectancy—which also is called Healthy Life Years (HLY)—measures the number of remaining years that a person of a certain age is supposed to live without disability. HLY is used to distinguish between years of life free of any activity limitation and years experienced with at least one activity limitation. The emphasis with the measure HLY is also on quality of life rather than duration, which is the focus when measuring life expectancy.

Life expectancy has risen continuously over the last 2 centuries, for example the female life expectancy has increased 3 months per year in 160 years (from an average of 45 years in 1840 to 85 years of age in 2010). Americans are living longer than ever before, yet their life expectancies lag behind those of other developed nations.

It is sometimes discussed that life expectancy has reached its limits, but there is no evidence for that. If the current trend of life expectancy increasing by 2.5 years per decade persists, the average lifespan may be 100 years by 2070.[10(p57)] However, now that chronic diseases are replacing infectious diseases as population health concerns, illness is not only associated with mortality risk but also to the risk of living with a chronic illness. Thus, it is not sufficient to monitor the increase in life expectancy to understand population health, the impact of chronic illness and disability associated with aging must also be estimated. Therefore, the indicator healthy life years is also used.

There are also gender differences in healthy life years. In Europe, men were expected to live 80% of their life without disabilities while women could expect to live 75% of their lives without disability, owing partly to a longer life expectancy than men. Surveys confirm that in many countries both life expectancy and healthy life years

is lower for elderly people who were blue collar workers.[11] The level of education also has a strong positive impact on life expectancy and on healthy life years, and social support and informal relations with the family seem to be important for successful aging as well.

An improvement in expected healthy life years and overall quality of life is the main health goal in the European Union, and that overall goal is also set by the National Institute on Aging.[12] Research and intervention efforts focus on preventing or reducing age-related diseases or disabilities, maintaining physical health and function, enhancing older adults' societal roles and personal support, and reducing social isolation.[12]

The Survey of Health, Ageing, and Retirement in Europe (SHARE) is a multidisciplinary and cross-national panel database of micro data on health, socioeconomic status, and social and family networks of more than 45,000 individuals aged 50 or over. These data provide useful socioeconomic demographics for analyses of population health.

These analyses show that morbidity is increasing and is more prevalent in females than in males. More than 66% have had at least 1 chronic disease diagnosed during their lifetime and around 40% have had 2 or more chronic diseases diagnosed. The most commonly reported diseases include arthritis, diabetes, heart disease, and hypertension.[13] Large proportions of older Americans report a variety of chronic health conditions, such as hypertension and arthritis. The prevalence of certain chronic conditions differs by sex. Women report higher levels of arthritis than men (55% vs 42%). Men report higher levels of heart disease (38% vs 27%) and cancer (24% vs 21%).[8] Despite these and other conditions, the rate of functional limitations among older people has declined in recent years.

Older adults often live active lives until their 80s, when several start to have difficulties performing everyday occupations and the need for support and assistance increase.[14] The ability to perform ADL gets more limited in older age for both men and women, but the decline is greater in women. In the group of individuals from 50 years of age and over, 90% reported having no disability in personal ADL. Around 17% report one or more limitations in IADL. For IADL as well as for personal ADL, the limitations increase with advancing age groups.[13] However, in the age group 85 years and over more than two-thirds are independent in ADLs, indicating that a large proportion of the oldest old are not disabled. Mobility limitations of some kind were found in up to a third of the population.

Older adults in Europe and in the United States contribute to society by being productive in different ways. Many are still working in the labor market after 65 years of age (Europe/United States: Men 9%/18%; Women 6%/10%). Almost one-fourth of the older adults provide help to relatives or friends outside their own household.

They assist with activities as personal care, practical household help, or paperwork.

As many as 25% of the older adults in Europe and almost 30% in the United States that are grandparents take care of grandchildren often, usually about once a week. Older adults are also moderately involved in social activities, such as doing voluntary or charity work, going to sports or other kind of clubs, or participating in various kinds of organizations. Some attend educational or training courses. The proportion of leisure time that older Americans spend on socializing declines with age.[8] Time spent in a typical day varies significantly, however, between countries, gender, and age groups. Despite this variation, the amount of time spent helping others and taking care of grandchildren is not trivial, and the economic value of these non-market activities is high.[15,16]

Activity Patterns of Older Adults

Patterns of activities commonly performed may change over the lifespan. In a European study on activity patterns of older adults, 3 main types of activities were identified[17]:

1. Home-based, family-oriented activities

2. Individual activities outside the home

3. Participation in the local community

The first type (home-based, family-oriented activities) refers to activities such as media use, housekeeping, social activities at home, hobbies, and outdoor activities. The older adults participated to a high degree in these activities in all age groups from 50 to 90 years of age. About 70% participated in these types of activities even at the age of 90, except for outdoor activities, which were performed by about half of the individuals that were 80 years and older. Media use, however, increased with age. In the second type of activities, individual activities outside the home, activities such as paid work, sports, cultural activities and entertainment, and traveling were typical. The results showed a decrease in these activities in the older adults after the age of 65 and at the age of 90; only 20% were active in these types of activities.

The overall involvement in the third category of activities, participation in the local community, was lower than in the other types of activities. Providing assistance, for example, was performed by half of those aged 50, but decreased to below 20% at the age of 85. Civic activities were performed by about 40% of the participants at all ages. Other studies on activity patterns among older adults in Western cultures support the results from this study; revealing that activities requiring a low level of physical activity, such as watching television and listening to music, increase in old age.[18,19] In contrast, participation in home maintenance and social activities remains stable in older age.[19]

A cross-cultural analysis of the main activities of older adults in both Eastern and Western countries also validated the activity patterns revealed previously by identifying the main activities as being IADL activities, low demand leisure activities, and social activities.[20] This cross-cultural analysis revealed interesting differences and similarities between the samples from Asian and Western countries. The Asian countries surveyed included Hong Kong, Singapore, and Korea; while the Western countries included the United States, Australia, Israel, The Netherlands, and Puerto Rico. Overall, 558 persons had responded to a culturally relevant version of the Activity Card Sort (ACS).[21] To be able to describe occupations across countries, the 8 different ACS versions were integrated and recoded. When this process was accomplished, the integrated ACS version comprised 105 activities.

Ten of those 105 activities were central to the older adults participating in the study across all cultures. These activities were shopping in a store, shopping for groceries, doing dishes, doing laundry, reading magazines/books, sitting and thinking, watching television, listening to radio/music, visiting with friends/relatives, and talking on the telephone. An activity was classified as central if more than 50% in all samples reported that they performed the activity. In a similar way, central activities in Eastern and Western cultures were identified. An activity was classified as central for a Western or an Asian culture if it was performed by more than 50% of the participants in the countries in a group and if less than 50% of the participants in the countries representing the other group performed the activity. There were 16 activities that were central in the Asian countries, equally distributed on IADLs and social and leisure activities. For the Western countries, 17 activities were identified as central and those were mainly leisure activities.

Most of those activities central in a Western culture were leisure activities, and the absolute majority of those did not require a high level of physical activity. This is in accordance with findings from a study on 9 Western countries[19] revealing that after the age of 74, a decrease was seen concerning time use in physically demanding activities. Albert and colleagues[18] found that in the United States, the most frequent and easiest to perform activities among older adults were watching television, taking out trash, listening to music, attending family gatherings, watching movies, reading magazines or books, and visiting with friends.

Activity patterns of older adults may also be viewed from the perspective of time use. According to surveys of time use, as people age they spend varying proportions of time in paid work, family care, personal care, and free time. Most of the variation comes from a decrease in time spent working, not from any demonstrable effects of aging. People who are still in the labor force after age 65 have time use patterns similar to those of younger people. So it seems that social structures, not age itself, might determine the uses of time in later life. Studies of old adults' time use from Canada,[22] the United Kingdom,[23] and Australia[24] showed that community-dwelling older adults (on average) spent about 11 hours in self-care (including sleep), 8 hours in leisure, more than 4 hours in domestic activities, and only a half hour per day in work activities.

In 2000, the project MOBILATE was carried out in 5 European countries (Finland, Germany, Hungary, Italy, and The Netherlands) with 3950 people aged over 55.[25] One part of the project focused on the analysis of the temporal aspects of out-of-home activities and also upon the differences between different groups of people. In the urban areas, more time is spent outdoors than in rural areas. It may be that the better availability of facilities in urban environments is a part of the explanation for their greater use. Furthermore, men go out more than women and older people stay at home more than younger adults.

The study showed interesting variability among countries with respect to patterns of mobility away from home during different periods of the day. Additionally, certain activities were associated with particular times during the day, reflecting the influences of universal rest-activity patterns, as well as culturally specific and geographic lifestyle differences.[25]

Section Summary: Activity Patterns of Elders

In this section we have described activity patterns of older adults. One conclusion that can be made is that older adults' activity patterns cannot be explained as typical, based on membership in an age group over a certain numeric ceiling. Nowadays, old age can span 30 or 40 years; thus, sweeping generalizations about activity participation based on age are simply not supported by empirical evidence.

Not all older people are frail and impaired. Getting along with rising life expectancy, more and more older persons feel they still have a lot to give and to experience even after they have reached an advanced age. When examining data on activity patterns and changes over the lifespan, it seems that activities requiring a low level of physical activity, such as watching television and listening to music, increase in old age and that outdoor activities such as participating in the local community may decrease. These decreases may be a consequence of mobility restrictions or economic constraints. Cultural factors might also have an impact on older adults' activity patterns. Environmental issues can also have an impact on older adults' activity patterns, such that those living in environments with better access or availability to recreational spaces may also spend more time outdoors.

Retirement as the First Step Into the Third Age

When retirement became institutionalized, it was a transformative event in the last years of an older person's life. For example, in Sweden the average age at retirement in the late 1950s was 3 to 5 years above the age that policymakers determined for the official retirement age (67 years).[26] Theories of aging started with retirement and outlined disengagement as the natural process where both social interaction and engagement in activities decreased in the very last years.[27] A well-earned rest after a long and hard life as a worker was the explanation for this activity decline. One may question if this theory mirrored most peoples' retirement experiences at the time; but most certainly the theory must be viewed differently today, as longevity has increased dramatically in most countries in the world.

Consider a woman in Sweden, where the retirement age is about 62 to 63 years on average.[14] This means that she will spend over one-third of her adult life as retiree (22 to 24 years). Given this increase in the period of retirement, how will retirees spend their time? Will they be inactive, choosing to rest and pursue what amounts to a very long vacation? Interesting retirement cards that people receive on their retirement day, for example from working colleagues, sometimes reflect this cultural view of doing nothing during retirement.

A longitudinal research project in Sweden studied retirement from an occupational perspective by following participants from when they were workers to becoming established retirees.[2,28] Narratives were collected and analyzed among 30 participants at 3 points: as workers, as persons who were newly retired, and as persons who had been retired for a longer period.[29] In these narratives, statements about doing nothing in retirement were found among the participants. For example one participant said: "I don't do anything, not a damn thing!"[28(p223)] However, this was not a description of a good life as a retiree; in fact, it was quite the opposite. It was a description of an activity void, of endless time that one had to kill and a life deprived of occupation. One participant said, "It is a whole new experience. It's like life itself sort of ends!"[28(p223)]

Perceived freedom was an experience shared by most of the participants following retirement. Yet freedom to do nothing was paradoxically experienced as a burden. The responsibility for planning a day and organizing daily occupations had now shifted from an employer to the retiree (and his or her partner). External demands and expectations decreased. So, this total freedom was not experienced as freedom. The paradox appeared that real freedom was to give away part of the freedom and to be involved in something that you found interesting and engaging. A man described his view of freedom: "I have my time, it is my own. I can use it, and I don't want to use it as just free time. I want to use it actively, and it's a very nice feeling. Yes, that's freedom."[30(p34)]

Narratives about a good life in retirement were stories about commitment and engagement. In the analysis, this was conceptualized as a specific type of occupation called *engaging occupation*. Engaging occupation had characteristics of being highly meaningful, was performed regularly, had developed to a commitment, and involved social community with people that shared the common interest. Inhabiting the broad role of a retiree, these engaging occupations also gave a complementary identity for the participants. Engaging occupation was not connected to a specific area in occupation. It could be that the participants continued in their former work, either fully or partly. It could be that they developed a leisure interest both new or continued, but increased after retirement. It could also be in the family arena, such as taking regular care of grandchildren or helping an older relative. The same type of activity (eg, fishing) could be viewed both as an engaging occupation or more as a time-killing occupation in a narrative that was characterized more as occupational deprivation. The concept of engaging occupation raises important questions for an occupational perspective on well-being, since it places emphasis on the experience and process of engagement rather than only on the type of occupation in which a person engages.

EARLY THEORIES OF AGING AND THE THIRD AGE

The theory of disengagement, which proposed that progressive social isolation and inactivity were characteristic of the aging process,[27] has been difficult to apply within contemporary views of aging. In contrast, Atchley's Continuity and Adaption Theory has been referred to in connection to the ideas of engaging occupations.[31] Continuity Theory proposes that older adults typically maintain the same activities, personal preferences, and social relationships as they did in their earlier years.

In the following paragraphs we will propose that a theory that might provide a useful framework for understanding current retirement trends is Laslett's Theory on the Third and Fourth Ages.[32,33] In Laslett's view, the third age can be seen as the culmination of certain obligatory roles and the beginning of a potential period of fulfilment. The responsibility of raising a family and earning a living steps back, and lifelong dreams can be pursued and fulfilled. Commitments and engagements in the community by life-experienced persons after retirement can be a win/win situation. This view is consistent with the Swedish longitudinal study of retirement, which showed

that engaging occupation was often a prerequisite for the experience of a good and rewarding life as a retiree. In Laslett's view, this could represent 20 to 30 years of engagement before what he called the fourth age—a period where disability becomes dominant and engagement recedes. Importantly, from an occupational therapy perspective, the presence of a disability does not necessarily mean that engagement and commitment cannot be present in an older person's life. Several studies within occupational therapy about older persons who are frail or live with the presence of disability show that as long as they can continue to perform some type of engaging occupation, people can experience what Hertha described in her opening narrative as "being old without feeling old."[4,30,34]

Thus, returning to the narrative of Hertha presented earlier in the chapter, we are able to illustrate several of the concepts presented in this section. First, Hertha's transformation to retirement at the early age of 58 was both unexpected and undesired, causing some disturbance in her life. However, because Hertha described herself as one who has become adept at confronting challenging situations, she typifies the third age as identified by Laslett, described as a period of possible fulfilment. Hertha manages to continue a valued (but not recently performed) occupation as a writer, an activity that became an engaging occupation for her. As the aging process continued for her, decreasing energy required that she abandon some of her valued occupations, but she continued to perform others—often with significant engagement despite facing challenging situations due to her disability. Yet, Hertha is now in the phase of realizing that her disability will become more dominant, and that she soon might enter what Laslett call the fourth age. Yet, she retains her writing as a valued and engaging occupation.

Continuity, Engagement, and Aging Without Feeling Old

In the following section, we discuss how knowledge from occupational therapy and occupational science and Atchley's Continuity Theory can be used to better understand the role and function of occupation during the aging process. A short introduction to Atchley's Continuity Theories is provided and Hertha's[4] story is linked to it.

Positive aspects on aging should be highlighted in occupational therapy practice and research. Theories from the field of gerontology can contribute to a better understanding of the process of aging. Nevertheless, theories cannot capture complex phenomena entirely, and the subjective experiences of older people do not fit to the theoretical assumptions.[35] It can be expected that the experiences of older women are different from those of older men, because gender and social classes are used very early in life by "various gatekeepers" and influence people's access to education and occupational roles.[31]

More recent publications in the field of gerontology prefer using the term *development* instead of *aging* to highlight the potential of growth in later adulthood.[36] The changes associated with aging are described differently in these theories. Examples are the theory of selective optimisation and compensation by Baltes & Baltes,[37] Laslett's theory about the Third and Fourth Ages[32] and Atchley's Continuity Theory.[31,38,39] In Continuity Theory, a stability or consistency of ideas and lifestyles is central to the process of adult development in later life and is described as a common strategy for coping with changes.[31] Its central idea is that there is an active "construction and use of enduring patterns to enhance life satisfaction and adaptation to change."[31(p7)] Atchley developed the Continuity Theory based on existing research findings and longitudinal research with 1.271 participants in a period of over 20 years from 1975 to 1995. A starting point was the fact that many older adults show "considerable consistency over time in their patterns of thinking, activity profiles, living arrangements and social relationships."[31] He also wanted to explore why many older adults did not experience retirement negatively, as theories like the disengagement theory in that time would have supposed. Concepts used by Atchley[31(p4)] for example are *life experience;* he also speaks of *activity patterns* that last over adulthood and old age. He described that people use life experience to "evaluate, refine, or revise both the initial pattern and the process of making behavioural choices."[31] Due to the quantitative nature of his research, a deeper understanding of how this feedback to modify personal constructs works was still to explore.[31(p156)] Atchley created the term *occupational identity,* meaning the same as work-identity, describing women in their retirement process. Positive effects of retirement are traced back to the fact that the women continued their occupational identities into retirement. The role of occupation in the aging process seems to be crucial; as in most gerontological theories, activity or active engagement in occupation is important. However, gerontological literature does not focus on the mechanisms and experiences of occupational changes in aging.

Seen from an occupational perspective, the aging process can be described as gradual changes during which the person experiences decline in physical ability, energy, and strength.[34,40-42] Struggling against and adapting to this decline by using resources and strategies can be possible reactions from the older person. Trying to prevent the decline can be seen as struggling; adapting to it can be described in giving up familiar occupations, or finding new strategies for doing them. Occupational adaptation has been described as the "series of actions, internal to the individual, which unfolds as the individual is faced with an occupational challenge."[43(p474)] Schultz and Schkade have highlighted that the individual engages in this process of adaptation with the intention to produce a response that should result in an experience of "relative mastery over the challenge."[43(p474)] Meaning, engagement, and involvement are key concepts in research about the elderly from an occupational perspective.[34,40,44] Personally meaningful occupations are described as "most beneficial" for adaptation. Adaptation in the context of aging can also be understood as finding new occupations or finding new meanings in old occupations.[4]

In occupational therapy and occupational science theory, engagement in occupation is essentially linked to well-being and health and makes one's life meaningful.[45,46] It has been suggested, that occupations that convey meaning are central to identity.[47,48] Christiansen[47] argued that people shape their identities through daily occupations and that identity could provide an important link in understanding the fundamental relationship between occupation and well-being. Therefore, the loss or change of occupation related to identity can thus be seen as a particular challenge during aging and may result in illness. Jonsson et al[49] revealed the possible occupational changes people experience when dealing with the life-transitioning processes of retirement with possible losses, as well as gains of regular and meaningful occupation. Jonsson et al[41(p428)] identified engaging occupation as "a main determinant" of whether aged persons experience their lives as positive. The key features of engaging occupation are that it embodies "intensity" and "goes beyond personal pleasure," involved "occupational community," and has "analogues for work." The presence or absence of engaging occupation is often the difference between feeling that you are the same and not feeling old, which was described by Hurd.[50] Engaging in occupation is thus an *identity-saver.*

In the context of Continuity Theory, occupation can be paradoxically viewed as both the means for creating continuity and adaptation. Atchley[31(p156)] points out the lack of research on "factors, that address the use of feedback to modify personal constructs." Engaging occupation can be understood as this "missing link." From an integrative point of view of occupational therapy/occupational science and in his theory, occupation functions as an important factor for feedback. It is used for "identity-testing" to see, if continuation is still possible or if the result of adaptation still fits to the older self. Occupation is thus like a litmus test of one's identity and capacities and is used as a measure for change while aging.

Atchley[31] found in his longitudinal data that more than half of the participants experienced continuity in their activity level, and that the prior activity level of his participants was the strongest predictor of the current activity level. Hertha herself explains her successful struggle with aging and chronic disease by her prior active engagement. In

Hertha's words: "It is some sort of exercise. If one over a longer period had to overcome obstacles, it's certainly easier... If I had been a 'princess and a pea' all my life. And then I have a problem."[4(pp138-149)] She describes her pattern of dealing with difficulties by what Atchley calls "coping."

Successful struggle and adaptation is expressed in Hertha's knowledge that she is old in age, but that she does not feel old. Aging has influenced her occupations significantly. To Hertha, occupation is both the means to test if she is still the same person, but also the way to transformation. The stories of "still doing it" and challenges in their everyday lives seem to be particularly useful to maintain a sense of self through occupation.[4,51]

Occupation as a Predictor of Survival in Old Age

"Occupation is as necessary to life as food and drink. Every human being should have both physical and mental occupations. All should have occupations which they enjoy, or hobbies."[52(p10)]

Occupations change through the lifespan; new is introduced and others slowly fade out or will suddenly disappear due to a variety of reasons. In the aging process, disappearance might be due to external circumstances (like retirement) or physical occupations that fade out due to health decline. However, an aspect of continuity in occupations is a common pattern.[53] It seems to be a vital part of keeping ones identity and experience—what can be called growing older without feeling old, as Hertha express in her occupational narrative and illustrates with her example of the visit to the theater. That is why we fully can endorse what one of our professions founders said almost 100 years ago, "occupation is as necessary to life as food and drink."[52(p10)]

In a study of very old persons (over 80 years), experience of participation[34] was expressed in engaging in occupations and feeling togetherness with others. A clear connection in activity level and survival in old age is found in several population studies conducted in the United States, Sweden, Canada, United Kingdom, and Germany.[53-58]

In the Swedish study that followed older people for 12 years,[53] the mortality risk was almost doubled when activity performance was rated 0-1 activity as compared to rated 4-6 activities (controlled for confounding factors). The same type of results was seen in a 13-year longitudinal study of elderly Americans that looked for performance level in 3 types of activities: social, productive, and physical activities.[54] The authors conclude:

> All 3 types of activity were independently associated with survival after age, sex, race/ethnicity, marital status, income, body mass index, smoking, functional disability, and history of cancer, diabetes, stroke, and myocardial infarction were controlled for... Social and productive activities that involve little or no enhancement of fitness lower the risk of all-cause mortality as much as fitness activities do. This suggests that in addition to increased cardio-pulmonary fitness, activity may confer survival benefits through psychosocial pathways.[54(p478)]

Productive activity was actually the strongest predictor of the 3 types of activities. Reasons for that might be that it commonly includes both physical and social aspects. But even more important might be that it includes engagement and commitment for the participants. This type of occupation has been named *engaging occupation,* and has been described as a key concept in relation to occupation and the experience of a good life as a retiree.[2] A study in a Swedish representative sample of people 77 years and older found that the psychological aspects, as a sense of purposefulness or motivation for engaging in activities, were the key factors in the promotion of health in late life—supporting the concept of engaging occupations.[2] Lennartsson et al[58] concluded that taking part in activities, not explicitly including social aspects, is a strong predictor for survival in old age.

In addition to improving health, being occupied also improves cognitive and physical performance. Extensive evidence shows that physically demanding leisure activities lower the rates of heart disease[59] and cognitive decline.[60] Participating in cognitively demanding activities have shown to be a predictor for physical functioning in elderly people,[57] as well as for cognitive functioning.[61] If one relates these findings to Hertha's story, they seem to harmonize. Hertha had challenged herself with cognitively demanding activities, as being a teacher in art history and as a journalist after her retirement, and she was cognitively well preserved late in life.

PREVENTIVE OCCUPATION-BASED INTERVENTIONS FOR WELL ELDERLY PERSONS

As the elderly population is both growing and on average also gets older, effective prevention and wellness programs become more important in public health. Older persons become frailer and exposed to risks within the environment. For example in Sweden, the risk for having a fall injury for women over 80 years is 50%.[62] These types of risks might result in loss of independence and withdrawal from valued occupations, leading to diminished health and occupational deprivation.[63] The good news, however, is that many threats to health and wellness can be averted through effective intervention programs targeted toward the elderly population. Such programs can promote healthy habits and lifestyles during old age so that elderly persons can continue to experience reasonable physical fitness, active engagement, and community participation. Hertha characterized this in her narrative as "being old without feeling that you are old."[4] In the following section, 4 examples of occupation-based interventions within different countries and targeted toward different groups of elderly persons are described.

The Well Elderly Studies: United States

A controlled study examining an occupation-based intervention targeted toward community dwelling well elderly persons was launched by the occupational science group at the University of Southern California in the mid 1990s.[64] A 9-month intervention program described as Lifestyle Redesign was created.[65] The intervention was conceptually founded on occupational science assumptions about occupation and health, and included group as well as participatory individual and group educational sessions. Themes included Transport and Occupation, Physical and Mental Activity, and Home and Community Safety. Independent living elderly in subsidized housing were recruited in a RCT with control groups. The results showed benefits in many health and well-being variables for the intervention group.[64] In a follow-up after 6 months, the results showed the same pattern in favor of the intervention group.[66] The studies were highly appreciated in the occupational therapy community worldwide, leading to the 3 studies described following. Results were also reported by news media as an example of innovative, community-based approaches for providing cost-effective preventive health services for the elderly. In a follow-up investigation called the Well Elderly 2 Study, a larger group of ethnically diverse elderly persons (including a large group of African Americans and Hispanics) were recruited to participate in a 6-month intervention.[67] This study was also a RCT, and the results showed favorable changes for the occupation-based intervention group on body pain, vitality, social function, life satisfaction, and depressive symptoms. These studies illustrated that occupation-based interventions for elderly persons can effectively improve or maintain functional status and social participation for older adults, and can be used as cost-effective preventive interventions to enhance health and subjective well-being in this group.

Do It Now Project: Australia

This project was conducted in Shoalhaven, a small community in New South Wales, Australia.[68] It was supported by the city of council, as well as through funding from the Australian Government. The intervention was inspired by the Well Elderly Study in the United States, as well as research about retirement from an occupational perspective conducted in Sweden.[69] The "Do it Now" project aimed to educate residents aged 55 and over about the importance of planning for what they were going to do in retirement, to have engaging occupations, and about opportunities to stay involved in the community. Twenty programs were conducted with a total of 171 residents. The program included several group sessions, covering concepts about engaging occupation and its relationship to health and life satisfaction in retirement, as well as information about local community resources that were available to support participation during retirement. The program also included the use of nonverbal creative activities. Evaluation showed that a large majority of program participants valued the intervention positively, became more aware of factors influencing their health, and planned to increase their involvement in the community.

Lifestyle Matters: United Kingdom

The Lifestyle Matters project was inspired by the US Well Elderly Study and was adapted to be suitable for elderly persons in the United Kingdom.[70] An 8-month intervention was designed and 2 intervention groups were formed with 28 participants. Quantitative measures of change showed an upward trend, but did not show significance in this small sample. A number of participants were followed with qualitative interviews and the participants reported that they were able to engage in new occupations as well as re-engage in old occupations as a result of the intervention.[71] Studies with larger samples are needed to generalize and confirm the results.

The Active Lifestyle All Your Life Intervention Program: Sweden

The Active Lifestyle All Your Life Intervention Program is an ongoing RCT designed to determine if occupation-based intervention can prevent falls among elderly persons at risk. In the study, subjects at risk are defined as elderly persons with a history of one or more falls, whether or not leading to injury. The literature clearly shows that the experience of a fall incident and/or injury tends to diminish a person's occupational repertoire and hinders involvement and engagement. The intervention used in this project was also inspired by the Well Elderly Study and is based on an occupational perspective.[72] The intervention builds on the assumption that, with knowledge and adaptive strategies, it is possible for elderly persons to maintain active lifestyles characterized by engagement in valued occupations, even if such persons are frail and/or have functional limitations. However, this project also pairs occupation-based strategies with interventions from other disciplines based on a meta-analysis of fall-prevention approaches, thus providing a range of interventions that can target fall risks on a broad scale within a primary care perspective.[73,74] The project is designed using a 6-month group-based intervention with individual sessions, and involves about 130 participants assigned to both intervention and control groups. Evaluation includes both quantitative and qualitative measures. Readers may wish to consult clinicaltrials.gov for reports on the outcome of this study conducted under the auspices of the Karolinska Institutet in Stockholm.

OCCUPATIONAL PERFORMANCE DEFICITS AND OLDER ADULTS

In this section we first present aging and occupational performance deficits, and then outline assessing and evaluating for planning interventions.

Aging and Occupational Performance Deficits

Empirical studies investigating aging and everyday life for older adults have found that problems in occupational performance increase gradually as a consequence of aging, including reduced performance capacity through decreased health.[75-77] In a systematic literature review by Stuck and colleagues,[78] risk factors for reduced ability to perform everyday life tasks for community-living older adults were investigated. They identified that personal factors, such as cognitive impairment, depression, isolation, poor self-rated health, and low levels of physical activity, impacted on the older adults' ability to perform everyday occupations. Furthermore, studies conducted in both Sweden and Denmark have found that a reduced physical performance capacity, such as pain and fatigue, are common for older adults and have large impacts on their occupational performance.[75,79] Research has also found that people who live with impairments in body functions and experience an early onset of chronic conditions incur age-related disability earlier than people who experience the process of normal health decline associated with aging.[80,81] This accelerated aging indicates that a person with chronic conditions, such as polio or rheumatoid arthritis, can experience symptoms of early aging such as osteoarthritis, respiratory disease, and circulatory disorders in adult life, 20 to 25 years earlier than people who experience a later onset of chronic health conditions.

Occupational performance deficits may not only be a consequence of the person's reduced performance capacities; they may also be related to barriers and inaccessible environments. Research has found that the home environ-ment has a vital role for older adults' abilities to perform everyday life tasks.[82-85] The ENABLE-AGE Project (by Oswald et al[84]) is a large, cross-national, interdisciplinary European project including 5 countries. It aims at increasing understanding of the relationship between housing, health, and everyday life in the aging process. Findings from this project showed that both objective and self-reported housing satisfaction was related to both well-being and the ability to perform everyday occupations for older people in 5 countries. Older adults who perceived their housing as useful had greater well-being and were more independent in their everyday life tasks.[84] Furthermore, researchers have found that many older adults with disabilities have barriers in their home environments that hinder their occupational performance. The barriers are often physical and are mostly found in stairways and bathrooms.[86-89]

Problems with performing everyday occupations are experienced differently by older adults. The problems may be shown as increased dependency, greater difficulty, lack of safety, or as a reduced efficacy in performing a task. Older adults that experience difficulty in occupational performance have an increased risk of developing disability, dependency, and thus have greater health care needs as well as a higher risk for future dependency and disability.[76,90,91] Furthermore, occupational performance deficits can also lead to a lower levels of self-rated health, as well as a higher degree of depression and social isolation.[92] Martin and colleagues[93] found that difficulty in the performance of everyday life tasks increased people's fear of falling. Similarly, experiencing unsafe conditions has been shown to decrease involvement in the performance of everyday life tasks for older adults,[94-96] and to advance disability.[97] It is also one of the most common reasons for dependency and placement in nursing homes.[98,99]

Older adults often experience problems in occupational performance due to a combination of intrinsic and extrinsic factors. Therefore, occupational therapy practitioners should base intervention decisions on assessments that consider factors related to both the person and the environment. An understanding of the client's story is essential, since the narrative context reveals important relationships between occupational performance and the values, roles, habits, meaningful occupations, and overall lifestyle of the client.

SUMMARY

This chapter has introduced occupations and occupational performance problems among older adults. Beginning with a narrative account of an older woman, the chapter reviewed key theories of aging to illustrate developmental and psychosocial influences on occupational engagement during the later stages of life. Using data from studies of time use and participation involving elderly persons, the chapter illustrated that cultural and geographical factors can influence what elderly people do, and when and where they do it.

Although recognizing that advancing age often leads to diminished occupational engagement due to chronic illness or frailty, the chapter also showed the importance of recognizing that there is large variability among individuals in their capacity to remain actively engaged despite advancing age. Making assumptions about elderly persons based on age is itself a type of discriminatory ageism that should be steadfastly avoided. The gerontological literature, including material from occupational science and occupational therapy, shows clearly that maintaining active occupational engagement through participation in valued occupations is an important component of health and well-being during elderhood, in effect enabling people "to be old without feeling old."

REFERENCES

1. Liang J, Luo B. Toward a discourse shift in social gerontology: from successful aging to harmonious aging. *Journal of Aging Studies*. 2012;26(3):327-334.

2. Jonsson H. A new direction in the conceptualization and categorization of occupation. *Journal of Occupational Science*. 2008;15(1):3-8.

3. Krekula C. Age coding: on age-based practices of distinction. *International Journal of Ageing and Later Life*. 2009;4(2):7-31.

4. Tatzer VC, van Nes F, Jonsson H. Understanding the role of occupation in ageing: four life stories of older Viennese women. *Journal of Occupational Science*. 2012;19(2):138-149.

5. World Health Organization. *Aging and Life Course*. World Health Organization. http://www.who.int/ageing/en/. Updated 2013. Accessed September 14, 2013.

6. United Nations: Department of Social and Economic Affairs: *Population Division*. World Population Ageing. United Nations. http://www.un.org/esa/population/publications/WPA2009/WPA2009_WorkingPaper.pdf. Published 2009. Accessed September 14, 2013.

7. Andersen-Ranberg K, Petersen I, Robine J-M, Christensen K. Who are the oldest-old? In: Börsch-Supan A, ed. *Who Are Our 50+ Olds? SHARE—Survey of Health, Ageing and Retirement in Europe*. http://www.share-project.org. Published 2012. Updated 2013. Accessed September 17, 2013.

8. Federal Interagency Forum on Aging-Related Statistics. *Older Americans 2012: Key Indicators of Well-Being*. Federal Interagency Forum on Aging-Related Statistics. Washington, DC: US Government Printing Office; 2012. http://www.agingstats.gov. Published June 2012. Accessed September 16, 2013.

9. European Commission: Eurostat. *Eurostat: Statistics Explained: Population Structure and Aging*. European Commission: Eurostat: Statistics Explained. http://epp.eurostat.ec.europa.eu/statistics_explained/index.php/Main_Page. Published 2011. Accessed September 16, 2013.

10. European Commission. Indicators: Healthy Life Years. *European Commission: Public Health*. http://ec.europa.eu/health/indicators/healthy_life_years/hly. Published 2011. Updated September 16, 2013. Accessed September 16, 2013.

11. Grammenos S. Implications of demographic ageing in the enlarged EU in the domains of quality of life, health promotion and health care. *Contract*. 2004;105:0076.

12. National Institute of Ageing. *Health Disparities Strategic Plan: Fiscal Years 2009-2013*. NIH: National Institute of Ageing: About NIA. http://www.nia.nih.gov/about/health-disparities-strategic-plan-fiscal-years-2009-2013. Published 2009. Accessed September 16, 2013.

13. Mackenbach J, Avendano M, Andersen-Ranberg K, Aro A. Physical health. In: Mackenbach J, ed. *3: Health and Health Care. SHARE—Survey of Health, Ageing and Retirement in Europe*. http://www.share-project.org/fileadmin/pdf_documentation/FRB1/CH3.pdf. Published 2011. Updated 2013. Accessed September 17, 2013.

14. Socialstyrelsen: National Institute of Health and Welfare. *Folkhälsorapport 2009, Äldres hälsa [in Swedish]. Socialstyrelsen*. www.socialstyrelsen.se. Updated 2013. Accessed September 16, 2013.

15. Croda E, Gonzalez-Chapela J. How do European older adults use their time? In: Börsch-Supan A, ed. *Health, Ageing and Retirement in Europe—First Results from the Survey of Health, Ageing and Retirement in Europe*. Mannheim, Germany: Mannheim Research Institute for the Economics of Aging (MEA);2005:265-271.

16. Gist Y, Hetzel L, US Department of Commerce Economics and Statistics Administration, US Census Bureau. *We the People: Aging in the United States*. Census 2000 Special Reports. 2004;CENSR-19:1-16. https://www.census.gov/prod/2004pubs/censr-19.pdf. Published 2004. Accessed September 16, 2013.

17. Droogleever Fortuijn J, Van der Meer M, Burholt V, et al. The activity patterns of older adults: a cross-sectional study in six European countries. *Population, Space and Place*. 2006;12(5):353-369.

18. Albert SM, Bear-Lehman J, Burkhardt A. Lifestyle-adjusted function: variation beyond BADL and IADL competencies. *The Gerontologist*. 2009;49:767-777.

19. Gauthier AH, Smeeding TM. Time use at old ages: cross-national differences. *Research on Aging*. 2003;25:247-274.

20. Eriksson G, Chung J, Beng L, et al. Describing occupations of older adults: a cross cultural description. *OTJR: Occupation, Participation and Health*. 2011;31(4):182-192.

21. Baum CM, Edwards DF. *Activity CARD Sort Test Manual*. St. Louis, MO: Penultima Press; 2001.

22. McKinnon AL. Time use for self-care, productivity, and leisure among elderly Canadians. *Canadian Journal of Occupational Therapy*. 1992;59(2):102-110.

23. Chilvers R, Corr S, Singlehurst H. Investigation into the occupational lives of healthy older people through their use of time. *Australian Occupational Therapy Journal*. 2010;57(1):24-33.

24. McKenna K, Broome K, Liddle J. What older people do: time use and exploring the link between role participation and life satisfaction in people aged 65 years and over. *Australian Occupational Therapy Journal*. 2007;54(4):273-284.

25. Tacken M, Marcellini F, Heidrun M, Ruoppila I, Szeman Z. Temporal aspects of the out-of-home activities of elderly people: the international MOBILATE survey: enhancing mobility in later life. In: *10th International Conference on Travel Behaviour Research*. Lucerne, Switzerland; 2003.

26. Senior 2005. *Riv Åldertrappan: Livslopp I Förändring (Tear Down the Stairs of Aging: Life Courses in Change)*. Stockholm, Sweden: Nordstedts; 2005.

27. Cummings E, Henry W. *The Process of Disengagement*. New York, NY: Basic Books; 1961.

28. Jonsson H. Occupational transitions: work to retirement. In: Christiansen C, Townsend E, eds. *Introduction to Occupation: The Art and Science of Living.* 2nd ed. Upper Saddle River, NJ: Prentice Hall; 2010:211-230.

29. Jonsson H, Josephsson S, Kielhofner G. Narratives and experience in an occupational transition: a longitudinal study of the retirement process. *American Journal of Occupational Therapy.* 2001;55(4):424-432.

30. Jonsson H. The first step into the third age: the retirement process from a Swedish perspective. *Occupational Therapy International.* 2011;18:32-38.

31. Atchley RC. *Continuity and Adaption in Aging: Creating Positive Experiences.* Baltimore, MD: The John Hopkins University Press; 1999.

32. Laslett P. *A Fresh Map of Life.* London, UK: Weidenfeld and Nicolson; 1989.

33. Laslett P. Interpreting the demographic changes. *Philosophical Transactions of the Royal Society: Biological Sciences.* 1997;352:1805-1809.

34. Haak M, Ivanoff DS, Fänge A, Sixsmith J, Iwarrsson S. Home as the locus and origin for participation: experiences among very old Swedish people. *OTJR: Occupation, Participation and Health.* 2007;27:95-103

35. Oberg P, Tornstam L. Body images among men and women of different ages. *Ageing and Society.* 1999;19(5):629-644.

36. Backes G, Clemens W. *Zukunft der Soziologie des Alter(n)s.* Opladen, Germany: Leske + Budrich; 2002.

37. Baltes PB, Baltes MM. Gerontologie: Begriff, Herausforderungen und Brennpunkte. In: Baltes PB, Mittelstraß J, Staudinger UM, eds. *Alter und Altern: Ein Interdisziplinärer Studientext zur Gerontologie.* Berlin, Germany: Walter de Gruyter; 1994:1-34.

38. Atchley RC. A continuity theory of normal aging. *Gerontologist.* 1989;29(2):183-190.

39. Kelly JR, ed. *Continuity Theory and the Evolution of Activity in Later Adulthood.* Newbury Park, CA: SAGE Publications Incorporated; 1993.

40. Jackson J. Living a meaningful existence in old age. In: Zemke R, Clark F, eds. *Occupational Science: The Evolving Discipline.* Philadelphia, PA: Davis Company; 1996:339-361.

41. Jonsson H, Josephson S, Kielhofner G. Narratives and experience in an occupational transition: a longitudinal study of the retirement process. *American Journal of Occupational Therapy.* 2001;55:424-432.

42. Häggblom-Kronlöf G, Hultberg J, Eriksson BG, Sonn U. Experiences of daily occupations at 99 years of age. *Scandinavian Journal of Occupational Therapy.* 2007;14:192-200.

43. Schultz S, Schkade J. Adaptation. In: Christiansen CH, Baum C, eds. *Enabling Function and Well-Being.* 2nd ed. Thorofare, NJ: SLACK Incorporated; 1997:458-482.

44. Van't Leven N, Jonsson H. Doing and being in the atmosphere of the doing: environmental influences on occupational performance in a nursing home. *Scandinavian Journal of Occupational Therapy.* 2002;9(4):148-155.

45. Meyer A. The philosophy of occupational therapy. *American Journal of Occupational Therapy.* 1922/1977;31(10):633-641.

46. Wilcock AA. *An Occupational Perspective of Health.* Thorofare, NJ: SLACK Incorporated; 1998.

47. Christiansen CH. Defining Lives: Occupation as identity: an essay on competence, coherence and the creation of meaning. *American Journal of Occupational Therapy.* 1999;53:547-558.

48. Laliberte-Rudman D. Linking occupation and identity: lessons learned through qualitative exploration. *Journal of Occupational Science: Australia.* 2002;9(1):12-19.

49. Jonsson H, Josephsson S, Kielhofner G. Evolving narratives in the course of retirement: a longitudinal study. *American Journal of Occupational Therapy.* 2000;54(5):463-470.

50. Hurd L. "We're not old!" Older women's negotiation of ageing and oldness. *Journal of Ageing Studies.* 1999;13:419-439.

51. Stamm T, Lovelock L, Stew G, et al. I have a disease but I am not ill: a narrative study of occupational balance in people with rheumatoid arthritis. *OTJR: Occupation, Participation and Health.* 2009;29(1):32-39.

52. Dunton WRJ. *Reconstruction Therapy.* Philadelphia, PA: WB Saunders; 1919.

53. Aghai N, Ahacic K, Parker MG. Continuity of leisure participation from middle age to old age. *Journal of Gerontology: Social Sciences.* 2006;61B(6):340-346.

54. Glass TA, de Leon CM, Marottoli R, Berkman L. Population based study of social and productive activities as predictors of survival among elderly Americans. *British Medical Journal.* 1999;319:478-483.

55. Klumb PL, Baltes MM. Time use of old and very old Berliners: productive and consumptive activities as functions of resources. *Journals of Gerontology: Series B, Psychological Sciences and Social Sciences.* 1999;54(4):273-284.

56. Menec VH. The relation between everyday activities and successful aging: a 6-year longitudinal study. *Journal of Gerontology: Social Sciences.* 2003;58B(2):74-82.

57. Warr P, Butcher V, Robertson I. Activity and psychological well-being in older people. *Aging and Mental Health.* 2004;8(2):172-183.

58. Lennartsson C, Silverstein M. Does engagement with life enhance survival of elderly people in Sweden? The role of social and leisure activities. *Journal of Gerontology: Social Sciences.* 2001;56B:S335-S342.

59. Blair SN, Morris JN. Healthy hearts—and the universal benefits of being physically active: physical activity and health. *Annals of Epidemiology.* 2009;19:253-256.

60. Pignatti F, Rozzini R, Trabucchi M. Physical activity and cognitive decline in elderly persons. *Archives of Internal Medicine.* 2002;162:361-362.

61. Newson RS, Kemps EB. General lifestyle activities as a predictor of current cognition and cognitive change in older adults: a cross-sectional and longitudinal examination. *Journal of Gerontology: Psychological Sciences.* 2005;60B:113-120.

62. Socialstyrelsen. *Vård och omsorg om äldre- lägesrapport 2004 (Care for the Elderly, State of the Art 2004).* Stockholm, Sweden: Socialstyrelsen (National Board for Health and Welfare); 2005.

63. Whiteford G. Occupational deprivation: global challenge in the new millennium. *British Journal of Occupational Therapy.* 2000;63(5):200-204.

64. Clark F, Azen S, Zemke R, et al. Occupational therapy for independent-living older adults. *Journal of American Medical Association.* 1997;278(16):1321-1326.

65. Mandel D, ed. *Lifestyle Redesign: Implementing the Well Elderly Program.* Bethesda, MD: AOTA Press; 1999.

66. Clark F, Azen SP, Carlson M, et al. Embedding health-promoting changes into the daily lives of independent-living older adults: long-term follow-up of occupational therapy intervention. *Journals Of Gerontology: Series B, Psychological Sciences and Social Sciences.* 2001;56(1):60-63.

67. Clark F, Jackson J, Carlson M, et al. Effectiveness of a lifestyle intervention in promoting the well-being of independently living older people: results of the Well Elderly 2 Randomised Controlled Trial. *Journal of Epidemiology and Community Health.* 2012;66(9):782-790.

68. Wicks A. *Do It Now: Promoting Participation in Engaging Occupations During Retirement.* Shoalhaven, Australia: Australasian Occupational Science Centre, University of Wollongong; 2006. University of Wollengong. http://ahsri.uow.edu.au/content/groups/public/@web/@chsd/@aosc/documents/doc/uow094082.pdf. Published December 2006. Accessed March 1, 2012.

69. Jonsson H. *Anticipating, Experiencing and Valuing the Transition from Worker to Retiree: A Longitudinal Study of Retirement as an Occupational Transition.* Stockholm, Sweden: Department of Clinical Neuroscience, Occupational Therapy and Elderly Care Research, Division of Occupational Therapy, Karolinska Institutet; 2000.

70. Mountain G, Mozley C, Craig C, Ball L. Occupational therapy led health promotion for older people: feasibility of the Lifestyle Matters programme. *British Journal of Occupational Therapy.* 2008;71(10):406-413.

71. Mountain G, Mozley C, Craig C. The lived experience of redesigning lifestyle post-retirement in the UK. *Occupational Therapy International.* 2011;18:48-58.

72. CeFam. *Aktiv livsstil hela livet: Studiecirkel för att förebygga fall och fallskador. (Active life-style all your life: A study-material to prevent falls and fall-injuries).* CeFam: Cetrum för allmänmedicin (Centre for Family Medicine). http://www.cefam.se/index.php?option=com_resource&controller=article&article=710&category_id=4&Itemid=176&lang=en. Published 2011. Accessed October 20, 2012.

73. Gillespie LD, Gillespie WJ, Robertson MC, Lamb SE, Cumming RG, Rowe BH. Interventions for preventing falls in elderly people (review). *Cochrane Database of Systematic Reviews.* 2009;1-289.

74. Chang J, Morton S, Rubenstein L, et al. Interventions for the prevention of falls in older adults: systematic review and meta-analysis of randomised clinical trials. *British Medical Journal.* 2004;328(7441):680.

75. Ahacic K, Kåreholt I, Thorslund M, Parker MG. Relationships between symptoms, physical capacity and activity limitations in 1992 and 2002. *Aging Clinical and Experimental Research.* 2007;19(3):187-193.

76. Jagger C, Arthur AJ, Spiers NA, Clarke M. Patterns of onset of disability in activities of daily living with age. *Journal of the American Geriatrics Society.* 2001;49(4):404-409.

77. Bravell ME, Berg S, Malmberg B. Health, functional capacity, formal care, and survival in the oldest old: a longitudinal study. *Archives of Gerontology and Geriatrics.* 2008;46(1):1-14.

78. Stuck AE, Walthert JM, Nikolaus T, Büla CJ, Hohmann C, Beck JC. Risk factors for functional status decline in community-living elderly people: a systematic literature review. *Social Science & Medicine.* 1999;48(4):445-469.

79. Avlund K, Vass M, Hendriksen C. Onset of mobility disability among community-dwelling old men and women: the role of tiredness in daily activities. *Age and Ageing.* 2003;32:579-584.

80. Campbell ML, Sheets D, Strong PS. Secondary health conditions among middle-aged individuals with chronic physical disabilities: implications for unmet needs for services. *Assistive Technology: The Official Journal of RESNA.* 1999;11(2):105-122.

81. Putnam M. Linking aging theory and disability models: increasing the potential to explore aging with physical impairment. *The Gerontologist.* 2002;42(6):799-806.

82. Gitlin LN. Conducting research on home environments: lessons learned and new directions. *The Gerontologist.* 2003;43(5):628-637.

83. Iwarsson S. A long-term perspective on person-environment fit and ADL dependence among older Swedish adults. *The Gerontologist.* 2005;45(3):327-336.

84. Oswald F, Wahl H-W, Schilling O, et al. Relationships between housing and healthy aging in very old age. *The Gerontologist.* 2007;47(1):96-107. http://hdl.handle.net/2173/86131. Published Feburary 2007. Accessed September 17, 2013.

85. Petersson I, Kottorp A, Lilja M, Bergstrom J. Longitudinal changes in everyday life after home modifications for people aging with disabilities. *Scandinavian Journal of Occupational Therapy.* 2009;16(2):78-87.

86. Gitlin L, Mann W, Tomit M, Marcus S. Factors associated with home environmental problems among community-living older people. *Disability and Rehabilitation.* 2001;23(17):777-787.

87. Johansson K, Lilja M, Petersson I, Borell L. Performance of activities of daily living in a sample of applicants for home modification services. *Scandinavian Journal of Occupational Therapy.* 2007;14(1):44-53.

88. Lilja M, Borell L. Elderly people's daily activities and need for mobility support. *Scandinavian Journal of Caring Sciences.* 1997;11(2):73-80.

89. Stark S. Creating disability in the home: the role of environmental barriers in the United States. *Disability and Society.* 2001;16(1):37-49.

90. Fried LP, Young Y, Rubin G, Bandeen-Roche K. Self-reported preclinical disability identifies older women with early declines in performance and early disease. *Journal of Clinical Epidemiology.* 2001;54(9):889-901.

91. Agree EM, Freedman VA. A comparison of assistive technology and personal care in alleviating disability and unmet need. *Gerontologist.* 2003;43(3):335-344.

92. Femia EE, Zarit SH, Johansson B. The disablement process in very late life: a study of the oldest-old in Sweden. *Journals of Gerontology: Series B, Psychological Sciences and Social Sciences.* 2001;56(1):12-23.

93. Martin FC, Hart D, Spector T, Doyle DV, Harari D. Fear of falling limiting activity in young-old women is associated with reduced functional mobility rather than psychological factors. *Age and Ageing.* 2005;34(3):281-287.

94. Mann WC, Hurren D, Tomita M, Bengali M, Steinfeld E. Environmental problems in homes of elders with disabilities. *Occup Ther J Res.* 1994;14(3):191-211.

95. Borell L, Lilja M, Carlsson-Alm S, Törnquist K, Stahl E. Community-based occupational therapy. *Scandinavian Journal of Occupational Therapy.* 1995;2:138-144.

96. Zimmer Z, Chappell NL. Receptivity to new technology among older adults. *Disability and Rehabilitation.* 1999;21(5-6):222-230.

97. Brenes GA, Guralnik JM, Williamson JD, et al. The influence of anxiety on the progression of disability. *Journal of the American Geriatrics Society.* 2005;53(1):34-39.

98. Cheek J, Ballantyne A, Roder-Allen G. Factors influencing the decision of older people living in independent units to enter the acute care system. *Journal of Clinical Nursing.* 2005;14:24-33.

99. Fonad E, Robins Wahlin T-B, Heikkila K, Emami A. Moving to and living in a retirement home: focusing on elderly people's sense of safety and security. *Journal of Housing for the Elderly.* 2006;20(3):45-60.

Ingela Petersson, RegOT, PhD, an original author of this chapter, is now deceased.

Chapter 12

OCCUPATIONS OF ORGANIZATIONS

Carol Haertlein Sells, PhD, OTR, FAOTA

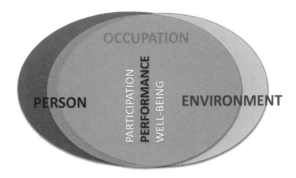

LEARNING OBJECTIVES

- Describe types of organizations and their roles in society.
- Identify tools that occupational therapy practitioners can use to determine the occupations of organizations.
- Differentiate the occupations in different types of organizations.
- Integrate concepts of the *Practice Framework* with the PEOP Model for organizations.
- Describe the PEOP Occupational Therapy Process for organization-centered interventions that are directed to individuals and populations served by organizations.
- Discuss the role of occupational therapy in providing occupation-centered interventions directly to organizations as clients.

KEY WORDS

- Board of directors
- Mission
- Nonprofit organization
- *Occupational Therapy Practice Framework*
- Organizational behavior
- Organizational culture
- Organizational structure
- Organizations
- PEOP Occupational Therapy Process

INTRODUCTION

A large, midwestern department store chain has recently employed an occupational therapy practitioner to do ergonomics evaluations and consultations for workers at its

Christiansen CH, Baum CM, Bass JD, eds.
Occupational Therapy: Performance, Participation, and Well-Being, Fourth Edition (pp 185-197).
© 2015 SLACK Incorporated.

warehouse and loading docks. The department store chain learns that the local university has an ergonomics certificate program; it contacts the university department to find out if there are faculty members who would evaluate the effectiveness of the ergonomic changes recommended by the occupational therapy practitioner. The ergonomics certificate program is located jointly within the university's biomedical engineering and occupational therapy departments; both engineering and occupational therapy faculty and students meet with the department store chain management to learn more about the program and determine its overall needs. It quickly becomes apparent from the narrative description of the organization and the challenges it has encountered in meeting its desired goals that occupational therapy services can be of benefit. Their benefits not only come from expert recommendations in the areas of ergonomics and safety assessment, but also from contributions in other areas. For example, occupational therapy practitioners can enhance accessibility for employees and customers with disabilities, including those with low vision; by recommending accessible and universal design changes to improve safety, prevent injury, and support the occupational performance of all workers. These recommendations may include modifications to buildings—accommodations in offices, warehouses, and meeting spaces and improvements in common areas, such as dining areas, rest rooms, parking garages, and hallways. Recommendations may also benefit the access and use of facilities by clients and customers in retail spaces, entry ways, merchandise aisles and walkways, and rest rooms. The company also has a daycare program for children, and there have been recent requests from employees for adult day care services.

The occupational therapy faculty members and their students are confident that they can provide the individual and population-centered interventions that would benefit the department store chain; they decide they need to learn much more about the organization's behavior, culture, mission, vision, structure, and other characteristics before they make a proposal of organization-centered interventions to meet the company's priorities and desired outcomes.

The *Occupational Therapy Practice Framework*, 3rd Edition[1] identifies organizations as one type of service recipient for occupational therapy services. This suggests that organizations may have improved health and participation as a result of occupational therapy services and, in fact, will have developed or improved their "engagement in occupation."[1(pS2)] The *Framework* also acknowledges the role of organizations in facilitating the occupational performance of individuals and populations via the organization's values, functions, structure, performance patterns, contexts, and environment. Finally, it notes that organizations have a role in the delivery of occupational therapy services.

Since the publication of the original *Occupational Therapy Practice Framework* in 2002[2] and the revised *Framework* in 2008 and 2014, there has been significant attention to the occupations, health, and participation of individuals and populations in the United States and international occupational therapy literature. There has been considerably less consideration devoted to the occupations of organizations. This chapter will build upon concepts about the occupations of organizations proposed by Baum, Bass Haugen, and Christiansen[3] in 2005. Types of organizations and their occupations and roles in society will be reviewed. The elements of organizations that either constrain or facilitate their occupations will be considered using the PEOP Occupational Therapy Process. The application of the PEOP Model for planning interventions by organizations to individuals and populations will be addressed, as well as the manner in which occupational therapy can serve organizations.

ORGANIZATIONS AND THEIR ROLES IN SOCIETY

A good place to start a discussion about organizations is to consider what they do, how they serve people, and their role in society. We will begin with a definition of an organization. The *Framework*[1] defines an organization as an "entity composed of individuals with a common purpose or enterprise, such as a business, industry, or agency."[1(pS44)] This definition may be somewhat limiting when we consider that we have all been a part of an organization from the beginning of life—membership in a family unit. So, although we may initially think of organizations as places where people work, go to school, or purchase items and services, organizations can have a much broader scope. Organizations have been described as socially constructed (created by humans), involving more than one person, having goals, structure, and boundaries.[4] Thus, a more complete and useful definition would be that organizations are "social entities brought into existence and sustained in an ongoing way by humans to serve some purpose, from which it follows that human activities in the entity are normally structured and coordinated towards achieving some purpose or goals."[4(p2)] This definition, which includes human activity that is structured and coordinated, helps us to consider organizations as both facilitators of occupational performance of individuals and populations, as well as recipients of occupational therapy services. In the following section, we will consider how organizations are classified and identify some of their common characteristics.

TYPES OF ORGANIZATIONS

The descriptions, categorizations, and systems for classifying organizations are as abundant as the books that depict them. For the purposes of better understanding organizations, 3 types of organizations in which occupational therapy practitioners might function or which might be served by occupational therapy will be described and used for examples: government, for-profit, and nonprofit.

- *Government Organizations:* Government (sometimes called public) organizations are controlled by national, state, or local governments and provide much of the education, health, and social services for designated jurisdictions. Other functions may include provision of defense, police and fire protection, water management, taxation, recreation, and social service programs. The mission of government organizations is to serve the public. Any profits or excess funds acquired through licenses or user fees must typically be reinvested in the organization to meet its mission or returned to the public treasury. There is often an overlap between government and private organizations in the provision of services (ie, education, health care, or security services), and government organizations may contract with private organizations to provide services (ie, a private landscaping firm may be hired to maintain county parks). Some selected examples where occupational therapy practitioners may provide services are at military facilities, state- or county-supported hospitals, libraries and museums, and in public school districts.

- *For-Profit Organizations:* Organizations that have a primary goal of making money for an owner or a group of investors are known as for-profit organizations. Most businesses are for-profit organizations, including those that occupational therapy practitioners own as private practitioners and those that employ occupational therapy practitioners to provide staffing for public schools. Occupational therapy practitioners may also be employed directly by clinics, hospitals, and private proprietary schools. Although they are primarily driven by a "bottom line" of profit, many for-profit organizations provide services for individuals who are unable to pay for service, or provide such services at a reduced rate.[5]

- *Nonprofit Organizations:* Nonprofit organizations can be large or small. They exist to serve the public good (ie, the YMCA), or the needs and interests of another defined entity (ie, members of a profession, for example the AOTA). Their status typically exempts them from paying taxes on most revenues, and they must demonstrate through independent accounting audits that their revenues are used to maintain the organization (eg, supporting salaries and operating costs) and improve itself (eg, building new facilities, buying new equipment, or offering new or enhanced services). They often rely upon funds from government grants, foundations, membership dues, and gifts and donations to support their work. Examples of nonprofits that employ occupational therapy practitioners include religiously-affiliated hospitals, health facilities, and schools; community-based programs for people with mental illness; senior centers; and many birth-to-3 (early intervention) programs.

Organizational Behavior

Regardless of size, profit orientation, or mission, all organizations will have defined organizational behaviors, specific structures, and unique cultures. Behavior in organizations has been studied over the past century,[4] and includes examination of social needs, motivation and human relations in the workplace, the analysis and impact of leadership, the functions of groups, and the effects of the nonhuman environment on organizational effectiveness. Organizational behavior is "a field of study devoted to understanding, explaining, and ultimately improving the attitudes and behaviors of individuals and groups within organizations."[6(p5)] The vast majority of organizational behavior research examines human behavior in the workplace, but draws upon knowledge from psychology, sociology, and economics. Consider the different types of organizations described earlier: What factors influence individuals to work for a private for-profit enterprise vs a nonprofit? How do groups of employees work together in small private practice compared to a large government hospital? Is leadership and decision making done in an autocratic, top-down manner or collaboratively? Each of these factors can influence the effectiveness of an organization to fulfill its mission, retain its employees, and continue to function and prosper. Research has found that the "best places to work," that is, companies that care about job satisfaction of employees, organizational integrity, employee development, participation in decision making, person-environment fit, and match of employee motivation to leadership demands, are more profitable than equivalent companies that did not have the desirable organizational behavior characteristics.[7]

Organizational Structure

The formal lines of communication, divisions of responsibility, and levels of responsibility or authority in an organization will be illustrated in its organizational structure. The simplest way this organization is typically communicated to interested parties is via an organizational chart with horizontal (functional or process) groupings

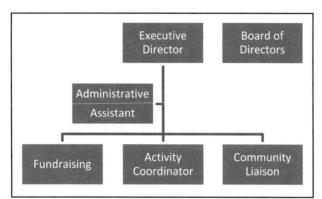

Figure 12-1. Example of organizational chart of small non-profit organization.

and vertical (communication and control) groupings.[4] See Figure 12-1 for an illustration.

An organizational chart will convey structure, but will lack the procedures and processes by which the work of the organization is accomplished; more information must be available about exactly who does what, when, and how. Typically, the larger an organization is, the more complex its structure. Large, highly structured organizations have been assumed to be less satisfying and creative places to work; however, effective structures can create smaller units within a large organization that are highly responsive to employees and foster originality.[8] An important characteristic of formal organizational structure is that it is relativity static or unchanging. Structures may change when leadership in an organization changes or its mission changes. By contrast, an informal organization or one that emerges from personal relationships within the organization rather than from the formal organizational structure and its suggested relationships, will be more fluid. Informal organizations are typically dependent upon the presence of one or more individuals, sometimes emanating from the influence of their personality. They use the "grapevine" method of communication, where information ranging from accurate and important to gossip is shared outside of formal lines of communication suggested by organizational structure. Interestingly, informal organizations (ie, the influential relationships) may stay intact even when formal organizational structures are altered.[8]

Organizational structure is relevant to any entity or individual intending to establish a new relationship with an organization. Consider the midwestern department store chain described at the beginning of the chapter that employs an occupational therapy practitioner in the company's wellness clinic to do ergonomics evaluations and consultations. The occupational therapy practitioner, a 35-year-old woman, recognizes many other areas of the organization in which she could make contributions. If she would like to make a proposal to the department store management to expand her role, it behooves her to carefully examine the organizational structure of the company to determine to whom the skills must be marketed. This proposal would identify the individuals and populations she would serve, as well as where her services might best fit into the organization.

Organizational Culture

Organizational culture is sometimes described as the characteristics of an organization that are intangible and difficult to classify, that is, "the way we do things." Evidence of an organization's culture will be found in shared values and norms, unwritten codes of conduct or rules of behavior, myths and rituals that are passed on to newcomers, and assumptions about the organization that are primarily unspoken but can be very powerful. Culture is communicated overtly via organizational vision and mission statements and standards of behavior set by leaders and managers (for example, punctuality at meetings and transparent decision-making processes). It is indirectly communicated by everyday actions of staff members, ways of thinking, and problem-solving approaches that are sometimes carried out without apparent reason—"the way we have always done things."[5] It has been suggested that organizational culture may be among the most influential features of the success of an organization and the most difficult to change during an organization's decline.[9]

Organizational culture may be influential in where one chooses to work or receive products and services. For example, parents may want their child with a disability to attend private religious schools because of their agreement with the values and mission of those institutions. However, they may find themselves in a cultural dilemma because the private school is less able to support the learning needs of their child as compared to the large public school. They decide to work alongside the occupational therapy practitioner who contracts to the private school to advocate for increased therapy services, and thus they help the organization (ie, private school) to better meet the occupational performance needs of the population it could potentially serve (ie, children with disabilities).

All of the qualities of an organization, its size, how it functions, its structure, and the explicit and implicit culture, will influence how it provides services and meets its goals. In occupational terms, the characteristics of organizations will shape their ability to meet the occupational performance needs of individuals and populations. Some of the qualities of the organization itself may be very well suited to improvement through the services of occupational therapy practitioners.

Roles of Organizations

The roles of organizations, or the ways that they will function and purposes they will serve, will depend upon their vision, mission, strategic plan, leadership, financial support, and countless other factors. The role of organizations in modern Western society has been described as "the structure through which most critical societal needs are met."[5(p55)] A brief review of vision and mission is useful to understand their impact on the role of organizations. A vision statement conveys an organization's future aspirations; what it is that an organization wants to become. A mission focuses on the present state of the organization; what it is, who it serves, and how. The earlier example of organizational culture being exhibited through a private school's mission is an illustration of the "what it is" and "how it does things" part of a mission statement.

The organizations in which occupational therapy practitioners may work fall along the entire continuum of services in health care, education, industry, and community needs: hospitals, rehabilitation centers, skilled nursing facilities, senior centers, daycare, birth-to-3 programs, schools, shopping malls, manufacturing sites, community centers, and shelters (temporary in disasters, permanent for homeless, people with serious mental, victims of domestic violence, refugee camps). The individuals and populations whom they will serve include at-risk, those with disability, as well as healthy populations.

Considering that the role of organizations is to provide the "structure through which most critical societal needs are met," we can review examples of the influence of visions and missions using government organizations, for-profit organizations, and nonprofits as examples. The mission of a government organization, like a city school system, is to provide education to all segments of society; their vision is to prepare the future citizens of the nation and prepare them for postsecondary education and the nation's workforce. The mission of a private rehabilitation company will be to provide convenient and accessible therapy services to consumers, to provide secure employment with benefits to therapy providers (such as occupational therapy practitioners), and to create a profit for the company owners. The vision of a nonprofit may be to assure rights of people with disabilities; their mission is to identify populations with specific needs and gain access to services and opportunities through advocacy and legal expertise. It is clear that the different visions and missions will drive the strategic planning of the organization.

Organizational Theory

Just as the profession of occupational therapy is driven by theories that guide decision making and explain practice; the functions, behavior, and structures of organiza-tions can also be explained by theories. Theory can be defined as the relationships among various facts, principles, and experiences that explain and predict phenomena. Organizational theory from the early 20th century originated out the fields of scientific management, bureaucratic and administrative theory, and was originally focused on task performance, rewards, and punishment of workers and planning and control by managers.[8] More recent theoretical orientations have focused on processes underlying working with people as individuals and within groups, as well as understanding and explaining the impact of organizational structures and culture on human performance.[10] Systems theory (particularly those pertaining to dynamic systems) also contributes to modern organizational theory in explaining how organizations function within the complex systems of which they are a part, such as political, economic, science, and public systems.[11] The PEOP Model is based upon systems theory, which acknowledges the complex and dynamic interface among the person, the environment, the occupation, and its performance. Organizational theory has been elegantly used to explain the relationships among phenomena that can predict the restructuring and reengineering of long-standing, highly regarded blue-chip companies, such as what happened to AT&T in the mid-1990s.[12] Several theoretical perspectives offered explanations of the crisis that occurred in that company, and how ineffective management led to disastrous consequences. This illustrates the usefulness of organizational theory when trying to understand and divert or minimize crisis situations.

The complexity of most organizations should not be underestimated (Box 12-1). External influences, especially advances in technology and unpredictable changes in the economy, can lead to unexpected and sometimes undesired transformations in relatively brief time frames. The internal drivers of organizational complexity are its people, the organization's non-linear nature (especially within larger systems), and the process of self-organization. As people respond to external influences they may change their behavior, which impacts the informal organization. Changes within a smaller unit of an organization can often have an impact on a larger system (eg, consider the effect of altering one classroom within a larger school). The process of self-organization, a quick response that takes the least amount of effort in response to a pressing external influence, may occur in a manner that does not always sustain the original vision and mission of the organization. It is accurate to assume that the response and potential interventions to meet occupational needs in one organization will not have the same results in another. Thus, some familiarity with organizational theory may be of use for occupational therapy practitioners striving to serve occupational needs of organizations. See Tables 12-1 and 12-2 for suggested sources of information.

BOX 12-1

COMPLEXITY AND CHANGE IN ORGANIZATIONS

Most organizations (unless they are very small) are complex social systems, and how to make them function more effectively at a reasonable cost is a challenge that nearly every organizational leader is pursuing. Already, through personal computing and the Internet, digital technologies have accelerated the growth of knowledge, which leads to even faster change and adds to the complexity of understanding organizations and how to make them work more effectively.

As Plsek has pointed out, organizations are complex social systems that have a number of characteristics that make them hard to predict.[13] First, they involve people, who serve as important system elements (or agents). People gather information from the environment (both local and global) and they learn from this and change their behaviors over time, often in unpredictable ways. People are also capable of being rational, or making the best decision from a number of alternatives, but they are also influenced by values and other social rules of behavior that are influenced by the relationships of the networks of people interacting within the organization. As a consequence, complex organizations are non-linear, their boundaries are difficult to define, they are often nested within larger systems, and their states (conditions) can change unpredictably based on events. This unpredictable change, without control or design, cannot be predicted based on an analysis of a systems elements and is a characteristic known as *emergence*.[14] Complex systems also have a behavioral characteristic known as *self-organization*. This is the organizational response that occurs when the organization alters its structure to meet the demands of the immediate environment. Organizations have memories, shared values, and interactions that are typified by feedback and interdependency, and the internal reorganization process typically takes place in a manner that requires the least amount of effort. Organizational history is important, because people remember previous experiences, and values exist whether or not they have been explicitly identified within the organization. Each of these factors influence the state of a complex system at a given time and are important to changes in the system.

Complex systems can be described as possessing 1 of 3 possible states, based upon the strength and number of connections between their elements; a *stable* state has only a few weak connections between elements, and therefore change is less likely or more predictable. In *chaos*, or the chaotic state, the system has large numbers of weak and rapidly changing connections. The organization has no memory, as the elements respond to one novelty after another without learning from the experience. The third condition, located between the 2 extreme states, is known as the edge of chaos or the *zone of criticality*.[15] Systems in this state have a level of balance between chaos and order that gives them the fitness to adapt and respond to environmental conditions with efficiency.[16]

It is important to understand the characteristics and features of complex organizations in order to better appreciate the challenges inherent in changing them. It should be clear that traditional organizational management theories that emphasize the alignment of organizational elements based on the identification of externally determined goals are woefully inadequate to motivate change, because these are often based on expectations driven by rational, linear models of systems change.

Given the complexity of organizations, it is easier to understand why government efforts to align systems with the rapid changes in technology and the demands created by changing demographics have been slower to occur than would be optimal for serving the needs of populations, groups, and individuals. The *butterfly effect*, where small events lead to disproportionately large change, is a phenomenon that typifies the unpredictable nature of change in complex systems. An example given by Kernick is useful here.[17] When the late actor Christopher Reeve suffered a spinal injury while jumping his horse, there was a disproportionate shift in funding for spinal injury research programs in the United States. Examples of butterfly effects can probably be found in all complex organizations.

Table 12-1. *Evidence Table*

Ref #	Key Idea and Purpose	Research Design and Methods; Level of Evidence	Results and Conclusions	Take Home Message
7	Organizational behavior	Survey of employees 50 "best" and 50 matching companies (average of 136 employees/company); Level 2 evidence	"Best" companies had more stable levels of positive employee attitudes and better market performance over time compared to companies with less emphasis on employee relations.	Organizations perform better when attention is paid to employees and their job satisfaction.
21	Safety-related behavior	Surveys of 49 group leaders of a manufacturing plant; responses correlated with accident rates; Level 2 evidence	Perceived organizational support was related to safety communication from leaders to team; communication between managers-leaders-team was related to safety communication, safety commitment, and accidents.	Employees who perceive the organization as supportive with good leader/employee relationships are more likely to raise safety concerns, this is related to fewer accidents.
22	Positive affect and service quality	Three studies reported: study 1 was surveys of 122 customer-contact employees in a bank, study 2 was surveys of 238 insurance agents, study 3 was 612 customers of the insurance agents in study 2; all Level 2 evidence	Employee positive affect was positively related to organizational behavior that was altruistic, customer-oriented, and to service quality; it was negatively related to a sales-oriented behavior in the bank sample, but not in the insurance sample. Insurance customers' perceptions were negatively correlated between perceived service quality and sales-oriented behavior.	Employee behavior in service organizations has a direct relationship with perceived service quality provided by the organization. Training employees to be customer-oriented is of value to the organization.
23	Balancing work and family	Surveys and interviews of employees in management, unions, and non-supervisory roles in several industries (N = 8483); Level 2 evidence		
24	Family-friendly policy	Retrospective study on data from federal United States agencies from 2004 to 2007, assessing the relative impact of family-friendly policies on employee turnover rate and agency performance; Level 2 evidence	Childcare subsidy programs and alternative work schedules had positive impacts on agency performance; childcare subsidies had a positive impact on reducing turnover.	It is worthwhile to consider childcare subsidies and alternative work schedules to improve employee morale and thus organizational effectiveness; telework and paid leave for family care are less important.
25	Effects of light on sales	Comparison of "sales index" for retail chain stores with and without skylights; Level 2 evidence	Skylights had the largest positive effect on sales and was the third largest most powerful variable in predicting store sales performance.	The lighting in an environment is very important in influencing positive behavior.

Table 12-2. *Table of Resources*

Name of Organization/ Resource	Brief Description of Interprofessional Resource	Web Address or Publisher
Certificate in Ergonomics at the University of Wisconsin-Milwaukee	A formal program of study, training, and experience in ergonomics for post-baccalaureate students in occupational therapy, nursing, engineering, and related fields who wish to specialize in the area of ergonomics, applicable to a wide range of workplace settings, including industry, hospitals, nursing homes, office work, government, and academia. The program will also be very useful in preparing for the examination for Certified Professional Ergonomist (CPE).	http://www4.uwm.edu/ceas/ie/academics/graduate_programs/ergonomics_certificate.cfm
Organizational Theory: Modern, Symbolic, and Postmodern Perspectives. Hatch MJ and Cunliffe AL (2006).	This text offers a clear and comprehensive introduction to the study of organizations and organizing processes. It provides a useful and understandable background on the many different perspectives on organizations.	Oxford University Press; ISBN 0199260214
The Creative Power: Transforming Ourselves, our Organizations and our World. Smith WE (2009).	This book takes a very different approach to organizations and their empowerment; using a philosophy called appreciation, influence, and control, the author challenges leaders to take a more holistic and transformative approach to developing and changing their organizations. Spectacular illustrations and graphics!	Routledge; ISBN 0415393612
Risky Business: Psychological, Physical and Financial Costs of High Risk Behavior in Organizations. Edited by Burke RJ and Cooper CL (2010).	This book examines the cost of "risky" or undesirable behaviors, such as addictions, theft, and aggression on organizations and their employees. It reviews these often unaddressed topics in a candid and proactive manner. It is very useful for all managers and leaders who will eventually face these issues in their organizations.	Gower Publishing Ltd; ISBN 0566089157

INTERNATIONAL PERSPECTIVE ON ORGANIZATIONS AND THEIR ROLE IN SOCIETY

Just as state and national organizations develop to address societal needs beyond the scope of the family and local communities, technology and economic forces now interact to allow organizations to function across national and international lines. The industrial revolution in the 19th century was the precursor to national markets for organizations, and it was a short step to the internationalization of organizations in the 20th century.[4] Although many of the trends and issues relative to the globalization of organizations (ie, competition, rapid technological change, cultural diversity of employees) are particularly applicable to the profit-oriented business world, we have seen their effect on health care and education organizations in which occupational therapy practitioners function.

Occupational therapy is internationally organized by the World Federation of Occupational Therapists (WFOT), which has 69 member organizations worldwide and represents more than 350,000 occupational therapy practitioners.[18] The international community of occupational therapy, outside of the United States, closely follows the ICF,[19] a classification system that recognizes participation in activities within a social and physical environment as the primary determinants of health. Because of the different economic and health care structures in the world's countries, the education of occupational therapy practitioners and the practice of occupational therapy have varied tremendously over the past 50 years. The practice of occupational therapy in countries other than the United States has sometimes been located outside of the traditional health care system, with a greater emphasis on population-based interventions compared to the fee-for-service model of health care delivery in the United States. In 2008, WFOT adopted a core of "entry-level competencies for the practice of occupational therapy" to assure a standard of practice in WFOT member countries.[18] It is increasingly easy for occupational therapy practitioners educated in the United States to practice around the world and for internationally prepared occupational therapy practitioners to seek advanced education and job opportunities in the United States. The challenges in this cross-cultural world of occupational therapy have received little attention in the literature, yet they will influence the organizations in which occupational therapy practitioners are employed and provide services for decades to come.

Occupations have been defined in a variety of ways in the occupational therapy literature. For the purposes of this chapter, the term means "engagement in activities, tasks and roles for the purpose of productive pursuit, maintaining one's self in the environment, and for the purposes of relaxation, entertainment, creativity, and celebration; activities in which people are engaged to support their roles."[20(p548)] The *Framework* notes that "occupations are central to a client's (person, organization, or population) identity and sense of competence and have particular meaning and value to the client. They influence how clients spend time making decisions."[1(pS5)] The doing of occupations or occupational performance is described as "the complex interactions between the person and the environments in which he or she carries out activities, tasks, and roles that are meaningful or required of them."[21(p 46-71)] So what are the occupations of organizations? How do they prioritize them? How do they foster occupational performance of their employees and the people they serve?

The Occupations of Organizations and Occupational Performance

Using the 3 types of organizations described earlier—government, for-profit, and nonprofits—we can consider some examples of the occupations of organizations and their occupational performance. A large public university has 3 primary foci to its mission—education, research, and service—and its occupations must "support the tasks and activities" that define it. Activities that support research would include grant-writing and data analysis expertise for students and faculty. The university will invest in current technology in its classrooms and laboratories to foster education of students. The university may run a low-cost rehabilitation clinic for people whose health insurance has been exhausted; this provides a valuable service to the local community and also supports clinical education of students.

In contrast, a for-profit manufacturing company's primary mission is the creation of a quality product at the lowest possible cost. In addition, it is in the company's interest to foster the job satisfaction and safety of its employees, and thus maintain high employee retention and low workers' compensation costs. Included among the occupations to achieve this mission are workplace modifications to assure ergonomically designed workstations, implementation of an employee wellness program, and provision of an onsite rehabilitation clinic for work-related injuries.

A nonprofit organization could focus on the social and educational needs of children of military families who have lost a parent at war. Its mission is the support of those children and surviving family members. Its occupations are fundraising events and the collection of household goods, clothing, food, school supplies, and myriad other items for families and children in transition. It also gives grants for college educations and operates an annual camp for social and recreation activities for the children. As illustrated here, the occupations of an organization are guided and prioritized by its mission; the occupational performance will be directed by the organizational structure, organizational culture, decision-making of leaders, and financial support. The *Framework*[1] provides a wide array of potential capacities in which organizations can facilitate the occupational performance of the clients that they serve (eg, homeless populations, disadvantaged children, and injured workers) by just considering their needs in the areas of occupation; particularly applicable are IADL, work, play, leisure, and social participation.

Another aspect of the occupations of organizations is consideration of the occupational needs of the organization itself. How exactly does an organization operationalize its mission with its employees who carry out activities and tasks? How are the organization's policies and procedures developed that guide the organizational behavior? What is the person-environment fit within the organization's structure and culture? Again, the *Framework*[1] provides many useful tools for the consideration of the occupational needs of organizations as it does for all clients of occupational therapy services; "...occupational therapy practitioners provide interventions to support participation of those who are members of or served by the organization...."[1(S3)] Using the language of the *Framework,* it is helpful to consider the client factors of the organization: What are its values and beliefs as demonstrated by its mission and vision statements? What are its functions of planning, organizing, coordination, carrying out the mission, developing policy, financial and communication management, and productivity? How does the organization's structure illustrate the departmental relationships, leadership and management functions, and job title?

Next, what are the activity demands of the various functions of the organizations? Consider the tools and equipment used to do the work, the flow/timing of and sequence of the work, the demands of the physical and

Figure 12-2. Organization-Centered PEOP Occupational Therapy Process.

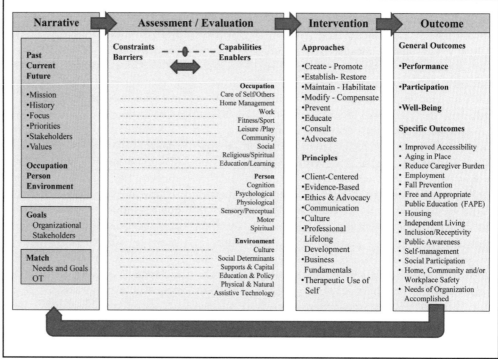

social environments, and how they can be adapted. Occupational therapy practitioners can also examine the performance patterns of the organization: how do the habits of employees, their daily routines, employees' roles outside of specific job title (eg, coordinates monthly birthday celebrations, manages the "sunshine club"), and overt (annual company awards banquet at which attendance is required) and covert ("voluntary" participation in the summer sports leagues) rituals impact the organization's effectiveness?

Finally, the contexts and environments can be addressed, including the ethnic and racial sensitivity, the health and wellness of employees, the effective use of technology throughout the organization, the natural and built environment, and the relationships among and between the various stakeholders. The *Framework* provides a rich resource if the occupational therapy profession wants to consider organizations as clients in the same way that we provide services to individuals and populations.

OCCUPATIONS OF ORGANIZATIONS: USE OF THE PERSON-ENVIRONMENT-OCCUPATION-PERFORMANCE OCCUPATIONAL THERAPY PROCESS

When the area of *evaluation* is considered within organizations, the first topic that often comes to mind is per-

formance evaluation or appraisal of personnel. Although an important function within an organization, performance appraisal is only one of many aspects of an organization to be considered in an evaluation or analysis. The evaluation of an organization must consider the individuals and groups who do its work, stakeholders who support it and benefit from its work, and countless other characteristics that will determine its effectiveness. According to the *Framework*,[1]

> …Using a client-centered approach, the practitioner gathers information to understand what is currently important and meaningful to the client (ie, what he or she wants and needs to do) and to identify past experiences and interests that may assist in the understanding of current issues and problems. During the process of collecting this information, the client, with the assistance of the occupational therapy practitioner, identifies priorities and desired targeted outcomes….[1(pS13)]

The PEOP Occupational Therapy Process is used to evaluate the constraints and enablers, within and outside of the organization, that impact its ability to meet the goals (Figure 12-2).

The PEOP Occupational Therapy Process of an organization starts with a process known as SWOT—an acronym describing the process of identifying Strengths, Weaknesses, Opportunities, and Threats—from which occupational performance issues can be determined and goals identified. Following the SWOT analysis, evidence-based interventions can be selected to assist the organization in addressing the necessary changes. Of course, the complexities of organizations can make achieving these changes a very involved and challenging process. Thus, a useful approach may be to apply the SWOT process in 3 stages: to the individuals within the organization, to the groups or teams of people organized around organizational functions, and to the organization itself.

A small nonprofit organization can be used as an example here. Consider that the organization is a local foundation whose mission is to serve the needs of local children who are diagnosed with cancer and their families. The organization is considering major changes, as the staff would like to expand its mission in meeting the health and community integration needs of newly arrived migrant workers' children. The staff is composed of an executive director, an administrative assistant (who manages the office), a fundraiser, and an outreach coordinator (implements the activities that meet the mission). There is also a board of directors composed of family members and friends of the child for whom the organization was founded and named. Additionally, the foundation has many, many volunteers who coordinate and run the various fundraising and outreach events.

The first step in the PEOP Occupational Therapy Process is learning the organization's "story" through a narrative process, essentially the creation of an occupational profile. At the individual level, this might involve interviews with stakeholders, such as staff and board members, and with individuals who have been served by the organization. The group or team level narrative may be determined by group interviews of the stakeholders, a review of meeting minutes of the staff and the board of directors, and with teams of volunteers who have implemented some of the events. The organization's narrative might be told through its mission and vision statements, policies and procedures, interviews with other organizations with whom it has collaborated (ie, local children's hospital), and its current focus and priorities. Once the perspectives from the 3 levels of the organization have been gathered and a complete narrative created, a preliminary SWOT analysis may be drafted. An important prerequisite for an occupational therapy practitioner doing a PEOP Occupational Therapy Process of an organization will be the practitioner's own expertise with the populations being served (in this case, children with cancer and their families, and needs of migrant workers' children).[3] A population-based PEOP Occupational Therapy Process may be needed, formal or informal, to assure the practitioner's ability to address the critical occupational performance issues, as well as ensure the organization's confidence in the practitioner's abilities.

Following development of the narrative and preliminary SWOT analysis, the next step in the PEOP Occupational Therapy Process will be a more formal assessment of the organization. The occupational therapy practitioner uses clinical reasoning to determine the needs of organization based upon an assessment of persons (to be served and who provide services), the environment (physical and social), occupations, and performance of occupations. Based upon the identified needs of the new population (migrant workers' children) as determined by the population-based PEOP Occupational Therapy Process, an assessment of the current capacity of the organization to meet these needs should be done.

The new population's needs may include IADL (eg, communication management, community mobility, and safety), educational preparation and participation, play exploration and participation, and social participation. Does the organization have the capacity within its current structure to evaluate and meet those needs? Environmental assessment will examine the natural and built environments in which new occupational performance will take place; occupational therapy expertise in person-environment[22] fit will determine current capacity and future needs. The social and cultural environment of staff, board of directors, volunteers, and collaborating organizations could also be assessed. Is there recognition of customs, beliefs, and values of the migrant worker population which will be served? Is language a barrier? Are collaborating organizations available to provide services (eg, preventive medicine) that are outside the scope of the nonprofit? Are resources available to support the occupational needs of the new population? Does it need to hire or contract with an occupational therapy practitioner to address these occupational performance issues?

As briefly illustrated here, the PEOP Occupational Therapy Process of an organization is an extremely complex process. The *Framework*[1] states that "…organizations serve as a mechanism through which occupational therapy practitioners provide interventions to support participation of those who are members of or served by the organization…."[1(pS3)] In fact, the potential contribution of occupational therapy to organizations goes beyond the needs of the individual or populations served to the organization itself.

The ultimate purpose of an organizational evaluation is to determine if the organization is effective in accomplishing its goals. *Organizational effectiveness* has been addressed in the management and business literature for decades, with many practices and concepts advanced by theorists such as Peter Drucker.[23] Criteria have been identified for fostering organizational effectiveness for a category of workers known as *knowledge workers*,[24] which are particularly applicable to occupational therapy practitioners who primarily work within the health and education domains. These criteria include establishing a climate of trust that gives people autonomy (organizational culture), creating vital work places (environment), and providing healthful physical support for individuals (ergonomics and wellness programs). Occupational therapy practitioners are well-equipped to help organizations develop and advance these elements of effective organizations, as well as to benefit from their presence as employees.

PROMOTING THE OCCUPATIONAL PERFORMANCE OF ORGANIZATIONS

Based on the PEOP Occupational Therapy Process, the occupational therapy practitioner is uniquely positioned to assist an organization and the people it serves to achieve desired outcomes; for the clients, patients, students, or consumers this will be improved health and participation through engagement in occupations. Like individuals and populations, the outcomes of an organization-centered intervention will be client-centered and based upon the organization's goals and priorities. They may be as general as improved organizational effectiveness or as specific as a percentage decrease in the number of work-related injuries and associated costs. These goals can be translated to improved "health and participation" of the organization when one considers that the organization will perform better to achieve its goals, have high job satisfaction and retention among employees, and maintain or improve itself financially. These are consistent with the outcomes of occupational therapy as described in the *Framework*,[1] which include occupational performance improvement or enhancement, adaptation, health and wellness, and participation.

Youngstrom and Brown[25] have outlined 5 principles of interventions they describe as applicable to individuals and populations; these are that interventions are client-centered, context driven, occupation-based, evidence-based, and interrelated with ongoing assessment. These principles can also be applied to interventions for organizations. As suggested in the first example in the chapter, the first step in planning interventions for the department store chain was to learn more about the goals and priorities of the company (client-centered). The planning of organization-centered interventions for the company may be directed to management, employees, customers, and the community in which it resides—each set of interventions will necessarily be context-driven for each targeted group and its contexts and environments. The occupation-based interventions for employees could involve workplace modifications and adaptations of routines and habits. Recommendations to management may be for changes in furniture and lighting to enhance employee comfort, and implementation of flexible work schedules and other family-friendly policies to better accommodate child and adult day care needs; this may lead to improved workplace morale and job satisfaction, and thus, increased productivity. There is evidence to demonstrate that when management expresses a high level of concern and support to employees, the workers reciprocate in ways that benefit the organization.[26-28] Likewise, employer efforts to address family responsibilities of employees, especially in the area of childcare, have been shown to reduce stress and employee turnover.[29]

Further recommendations to management may include changes in merchandise arrangements and lighting to accommodate customers with disabilities and improve sales.[30] The ongoing assessment of organization-centered interventions is accomplished with a regularly scheduled evaluation plan of desired outcomes (ie, increased sales, reduced use of sick time), specific indicators of outcomes that are created in advance, and determination of modifications of interventions if outcome indicators are not being reached.

There is a 2-decade history of organizational implementation of health promotion programs to enhance organization effectiveness.[31] These programs have traditionally focused on the development of fitness centers, smoking cessation programs, nutrition consultations, and stress management. Occupational therapy practitioners have the expertise to develop and implement such programs and bring the added value of expertise in ergonomics, family-life balance issues, accessibility and universal design, performance patterns, person-environment fit, as well as the treatment of traditional clinical issues like upper extremity injuries. Even though identified as a client in the *Framework*,[1] organizations may be under-recognized as the direct recipients of occupational therapy services, separate from the individuals and populations that they serve. It could be that occupation therapy services for organizations is in its infancy, just as it was for individuals (eg, TB patients) and at-risk populations (eg, immigrants) in the founding years of the profession in the 1920s. The time may be right for the profession to reconsider its role with organizations.

REFERENCES

1. AOTA. Occupational therapy practice framework: domain and process (3rd ed). *Am J Occup Ther.* 2014;68(Supplement 1:S1-S51.
2. AOTA. Occupational therapy practice framework: domain and process. *Am J Occup Ther.* 2002;56:609-639.
3. Baum CM, Bass Haugen J, Christiansen CH. Person-environment-occupation-performance: a model for planning interventions for individuals and organizations. In: Christiansen CH, Baum CM, Bass Haugen J, eds. *Occupational Therapy: Performance, Participation, and Well-Being.* 3rd ed. Thorofare, NJ: SLACK Incorporated; 2005:372-385.

4. Rollinson D, Edwards D, Broadfield A. *Organizational Behaviour and Analysis: An Integrated Approach.* New York, NY: Addison Wesley Longman, Inc; 2008.

5. Braveman B. Understanding and working within organizations. In: Braveman B, ed. *Leading and Managing Occupational Therapy Services: An Evidence-based Approach.* Philadelphia, PA: FA Davis; 2006:53-80.

6. Colquitt JA, LePine JA, Wesson, MJ. Organizational behavior: an overview. In: Colquitt JA, LePine JA, Wesson MJ. *Organizational Behavior: Essentials for Improving Performance and Commitment.* New York, NY: McGraw Hill; 2010:2-21.

7. Fulmer IS, Gerhart B, Scott, KS. Are the 100 best better? An empirical investigation of the relationship between being a "great place to work" and firm performance. *Pers Psych.* 2003;56:965-993.

8. Walonick DS. *Organizational Theory and Behavior: Classical Organization Theory.* StatPac Survey Research Library. http://statpac.org/walonick/organizational-theory.htm. Published 1993. Accessed September 21, 2013.

9. Broiody EK, Trotter RT, Meerwarth TL. *Transforming Culture: Creating and Sustaining a Better Manufacturing Organization.* New York, NY: Palgrave Macmillan; 2010.

10. Barzilai K. *Organizational Theory.* Case Western Reserve University. http://www.cwru.edu/med/epidbio/mphp439/Organizational_Theory.htm. Updated 2012. Accessed September 21, 2013.

11. Theis-Berglmair AM. *The Role of Organizations in the Modern Society: An Outlook From the Perspective of Systems Theory.* Paper presented at the 55th Annual Conference of the International Communication Association (ICA): *Communication: Questioning the Dialogue.* 2005;1-13. http://www.uni-bamberg.de/fileadmin/uni/fakultaeten/split_lehrstuehle/kommunikationswissenschaften_1/Dateien/Downloads/Veroeff/Anna_Maria_Theis_Berglmair/The_role_of_organizations.pdf. Published May 26, 2005. Accessed September 21, 2013.

12. Christen CT. The restructuring and reengineering of AT&T: analysis of a public relations crisis using organizational theory. *Pub Rel Rev.* 2005;31:239-251.

13. Plsek PE. Redesigning health care with insights from the science of complex adaptive systems. In: IOM Committee on Quality of Health Care in America. *Crossing the Quality Chasm: A New Health System for the 21st Century.* Washington, DC: National Academy Press; 2001.

14. Waldrop M. *Complexity: The Emerging Science on the Edge of Order and Chaos.* London, England: Penguin; 1992.

15. Lewin R. *Complexity: Life on the Edge of Chaos.* London, England: Phoenix; 1993.

16. Bak P. How nature works: the science of self organized criticality. *Nature.* 1996;383(6603):772-773.

17. Kernick, D. An introduction to complexity theory. In: Kernick, D, ed. *Complexity and Healthcare Organization.* Oxon, UK: Radcliffe Medical Press, Ltd; 2004:23-38.

18. World Federation of Occupational Therapists. *Member Organizations of WFOT.* WFOT: World Federation of Occupational Therapists. http://www.wfot.org/Membership/MemberOrganisationsofWFOT.aspx. Updated 2011. Accessed September 21, 2013.

19. World Health Organization. *International Classification of Functioning, Disability and Health (ICF).* World Health Organization. http://www.who.int/classifications/icf/en/. Updated 2013. Accessed September 21, 2013.

20. Christiansen CH, Baum CM, Bass Haugen J. *Occupational Therapy: Performance, Participation, and Well-Being.* 3rd ed. Thorofare, NJ: SLACK Incorporated; 2005.

21. Christiansen CH, Baum CM. Person-environment occupational performance: a conceptual mode for practice. In: Christiansen CH, Baum CM, eds. *Occupational Therapy: Enabling Function and Well-Being.* 2nd ed. Thorofare, NJ: SLACK Incorporated; 1997:46-71.

22. Stark SL, Sanford JA. Environmental enablers and their impact on occupational performance. In: Christiansen CH, Baum CM, Bass Haugen J, eds. *Occupational Therapy: Performance, Participation, and Well-Being.* 3rd ed. Thorofare, NJ: SLACK Incorporated; 2005:298-336.

23. Drucker P. *The Practice of Management.* New York, NY: Harper Business; 2006.

24. Herman Miller Inc. *Quantifying and Fostering Organizational Effectiveness.* Kansas State University. http://swat.gis.ksu.edu/documents/org_effectiveness.pdf. Published 2004. Accessed September 21, 2013.

25. Youngstrom MJ, Brown C. Categories and principles of interventions. In: Christiansen CH, Baum CM, Bass Haugen J, eds. *Occupational Therapy: Performance, Participation, and Well-Being.* 3rd ed. Thorofare, NJ: SLACK Incorporated; 2005:396-419.

26. Hofmann D, Morgeson F. Safety-related behavior as a social exchange: the role of perceived support and leadership-member exchange. *J Appl Psych.* 1999;84:286-296.

27. Kelley SW, Hoffman KD. An investigation of positive affect, prosocial behaviors and service quality. *J Retail.* 1997;73:407-427.

28. Berg P, Kallenberg, AL, Appelbaum, E. Balancing work and family: the role of high commitment environments. *Ind Rel: J Econ Soc.* 2003;2:168-188. doi: 10.1111/1468-232X.00286.

29. Lee S, Hong JH. Does family-friendly policy matter? Testing its impact on turnover and performance. *Pub Admin Rev.* 2011;71:870-879. doi: 10.1111/j.1540-6210.2011.02416.x.

30. Heschong L, Wright RL, Okura S. Daylighting impacts on retail sales performance. *J Illuminat Engr Soc.* 2002;2:21-25.

31. Lloyd PJ, Foster SL. Creating health, high-performance workplaces: strategies from health and sports psychology. *Cons Psych J: Prac Res.* 2006;1:23-39.

Chapter 13

OCCUPATIONS OF POPULATIONS

Julie D. Bass, PhD, OTR/L, FAOTA

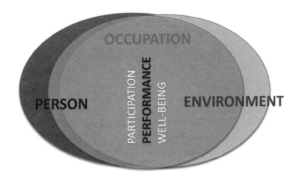

LEARNING OBJECTIVES

- Define the concept of a population and identify disciplines that contribute to an understanding of populations.
- Discuss definitions of population health and public health and how these definitions support occupational therapy's role in meeting population needs.
- Define terminology, concepts, and measures used in population health and public health that address the occupations of populations, including health behaviors, time use, quality of life (QOL), well-being, and patient-reported outcomes.
- Compare and contrast different international and national measures of population health and public health.
- Describe occupational therapy concepts that have been used to summarize occupational issues of

concern in populations and identify related interdisciplinary terminology.

- Identify current priorities for population health and public health, and sources of information on these priorities.

KEY WORDS

- Health behavior
- Health promotion
- Occupational justice
- Population
- Public health
- QOL
- Time use
- Well-being

Christiansen CH, Baum CM, Bass JD, eds.
*Occupational Therapy: Performance, Participation,
and Well-Being, Fourth Edition (pp 199-213).*
© 2015 SLACK Incorporated.

INTRODUCTION

Occupations of populations is mostly an unfamiliar phrase in occupational therapy. Occupational therapy practice, research, and education have traditionally focused on understanding the important and meaningful occupations of individuals that support performance, participation, and well-being. This emphasis on individuals is aligned with the biomedical approach of individual practitioners providing interventions to individual clients or patients. In recent years, population health and public health have had increased prominence in national and international conversations and initiatives designed to meet societal needs. Occupational therapy practitioners have opportunities during this critical period of our profession's history to develop the profession's knowledge related to the occupations of populations and contribute the unique knowledge, expertise, and perspectives of the field to improve population health. This chapter will introduce ideas related to population health and public health and identify the interdisciplinary terminology that serves as a bridge between occupational therapy and population-based programs.

DEFINING POPULATIONS

Population is a term that has been used by many disciplines and may be defined simply as the complete "body of persons or individuals having a quality or characteristic in common."[1(np)] Populations are typically defined or identified by individuals or organizations that have interest in the characteristics of a particular group of people. Thus, a population may be relatively small (eg, all students at a local university), moderate in size (eg, individuals with ALS [amyolateral sclerosis] in the United States), or large (eg, individuals at risk for heart disease in Europe). Traditionally, occupational therapy practitioners have sought to understand the occupations and occupational performance of individuals across the lifespan and defined their practice as one practitioner making a difference in the life of one person. As advances in knowledge about occupations were made, it became clear that descriptions of occupations, personal factors, and environmental factors needed to expand beyond the individual level. For example, the childhood games of tag or football cannot be correctly conceptualized as individual occupations. Similarly, religious worship at a church, synagogue, or mosque is an occupation of a community rather than an individual pursuit. Finally, the American Heart Association is rightfully concerned that Americans as a whole do not sufficiently engage in occupations that promote physical activity and fitness and thus reduce their risk for heart disease and stroke.

The PEOP Model and PEOP Occupational Therapy Process intend to support a broader understanding of occupations to include populations and organizations. A population approach to occupations requires evidence from disciplines that focus their research on the population level, including sociology, public health, economics, epidemiology, population studies, women's studies, geography, human ecology, political science, information technology, public policy, and planning. For example, the reader may likely have come to appreciate the enormous contributions that occupational therapy can make to an individual older adult who needs advice on mobility devices for the community. What additional information would a practitioner need to understand and contribute to community mobility initiatives at the population level? Knowledge from public policy, planning, architecture, engineering, and geography, to name a few, may be helpful in preparing to assist in designing transportation systems for the community mobility of an aging population. Population health and public health are important bridges for occupational therapy at the population level.

Population Health and Public Health

Although the term *population health* has been the basis for many research studies, it has often been introduced without a formal definition. Kindig and Stoddard proposed that any definition of population health should include both the determinants of health and outcomes of health; they introduced the definition of population health as "the health outcomes of a group of individuals, including the distribution of such outcomes within the group."[2(p381)] The Public Health Agency of Canada has emphasized doing in population health by defining it as the "capacity or resource for everyday living that enables us to pursue our goals, acquire skills and education, grow and satisfy personal aspirations."[3(p2)]

Public health is the commonly used term to refer to the predominant concerns of health that may be addressed at the population or community level. In 1920, Winslow defined public health as,

> ... the science and art of preventing disease, prolonging life, and promoting physical health and efficiency through organized community efforts for the sanitation of the environment, the control of community infections, the education of the individual in principles of personal hygiene, the organization of medical and nursing services for the early diagnosis and preventive treatment of disease, and the development of the social machinery, which will ensure to every individual in the community a standard of living adequate for the maintenance of health.[4(p183)]

This definition is still referenced and adapted by organizations today to differentiate public health from an individual-focused biomedical framework. In 1988, the Institute of Medicine's (IOM) Study of the Future of Public Health Committee defined public health as "fulfilling society's interest in assuring conditions in which people can be healthy."[5(p19)]

The WHO's Ottawa Charter for Health Promotion[6] started a movement to reshape the meaning of public health and health promotion, and strengthen the links to everyday performance, participation, and well-being for populations. Building upon the 1948 WHO definition of health as "a state of complete physical, mental, and social well-being and not merely the absence of disease or infirmity,"[7(np)] this charter proposed that achieving health requires individuals and populations "to identify and to realize aspirations, to satisfy needs, and to change or cope with the environment. Health is, therefore, seen as a resource for everyday life, not the objective of living."[6(np)] Similarly, the WHO's ICF[8] and the Disability Assessment Schedule[9] have begun to recognize the importance of person-environment-occupation in framing health aspects of performance, participation, and well-being for populations. In the ICF, health domains include body functions and structure, activities, participation, and environmental factors. The most recent version of the Disability Assessment Schedule (WHO DAS 2.0)[9] uses 6 domains to evaluate the impact of health and disability on participation, performance, and well-being: cognition, mobility, self-care, getting along, life activities, and participation. This assessment has been proposed as a tool to understand disability across clinical and population levels and across cultures.

OCCUPATION-BASED CONCEPTS FOR POPULATIONS: CONCEPTS AND MEASURES

In studies of populations and public health, the term *occupation* is typically only used to describe characteristics associated with work. Thus, occupational therapy practitioners who are interested in the full array of occupations for populations must learn terminology and concepts that are used by governmental agencies, international organizations, and disciplines that focus on populations. Several concepts will be introduced in this chapter: health behaviors, time use, QOL, well-being, and patient-reported outcomes. Each of these concepts is tracked at the population level and has specific measures that are used by governments and international agencies to document the health of target populations.

Health Behaviors

Health behavior is an interdisciplinary term used to describe individuals' positive and negative attributes associated with health. Health behaviors may be defined as:

... those personal attributes such as beliefs, expectations, motives, values, perceptions, and other cognitive elements; personality characteristics, including affective and emotional states and traits; and overt behavior patterns, actions, and habits that relate to health maintenance, to health restoration, and to health improvement.[10(p3)]

In this definition, Gochman[10] emphasized that health behavior includes thoughts and feelings about health as well as doing or observable actions, and consists of several categories: preventive or protective, illness, sick role, and societal health. Preventive or protective health behaviors include those medical (eg, routine preventive care) and nonmedical activities (eg, eating habits, physical activity, oral hygiene, spiritual activities) that individuals engage in to stay healthy; these behaviors are associated with cognition and emotional states, and shape lifestyle and risk behaviors. In addition, these behaviors may entail active choices regarding completion of an activity (eg, wearing a helmet while bicycling) or passive protection through public health initiatives (eg, drinking tap water that is chlorinated). Illness behaviors are characterized by the actions one takes when there are concerns about health and illness. These activities often entail seeking health information and care (eg, information seeking, primary care visits, alternative health remedies). Sick role behaviors include those activities associated with management of a diagnosed condition (eg, medication management, dietary changes) and how the activities are carried out (eg, adherence). Societal health behaviors are the actions and activities conducted by agencies and organizations to promote and maintain public health (eg, restaurant inspections, neighborhood clean-ups). This category broadens the definition of health behaviors to emphasize health education efforts in schools, neighborhoods and communities, work settings, homes, consumer products, and media campaigns that are provided by groups and organizations with goals to improve population health.[11]

The AOTA's third edition of the *Occupational Therapy Practice Framework: Domain and Process*[12] and the *Blueprint for Entry-Level Education*[13] identify several areas of occupation that are particularly relevant to health behaviors, for example personal hygiene and grooming, sexual activity, safety and emergency maintenance, health management and maintenance, and rest. The health promoting (or health limiting) performance patterns for these occupations may be observed in the health behaviors of individuals, organizations, and populations.

Measuring health behaviors documents the characteristics and contributing factors to population health. Measures of health behavior are commonly used by federal and state governmental agencies to document the current status and trends in public health; these data on health behaviors are collected through telephone, face-to-face, mail, or internet surveys.[14] The most common measures of health behavior in the United States are the Behavioral Risk Factor Surveillance System (BRFSS), the National Health and Nutrition Examination Survey (NHANES), the Pregnancy Risk Assessment Monitoring System (PRAMS), the Youth Risk Behavior Surveillance System (YRBSS), and the National Survey on Drug Use and Health (NSDUH).[14]

Health behaviors may be measured in terms of either positive and/or negative attributes. For example, current recommendations for adolescents include a nutritious diet, being active, and getting adequate sleep[15]; while the YRBSS surveys risk behaviors associated with injuries and violence; unintended pregnancies and sexually transmitted diseases; alcohol, drug, and tobacco use; unhealthy diets; and insufficient physical activity.[16] Similarly, adults are advised to adopt health behaviors that include only moderate alcohol use, no tobacco use, good nutrition, and regular physical activity[17] because risk behaviors related to alcohol, tobacco, nutrition, and physical activity are known to contribute to morbidity and mortality.

At first glance, an occupational therapy practitioner may believe that the current scope of practice has little to do with health behaviors. There are numerous examples, however, of opportunities to support health behavior recommendations by applying knowledge of person-environment-occupation-performance. For example, there is growing interest in using a broader array of occupations (eg, IADLs, leisure) to meet physical activity guidelines, because there is awareness that aerobic and strengthening goals can be met through activities other than exercise.[18]

Time Use

Time use has been studied for over a century and is of interest to governments (eg, US Bureau of Labor Statistics), international organizations (eg, United Nations Statistics Division), and in a variety of disciplines including social science, business, labor, economics, and health. Time use has also been referred to as time allocation and time budget by different research groups.

There are few conceptual models of time use in the literature. In the introduction to the inaugural edition of the electronic *International Journal of Time-Use Research* (eIJTUR), the editors proposed that the "things that we do with our time, regularly and repeatedly, on a daily, weekly, or monthly cycle, may add to our stock of personal capacities, and hence to the resources that determine

our life chances" and that "what we have done, determines who we become;"[19(pI)] this framework recognizes the social and economic implications of time use both at the individual and population level.

There are a number of approaches to measuring how people spend their time, including observation, structured questions, activity logs, and time diaries. However, there is general agreement that time diaries, capturing the flow and multiple dimensions of daily activity, may be the best approach to support understanding and theory development.[20] The International Association Time Use Research (IATUR)[21] summarizes international and national time use measures in common use.

Some countries administer their own time use surveys to meet specific needs. The US Bureau of Labor Statistics administers the American Time Use Survey (ATUS) that provides annual "estimates of how, where, and with whom Americans spend their time, and is the only federal survey providing data on the full range of nonmarket activities, from childcare to volunteering."[22] In 2011, the ATUS included 17 activity areas in its classification scheme. Statistics Canada administers the General Social Survey—Overview of the Time Use of Canadians on an annual basis.[23] There has been increasing efforts to develop international measures of time use to allow comparisons across different countries and regions. The United Nations Statistics Division identifies time use as an important measure of activities that may be used to explore "social change, division of labor, allocation of time for household work, the estimation of the value of household production, transportation, leisure and recreation, pension plans, and health-care programs, among others."[24] The draft of the International Classification of Activities for Time-Use Statistics (ICATUS)[24] represents a collaborative effort to identify activities that are part of everyday life across geographic areas. The Multinational Time Use Study (MTUS)[25] has data representing 25 countries. A comparison of the areas of occupation from the *Occupational Therapy Practice Framework*, 3rd edition[12] with these 4 measures of time use is provided in Table 13-1. It is evident that measures of time use have categories of activities that are similar to the *Practice Framework*, but have differing levels of emphasis within categories.

Much of the current information on time use comes from studies by governments, often gathered for the purposes of understanding productivity and economic trends. Some consumer research and studies by social scientists have also made useful contributions to the general understanding of how people spend their time. Data from time use studies collected for economic purposes are also used to discern cultural changes and patterns of work and leisure. According to information provided by the International Association of Time Use Research (IATUR), nearly 100 countries have sponsored studies of time use

Table 13-1. Comparison of the Practice Framework With National and International Measures of Time Use

OTPF Areas of Occupation[12]	Examples of Country-Specific Measures of Time Use		International Measures of Time Use	
	United States: American Time Use Survey (ATUS)[22]	Canada: General Social Survey—2010 Overview of the Time Use of Canadians (GSS)[23]	International Classification of Activities for Time-Use Statistics (ICATUS)[24]	Multinational Time Use Study (MTUS)[25]
Activities of daily living	• Personal care • Eating and drinking	• Sleep, meals, and other personal activities	• Personal care and maintenance	• Dress/personal care • Meals and snacks
Instrumental activities of daily living	• Household activities • Caring for, helping household members • Caring for, helping non-household members • Consumer purchases • Professional, personal care services • Household services • Religious and spiritual activities • Telephone calls	• Household work and related activities	• Providing unpaid domestic services for own final use within household • Providing unpaid caregiving services to household members • Providing community services and help to other households • Mass media	• Cook, wash up • Housework • Odd jobs • Gardening • Shopping • Childcare • Domestic travel • Consume personal services • Religious activities
Rest and sleep				• Sleep • Relax
Education	• Education	• Education and related activities	• Learning	• School, classes • Study, homework
Work	• Work and work-related activities	• Paid work and related activities	• Work for corporations/quasi-corporations, non-profit institutions, and government (formal sector work) • Work for household in primary production • Work for household in non-primary production activities • Work for household in construction activities • Work for household providing services for income	• Paid work • Paid work at home • Paid work, second job • Travel to/from work

(continued)

Table 13-1 (continued).   *Comparison of the Practice Framework With National and International Measures of Time Use*

OTPF Areas of Occupation[12]	Examples of Country-Specific Measures of Time Use		International Measures of Time Use	
	United States: American Time Use Survey (ATUS)[22]	Canada: General Social Survey—2010 Overview of the Time Use of Canadians (GSS)[23]	International Classification of Activities for Time-Use Statistics (ICATUS)[24]	Multinational Time Use Study (MTUS)[25]
Play, leisure	• Socializing, relaxing, and leisure • Sports, exercise, and recreation • Traveling	• Television, reading, and other passive leisure • Sports, movies, and other entertainment events	• Attending/visiting cultural, entertainment, and sports events/venues • Hobbies, games, and other pastime activities • Indoor and outdoor sports participation and related courses	• Free time travel • Excursions • Active sports participation • Passive sports participation • Walking • Cinema or theater • Dances or parties • Pubs • Restaurants • Listen to radio • Watch television or video • Listen to records, tapes, cds • Read books • Read papers, magazines • Knit, sew • Other leisure
Social participation	• Government services and civic obligations • Volunteer activities	• Civic and voluntary • Socializing including restaurant meals	• Socializing and community participation	• Civic activities • Social clubs • Visit friends at their homes • Conversation • Entertain friends at home

Table 13-2. Domains and Facets of the Centers for Disease Control Health-Related Quality of Life-14 Measure

Module	Questions
Healthy Days Core	• General Rating of Health: ◇ Number of days in past 30 days that physical health was not good ◇ Number of days in past 30 days that mental health was not good ◇ Number of days in past 30 days that poor health kept you from usual activities
Activity Limitations Module	• Limitations in any activities because of impairment or health problem • Major impairment or health problem limiting activities • Length of time activities have been limited • Need for help with personal cares from other persons • Need for help with routine needs from other persons
Healthy Days Symptoms Module	• Number of days in past 30 days that pain kept you from usual activities • Number of days in past 30 days with depression feelings • Number of days in past 30 days with anxious feelings • Number of days in past 30 days with not enough rest or sleep • Number of days in past 30 days feeling health and full of energy

Adapted from US Centers for Disease Control and Prevention. Health-Related Quality of Life. US Centers for Disease Control and Prevention. http://www.cdc.gov/hrqol/concept.htm. Updated March 17, 2011. Accessed June 10, 2013.

during the past 40 years; these studies are done for purposes of understanding economic and social trends and for informing public policy.[21] Other studies, done by social scientists or businesses, seek to understand the time use of individuals for behavioral analysis or marketing purposes.

Occupational therapy research has contributed to knowledge on time use for special populations; ie, studies on time use for individuals with serious mental illness,[26] older adults,[27] and mothers of preschool children[28] may help to further extend research on time use beyond its current focus on categories of activities to include its relationship to performance, participation, and well-being.

Quality of Life

Both QOL and health-related quality of life (HRQOL) are used to describe subjective evaluations of the multiple domains that contribute to positive or negative perceptions of life. For both of these concepts, the definitions and domains continue to evolve to reflect emerging knowledge. *QOL* is a broader term because it includes environmental factors (characteristics of community, schools, employment, homes, culture), personal factors (values, spirituality), as well as health.[29] In a study of over 1700 healthy males and females in Japan, 10 domains were associated with QOL: social and community life, hobbies and learning, standard of living, personal health, relationships with family, morale in daily living, relationships with friends, work, self-supported living, and religion or belief.[30]

HRQOL emphasizes the multidimensional aspects of health and includes both individual (physical, mental, social, functional, health risks, health conditions, socioeconomic) and community components (resources and services, policies and practices, conditions and characteristics).[29] Since 2000, Healthy People goals have included HRQOL as a priority goal.[31] A number of measures are used to assess HRQOL in populations. Some of these measures are disease-specific, while others are generic. In this section, a selection of generic measures will be described, recognizing that disease-specific QOL measures may be suitable for determining outcomes in populations with specific conditions.

The CDC HRQOL-14 Healthy Days Measure, consists of the Healthy Days Core Module (4 questions, used in the BRFSS, NHANES, Medical Outcomes Study Short Forms (MOS), the Activity Limitations Module (5 questions, used in the BRFSS), and the Healthy Days Symptoms Module (5 questions, used in the BRFSS) (Table 13-2).[29] Other measures of HRQOL include the Sickness Impact Profile and the Quality of Well-Being

Table 13-3. *Domains and Facets of the World Health Organization Quality of Life Measure (WHO QOL)*

Domain	Facets
Physical	Pain and discomfort, energy and fatigue, sleep and rest
Psychological	Positive feelings; thinking, learning, memory and concentration; self-esteem; body image and appearance; negative feelings
Level of independence	Mobility, activities of daily living, dependence on medication or treatments, working capacity
Social relationships	Personal relationships, social support, sexual activity
Environment	Physical safety and security, home environment, financial resources, health and social care, opportunities for acquiring new information and skills, participation in and opportunities for recreation and leisure, physical environment (pollution/noise/traffic/climate), transport
Spirituality/religion/personal beliefs	Spirituality/religion/personal beliefs

Adapted from World Health Organization. WHO Quality of Life-BREF (WHO QOL-BREF). World Health Organization. http://www.who.int/substance_abuse/research_tools/whoqolbref/en/. Updated 2013. Accessed June 10, 2013.

Scale. The WHO has developed a measure of QOL that includes 6 domains and 24 facets/concepts (Table 13-3).[32]

HRQOL is regarded as an important concept in population and public health. It fosters connections among diverse disciplines, guides development of health policy, and is used to track the impact of health issues and their risk factors.[29] Because HRQOL is based on subjective evaluations by individuals in a community, it enables identification of specific populations that may need targeted services and programs.[29] QOL has also been recommended as an outcome measure for occupational therapy and rehabilitation, but has not been routinely used in research or practice; overviews of definitions, measures, and issues have been provided to increase awareness of this concept.[33,34] Because QOL domains are related to occupational performance, participation, and well-being, there are growing opportunities to become involved in research that examines QOL, especially for special populations, and programs that address the factors influencing QOL.

Well-Being

Well-being is an integral part of the WHO's definition of health as "a state of complete physical, mental and social well-being and not merely the absence of disease or infirmity."[7] Well-being is often described as a positive, subjective experience that may be explored through people's perspectives regarding the quality of their lives in terms of "their relationships, their positive emotions, resilience, the realization of their potential, or their overall satisfaction with life."[35]

The Canadian Index of Well-Being defines well-being in terms of QOL as "the presence of the highest possible quality of life in its full breadth of expression focused on but not necessarily exclusive to: good living standards, robust health, a sustainable environment, vital communities, an educated populace, balanced time use, high levels of democratic participation, and access to and participation in leisure and culture."[36] It differentiates between positive activities that are assets (eg, volunteering) and harmful activities that are barriers (eg, smoking) to well-being.[36]

Well-being has been studied in a number of different disciplines and in terms of person factors (eg, physical well-being, emotional well-being, psychological well-being, life satisfaction, domain specific satisfaction), environment factors (eg, social well-being), and occupational performance (eg, development and activity, engaging activities and work).[35] In the United States, several self-report surveys are used to monitor components of well-being in the population, including the National Health Interview Survey (NHIS), BRFSS, the Porter Novelli Healthstyles Survey for adults,[35] the National Survey for Children's Health (NSCH), and the National Survey of Children with Special Needs (NSCSN) for children (Table 13-4).[37] Key indicators of well-being have been developed for 2 age groups in the United States population: children[37] and older adults[38] (see Table 13-4). Other

Table 13-4.   *Well-Being Concepts and Indicators: United States*

Components of Well-Being: Centers for Disease Control and Prevention[35]	US Children: Key National Indicators of Well-Being, 2012[37]	US Older Americans: Key Indicators of Well-Being, 2012[38]	US Well-Being Index[39]
Common Concepts			
Economic	Economic circumstances	Economic circumstances	—
Emotional	—	—	Emotional health
Social	Family and social environment	—	—
Physical	—	—	Physical health
—	Health care	Cost and use of health care services	Basic access
—	Behavior	Health risks and behaviors	Healthy behaviors
—	Health	Health status	—
Additional Concepts			
Development and activity	Education	Demographic characteristics	Daily pulse
Engaging activities and work	Physical Environment and Safety	End of life	Life evaluation
Psychological			Work environment
Life satisfaction			
Domain specific			

countries also measure well-being in their population. For example, comparisons of United States,[39] United Kingdom,[40] Canada,[41] and Australia[42] measures of well-being reflect differences in their societal views on factors related to well-being (Table 13-5).

Well-being is gaining momentum as an important indicator of the human condition at the population level. It is being used to analyze health, social circumstances, and economic conditions and inform policy and program decisions. For example, the Organization for Economic Co-Operation and Development (OECD), which consists of 34 member countries, has a mission to improve the "economic and social well-being of people around the world."[43] One of their strategies has been to create a Better Life Index of Well-Being, which allows comparisons across countries and by gender.[44] The index includes many of the same topics as other measures of well-being, including housing, income, jobs, community, education, environments, civic engagement, health, life satisfaction, safety, and work-life balance. The purpose of the index is to build a comprehensive population-based measure of well-being and support the work of policy makers as they

develop national and international priorities and programs.

Occupational therapy has had a long-standing interest in the well-being of individuals, but limited involvement at the population level to date. Occupational therapy's knowledge of person-environment-occupations as they support performance, participation, and well-being may improve the quality of the population data collected on well-being and the interpretation of current data, especially with regards to populations with special or unique conditions and needs, such as those with disabilities.

Patient-Reported Outcomes

Patient-reported outcomes (PRO) have recently been proposed as an important strategy for many areas of health research. PROs are direct reports from patients that convey their feelings and levels of function as these pertain to health conditions.[45,46] PROs are unique measures of population health because patients identify the concepts to be included and assist in developing questions as well as participate in the evaluation.[45] PROs may be developed as

Table 13-5.   *Domains in Measures of Well-Being: Four Countries*

United States Well-Being Index[39]	United Kingdom Measuring National Well-Being Programme[40]	Canada Areas of Well-Being[41]	Australian Unity Well-Being Index: Personal Well-Being Index (PWI)[42]
• Emotional health	• Health	• Learning	• Health
• Physical health	• What we do	• Work	• Personal relationships
• Basic access	• Personal finance	• Housing	• Feelings of safety
• Healthy behaviors	• Economy	• Family life	• Standard of living
• Daily pulse	• Natural environment	• Social participation	• Achievements in life
• Work environment		• Leisure	• Feeling part of community
• Life evaluation		• Health	• Future security
		• Security	
		• Environment	
		• Financial security	

measures that are disease-specific (eg, arthritis), condition-specific (eg, chronic pain, total hip replacement), or generic. In clinical research, PROs may include patient perspectives of symptoms, function, and feelings or concepts associated with general health status and QOL (eg, HRQOL, QOL, well-being).[45] The National Institutes of Health funds the Patient–Reported Outcome Measurement Information System (PROMIS) to coordinate information and resources on patient reported outcome measures for children and adults.[47] The *PROMIS Domain Framework* consists of multiple domains that are organized under 3 major components and their related subcomponents: physical health (symptoms, function), mental health (affect, behavior, cognition), and social health (relationships, function).[47] PROs are now proposed as critical aspects of clinical research and intervention evaluations.

OCCUPATIONAL ISSUES ASSOCIATED WITH POPULATION HEALTH

When occupational therapy practitioners learn about population issues related to health behaviors, time use, QOL, well-being, and PROs, it is natural that they also explore the person-environment-occupational performance factors that are associated with these problems. A number of terms have been proposed to characterize the nature of occupational concerns for a given population. Terms like *delay, deprivation, disparity,* and *imbalance* may help to communicate the underlying cause of the concern

and facilitate the exploration of remedies that will lead to improved occupational performance.

Developmental delay is evident when occupational development occurs on a schedule that is not typical. Delay is found in situations that "put off to a later time; defer; postpone" or "impede the process or progress of; retard; hinder"[48(p526)] opportunities for occupational performance. Occupational delay is generally associated with the lifespan period from infancy to young adulthood and is evident in children with developmental disabilities or from at-risk populations.

There were an estimated 10 million children ages 3 to 17 in 2006 to 2008 with developmental disabilities in the United States[49] according to parent report. The global incidence of developmental disabilities is believed to be enormous, but no reliable estimates are available.[50] The Developmental Disabilities Act and Bill of Rights Act of 2000 (DD Act) defines developmental disability as:

> ... a severe chronic, disability that is due to mental and/or physical impairment which manifest before age 22 and are likely to continue indefinitely. They result in substantial limitations in 3 or more areas: self-care, receptive and expressive language, learning, mobility, self-direction, capacity for independent living, and economic self-sufficiency, as well as the continuous need for individually planned and coordinated services.[51(np)]

This emphasizes the need for programs and services that promote self-determination, independence, productivity, and integration and inclusion.

Populations at risk for developmental delay include those groups of individuals who have a possible or probable risk of developing an undesirable trait or outcome. Examples of at-risk populations may include refugees, children from low-income families, and children from military families. At-risk populations are usually identified and described by regional, national, or international organizations as they develop projections and goals for various populations.

Occupational deprivation occurs when there is "deprivation of occupational choice and diversity because of circumstances beyond the control of individuals or communities."[52(p343)] External agencies and circumstances may include personal characteristics (eg, disease, body structure/function) and environmental characteristics (eg, finances, social network). Deprivation may be defined as an act or instance of taking something away from or withholding, especially the necessities of life or of healthful environmental influences[53] or "to remove or withhold something from the enjoyment or possession of (a person or persons)."[48(p535)] Deprivation may occur in preschool children living in poverty who do not have access to safe playgrounds, and in adults with mental illness who are unable to maintain a job because of medication problems.

Health disparities may be evident when measures of performance, participation, and well-being reflect inequalities across different populations. A disparity is a "lack of similarity or equality; inequality; difference."[48(p567)] Health disparities are often associated with complex factors that may include behavioral, economic, cultural, and political influences. Some disparities occur due to the different values and choices made by people. Other disparities occur due to unequal opportunities available for different populations.

When disparities in health and well-being are attributable to equity issues, conditions of occupational injustice may also be present. *Occupational justice* was defined by Wilcock in the previous edition of this text as a fairly recent term that refers to the "just and equitable distribution of power, resources, and opportunity so that all people are able to meet the needs of their occupational natures, and so experience health and well-being"[54(p134)]; thus, injustice is the lack of this characteristic. Injustice is also defined as a "violation of the rights of others, unjust or unfair action or treatment."[48(p983)] Injustice issues are identified and addressed by many national and international groups concerned with human rights issues. Some recent issues of concern are poverty in third world countries, refugee camps, and racism/classism in the United States.

Occupational imbalance:

...involves a state that occurs because people's engagement in occupation fails to meet their unique physical, social, mental, or rest needs and allows

insufficient time for their own occupational interests and growth, as well as for the occupations each feels obliged to undertake in order to meet family, social, and community commitments.[55(p138)]

Imbalance is unique to the individual because "capacities, interests, and responsibilities differ."[55(p138)] Imbalance may occur in children who have too many commitments and, thus, little unstructured play time; women who are trying to meet the needs of both their young children and their elderly parents (ie, the sandwich generation)[56]; workers who have jobs that require excessive repetition of the same tasks[57]; and individuals in the early stage of retirement.[58]

These definitions of delay, deprivation, disparities, and imbalance provide an introduction to occupational issues of concern that are often noted in at-risk populations. As occupational therapy practitioners work on interprofessional teams and with communities to address population health and public health in at-risk populations, it is important that they frame occupational issues in terms that are understandable by individuals outside the occupational therapy profession.

CURRENT PRIORITIES FOR POPULATION HEALTH AND PUBLIC HEALTH

Priorities for population health and public health are established by governments, international agencies, and nonprofit organizations to respond to societal needs, designate funding for specific programs, and guide research agendas. Occupational therapy practitioners keep abreast of these priorities because they help identify target populations for occupational therapy practice, education, and research, and alert the profession to emerging opportunities.

A population at risk is defined as "those in the population who are susceptible to a particular disease or condition."[59(p66)] In a rapidly changing world, the populations at risk for occupational concerns may vary over time. In the last century, interventions were targeted to specific populations to address their occupational needs. During the settlement movement of the early 1900s, creative occupations were used with various populations at risk, especially immigrants, to address individual and societal problems associated with poverty and industrialization.[60] During the first half of the 20th century, the mental hygiene movement, the philosophy of pragmatism, and the arts and crafts movement also supported the use of occupations with individuals having various maladies, including psychiatric illnesses and tuberculosis.[61] Occupations in the 20th century also were a primary means of restoring health and functional ability to individuals with disabilities secondary to medical conditions. Improvement in occupational performance was a primary goal in rehabilitation programs and special education programs. Specific populations having occupational interventions included veterans returning from wars with injuries or post-traumatic stress; individuals with medical conditions like stroke, spinal cord injury, or psychiatric diagnoses; and children with developmental disabilities. Many of these interventions were provided by occupational therapy practitioners. The education and practice of these professionals focused on occupational interventions and the supporting components of occupation. These examples from the history of occupational therapy illustrate past populations at risk for occupational performance problems.

The ICF framework of the WHO[8] provides an important tool for describing individuals and populations at risk for occupational concerns. The ICF dimensions of body structure, body function, and environment promote understanding of the specific personal and environmental characteristics that support and limit occupational performance. The ICF framework also includes activity and participation dimensions that illustrate the complete constellation of occupations important for understanding health and disease from the standpoint of everyday living.

In community health, the general characteristics of the population at risk: incidence, significance, and importance of the issue in the population, and related population factors, are examined in terms of human policies and the current political climate. Several dimensions are used to characterize at-risk populations: gender, age, health status, ethnic background, socioeconomic levels, education, and geographic residence. These dimensions are examined because occupational concerns are often found in specific populations. At-risk populations may be described in terms of positive attributes or assets (eg, health behavior,[10] social participation,[41]) and negative attributes or barriers (eg, risk behaviors,[16] participation restrictions[8])

Community health initiatives emphasize the importance of describing at-risk populations because of disparities in health status for different groups. *Healthy People 2020*[31] summarizes the national health priorities for the United States as identified by the Department of Health and Human Services. *Healthy People 2020* has established over-arching goals and measures that serve as indicators of progress toward the overall goals (Table 13-6) with a primary goal to "achieve health equity, eliminate disparities, and improve the health of all groups."[31(np)] There are still substantial differences in morbidity and mortality rates for different populations associated with race, income, and gender. Disparities are also found in populations having different educational levels, disabilities, geographic residences, and sexual orientations. Many of these health disparities are related to occupational issues and are believed to result from variations in personal characteristics, environmental factors, and health behaviors.

At-risk populations are identified by different governmental agencies. At a regional level, states or provinces often establish goals or priorities for populations with certain characteristics living in specific geographic, economic, and political environments. For example, one state might have a particularly large immigrant population that is adjusting to different social and cultural norms. Individual countries usually establish priorities for funding and programs that are linked with specific populations. For example, the United States has identified autism and dementia as priorities for both research and programs.

Populations with certain diseases or disabilities are often identified as those at greatest risk for occupational performance problems. However, there has been growing interest in the occupations of populations who are typically described as healthy. These issues may be initially targeted in public health and education prevention programs as a means of decreasing the incidence of major health problems and then popularized in magazines and talk shows. Some recent issues of discussion have included the brain injuries due to concussions from sports or recreation activities, community recovery and resilience after emergencies and natural disasters, and physical activity levels of youth at risk for obesity.

Management of chronic conditions has been identified as a critical population health issue for the coming years. Kaiser Permanente and other groups[62] have developed models of chronic care to document the type and level of care needed by populations with chronic conditions and to estimate the percentage of the population needing different types of care (Figure 13-1). For example, it has been estimated that 60% to 70% of the population with chronic conditions may be able to effectively manage health needs associated with their conditions through self-management programs, primary care, and supported care. Individuals who have high risks (15% to 20%) or complex health issues (3% to 5%) may need individualized disease management or specialty care programs. Preventive programs targeted toward populations also are important strategy to reduce risk factors associated with chronic conditions.

SOURCES OF INFORMATION

There are numerous community organizations that serve as valuable sources of information and provide projections and goals for the occupations of populations and specific populations at risk. These community organizations may be part of health, education, or social service arenas and classified as governmental, quasi-governmental, or non-governmental.[59] Governmental organizations are defined as those international and national agencies that are funded by taxes and managed by the government. Governmental organizations may exist at the federal,

Table 13-6. *Healthy People 2020 Goals and Measures Related to PEOP*

Healthy People 2020 Goals	Foundation Health Measures	Specific Health Measures	Selected Healthy People 2020 Topics and Objectives Related to PEOP
Attain high-quality, longer lives free of preventable disease, disability, injury, and premature death.	General health status	• Life expectancy • Healthy life expectancy • Years of potential life lost • Physical/mental unhealthy days • Self-assessed health status • Limitation of activity • Chronic disease prevalence	• Arthritis, osteoporosis, and chronic back condition • Dementias, including Alzheimer's disease • Diabetes • Mental health and mental disorders • Vision
Achieve health equity, eliminate disparities, and improve the health of all groups.	HRQOL and well-being	• Physical, mental, and social HRQOL • Well-being/satisfaction • Participation in common activities	• Early and middle childhood • Adolescent health • Older adults
Create social and physical environments that promote good health for all.	Determinants of health	• Personal factors • Social factors • Economic factors • Environmental factors	• Disability and health • Social determinants of health
Promote QOL, healthy development, and healthy behaviors across all life stages.	Disparities	• Race/ethnicity • Gender • Physical and mental ability • Geography	• Educational and community-based programs • Injury and violence prevention • Occupational safety and health • Physical activity • Preparedness

Reprinted from US Department of Health and Human Services. Healthy People 2020. HealthyPeople.gov. http://www.healthypeople.gov/2020/default.aspx. Updated August 28, 2013. Accessed September 22, 2013.

regional, state, or local level. Quasi-governmental organizations are defined as those agencies that receive some governmental funding but otherwise operate independently from governmental agencies (eg, Red Cross). Other funds are received from a variety of private sources, or public donations. Non-governmental organizations are defined as those agencies that are funded by private sources for a specific mission. Examples of non-governmental organizations include voluntary health agencies; professional associations; foundations; and other service, social, religious, and corporate organizations.

Summary

This chapter examined the occupations of populations through concepts and evidence from population and

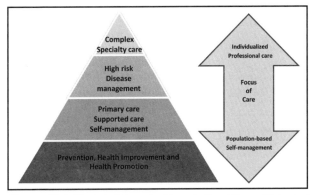

Figure 13-1. Model of Care for Chronic Conditions. (Adapted from Kaiser; The Scottish Government. *Improving the Health and Well-Being of People With Long Term Conditions on Scotland: A National Action Plan. The Scottish Government.* http://www.scotland.gov.uk/Publications/2009/12/03112054/4. Published 2009. Updated December 3, 2009. Accessed June 10, 2013.)

public health. Health behaviors, time use, QOL, well-being, and PROs were introduced as concepts that are used to describe person-environment-occupation factors that support performance, participation, and well-being for populations. Opportunities for occupational therapy in population health and public health programs, research, and education were discussed.

REFERENCES

1. Merriam-Webster. *Population*. Merriam-Webster. http://www.merriam-webster.com/dictionary/population. Updated 2013. Accessed June 6, 2013.
2. Kindig D, Stoddard G. What is population health? *American Journal of Public Health*. 2003;93:380-383.
3. Public Health Agency of Canada. *The Population Health Template: Key Elements and Actions That Define a Population*. Public Health Agency of Canada: what is the population health approach? http://www.phac-aspc.gc.ca/ph-sp/approach-approche/. Updated February 7, 2012. Accessed June 10, 2013.
4. Winslow CEA. The untilled field of public health. *Modern Medicine*. 1920;2:183-191.
5. National Research Council. *The Future of Public Health*. Washington, DC: The National Academies Press; 1988.
6. World Health Organization. *Health Promotion: the Ottawa Charter for Health Promotion*. World Health Organization. http://www.who.int/healthpromotion/conferences/previous/ottawa/en/. Published November 21, 1986. Updated 2013. Accessed June 6, 2013.
7. World Health Organization. *Preamble to the Constitution of the World Health Organization*. Adopted by the International Health Conference, New York, 19-22 June 1946; signed on 22 July 1946 by the representatives of 61 States (Official Records of the World Health Organization, no. 2, p. 100) and entered into force on 7 April 1948. World Health Organization. http://www.who.int/suggestions/faq/en/. Published 1946. Accessed September 22, 2013.
8. World Health Organization. *Classifications: International Classification of Functioning, Disability, and Health (ICF)*. World Health Organization. http://www.who.int/classifications/icf/en/. Published May 22, 2001. Updated 2013. Accessed June 6, 2013.
9. Üstün TB, Chatterji S, Kostanjsek N, et al. Developing the World Health Organization Disability Assessment Schedule 2.0. *Bulletin of the World Health Organization*. 2010;88:815-823. doi: 10.2471/BLT.09.067231.
10. Gochman DS. Health behavior research: definitions and diversity. In: Gochman DS, ed. *Handbook of Health Behavior Research I: Personal and Social Determinants*. New York, NY: Springer; 1997:1-20.
11. Glanz K, Rimer BK, Viswanath K. The scope of health behavior and health education. In: Glanz K, Rimer BK, Viswanath K, eds. *Health Behavior and Health Education: Theory, Research, and Practice*. 4th ed. New York, NY: John Wiley & Sons; 2008:1-18.
12. AOTA. Occupational therapy practice framework: domain and process (3rd ed). *Am J Occup Ther*. 2014;68(Supplement 1):S1-S51.
13. Baum C, Barrows C, Bass Haugen JD, et al. Blueprint for entry-level education. *American Journal of Occupational Therapy*. 2010;64:186-194.
14. Mokdad AH, Remington PL. Measuring health behaviors in populations. *Preventing Chronic Disease*. 2010; 7(4): A75. http://www.cdc.gov/pcd/issues/2010/jul/10_0010.htm. Published 2010. Accessed June 6, 2013.
15. US Department of Health and Human Services, Office of Adolescent Health. *Physical Health: Healthy Behavior*. US Department of Health and Human Services: Office of Adolescent Health. http://www.hhs.gov/ash/oah/adolescent-health-topics/physical-health-and-nutrition/healthy-behavior.html. Updated April 29, 2013. Accessed June 10, 2013.
16. US Centers for Disease Control and Prevention. Methodology of the youth risk behavior surveillance system—2013. *MMWR*. 2013;62 (RR-1):1-20.
17. Ford ES, Zhao G, Tsai J, Li C. Low-risk lifestyle behaviors and all-cause mortality: findings from the National Health and Nutrition Examination Survey III Mortality Study. *American Journal of Public Health*. 2011;101(10):1922-1929.
18. US Department of Health and Human Services. *2008 Physical Activity Guidelines for Americans*. US Department of Health and Human Services. http://www.health.gov/paguidelines/guidelines/default.aspx. Published June 2008. Updated March 11, 2013. Accessed June 6, 2013.
19. Gershuny J, Harvey AS, Merz J. Editors' introduction. *Electronic International Journal of Time Use Research*. 2004;1(No. 1):I-II. http://www.eijtur.org/pdf/volumes/eIJTUR-1-1-2_Editors_Introduction.pdf. Published 2004. Accessed June 6, 2013.
20. Robinson JP. The time-diary method. In: AS Pentland, Lawton MAM. *Time Use Research in the Social Sciences*. New York, NY: Kluwer Academic Plenum Publishers; 1999:47-89.
21. International Association Time Use Research. *International Association Time Use Research*. International Association Time Use Research: iatur.timeuse.org. http://iatur.timeuse.org. Accessed June 10, 2013.
22. US Department of Labor: Bureau of Labor Statistics. *American Time Use Survey: Overview*. US Department of Labor: Bureau of Labor Statistics. http://www.bls.gov/tus/overview.htm#1. Updated June 20, 2013. Accessed September 22, 2013.
23. Statistics Canada. *General Social Survey—2010 Overview of the Time Use of Canadians*. Statistics Canada. http://www.statcan.gc.ca/pub/89-647-x/89-647-X2011001-eng.pdf. Published July 2011. Accessed June 10, 2013.
24. United Nations Statistics Division. *Allocation of Time and Time Use*. United Nations. http://unstats.un.org/unsd/demographic/sconcerns/tuse/default.aspx. Updated 2013. Accessed June 10, 2013.
25. Centre for Time Use Research. *Multinational Time Use Study*. Centre for Time Use Research. http://www.timeuse.org/mtus. Accessed June 10, 2013.
26. Leufstadius C, Erlandsson LK, Eklund M. Time use and daily activities in people with persistent mental illness. *Occupational Therapy International*. 2006;13(3):123-141.
27. McKenna K, Broome K, Liddle J. What older people do: time use and exploring the link between role participation and life satisfaction in people aged 65 years and over. *Australian Occupational Therapy Journal*. 2007;54(4):273-284.
28. Crowe TK, Florez SI. Time use of mothers with school-age children: a continuing impact of a child's disability. *American Journal of Occupational Therapy*. 2006;60(2):194-203.
29. US Centers for Disease Control and Prevention. *Health-Related Quality of Life*. US Centers for Disease Control and Prevention. http://www.cdc.gov/hrqol/concept.htm. Updated March 17, 2011. Accessed June 10, 2013.

30. Tarumi K, Imanaka Y, Isshiki Y, Morimoto K. Quality of life domains in the healthy public: a trial investigation using attendants for an annual health checkup. *Environmental Health and Preventive Medicine*. 1999;4:39-48.

31. US Department of Health and Human Services. *HealthyPeople.gov*. HealthyPeople.gov. http://www.healthypeople.gov/2020/default.aspx. Updated August 28, 2013. Accessed September 22, 2013.

32. World Health Organization. *WHO Quality of Life-BREF (WHO QOL-BREF)*. World Health Organization. http://www.who.int/substance_abuse/research_tools/whoqolbref/en/. Updated 2013. Accessed June 10, 2013.

33. Liddle J, McKenna K. Quality of life: an overview of issues for use in occupational therapy outcome measurement. *Australian Occupational Therapy Journal*. 2000;47(2):77-85.

34. Bergland A, Narum I. Quality of life: diversity in content and meaning. *Critical Reviews in Physical and Rehabilitation Medicine*. 2007;19(2):115-140.

35. US Centers for Disease Control and Prevention. *Health-Related Quality of Life (HRQOL): Well-Being Concepts*. US Centers for Disease Control and Prevention. http://www.cdc.gov/hrqol/wellbeing.htm. Updated March 6, 2013. Accessed June 10, 2013.

36. University of Waterloo. *Canadian Index of Well-Being*. University of Waterloo. https://uwaterloo.ca/canadian-index-wellbeing/. Accessed June 10, 2013.

37. Federal Interagency Forum on Child and Family Statistics. *America's Children: Key National Indicators of Well-Being*. Childstats.gov: Forum on Child and Family Statistics. http://www.childstats.gov/. Published 2012. Accessed June 10, 2013.

38. Federal Interagency Forum on Aging-Related Statistics. *Older Americans 2012: Key Indicators of Well-Being*. Agingstats.gov: Federal Interagency Forum on Aging-Related Statistics. http://www.agingstats.gov/Main_Site/Data/2012_Documents/Highlights.aspx. Published 2012. Accessed June 10, 2013.

39. Gallup Healthways. *Well-Being Index*. Gallup Healthways. http://www.well-beingindex.com/overview.asp. Updated 2008. Accessed June 10, 2013.

40. UK Office for National Statistics. *National Well-Being: Measuring What Matters*. UK Office for National Statistics. http://www.ons.gov.uk/ons/guide-method/user-guidance/well-being/index.html. Accessed June 10, 2013.

41. Human Resources and Skills Development Canada. *Indicators of Well-Being in Canada*. Human Resources and Skills Development Canada. http://www4.hrsdc.gc.ca/h.4m.2@-eng.jsp. Updated September 22, 2013. Accessed September 22, 2013.

42. Australian Unity. *What is Well-Being?* Australian Unity. http://www.australianunity.com.au/about-us/Wellbeing/What-is-wellbeing. Accessed June 10, 2013.

43. Organization for Economic Co-Operation and Development (OECD). *About the OECD*. OECD: Better Policies for Better Lives. http://www.oecd.org/about/. Accessed June 10, 2013.

44. Organization for Economic Co-Operation and Development (OECD). *Better Life Index: Create Your Better Life Index*. OECD. http://www.oecdbetterlifeindex.org/. Updated 2013. Accessed June 10, 2013.

45. Patrick D, Guyatt GH, Acquadro C. Chapter 17: Patient-reported outcomes. In: Higgins JPT, Green S, eds. *Cochrane Handbook for Systematic Reviews of Interventions*. Version 5.0.1 (updated September 2008). England: John Wiley & Sons, Ltd/the Cochrane Collaboration; 2008. http://hiv.cochrane.org/sites/hiv.cochrane.org/files/uploads/Ch17_PRO.pdf. Published 2008. Updated September 2008. Accessed September 22, 2013.

46. National Quality Forum. *Patient-Centered Measures = Patient-Centered Results*. National Quality Forum. http://www.qualityforum.org/Measuring_Performance/ABCs/Patient-Centered_Measures_=_Patient-Centered_Results.aspx. Updated 2013. Accessed June 11, 2013.

47. National Institutes of Health. *PROMIS Domain Framework*. PROMIS: Dynamic Tools to Measure Health Outcomes from the Patient Perspective. http://www.nihpromis.org/default#1. Accessed June 10, 2013.

48. Flexner SB, ed. *The Random House Dictionary of the English Language*. 2nd ed. New York, NY: Random House; 1987.

49. Boyle A, Boulet S, Schieve LA, et al. Trends in the prevalence of developmental disabilities in US children, 1997–2008. *Pediatrics*. 2011;127:1034-1042.

50. Institute of Medicine, Committee on Nervous System Disorders in Developing Countries and Board of Global Health. *Neurological, Psychiatric, and Developmental Disorders: Meeting the Challenge in the Developing World*. Washington, DC: National Academy Press; 2001. http://books.nap.edu/books/0309071925/html/. Published 2001. Accessed September 29, 2002.

51. US Department of Health and Human Services: Administration on Intellectual and Developmental Disabilities. *History of the DD Act*. US Department of Health and Human Services: Administration for Children and Families. http://www.acf.hhs.gov/programs/aidd/resource/history-of-the-dd-act. Updated July 9, 2012. Accessed June 10, 2013.

52. Wilcock A. *An Occupational Perspective on Health*. 2nd ed. Thorofare, NJ: SLACK Incorporated; 2006.

53. Mish F, ed. *Webster's Ninth New Collegiate Dictionary*. Springfield, MA: Merriam-Webster Inc; 1988.

54. Wilcock A. Relationship of occupations to health and well-being. In: Christiansen C, Baum C, Bass J, eds. *Occupational Therapy: Performance, Participation, and Well-Being*. Thorofare, NJ: SLACK Incorporated; 2005:134-157.

55. Wilcock A. *An Occupational Perspective on Health*. Thorofare, NJ: SLACK Incorporated; 1998.

56. Brody E. "Women in the middle" and family help to older people. *Gerontologist*. 1981;21:471-479.

57. US Centers for Disease Control and Prevention, National Institute for Occupational Safety and Health. *Work-related Musculoskeletal Disorders* (CDC Document # 705005). US Centers for Disease Control and Prevention. http://www.cdc.gov/niosh/muskdsfs.html. Published 1997. Accessed September 29, 2002.

58. Jonsson H, Staffan J, Kielhofner G. Narratives and experience in an occupational transition: a longitudinal study of the retirement process. *American Journal of Occupational Therapy*. 2000;55:424-432.

59. McKenzie J, Pinger R, Kotecki J. *An Introduction to Community Health*. 3rd ed. Boston, MA: Jones and Bartlett; 1999.

60. Addams J. *Twenty Years at Hull-House: With Autobiographical Notes*. New York, NY: Signet; 1961.

61. Clark F, Wood W, Larson E. Occupational science: occupational therapy's legacy for the 21st century. In: Neistad M, Crepeau EB, eds. *Willard and Spackman's Occupational Therapy*. 9th ed. Philadelphia, PA: Lippincott; 1998:13-21.

62. The Scottish Government. *Improving the Health and Well-Being of People With Long Term Conditions on Scotland: A National Action Plan*. The Scottish Government. http://www.scotland.gov.uk/Publications/2009/12/03112054/4. Published 2009. Updated December 3, 2009. Accessed June 10, 2013.

PERSON FACTORS THAT SUPPORT OCCUPATIONAL PERFORMANCE

PEOP: Enabling Everyday Living

THE NARRATIVE
The past, current and future perceptions, choices, interests, goals and needs that are unique to the Person, Organization, or Population

PERSON
- Cognition
- Psychological
- Physiological
- Sensory
- Motor
- Spirituality

OCCUPATION
- Activities
- Tasks
- Roles

ENVIRONMENT
- Culture
- Social Determinants
- Social Support and Social Capital
- Education and Policy
- Physical and Natural
- Assistive Technology

Personal Narrative
- Perception and Meaning
- Choices and Responsibilities
- Attitudes and Motivation
- Needs and Goals

Organizational Narrative
- Mission and History
- Focus and Priorities
- Stakeholders and Values
- Needs and Goals

Population Narrative
- Environments and Behaviors
- Demographics and Disparities
- Incidence and Prevalence
- Needs and Goals

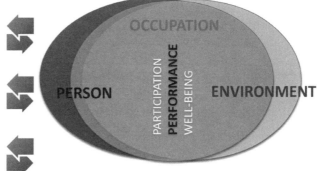

Section III provides an overview of the critical person factors that support occupational performance, participation, and well-being. The PEOP Model has "P" for Person as its first letter. Even though occupational performance is a focus of this model, it is not an accident that the "P" for person comes first. After all, practice models are designed to help us in our work with people. If our practice is targeted at people, then we must understand the person.

The PEOP Model includes 6 primary person factors: psychological, cognition, sensory, motor, physiological, and meaning/sensemaking/spiritual. Each factor has many subfactors that provide more detail about personal characteristics or characteristics that are intrinsic to the person. So, the PEOP Model is a starting point for your learning about the person. You will continue to build knowledge about personal factors over your entire professional life. At this point, it is sufficient to get the big picture and some specific examples of the level of detail you will learn along the way.

Upon completion of this section, you will begin to appreciate the many, complex person factors that influence occupational performance. These factors are important to consider as information is gathered in a particular situation and used to develop intervention plans for individuals, families, groups, organizations, communities, and populations. As an occupational therapy practitioner, you will continue to learn about person factors throughout your career. This knowledge will be important not only in your practice but in your personal life as well.

Chapter	Title	FAQ
14	*Person Factors: Psychological* (Brown, Stoffel)	• Why are personal narratives so important in gathering information about psychological factors? • How are intervention approaches that originated in psychology used to support occupational performance, participation, and well-being?
15	*Person Factors: Cognition* (Maeir, Rotenberg-Shpigelman)	• What is the role of different mental processes in everyday life and how do these processes interact to support performance? • What intervention approaches are used to restore cognitive factors and/or compensate for deficits as a means to enable participation?
16	*Person Factors: Sensory* (Carey)	• How do vision, audition, somatosensation, vestibular, olfactory, and gustatory senses support occupational performance? • What clinical conditions often have sensory impairments that limit occupational performance?
17	*Person Factors: Motor* (Dutton, Bass)	• What motor factors contribute to effective movement during occupational performance? • How do current intervention approaches use task performance to address motor impairments?
18	*Person Factors: Physiological* (Rogers)	• What aspects of physiological function support performance of daily occupations? • What limitations in physiological function should be considered in occupational therapy evaluations and interventions?
19	*Person Factors: Meaning, Sensemaking, and Spirituality* (Eakman)	• Why is meaning, sensemaking, and spirituality critical in supporting performance, participation, and well-being? • Why do client-centered approaches support development of meaning, sense-making, and spirituality?

Chapter 14

PERSON FACTORS
Psychological

Catana Brown, PhD, OTR/L, FAOTA and Virginia C. Stoffel, PhD, OT, BCMH, FAOTA

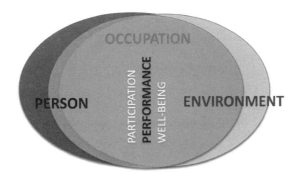

LEARNING OBJECTIVES

- Identify and define the primary psychological factors that influence performance and participation.
- Describe how strengths/affordances as well as constraints/barriers in psychological factors may affect a person's performance, participation, and well-being.
- Identify major health conditions or disabilities in which psychological factors could influence performance, participation, and well-being.
- Demonstrate your understanding of psychological factors in occupational performance through structured observation and task analysis.
- Identify established assessments that are evidence-based and measure psychological capabilities and limitations related to occupational performance.
- Identify intervention principles to address psychological factors that promote occupational performance.
- Describe 3 to 5 intervention approaches that strengthen psychological factors to support performance, participation, and well-being.

- Recognize the complexity of how psychological factors interact with other person and environment factors to influence performance in everyday life.

KEY WORDS

- Affect
- Coping
- Emotional regulation
- Identity
- Life balance
- Mood
- Motivation
- Self-concept
- Self-efficacy
- Self-esteem
- Well-being

Christiansen CH, Baum CM, Bass JD, eds.
Occupational Therapy: Performance, Participation, and Well-Being, Fourth Edition (pp 217-232).
© 2015 SLACK Incorporated.

INTRODUCTION

The PEOP Model, as a transactive systems model, focuses on the person; their personal, family, and community context (environment); and the occupations they hold to be important as 3 relevant domains affecting the performance of their everyday occupations. As a model guiding occupational therapy practitioners, the PEOP approach is applied to working with persons, populations, and organizations using a client-centered approach so that the goals are actively driven by the client and ultimately meet what the client defines as important. Full participation (as defined by the client) in everyday life in communities of their choice is associated with health and well-being.[1] This chapter will primarily use the lens of persons and their life narratives, although these concepts can be applied to an aggregate understanding of populations and organizations.

Planning interventions that support performance, participation, and well-being are, at best, client-centered and begin with a clear understanding of the occupational history, needs, and preferences of the individual. Eliciting the perspectives of the client to gain their world view allows the occupational therapy practitioner to begin to build an understanding of the meanings associated with valued occupational roles, habits, and routines that are a part of the individual's everyday life activities. Having the person share stories about a typical day, a particularly important time where he or she felt challenged, a time where he or she felt most successful, and a description of what he or she hopes the future holds will uncover a personal framework of factors such as occupational identity, self-concept, self-efficacy, and coping strategies. Careful listening to personal narratives will also reveal aspects of the person's environment that support or impede their occupational performance and contribute to their sense of well-being.

This chapter will explore the psychological factors that impact occupational performance, participation, and well-being, including such concepts as identity, self-concept, self-efficacy, mood and emotion regulation, motivation, coping, and perspectives on the connections between these psychological factors and such outcomes as well-being and life balance. Several personal narratives will highlight the deeper understanding of psychological factors that will enable the occupational therapy practitioner to plan interventions that meet the needs, goals, level of participation, and well-being as defined by the client. Assessment tools addressing psychological factors that might promote or limit occupational performance, typically self-report and observation, will be reviewed. Intervention principles and approaches will be described to illustrate how they can be effectively used to enable participation and achievement of the client-determined outcomes. Interventions at the person level and the environment level will be reviewed as they impact the person's participation in their meaningful life routines. This chapter will close with an exploration of how participation results in significant health and well-being outcomes, as well as life balance.

NARRATIVE AND BACKGROUND LITERATURE

When I think about my life after my aortic dissection and stroke, I try to focus on what I can do and how important my family, grandchildren, and friends are instead of feeling sorry for myself. Although I landed my dream job just a year before, one that I no longer can function in, I remind myself that I am lucky to be alive and take each day, one at a time, to cherish and find meaning in helping others.

    JJ, age 59

I found out about my breast cancer 4 years ago and I decided that I would aggressively pursue any cancer treatment that would allow me more time with my husband, children, and grandchildren. I continue to work in my greenhouse with my husband and 2 children, make beautiful floral arrangements for weddings, raise our 6 grandkids who come to the greenhouse each day, and make time for trips to warm and relaxing places that I enjoy with my husband. Although some days are emotional roller coasters, I cope with my feelings by working in the greenhouse, cooking meals, and sewing beautiful outfits that my granddaughters wear at the holidays. My greenhouse customers have gotten used to seeing me with and without hair… pink has become my favorite color for jewelry and clothes… I am a cancer survivor!

    ES, age 55

Recovery from alcohol and drugs is something that I am working on, with the help of my parents and occupational therapist, each day. Although there are times that I wonder if I really can make it through the day without succumbing to my cravings for almost anything that changes my feelings, I am finally getting a sense that I really do have the skills to make it in life without drugs. My girlfriend and I actually are finding ways to have fun without using, and I am finally doing better in school. I am still working on my perfectionism that affects my schoolwork (I don't turn in papers unless I feel they are perfect), my art (I keep working on things far longer than needed as I'm never sure when I'm done), and my guitar playing, but I think that I can learn how to manage these down the road.

    MP, age 17

As you read the personal narratives, consider the people, their environments, and the occupations in which they engage. Identify issues around psychological factors, such as coping with the loss of a treasured job; finding meaning and motivation in relationships; gaining a positive sense of self by focusing on what one can do (vs what one can no longer do); discovering a new identity; and gaining a sense that one can cope, change, and find new ways to be balanced in life. Be aware that by engaging clients in sharing personal narratives, you will be far more able to construct meaningful and realistic intervention plans based on a clear understanding of the client's world, their current situation, the meaning they attribute to what they can do and are limited in doing, their choices and responsibilities, their attitudes and motivations toward their desired outcomes, and what it will take to get there, and ultimately how they define well-being and life balance as outcomes they hope to achieve.

The psychological and occupational therapy literature inform our understanding of the psychological factors that support occupational performance, participation, and well-being. These constructs are defined in Table 14-1, linked to examples extracted from the personal narratives.

Note that while psychological factors are the focus of this chapter, they are also affected by other factors intrinsic to the person, such as physiological, cognitive, sensory/perceptual, motor, and spiritual factors (all chapters in this book). For example, a person imbued with many physiological strengths combined with motor and cognitive strengths that allow the person to pursue their dream of being an elite athlete, gifted musician, or skilled dancer will impact such psychological factors as motivation toward excellence (based on self-efficacy and a record of achievement as an athlete, musician, or dancer); identity in their chosen occupations of athlete, musician, or dancer; and affect experienced while engaging in desired occupations (joy, frustration, flow). Well-being could also be defined differently by each, based on their self-expectations and expectations by others (coaches, teachers, fans, other experts). Spiritual factors might also interact to promote well-being, such as feeling like one is carrying out a life worth living, or may hinder well-being when feeling empty spiritually. Environmental aspects extrinsic to the person will also interact to support or inhibit occupational participation and performance, such as having access to a skilled coach; time to be able to participate; resources to access the equipment and technology needed to carry out the occupation; and social support offering encouragement, resilience, and assistance meeting basic human needs for food, water, and shelter wherever the practice and performance space for sports, concert, or recital is conducted.

ASSESSMENTS AND EVALUATIONS

The internal nature of psychological factors makes them difficult to observe. To gather information about identity, self-concept/efficacy, mood/emotion regulation, motivation, coping, and life balance, you typically need to rely on the perspective of the individual. Consequently, most measures of psychological factors use a self-report method. Because individuals usually want to present themselves in the best light possible, self-reports may be biased; however, evidence suggests that the unreliability of self-reports has been overstated.[14,15] In addition, there are methods that an occupational therapy practitioner can use to increase the reliability of self-report, such as:

- Making sure the respondent understands the questions
- Asking the questions in such a way that memory is less likely to be a problem (for example, a respondent will be more accurate in reporting how many times he or she felt depressed in the past month as opposed to how many times he or she felt depressed in the past year)
- Insuring the confidentiality of the response so that others (eg, family members, employers) do not have access to the responses
- Establishing rapport and developing a partnership with the individual and informing him or her that honest responses will be useful in the development of an effective intervention plan

There are many standardized measures available for measuring psychological factors. Table 14-2 provides examples of measures an occupational therapy practitioner may use for assessing each of the psychological factors. Note that several of the measures assess more than one psychological factor. The occupational therapy practitioner has the tool of an *occupational profile* that adds an important dimension to how the psychological issue is impacting the person's everyday life.

INTERVENTIONS

When providing interventions to enhance psychological factors, it is difficult to separate the individual factors because they overlap. Interventions that address one aspect of psychological functioning are likely to have positive benefits for multiple areas. For example, an increase in self-efficacy is likely to be motivating, improve emotion regulation, and enhance overall well-being. Therefore, interventions will not focus on individual psychological factors, but are categorized only at the level of person, environment, and occupation approaches (Table 14-3).

Intervention at the Person Level

Interventions at the person level are directed at enhancing specific psychological factors. Several approaches that

Table 14-1. *Glossary of Terms Associated With Psychological Factors*

Term	Definition	Examples from Personal Narratives
Psychological Factors		
Identity	"A composite definition of the self and includes an interpersonal aspect… an aspect of possibility or potential (who we might become), and a values aspect (that suggests importance and provides a stable basis for choices and decisions)…Identity can be viewed as the superordinate view of ourselves that includes both self-esteem and self-concept, but also importantly reflects and is influenced by the larger social world in which we find ourselves."[2(pp548-549)]	• JJ: "I focus on what I can do…and find meaning in helping others." JJ's identity significantly changed because of his aortic dissection and stroke from having his "dream job" to reminding himself of his important family relationships and finding new ways to help others. • ES: "I am a cancer survivor" is a clear part of her identity, in addition to being a wife, mother, grandmother, employer in her greenhouse, and pursuing her cooking and sewing occupations. She found a way to pursue those meaningful occupations while at the same time fitting in her active cancer treatment and recovery.
Self-concept/ self-esteem	Composite of beliefs and feelings about oneself, the evaluative component as positive or negative	• MP: "I am still working on my perfectionism, which affects my schoolwork (I don't turn in papers unless I feel they are perfect), my art (I keep working on things far longer than needed as I'm never sure when I'm done), and my guitar playing, but I think that I can learn how to manage these down the road." His self-concept is changing toward one that will support his ongoing recovery, and one that is growing based on his increased self-efficacy.
Self-efficacy	A primary driver impacting motivation based on a belief in one's capability[3]	
Affect	Display of a subjectively experienced feeling state (or the absence of such)	• JJ: "I try to focus on what I can do and how important my family, grandchildren, and friends are instead of feeling sorry for myself. Although I landed my dream job just a year before, one that I no longer can function in, I remind myself that I am lucky to be alive and take each day, one at a time, to cherish and find meaning in helping others." His affective response to his changed life narrative demonstrates effective emotional regulation after experiencing his significant life losses, reframing his focus on the positives central to his life. • MP: "Although there are times that I wonder if I really can make it through the day without succumbing to my cravings for almost anything that changes my feelings, I am finally getting a sense that I really do have the skills to make it in life without drugs. My girlfriend and I actually are finding ways to have fun without using, and I am finally doing better in school." MP used to seek out drugs to change his affective state and mood, and is now finding new ways to regulate his emotions while staying chemically free.
Mood	A pervasive and sustained emotion such as happiness, optimism, depression, anxiety, and hopefulness	
Emotional regulation	Actions or behaviors one can use to identify, manage, and express feelings while engaging in activities or interacting with others, including those that can be done before or after an activity occurs (such as reframing the meaning of an event or putting an event into perspective)[4,5]	

(continued)

Table 14-1 (continued).   *Glossary of Terms Associated With Psychological Factors*

Term	Definition	Examples from Personal Narratives
Motivation	Can be understood as a continuum that guides engagement in occupations, from exploration to competency, and ultimately seeks achievement with new challenges[6]; important factor in the change process[7]	• JJ: "I remind myself that I am lucky to be alive and take each day, one at a time, to cherish and find meaning in helping others." JJ has newfound areas that he finds motivating: helping others who may not be aware of their own medical family history to uncovering possible predispositions to negative health events, like his experience with aortic dissection and stroke. • MP: "Recovery from alcohol and drugs is something that I am working on, with the help of my parents and occupational therapist, each day." MP has found that he needs others as active supports to help keep his motivation to change high on his list of daily routines.
Coping	A process that includes adjustment to the stressful demands and opportunities presented in everyday life[8]	• ES: "Although some days are emotional roller coasters, I cope with my feelings by working in the greenhouse, cooking meals, and sewing beautiful outfits that my granddaughters wear at the holidays. My greenhouse customers have gotten used to seeing me with and without hair…pink has become my favorite color for jewelry and clothes…I am a cancer survivor!" ES demonstrates great resilience in coping with the changes in her feelings, her appearance, and her overall role performance as a cancer survivor, wife, mother, grandmother, and greenhouse owner.

Outcomes From Psychological Factors

Term	Definition	Examples from Personal Narratives
Well-being	An outcome associated with self-acceptance, positive relationships, autonomy for self-regulation and being true to one's identity, environmental mastery, purpose in life and personal growth,[9,10] as well as other psychological states (such as curiosity; hardiness; sense of coherence; vitality; commitment, happiness; and low level of anger, fear, and depression)[11]	• JJ: His narrative is one that suggests that he is currently experiencing aspects of well-being, such as self-acceptance, positive relationships, commitment, and purpose in life—all important aspects of well-being. • ES: Her narrative demonstrates well-being in terms of her overall level of engagement in everyday life, self-acceptance, hardiness, and purpose in life. She has clarity of thinking about how she hopes to live life to its fullest for as long as she has her health. • MP: His narrative demonstrates that he seems on a road that could lead to his well-being. He is working on building a sense of self-acceptance and positive relationships. As a 17-year-old, he is clearly working on his autonomy and discovering his true identity.
Life balance	An outcome associated with "a satisfying pattern of daily activity that is healthful, meaningful, and sustainable to an individual within the context of his or her current life circumstances,"[12(p11)] that meets one's needs of health, relationships, challenges, and identity with the skills to "organize time and energy in ways that enable them to meet important personal goals and renewal"[13]	• JJ: Although his narrative does not contain enough details to definitively confirm life balance, he seems satisfied with how he spends his time and seems to meet his needs related to his health, relationships, challenges and identity. As this is an outcome that is being defined by current researchers, we can look to future work that will better define outcome measures of life balance.

Table 14-2. *Assessments of Psychological Factors*

Assessments	Area of Function	Description of the Measure
Occupational Performance History Interview—II[16]	Identity, self-concept, and self-efficacy	Suggested interview questions organized in areas of occupational roles, daily routine, occupational behavior settings, activity/occupation choices, and critical life events—includes qualitative and quantitative data
Multidimensional Health Locus of Control Scale[17]		Evaluates perceived self-efficacy or locus of control over one's own health
Self-Efficacy Gauge[18]		Measures confidence with which people with occupational performance impairments believe they carry out self-care, productivity, and leisure activities
Beck Depression Inventory[19]	Mood and emotion regulation	Self-reported depression scale
Patient Health Questionnaire—9 (PHQ-9)[20]		Brief screening of depression
Center for Epidemiological Studies—Depression Scale (CES-D)[21]		Assesses the severity of symptoms of depression
Spielberger State—Trait Anxiety Inventory for Adults[22]		Measures current feelings of anxiety (state) as well as long-standing anxiety
Difficulties in Emotional Regulation Scale[23]		Includes items examining acceptance of negative emotions, engagement in goal-directed behavior, controlling impulsive behavior, emotion regulation strategies, emotional awareness, and emotional clarity
University of Rhode Island Change Assessment[24]	Motivation	Uses the transtheoretical model to assess an individual's readiness to change
Volitional Questionnaire[25] and Pediatric Volitional Questionnaire[26]		An observational assessment rates the individual in terms of volitional development in the stages of exploration, competency, and achievement. Includes an assessment of the environment's effect on motivation
Ways of Coping Questionnaire[27]	Coping	Determines most commonly used coping processes: confrontive, distancing, self-controlling, seeking social support, accepting responsibility, escape-avoidance, planful problem solving, positive reappraisal
Resilience Quotient[28]		Measures emotional regulation, impulse control, optimism, causal analysis, empathy, self-efficacy, and reaching out and provides on overall resilience quotient
Hope Scale[29]	Well-being and life balance	Assesses hope as goal-directed energy and planning to meet goals
Day Reconstruction Method[30]		Uses a diary that reports the individual's experiences during the day and associated emotions
Satisfaction with Life Scale[31]		Brief measure of overall life satisfaction
Kawa River Model Assessment[32]		Uses the metaphor of life as a river and has individual depict current life circumstances including supports, difficulties, assets, and occupations

Table 14-3. *Intervention Table*

Interventions	Level	Examples
• Cognitive behavioral therapy • Dialectical behavior therapy • Motivational interviewing	Person	• Keeping a diary of positive experiences in the work place • Practice providing feedback to a co-worker in a manner that demonstrates control of one's emotions • Identifying personal values that are compromised during parenting due to drug use
• Occupations that provide mastery experiences • Occupations that enhance mood • Interventions to return to desired or discover new occupations to restore healthy identity	Occupation	• Use of graded activities as individual learns new job responsibilities • Adjusting daily routine to include more time for leisure pursuits • Using adaptive equipment to return to prominent role as meal preparer at home
• Support groups • Peer support services • Interventions to enhance social networks and increase social contact	Environment	• Meeting for lunch with other stroke survivors • Using a peer coach to encourage regular swimming • Joining a neighborhood book club after a recent relocation

originated in psychology for use in counseling (eg, cognitive behavioral therapy, dialectical behavior therapy, and motivational interviewing) all are strategies that the occupational therapy practitioner uses to enable the skills for daily life. When occupational therapy practitioners use these approaches, they are implemented with an occupational performance perspective. In other words, psychological skills are addressed within the context of everyday life with the goal of promoting satisfying and successful occupational performance.

CBT is based on the theory that distortions in thinking can lead to unpleasant moods and maladaptive behaviors.[33] For example, an individual that sees him or herself as incompetent may become anxious during occupational performance and may avoid certain situations to prevent those feelings. The first step in CBT involves identifying the core cognitive distortions used by the person. Occupational therapy practitioners have the opportunity to observe faulty thinking as it occurs in everyday life. For example, the person with a spinal cord injury in the rehabilitation hospital may overgeneralize a challenging day in therapy by commenting, "I'm not getting any better. I might as well give up." Another occupational therapy practitioner might observe a child in school jumping to the conclusion that no one will pick him or her for a team because he or she has a disability. After identifying and pointing out the distortion, the occupational therapy prac-

titioner collaborates with the person to challenge distorted thinking by gathering evidence to the contrary, and helps the person develop strategies to enable successful performance of the activity. For example, in the first scenario, the practitioner might point out that the individual with a spinal cord injury is now able to eat independently, which was not true a few weeks earlier, and that similar gains can be expected. In the second case, the practitioner might ask the child to make a list of situations in which she was included in team or group activities.

Dialectical behavior therapy (DBT) was initially developed as a treatment for individuals with borderline personality disorder.[34] More recently, DBT has been applied to other psychiatric conditions, and components of the approach are used more broadly to address psychological factors, particularly *emotion dysregulation*. DBT typically includes both individual and group formats. It is the group component, with a focus on self-management and skills training, that is most suitable for occupational therapy practice.[35] The skills and strategies that are taught include core mindfulness, interpersonal effectiveness, emotion regulation, and distress tolerance and learning to plan and carryout strategies that will meet their goals. Occupational therapy practitioners can contribute their unique expertise to DBT skills training by embedding the training within the real-life occupations of the group participants. For example, instead of lecturing on the topic of attending to positive experiences, the group might participate in pleasant activities of their choosing and practice mindfulness and share their strategies during the event. For example, the group may find that many enjoy spending time outside, so the group goes for a walk at a park and are encouraged to pay attention to the present and focus on positive feelings while walking.

Motivational interviewing (MI) is a skilled method of communication that is used to elicit change by resolving ambivalence about that change.[36] Originally developed to address addictions, it is now widely employed in rehabilitation. MI is applicable to virtually all occupational therapy practice areas, because behavioral change is often a component of the occupational therapy process (see the occupational therapy process at the person, organization, and population levels in Chapter 5). Characteristics of MI include collaboration instead of confrontation, an evocative approach to having the person identify his or her own reasons for change, and an appreciation for the person's autonomy to make his or her own decisions. Occupational therapy practitioners might use motivational interviewing for a client that needs to change spending habits to avoid eviction, a child that is not turning in classroom assignments, or a client in a rehabilitation setting that is refusing therapy. By knowing the person's activity profile, it would be possible to find out what they did or wished they could do.

Intervention at the Occupation Level

When people engage in occupations, the resulting experience is personal evoking thoughts, such as, "This is boring," "This makes me happy," "I'm really good at this," or maybe even "I'll never do this again." Occupational therapy practitioners use occupations as a means to enhance psychological factors. This is achieved by utilizing a favorable person-occupation match to advance positive outcomes. Theory can be useful in helping occupational therapy practitioners make the best person-occupation match.

Many people seen in occupational therapy experience multiple failures in occupational performance as they adjust to a new disability, live with a chronic condition, or find themselves challenged by difficult life circumstances. According to Bandura's[3] Self-Efficacy Theory, failure contributes to a negative sense of self while mastery is the strongest and most enduring source of self-efficacy. Similarly, the MOHO[37] suggests that when the components of the volitional subsystem are maximized (interests, values, and personal causation), occupational performance will be enhanced. The PEOP Model guides the importance of the person-environment fit that enables the person to do what he or she needs to do to support their performance, participation, and well-being. Occupational

therapy intervention promotes a positive self-concept and a belief in one's own ability by creating opportunities for mastery during occupational performance. For example, an occupational therapy practitioner working with a person adjusting to a stroke who is also a proficient cook can set up a situation where the stroke survivor works on upper extremity function, while teaching the practitioner and other interested clients how to prepare a favorite dessert. Or, in a school setting, the occupational therapy practitioner could help the teacher create assignments that take advantage of an autistic child's deep knowledge of geology.

Occupations can also be used to help regulate emotions. What we do influences how we feel. Csikszentmihalyi[38] coined the term *flow* to refer to the optimal experience of losing oneself in an intensely rewarding activity. A person is most likely to experience flow when the activity provides the ideal match of challenge and skill (Figure 14-1). Although this optimal experience may only occur infrequently, people can improve their mood by increasing their participation in activities with a high or moderate challenge, consistent with the individual's skill level. Conversely, the individual should avoid activities where the challenge is too much, can result in anxiety, or where the challenge is too little and the individual is bored. One way to identify mood-enhancing activities is to keep a mood diary that tracks daily activities along with a mood rating. Using the diary, one can identify those activities associated with a positive mood and those associated with a negative mood and modify one's day accordingly. Figure 14-1 can be a helpful tool in discussing activity choices and how they make the person feel, especially when the person is trying to develop more healthy activity choices for health reasons.

In his Eleanor Clark Slagle lecture, Christiansen[2] discussed the link between occupation and identity. Our impression of who we are is created from an interpretation of what we do as influenced by the social world. Identity then provides coherence and meaning for everyday life. People with disabilities may find their identity disrupted when they can no longer engage in desired occupations at their previous level of competence. Occupational therapy practitioners can work to restore a healthy identity by providing interventions that allow people to return to desired occupations or to discover new occupations that create a meaningful life.

Environmental Interventions

Interventions to address psychological factors may also target the environment, particularly the social environment. Constructive interaction and connection with others are essential to a positive self-concept and are important in promoting other psychological factors, such as coping and motivation. Generally speaking, social contact is protective

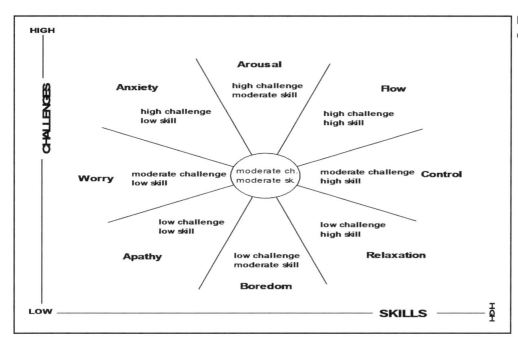

Figure 14-1. Flow in daily life: quality of life.

of psychological factors. For example, one study found that people who spend less time with those they are close to tend to be more depressed.[39] In addition, people with disabilities often have smaller social networks; the acquisition of a disability, such as a stroke, can cause people to lose friends.[40]

One example of an intervention directed at the social environment is the *support group*. Individuals with disabilities or persons dealing with difficult life circumstances may find that the people they typically turn to for support are not able to relate to their situation. A support group provides an opportunity for people with similar life experiences to relate to one another. For example, occupational therapy practitioner Sharon Schwartzberg[41] describes a support group for people with brain injury that she co-facilitated. This particular group helped participants legitimize what is often felt to be a hidden disability while providing validation, a place to laugh, grieve, and opportunities to be oneself. In another program, an occupational therapy practitioner facilitated the development of a peer-driven community within a program for individuals with substance abuse and chronic homelessness.[42] The occupational therapy practitioner provided group leaders with training in organizational leadership, group communication, and group facilitation. The program promoted participation and support among the group members. A specific type of support group for people with serious mental illness and their families, called *psychoeducation,* can reduce relapse and rehospitalization and improve family burden and relationships.[43] Typically family members and individuals with mental illness meet in separate groups. Effective psychoeducation programs include illness educa-

tion, crisis intervention, emotional support, and training in managing family problems.

Peer support is not only available in support groups, but may be provided in other formats such as 1:1 support, peer run agencies, or even on-line services. Peers can play a significant role in illness self-management (see Chapter 27). Peers with similar lived experiences may be useful in sharing both knowledge and coping strategies. In addition, peers provide models and success stories that can serve as powerful motivators for change.

The use of peers as service providers is becoming common in many programs for people with psychiatric disabilities. For example, peers have been used to provide wellness coaching to individuals with serious mental illness that are interested in addressing health and wellness concerns.[44] Some agencies are run primarily or exclusively by individuals who also experience a disability. These programs, which may be referred to as consumer-operated services, typically offer socialization, education, and opportunities to participate in meaningful occupations.[44] A primary principle of consumer-operated services is that both the helper and helpee receive benefits from the relationship. One study compared consumer-operated services utilized in combination with traditional community mental health agency services to community mental health services provided alone,[45] and found that the combined services resulted in greater empowerment, self-efficacy, and social integration.

Occupational therapy practitioners can assume several roles in promoting social support. Occupational therapy practitioners may make referrals to support groups or to consumer-operated programs. They may co-facilitate groups or provide training to peers that will serve as group leaders or staff at agencies. Occupational therapy practitioners may look within an individual's existing social network and provide education or training to friends and family to maintain positive relationships. In addition, the importance of maintaining social contact can be emphasized when working with clients, and occupational therapy practitioners can help the client figure out ways to establish or maintain positive and regular social contact.

OUTCOMES

By addressing psychological factors and recognizing the impact they have on the goals, hopes, and desires of the person engaged in the occupational therapy process, outcomes are expected to move the person toward a state of well-being and life balance (Table 14-4). Although there are many external factors that impact whether a person is able to achieve a stable state of well-being and life balance, active engagement in everyday occupations that a person wants and needs to do will likely enhance a person's state of health, well-being, and life balance. The goal-setting process begins by eliciting the person's narrative and helping them to identify the important and meaningful changes they hope to attain. Having a clear image of what the person hopes to attain, a clear image of their natural occupational environments, and a clear image of their opportunities and challenges will allow the occupational therapy practitioner to explore with the client which, if any, psychological factors might impinge or enhance their goals. For example, an awareness of how one's mood and emotional regulation strategies might help meet key goals in returning to active family and work roles after a traumatic injury may increase the likeliness that such a goal may be reached. Psychological factors, such as motivation and strong coping skills, may allow an individual to achieve far more than what is perceived by others to be possible. The occupational therapy practitioner who serves by enhancing the sense of hopefulness and realistic efficacy, and clarifying the meaningfulness of goals, is one who can facilitate participation and well-being, and move the person toward finding ways to balance their lifestyle to support optimum health. Table 14-5 lists resources practitioner can use to help their clients, and additionally suggests journals that practitioners can use to keep abreast of changes in this area.

SUMMARY

Psychological factors enhance a person's ability to reengage in everyday life, participate more fully in meaningful life roles, and move a person toward well-being and life balance. Using a PEOP approach to goal setting and intervention planning; addressing motivation, identity, coping, and emotional regulation so that the person can use those strategies to build a lifestyle balanced across important life roles; sleep and rest; and engendering a sense of hopefulness about oneself will create the greatest likelihood for well-being.

Table 14-4. Psychological Factors Evidence Table

Study and Reference	Aim of Study	Methods	Participants	Results and Outcome(s)	Conclusion(s) and Implications	Level or Type of Evidence	Statistical Probability or Effect Size
Performance in Leisure Time Physical Activities and Self-Efficacy in Women with Rheumatoid Arthritis[46]	To examine leisure-time physical activities (LPTA) and their association with self-efficacy in females with rheumatoid arthritis	Cross-sectional and retrospective design using self-reported performance in LTPAs was measured by the Interest Checklist and efficacy beliefs by using the Arthritis Self-Efficacy Scales.	238 females with a diagnosis of rheumatoid arthritis for more than 2 years between the ages of 20 and 79, treated in Norway	Active individuals performed vigorous activities more often, had higher education, worked more, reported better function, had higher self-efficacy, and less joint pain and fatigue	Partaking in a high amount of LTPAs was related to less fatigue and higher efficacy beliefs.	Level IV: Descriptive study examining analysis of outcomes	Multivariate analyses showed high LTPA independently related to less fatigue (OR=0.98; $P=.004$); positive self-efficacy in coping with RA (OR=1.03; $P=.0015$), and higher employment level (OR=.42; $P=.039$)
Wellness Coaching: A New Role for Peers[44]	To define a framework for a peer wellness coach role in meeting the needs of persons with serious mental illness	Review of the literature and collective experiences by the authors in this new practice approach, addressing a collaborative approach to coping with everyday health needs	A peer wellness coaching curriculum developed, 33 peer recovery specialists completed it	Addresses issues such as metabolic syndrome, nutrition, smoking cessation, lifestyle factors, exercise, oral health	Ongoing development of the role and curriculum will be studied, as well as impact of the peer wellness coaching programs	Level V: Expert opinion and literature review	NA
Helping Factors in a Peer-Developed Support Group for Persons With Head Injury: Part 1: Participant Observer Perspective[41]	Ethnographic study of a peer-developed support group for persons with head injury as to processes of self-help and peer-group experiences	Empirical and theoretically grounded, used participant observation, audiotapes, and videotapes of groups carried out over a 16-month period	13 group members with a head injury participated in the support group over a 16-month period	Factors were qualitatively analyzed as to the contribution to a positive group experience, such as believing and feeling part of a group who shares a common problem; offer input validating the effect of living with a brain injury	Legitimization for the participants led to accepting the head injury as real (related to psychological factor of self-concept)	Level V: Ethnographic qualitative analysis	NA

(continued)

Table 14-4 (continued).   *Psychological Factors Evidence Table*

Study and Reference	Aim of Study	Methods	Participants	Results and Outcome(s)	Conclusion(s) and Implications	Level or Type of Evidence	Statistical Probability or Effect Size
Level of Motivation in Mastering Challenging Tasks in Children With Cerebral Palsy[47]	To describe and identify factors associated with motivation in children with cerebral palsy (CP)	Cross-sectional study using the Leiter Intelligence Test, Gross Motor Function Measure, and Vineland Adaptive Behavior Scale with the children; Dimensions of Mastery Questionnaire with parent	Parents of 74 children with CP (46 males, 28 females (mean age 9 years 2 months; range 5 years 10 months to 12 years 11 months) with most common diagnoses of spastic hemiplegia and quadriplegia (23 each) and 14 with diplegia	Related to motivation, highest scores were for the dimensions of mastery, pleasure, and social persistence, and lowest for persistence with motor or cognitive tasks. Higher IQ ($r = .41$), better motor ability ($r = .43$), and fewer limitations in self-care, communication, and socialization ($r = .44$-$.53$) were positively associated with motivation total score. Negative impact of the child's disability was associated with lower motivation	Fewer activity limitations, behavioral problems and reduced family burden were associated with higher motivation. Should low motivation exist, the child's functional potential and overall effectiveness of the interventions might be compromised. Practitioners should use strategies that enhance mastery, motivation, and provide the just right challenge to empower the child, structure the environment, connect with peers, and ensure initial successes	Level IV: Cross-sectional descriptive study	

(continued)

Table 14-4 (continued).   Psychological Factors Evidence Table

Study and Reference	Aim of Study	Methods	Participants	Results and Outcome(s)	Conclusion(s) and Implications	Level or Type of Evidence	Statistical Probability or Effect Size
Level of Motivation in Mastering Challenging Tasks in Children With Cerebral Palsy[47]	To describe and identify factors associated with motivation in children with cerebral palsy (CP)	Cross-sectional study using the Leiter Intelligence Test, Gross Motor Function Measure, and Vineland Adaptive Behavior Scale with the children; Dimensions of Mastery Questionnaire with parent	Parents of 74 children with CP (46 males, 28 females [mean age 9 years 2 months; range 5 years 10 months to 12 years 11 months] with most common diagnoses of spastic hemiplegia and quad-riplegia (23 each) and 14 with diplegia	Related to motivation, highest scores were for the dimensions of mastery, pleasure, and social persistence, and lowest for persistence with motor or cognitive tasks. Higher IQ ($r = .41$), better motor ability ($r = .43$), and fewer limitations in self-care, communication, and socialization ($r = .44-.53$) were positively associated with motivation total score. Negative impact of the child's disability was associated with lower motivation	Fewer activity limitations, behavioral problems and reduced family burden were associated with higher motivation. Should low motivation exist, the child's functional potential and overall effectiveness of the interventions might be compromised. Practitioners should use strategies that enhance mastery, motivation, and provide the just right challenge to empower the child, structure the environment, connect with peers, and ensure initial successes	Level IV: Cross-sectional descriptive study	

(continued)

Table 14-4 (continued).   Psychological Factors Evidence Table

Study and Reference	Aim of Study	Methods	Participants	Results and Outcome(s)	Conclusion(s) and Implications	Level or Type of Evidence	Statistical Probability or Effect Size
The 12-Month Effects of Early Motivational Interviewing After Acute Stroke: A RCT[48]	To determine if motivational interviewing can improve mood after a stroke.	RCT measuring mood with the General Health Questionnaire, motivational interviewing was compared to usual care 12 months post-stroke. Intervention group received up to 4 sessions of MI, focused on adjustment to stroke and goals for recovery reinforcing optimism and self-efficacy	394 individuals admitted consecutively to the stroke unit of a hospital	48% of participants in the intervention group had normal mood compared to 37.7% in the control group; there was also a reduction in mortality, with a mortality rate of 6.5% in the intervention group compared to 12.8% in the control group	Motivational interviewing can improve mood and reduce mortality among individuals with stroke	Level I: RCT	For mood P=.02, OR=1.66, for mortality P=.035, OR=2.14.
Mindfulness Meditation for the Treatment of Chronic Low Back Pain in Older Adults: A Randomized Controlled Pilot Study[49]	A pilot study to examine the efficacy of mindfulness meditation (an approach associated with emotion regulation) on chronic low back pain	RCT of individuals receiving mindfulness meditation, compared to a wait list control group	37 community dwelling older adults with chronic low back pain	Individuals receiving mindfulness meditation experienced significant improvement when compared to the control group in the areas of physical function and activities engagement	Mindfulness meditation may reduce chronic pain in older adults	Level I: RCT	For activities engagement P=.004, for physical function P=.03

Table 14-5. *Organizations and Journals That Focus on Psychological Factors for Performance*

Organization or Journal	Description	Web Address
American Psychological Association	Scientific and professional organization representing psychology in the United States. Seeks to advance the creation, communication, and application of psychological knowledge to benefit society and improve people's lives.	http://www.apa.org
Society for Personality and Social Psychology	Society promotes scientific research in personality and social psychology through the publication of scientific journals, an annual conference, and sponsoring activities that foster professional development among students and faculty.	http://www.spsp.org
National Institute of Mental Health	Conducts and supports research on mental disorders and the underlying basic science of brain and behavior. Supports the training of more than 1000 scientists each year to carry out basic and clinical mental health research.	http://www.nimh.nih.gov/index.shtml
PsycTESTS	A research database that provides access to psychological tests, measures, scales, surveys, and other assessments as well as descriptive information about the test and its development and administration.	http://www.apa.org/pubs/databases/psyctests/index.aspx
National Alliance on Mental Illness (NAMI)	Grassroots mental health organization in the United States. Advocates for access to services and treatment, supports and conducts research, and is committed to educating and raising awareness in the community regarding mental illness.	http://www.nami.org/
e-Source: Behavioral and Social Science Research	Contributions from international experts on methodological questions of behavioral and social science research.	http://www.esourceresearch.org/
Routledge Mental Health	Provides resources on the broad topics related to mental health.	http://www.routledge-mentalhealth.com/
Journal of Personality and Social Psychology	Publishes papers in areas of personality and social psychology regarding attitudes and social cognition, interpersonal relations and group processes, and personality processes and individual differences.	http://www.apa.org/pubs/journals/psp/index.aspx
Social Behavior and Personality: An International Journal	Publishes papers on all aspects of social, personality, and developmental psychology.	http://www.sbp-journal.com/index.php/sbp
American Journal of Psychology	Explores the science of the mind and behavior; publishing reports of original research in experimental psychology, theoretical presentations, combined theoretical and experimental analyses, historical commentaries, and in-depth reviews of significant books.	http://www.press.uillinois.edu/journals/ajp.html

REFERENCES

1. Christiansen C, Baum, MC, Bass, JD. The Person-Environment-Occupational Performance (PEOP) Model. In: Christiansen CH, Baum CM, Bass JD, eds. *Occupational Therapy: Performance, Participation, and Well-Being.* 4th ed. Thorofare: SLACK Incorporated; 2015.

2. Christiansen CH. Defining lives: occupation as identity: an essay on competence, coherence & the creation of meaning, 1999 Eleanor Clark Slagle lecture. *Am J Occup Ther.* 1999;53:547-558.

3. Bandura A. Self-efficacy: toward a unifying theory of behavioral change. In: Baumeister RF, ed. *The Self in Social Psychology.* New York, NY: Psychology Press; 1999:285-298.

4. AOTA. Occupational therapy practice framework: domain and process. 2nd ed. *Am J Occup Ther.* 2008;62:625-683.

5. Scheinholz, M. Emotion regulation. In Brown C, Stoffel VC, eds. *Occupational Therapy in Mental Health: A Vision for Participation.* Philadelphia, PA: FA Davis, Inc; 2011:345-357.

6. de lasHeras CG, Llerena V, Kielhofner G. *The Remotivation Process, Version 1.0.* Chicago, IL: Model of Human Occupation Clearinghouse; 2003.

7. Miller WR, Rollnick S. *Motivational Interviewing: Preparing People for Change.* 2nd ed. New York, NY: Guilford Press; 2002.

8. Haertl K, Christiansen C. Coping skills. In: Brown C, Stoffel VC, eds. *Occupational Therapy in Mental Health: A Vision for Participation.* Philadelphia, PA: FA Davis, Inc; 2011:313-329.

9. Ryff CD, Singer, B. The contours of positive human health. *Psych Inq.* 1998;9:1-28.

10. Deci EL, Ryan RM. The "what" and "why" of goal pursuits: human needs and the self-determination of behavior. *Psych Inq.* 2000;11:227-268.

11. Diener E, Chan MY. Happy people live longer: subjective being contributes to health and longevity. *App Psych: Health and Well-Being.* 2011;3(1):1-43.

12. Matuska KM, Christiansen CH. A proposed model of lifestyle balance. *J Occ Sci.* 2008;15(1):9-19.

13. Matuska K. Description and development of the Life Balance Inventory. *OTJR.* 2012;32(1):220.

14. Brener ND, Billy JOG, Grady WR. Assessment of factors affecting the validity of self-reported health-risk behavior among adolescents: evidence from the scientific literature. *J Adol Health.* 2003;33:436-457.

15. Chan D. So why ask me? Are self report data really that bad? In: Lance CE, Vandenberg RJ, eds. *Statistical & Methodological Myths and Urban Legends: Doctrine, Verity & Fable in the Organizational and Social Sciences.* New York, NY: Routledge; 2009:309-335.

16. Kielhofner G, Mallinson T, Crawford C, Nowak M, Rigby M, Henry A. *User's Manual for the Occupational Performance History Interview—II (OPHI-II).* Chicago, IL: Model of Human Occupation Clearinghouse, University of Illinois; 2004.

17. Wallston KA. *Multidimensional health locus of control scale.* www.vanderbilt.edu/nursing/kwallston/mhlcscales.htm. Accessed June 14, 2013.

18. Gage M, Noh S, Polatajko HJ, Kaspar V. Measuring perceived self-efficacy in occupational therapy. *Am J Occup Ther.* 1994;48:783-790.

19. Beck AT, Steer RA, Brown GK. *Beck Depression Inventory – II.* San Antonio, TX: Pearson Education; 1996.

20. Kroenke K, Spitzer R, Williams W. The PHQ-9: validity of a brief depression severity measure. *J Gen Int Med.* 2001;16:606-616.

21. Radloff LS. The CES-D Scale: a self reported depression scale for research in the general population. *Appl Psychol Measurement.* 1977;1:385-4-1

22. Spielberger CD. *State-Trait Anxiety Inventory for Adults.* Menlo Park, CA: Mind Garden Inc; 1982.

23. Gratz KL, Roemer L. Multidimensional assessment of emotion regulation and dysregulation: development, factor structure and initial validation of the Difficulties with Emotion Regulation Scale. *J Psychopathol Behav Assess.* 2004;41-54.

24. McConnaughy EA, Prochaska JO, Velicer WF. Stages of change in psychotherapy: measurement and sample profiles. *Psychother: Theory, Res Prac.* 1983;20:368-375.

25. Chern J, Kielhofner G, de lasHeras C, Magalhaes L. The Volitional Questionnaire: psychometric development and practical use. *Am J Occup Ther.* 1996;50:516-525.

26. Andersen S, Kielhofner G, Lai JS. An examination of the measurement properties of the Pediatric Volitional Questionnaire. *Phys Occup Ther Ped.* 2005;25:39-57.

27. Folkman S, Lazarus RS. *Ways of Coping Questionnaire.* Menlo Park, CA: Mind Garden, Inc; 1988.

28. Reivich K, Shatte A. *The Resilience Factor: 7 Essential Skills for Overcoming Life's Inevitable Obstacles.* New York, NY: Broadway Books; 2002.

29. Snyder CR, Harris C, Anderson JR, et al. The will and the ways: development and validation of an individual difference measure of hope. *J Pers Soc Psychology.* 1991;60:570-585.

30. Kahneman D, Krueger AB. Developments in the measurement of subjective well-being. *J Economic Persp.* 2006;20:3-24.

31. Diener E, Emmons RA, Larson RJ, Griffin S. The satisfaction with life scale. *J Pers Assess.* 1984;49:71-75.

32. Iwama MK. *The Kawa Model: Culturally Relevant Occupational Therapy.* Philadelphia, PA: Elsevier; 2006.

33. Beck JS. *Cognitive Behavior Therapy: Basics and Beyond.* 2nd ed. New York, NY: Guilford Press; 2011.

34. Linehan MM. *Skills Training Manual for Treating Borderline Personality Disorder.* New York, NY: The Guilford Press; 1993.

35. Linehan MM. *Cognitive Behavioral Treatment for Borderline Personality Disorder.* New York, NY: The Guilford Press; 1993.

36. Miller WR, Rollnick S. Ten things that motivational interviewing is not. *Beh Cog Ther.* 2009;37:129-140.

37. Kielhofner G. *Model of Human Occupation: Theory and Application.* 4th ed. Baltimore, MD: Lippincott Williams & Wilkins; 2008.

38. Csikszentmihalyi M. *Beyond Boredom and Anxiety: Experiencing Flow in Work and Play.* San Francisco, CA: Jossey-Bass; 2000.

39. Brown JH, Strauman T, Barrantes VN, Silvia PJ, Kwapil, TR. An experience sampling study of depressive symptoms and their social context. *J Nerv Ment Dis.* 2011;199:403-409.

40. Northcott S, Hilari K. Why do people lose their friends after stroke? *Int J Language Communication Dis.* 2011;46:524-534.

41. Schwartzberg SL. Helping factors in a peer-developed support group for persons with head injury: part 1: participant observer perspective. *Am J Occup Ther.* 1994;48:297-304.

42. Boisvert RA, Martin LM, Grosek M, Clarie, AJ. Effectiveness of a peer-support community in addiction recovery: participation as intervention. *Occup Ther Int.* 2008;15:205-220.

43. Kreyenbuhl J, Buchanan RW, Dickerson FB, Dixon LB. The Schizophrenia Patient Outcomes Research Team (PORT): updated treatment recommendations 2009. *Schiz Bull.* 2009;36:94-103.

44. Swarbrick M, Murphy AA, Zechner M, Spagnolo AB, Gill KJ. Wellness coaching: a new role for peers. *Psych Rehabil J.* 2011;34:328-331.

45. Segal SP, Silverman CJ, Temkin TC. Self-help and community mental health agency outcomes: a recovery focused randomized controlled trial. *Psych Serv.* 2010;61:905-910.

46. Reinseth L, Uhlig T, Kjeken I, SveanKoksvik H, Skomsvoll JF, Espness GA. Performance in leisure time physical activities and self-efficacy in women with rheumatoid arthritis. *Scand J Occup Ther.* 2011;18:210-218.

47. Majnemer J, Shevell M, Law M, Poulin C, Rosenbaum P. Level of motivation in mastering challenging tasks in children with cerebral palsy. *Dev Med Child Neurol.* 2010;52:1120-1126.

48. Watkins CL, Wathan JV, Leathley MJ, et al. The 12-month effects of early motivational interviewing after acute stroke: a randomized controlled trial. *Stroke.* 2011;42:1956-1961.

49. Morone NE, Greco CM, Weiner DK. Mindfulness meditation for the treatment of chronic low back pain in older adults: a randomized controlled pilot study. *Pain.* 2008;134:310-319.

Chapter 15

PERSON FACTORS
Cognition

Adina Maeir, PhD, OT and Shlomit Rotenberg-Shpigelman, MSc, OT

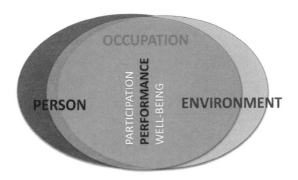

LEARNING OBJECTIVES

- Identify and define the primary cognitive factors that influence performance and participation.
- Describe how cognitive constraints and barriers may affect a person's performance, participation, and well-being.
- Identify major health conditions or disabilities in which cognitive factors could influence performance, participation, and well-being.
- Demonstrate your understanding of cognitive factors in occupational performance through structured observation and task analysis.
- Identify established assessments that are evidence-based and measure cognitive capabilities and limitations related to occupational performance.
- Identify intervention principles to address cognitive factors that are limiting occupational performance.

- Describe 3 to 4 intervention approaches that would address limitations associated with cognitive factors.
- Recognize the complexity of how cognitive factors interact with other person and environment factors as they relate to performance in everyday life.

KEY WORDS

- Attention
- Awareness/insight
- Cognitive-functional assessment
- Communication
- Executive function
- Learning
- Memory
- Social awareness (theory of mind)

Christiansen CH, Baum CM, Bass JD, eds.
Occupational Therapy: Performance, Participation, and Well-Being, Fourth Edition (pp 233-247).
© 2015 SLACK Incorporated.

INTRODUCTION

The PEOP Model provides a comprehensive understanding of interactions among person, environment, and occupation in order to explain the complexity of occupational performance. This chapter will focus on the cognitive factors in the person as they interact with the other factors in the model. Cognition is defined as the mental processes used to acquire, process, and use information to direct and adapt our actions toward desired goals. Cognitive processes include basic cognitive skills, such as attention and memory, as well as higher level cognitive functions including executive function and awareness that interplay to enable us to adapt to the world around us. Cognition is involved in all areas of everyday life, and as such has a significant influence on occupational performance.[1] Cognitive disabilities of varied types and severity are highly common among populations with health conditions that are in need of occupational therapy service. Cognitive factors are typically affected in developmental or acquired neurological and psychiatric health conditions across the lifespan. However, occupational therapy defines a unique intervention perspective and clinical reasoning that is guided by the implications of these health conditions and is not diagnostic specific. For example, an individual with a diagnosis of acquired mild Traumatic Brain Injury (mTBI) may be facing similar cognitive deficits to an individual with Attention Deficit Hyperactivity Disorder (ADHD). Furthermore, 2 individuals with the same diagnosis (eg, stroke) and the same cognitive profile may differ in their occupational performance. This unique occupational therapy perspective maintains that occupational performance cannot be explained by cognitive factors in isolation, but rather as they interact with the whole person in context. The following narratives will illustrate how cognitive factors may interact with occupational performance.

NARRATIVE

When I woke up after the accident, I was so grateful to be alive and so relieved that I was able to walk and go to the bathroom on my own. I was discharged from the hospital after 10 days and was thrilled to be home with my family. I tried to prepare one of my specialty dishes for the family in order to celebrate my return home. I was surprised and confused when it took me 5 hours to make my famous homemade pizza. I couldn't locate all the items in my own kitchen and couldn't follow the directions on the recipe. Later on, I felt extremely overwhelmed when driving downtown in a traffic jam. My wife noticed and suggested she take the wheel. When I went back to work everyone said I looked great, yet when

I tried to begin my work tasks I realized that something in me is different and I can't go back to doing things the way I used to. I have learned about these "invisible problems" that are called cognitive problems. I now understand how much I took cognition for granted when it was all there.

YT, age 35, suffered a head injury 6 months ago

I have always had a great memory, and I perceive memory and intelligence as the essence of a persons' worth. I used to be able to name all my students even after they finished school. A few months ago, when one of my former students approached me in the supermarket, I was so embarrassed that I couldn't remember his name that I pretended not to see him. I couldn't believe this was happening to ME. If you forget someone's name it means you don't care about them, because people remember the important things. I'm better off not going to places where I could make a fool of myself and insult other people.

RM, age 69, diagnosed with mild cognitive impairment (MCI), lives alone, with pronounced withdrawal from social participation

I don't let my memory problems hold me back from anything. I write down all my events and dates in my calendar, but I still encounter occasional mishaps. I know a lot of other people my age who have similar problems and we make jokes about them. I enjoy all the activities I participate in, even if I don't remember all the details. I focus on my feelings and the sense of connection I have with my community. When I started forgetting things I was very scared but my friends encouraged me, and I realized that as long as I write down the important things, and maintain my sense of humor I can cope with this.

TB, age 70, diagnosed with MCI, lives in an assisted living community

I am not the same person I used to be. I am making a big effort to act like nothing has changed since my stroke. I can't let my employees discover my problems because they would never trust me to be their boss. My wife has told me that I shouldn't make a big deal out of this, and thank the Lord it was just a mild stroke. She is used to relying on me and I can't let her down. My children are worried about me and I have to show them that I am strong.

JL, age 52, 3 months after his mild stroke

These examples illustrate the complex interactions between cognitive factors and the PEOP components. The discovery of cognitive problems is often elusive and difficult to grasp. Cognition is typically highly valued by individuals as an expression of their self-worth, and negative beliefs may trigger severe occupational withdrawal.

On the other hand, positive beliefs and social support may enable constructive coping and limit the negative impact on occupational performance. Finally, the occupational demands and social context significantly mediate the impact of cognitive deficits in everyday life. This chapter will define key cognitive factors, their impact on occupational performance and occupational therapy assessment, and treatment approaches.

BACKGROUND LITERATURE

A significant amount of evidence supports the relationship between cognitive impairment and occupational performance. Developmental or acquired impairments in cognitive factors may lead to functional deficits in all areas of occupation. The following section will define primary cognitive factors and their potential impact on occupational performance. The cognitive factors described henceforth all represent broad concepts with definitions that may vary across professional disciplines and paradigms. This section will provide a definition that best fits to explain the effect of cognitive factors on occupational performance.

Attention

Attention can be conceptualized as the process of selecting some information for further processing while inhibiting irrelevant or distracting information from being processed.[2,3] A clinical model of attention described by Sohlberg and Mateer[4] includes 5 components that describe the clinical manifestation of attention deficits:

1. Focused attention, the basic ability to respond to target stimuli
2. Sustained attention, the ability to maintain a consistent level of focus on a target stimulus over time
3. Selective attention, the ability to attend to a target stimulus and not be distracted by competing stimuli
4. Alternating attention, the ability to shift attention from one target stimulus to another as needed
5. Divided attention, the ability to attend to 2 or more target stimuli at the same time

Attention deficits may influence all aspects of daily life. Difficulty in focused attention is typical in the acute phase following acquired brain injury (ABI),[4] while the other components may affect occupational performance in all developmental or acquired neurological and psychiatric health conditions. Problems in sustained attention may create a difficulty for a child with ADHD or with autism to fully comprehend information in class, or may make it hard for adults with ABI to keep track of a plot in a book

they're reading or follow a set of instructions in order to operate an electric appliance. Difficulties in selective attention make a person highly distractible, creating difficulty for a student to attend to a lecture when other students are whispering or when he or she is preoccupied by other concerns. Problems with divided attention can cause great frustration for a person attempting to cook while speaking on the phone, and creates potential danger for an elderly person with MCI who is crossing the street while having a casual conversation with a friend. Deficits in alternating attention may put drivers at risk for vehicle accidents because of difficulty to shift their attention to an unexpected occurrence that calls for an immediate change in automatic driving patterns.

Memory and Learning

Memory, like attention, is a multifaceted and complex process. Most memory models include 3 interacting stages: encoding, storage, and retrieval. Long-term memory refers to the encoding of information in the course of an experience and the ability to retrieve it long after the experience is past.[3] Encoding is the initial stage of memory that includes analysis of input in a verbal or visual system.[4] Craik and Lockhart[5] highlight the importance of encoding to improve retrieval, and suggest that a deeper level of encoding (based on meaning) will improve the ability to recall information. Storage refers to the transfer of information for permanent retention in the brain. Retrieval relates to searching for and activating previously encoded memories, and includes monitoring the accuracy and appropriateness of the information retrieved.[3] The issue of short-term retention and manipulation of information can be conceptualized as a process that combines attention and memory. The widely accepted Baddeley-Hitch model[6] refers to this process as "working memory." In this model, working memory is a dynamic concept that consists of 2 short-term stores (phonological and visuospatial) and an executive control system that oversees the deposition and removal of information to and from the short-term storage.[3]

Memory is the basis for learning from experience and can be classified into declarative (explicit) and nondeclarative (implicit) processes. Declarative memory comprises semantic memory for facts (eg, remembering historic dates, names) and episodic memory for autobiographic events in context (eg, what happened, where, when, how I felt?). Declarative memory is characterized by conscious recollection whereas nondeclarative memory involves acquiring and storing knowledge that is unconsciously or implicitly expressed. The nondeclarative systems support skilled behavior, the acquisition of stimulus-response habits, and the formation and expression of conditioned associations.[3] These implicit learning processes are much less vulnerable to neurological impairment and enable skill acquisition, even in clients with impaired explicit learning abilities including those with Alzheimer's disease.

An additional important aspect of memory is metamemory, which refers to the person's awareness to memory abilities, related beliefs, and strategy knowledge and use. Metamemory plays an important role in understanding the variance among individuals' adaptation to memory deficits.[7] For example, RM and TB (quoted in the narratives) both have a similar memory profile, yet they differ in their beliefs regarding their memory problems, as well as strategy, knowledge and use, and consequent levels of participation.

Memory problems are the most common complaint in clients with suspected cognitive deficits. Clients often mistakenly perceive attention and executive function deficits as problems in their memory. Furthermore, memory deficits tend to be associated with low self-worth, negative beliefs, and occupational withdrawal.

Social Awareness (Theory of Mind)

Social awareness involves the interpretation of verbal and nonverbal cues in social context in order to understand other people's emotions and intentions. Social awareness is an integral aspect of social cognition and includes attending to and recognizing linguistic and paralinguistic information (eg, intonation), nonverbal behaviors (eg, facial expression and gesture), and contextual information such as knowledge of the type of relationships (eg, student-teacher, manager-employee).[8] These higher level cognitive functions are also termed *Theory of Mind*, as they entail obtaining a perspective of the other's mental state as separate than one's own. Social awareness enables apt responses that support occupational performance in the dynamic context of human interaction. Theory of Mind is present in many chronic neurological and psychiatric conditions, and has become a major area of concern in the autism spectrum disorders.

Communication and Social Skills

Communication and social skills are defined as actions or behaviors (verbal and nonverbal) a person uses to communicate and interact with others in an interactive environment. These skills are used for sending, receiving, and interpreting information in a social context.[9] The main categories of interaction skills include initiating and terminating social interaction (eg, starting, greeting), producing social interaction (eg, communicating with speech and gestures), physically supporting social interaction (eg, making eye contact, positioning oneself in relation to others), shaping content of social interaction (eg, asking questions, expressing opinions), maintaining flow of interactions (eg, responding at the right time), and adapting social interaction (eg, solving problems in social interaction).[10] Communication skills are necessary for supporting all occupations that occur in a social context and therefore have a significant impact on participation. For example, a client with Asperger's syndrome may encounter problems communicating with coworkers due to difficulties in placing himself in the appropriate distance from others, maintaining eye contact, and responding in a timely manner.

Executive Functions

Executive functions is an umbrella term to describe goal-oriented nonautomatic behavior in daily life.[11] Various higher-level cognitive skills that control and regulate cognition, affect, and behavior have been defined as executive functions, including inhibition, working memory, emotional regulation, and planning.[12,13] Ylvisaker, Szekeres, and Feneey[14] suggested an operational definition of executive functions from a clinical and ecological perspective, consisting of goal selection, planning steps to achieve goals, initiation of behavior toward implementing a plan, inhibition of behavior that would interfere with goal achievement, monitoring and evaluating performance in relation to the goals, and strategic problem solving in the face of obstacles. Therefore, executive functions are necessary to support all areas of occupation in nonroutine, unstructured, and dynamic situations (such as novel, conflicting, or complex tasks).[13,15] Executive function deficits are highly common in developmental and acquired neurological and psychiatric heath conditions across the lifespan and have been shown to be significant and unique predictors of complex activity participation, beyond other disease-related person factors (eg, motor deficits).[16,17] Executive functions are challenged when a person starts a new job or moves to a new residence, and also in daily disruptions of routine (such as unexpected guests, a traffic jam, or a broken appliance). Such changes require identifying the problem, inhibiting habitual behavior, formulating an alternative plan, and monitoring its implementation. YT's narrative demonstrates the impact of impaired executive functions after brain injury that impeded his reintegration to his previous roles. Since executive functions are manifested in dynamic and complex tasks, occupational therapy practitioners play a unique role in understanding these problems as they occur in context and in implementing interventions to improve the lives of clients that are affected by them.[15]

Awareness (Insight)

Awareness is a metacognitive process integrating both thoughts and feelings pertaining to the self, the task, or to strategies.[18,19] Understanding one's abilities in relation to task requirements is a prerequisite for strategy recruitment that supports occupational performance. Therefore, awareness is an important predictor of adaptation to health conditions, by enabling the client to compensate for deficits in person factors. On the other hand, deficits in awareness (also termed *unawareness* or *anosognosia)* have been found to be a negative predictor of safety and participation after acquired brain injury.[20] Awareness phenomena in clients that are living with health conditions should be examined in relation to the object of awareness (ie, awareness to what?), the context of awareness (ie, during task performance or general knowledge), and the cause of unawareness (ie, neurogenic, psychogenic). The objects of awareness include awareness to the injury/health condition, to the associated impairment, and to the functional consequences. The context of awareness differentiates between intellectual awareness, the static knowledge regarding one's abilities and capacities, and online awareness, which is activated during task performance (also termed *emergent awareness)*.[21] Unawareness can be attributed to psychogenic causes, such as defense mechanisms, or neurogenic causes, such as inattention and poor initiation, which may impede discovery of difficulties.[22-24]

Deficits in the various aspects of awareness described previously pose potential hazards to safe and fulfilling occupational performance. For example, YT's unawareness of the implications of his brain injury led him to attempt driving, which threatened his safety. A student with ADHD who demonstrates poor awareness of inattentive errors in written assignments (eg, does not detect mistakes, does not review his performance) does not understand why he is failing and therefore does not employ effective compensatory strategies. This negative cycle of failures and poor awareness may have long-term consequences on the student's self-esteem and occupational choices.

Assessments and Evaluations

The unique role of occupational therapy practitioners in the assessment of cognitive factors is to depict the clients' cognitive profile in relation to occupation.[25] The purpose of the assessment is to determine the client's capacity to live in his or her home, work, or do any daily task that is important and meaningful for him or her in a safe and efficient manner. The evaluation is a multi-stage process that incorporates self and informant reports, as well as performance-based measures. The evaluation begins with the clients' occupational narrative as depicted in the examples previously, and continues with performance measures. Each of these 2 methods (narrative-based and performance-based) contributes a distinctive facet to the understanding of the clients' cognitive profile and its impact on occupational performance.

A detailed investigation of the clients' occupational performance over time contributes to understanding the presence of cognitive deficits in daily functioning, associated perceptions and beliefs, and environmental factors that facilitate or impede occupational functioning. This narrative-based method of evaluation (based on interviews with client and informant) is particularly valuable in detecting mild cognitive deficits that may not appear in performance-based assessments, which provide structure and implicit support. For example, the structure of a performance test with explicit instructions and cues regarding when to start and when to end may compensate for difficulties in initiation, planning, and self-regulation, and mask the presence of executive function deficits that appear in real-life contexts over time. The occupational therapy practitioner should also obtain a perspective on the client's occupational performance from someone who knows the client well, since many clients with cognitive deficits are not sufficiently aware of their problems. This stage of the evaluation process utilizes interviews and structured verbal or pictorial assessments, such as the Occupational Questionnaire (OQ),[26] the Activity Card Sort,[27] the Self-Awareness of Deficits Interview (SADI),[28] the Everyday Memory Questionnaire (EMQ),[29] and the Behavior Rating Inventory of Executive Function (BRIEF),[30] as seen in Table 15-1.

The second performance-based evaluation method includes cognitive-functional observations as well as cognitive tests. Global observations of cognition in function are designed to examine cognitive skills in relatively complex tasks such as IADLs (see Table 15-1). They typically provide scores pertaining to cognitive skills (ie, attending to task demands, spatial and temporal organization), performance (ie, completion of steps and quality of output), and assistance necessary for task completion (ie, general and specific cues). Cognitive tests include general cognitive status and domain specific tests. Occupational therapy practitioners use tests that other health professions use to screen for cognitive deficits (eg, physicians, psychologists, and speech and language pathologists). General cognitive screening tests that are widely used by many health professionals include the Mini Mental Status Examination (MMSE),[36] the Clock Drawing Test (CDT),[46] and the Montreal Cognitive Assessment (MoCA),[37] which provide norm-referenced evidence pertaining to the presence of cognitive deficits. As seen in Table 15-1, this baseline information may indicate a need for further evaluation of specific cognitive factors using domain-specific tests of attention, memory, and executive functions. When safety concerns arise, an observation of the client in his or her natural context is indicated to determine whether he or

Table 15-1.   *Assessment of Cognitive Factors*

Assessment	Cognitive Factor Assessed	Description
Routine Task Inventory Expanded (RTI-E)[31,32]	Global cognitive factors in occupation	• Client, caregiver, and occupational therapy practitioner rating • ADL, IADL, communication, and work readiness scales • Scores reflect the Allen cognitive levels of performance (level 1.0 to 6.0)
Everyday Memory Questionnaire (EMQ)[29]	Memory in daily life	• Self-rating questionnaire • 28 items describing memory failures, rated for frequency
Multifactorial Memory Questionnaire (MMQ)[33]	Memory and meta-memory	• Self-rating questionnaire • 57 items that assess 3 aspects of subjective memory appraisal: contentment (feelings about memory), ability (impressions of memory capability), and strategy (reported frequency of use of memory aids)
Self-Awareness of Deficits Interview (SADI)[28]	Intellectual awareness	• Semi-structured interview • 3 indices: awareness of deficits, awareness of functional consequences of deficits, and ability to set realistic goals for the future
Self-Regulation Skills Interview (SRSI)[34]	Self-regulation skills	• Semi-structured interview • 6 questions that apply to an area of difficulty in everyday living identified by the client • Three indices: awareness, readiness to change, strategy behavior
Behavior Rating Inventory of Executive Function— Adult version (BRIEF-A)[30]	Executive functions in daily life	• Self-rating or informant questionnaire • 75 items scored on 9 EF scales (inhibition, shifting, emotional regulation, self-monitoring, initiation, working memory, planning, task monitoring, organization of materials • Versions: children, adolescent
Dysexecutive Questionnaire (DEX)[35]	Executive functions in daily life	• Self-rating or informant questionnaire • 20 items recording behavioral symptoms in daily functioning associated with dysexecutive syndrome, in areas of emotional or personality, motivational, behavioral, and cognitive changes
The Mini Mental State Examination (MMSE)[36]	Global cognitive status	• Screening test • Designed to detect cognitive deficits in orientation, registration, attention, memory, language, and spatial relationships • 30 items, with a total possible score of 30. A score below 24 is typically used to describe people who could be experiencing cognitive deficits that would interfere with daily living • Used extensively as screening tools for dementia
Montreal Cognitive Assessment (MoCA)[37]	Global cognitive status	• Screening test • 30-point test including short-term memory recall task, visuo-spatial abilities, executive functions, attention, working memory, language and orientation • Sensitive to the presence of MCI

(continued)

Table 15-1 (continued). *Assessment of Cognitive Factors*

Assessment	Cognitive Factor Assessed	Description
Neurobehavioral Cognitive Status Examination[38]	Global cognitive status; a profile of cognitive performance by domain	• Screening test • Employs graded series of tasks in orientation, attention, language, construction, memory, calculations, and reasoning. • Sensitive to presence of cognitive impairments in specific domains
Loewenstein Occupational Therapy Cognitive Assessment (LOTCA)[39]	Orientation, perception, praxis, and thinking	• Developed by occupational therapy practitioners to assess cognitive skills that underlie everyday functioning • Employs graded series of tasks in orientation, visual and spatial perception, praxis, visuomotor construction, and thinking operations • Provides a profile of the domains above • Developed for adults with ABI • Versions: elderly, children, and dynamic
Cognitive Performance Test (CPT)[40]	Cognitive level in ADL	• Occupation-based test • 6 tasks: dress, shop, toast, phone, wash, and travel • Scoring based on the Allen cognitive levels • Designed to predict level of cognitive performance in daily life
Kettle Test[41]	Cognition in complex task performance	• Occupation-based test • Preparing 2 hot beverages in complex conditions (empty disassembled electric kettle and distractors in kitchen setting) • Challenges attention, working memory, problem-solving skills, and safety judgment • 13 steps scored by level of cuing needed to complete the task • Designed to predict need for assistance in daily living at home
Behavioral Inattention Test (BIT)[42]	Visual attention and unilateral spatial neglect	• "Paper and pencil" and simulated everyday tasks • 2 parts: *conventional* (line crossing, letter cancellation, star cancellation, figure and shape copying, line bisection, and representational drawing) and *behavioral* (picture-scanning, phone dialing, menu reading, article reading, telling and setting time, coin sorting, address and sentence copying, map navigation, and card sorting) • Designed to detect unilateral spatial neglect and its functional implications
Color Trails Test[43]	Visual attention and mental flexibility	• "Paper and pencil" assessment • 2 subtests: CTT-1 connecting numbers in ascending order and CTT-2 alternating between numbers and 2 colors • Sensitive to driving competence
Contextual Memory Test (CMT)[7]	Metamemory and visual memory in daily contexts	• Awareness of memory strategy use, recall, and learning potential • Static (no mediation) and dynamic (structured cueing) recall of pictures in restaurant and morning context • Scores for recall, strategy use, online awareness (discrepancy between prediction and performance), and learning potential (discrepancy between static and dynamic performance)

(continued)

Table 15-1 (continued). *Assessment of Cognitive Factors*

Assessment	Cognitive Factor Assessed	Description
Rivermead Behavioral Memory Test-Third Edition (RBMT-3)[44]	Everyday memory	• Simulated everyday tasks • 14 subtests assessing aspects of episodic, semantic, and prospective memory in verbal, spatial, and pictorial recall and recognition tasks • Designed to predict memory problems in daily life • Versions: elderly, extended, children
The Awareness of Social Inference Test (TASIT)[8]	Social perception	• Videotaped vignettes of everyday social interactions • 3 parts: Part 1, Emotion Evaluation Test (EET) assesses recognition of spontaneous emotional expression. Parts 2 and 3 assess the ability to interpret conversational remarks meant literally (ie, sincere remarks and lies) or non-literally (ie, sarcasm), as well as the ability to make judgments about the thoughts, intentions, and feelings of speakers • Performance is assessed via 4 standard questions per item regarding emotions, intentions, beliefs, and meanings of the speakers
The Evaluation of Social Interaction (ESI)[45]	Social interaction skills	• Occupation-based assessment • Observation of social interaction in the natural context • 27 interaction skills that evaluate how a person begins, supports and maintains, and ends social interactions with others (eg, approaches/starts, gesticulates, turns toward, takes turns, clarifies) • Scoring uses criteria rating how competently, socially polite, and timely the person performs
Clock drawing tests (CDT)[46]	Visual-motor abilities and executive functions	• "Paper and pencil" screening test • Employs a single task of drawing a clock with all its numbers and with hands showing time as directed (commonly 11:10) • Several versions of administration and scoring
Executive Function Performance Test (EFPT)[47]	Executive functions in task performance	• Observational assessment • 4 IADL tasks: preparing oatmeal, using the telephone, taking medication, and paying bills. • Scores on initiation, execution (organization, sequencing, judgment, and safety), and level of cueing required • Designed to determine which executive functions are impaired, capacity for independent functioning, and the type of assistance necessary for daily living at home
Behavioral Assessment of the Dysexecutive Syndrome (BADS)[35]	Executive functions	• Simulated everyday tasks • 6 tests measuring planning, organizing, and behavior monitoring • Designed to predict dysexecutive syndrome in daily life

(continued)

Table 15-1 (continued).   *Assessment of Cognitive Factors*

Assessment	Cognitive Factor Assessed	Description
Multiple Errand Test (MET)[48]	Executive functions in multi-tasking performance	• 12 tasks, including 6 errands (purchasing 3 items, using the telephone, sending a letter, collecting an item from an office), obtaining 4 items of information, meeting the assessor at a designated place and time, and informing the assessor when finishing the test • The participant is required to perform these tasks while adhering to a list of 9 rules, such as money spending limits, not exiting the boundaries of the building, and not entering a room twice • MET scores represent errors in the following categories: inefficiencies, rule breaks, interpretation failures, and task failures • Designed to examine executive functions in multitasking context and predict participation in complex areas of occupation

she can live alone and what type of supports will enable optimal occupational performance and well-being. Occupational therapy practitioners have developed performance-based tests of cognition to understand how the individuals' cognition is affecting their abilities to plan, organize, and carry out tasks. Such tests are important to use when the issue of safety or need for supervision is being addressed. Tests like the Kettle Test,[41] the Executive Function Performance Test,[47] and the Multiple Errands Test[48] fit into this category of testing (see Table 15-1 for more detail).

The product of the evaluation is a cognitive functional profile that provides a description of cognitive strengths and weaknesses and their implications for occupational performance. This includes recommendations concerning the type and amount of assistance currently required for safe and meaningful occupational performance, and affords the basis for clinical reasoning in selecting the approach to treatment.

INTERVENTIONS

Interventions for rehabilitation of individuals with impaired cognitive factors employ several occupational therapy approaches designed to improve participation and well-being.[49] These approaches can be classified according to their treatment methods, their hypothesized change mechanisms (neuroplasticity, declarative learning, procedural learning, and environmental resources) and their expected outcomes. Participation is enabled by means of restoring cognitive factors and/or compensating for cognitive deficits via metacognitive learning, task specific learning, and adapting occupation or environment. The

treatment plan is tailored to the client's profile and is geared toward maximizing personal and environmental resources. The treatment may be based on a single approach or an integrative approach that will harness multiple enabling pathways. The following is a brief review of the treatment approaches; Table 15-2 summarizes this information with references of evidence in the literature.

The Restorative Approach

The restorative approach focuses on ameliorating cognitive deficits through hierarchical intensive training of specific cognitive factors. This approach is best delivered by Computerized Cognitive Training (CCT) that targets isolated cognitive factors, such as attention, working memory, and response inhibition. Restorative training assumes that cognitive factors can improve due to neuroplasticity and, therefore, will lead to spontaneous improvement in occupational performance. There is some supporting evidence for the impact of cognitive training in improving mild deficits such as those found in healthy elderly, individuals with ADHD, and mild ABI.[50-52,66] There continues to be a question of transfer to daily life situations with this approach, and therefore it should not be used as a stand-alone method in occupational therapy.

The Metacognitive Treatment Approach

The metacognitive treatment approach focuses on acquiring cognitive strategies that bypass or overcome the cognitive deficits in occupational performance.[53] The hypothesized underlying mechanisms of change are awareness and strategy competence that facilitate top-down controlled behavior in multiple contexts. This

Table 15-2. Occupational Therapy Treatment Approaches for Clients With Deficits in Cognitive Factors

Treatment Approach	Methods	Hypothesized Change Mechanisms	Expected Outcomes	Research Examples
Restorative/remedial	• Hierarchical intensive training of discrete cognitive areas • Computerized cognitive training packages	• Behavior-induced neuroplasticity • Automatic transfer of training to daily life	• Cognitive abilities • Occupational performance	• Computerized training of working memory in patients with acquired brain injury[50] • Computerized training of working memory in children with ADHD[51,52]
Metacognitive strategy acquisition	• The Multicontext Treatment Approach[53]: mediated discovery of strategies that compensate for cognitive deficits, practice, and transfer to multiple tasks and contexts	• Declarative learning processes; strategy knowledge and use in multiple contexts that guide behavior in occupational performance	• Strategy knowledge and use • Online awareness • Occupational performance • Self-efficacy	• Multi-context approach promoting learning and transfer of strategies and self-regulation after brain injury[54,55] • CO-OP approach with adults with executive dysfunction following TBI[56] • Occupational goal intervention for clients with schizophrenia[57]
Task-specific learning	• Neurofunctional Treatment approach[58] • Behavioral, errorless learning techniques • No transfer assumed to non-learned tasks	• Implicit learning processes, specific behavioral learning of tasks with high significance to client or caregiver	• Occupational performance in designated trained tasks • Self-efficacy	• ADL retraining program for adults with brain injury[59,60] • Neurofunctional treatment targeting participation among chronic stroke survivors[61]
Environmental adaptation	• Adapting task, environment • Providing support to match clients cognitive profile[62]	• Improving person-environment fit, reducing frustration, and enabling participation	• Occupational performance • Reduction of negative behaviors • Well-being	• Community Aging in Place, Advancing Better Living for Elders: Bio-Behavioral-Environmental intervention for disabled older adults[63] • Biobehavioral home-based intervention for patients with dementia and their caregivers (COPE)[64] • Home-based electronic memory aid for persons with memory impairments to support everyday activities[65]

approach relies on declarative learning abilities and language skills to enable strategy acquisition. In addition, some level of awareness to occupational limitations is required to motivate the effortful learning process. The occupational therapy practitioner provides the necessary mediation to discover, practice, and transfer strategies to life situations. The designated strategies are selected in relation to the client's occupational needs and preferences. This treatment utilizes general strategies, such as an executive strategy like "Goal, Plan, Do, Review," that supports a wide array of complex occupations and specific strategies, such as "systematic visual scanning" or "repeating a verbal communication out loud," that are relevant to certain occupations only. Mediation of strategy learning and transfer to occupational goals is a central part of the treatment. This approach is gaining validation in improving occupational performance in individuals with mild to moderate cognitive deficits across the lifespan.[43-46] The metacognitive treatment approach may be used in conjunction with the cognitive-behavioral approach that targets lack of knowledge and distorted beliefs about cognition and health (see Chapter 18).

Task-Specific Learning

Task-specific learning is focused on achieving specific functional goals while employing primarily behavioral learning techniques. The targeted functional task is broken down to small chunks; probability of errors largely reduced, behaviors practiced, reinforced, and "over-learned." As opposed to metacognitive treatment, task-specific learning is designed to minimize effort and enable relatively rapid success in designated tasks that are of high motivational significance to the client and/or family. Learning is task specific and there is no expectation of skill transfer to other tasks; yet an improvement in self-efficacy and other volitional factors is often found. The underlying change mechanisms are implicit procedural learning processes that bypass the cognitive deficit area, as well as the recruitment of motivational resources. Both of these mechanisms foster the attainment of predefined functional goals.[47,48] This approach is typically recommended for clients with severe deficits in cognitive factors, such as clients with dementia, in order to obtain functional goals. However, due to the positive impact on volition, task-specific training is also recommended for clients with more mild cognitive deficits that do not currently possess the emotional resources for the more demanding approaches. For example, task-specific training to learn the use of a computerized telephone (eg, Skype) may be a first-stage intervention for a client with mild cognitive deficits and depression who wants to communicate long distance with her family.

Environmental Adaptations

Environmental adaptations for individuals with cognitive disabilities concentrate on enabling function and participation through modifying factors that are external to the individual.[49] The physical and human factors in the clients' environment are adapted to the cognitive profile of the individual, based on theories of cognitive task analysis and understanding of the person-environment interface. The hypothesized mechanism of change is the suitability of the adaptation (ie, environment-person fit) and to the potential impact of environmental factors on health and well-being. Adaptations depend on the presence and availability of environmental resources (eg, family members, practitioner access to home or work environment) to implement them. This approach is typically recommended for clients with severe cognitive deficits, yet it should be used to ameliorate environmental barriers and enable occupational performance in all clients, even with mild deficits. For example, modifying a spouse's expectations of a client's occupational performance after a mild brain injury (see JL's narrative), or teaching a parent how to communicate with a child with working memory deficits may be critical components of the enabling process and supplement other treatment approaches.

The following case study will demonstrate an integrative approach that will harness multiple enabling pathways. DH is a 38-year-old woman who sustained mTBI in a motor vehicle accident. She was discharged from a hospital neurology ward 2 days after her injury and referred to community-based neurorehabilitation. DH lives with her husband and 2 children (ages 7 and 9) and works part-time as a legal secretary. On weekdays, her husband works late hours and typically arrives home after the children are asleep, and she is responsible for the childcare and homemaking. She lives close to her younger sister, whom she considers her best friend, and before the accident used to enjoy her company in the evenings.

The occupational therapy practitioner conducted an intake interview 6 weeks after the injury. DH was very distressed and reported that she had serious memory problems and was making many mistakes at home and in work. She could not keep track of the children's extracurricular activities, like soccer practice schedule, and her son came home crying after going to school without his sports gear. She was feeling impatient with her children in the afternoons and described dinner and bedtime as hell. She experienced difficulties and frustration at work because she couldn't remember clients' names as she did before the accident, and sometimes forgot to perform a task or got confused regarding instructions she received from her bosses. She tried to hide her difficulties and was worried she would lose the respect she had gained over years of hard work. Her sister validated DH's description of her forgetfulness and reported that DH seemed overwhelmed and tired, yet was reluctant to accept her offers to help out at home. Results of performance-based assessments revealed mild deficits in attention, memory, and executive functions that posed barriers to complex occupational functioning (IADL and work).

The occupational therapy practitioner employed an integrative approach. Environmental supports were suggested, relying on her sister and husband as willing resources to alleviate the burden she was experiencing at home. In order for DH to accept their help, the practitioner assisted in identifying and modifying her beliefs from "accepting help symbolizes weakness" to "accepting help will enable me participate in life roles that are so important to me." Compensatory strategies were discovered and practiced in therapy, and transfer was mediated to home and work tasks. The targeted strategies were: global executive strategy, prioritizing, verbal guidance of behavior, attending to one task at a time, and use of external memory aids. Task-specific errorless training was employed so that DH could rapidly master the operation of an electronic organizational aid (in her cell phone) that was so needed to reliably compensate for her cognitive problems. These treatment methods were used in an integrative manner, guided by PEOP clinical reasoning, addressing the interactions between DH's cognitive deficits and her occupational preferences in her family and work environment. In the 3 months of treatment (one session per week), strategy implementation was monitored and level of supports were adjusted to DH's changing needs. DH reported improved occupational performance and satisfaction and was gaining confidence in her abilities to overcome her cognitive deficits and participate in her life roles. She demonstrated independent use of strategies and the ability to generate new ones as needed. In DH's words: "It's not easy, but I know that there is always something I can do."

SUMMARY

This chapter introduced central concepts for understanding cognitive factors in occupational performance. Cognitive deficits are consequential to many health conditions, are significant barriers to participation, and therefore are relevant in all occupational therapy practice areas. Occupational therapy practitioners assess the impact of cognitive factors on occupation in context and perform clinical reasoning that is guided by the interactions among the cognitive factors—with other person factors, occupation, and environment factors. The treatment process focuses on enabling participation by integrating multiple change mechanisms of neuroplasticity, explicit, and implicit learning and environmental adaptation. Treatment outcomes are measured at the occupation level and may or may not include changes in cognitive factors. The commitment to occupational outcomes is at the core of the occupational therapy approach to cognitive factors. Table 15-3 provides resources to help the practitioner stay abreast of the literature and lists major organizations that provide help to patients and their families.

Table 15-3. *Organizations and Journals That Focus on Cognitive Factors for Performance*

Organization or Journal	Description	Web Address
Society for Cognitive Rehabilitation	Promote interdisciplinary dialogue among these different professions, engaged directly or indirectly in the practice of cognitive rehabilitation toward the creation of consensus; endorsed by those professions.	http://www.societyforcogniti-verehab.org/
Cognitive Science Society	Society promotes scientific interchange among researchers in disciplines comprising the field of cognitive science, including artificial intelligence, linguistics, anthropology, psychology, neuroscience, philosophy, and education.	http://cognitivesciencesociety. org/index.html
Alzheimer's Foundation of America	Dedicated to meeting the educational, social, emotional, and practical needs of individuals with Alzheimer's disease and related illnesses and their caregivers and families.	http://www.alzfdn.org/?gclid=C PDIrty4qrUCFcpDMgodJxAA3Q
American Stoke Association	A resource for professionals and families.	http:// http://www.strokeas-sociation.org/STROKEORG/ Professionals/Stroke-Resources-for-Professionals_UCM_308581_ SubHomePage.jsp
Brain Injury Association of America	Dedicated to advancing brain injury prevention, research, treatment, and education and to improve the quality of life for all people affected by brain injury. Has a network of state affiliates, local chapters and support groups.	http://www.biausa.org/
Stroke Engine	Resource for individuals who have experienced stroke, their families, and health professionals who work in the field of stroke rehabilitation. Supports the use of evidence-based stroke rehabilitation in clinical practice. Recognized for its scientific rigor.	http://strokengine.ca/
Journal of Cognitive Psychology	Publishes and encourages the exchange and integration of ideas and research in cognitive psychology from experimental cognitive psychologists and cognitive neuroscientists.	http://www.escop.eu/about_us/ journal/
Journal of Cognitive Neuroscience	Investigates brain–behavior interaction and promotes lively interchange among the mind sciences.	http://www.mitpressjournals. org/loi/jocn

REFERENCES

1. Katz N, Baum C, Maeir A. Introduction to cognitive intervention and cognitive functional evaluation. In Katz N, ed. *Cognition, Occupation, and Participation Across the Life Span: Neuroscience, Neurorehabilitation, and Models of Intervention in Occupational Therapy.* 3rd ed. Bethesda, MD: AOTA Press; 2011:3-12.

2. Levy LL. Cognitive information processing. In Katz N, ed. *Cognition, Occupation, and Participation Across the Life Span: Neuroscience, Neurorehabilitation, and Models of Intervention in Occupational Therapy.* 3rd ed. Bethesda, MD: AOTA Press; 2011:93-116.

3. Smith EE, Kosllyn SM. *Cognitive Psychology: Mind and Brain.* Upper Saddle River, NJ: Pearson Prentice Hall; 2007.

4. Sohlberg MM, Mateer CA. *Cognitive Rehabilitation.* New York, NY: Guilford Press; 2001.

5. Craik FM, Lockhart RS. Levels of processing: a framework for memory research. *J Verb Learn Verb Be*. 1972;11:671-684.

6. Baddeley A. Exploring the central executive. *Q J Exp Psychol*. 1996;49A:5-28.

7. Toglia JP. *Contextual Memory Test Manual*. San Antonio, TX: The Psychological Corporation; 1993.

8. McDonald S, Bornhofen C, Shum D, Long E, Saunders C, Neulinger K. Reliability and validity of The Awareness of Social Inference Test (TASIT): a clinical test of social perception. *Disabil Rehabil*. 2006;28:1529-1542.

9. AOTA. Occupational therapy practice framework: domain and process. 2nd ed. *Am J Occup Ther*. 2008;62:625-683.

10. Simmons CD, Griswold LA, Berg B. Evaluation of social interaction during occupational engagement. *Am J Occup Ther*. 2010;64:1010-1017.

11. Lezak MD, Howieson DB, Loring DW, Hannay HJ, Fischer JS. *Neuropsychological Assessment*. 4th ed. New York, NY: Oxford University Press; 2004.

12. Connor L, Maeir A. Putting executive performance in a theoretical context. *Occup Ther J Res*. 2011;31:S3-S8.

13. Katz N, Maeir A. Higher level cognitive functions: awareness and executive functions. In Katz N, ed. *Cognition, Occupation, and Participation Across the Life Span: Neuroscience, Neurorehabilitation, and Models of Intervention in Occupational Therapy*. 3rd ed. Bethesda, MD: AOTA Press; 2011:13-40.

14. Ylvisaker M, Szekeres SF, Feneey TJ. Cognitive rehabilitation: executive functions. In Ylvisaker M, ed. *Towards Brain Injury Rehabilitation: Children and Adolescents*. Boston, MA: Butterworth-Heinemann; 1998:221–269.

15. Baum CM, Katz, N. Guest editorial: introduction to the special issue on cognition and executive function. *Occup Ther J Res*. 2011;31:S2.

16. Foster ER, Hershey T. Everyday executive function is associated with activity participation in Parkinson's disease without dementia. *Occup Ther J Res*. 2011;31:S16-S22.

17. Ownsworth T, Shum D. Relationship between executive functions and productivity outcomes following stroke. *Disabil Rehabil*. 2007;30:531-540.

18. Flavell JH. *Cognitive Development*. Englewood Cliffs, NJ: Prentice Hall; 1985.

19. Prigatano GP. *The Study of Anosognosia*. New York, NY: Oxford University Press; 2010.

20. Hartman-Maeir A, Soroker N, Oman SD, Katz N. Awareness of disabilities after stroke. *Disabil Rehabil*. 2003;25:35-44.

21. Toglia JP, Kirk U. Understanding awareness deficits following brain injury. *Neurorehabil*. 2000;15:57-70.

22. Lewis L. Role of psychological factors in disordered awareness. In Prigatano GP, Schacter DL, eds. *Awareness of Deficits After Brain Injury: Clinical and Theoretical Issues*. New York, NY: Oxford University Press; 1991;223-39.

23. Kortte KB, Wegener T. Denial of illness in medical rehabilitation populations: theory, research and definition. *Rehabil Psychol*. 2004;49:187-99.

24. Heilman KM, Barrett, AM, Adair JC. Possible mechanisms of anosognosia: a defect in self-awareness. *Philos T Roy Soc B*. 1998;353:1903-1909.

25. Hartman-Maeir A, Katz N, Baum C. Cognitive functional evaluation (CFE) for individuals with suspected cognitive disabilities. *Occup Ther Health Care*. 2009;23:1-23.

26. Smith NR, Kielhofner G, Watts JH. The relationships between volition, activity pattern, and life satisfaction in the elderly. *Am J Occup Ther*. 1986;40:278-283.

27. Baum CM, Edwards D. *Activity Card Sort*. 2nd ed. Bethesda, MD: AOTA, Inc; 2008.

28. Fleming JM, Strong J, Ashton R. Self-awareness of deficits in adults with traumatic brain injury: How best to measure? *Brain Inj*. 1996;10:1-15.

29. Sunderland A, Harris JE, Gleave J. Memory failures in everyday life following severe head injury. *J Clin Neuropsychol*. 1984;6:125-141.

30. Roth RM, Isquith PK, Gioia GA. *Behavior Rating Inventory of Executive Function—Adult Version*. Lutz, FL: Psychological Assessment Resources, Inc; 2005.

31. Allen CK, Heimann NE, Yerxa, EJ. The Routine Task Inventory: a tool for describing the functional behavior of the cognitively disabled. *OT Practice*. 1989;1:67-74.

32. Katz N. *Routine Task Inventory—RTI-E manual*. http://www.allen-cognitive-network.org/images/stories/pdf_files/rtimanual2006.pdf. Accessed May 28, 2012.

33. Troyer AK, Rich JB. Psychometric properties of a new metamemory questionnaire for older adults. *J Gerontol*. 2002;57:19-27.

34. Ownsworth TL, McFarland K, Young R. Development and standardization of the Self-Regulation Skills Interview (SRSI): a new clinical assessment tool for acquired brain injury. *Clin Neuropsychol*. 2000;14:76-92.

35. Wilson BA, Alderman N, Burgess PW, Emslie H, Evans, JJ. *Behavioural Assessment of the Dysexecutive Syndrome*. Bury St. Edmund, UK: Thames Valley Test Co; 1996.

36. Folstein M, Folstein SE, McHugh PR. "Mini-Mental State" a practical method for grading the cognitive state of patients for the clinician. *J Psychiatr Res*. 1975;12:189-198.

37. Nasreddine ZS, Phillips NA, Bédirian V, et al. The Montreal cognitive assessment (MoCA): a brief screening tool for mild cognitive impairment. *J Am Geriatr Soc*. 2005;53:695-699.

38. Mueller J, Kierman R, Langston JW. *Cognistat Manual*. Fairfax, CA: The Northern California Neurobehavioral Group; 2007.

39. Elazar B, Itzkovich M, Katz N. *Loewenstein Occupational Therapy Cognitive Assessment: Geriatric Version (LOTCA-G) Battery*. Pequannock, NJ: Maddak Inc; 1996.

40. Burns T. *Cognitive Performance Test (CPT)*. Pequannock, NJ: Maddak; 2006.

41. Hartman-Maeir A, Harel H, Katz N. Kettle Test—a brief measure of cognitive functional performance: reliability and validity in stroke rehabilitation. *Am J Occup Ther*. 2009;64:592-599.

42. Wilson BA, Cockburn J, Halligan PW. *Behavioural Inattention Test Manual*. Fareham, England: Thames Valley Test Co; 1987.

43. D'Elia LF, Satz P, Uchiyama CL, White T. *Color Trails Test (CTT)*. Lutz, FL: Psychological Assessment Resources Inc; 1994.

44. Wilson BA, Cockburn J, Baddley A. *The Rivermead Behavioral Memory Test*. Reading, England: Thames Valley Test Co; 1985.

45. Fisher AG, Griswold LA. *Evaluation of Social Interaction, Research Edition IV*. Fort Collins, CO: Three Star Press; 2009.

46. Freedman M, Leach L, Kaplan E, Winocur G, Shulman K, Delis DC. *Clock Drawing: A Neuropsychological Analysis*. New York, NY: Oxford University Press; 1994.

47. Baum C, Morrison T, Hahn, M, Edwards, D. *Executive Function Performance Test: Test Protocol Booklet*. St. Louis, MO: Program in Occupational Therapy, Washington University School of Medicine; 2007.

48. Dawson DR, Anderson ND, Burgess P, Cooper E, Krpan KM, Stuss D. Further development of the multiple errands test: standardized scoring, reliability, and ecological validity for the Baycrest version. *Arch Phys Med Rehab*. 2009;90:s41-s51.

49. Katz N. *Cognition, Occupation, and Participation Across the Life Span: Neuroscience, Neurorehabilitation, and Models of Intervention in Occupational Therapy*. 3rd ed. Bethesda: AOTA Press; 2011.

50. Lundqvist A, Grundstrm K, Samuelsson K, Rönnberg J. Computerized training of working memory in a group of patients suffering from acquired brain injury. *Brain Inj.* 2010;24:1173-1183.

51. Klingberg T, Fernell E, Olesen P, et al. Computerized training of working memory in children with ADHD—a randomized, controlled trial. *J Am Acad Child Psy.* 2005;44:177-86.

52. Shalev L, Tsal Y, Mevorach C. Computerized Progressive Attentional Training (CPAT) program: effective direct intervention for children with ADHD. *Child Neuropsychol.* 2007;13:382-388.

53. Toglia JP. The dynamic interactional model of cognition in cognitive rehabilitation. In Katz N, ed. *Cognition, Occupation, and Participation Across the Life Span: Neuroscience, Neurorehabilitation, and Models of Intervention in Occupational Therapy.* 3rd ed. Bethesda, MD: AOTA Press; 2011:161-202.

54. Toglia JP, Goverover Y, Johnston MV, Dain B. Application of the multicontextual approach in promoting learning and transfer of strategy use in an individual with TBI and executive dysfunction. *Occup Ther J Res.* 2011;31:S53-S60.

55. Toglia JP, Johnston MV, Goverover Y, Dain B. A multicontext approach to promoting transfer of strategy use and self regulation after brain injury: an exploratory study. *Brain Inj.* 2010;24:664-677.

56. Dawson DR, Gaya A, Hunt A, Levine B, Lemsky C, Polatajko HJ. Using the Cognitive Orientation to Occupational Performance (CO-OP) approach with adults with executive dysfunction following traumatic brain injury. *Can J Occup Ther.* 2009;76:115-127.

57. Katz N, Keren N. Effectiveness of occupational goal intervention for clients with schizophrenia. *Am J Occup Ther.* 2011;65:287-296.

58. Giles GM. A neurofunctional approach to rehabilitation following severe brain injury. In Katz N, ed. *Cognition, Occupation, and Participation Across the Life Span: Neuroscience, Neurorehabilitation, and Models of Intervention in Occupational Therapy.* 3rd ed. Bethesda, MD: AOTA Press; 2011:351-382.

59. Giles GM, Ridley JE, Dill A, Frye S. A consecutive series of adults with brain injury treated with a washing and dressing retraining program. *Am J Occup Ther.* 1997;51:256-266.

60. Parish L, Oddy M. Efficacy of rehabilitation for functional skills more than 10 years after extremely severe brain injury. *Neuropsychol Rehabil.* 2007;17:230-243.

61. Rotenberg-Shpigelman S, Erez AB, Nahaloni I, Maeir A. Neurofunctional treatment targeting participation among chronic stroke survivors: a pilot randomised controlled study. *Neuropsychol Rehabil.* 2012;22(4):532-549.

62. McCraith DB, Austin SL, Earhart CA. The cognitive disabilities model in 2011. In Katz N, ed. *Cognition, Occupation, and Participation Across the Life Span: Neuroscience, Neurorehabilitation, and Models of Intervention in Occupational Therapy.* 3rd ed. Bethesda, MD: AOTA Press; 2011:383-406.

63. Szanton SL, Thorpe RJ, Boyd C, et al. Community aging in place, advancing better living for elders: a bio-behavioral-environmental intervention to improve function and health-related quality of life in disabled older adults. *J Am Geriatr Soc.* 2011;59:2314-2320.

64. Gitlin LN, Winter L, Dennis MP, Hodgson N, Hauck WW. A biobehavioral home-based intervention and the well-being of patients with dementia and their caregivers. *JAMA.* 2010;304:983-991.

65. Boman IL, Bartfai A, Borell L, Tham K, Hemmingsson H. Support in everyday activities with a home-based electronic memory aid for persons with memory impairments. *Disabil Rehabil.* 2010;5:339-350.

66. Smith GE, Housen P, Yaffe K, et al. A cognitive training program based on principles of brain plasticity: results from the improvement in memory with plasticity-based adaptive cognitive training (IMPACT) study. *J Am Geriatr So.* 2009;57:594-603.

67. Polatajko HJ, Mandich A, McEwen SE. Cognitive Orientation to Daily Occupational Performance (CO-OP): a cognitive-based intervention for children and adults. In Katz N, ed. *Cognition, Occupation, and Participation Across the Life Span: Neuroscience, Neurorehabilitation, and Models of Intervention in Occupational Therapy.* 3rd ed. Bethesda, MD: AOTA Press; 2011:299-321.

Chapter 16

PERSON FACTORS
Sensory

Leeanne M. Carey, BAppSc(OT), PhD, FAOTA

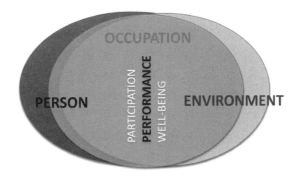

LEARNING OBJECTIVES

- Identify and define the sensory factors, including vision, audition, and somatic sensation that influence performance and participation.

- Describe how constraints and barriers in sensory factors may affect a person's performance, participation, and well-being.

- Identify major health conditions or disabilities in which sensory factors could influence performance, participation, and well-being (Table 16-1).

- Demonstrate your understanding of the influence of sensory factors on occupational performance through structured observation and task analysis.

- Identify established assessments of sensation that are evidence-based and measure capabilities and limitations related to occupational performance (Table 16-2).

- Identify intervention principles to address sensory factors that are limiting occupational performance.

- Describe 3 to 5 intervention approaches that would address limitations associated with sensory factors.

- Recognize the complexity of how sensory factors interact with other person and environment factors as it relates to performance in everyday life.

KEY WORDS

- Audition
- Detection
- Discrimination
- Gustatory
- Multisensory
- Olfactory
- Perception[7]
- Proprioceptive
- Recognition
- Sensory processing

Christiansen CH, Baum CM, Bass JD, eds.
*Occupational Therapy: Performance, Participation,
and Well-Being, Fourth Edition* (pp 249-265).
© 2015 SLACK Incorporated.

Table 16-1. *Major Health Conditions or Disabilities in Which Sensory Factors Could Influence Performance, Participation, and Well-Being*

Condition	Vision	Audition	Tactile	Proprio-ceptive	Vestibular	Olfactory and Gustatory	Multisensory Processing
Cerebral palsy	X	X	X	X	X	X	X
Developmental coor-dination disorder	X			X			X
Autism	X						X
Mental retardation							X
Orthopedic injury				X			
Hand injury			X				
Spinal cord injury			X	X			
Multiple sclerosis	X	X	X	X	X	X	
Stroke	X	X	X	X	X	X	X
Parkinson's			X			X	
Dementia							X
Schizophrenia							X
Elderly	X	X	X	X	X	X	X
Head injury	X	X	X	X	X	X	X

- Somatosensory[8]
- Tactile
- Vestibular
- Vision

INTRODUCTION

Understanding Our Senses Within the Person-Environment-Occupation-Performance Model

Sensation is everywhere. Sensory factors are one of the categories of person factors that underpin the capacity of an individual to perform everyday occupations. Sensory factors refer to an individual's capacity to see, hear, touch, smell, and taste. These factors influence the individual's ability to interact with their environment and participate in meaningful life occupations. Sensation is part of everything we do.

There are 3 levels at which we may view the influence of sensation.[9,10]

Sensation for Perception

Without our senses we can't process the world around us. Sensation is important in its own right and important for whom we are as human beings. We want to feel, see, taste, and interact with the world around us. It allows us to experience pleasure and be alerted to danger. Senses are also part of the way we learn and adapt.

Sensation for Action

Sensation influences our ability to move around safely in our environment and to engage in the day to day activities that are important to us all. For example, vision is important to maneuver safely around the home, while touch is important to grip and manipulate objects and to sustain and adapt forces when using objects.

Sensation for Occupational Performance and Life Roles

Sensation is important for a number of life roles. Loss of sensations may affect the client's ability to return to previous life roles as a parent or worker; it may impact on safety, social roles, and participation in personal and domestic ADL.

Table 16-2. *Evidence-Based Formal Assessments of Sensation*

Sense	Recommended Assessments	Comment/Reference
Vision	Visual acuity: The ETDRS visual acuity test is a standardized instrument designed to evaluate visual acuity. ETDRS stands for Early Treatment Diabetic Retinopathy Study. The ESV-3000 ETDRS testing device has self-calibrated test lighting.	ETDRS acuity testing has become the worldwide standard for visual acuity testing.
	Visual fields: Visual fields are measured by mapping out blind or visually impaired areas in visual space.	Visual field detection is usually measured with a motion perimetry instrument.
	Vision impact: National Eye Institute's Visual Function Questionnaire (NEI VFQ) or Impact of Vision Impairment (IVI) questionnaire.	
Audition	Pure tone audiometry, bone conduction hearing test, and standardized linguistic related hearing tests; including Hearing Thresholds and Hearing Handicap Inventory for Adults—Short Form	Tests are most often performed by an audiologist. http://en.wikipedia.org/wiki/Hearing_test
Touch	Detection of light touch and deep pressure: Semmes-Weinstein monofilaments or Weinstein Enhanced Sensory Test (WEST) hand monofilaments	1
	Texture discrimination: Tactile Discrimination Test (TDT)	2
	Shape discrimination: Manual Form Perception Test	3
	Sensory function: Modified Moberg pick up test	4
Proprioception	Limb position sense: Wrist Position Sense Test	5
	Movement sense: Kinesthesia Test	6
Vestibular	Angular vestibulo-ocular reflex (eg, gaze stabilization): Dynamic Visual Acuity test	http://www.nihtoolbox.org/WhatAndWhy/Sensation/Vestibular/Pages/default.aspx
	Performance dependent upon vestibulospinal output (eg, postural control output or balance ability)	
Olfaction	Odor Identification Test	http://www.nihtoolbox.org/WhatAndWhy/Sensation/Olfaction/Pages/default.aspx
Gustatory	Regional Taste Test	http://www.nihtoolbox.org/WhatAndWhy/Sensation/Taste/Pages/default.aspx
Multisensory	Sensory Profile, Sensory Profile School Companion, Infant/Toddler Sensory Profile, Adolescent/Adult Sensory Profile	http://www.pearson-clinical.com/therapy/products/100000822/sensory-profile-2.html?Pid=076-1638-008&Mode=summary

The environmental consequence of loss of sensory factors will also be influenced, at least in part, by the surrounding environment. For example, low vision will impact most when lighting is poor in the home or when the person needs to move around at night. Thus, environment-related resources and barriers need to be considered when understanding the impact of the sensory loss and how to enable your clients to perform the particular occupations that are important to them. It may also be influenced by the particular demands of the occupations they choose to engage in. For example, a person who works in the textile industry may be particularly impacted by impaired touch discrimination ability.

The relationship between our senses and interface with the environment is dynamic, reciprocal, and consistent with the PEOP Model. Importantly, we need to recognize and integrate the individual's abilities and strengths when working out the most optimal strategies to use under the sensory-impaired conditions. Interventions may be directed at remediating the lost sensation or may be more compensatory in nature, taking into account how the environment may be adapted. The decision of the most appropriate approach to take will be influenced by the individual, as well as evidence of the potential for change and current evidence of effective interventions.

NARRATIVE AND BACKGROUND LITERATURE

We are all sensory beings, yet our experiences are unique.[11] Sensation is everywhere. We are surrounded by sounds, textures, tastes, smells, and an ongoing range of things to see. Sensation is the brain's source of information. Many of our memories are based on and recalled in the context of sensations. Each of us operates best with different amounts of sensory information.[11]

Loss of one's senses can have a major personal and functional impact on an individual. It can be difficult for us to appreciate what that might be like. Below are some quotes from people who experience loss of body sensations after a stroke. Note the impact at multiple levels; personal through to activity and participation levels. The impact is evident in relation to one's perceptions, motivations, goals, and responsibilities.

> *"I may look alright but I feel all left... and half lost."*[12]

> *"To reach out, connect and make contact with another person is to feel alive and part of the human race."*[12]

> *"My right side cannot discriminate rough or smooth, rigid or malleable, sharp or blunt, heavy or light. It cannot tell if that which touches it is a hand or a tennis racket... disconcerting also to search around for that book to read in bed, only to discover that it is wedged, unfelt, under one's right side... better to feel something, however bizarre, than nothing."*

> *"The dullness of sensation and absence of knowledge of my body's right-sided perimeters, combined with the changeableness and strength of the 'internal' sensations, makes it frustratingly difficult to control or feel relaxed about any right-sided movement."*

> *"How does one trust a leg that 'feels' as though it is floating within the skin or a foot that 'feels' as though it has no real connection with the earth?"*

> *"Searching for anything in my bag with my right hand was hazardous."*[12]

> *"After my stroke I had quite good movement in my stroke-affected hand, but very little sense of touch. My hand felt like it was blind. Everyday tasks were very clumsy and required so much concentration. Things like picking up and using a fork were labored and tasks where my hand was out of sight, like doing up a bra, putting on jewelry, and tying up my hair, were beyond me."*

> *"Doing dishes can take me up to an hour, even sometimes 2 hours. Because my hand, I can't feel things in my hand... and I can break glasses in my hand."*

> *"You just don't feel confident in anything you do and you get depressed. Like changing my daughter's nappies, 'cause I cannot feel them and I cannot feel her in my hands, I can hurt her and I can bruise her with my hand, and I've done that in the past week."*

Knowing a client's story is essential for planning effective and relevant interventions. For example, as one stroke survivor said, "I want to be the best I can be." While there are compensatory approaches, and for some individuals these are most appropriate, there is also hope and evidence of effective remediation approaches. It is critical that the practitioner is aware of these and able to facilitate an appropriate level of intervention for their client.

Sensory Factors: Overall Definition, Role, and Impact

Sensory perception refers to the ability to detect, discriminate, and recognize sensory stimuli around us. Sensory stimuli may be detected through vision, touch, or other sensory systems. This involves processing of sensory information from the periphery (sensory receptors) through to perception via brain networks.[8]

Our senses tell us about the edge of our body (touch); where body parts are in space (proprioception); where we are in space (movement sensors); flavors, textures, and temperatures (oral sensations); a map of the space and world around us (visual senses); the distance around us (auditory sensations); and smells of objects and the world around us (smell).[11]

Sensory perception is part of our conscious experience of who we are in our environment. Our sensory systems and sensory preferences help define who we are as individuals. Individual sensory patterns can affect the way we react to everything that happens to us throughout the day.[11] One of the major roles of our senses is for perception—to sense and appreciate ourselves in the world around us. These perceptions are constantly being used and updated in the context of actions and in response to our environment. Sensations affect behavior in everyday life, from when we put our feet on the ground when we get out of bed in the morning to what we choose to wear.[9,11]

To understand sensory factors fully, we need to appreciate the totality of their impact: the interaction between person-level sensory factors, other person-level factors, the person's situation (ie, extrinsic factors), and the occupations of importance to the person's well-being (eg, activities, tasks, and role). Sensory factors interact with other person-level factors, such as movement and cognition. For example, upper limb function involves controlled, goal-directed movements of the upper limb that are guided and updated by vision and somatosensations. Sensory factors also interact with cognitive functions. Attention is critical to how we selectively attend to and perceive sensory information, and our senses form the basis for more complex cognitive functions, including remembering, producing and understanding language, solving problems, and making decisions.

These personal characteristics of the individual are further influenced by the unique environment in which the individual performs their tasks and activities, and the nature and meaning of the actions, tasks, and roles to the individual.[13] Impairment in sensory factors can have a major and ongoing impact on performance and lead to occupational deprivation, social isolation, or occupational gaps, as outlined in the following text.

Key knowledge, anatomical, physiological, and neuroscience, related to understanding our senses is outlined hereafter for each of our major senses. The role of these senses in supporting the occupational performance of an individual and how limitations might challenge a person's performance, participation, and well-being are then briefly discussed.

VISION

Key Knowledge: Anatomical, Physiological, Neuroscience

Vision is a complex sensation that provides information about our surrounding environment. The process giving rise to vision begins when the cornea and lens refract light from objects and surfaces in the world to form a panoramic hemispheric image on the retina, the thin layer of nerve cells that lines the inside surface of the eye (http://www.nihtoolbox.org/WhatAndWhy/Sensation/Vision/Pages/default.aspx).

The human visual system is a complex sensory system. The anatomy of the visual system is composed of photo-receptors in the outer layer of the retina, optic nerve, optic tract, extrageniculostriate pathway (involving the superior colliculi, pulvinar, and posterior parietal cortex), and retinogeniculstriate pathway (involving the lateral geniculate nuclei, striate cortex, and interior temporal cortex). Its widely distributed nature renders it vulnerable to insults along its long pathways.[14]

The human visual system, despite or because of its complexity, now appears to be extraordinarily plastic. Neural plasticity can improve vision leading to visual recovery. There is now good evidence that this can occur many years after brain injury, at any age, and in a range of visual pathway injuries.[14]

How Vision Supports the Occupational Performance of an Individual

Intact vision supports occupational performance particularly in areas such as reading, mobility (including driving), visual information processing (or "seeing"), and visually guided motor behavior (or manipulation) (http://www.nihtoolbox.org/WhatAndWhy/Sensation/Vision/Pages/default.aspx).

Using the Activity Inventory (AI), visual ability was defined as a composite variable with 2 factors; one most heavily influences reading function and the other most heavily influences mobility function.[15]

How Limitations Might Challenge a Person's Performance, Participation, and Well-Being

Loss of vision or blindness, due to disease or disorders of the visual system, may limit a person's ability to perform the occupational tasks outlined previously, and may impact on one's quality of life. The loss may be experienced as problems with resolution of detail; field of view; appearance of contrast, colors, and motion; depth perception; seeing in dim light; and disablement from glare. Visual acuity and visual field impairments are key features of vision loss that are commonly encountered in clinical settings. In community settings, many aspects of vision are seen as central to performance by occupational therapy practitioners working specifically with individuals with low vision.

Investigation of the determinants of participation in people with impaired vision found the areas of greatest restriction of participation were associated with reading, outdoor mobility, participation in leisure activities, and shopping.[16] Loss of vision can also impact on an individual's psychological well-being and quality of life. For example, in older people living in residential care, the quality of life aspects most affected by vision loss were related to general vision, reading, hobbies, emotional well-being, and social interaction.[17] Compromised vision also significantly increases the risk of having depression and hip fractures, needing community and/or family support, nursing home placement, and a low self-rating of health.[18] Non-correctable unilateral vision loss was associated with issues of safety and independent living, while non-correctable bilateral vision loss was associated with nursing home placement, emotional well-being, use of community services, and activities of daily living.[19]

In older adults, even mild levels of decreased vision were associated with lower participation in instrumental, leisure, and social activities.[20] Older spouses' vision impairment also negatively impacts on partner depression, physical functioning, well-being, social involvement, and marital quality; these effects were not greatly different in magnitude from those associated with the partners' own vision impairment.[21] Thus the impact of visual impairment on occupation and participation is highlighted.

AUDITION

Key Knowledge: Anatomical, Physiological, Neuroscience

Hearing is an obligatory, ongoing sensory function (ie, it cannot be turned off) (http://www.nihtoolbox.org/WhatAndWhy/Sensation/Audition/Pages/default.aspx).

The auditory system processes acoustic energy (sound) in order to allow us to hear. Sound enters the outer ear and travels down the ear canal to stimulate the eardrum, which transduces acoustic energy into mechanical energy. This mechanical energy is transmitted into electrochemical energy to activate the 8th cranial nerve (the auditory nerve). The neural signal is then transmitted through the brainstem to the midbrain, the thalamus, and the cortex where "perception" occurs. The auditory system has high sensitivity, sharp frequency tuning, fast temporal resolution, and a wide dynamic range (http://www.nihtoolbox.org/WhatAndWhy/Sensation/Audition/Pages/default.aspx).

How Audition Supports the Occupational Performance of an Individual, and How Limitations Might Challenge a Person's Performance, Participation, and Well-Being

Hearing is critical to be aware of and perceive elements of our environment from a distance; for example, to hear the approaching sound of a train at a railway crossing or to hear one's baby crying in another room. This has important implications for safety and performance of life roles. Hearing also has an important role in the development of language and speech. Children who experience long periods of auditory deprivation are susceptible to large-scale reorganization of auditory cortical areas responsible for the perception of speech and language.

SOMATOSENSATION, INCLUDING TOUCH (TACTILE) AND PROPRIOCEPTION

Key Knowledge: Anatomical, Physiological, Neuroscience

Somatic (body) sensation takes a number of forms, including touch, pressure, vibration, temperature, itch, tickle, and pain. The somatosensory system allows us to interpret sensory messages received from our body, and consists of sensory receptors located in the skin, tissues and joints, the nerve cell tracts in the body and spinal cord, and brain centers that process and modulate incoming sensory information.[8] Major brain regions involved in processing somatosensory information include the primary somatosensory cortex (SI), secondary somatosensory cortex (SII), thalamus, insula, posterior parietal cortex, and cerebellum.[22,23]

Sensory brain regions have varying roles in relation to information processing.[22] For example, SI is primarily involved in feature detection and remains somewhat modality-specific, although higher level processing also begins to take place in SI. SII is implicated in texture discrimination and tactile object recognition, and is considered to be specialized for tactile learning and tactile working memory.[22,24,25] The thalamus has an important role in gating of sensory information. A model of somatosensory information processing has been proposed by Dijkerman and de Haan[23] that relates to the purpose of the information processing: sensation for perception and sensation for action.

Key features of central processing of somatosensory information are critical in understanding the nature of somatosensory processing deficits after central nervous system lesions, as well as the potential for neural plasticity and recovery. These include parallel and serial processing, multiple and multimodal representations of sensory maps, functional and structural interhemispheric connections, and top-down and bottom-up influences on information processing.[22] Interactions with related networks such as attention and vision are also critical in understanding the central processing of somatosensory information.[26] Finally, there is increasing evidence of plasticity within the somatosensory system. Neural correlates of sensory recovery after stroke have been described.[27-29] These findings have implications for occupational therapy practitioners.

How Somatosensation Supports the Occupational Performance of an Individual

Somatosensations are important for perception and for action.[30] We need our body sensations to sense our environment and make quick adjustments. Sensation for perception involves characterizing and localizing touch and pain, sensing the position of different parts of the body with respect to one another, recognition of objects through the sense of touch, and memory of those perceptions.[30] It allows us to explore and interact with the world and others, to experience pleasure, and to be alerted to danger.[22]

Sensation also has an important role for action, particularly in relation to control of pinch grip,[31,32] ability to sustain and adapt appropriate force without vision,[33,34] object manipulation,[35] combining component parts of movement such as transport and grasp,[36] and adjustment to sensory conflict conditions (eg, rough surface).[22,37] Somatosensation, in particular proprioception, is also important in the learning of any new movement or skill. Proprioception is, in essence, a feedback mechanism; that is, the body moves (or is moved) and then the information about this is returned to the brain, whereby subsequent adjustments could be made. Somatosensory loss cannot be adequately compensated for by sight.

How Limitations Might Challenge a Person's Performance, Participation, and Well-Being

Somatosensory loss can have an ongoing and negative impact on individuals in their daily lives. Deficits in occupational performance outlined previously will have a negative impact on the ability to perform routine activities of daily living, such as dressing, doing up buttons, donning a bra at back, toileting and adjusting clothing, using a knife or fork, washing dishes, cooking, making the bed, writing or using a computer, sewing, wallet use, or turning key in lock as described by stroke survivors.[9,38] Moreover, the affected limb may not be used spontaneously, despite adequate movement abilities. This may contribute to a learned non-use of the limb and further deterioration of motor function.[9,38] Further, if holding a fork is labored and clumsy due to tactile loss, the individual may not engage in social activities, such as eating out with friends. The personal narratives included highlight the ongoing impact of sensory loss in terms of a person's performance, participation, and well-being. The impact of somatosen-

sory loss is hard to understand and is often under-rated.[9,39]

VESTIBULAR

Key Knowledge: Anatomical, Physiological, Neuroscience

The vestibular system is the sensory system that provides key information about movement and sense of balance. It comprises the labyrinth of the inner ear and the cochlea (a part of the auditory system). The system is used to indicate rotational movements (via the semicircular canal system) and linear accelerations (via the otoliths). The vestibular system sends signals that control our eye movements and projections to muscles that keep us upright. The vestibulo-ocular reflex (VOR) is a reflex eye movement that stabilizes images on the retina during head movement. It does not depend on visual input, and works when the eyes are closed and in total darkness. Since slight head movements are present all the time, the VOR is very important for stabilizing vision. When the vestibular system is stimulated without any other inputs, one experiences a sense of self-motion.

The system includes a complex multisensory interplay between the cortex, cerebellum, brainstem, spinal cord, eye, inner ear, and somatosensory inputs. It is a bilateral system with optimal interpretation of stimuli dependent upon input form left and right sides. Information processed by the vestibular system is, for the most part, concerned with automatic, subcortical control.

How Vestibular Function Supports the Occupational Performance of an Individual

The vestibular system is required for clear vision and to keep us upright. People whose VOR is impaired find it difficult to read because they cannot stabilize the eyes during small head movements. Vestibular function is also important for balance and equilibrium, and has an influence on motor and balance development.[40] When subjects stand on an unstable or compliant support surface, rather than a stable one, vestibular information becomes more important for the control of posture.

How Limitations Might Challenge a Person's Performance, Participation, and Well-Being

Diseases of the vestibular system usually induce vertigo and instability, often accompanied by nausea. People who experience impaired vestibular function and balance may lose the confidence to go outside, go to work, and perform domestic activities such as shopping and cooking.

OLFACTORY AND GUSTATORY

Key Knowledge: Anatomical, Physiological, Neuroscience

The sense of smell is mediated by specialized sensory cells of the nasal cavity in humans. Olfaction along with taste are referred as the chemosensory senses, because both transduce chemical senses into perception. The olfactory system comprises 2 distinct parts: a main olfactory system and an accessory olfactory system. The main olfactory system detects volatile, airborne substances, while the accessory olfactory system senses fluid-phase stimuli.

Humans receive tastes through sensory organs called taste buds that are concentrated on the top of the tongue, but are also throughout the oral cavity. The taste molecules that interact with these receptors can be separated into 5 primary taste qualities: sweet, salty, sour, bitter, or umami. The interaction between taste and smell is bidirectional.[41]

How the Sense of Smell and Taste Support the Occupational Performance of an Individual, and How Limitations Might Challenge a Person's Performance, Participation, and Well-Being

The ability to detect odors, to recognize and discriminate odor quality, and to identify the source of odors are primary functions of the olfactory system (http://www.nihtoolbox.org/WhatAndWhy/Sensation/Olfaction/Pages/default.aspx).

Olfaction is important in humans to detect and perceive volatile airborne chemicals that provide information about our environment and food quality that is critical to our health: a nutritious diet and psychological well-being.

MULTISENSORY PROCESSING

Key Knowledge: Anatomical, Physiological, Neuroscience

Multimodal integration, also known as *multisensory integration*, is the study of how information from the different sensory modalities, such as sight, sound, touch, smell, self-motion, and taste, may be integrated by the nervous system. Indeed, multisensory integration is central to adaptive behavior because it allows us to perceive a world of coherent perceptual entities.[42] Multimodal integration also deals with how different sensory modalities interact with one another and alter each other's processing. Multisensory integration can occur across various stages of stimulus processing that are linked to, and can be modulated by attention.[43]

Combining information across modalities can affect sensory performance. For example, there is evidence of multisensory enhancement of detection sensitivity for low-contrast visual stimuli by co-occurring sounds.[44] Multisensory convergence and integration take place at a number of brainstem and cortical sites. Key brain regions involved with multisensory processing include superior temporal sulcus (STS) and superior colliculus (SC).[45] It is thought that development of multisensory integration may be tied to sensory experiences acquired during postnatal life.[46]

How Multisensory Processing Supports the Occupational Performance of an Individual, and How Limitations Might Challenge a Person's Performance, Participation, and Well-Being

In conditions affected by problems with multisensory processing the individual may have difficulty adequately processing information in complex, multisensory environments. For example, children with developmental coordination disorder (DCD) experience difficulty participating in the typical activities of childhood and are known to have a more sedentary pattern of activities than their peers.[47] Developmental disorders and social functioning may also be affected by problems with multisensory processing, as is the case in autism spectrum disorders.[48] Elderly with multisensory processing problems may have difficulty moving safely and efficiently in their environment.

COMMON POPULATIONS/CONDITIONS AFFECTED BY SENSORY IMPAIRMENT

Cerebral Palsy

Children with cerebral palsy may experience impairment of one or more sensory modalities, and have difficulty with multisensory processing. Vision or ocular defects have been reported in 86% of children with cerebral palsy (see Table 16-1).[49]

Autism

There is a growing body of evidence that unusual sensory processing is at least a concomitant, and possibly the cause, of many of the behavioral signs and symptoms of autism spectrum disorders.[48] In a sample of 281 children with autism, 95% had difficulty with sensory processing.[50] Multisensory temporal processing is significantly altered in autism.[51] Cognitive neuroscience theory of multisensory integration has also been described in relation to autism.[52] Further, evidence suggests alterations in visual perception.[53]

Hand Injury

Somatosensory impairment may be caused by peripheral nerve injury or a peripheral neuropathy involving peripheral nerves of the somatosensory system. This may present as numbness or paresthesia. Changes in somatosensation may also be found in people who have a limb amputated. This may include hypersensitivity at the amputation site and a confused sense of that limb's existence on their body, known as phantom limb syndrome.

Spinal Cord Injury

People with spinal cord injury can experience loss of body sensation from the site of the lesion down. This can often be accompanied by paralysis, thus exacerbating the problem.

Multiple Sclerosis

Impairment in low-contrast vision has been described in multiple sclerosis.[54] People with multiple sclerosis may also experience impaired somatosensations.

Stroke

A stroke may lead to impairment in any of the senses. One in 2 stroke survivors lose the sense of touch and other body sensations after a stroke.[55] The types of visual impairment following stroke are wide ranging and included eye alignment/movement impairment (68%), visual field impairment (49%), low vision (26.5%), and perceptual difficulties (20.5%) in a prospective sample (N = 323) with suspected visual difficulty.[56] A substantial proportion of patients may also experience auditory functional limitations not limited to speech sounds after stroke of the auditory brain.[57]

Somatosensory loss following stroke contributes to inferior results in level of function and independence, mobility, activity performance, quality of life, longer rehabilitation, and discharge destination.[9,58] Patient groups with hemiparesis, hemihypesthesia, and/or hemianopia compared to hemiparesis alone show significantly poorer function[59] and time to maximal recovery.[60,61] Loss of sensation also negatively impacts personal safety, return to sexual and leisure activities, and reacquisition of skilled movements.[9,58,62]

Head Injury

Traumatic brain injury (TBI) patients may have sensory problems, especially problems with vision; they may not be able to register what they are seeing or may be slow to recognize objects. Also, TBI patients often have difficulty with hand-eye coordination, causing them to seem clumsy or unsteady. Other sensory deficits include problems with hearing, smell, taste, or touch. Post-concussive symptoms have been associated with sensory gating impairment.[63]

Elderly

Deterioration in the senses is evident with aging. Many individuals experience loss of vision and hearing in old age, in an increasing proportion from age 80 onward.[64] Age-related decline in somatosensory function, particularly in individuals 65 years and over, is well established and includes touch and proprioception.[65,66]

Visual impairment remains a major form of disability in individuals living in residential care facilities, and affects vision-specific functioning and socioemotional aspects of daily living.[17] Impaired somatosensory and/or vestibular function may impact on the high incidence of falls, which are a leading cause of death from injury.[67,68] Problems with multisensory processing are also linked with dementia and falls.

ASSESSMENTS AND EVALUATIONS

The purpose of assessment is to inform an understanding of the person's sensory information processing capacities and the impact of these on occupational performance, life roles, and well-being. The therapist uses this information to determine the person's capabilities and enablers and identify barriers and constraints to be considered in an intervention plan. This will involve using different types of assessments, as follows.

Personal Narrative and Occupational Goals

Occupational History

This is the opportunity to get to know the client, his or her perceptions, responsibilities, etc, and how the current situation and sensory factors impact on him or her. It is critical to appreciate the person's perceptions of the situation and the meaning they attribute to what they can or are limited in doing. What are the occupational performance problems identified by the client? What is the nature of the sensory deficit and how does it impact the client?

Current Situation

It is important to begin by asking the person about his or her awareness of any sensory changes and his or her perception of the impact of these changes on what he or she can do and what they need to do. Also identify your client's strengths and capacities. These may include motivation and attentional capacities to be involved in an intensive learning-based training program, or problem-solving abilities to be able to work through different challenges in different environments.

Client Goals

Because occupational therapy and the PEOP Model are based on a partnership with the client, it is important that you take time to understand your client's goals in relation to their sensory capacities. Understand how the impaired sensory capacities impact on the person (mind, brain, and body). The COPM is a useful tool to help assess occupational tasks impacted by the sensory impairment. Ask clients to identify occupational performance tasks that they think have been impacted by their sensory loss and are important to them, and then self-rate their performance and perceived satisfaction. Using this information, you can then match the client's needs and goals with knowledge of evidence-based interventions that may be appropriate. Determine with the client what will be the primary outcomes of interest; from performance to participation.

PEOP Occupational Therapy Process

The PEOP Occupational Therapy Process will bring together information from the narrative, formal assessments, observation, and testing of the impact of the loss in daily activities in the context of potential interventions and the client's expectations and goals regarding outcome. Together, these will help to summarize the client's perspectives and values.

Evidence-Based Formal Assessments

The directive to follow evidence-based practice demands that clinicians employ quantitative measures that are valid and reliable. Measurement of sensation spans multiple levels: from sensory thresholds of single modalities, defined using controlled psychophysical methods; through to functional sensibility, where the focus is on

measuring sensation that may include integration of more than one modality; to evaluation of performance on a task with specific sensory demands.[1-6,69] Changes in sensation at the receptor and threshold level do not necessarily have a direct relationship with change in functional sensibility, thus assessment across levels is typically required. The National Institute of Health Toolbox project has recently undertaken a major review of current measures to assess neurological and behavioral functions across the lifespan. A number of the suggestions following are based on recommendations from that group, as sourced on their website (http://www.nihtoolbox.org/WhatAndWhy/Sensation/Pages/default.aspx).

Vision

Visual acuity and visual fields are key aspects of vision that are commonly tested in clinical settings. Visual acuity is measured as the ratio of the viewing distance to the size of the smallest letters that can be read, or smallest symbols that can be recognized on a standard vision chart (http://www.vectorvision.com/html/educationETDRSAcuity.html). In assessing vision, one must also be aware of the impact of the environment and lighting. Performance on clinical measures of visual function were found to be better in the clinic than in the home in glaucoma and normal participants.[70] Illumination was substantially higher in the clinic than home.

The impact of vision loss on functional abilities and well-being are often assessed by using questionnaires such as the National Eye Institute's Visual Function Questionnaire (NEI VFQ) or Impact of Vision Impairment (IVI) questionnaire.[69] The instruments typically use a list of statements about specific activities that are answered in terms of frequency of occurrence, level of agreement, perceived difficulty, or some other response to each item using a categorical response rating scale (http://www.nihtoolbox.org/WhatAndWhy/Sensation/Vision/Pages/default.aspx). There are also Vision-Related Quality of Life Scales.

Vision may also need to be assessed in the context of particular occupations, such as driving, and in relation to specific driving conditions, such as at night, in the rain, on high traffic roads on highways, and in rush hour traffic—given associations with increasing visual loss.[71] The WHO uses a taxonomy to classify visual impairment as socially significant visual impairment, visual impairment, severe visual impairment, or blindness.[69]

Audition

A variety of techniques are available to assess and quantify hearing, including behavioral, psychophysical, and electrophysiological measures. Measures of hearing can be conducted on the right and left ears separately or on both ears at the same time (binaural hearing) (http://www.

nihtoolbox.org/WhatAndWhy/Sensation/Audition/Pages/default.aspx).

The range of sounds that can be heard varies across parameters of complexity, intensity, frequency, and temporal characteristics. The ability to determine where a sound is coming from and the direction of sound movement is also part of hearing. Hearing can be assessed in response to linguistic (eg, words) and nonlinguistic (tones, clicks) stimuli, and under optimal (quiet) and challenging (with competing sounds) conditions (http://www.nihtoolbox.org/WhatAndWhy/Sensation/Audition/Pages/default.aspx).

Sound repetition screening tests have been used as a bedside clinical test for stroke.[72] Hearing, communication function, and consequences of hearing loss should be assessed through self-report and reports of others, such as family members and caretakers. A hearing questionnaire may help identify patients who require more extensive assessment to inform rehabilitation plans.

Somatosensory Function

Numerous tests have been developed to evaluate the various qualities of sensibility, including touch, pressure, temperature, pain, proprioception, and tactual object recognition.[4,9,73] Quantitative tests of specific sensory functions that have been developed and empirically tested for use in clinical and research settings include:

- Semmes-Weinstein monofilaments and Weinstein Enhanced Sensory Test (WEST) hand monofilaments[1] to assess detection of light touch and deep pressure
- 2-point Disk-Criminator[74]
- Tactile Discrimination Test (TDT) to assess texture discrimination[2]
- Grating orientation discrimination test[75]
- AsTex test of touch sensibility[76]
- Shape/texture identification test (STI)[77]
- The Manual Form Perception Test[3]
- Pfizer (New York, NY) thermal tester and tuning fork or vibrometer[4]
- Wrist Position Sense Test[5]
- Kinesthesia Test[6]
- Hand Active Sensation Test[78]
- Functional Tactile Object Recognition Test (fTORT)[79]
- Modified Moberg pick up test[4]

The Hand Function survey[80] and Jebsen Taylor Hand Function Test[81] may be useful clinical measures, as they are associated with quantitatively defined sensory impairment and pinch grip deficit after stroke.[82]

Vestibular Function

Vestibular function should be assessed in relation to the angular vestibulo-ocular reflex (eg, gaze stabilization) and on performance dependent upon vestibulospinal output (eg, postural control output, or balance ability) (http://www.nihtoolbox.org/WhatAndWhy/Sensation/Vestibular/Pages/default.aspx).

Olfactory and Gustatory Function

Odor detection is evaluated by measuring the lowest concentration of an odorant at which an individual (a) can just detect the odor's presence or (b) can discriminate it from a sample of odorless air. Odor identification is evaluated by presenting individuals with a variety of recognizable smells at supra-threshold concentrations and requiring them to choose what the odor is from a set of possible names or pictures. Performance can be compared with age-adjusted and gender-adjusted norms.

Psychophysical measures of taste include measures of sensitivity, such as thresholds, just noticeable differences, intensity judgments, and sensory adaption, as well as estimates of liking or preference (http://www.nihtoolbox.org/WhatAndWhy/Sensation/Taste/Pages/default.aspx).

Multisensory Processing

One of the most basic measures of multisensory integration is intersensory facilitation of reaction times (RTs), in which bimodal targets, with cues from 2 sensory modalities, are detected faster than unimodal targets.[83] The Sensory Profile family of products, developed by Dunn and colleagues, is available to determine how individuals process sensory information (http://psychcorp.pearsonassessments.com/HAIWEB/Cultures/en-us/Productdetail.htm?Pid=076-1638-008&Mode=summary).

Observation in Occupational Tasks

Systematic observation of the impact of sensory capacities/limitations on occupational performance is critical. This will involve observation of occupational performance difficulties in tasks relevant to the patient and under conditions of variable sensory demand. For example, assessment of the impact of somatosensory impairment may be observed in the context of tasks, such as using a fork, which have a high somatosensory demand.[9] Further, as effective use of our senses is influenced by the environment, the client's current environment and social circumstances also need to be carefully evaluated.

INTERVENTIONS

Interventions for sensory factors may be part of a person-centered intervention plan. Evidence-based interventions

Table 16-3. *Evidence-Based Interventions for Sensation*

Recommended Interventions	Sense	Comment/Reference
Multidisciplinary low-vision rehabilitation program	Vision	18
Low vision aids		84
Boundary marking and scanning therapy for visual field deficits		http://www.eyeassociates.com/
Visual field perceptual training		85
Screen for visual impairment and improve lighting for older adults		20
Sensory re-education for peripheral nerve lesions	Touch	4
SENSe perceptual learning approach to sensory rehabilitation for stroke survivors	Touch, proprioception and tactile object recognition	86
Vestibular Rehabilitation Therapy	Vestibular	87
Applied Behavioural Analysis (ABA), Relationship Development Intervention (RDI) for autism	Multisensory	88, 89, 90
Sensory processing and integration		91, 92
Cognitive Orientation to Occupational Performance (CO-OP) intervention for DCD and stroke		93, 94

may be applied to the individual in the context of activities and goals identified by the client as being important. Interventions may include perceptual learning approaches, sensory stimulation, activity analysis, use of assistive technology, environmental strategies, and self-management strategies. Specific evidence-based approaches are outlined in the following text for each of the major sensory functions treated by occupational therapy practitioners. It is often the person-level factors that practitioners speak about when they are using an intervention to support recovery.[13]

Population-centered intervention plans may also be used to addressing sensory problems; for example, optimizing lighting levels in residential accommodation. Interventions developed at an organization level may target special groups, such special perceptual motor training for children with multisensory integration problems. Evidence-based interventions for sensory functions, focused on person-centered intervention plans, are outlined in Table 16-3.

Vision

Significant improvements in overall quality of life, emotional well-being, and 2 areas of daily living (reading and accessing information) were found in people with low vision following a multidisciplinary low-vision rehabilitation program that included occupational therapy practitioners, orientation and mobility, orthoptics, and welfare specialists.[18] Low-vision rehabilitation involves the provi-

sion of devices or training techniques for the enhancement of residual vision and devices or techniques for performing tasks without reliance on vision. The magnitude and clinical significance of the rehabilitation-induced gains were modest. It has been estimated that 90% of individuals with vision impairment have useful residual vision, which could benefit from low-vision rehabilitation programs.[18] Low-vision aids are an effective means of providing visual rehabilitation, helping almost 9 out of 10 patients with impaired vision to read.[84] Self-management programs for adults with low vision may include vision-specific strategies, training in generic problem-solving and goal setting skills, and how to cope with emotional reactions to vision impairment. However, barriers to participation were noted.[95] Involvement of spouses and other family members in rehabilitation may be important given the negative impact of the visual impairment on them, in addition to the visually impaired individual.[21]

Treatment of the hemianoptic patient, a common condition following stroke, includes the following:

- Teaching the patient basic strategies to overcome the hemianopsia (such as boundary marking, use of the finger or sticky note to mark edge of print) and encouraging the client to first look in the direction of the field loss before trying to search for an object
- Use of optical devices to shift the visual field over, including the Gottlieb Visual Field Awareness System

- Scanning therapy to train the patient to better compensate for the loss of visual field

At a population level, a low-cost public health intervention that involves screening for visual impairment in older adults, increasing levels of luminance in the home, and getting new glasses is recommended to improve activity participation and quality of life in older adults living in the community.[20]

Touch, Proprioception, and Tactile Object Recognition

Sensory re-education of patients with peripheral nerve disorders employ principles of direct, repeated sensory practice; feedback through vision; subjective grading of stimuli, such as texture and objects; verbalization of sensations; and comparison of sensations experienced across hands. Evidence for the effectiveness of sensory training following peripheral lesions is reviewed in Dellon.[4] Some programs are directed to localization of sensation and regeneration of specific nerve fibers. However, the need to focus on interpretation of altered stimuli at a cortical level based on evidence of neural plasticity is highlighted.[4]

There are a few documented and tested sensory retraining programs designed for use with stroke patients.[9,10,86,96,97] Yekutiel and Guttman[98] reported significant gains in 20 chronic stroke patients, based on a program that included focus on the hand, attention and motivation, guided exploration of the tactics of perception, and use of the "good" hand. Byl et al[99] described a program aimed to improve accuracy and speed in sensory discrimination and sensorimotor feedback. Principles included matching tasks to ability of the subject, attention, repetition, feedback on performance, and progression in difficulty. Carey et al developed and investigated the effectiveness of two different approaches to sensory discrimination training focused on the upper limb: Stimulus Specific Training (SST)[100] and Stimulus Generalization Training (SGT).[86,101] The approach is founded on principles of neural plasticity and perceptual learning, and includes attentive exploration with vision occluded, feedback on accuracy and method of exploration, internal calibration of the altered sensation via the other hand and vision, anticipation trials, intensive training, progression from easy to difficult discriminations, and variety of stimuli to facilitate transfer. Training involves discrimination of a variety of sensory attributes, such as roughness, limb position sense, and tactile object recognition across a matrix of sensory tasks including common textures, quantitative limb positions, and everyday objects. Improvement in functional sensory discrimination capacity was demonstrated in the randomized controlled trial Study of the Effectiveness of Neurorehabilitation on Sensation (SENSe).[86]

Vestibular

Although rehabilitation has been shown to facilitate recovery of vestibular-related impairments of balance, its success is dependent upon appropriate identification of the vestibular function (http://www.nihtoolbox.org/WhatAndWhy/Sensation/Vestibular/Pages/default.aspx).

Vestibular rehabilitation therapy (VRT), or more generally "balance rehabilitation," in a variety of conditions associated with dizziness has been advocated based on double-blinded placebo controlled trials.[87] Vestibular stimulation has also been used in the context of sensory integration.

Multisensory

Everyday experience affords us many opportunities to learn about objects through multiple senses using physical interaction. A range of interventions have been developed for use with children with autism. Review of these approaches and evidence to support them has been undertaken. The most researched is applied behavioral analysis.[89] Other approaches include developmental interventions focusing on relationship development; therapy interventions focusing on communication, social, and/or sensorimotor development; and combined interventions.[88] Reviews of sensory and motor interventions are available.[91,92] Intervention based on visual processing has also been described.[53]

Evidence indicates that active motor learning modulates the processing of multisensory associations.[102] *Dynamic Performance Analysis* is learned by children with DCD during CO-OP intervention.[93] The CO-OP intervention is a task-oriented approach that involves strategy use and guided discovery, rather than using direct skill training.[103]

There is some suggestion that a occupational therapy group using a sensory integration approach (OT-SI), compared to the other 2 groups, made significant gains on goal attainment scaling in children with sensory modulation disorder.[104]

The introduction of a motor and multisensory-based approach in care routines may improve residents' engagement and attention to the environment.[105] Systematic review on the effect of multisensory therapy in adult clients with developmental disabilities demonstrates a beneficial effect of multisensory therapy in promoting participants' positive emotions and behavior.[106]

OUTCOMES

Outcomes for individuals with sensory dysfunction will primarily be focused at a personal level. This may include

Table 16-4. *Organizations and Journals That Focus on Sensory Factors for Performance*

Organization or Journal	Description	Web Address
Society for Sensory Professionals	A nonprofit organization devoted to developing and promoting the field of sensory science. Creates forums for sharing research, provides mentoring in the field, provides training courses and educational seminars, and links with existing organizations that serve the sensory and consumer research community.	http://www.sensorysociety.org/
Sensory Processing Disorder Foundation	A world leader in research, education, and advocacy for Sensory Processing Disorder (SPD). Conducts research; educates caregivers, pediatric professionals, and educators; and empowers scientists to study the diagnosis and treatment of SPD.	http://spdfoundation.net/index.html
American Journal of Occupational Therapy	Peer-reviewed journal focuses on research, practice, and health care issues in the field of occupational therapy, and covers issues regarding sensory issues faced by people served by occupational therapy.	http://ajot.aota.org/

improvement in sensory capacity, such as texture discrimination; following an active perceptual learning-based approach; and improved performance in tasks requiring use of sensory information, such as using a fork without dropping it from grip. In turn, this is likely to impact on the person's confidence and ability to participate in tasks that are important to them, such as independently using cutlery at mealtimes and socializing with friends at a restaurant. Improvement in occupational tasks that are important to the client and active participation in life activities are all critical to good health and well-being. One stroke survivor who participated in an active learning-based neuroscience approach to sensory rehabilitation known as SENSe[86] made the following comment after training:

> Since undertaking sensory retraining, all tasks using my stroke-affected hand are easier and require less concentration. It still doesn't feel as though I have as much sense of touch in my stroke affected hand, but obviously my brain is making sense of a lot of information, as I am now quite competently performing most tasks. Because things require less concentration, I am less frustrated and fatigued, leaving more brain space and energy for enjoying life and assisting others. I am able to celebrate more things I can do rather than feel the setbacks of the things I can't do or struggle with.

Other outcomes that may also be important to match the needs and goals of individuals are to adapt the way certain tasks are achieved within the barriers imposed by the sensory loss. For example, a person who is blind may use special equipment when cooking, and low-vision aids may be used to assist an elderly person to remain independent in their home. Assisting the client to adapt their environment (eg, better lighting in the home) may also ensure success and participation in activities that the client enjoys, such as reading or doing crossword puzzles. As previously discussed, outcomes may also be important at a population level, such as using Braille signs in public places and improving lighting in residential care settings.

SUMMARY

The impact of sensory factors on performance, participation, and well-being have been described and personal insights provided. Occupational therapy practitioners will encounter sensory factors as being important for a number of major health conditions, as identified. Established, quantitative assessments may be used to detect and understand the nature of the sensory processing dysfunction in the context of the client's goals and environment. A number of approaches have been developed and tested to address the sensory processing deficits and associated limitations. The task of the practitioner is to work in partnership with their client to identify appropriate evidence-based interventions that match the client's goals (Table 16-4).

REFERENCES

1. Weinstein S. Fifty years of somatosensory research: from the Semmes-Weinstein monofilaments to the Weinstein Enhanced Sensory Test. *Journal of Hand Therapy.* 1993;Jan-Mar:11-28.

2. Carey LM, Oke LE, Matyas TA. Impaired touch discrimination after stroke: a quantitative test. *Neurorehabilitation and Neural Repair.* 1997;11(4):219-232.

3. Ayres AJ. *Southern California Sensory Integration Tests.* Rev ed. Los Angeles, CA: Western Psychological Services; 1980.

4. Dellon AL. *Somatosensory Testing and Rehabilitation.* Baltimore, MD: Institute for Peripheral Nerve Surgery; 2000.

5. Carey LM, Oke LE, Matyas TA. Impaired limb position sense after stroke: a quantitative test for clinical use. *Archives of Physical Medicine and Rehabilitation.* 1996;77(12):1271-1278.

6. Ayres AJ. *Southern California Sensory Integration Tests: Manual.* Los Angeles, CA: Western Psychological Services; 1972.

7. Pomerantz JR. Perception: overview. In: Nadel L, ed. *Encyclopedia of Cognitive Science.* Vol 3. London, UK: Nature Publishing Group; 2003:527-537.

8. Puce A, Carey L. Somatosensory function. In: Weiner IB, Craighead WE, Nemeroff CB, eds. *The Corsini Encyclopedia of Psychology.* 4th ed. New York, NY: John Wiley & Sons, Inc; 2010.

9. Carey LM. Somatosensory loss after stroke. *Critical Reviews in Physical and Rehabilitation Medicine.* 1995;7(1):51-91.

10. Carey LM. Loss of somatic sensation. In: Selzer M, Clarke S, Cohen L, Duncan P, Gage FH, eds. *Textbook of Neural Repair and Rehabilitation. Vol II. Medical Neurorehabilitation.* Cambridge, UK: Cambridge University Press; 2006:231-247.

11. Dunn W. Living *Sensationally: Understanding Your Senses.* London, UK: Jessica Kingsley Publishers; 2008.

12. Lyons W. *Left of Tomorrow.* Glen Waverley, Australia: Sid Harta Publishers; 2010.

13. Lou JQ, Lane SJ. Personal performance capabilities and their impact on occupational performance. In: Christiansen CH, Baum CM, Bass-Haugen J, eds. *Occupational Therapy: Performance, Particpation, and Well-Being.* 3rd ed. Thorofare, NJ: SLACK Incorporated; 2005.

14. Brodtmann A. Vision. In: Carey LM, ed. *Stroke Rehabilitation: Insights from Neuroscience and Neuroimaging.* New York, NY: Oxford University Press; 2012:173-190.

15. Massof RW, Ahmadian L, Grover LL, et al. The activity inventory: an adaptive visual function questionnaire. *Optometry and Vision Science.* 2007;84(8):763-774.

16. Lamoureux EL, Hassell JB, Keeffe JE. The determinants of participation in activities of daily living in people with impaired vision. *American Journal of Ophthalmology.* 2004;137(2):265-270.

17. Lamoureux EL, Fenwick E, Moore K, Klaic M, Borschmann K, Hill K. Impact of the severity of distance and near-vision impairment on depression and vision-specific quality of life in older people living in residential care. *Investigative Ophthalmology and Visual Science.* 2009;50(9):4103-4109.

18. Lamoureux EL, Pallant JF, Pesudovs K, Rees G, Hassell JB, Keeffe JE. The effectiveness of low-vision rehabilitation on participation in daily living and quality of life. *Investigative Ophthalmology and Visual Science.* 2007;48(4):1476-1482.

19. Vu HTV, Keeffe JE, McCarty CA, Taylor HR. Impact of unilateral and bilateral vision loss on quality of life. *British Journal of Ophthalmology.* 2005;89(3):360-363.

20. Perlmutter MS, Bhorade A, Gordon M, Hollingsworth HH, Baum MC. Cognitive, visual, auditory, and emotional factors that affect participation in older adults. *American Journal of Occupational Therapy.* 2010;64(4):570-579.

21. Strawbridge WJ, Wallhagen MI, Shema SJ. Impact of spouse vision impairment on partner health and well-being: a longitudinal analysis of couples. *Journals of Gerontology Series B: Psychological Sciences and Social Sciences.* 2007;62(5):S315-S322.

22. Carey LM. Touch and body sensations. In: Carey LM, ed. *Stroke Rehabilitation: Insights from Neuroscience and Imaging.* New York, NY: Oxford University Press; 2012:157-172.

23. Dijkerman HC, de Haan EH. Somatosensory processing subserving perception and action: dissociations, interactions, and integration. *Behavioral and Brain Sciences.* 2007;30(2):224-230.

24. Kandel ER, Jessell TM. Touch. In: Kandel ER, Schwartz JH, Jessell TM, eds. *Principles of Neural Science.* 3rd ed. London, UK: Prentice Hall; 1991.

25. Burton H, Sinclair RJ, Wingert JR, Dierker DL. Multiple parietal operculum subdivisions in humans: tactile activation maps. *Somatosensory and Motor Research.* 2008;25(3):149-162.

26. Corbetta M. Functional connectivity and neurological recovery. *Developmental Psychobiology.* 2011.

27. Rossini PM, Altamura C, Ferreri F, et al. Neuroimaging experimental studies on brain plasticity in recovery from stroke. *Europa Medicophysica.* 2007;43:241-254.

28. Staines WR, Graham SJ, Black SE, McIlroy WE. Task-relevant modulation of contralateral and ipsilateral primary somatosensory cortex and the role of prefrontal-cortical sensory gating systems. *Neuroimage.* 2002;15(1):190-199.

29. Carey LM, Abbott DF, Harvey MR, Puce A, Seitz RJ, Donnan GA. Relationship between touch impairment and brain activation after lesions of subcortical and cortical somatosensory regions. *Neurorehabilitation and Neural Repair.* 2011;25(5):443-457.

30. Dijkerman HC, de Haan EH. Somatosensory processes subserving perception and action. *Behavioral and Brain Sciences.* 2007;30(2):189-201.

31. Johansson RS, Westling G. Roles of glabrous skin receptors and sensorimotor memory in automatic control of precision grip when lifting rougher or more slippery objects. *Experimental Brain Research.* 1984;56:550-564.

32. Blennerhassett JM, Matyas TA, Carey LM. Impaired discrimination of surface friction contributes to pinch grip deficit after stroke. *Neurorehabilitation and Neural Repair.* 2007;21(3):263-272.

33. Blennerhassett JM, Carey LM, Matyas TA. Grip force regulation during pinch grip lifts under somatosensory guidance: comparison between people with stroke and healthy controls. *Archives of Physical Medicine and Rehabilitation.* 2006;87(3):418-429.

34. Jeannerod M, Michel F, Prablanc C. The control of hand movements in a case of hemianaesthesia following a parietal lesion. *Brain.* 1984;107:899-920.

35. Hermsdörfer J, Hagl E, Nowak D, Marquardt C. Grip force control during object manipulation in cerebral stroke. *Clinical Neurophysiology.* 2003;114:915-929.

36. Gentilucci M, Toni I, Daprati E, Gangitano M. Tactile input of the hand and the contol of reaching to grasp movements. *Experimental Brain Reseach.* 1997;114:130-137.

37. Wing AM, Flanagan JR, Richardson J. Anticipatory postural adjustments in stance and grip. *Experimental Brain Reseach.* 1997;116(1):122-130.

38. Mastos M, Carey L. Occupation-based outcomes associated with sensory retraining post-stroke. *International Journal of Stroke.* 2010;(Suppl 1, Sept).

39. Robles-De-La-Torre G. The importance of the sense of touch in virtual and real environments. *IEEE Multimedia.* 2006;13(3):24-30.

40. Rine RM, Cornwall G, Gan K, et al. Evidence of progressive delay of motor development in children with sensorineural hearing loss and concurrent vestibular dysfunction. *Perceptual and Motor Skills.* 2000;90:1101-1112.

41. Yeshurun Y, Sobel N. Multisensory integration: an inner tongue puts an outer nose in context. *Nature Neuroscience.* 2010;13(2):148-149.

42. Lewkowicz DJ, Ghazanfar AA. The emergence of multisensory systems through perceptual narrowing. *TRENDS in Cognitive Sciences*. 2009;13(11):470-478.

43. Talsma D, Senkowski D, Soto-Faraco S, Woldorff MG. The multifaceted interplay between attention and multisensory integration. *TRENDS in Cognitive Sciences*. 2010;14(9):400-410.

44. Noesselt T, Tyll S, Boehler CN, Budinger E, Heinze HJ, Driver J. Sound-induced enhancement of low-intensity vision: multisensory influences on human sensory-specific cortices and thalamic bodies relate to perceptual enhancement of visual detection sensitivity. *Journal of Neuroscience*. 2010;30(41):13609-13623.

45. Ursino M, Cuppini C, Magosso E, Serino A, di Pellegrino G. Multisensory integration in the superior colliculus: a neural network model. *Journal of Computational Neuroscience*. 2009;26(1):55-73.

46. Wallace MT. The development of multisensory processes. *Cognitive Processes*. 2004;5:69-83.

47. Mandich AD, Polatajko HJ, Rodger S. Rites of passage: Understanding of children with developmental coordination disorder. *Human Movement Science*. 2003;22(4-5):583-595.

48. Simmons DR, Robertson AE, McKay LS, Toal E, McAleer P, Pollick FE. Vision in autism spectrum disorders. *Vision Research*. 2009;49(22):2705-2739.

49. Lo Cascio GP. A study of vision in cerebral palsy. *American Journal of Optometry and Physiological Optics*. 1977;54(5):332-337.

50. Tomchek SD, Dunn W. Sensory processing in children with and without autism: a comparative study using the short sensory profile. *American Journal of Occupational Therapy*. 2007;61(2):190-200.

51. Kwakye LD, Foss-Feig JH, Cascio CJ, Stone WL, Wallace MT. Altered auditory and multisensory temporal processing in autism spectrum disorders. *Frontiers in Integrative Neuroscience*. 2011;4:Article 129.

52. Iarocci G, McDonald J. Sensory integration and the perceptual experience of persons with autism. *Journal of Autism and Developmental Disorders*. 2006;36(1):77-90.

53. Carey LM. Loss of somatic sensation. In: Selzer N, Clarke S, Cohen L, Kwakkel G, Miller R, eds. *Textbook of Neural Repair and Rehabilitation. Vol II: Medical Neurorehabilitation*. 2nd ed. Cambridge, UK: Cambridge University Press; 2012.

54. Balcer LJ, Baier ML, Pelak VS, et al. New low-contrast vision charts: reliability and test characteristics in patients with multiple sclerosis. *Multiple Sclerosis*. 2000;6(3):163-171.

55. Carey LM, Matyas TA. Frequency of discriminative sensory loss in the hand after stroke. *Journal of Rehabilitation Medicine*. 2011;43(3):257-263.

56. Rowe F, Brand D, Jackson CA, et al. Visual impairment following stroke: do stroke patients require vision assessment? *Age and Ageing*. 2009;38(2):188-193.

57. Bamiou D-E, Werring D, Cox K, et al. Patient-reported auditory functions after stroke of the central auditory pathway. *Stroke*. 2012;43(5):1285-1289.

58. Sullivan JE, Hedman LD. Sensory dysfunction following stroke: incidence, significance, examination, and intervention. *Topics in Stroke Rehabilitation*. 2008;15(3):200-217.

59. Han L, Law-Gibson D, Reding M. Key neurological impairments influence function-related group outcomes after stroke. *Stroke*. 2002;33(7):1920-1924.

60. Reding MJ, Potes E. Rehabilitation outcome following initial unilateral hemispheric stroke: life table analysis approach. *Stroke*. 1988;19:1354-1358.

61. Dromerick AW, Reding MJ. Functional outcome for patients with hemiparesis, hemihypesthesia, and hemianopsia. Does lesion location matter? *Stroke*. 1995;26(11):2023-2026.

62. Schaechter JD, Moore CI, Connell BD, Rosen BR, Dijkhuizen RM. Structural and functional plasticity in the somatosensory cortex of chronic stroke patients. *Brain*. 2006;129(10):2722-2733.

63. Kumar S, Roa SL, Nair RG, Pillai S, Chandramouli BA, Subbakrishna DK. Sensory gating impairment in development of post-concussive symptoms in mild head injury. *Psychiatry and Clinical Neurosciences*. 2005;59:466-472.

64. Bergman B, Rosenhall U. Vision and hearing in old age. *Scandinavian Audiology*. 2001;30(4):255-263.

65. Wickremaratchi M, Llewelyn JG. Effects of ageing on touch. *Postgraduate Medical Journal*. 2006;82:301-304.

66. Ribeiro F, Oliveira J. Aging effects on joint proprioception: the role of physical activity in proprioception preservation. *European Review of Aging and Physical Activity*. 2007;4(2):71-76.

67. Stevens J, Olsen S. *Reducing Falls and Resulting Hip Fractures Among Older Women*. National Center for Injury Prevention and Control, Division of Unintentional Injury. http://www.cdc.gov/mmwr/preview/mmwrhtml/rr4902a2.htm. Published 2000. Accessed March 5, 2012.

68. Shaffer SW, Harrison AL. Aging of the somatosensory system: a translational perspective. *Physical Therapy*. 2007;87(2):193-207.

69. Lamoureux EL, Pallant JF, Pesudovs K, Hassell JB, Keeffe JE. The impact of vision impairment questionnaire: an evaluation of its measurement properties using Rasch analysis. *Investigative Ophthalmology and Visual Science*. 2006;47(11):4732-4741.

70. Bhorade AM, Perlmutter MS, Chang ST, et al. The relationship between lighting and clinical measures of visual function at home and in the clinic in normal and glaucoma participants. *Investigative Ophthalmology and Visual Science*. 2009;50:E-abstract 3776.

71. Bhorade AM, Perlmutter MS, Wilson BS, et al. The impact of glaucoma severity on driving difficulty. *Investigative Ophthalmology and Visual Science*. 2010;51:E-abstract 943.

72. Edwards DF, Hahn MG, Baum CM, Perlmutter MS, Sheedy C, Dromerick AW. Screening patients with stroke for rehabilitation needs: validation of the post-stroke rehabilitation guidelines. *Neurorehabilitation and Neural Repair*. 2006;20(1):42-48.

73. Shy ME, Frohman EM, So YT, et al. Quantitative sensory testing—report of the therapeutics and technology assessment subcommittee of the American Academy of Neurology. *Neurology*. 2003;60(6):898-904.

74. Mackinnon SE, Dellon AL. Two point discrimination tester. *Journal of Hand Surgery*. 1985;10:906-907.

75. Van Boven RW, Johnson KO. The limit of tactile spatial resolution in humans: grating orientation discrimination at the lip, tongue, and finger. *Neurology*. 1994;44(12):2361-2366.

76. Miller KJ, Phillips BA, Martin CL, Wheat HE, Goodwin AW, Galea MP. The AsTex: clinimetric properties of a new tool for evaluating hand sensation following stroke. *Clinical Rehabilitation*. 2009;23(12):1104-1115.

77. Rosen B, Lundborg G. A new tactile gnosis instrument in sensibility testing. *Journal of Hand Therapy*. 1998;11:251-257.

78. Williams PS, Basso M, Case-Smith J, Nichols-Larsen DS. Development of the hand active sensation test: reliability and validity. *Archives of Physical Medicine and Rehabilitation*. 2006;87:1471-1477.

79. Carey LM, Nankervis J, LeBlanc S, Harvey L. *A New Functional Tactual Object Recognition Test (Ftort) for Stroke Clients: Normative Standards and Discriminative Validity*. Paper presented at: 14th International Congress of the World Federation of Occupational Therapists; Sydney, Australia; July 23-28, 2006.

80. Blennerhassett JM, Avery RM, Carey LM. The test-retest reliability and responsiveness to change for the Hand Function Survey during stroke rehabilitation. *Australian Occupational Therapy Journal*. 2010;57:355-446.

81. Jebsen R, Taylor N, Trieschmann R, Howard L. An objective and standardized test of hand function. *Archives of Physical Medicine and Rehabilitation.* 1969;50(6):311-319.

82. Blennerhassett JM, Carey LM, Matyas TA. Clinical measures of handgrip limitation relate to impaired pinch grip force control after stroke. *Journal of Hand Therapy.* 2008;21(3):245-252.

83. Williams LE, Light GA, Braff DL, Ramachandran VS. Reduced multisensory integration in patients with schizophrenia on a target detection task. *Neuropsychologia.* 2010;48(10):3128-3136.

84. Margrain TH. Helping blind and partially sighted people to read: the effectiveness of low vision aids. *British Journal of Ophthalmology.* 2000;84(8):919-921.

85. Zihl J, Von Cramon D. Restitution of visual function in patients with cerebral blindness. *Journal of Neurology, Neurosurgery, and Psychiatry.* 1979;42:312-322.

86. Carey LM, Macdonnell R, Matyas T. SENSe: study of the effectiveness of neurorehabilitation on sensation: a randomized controlled trial. *Neurorehabilitation and Neural Repair.* 2011;25:304-313.

87. Hillier SL, McDonnell M. Vestibular rehabilitation for unilateral peripheral vestibular dysfunction to improve dizziness, balance, and mobility. *Cochrane Database of Systematic Reviews.* 2011;2:CD005397.

88. Prior M, Roberts JMA, Rodger S, Williams K, Sutherland R. A review of the research to identify the most effective models of practice in early intervention of children with autism spectrum disorders. Greenway, Canberra, Australia: Australian Government Department of Families, Housing, Community Services and Indigenous Affairs; 2011.

89. Spreckley M, Boyd R. Efficacy of applied behavioural intervention in preschool children with autism for improving cognitive, language, and adaptive behavior: a systematic review and meta-analysis. *Journal of Pediatrics.* 2009;154:338-344.

90. Gutstein SE, Burgess AF, Montfort K. Evaluation of the relationship development intervention program. *Autism.* 2007;11(5):397-411.

91. Dawson G, Watling R. Interventions to facilitate auditory, visual, and motor integration in autism: a review of the evidence. *Journal of Autism and Developmental Disorders.* 2000;30(5):415-421.

92. Baranek GT. Efficacy of sensory and motor interventions for children with autism. *Journal of Autism and Developmental Disorders.* 2002;32(5):397-422.

93. Hyland M, Polatajko HJ. Enabling children with developmental coordination disorder to self-regulate through the use of dynamic performance analysis: evidence from the CO-OP approach. *Hum Mov Sci.* 2012;31(4):987-998.

94. Henshaw E, Polatajko H, McEwen S, Ryan JD, Baum CM. Cognitive approach to improving participation after stroke: two case studies. *American Journal of Occupational Therapy.* 2011;65(1):55-63.

95. Rees G, Saw CL, Lamoureux EL, Keeffe JE. Self-management programs for adults with low vision: needs and challenges. *Patient Education and Counseling.* 2007;69(1-3):39-46.

96. Doyle S, Bennett S, Fasoli SE, McKenna KT. Interventions for sensory impairment in the upper limb after stroke. *Cochrane Database of Systematic Reviews.* 2010;6:CD006331.

97. Schabrun SM, Hillier S. Evidence for the retraining of sensation after stroke: a systematic review. *Clinical Rehabilitation.* 2009;23(1):27-39.

98. Yekutiel M, Guttman E. A controlled trial of the retraining of the sensory function of the hand in stroke patients. *Journal of Neruology, Neurosurgery, and Psychiatry.* 1993;56:241-244.

99. Byl N, Roderick J, Mohamed O, et al. Effectiveness of sensory and motor rehabilitation of the upper limb following the principles of neuroplasticity: patients stable poststroke. *Neurorehabilitation and Neural Repair.* 2003;17:176-191.

100. Carey LM, Matyas TA, Oke LE. Sensory loss in stroke patients: effective training of tactile and proprioceptive discrimination. *Archives of Physical Medicine and Rehabilitation.* 1993;74(6):602-611.

101. Carey LM, Matyas TA. Training of somatosensory discrimination after stroke: facilitation of stimulus generalization. *American Journal of Physical Medicine and Rehabilitation.* 2005;84(6):428-442.

102. Butler AJ, James TW, James KH. Enhanced multisensory integration and motor reactivation after active motor learning of audiovisual associations. *Journal of Cognitive Neuroscience.* 2011;23(11):3515-3528.

103. Polatajko HJ, Mandich A. *Enabling Occupation in Children: The Cognitive Orientation to Daily Occupations Performance (CO-OP) Approach.* Ottawa, ON: CAOT Publications ACE; 2004.

104. Miller LJ, Coll JR, Schoen SA. A randomized controlled pilot study of the effectiveness of occupational therapy for children with sensory modulation disorder. *American Journal of Occupational Therapy.* 2007;61(2):228-238.

105. Cruz J, Marques A, Barbosa AL, Figueiredo D, Sousa L. Effects of a motor and multisensory-based approach on residents with moderate-to-severe dementia. *American Journal of Alzheimer's Disease and Other Dementias.* 2011;26(4):282-289.

106. Chan SWC, Thompson DR, Chau JPC, Tam WWS, Chiu IWS, Lo SHS. The effects of multisensory therapy on behaviour of adult clients with developmental disabilities-A systematic review. *International Journal of Nursing Studies.* 2010;47(1):108-122.

Chapter 17

PERSON FACTORS
Motor

Lisa L. Dutton, PhD, PT and Julie D. Bass, PhD, OTR/L, FAOTA

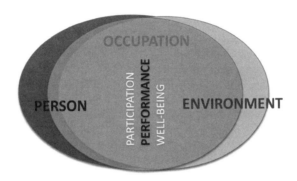

LEARNING OBJECTIVES

- Identify and define the primary motor factors that influence performance and participation.
- Describe how constraints/barriers in motor factors may affect a person's performance, participation, and well-being.
- Identify major health conditions or disabilities in which motor factors could influence performance, participation, and well-being.
- Demonstrate your understanding of motor factors in occupational performance through structured observation and task analysis.
- Identify established assessments that are evidence-based and measure capabilities and limitations related to occupational performance.
- Identify intervention principles to address motor factors that are limiting occupational performance.
- Describe 3 to 5 intervention approaches that would address limitations associated with motor factors.

- Recognize the complexity of how factors interact with other person and environment factors as it relates to performance in everyday life.

KEY WORDS

- Abnormal synergy
- Associated movement
- Athetosis
- Balance
- Blocked practice
- Bradykinesia
- Chorea
- Coordination
- Distributed practice
- Dysdiadochokinesis
- Extrinsic or augmented feedback
- Hypermetria

Christiansen CH, Baum CM, Bass JD, eds.
Occupational Therapy: Performance, Participation, and Well-Being, Fourth Edition (pp 267-287).
© 2015 SLACK Incorporated.

- Hypometria
- Intrinsic feedback
- Massed practice
- Motor control
- Motor learning
- Muscle tone
- Reflex
- Rigidity
- Spasticity
- Strength
- Tremors
- Variable practice

INTRODUCTION

The ability to move is essential for independent performance of basic activities, such as eating, communicating, and walking, and provides a foundation for full participation in life roles, such as family, work, and community engagement. Consider a recent client receiving outpatient rehabilitation services following a stroke. This individual is a retired high school music teacher who now, in addition to a mild cognitive impairment, has limited use of his left upper and lower extremity. His inability to generate skilled movement impacts his independent participation in previously important activities; tasks; and roles, such as self-care, transfers, gait, volunteer work, and leisure pursuits, including musical expression and woodworking. Furthermore, his social context and self-image as a father are altered, in that he now lives with and relies on his daughter for assistance. He expresses his most immediate goal as a desire to move back to his home. Accomplishing this goal requires independent performance of transfers and activities to support his daily living, both of which require him to generate movement.

Theories of Motor Control

As illustrated previously, movement is essential for performance of daily activities, as well as participation in everyday life. Motor control has been defined as "the ability to regulate or direct the mechanisms essential to movement."[1(p3)] Theories of motor control influence how movement and movement dysfunction are conceptualized and addressed. For example, one theory of motor control is the Reflex Model. This model, which is attributed to Sir Charles Sherrington, suggests that reflexes form the basis of all movement and, as such, sensory input is directly linked to motor output.[2] An occupational therapy practi-

tioner operating from this perspective might focus his or her examination on reflex testing as a measure of motor integrity. Another historically influential model is the Hierarchical Model. The Hierarchical Model was first suggested by Hughlings Jackson, and posits that the nervous system is organized in a top-down manner from the cortex to the spinal cord, with higher centers responsible for inhibiting lower centers.[3] More recently, the Systems Model has emerged as a dominant theory of motor control. In this model, described by Shumway-Cook and Woollacott, movement arises out of interplay between the individual, the task, and the environment.[1] Individual or person-oriented factors that contribute to movement include systems related to perception, action, and cognition. The amount of transport and level of manipulation involved in an activity are important considerations associated with the task and environmental factors, and include conditions to which the movement must conform (regulatory) as well as non-regulatory conditions, such as noise or other distractions.[4]

Motor Control Within the Person-Environment-Occupational Performance Model

The Systems Model can be viewed from the perspective of the PEOP Model. The individual in the Systems Model is equivalent to the person in the PEOP Model, although the PEOP Model extends this concept to include spirituality/meaning as an intrinsic aspect of the individual—which is not discussed in the motor control literature, but is important in motivating an individual to do the tasks that are meaningful to them. The task can be seen as part of occupation within the PEOP Model; the environment in systems theory addresses the physical environment, which is one aspect of environment in the PEOP Model. In the Systems Model, movement arises from the interaction of the individual, task, and environment. The PEOP Model describes this in broader terms, with the movement of the Systems Model being a component of the performance of occupation (doing) that is described in the PEOP Model. This occupational performance then gives rise to participation (engagement) and sense of well-being (satisfaction). From a Systems Model perspective, the focus of this chapter will be on individual factors related to action or motor output. This includes person motor factors in the PEOP Model, such as reflexes, tone, strength, motor control, motor planning, coordination, and postural control. See Figure 17-1 for a depiction of the interface between the systems and the PEOP Models.

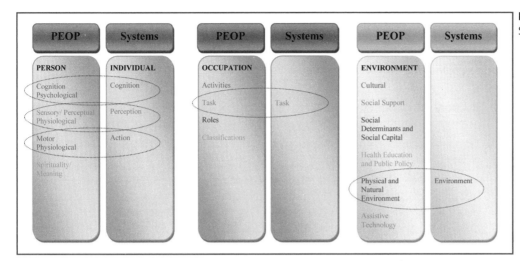

Figure 17-1. PEOP and Systems models.

Common Health Conditions, Motor Control, and Occupational Performance

Impaired motor function can occur secondary to both congenital and acquired health conditions, and these conditions can be classified as progressive or non-progressive. How a condition is classified may significantly impact the client's narrative. For example, a client with amyotrophic lateral sclerosis (ALS), which is an acquired, progressive condition, may have different needs and goals than an individual with Guillain-Barré syndrome (GBS), which is an acquired, non-progressive condition. Specifically, the individual with ALS is likely to experience ongoing decline of motor performance and may be interested in compensation and environmental modification to support his or her ongoing participation in everyday life. In contrast, the individual with GBS is likely to anticipate improvement in motor performance and may be more interested in pursuing restoration of motor function and realizing full recovery of previous levels of participation. For neuromuscular disorders, classification can also include differentiation between central and peripheral disorders. This distinction can guide occupational therapy examination and intervention. For example, one would not expect increased tone or abnormal movement patterns in an individual with a peripheral disorder, whereas this might be expected in an individual with a condition that affects the central nervous system (CNS). For a summary of common health conditions likely to result in motor dysfunction, please refer to Table 17-1.

ASSESSMENTS AND EVALUATIONS

Reflexes

"A reflex is an involuntary, stereotyped response to a particular stimulus."[15(p170)]

The stretch reflex is a spinal level reflex that occurs in response to muscle stretch. During an occupational therapy examination, this reflex is most commonly elicited by tapping on the muscle tendon with a reflex hammer. The expected response is a slight contraction of the muscle that was tapped, and these reflex responses are often graded on the following scale[16]:

- 0 = No response
- 1+ = Present but depressed, low normal
- 2+ = Average, normal
- 3+ = Increased, brisker than average; possibly but not necessarily abnormal
- 4+ = Very brisk, hyperactive, with clonus; abnormal

A description of the examination procedure for selected stretch reflexes is provided in Table 17-2. Low or depressed reflex responses are indicative of possible nerve impingement, as might be observed in carpal tunnel syndrome. An increased or hyperactive response is suggestive of a CNS condition.

Primitive reflexes are brainstem level reflexes that are present at birth. In typically developing infants, primitive reflexes are difficult to elicit after 6 months of age because these responses are inhibited as the CNS develops.[19,20] Children with CNS conditions, such as CP, may exhibit a delay in the onset and subsequent persistence of these

Table 17-1. *Common Conditions Associated With Impaired Motor Function*

Common Conditions	Brief Description of Condition
Amyotrophic lateral sclerosis	Amyotrophic lateral sclerosis is a progressive disease of unknown etiology in which the upper and lower motor neurons that control voluntary muscle action waste away or die resulting in the development of weakness throughout the body.[5]
Cerebral palsy	CP is a disorder of movement and posture that is caused by a nonprogressive abnormality of the immature brain.[6]
Guillain-Barré syndrome	Also known as acute inflammatory demyelinating polyneuropathy, GBS is generally believed to be an autoimmune disorder directed against myelin and/or peripheral nerve axons.[7] The initial onset is rapid and symptoms include paralysis, areflexia, and distal sensory loss. After the acute stage, the syndrome is nonprogressive and most individuals experience at least partial recovery.
Multiple sclerosis	Multiple sclerosis is a chronic disease in which the immune system attacks the body's myelin in the central nervous system, resulting in impaired nerve conduction. Common symptoms, presentation, and progression vary widely and may include visual deficits, paresthesias, cognitive impairments, extremity weakness, fatigue, and loss of postural control.[8,9]
Myasthenia gravis	Myasthenia gravis is a chronic autoimmune disorder affecting the neuromuscular junction resulting in muscle weakness and fatigue that worsens with use.[10]
Parkinson's disease	Parkinson's Disease occurs secondary to the progressive loss of dopamine-generating cells in the substantia nigra, which results in tremor, rigidity, bradykinesia, impaired coordination, and balance deficits.[9,11]
Spinal cord injury	Spinal cord injuries occur due to direct or indirect trauma to the spinal cord and result in a loss of motor and sensory function below the level of the lesion; can range from complete (absence of all sensory and motor function) to incomplete (partial preservation of function).[12]
Stroke	A stroke occurs when blood vessels bringing oxygen to the brain are either blocked (ischemic) or rupture (hemorrhagic) leading to tissue death and loss of motor, sensory, and/or cognitive function.[13]
Traumatic brain injury	TBI occurs when there is an insult to the brain as the result of an external force. Symptoms may range from mild to severe and may include loss of consciousness, weakness, impaired coordination, difficulty with balance, diminished sensation, and cognitive deficits.[14]

responses beyond the age at which they disappear in typically developing children. In adults, the presence of primitive reflexes is indicative of a condition affecting the CNS and suggests possible cortical disinhibition.[20] Occupational therapy practitioners examining these reflexes should observe the degree to which reflex responses are obligatory and sustained. These reflexes have also been incorporated into intervention approaches as a means of eliciting motor activity in very weak or inactive muscles.[21] Refer to Table 17-3 for a summary of primitive reflexes that are commonly assessed and/or used in intervention approaches.

Tone, Spasticity, and Rigidity

Muscle tone has been defined as resistance to passive stretch,[24] and increased muscle tone in individuals with neuromuscular disorders can be related to both changes in the intrinsic properties of muscle, tendon, and connective tissue, as well as hyperactive stretch reflexes.[25] There are 2 types of increased tone or hypertonicity: these are spasticity and rigidity. Spasticity is characterized by a velocity-dependent increase in tonic stretch reflexes accompanied by exaggerated tendon jerks.[26] In contrast, while rigidity is

Table 17-2. Examination of Selected Stretch Reflexes[17,18]

Stretch Reflex	Nerve (Nerve Roots)	Stimulus	Response
Biceps	Musculo-cutaneous nerve (C5, C6)	Patient is sitting with arm flexed and supported. Examiner's thumb places slight tension on the biceps tendon and examiner taps his or her thumb with the reflex hammer.	Slight contraction of elbow flexors.
Brachioradialis	Radial nerve (C5, C6)	Patient is sitting with arm flexed and supported. Thumb or finger is placed over the brachioradialis tendon at the musculotendinous junction. Examiner grips reflex hammer loosely and taps his or her thumb.	Slight contraction of elbow flexors, slight wrist extension or radial deviation.
Triceps	Radial nerve (C6, C7)	Patient is sitting with arm supported in shoulder abduction and internal rotation with the elbow flexed. Examiner taps directly on triceps tendon with the reflex hammer, just above the olecranon.	Slight contraction of elbow extensors.

Table 17-3. Primitive Reflexes[22,23]

Reflex	Position	Method	Response	Age at Disappearance
Asymmetric tonic neck	Supine	Rotate head to one side	Extension of the arm on the chin side, flexion of the arm on the skull side	3 to 6 months
Symmetric tonic neck	Sitting	Flex or extend the head	*Head flexion:* flexion of upper extremities and extension of lower extremities *Head extension:* extension of upper extremities and flexion of lower extremities	3 to 6 months
Symmetric tonic labrinthine	Supine or prone	Position in supine or prone	*Supine:* extension of extremities or increase in extensor tone *Prone:* flexion of extremities or increase in flexor tone	3 to 6 months
Babinski	Supine	Stroke lateral aspect of plantar surface of the foot from the heel to the head of the fifth metatarsal	Dorsiflexion of the great toe and extension of remaining toes	Presence always abnormal

also characterized by resistance to passive stretch, this resistance is independent of the direction or velocity of the stretch.[27]

Individuals with hypertonicity often report difficulty with basic ADL and other tasks that support their daily lives. They find that increased tone may lead to muscle contracture, reduced joint mobility, and subsequent difficulty with activities such as dressing or bathing.[25] Significant contractures, in the hand for example, can also lead to other complications, such as skin breakdown. As such, increased tone and spasticity can limit participation in life roles that are important to clients. In a study of more than 1500 individuals with traumatic spinal cord injury, spasticity was negatively correlated with home life satisfaction, global satisfaction, and quality of life.[28] Furthermore, in a study of occupational therapy practitioners, severity of spasticity in individuals with CP was found to be the most important clinical factor in practitioners' decisions to pursue more invasive treatment approaches, such as casting, referral for Botulinum Toxin, or surgery.[29] As such, an understanding of hypertonicity is important in order for occupational therapy practitioners to address the needs and goals identified by their clients and to assess and re-assess outcomes associated with their interventions for hypertonicity.

The most commonly used clinical measure of muscle tone is the Modified Ashworth Scale (MAS).[30] This 6-point scale allows muscle tone to be graded based on resistance to passive movement on the following scale[30]:

- 0 = No increase in muscle tone
- 1 = Slight increase in muscle tone, manifested by a slight catch and release or by minimal resistance at the end of the ROM when the affected part is moved in flexion or extension
- 1+ = Slight increase in muscle tone, manifested by a catch, followed by minimal resistance throughout the remainder (less than half) of the ROM
- 2 = More marked increase in muscle tone through most of the ROM, but affected part(s) easily moved
- 3 = Considerable increase in muscle tone, passive movement is difficult
- 4 = Affected part(s) rigid in flexion or extension

Reported inter-rater reliability for the MAS is variable and can differ based on both the patient population and muscle group under study. For example, in 2 separate studies examining the inter-rater reliability of the MAS for individuals with acute stroke, Gregson et al reported kappa values of .84 at the elbow and .51 at the knee.[31,32] In another study of persons with profound intellectual and multiple disabilities, researchers reported strong inter-rater reliability for both the arm (ICC = .894) and leg (ICC = -.895).[33] Other studies have reported insufficient inter-rater reliability.[34-36] For example, Ansari et al reported a Kappa value of .21 for the MAS at the elbow in patients with acute stroke.[36]

A more recently suggested alternative to the MAS is the Modified Tardieu Scale (MTS). The MTS quantifies the angle at which a "catch" occurs during slow and fast passive movements, and also assigns a qualitative score to the fast movement. Researchers have suggested that the angle of "catch" at slow speeds is reflective of contracture whereas the "catch" at fast speeds is more reflective of spasticity.[37] As such, if there is a large difference in the angle of "catch" between slow and fast speeds, this is indicative of spasticity. If there is little difference based on

speed, this is more indicative of contracture. In this way, the MTS allows for greater differentiation between musculoskeletal contributions to hypertonicity vs neurologic contributions. This, in turn, has the potential to provide greater guidance for selection of intervention approaches. Reported reliability for the MTS also ranges from moderate to good.[38,39] In conclusion, although more reliable measures of tone and spasticity are desirable, the MAS is the most commonly used and has the most data evaluating its reliability and validity. The MTS is emerging as a viable option, particularly when differentiation between spasticity and contracture is desired.

Strength

Strength can be defined as "the force generated by a single maximal isometric contraction."[40(p243)] The ability to generate muscle power is related to both intrinsic muscle properties and the neural activation of that muscle.[1] For example, an individual may demonstrate weakness because of deconditioning, loss of peripheral nerve innervation, or decreased input from the cerebral cortex, as occurs with a stroke. Strength can be reliably assessed in individuals with musculoskeletal and neuromuscular conditions through isometric, isokinetic, and functional measures.[41-43] Historically, it has been suggested that spasticity may prevent reliable and valid assessment of strength in individuals with upper motor neuron disorders.[44,45] Specifically, it was proposed that excessive co-contraction by spastic antagonists masked true agonist muscle strength and resulted in the appearance of weakness, when in fact, muscle strength was intact. Despite this persistent clinical belief, it has been demonstrated in patients with strokes that inadequate recruitment of agonist muscles is not related to spasticity in the antagonist.[46] Furthermore, strength testing has been shown to be reliable in individuals with a variety of neuromuscular diagnoses, including CP,[47,48] TBI,[42] stroke,[49] and spinal cord injury.[50]

Manual muscle testing (MMT) is the most widely used method of examining strength in rehabilitation settings.[51] This examination technique grades muscle strength on an ordinal scale relative to gravity (grades 0 to 2+) and relative to the clinician's judgment of normal strength values for gender, age, and activity level (grades 3 to 5).[52,53] Table 17-4 describes each manual muscle test grade and its definition. The intrarater and inter-rater reliability of manual muscle testing is generally good, particularly in studies where standardized protocols are used.[55-57] On the other hand, while muscle grades can be reliably reproduced, manual muscle testing has been criticized for having relatively poor ability to detect smaller strength changes over time and for having a ceiling effect.[58] For example, in a study examining 3 methods of assessing shoulder strength, individuals graded as 5 by manual

Table 17-4. *Manual Muscle Test Grades*[54]

Number	Word Grade	Definition
0	Zero	No evidence of contraction by vision or palpation
1	Trace	Slight contraction; no motion
2-	Poor minus	Movement through partial test range in gravity eliminated position
2	Poor	Movement through complete test range in gravity-eliminated position
2+	Poor plus	Movement through complete test range in gravity-eliminated position and through up to one-half of test range against gravity
3-	Fair minus	Movement through complete test range in gravity eliminated position and through more than one-half of test range against gravity
3	Fair	Movement through complete test range against gravity
3+	Fair plus	Movement through complete test range against gravity and able to hold against minimum resistance
4	Good	Movement through complete test range against gravity and able to hold against moderate resistance
5	Normal	Movement through complete test range against gravity and able to hold against maximum resistance

muscle testing had strength values that ranged from 50 to 175 Newtons (N) when tested with hand-held dynamometry.[51]

As such, hand-held dynamometry has been proposed as an alternative to MMT. In this examination approach, the dynamometer is positioned perpendicularly to the limb segment and stabilized while the individual being tested is asked to exert an isometric force into the dynamometer. The exerted force is then measured in Newtons. Studies indicate that measurements taken with hand-held dynamometers are correlated with MMT at grades below 4, but provide a more accurate evaluation of muscle strength for grades 4 and 5.[59-61] Hand-held dynamometers are also used to measure grip strength. The American Society of Hand Therapists recommends the following test position for measuring grip strength: seated with feet flat on the floor, shoulders adducted and neutrally rotated, with 90 degrees of elbow flexion and neutral forearm and wrist position.[62] In addition, the average of 3 trials is typically recorded. Alterations to wrist position, such as ulnar or radial deviation,[63] as well as visual feedback,[64] have been shown to impact grip strength and therefore it is important to maintain a consistent position and procedure across tests.

Motor Control

Abnormal movement patterns, or *abnormal synergies,* have been described after CNS conditions such as stroke, CP, and TBI.[25] Abnormal synergies are stereotypic patterns of movement that limit an individual's ability to dissociate movement at one joint from movement at another and to generate a variety of movement patterns in response to task demands.[1] For example, when asked to raise his arm, the client with an abnormal flexor synergy in the upper extremity may be unable to flex his shoulder without shoulder elevation, shoulder abduction, and elbow flexion accompanying the movement. The abnormal extensor synergy in the upper extremity consists of shoulder adduction, elbow extension, forearm pronation, and wrist and finger extension. The abnormal flexor synergy for the upper extremity includes shoulder abduction, elbow flexion, forearm supination, and wrist and finger flexion.[21]

The most common measure of motor recovery in stroke patients is the Fugl-Meyer Assessment.[65,66] This test is based on the motor recovery sequence described by Brunnstrom,[21] in which reflex activity returns first, followed by volitional movement dominated by abnormal synergy patterns, and subsequent progressive isolation of movement outside of the synergy pattern. Thus, the motor recovery portion of the Fugl-Meyer Assessment includes measurement of the patient's ability to move in and out of synergy with the upper and lower extremities. Sample upper extremity tasks on the of the Fugl-Meyer Assessment that indicate beginning ability to combine synergies include the ability to flex the shoulder to 90 degrees with the elbow extended and the ability to pronate and supinate the forearm with the shoulder at 0 degrees and the elbow at 90 degrees. The validity and reliability of this assessment tool are well established.[66]

Balance and Postural Control

Balance is a multidimensional construct that has been described as including the ability to maintain one's position in space, stabilize in anticipation of voluntary movement, and respond to external perturbations.[67,68] *Static balance* can be described as the ability to maintain the body's center of mass over its base of support when the body is at rest, and *dynamic balance* can be described as the ability to maintain the body's center of mass over its base of support when the body is in motion. Static and dynamic balance can also be assessed in different positions, such as sitting or standing.

In stance, the coordination of balance is simplified through the use of patterns of muscular activation that vary based on task and environmental constraints.[69,70] The 3 primary strategies include the ankle, hip, and stepping strategies. Ankle strategies are used for controlling backward and forward sway, and include sequential activation from distal to proximal of the gastrocnemius, hamstring, and paraspinal muscles in response to forward sway and activation of tibialis anterior, quadriceps, and abdominal muscles in response to backward sway. Ankle strategies are most commonly used when the perturbation is small and/or the support surface is large and firm.[1] These strategies are observed both in response to a displacement (reactive balance control) as well as in anticipation of a potential displacement (anticipatory balance control). In other words, if an individual was getting ready to pull on a heavy door, in anticipation of being pulled forward the posterior ankle strategy fires prior to pulling the door handle. The hip strategy involves flexion and extension of the trunk around the hip and is used in response to large or rapid displacements or when the support surface is small. Stepping strategies are used in response to large movements of the body's center of mass outside of the base of support.

A variety of tests and measures have been developed that examine one or more of the different components of balance. These include scales such as the Romberg, Functional Reach Test (FRT), Timed Up and Go (TUG), and the Berg Balance Scale (BBS) (Table 17-5).

For the Romberg test, individuals are asked to stand with their eyes open and their eyes closed for 20 to 30 seconds. If the individual falls or loses his or her balance in either condition, the test is considered positive. This test assesses static balance and in the eyes closed condition provides a general assessment of visual contributions to balance.[16]

The FRT is designed to examine the ability to reach outside of one's base of support.[101] In standing, the individual being tested is asked to stand near a wall upon which a yardstick has been placed at the level of his acromion. The individual is then instructed to raise his arm to 90 degrees and reach forward as far as he can without taking a step or losing his balance. The distance reached is measured and can be compared to normative values.[101] The test can also be performed to assess the ability to move outside of one's base of support in a backward or sideways direction, and norms for the multidirectional FRT have also been published.[102] In addition, this test has been modified for use in sitting.[103,104]

The TUG assesses dynamic balance and is more functional in nature.[105] In this test, individuals are asked to stand from a chair, walk 3 meters, turn around, and return to the chair. They are instructed to walk as quickly and safely as they can and are allowed to use an assistive device. The test is timed and most healthy adults are able to complete it in less than 10 seconds.

Finally, the BBS includes multiple items which address static and dynamic balance.[106,107] It also allows for the examination of both postural adjustments to voluntary movement as well as reaction to external disturbances. Sample items range from static sitting without use of the arms to turning 360 degrees, toe-tapping on a step-stool, and standing on one leg. Each item is rated from 0 to 4 and the total possible score is 56 points. This test is widely used across a variety of patient populations and has well-established validity and reliability.[106,108]

Coordination

Impaired coordination can be related to deficits in motor activation and sequencing, scaling, and/or timing. For example, the abnormal synergy patterns described earlier are an example of impaired coordination related to activation and sequencing. In this case, there are a reduced number of options for muscle activation and sequencing available to the individual. Similarly, abnormal co-contraction of agonist and antagonist muscles during functional tasks, such as is observed during gait in individuals with CP, is another example of impaired muscle activation and sequencing. *Dysdiadochokinesis* is a term used to refer to impaired ability to perform rapid alternating movements, such as forearm pronation and supination. Other problems of coordination include those related to the scaling of movement. Individuals who over-reach (hypermetria) or under-reach (hypometria) targets are displaying coordination deficits related to scaling. Difficulties with scaling are commonly observed in individuals with cerebellar conditions. Finally, issues of timing can impact coordination. For example, individuals with the diagnosis of Parkinson's Disease often have difficulty initiating movement and may exhibit "freezing" of movement. Similarly, their movement may be slowed or bradykinetic. In contrast, some individuals (such as those with Huntington's disease) display too much movement or difficulty with terminating movement. Coordination is typically assessed through observation of

Table 17-5. *Assessment Table*

Assessment	Motor Factor Assessed	Description	Where It Can Be Obtained
Reflex Testing	Reflexes	• Measure of motor system integrity • Measurement qualities: expert opinion	Textbooks[71]
Modified Ashworth Scale	Muscle tone	• Clinical measure of muscle tone • Six point scale • Measurement qualities: reliability dependent on standard procedures	http://www.rehabmeasures.org/[72-76]
Modified Tardieu Scale	Muscle tone	• Clinical measure of muscle tone • Measures angle of "catch" in passive movement • Measurement qualities: moderate reliability	[77-79]
Manual Muscle Testing	Strength	• Clinical measure of strength. • Ordinal scale (0 to 5) • Measurement qualities: moderate reliability when standard procedures used	Textbooks[80-84]
Hand-Held Dynamometry	Strength	• Clinical measure of hand strength • Equipment required • Measurement qualities: strong reliability and validity, normative data	Textbooks[85-87]
Fugl-Meyer Assessment	Movement patterns and motor recovery	• Measures recovery post-stroke • Widely used clinical and research measures • Measurement qualities: moderate to strong reliability and validity	http://www.rehabmeasures.org/[88]
Functional Reach Test	Balance, motor function	• Assesses ability to reach forward during standing and sitting • Populations: stroke, Parkinson's, SCI, elders • Measurement qualities: excellent reliability and moderate validity, normative data	http://www.rehabmeasures.org/[89]
Timed Up and Go	Balance	• Assesses mobility, balance, walking ability, and fall risk • Measurement qualities: moderate to strong reliability and validity, normative data	http://www.rehabmeasures.org/[90]
Berg Balance Scale	Balance	• Assesses standing balance and fall risk using 14 items • Populations: multiple • Measurement qualities: excellent reliability and validity, normative data	http://www.rehabmeasures.org/[91,92]
Motor Assessment Scale (MAS)	Motor behavior and motor function	• Assesses everyday motor function on 8 tasks • Measurement qualities: moderate to strong reliability and validity, normative data	http://www.rehabmeasures.org/[93]

(continued)

Table 17-5 (continued).   *Assessment Table*

Assessment	Motor Factor Assessed	Description	Where It Can Be Obtained
Arm Motor Ability Test (AMAT)	Functional ability and quality of movement	• Assesses performance difficulties on 13 activities of daily living • Population: multiple • Measurement qualities: excellent reliability, moderate to strong validity	http://www.rehabmeasures.org/94
Wolf Motor Function Test (WFMT)	Upper extremity movement in functional tasks	• Assesses functional ability, strength, and movement quality in 17 tasks • Populations: stroke and brain injury • Measurement qualities: excellent reliability, moderate to strong validity	http://www.rehabmeasures.org/95
Motor Activity Log	Self-reported use of upper extremity in functional tasks	• Assesses self-reported functional use of upper extremity in the natural environment • Population: stroke • Measurement qualities: moderate to strong reliability and validity	96-98
Action Research Arm Test (ARA)	Upper extremity function and performance	• Assesses upper extremity function on 19 tasks and 4 domains: grasp, grip, pinch, and gross arm movement Populations: stroke, brain injury, and MS • Measurement qualities: strong reliability and validity, normative data	http://www.rehabmeasures.org/99
Assessment of Motor and Process Skills (AMPS)	Motor behavior and motor function	• Quality of performance in ADL effort, efficiency, safety, and independence • Special training required • Populations: multiple • Measurement qualities: reported reliability and validity	http://www.innovativeot-solutions.com/content/amps/100
Box and Block Test	Dexterity and coordination	• Assesses speed in moving blocks within time limit • Populations: multiple • Measurement qualities: strong reliability and validity, normative data for children and adults	http://www.rehabmeasures.org/

functional tasks and through specific non-equilibrium coordination tests.[109] These tests include tasks such as asking the individual to move his or her finger to the practitioner's finger, rapid forearm pronation and supination, and finger opposition (touching the tip of the thumb to the tip of each finger in sequence).

Some conditions result in involuntary movements. For example, tremors are associated with both cerebellar disorders and Parkinson's disease. They are defined as involuntary, rhythmic movements and are typically examined through observation.[109] Tremors can also be described based on whether they occur at rest (resting tremor) or

with movement (intention tremor), based on the body part(s) involved, and their intensity. The term *athetosis* is used to describe involuntary, slow, writhing movements that may include movement between hyperextension and flexion of the wrist and fingers, but can also include other parts of the body such as the neck, face, and trunk.[109] *Chorea* is characterized by involuntary, rapid, irregularly timed movements involving multiple joints; these movements cannot be inhibited and are associated with Huntington's disease.[109] Associated movements involve unintentional movement of one limb during intentional movement of another limb.[25] One commonly observed

Table 17-6. *Intervention Table*

Construct, Mechanism, or Factor	Intervention and Reference	How Motor Interventions Relate to PEOP
Performance of meaningful and functional tasks Motor learning	Task-oriented approaches	Task-oriented approaches are complementary to the PEOP Model because the focus is on optimal performance of meaningful occupations using both personal and environmental factors[110-114]
Motor performance and function	Constraint-induced movement training (CIMT)	CIMT supports motor performance of occupations, especially those that entail bilateral coordination for individuals with hemiplegia
Tone, spasticity, rigidity	Stretching	Stretching may be a necessary prerequisite for addressing impairments that limit occupational performance[115]
Strengthen and function	Strength training	Strength training may improve motor factors to support performance of some meaningful occupations that require increased strength[116-119]
Balance	Balance training	Balance in standing and sitting supports optimal performance and contributes to self-efficacy in participation[120-123]

example of this is progressive flexing of the hemiparetic elbow that may occur during ambulation in individuals with stroke.

INTERVENTIONS

Motor Learning

Schmidt and Lee define motor learning as "a set of processes associated with practice or experience leading to relatively permanent changes in the capability for skilled movement"[124(p327)] (Table 17-6). Because motor learning is a process, it is often described as occurring in stages or along a continuum. Fitts and Posner described a 3-stage model that includes the cognitive, associative, and autonomous stages.[125] The *cognitive stage* occurs early in motor learning. In this stage, increased attention to the motor task is required and individuals often verbalize what they are doing. Performance is highly variable, but improvements are rapid. As learning progresses, individuals begin to solidify and refine their movement patterns. Fewer errors are made and improvements continue in a gradual fashion. This middle stage is called the *associative stage.* Finally, as individuals become skilled with their movements, they no longer need to consciously think about what they are doing and the motor task becomes very *automatic.* This, for example, allows one to walk and carry

on a conversation at the same time because active attention does not need to be directed toward walking. Because motor learning is associated with relatively permanent changes in skilled movement, it is important to distinguish learning from performance. As such, changes in motor behavior that occur immediately after practice are indicative of improved performance, but are not generally considered evidence of motor learning. Changes in motor behavior that are retained after a period of time are considered to reflect motor learning. Clinically, if an occupational therapy practitioner observes an improvement in coordinated reaching ability immediately following a treatment session, he or she can not necessarily infer that learning has occurred unless that same improvement is retained at the next treatment session, for example.

The two most important factors impacting motor learning are feedback and practice. Feedback can be described in 2 ways, *intrinsic* and *extrinsic.* When individuals use information from their sensory system to refine movement, they are using intrinsic feedback. For example, individuals use proprioceptive and visual information to refine their movement patterns when throwing a ball. Extrinsic or augmented feedback is feedback that is provided externally and serves as a supplement to intrinsic feedback.[124] Examples of augmented feedback that might be used in occupational therapy include verbal or manual cues, mirrors, or demonstration. This type of feedback can be classified as involving knowledge of results (KR), which is feedback about the outcome of the movement, or knowledge of performance (KP), which is related to the movement pattern used to achieve that result.[4] For example, if a child is learning to throw a ball, he can be given feedback about the accuracy of his throw (KR) or about the positioning of his shoulder during the throw (KP). These types of augmented feedback are distinct from motivational feedback and can be provided concurrently with the motor task, immediately following the task, or after a period of delay.[126]

The impact of augmented feedback on both the performance of motor skills and motor learning has been studied in individuals with and without neurological deficit. In terms of frequency, a number of different methods for varying the frequency of feedback have been examined in the literature. These include absolute frequency (providing feedback after each practice trial or 100%), relative frequency (feedback after a fixed number of trials, eg, every other trial or 50%),[127] bandwidth frequency (feedback if the results or performance fall outside of a pre-determined range),[128] summary feedback (feedback that summarizes multiple trials, eg, after 10 trials),[129,130] and fading feedback (reducing the amount of feedback as practice progresses).[131] Across these different feedback paradigms, a number of researchers have demonstrated that less frequent provision of feedback is detrimental to initial performance, but enhances learning on retention tests. For example, in 2 studies of summary feedback, groups of college students were trained in an upper extremity task that involved using a lever to backswing, intersect a moving light at a specific point, and follow through.[129,130] Participants were provided a skill score based on the velocity of the lever or "bat" at the time of contact with the light and minimization of spatial errors. Those participants receiving summary feedback made more errors while learning the motor task than did subjects who received knowledge of results after every trial. But when subjects were tested for retention at a later date, those who received summary feedback made fewer errors. Similarly, in another study with 25 adults without disabilities that compared feedback during every trial (100%) and feedback after every other trial (50%) on a task requiring modulation of isometric elbow extension force, researchers found that while performance was best during acquisition in the 100% group, on retention tests the group receiving feedback every other trial exhibited the fewest errors.[127] Furthermore, in a study with 136 graduate students when KR was provided on a faded schedule, with more feedback provided in the early phases of learning and gradually less feedback provided in the later phases, superior motor learning occurred in the faded practice condition.[131] Similar results have also been found with physical guidance feedback.[132] Specifically, 40 individuals learning an upper extremity motor task had the poorest retention when they received high frequency physical guidance as opposed to faded physical or verbal feedback. Furthermore, high frequency physical guidance resulted in poorer learning outcomes than verbal knowledge of results feedback provided with the same frequency. As such, in addition to the frequency of feedback, the type of feedback may also affect motor learning. Finally, the timing of feedback is also critical. Research involving subjects without neuromuscular conditions suggests that immediate feedback adversely impacts motor learning because it interferes with the individual's self-assessment of performance.[133] In a study by Swinnen et al,[133] learning was facilitated with a 3- to 4-second delay in the provision of KR. Similarly, other researchers have demonstrated that the provision of feedback concurrently with a motor task supports performance but is detrimental to motor learning.[127,134] On the other hand, learning improves if the relative frequency of trials in which concurrent feedback is provided is reduced.[135]

The most significant variable in regard to practice is the amount. This effect on learning is called the *law of practice* and, in general, more learning occurs as the number of practice trials increase.[124] The importance of practice dose has been reinforced in studies of neuroplasticity.[136,137] In these studies, it has been demonstrated that somatosensory and motor maps in the cerebral cortex are altered by practice experience, but many practice trials are needed. For example, in one study, animals demonstrated an increased number of synapses in the motor cortex after 400 trials of a skilled reaching task, whereas after 60 trials they did not.[138]

The scheduling of practice can be described as *blocked* or *variable*. In blocked practice, all of the trials for a given motor task are practiced together. For example, a client might practice reaching for a defined target 10 times and then complete 10 trials of a fine motor task, such as turning playing cards. In variable practice, different motor tasks are practiced throughout a session. In this practice schedule the individual might practice a trial of reaching for a target, then a trial of turning cards, and then a trial of buttoning a shirt. Although initial acquisition and performance of a motor skill may be best when a blocked practice paradigm is incorporated, learning (as measured by retention of the motor skill) is improved when healthy subjects engage in random practice.[139] Similarly, in a RCT with 24 individuals post-stroke, the group that alternated practice of the experimental task with other tasks (random practice) performed better than the group that practiced the experimental task for multiple consecutive repetitions.[140] One reason for this may be because more active engagement is required when moving from task to task.

Practice can also be considered in terms of distribution. From this perspective, one can have massed practice in which the time spent practicing is greater than that spent resting, or distributed practice in which a greater amount

Table 17-7. *Evidence Table for Task-Oriented Approaches*

Study and Reference	Aim of Study	Methods	Participants	Results and Outcome(s)
177	Examine evidence for task-oriented training for stroke	Systematic review	Total articles: 42 Systematic reviews: 9 RCTs: 33	Results support task-oriented training for improving balance, sit to stand, walking, and arm use.
178	Identify and examine characteristics of task-oriented training components for stroke	Systematic review	Total articles: 362 Articles meeting inclusion criteria: 16	Evidence supports distributive practice and feedback for post-intervention effect size, and feedback and clear functional goals in follow-up effect size.
179	Identify practice guidelines for stroke rehabilitation	Practice guideline	Review of evidence on stroke rehabilitation	Functional goals should guide the rehabilitation process. Measures should examine task-specific function on areas important for well-being.

of time is spent resting in comparison to time in practice. In general, distributed practice appears to be more beneficial than massed for motor learning, as it may assist with memory consolidation.[141] *Part practice,* or the breaking up of a motor task into parts, has also been examined in the literature. In general, the effectiveness of part practice depends on the type of action being learned. Specifically, part practice appears to be most effective for serial tasks in which the task incorporates multiple, discrete tasks; and less effective for continuous tasks in which the coordination of individual parts is an essential component of completing the task.[124]

Consideration of Task and Environment

Gentile's Taxonomy of Movement Tasks is often used as a framework for environmental and task analysis for the purpose of guiding examination and intervention.[4] In this taxonomy, functional activities are evaluated based on the environmental context of the task and its functional role. Specifically, regulatory conditions, or those elements of the environment to which a task must conform, are conceptualized as being either stationary or in motion, and presenting with or without inter-trial variability. For example, if one were to practice writing at a desk, the regulatory conditions (the desk, the pencil) would be stationary and, assuming one used the same pencil, present no inter-trial variability. This is considered a closed task. On the other hand, if one were to practice catching a ball, the regulatory conditions (the ball) would be in motion and that motion would be variable from trial to trial. This is considered an open task. One can also analyze the function of the task.

From this perspective, Gentile[4] suggested considering whether or not the task required body stability or transport and whether the upper extremities were used primarily for stability or manipulation.

Task-Oriented Approaches

The task-oriented approaches suggested by Carr and Shepherd,[142,143] Shumway-Cook and Woollacott,[1] and Bass-Haugen et al[144] are based on scientists' current understanding of how movement arises from the interaction between systems at the level of the individual, the environment, and the task (Table 17-7). In addition, these approaches more fully incorporate emerging knowledge regarding neural plasticity and motor learning and take into consideration the implications of research in the areas of environmental and task analysis, feedback, and practice. Bass-Haugen et al describe the Occupational Therapy Task-Oriented Approach as incorporating the following principles[144]:

- Client-centered focus
- Occupation-based focus
- Person and environment
- Practice and feedback
- General treatment goals

As part of this framework, the Occupational Therapy Task-Oriented Approach focuses intervention on meaningful, functional tasks. Emerging evidence in neuroscience and motor learning also supports these principles.[137] For example, in both animal and human models, it has been demonstrated that motor learning is highly task-specific. The importance of specificity relates both to the actual task practiced[145-148] as well as its context and parameters.[149,150] This was illustrated in a study that used different speeds of body weight-supported treadmill training for individuals with diagnoses of stroke.[149] Although all groups received the same amount of intervention, the group practicing at the highest speed, which was closest to normal walking speed, showed the greatest improvement in over-ground gait velocity. Similarly, Boyd et al demonstrated that individuals with diagnoses of mild stroke were able to make greater motor learning gains on functional hand tasks, in comparison to serial reaction time tasks. This result supports both the need to incorporate functional tasks into treatment, as well as the potential importance of salience or meaning for motor learning.[148] Winstein et al also demonstrated greater increases in Fugl-Meyer motor scores and strength post-treatment for individuals with recent stroke diagnoses who participated in an upper-extremity rehabilitation program focused on functional tasks, when compared to a group that received standard care (ie, muscle facilitation with neurodevelopmental treatment (NDT) focus, electrical stimulation, stretching, ADL).[147]

In addition to selecting tasks that are meaningful to the client and focused on function, occupational therapy practitioners should also consider the characteristics of the task. As noted previously, the motor learning literature indicates that the context and parameters of selected tasks are important for motor learning. As such, consideration of Gentile's taxonomies and, in particular, whether tasks are open or closed is also essential.[4] More specifically, when functioning in a closed environment, motor patterns become consistent and over time require less attention, whereas open environments demand variable motor patterns, predictive abilities, and greater attention.[1] For example, when turning on a light switch in the home, one can use the same motor pattern each time as the regulatory conditions (the position of the switch) are stable and invariant. Thus, refinement of a consistent motor pattern will allow for successful performance of this task. In contrast, when relearning to drive a car, the regulatory conditions (eg, other cars, the road surface) are in motion and highly variable. Thus, a diversity of motor plans and the ability to anticipate and predict the actions of other drivers are needed for successful performance.

Next, from the perspective of the person and motor factors, underlying deficits that are identified in the occupational therapy assessment and may contribute to motor performance or participation deficits should be addressed. Those factors highlighted in the assessment portion of this chapter are discussed in the following section.

Interventions for Tone, Spasticity, and Rigidity

Specific interventions for tone, spasticity, and rigidity include approaches such as stretching, splinting, casting, active movement, and positioning.[151] Although there is a correlation between spasticity and contracture,[152] the literature supporting passive movement and stretching as an effective intervention is mixed. In a recent systematic review by Katalinic et al, stretching, which included the use of splints, casts, and positioning, was found to have no benefit for spasticity, a small immediate effect for joint mobility, and no long-term effects on joint mobility.[153] A review of sustained stretch through casting for individuals with TBI also found limited evidence that this was effective in decreasing spasticity, but did find evidence that it resulted in improved passive range of motion.[154] Both transcutaneous and functional electrical stimulation (FES) have also been incorporated as means of decreasing spasticity and tone.[151,155] It is postulated that cutaneous stimulation of spastic muscles may alter afferent sensitivity and/or depress spinal interneural activity, and functional electrical stimulation (FES) to the antagonist may decrease spasticity through reciprocal inhibition.[155] In an RCT of 46 patients with diagnoses of acute stroke and moderate spasticity, 15 30-minute sessions of FES to the ankle dorsiflexors led to significantly smaller increases in spasticity over 8 weeks when compared to groups receiving placebo FES or standard care.[156]

Interventions for Strength

In general, exercise-based or activity-based programs that incorporate progressive resistance activities are effective for increasing strength.[157-160] The literature supporting their relationship to improvements in performance and participation is mixed.[157,159-161] For example, in a systematic review by Morris et al, both positive effects and no improvement were reported related to the effect of strengthening on sit-to-stand, walking speed, and stair climbing for patients with stroke.[157] In contrast, Goodwin et al reported positive benefits for exercise related to balance, gait speed, and quality of life in a systematic review of exercise for individuals with diagnoses of Parkinson's disease,[160] and Dibble et al found that strengthening resulted in improved balance in this same population.[102] Key elements of progressive resistance strength training programs include the following[157]:

- Sufficient load
- Regular re-examination and progression
- Adequate duration

When determining sufficient load, the American Heart Association recommends using 70% of the individual's one repetition maximum.[162] Another method for determining sufficient load is to identify the maximum load for which 10 to 12 repetitions can be completed.[157]

Interventions for Motor Control and Coordination

Interventions for impaired motor control and coordination are typically integrated into the functional activities associated with the neurofacilitation or task-oriented approaches described earlier. In this way, individuals with motor control or coordination deficits are challenged to refine the timing, sequencing, and activation of groups of muscles during the performance of functional tasks. Augmented feedback, as previously described, can also be incorporated to assist clients to generate movements that are more accurate in their timing, sequencing, and activation. This may include physical cues to provide increased sensory input, such as joint approximation or the inclusion of weight-bearing activities. In addition, some nonfunctional tasks, such as those included in typical coordination testing (eg, rapid, alternating forearm pronation and supination), may be incorporated into treatment. Intervention for involuntary movements is typically focused on teaching compensatory strategies.[1]

Interventions for Balance and Postural Control

From a motor perspective, interventions for balance involve addressing problems with alignment, movement strategies, and any underlying motor factors that may be contributing to decreased postural control. For static and dynamic postural control, augmented feedback (such as the use of mirrors or biofeedback) can be used to provide clients with feedback about their position in space when standing or weightshifting.[163-165] It is important to note that in many of these studies, participants improved their static and dynamic postural control in standing, but there was little carry-over to gait. This, again, speaks to the need to incorporate task-specific training in occupational therapy intervention. The movement strategies for balance can be addressed through the inclusion of functional activities in intervention. Tasks should be structured to address the multiple contexts in which balance may be challenged, and include opportunities to practice both anticipatory and reactive balance control. Common activities associated with these treatment protocols include those that require individuals to move outside of their base of support, react quickly to changing surfaces, or anticipate potential disturbances to balance and may include reaching, catching,

throwing, kicking, or lifting objects. Tasks can be progressed according to Gentile's taxonomy. For example, the occupational therapy practitioner might begin by reaching for an object from a shelf, progress to reaching for different objects, and then proceed to catching objects that are moving. Activities that encourage single-leg stance and increased speed of movement will also challenge balance. Different standing and walking surfaces will change the sensory input available for balance, and will also provide a challenge to balance within an intervention session. There is significant evidence that the practice of functional tasks can improve balance across a range of conditions.[161,166-169]

Interventions That Use Strategies From Neurodevelopmental Approaches

Neurodevelopmental approaches, such as proprioceptive neuromuscular facilitation (PNF)[170] and NDT,[171,172] are approaches that are associated with the historical reflex and hierarchical models of motor control.[24] The emphasis of the strategies used in these intervention approaches was on facilitation of normal movement patterns, while inhibiting abnormal synergies to optimize function and promote motor recovery in a predictable sequence.[24,173,174] These approaches have limited evidence to support their use in addressing motor problems and improving performance. In recent years, findings from neuroscience and motor learning research, along with an increased focus on functional outcomes in rehabilitation, has provided support for adoption of task-oriented approaches.

OUTCOMES

The intended outcomes of interventions for motor impairments are reflected in improved performance, participation, and well-being. Selection of specific outcome measures depends in part on the severity of the motor problems, the targeted stakeholder groups, and the practice settings.[175] In rehabilitation, an outcome has been defined as "the expected or looked-for change in some measure or state" that is "concerned with changes in those aspects of quality of life (QOL) or activities that are due to or caused by the treatment more than QOL or activities as a whole."[175(pS27)]

For the individual with motor impairments, the outcomes of interest are identified by the client and measure the client's ability to perform roles, responsibilities, and interests, as well as achieve optimal participation in everyday life. Wade[175] suggested that activity performance be adopted as the primary measure of rehabilitation outcomes as it documents change that is meaningful to the client and family. Other outcome measures that evaluate role performance, life satisfaction, and QOL are important

Table 17-8. *Organizations and Journals That Focus on Motor Factors for Performance*

Organization or Journal	Description	Web Address
The Movement Disorder Society	Advance neurological sciences related to movement science through diagnosis and treatment, research, education, forums, collaborations	http://www.movementdisorders.org
Rehab Measures Database	Provides a database to summarize reliable and valid instruments of assessments and patient outcome measures during all stages of rehabilitation	http://www.rehabmeasures.org/
American Stroke Association	Provides resources and evidence on interventions for movement problems associated with stroke	http://www.strokeassociation.org/STROKEORG/
Journal of Motor Behavior	Multidisciplinary journal of movement neuroscience to advance basic understanding of motor control	http://www.tandfonline.com/toc/vjmb20/current
Stroke: A Journal of Cerebral Circulation	Reports of clinical and basic research of any aspect related to stroke from many disciplines, including rehabilitation	http://stroke.ahajournals.org/
Clinical Rehabilitation	Combines clinical application of scientific results and theoretical components; effectiveness of therapeutic interventions and the evaluation of new techniques and methods	http://cre.sagepub.com/
Archives of Physical Medicine and Rehabilitation	Summarizes physical, behavioral, and pharmaceutical therapies used in comprehensive care for individuals with chronic illness and disabilities	http://www.archives-pmr.org/home

as they address the end-products of interventions designed to improve motor and occupational performance, but may be problematic because measures have not been adequately developed.

For organization-based and population-based programming, the outcomes of interest may relate to the value of interventions in terms of use of resources and priorities for services.[175] Cost-benefit analyses may measure cost in terms of practitioner direct services, indirect clinic costs, equipment and resources, and objective impact on the client and family. Benefits of interventions may be documented as cost savings over time, objective improvement in performance, as well as perceived changes in QOL.

Further development of outcome measures is important to support evidence-based practice on interventions for motor problems. Although some measures of body function and activity level have strong psychometric properties, additional outcomes measures are needed, particularly for measuring participation, well-being, and value. A table to guide the learner to resources for their clients and to keep abreast of new knowledge in motor control and motor learning can be found in Table 17-8.

SUMMARY

This chapter described the importance of motor factors for occupational performance. Foundational knowledge in motor control, motor learning, and task performance influences our contemporary intervention approaches to address motor problems that stem from central or peripheral nervous system disorders, inactivity, and disuse. Motor factors interact with other person factors and environmental factors to support occupational performance, participation, and well-being.

REFERENCES

1. Shumway-Cook A, Woollacott M. *Motor Control: Translating Research into Clinical Practice.* 4th ed. Baltimore, MD: Lippincott Williams & Wilkins; 2012.

2. Sherrington C. *The Integrative Action of the Nervous System.* 2nd ed. New Haven, CT: Yale University; 1947.

3. Foerster O. The motor cortex in man in the light of Hughlings Jackson's Doctrines. In: Payton OD, Hirt S, Nesman R, eds. *Scientific Bases for Neurophysiologic Approaches to Therapeutic Exercise.* Philadelphia, PA: FA Davis; 1977.

4. Gentile A. Skill acquisition: action, movement, and neuromotor processes. In: Carr J, Shepherd R, eds. *Movement Science: Foundations for Physical Therapy in Rehabilitation.* 2nd ed. Gaithersburg, MD: Aspen; 2000.

5. National Institute of Neurological Disorders and Stroke. *NINDS ALS (Amyotrophic Lateral Sclerosis) Information Page.* http://www.ninds.nih.gov/disorders/amyotrophiclateralsclerosis/ALS.htm. Accessed January 3, 2012.

6. Pellegrino L. Cerebral palsy. In: Batshaw ML, ed. *Children with Disabilities.* 5th ed. Baltimore, MD: Paul H. Brookes Publishing Co; 2002:443-466.

7. National Institute of Neurological Disorders and Stroke. *Guillain-Barré Fact Sheet.* http://www.ninds.nih.gov/disorders/gbs/detail_gbs.htm?css=print. Accessed January 3, 2012.

8. National Institute of Neurological Disorders and Stroke. *NINDS Multiple Sclerosis Information Page.* http://www.ninds.nih.gov/disorders/multiple_sclerosis/multiple_sclerosis.htm. Accessed January 3, 2012.

9. Forwell SJ, Copperman LF, Hugo L. Neurodegenerative diseases. In: Radomski MV, Trombly Latham CA, eds. *Occupational Therapy for Physical Dysfunction.* 6th ed. Baltimore, MD: Lippincott Williams & Wilkins; 2008:1080-1105.

10. Armstrong SM, Schumann L. Myasthenia Gravis: diagnosis and treatment. *J Am Acad Nurse Pract.* 2003;12:72-78.

11. Dirette DK. Progressive neurological disorders. In: Atchison BJ, Dirette DK, eds. *Conditions in Occupational Therapy: Effect on Occupational Performance.* 3rd ed. Baltimore, MD: Lippincott Williams & Wilkins; 2007:261-274.

12. Atkins MS. Spinal cord injury. In: Radomski MV, Trombly Latham CA, eds. *Occupational Therapy for Physical Dysfunction.* 6th ed. Baltimore, MD: Lippincott Williams & Wilkins; 2008:1172-1213.

13. Centers for Disease Control and Prevention. *About Stroke.* http://www.cdc.gov/stroke/about.htm. Accessed January 3, 2012.

14. Radomski MV. Traumatic brain injury. In: Radomski MV, Trombly Latham CA, eds. *Occupational Therapy for Physical Dysfunction.* 6th ed. Baltimore, MD: Lippincott Williams & Wilkins; 2008:1042-1078.

15. Mathiowetz V, Bass Haugen JB. Evaluation of motor behavior: traditional and contemporary views. In: Trombly CA, ed. *Occupational Therapy for Physical Dysfunction.* 4th ed. Philadelphia, PA: Lippincott Williams & Wilkins; 1995:157-185.

16. O'Sullivan SB. Examination of motor function: motor control and motor learning. In: O'Sullivan SB, Schmitz TJ, eds. *Physical Rehabilitation.* 5th ed. Philadelphia, PA: FA Davis; 2007: 227-271.

17. O'Sullivan SB. Examination of motor function: motor control and motor learning. In: O'Sullivan SB, Schmitz TJ, eds. *Physical Rehabilitation.* 5th ed. Philadelphia, PA: FA Davis; 2007:237.

18. DeMyer WE. *Technique of the Neurologic Examination.* 5th ed. New York, NY: McGraw Hill; 1994:294.

19. Blasco P. Primitive reflexes: their contribution to the early detection of cerebral palsy. *Clin Ped.* 1994;33:388-397.

20. Zafeiriou DI. Primitive reflexes and postural reactions in the neurodevelopmental examination. *Pediatr Neurol.* 2004;31:1-8.

21. Sawner K, LaVigne JM. *Brunnstrom's Movement Therapy in Hemiplegia: A Neurophysical Approach.* Philadelphia, PA: JB Lippincott Company; 1992.

22. Mathiowetz V, Bass Haugen JB. Evaluation of motor behavior: traditional and contemporary views. In Trombly CA, ed. *Occupational Therapy for Physical Dysfunction.* 4th ed.

23. Zafeiriou DI. Primitive reflexes and postural reactions in the neurodevelopmental examination. *Pediatr Neurol.* 2004;31:1-8.

24. Horak FB. Assumptions underlying motor control for neurologic rehabilitation. In: Lister MJ, ed. *Contemporary Management of Motor Control Problems: Proceedings of the II STEP Conference.* Fredricksberg, VA: Foundation for Physical Therapy; 1991.

25. Sheean G. The pathophysiology of spasticity. *Eur J Neurol.* 2002;9(Suppl 1):3-9.

26. Lance JW. What is spasticity? *Lancet.* 1990;335:606.

27. Lundy-Ekman L. *Neuroscience: Fundamentals for Rehabilitation.* 3rd ed. St. Louis, MO: Elsevier; 2007.

28. Westerkam D, Saunders LL, Krause JS. Association of spasticity and life satisfaction after spinal cord injury. *Spinal Cord.* 2011;49:990-994.

29. Rassafiani M, Ziviani J, Rodger S, Dalgleish L. Occupational therapists' decision-making in the management of clients with upper limb hypertonicity. *Scand J Occup Ther.* 2008;15:105-115.

30. Bohannon RW, Smith MB. Interrater reliability of a Modified Ashworth Scale of muscle spasticity. *Phys Ther.* 1987;67:206-207.

31. Gregson JM, Leathley M, Moore P, et al. Reliability of the Tone Assessment Scale and the Modified Ashworth Scale as clinical tools for assessing poststroke spasticity. *Arch Phys Med Rehabil.* 1999;80:1013-1015.

32. Gregson JM, Leathley M, Moore P, et al. Reliability of measurements of muscle tone and muscle power in stroke patients. *Age Ageing.* 2000;29:223-228.

33. Waninge A, Rook RA, Dijkhuizen A, et al. Feasibility, test-retest reliability, and interrater reliability of the Modified Ashworth Scale and Modified Tardieu Scale in persons with profound intellectual and multiple disabilities. *Res Dev Disabil.* 2001;32:613-620.

34. Sloan RL, Sinclair E, Thompson J, et al. Inter-rater reliability of the Modified Ashworth Scale for spasticity in hemiplegic patients. *Int J Rehabil Res.* 1992;15:158-161.

35. Blackburn M, van Vliet P, Mockett SP. Reliability of measurements obtained with the Modified Ashworth Scale in the lower extremities of people with stroke. *Phys Ther.* 2002;82:25-33.

36. Ansari NN, Jaghdi S, Moammeri H, et al. Ashworth Scales are unreliable for the assessment of muscle spasticity. *Physiother Theory Pract.* 2006;22:119-125.

37. Patrick E, Ada L. The Tardieu Scale differentiates contracture from spasticity whereas the Ashworth Scale is confounded by it. *Clin Rehabil.* 2006;20(2):173-182.

38. Ansari NN, Jaghdi S, Hasson S, et al. The Modified Tardieu Scale for the measurement of elbow flexor spasticity in adult patients with hemiplegia. *Brain Inj.* 2008;22:1007-1012.

39. Merholz J, Wagner K, Meissner D, et al. Reliability of the Modified Tardieu Scale and the Modified Ashworth Scale in adult patients with severe brain injury: a comparison study. *Clin Rehabil.* 2005;19:751-759.

40. Jacobs K, Jacobs L. *Quick Reference Dictionary for Occupational Therapy.* 5th ed. Thorofare, NJ: SLACK Incorporated; 2009:243.

41. Armstrong LE, Winant DM, Swasey PR, et al. Using isokinetic dynamometry to test ambulatory patients with multiple sclerosis. *Phys Ther.* 1983;63:1274-1273.

42. Tripp EJ, Harris SR. Test-retest reliability of isokinetic knee extension and flexion torque measurements in persons with spastic hemiparesis. *Phys Ther.* 1991;71:290-296.

43. Watkins MP, Harris BS, Koslowski BA. Isokinetic testing in patients with hemiparesis. *Phys Ther.* 1984;2:1185-1189.

44. Boabth B. *Adult Hemiplegia: Evaluation and Treatment.* 3rd ed. Oxford, UK: Heinemann Medical Books; 1990.

45. Davies PM. *Steps to Follow: A Guide to the Treatment of Adult Hemiplegia.* New York, NY: Springer-Verlag; 1985.

46. Sahrmann SA, Norton BS. The relationship of voluntary movement to spasticity in the upper motor neuron syndrome. *Ann Neurol.* 1977;2:460-465.

47. Kingels K, De Cock P, Molenaers G, et al. Upper limb motor and sensory impairments in children with hemiplegic cerebral palsy. Can they be measured reliably? *Disabil Rehabil.* 2010;32:409-416.

48. Dyball KM, Taylor NF, Dodd KJ. Retest reliability of measuring hip extensor muscle strength in different testing positions in young people with cerebral palsy. *BMC Pediatr.* 2011;11:42-49.

49. Bohannon RW, Walsh S. Nature, reliability, and predictive value of muscle performance measures in patients with hemiparesis following stroke. *Arch Phys Med Rehabil.* 1992;73:721-725.

50. Sisto SA, Dyson-Hudson T. Dynamometry testing in spinal cord injury. *J Rehab Res Dev.* 2007;44:123-136.

51. Hayes K, Walton JR, Szomor ZL, Murrell GA. Reliability of 3 methods for assessing shoulder strength. *J Shoulder Elbow Surg.* 2002;80:1072-1076.

52. Hislop JH, Montgomery J. *Daniels and Worthingham's Muscle Testing.* 7th ed. Philadelphia, PA: BW Saunders; 1995.

53. Kendall FP, McCreary EK, Provance PG. *Muscles: Testing and Function.* 4th ed. Baltimore, MD: Williams & Wilkins; 1993.

54. Reese NB. *Muscle and Sensory Testing.* 2nd ed. St. Louis, MO: Elsevier; 2005:16.

55. Kleyweg RP, Van Der Meché FGA, Schmitz PIM. Interobserver agreement in the assessment of muscle strength and functional abilities in Guillain-Barré syndrome. *Muscle Nerve.* 1991;14:1103-1109.

56. Brandsma JW, Schreuders TAR, Birk JA, et al. Manual muscle strength testing: intraobserver and interobserver reliabilities for the instrinsic muscles of the hand. *J Hand Ther.* 1995;8:185-190.

57. Escolar DM, Henricson EK, Mayhew J, et al. Clinical evaluator reliability for qualitative and manual muscle testing measures of strength in children. *Muscle Nerve.* 2001;24:787-793.

58. Kolber MJ, Cleland JA. Strength testing using hand-held dynamometry. *Phys Ther Rev.* 2005;10:99-112.

59. Kimura I, Jefferson L, Gulick D, Coll R. Intra- and intertester reliability of Chatillon and MicroFet hand-held dynamometers in measuring force production. *J Sports Rehabil.* 1996; 5:197-205.

60. Bohannon RW, Andrews AW. Interrater reliability of hand-held dynamometry. *Phys Ther.* 1987;67:931-933.

61. Fenter P, Bellew J, Pitts T, et al. A comparison of 3 hand-held dynamometers used to measure hip abduction strength. *J Strength Cond Res.* 2003;17:531-535.

62. Fess EE. Grip strength. In: Casanova JS, ed. *Clinical Assessment Recommendations.* 2nd ed. Chicago, IL: American Society of Hand Therapists; 1992: 41-45.

63. Su CY, Lin JH, Chien TH et al. Grip strength in different positions of elbow and shoulder. *Arch Phys Med Rehabil.* 1994;75:812-815.

64. Weinstock-Zlotnick G, Bear-Lehman J, Yu TY. A test case: does the availability of visual feedback impact grip strength scores when using a digital dynamometer? *J Hand Ther.* 2011;24:266-276.

65. Fugl-Meyer AR, Jaasko L, Leyman I, et al. The post-stroke hemiplegic patient. I. A method for evaluation of physical performance. *Scand J Rehabil Med.* 1975;7:13-31.

66. Gladstone DJ, Danells CJ, Black SE. The Fugl-Meyer Assessment of Motor Recovery after stroke: a critical review of its measurement properties. *Neurorehabil Neural Repair.* 2002;16:468-477.

67. Berg KO, Maki BE, Holliday PJ, et al. Clinical and laboratory measures of postural balance in an elderly population. *Arch Phys Med Rehabil.* 1992;73:1073-1080.

68. Horak FB, Henry SM, Shumway-Cook A. Postural perturbations: new insights for treatment of balance disorders. *Phys Ther.* 1997;77:517-533.

69. Nashner LM. Fixed patterns of rapid postural responses among leg muscles during stance. *Exp Brain Res.* 1977; 30:13-24.

70. Horak F, Nashner L. Central programming of postural movements: adaptation to altered support surface configurations. *J Neurophysiol.* 1986;55:1369-1381.

71. O'Sullivan SB. Examination of motor function: motor control and motor learning. In: O'Sullivan SB, Schmitz TJ, eds. *Physical Rehabilitation.* 5th ed. Philadelphia, PA: FA Davis; 2007:227-271.

72. Gregson JM, Leathley M, Moore P, et al. Reliability of measurements of muscle tone and muscle power in stroke patients. *Age Ageing.* 2000; 29:223-228.

73. Waninge A, Rook RA, Dijkhuizen A, et al. Feasibility, test-retest reliability, and inter-rater reliability of the Modified Ashworth Scale and Modified Tardieu Scale in persons with profound intellectual and multiple disabilities. *Res Dev Disabil.* 2001;32:613-620.

74. Sloan RL, Sinclair E, Thompson J, et al. Inter-rater reliability of the Modified Ashworth Scale for spasticity in hemiplegic patients. *Int J Rehabil Res.* 1992;15:158-161.

75. Blackburn M, van Vliet P, Mockett SP. Reliability of measurements obtained with the Modified Ashworth Scale in the lower extremities of people with stroke. *Phys Ther.* 2002;82:25-33.

76. Ansari NN, Jaghdi S, Moammeri H, et al. Ashworth Scales are unreliable for the assessment of muscle spasticity. *Physiother Theory Pract.* 2006;22:119-125.

77. Patrick E, Ada L. The Tardieu Scale differentiates contracture from spasticity whereas the Ashworth Scale is confounded by it. *Clin Rehabil.* 2006;20(2):173-182.

78. Ansari NN, Jaghdi S, Hasson S, et al. The Modified Tardieu Scale for the measurement of elbow flexor spasticity in adult patients with hemiplegia. *Brain Inj.* 2008;22:1007-1012.

79. Merholz J, Wagner K, Meissner D, et al. Reliability of the Modified Tardieu Scale and the Modified Ashworth Scale in adult patients with severe brain injury: a comparison study. *Clin Rehabil.* 2005;19:751-759.

80. Tripp EJ, Harris SR. Test-retest reliability of isokinetic knee extension and flexion torque measurements in persons with spastic hemiparesis. *Phys Ther.* 1991;71:290-296.

81. Kingels K, De Cock P, Molenaers G, et al. Upper limb motor and sensory impairments in children with hemiplegic cerebral palsy. Can they be measured reliably? *Dis Rehabil.* 2010;32:409-416.

82. Dyball KM, Taylor NF, Dodd KJ. Retest reliability of measuring hip extensor muscle strength in different testing positions in young people with cerebral palsy. *BMC Pediatr.* 2011;11:42-49.

83. Bohannon RW, Walsh S. Nature, reliability, and predictive value of muscle performance measures in patients with hemiparesis following stroke. *Arch Phys Med Rehabil.* 1992;73:721-725.

84. Sisto SA, Dyson-Hudson T. Dynamometry testing in spinal cord injury. *J Rehabil Res Dev.* 2007;44:123-136.

85. Kimura I, Jefferson L, Gulick D, Coll R. Intra- and intertester reliability of Chatillon and MicroFet hand-held dynamometers in measuring force production. *J Sports Rehabil.* 1996;5:197-205.

86. Bohannon RW, Andrews AW. Interrater reliability of hand-held dynamometry. *Phys Ther.* 1987;67:931-933.

87. Fenter P, Bellew J, Pitts T, et al. A comparison of 3 hand-held dynamometers used to measure hip abduction strength. *J Strength Cond Res.* 2003;17:531-535.

88. Gladstone DJ, Danells CJ, Black SE. The Fugl-Meyer Assessment of Motor Recovery after stroke: a critical review of its measurement properties. *Neurorehabil Neural Repair.* 2002;16:468-477.

89. Duncan P, Studenski S, Chandler J, Prescott B. Functional reach: a new clinical measure of balance. *J Gerontol.* 1990;45:M192-M197.

90. Podsiadlo D, Richardson S. The timed "up and go" test: a test of basic functional mobility for frail elderly persons. *J Am Geriatr Soc.* 1991;39:142-148.

91. Berg K, Wood-Dauphinee S, Williams J, et al. Measuring balance in the elderly: preliminary development of an instrument. *Physiother Can.* 1989;41:304-308.

92. Berg K, Wood-Dauphinee SL, Williams JT. Measuring balance in the elderly: validation of an instrument. *Can J Public Health.* 1992;83:S9-S11.

93. Carr JH, Shepherd RB, Nordholm L, Lynne D. Investigation of a new Motor Assessment Scale for stroke patients. *Phys Ther.* 1985;65:175-180.

94. Kopp B, Kunkel A, Flor H, et al. The Arm Motor Ability Test: reliability, validity, and sensitivity to change of an instrument for assessing disabilities in activities of daily living. *Arch Phys Med Rehabil.* 1997;78:615-620.

95. Wolf SL, Catlin PA, Ellis M, Archer AL, Morgan B, Piacentino A. Assessing Wolf Motor Function Test as outcome measure for research in patients after stroke. *Stroke.* 2001;32:1635-1639.

96. Taub E, Miller NE, Novack TA, et al. Technique to improve chronic motor deficit after stroke. *Arch Phys Medicine and Rehabilitation.* 1993;74:347-354.

97. Uswatte G, Taub E, Morris D, Light K, Thompson PA. The Motor Activity Log-28: assessing daily use of the hemiparetic arm after stroke. *Neurology.* 2006;67:1189-1194.

98. Uswatte G, Taub E, Morris D, Vignolo M, McCulloch K. Reliability and validity of the upper-extremity Motor Activity Log-14 for measuring real-world arm use. *Stroke.* 2005;36:2493-2496.

99. Lyle RC. A performance test for assessment of upper limb function in physical rehabilitation treatment and research. *Int J Rehabil Res.* 1981;4:483-492.

100. Fisher AG. *AMPS, Assessment of Motor and Process Skills. Development, Standardization and Administration Manual.* 5th ed. Fort Collins, CO: Three Star Press; 2003.

101. Duncan P, Studenski S, Chandler J, Prescott B. Functional reach: a new clinical measure of balance. *J Gerontol.* 1990;45:M192-M197.

102. Newton J. Validity of the Multi-Directional Reach Test: a practical measure for limits of stability in older adults. *J Gerontol: Med Sci.* 2001:M248-M252.

103. Thompson M, Medley A. Forward and lateral sitting functional reach in younger, middle-aged, and older adults. *J Geriatr Phys Ther.* 2007;30:43-48.

104. Katz-Leurer M, Fisher I, Neeb M, et al. Reliability and validity of the modified functional reach test at the sub-acute stage post-stroke. *Disabil Rehabil.* 2009;31(3):243-248.

105. Podsiadlo D, Richardson S. The timed "up and go" test: a test of basic functional mobility for frail elderly persons. *J Am Geriatr Soc.* 1991;39:142-148.

106. Berg K, Wood-Dauphinee S, Williams J, et al. Measuring balance in the elderly: preliminary development of an instrument. *Physiother Can.* 1989;41:304-308.

107. Berg K, Wood-Dauphinee SL, Williams JT. Measuring balance in the elderly: validation of an instrument. *Can J Public Health.* 1992;83:S9-S11.

108. Berg KO, Maki BE, Holliday PJ, et al. Clinical and laboratory measures of postural balance in an elderly population. *Arch Phys Med Rehabil.* 1992;73:1073-1080.

109. Schmitz TJ. Examination of coordination. In O'Sullivan SB, Schmitz TJ, eds. *Physical Rehabilitation.* 5th ed. Philadelphia, PA: FA Davis; 2007:193-226.

110. Kwakkel G, Wagenaar RC, Twisk J, et al. Intensity of leg and arm training after primary middle-cerebral artery stroke: a randomized trial. *Lancet.* 1999; 354: 189-194.

111. Winstein CJ, Rose DK, Tan SM, et al. A randomized controlled comparison of upper-extremity rehabilitation strategies in acute stroke: a pilot study of immediate and long-term outcomes. *Arch Phys Med Rehabil.* 2004;85:620-628.

112. Boyd LA, Quaney BM, Pohl PS, et al. Learning implicitly: effects of task and severity after stroke. *Neurorehabil Neural Repair.* 2007;21:444-454.

113. Sullivan KJ, Knowlton BJ, Dobkin BH. Step training with body weight support: effect of treadmill speed and practice paradigms on poststrokelocomotor recovery. *Arch Phys Med Rehabil.* 2002;83:683-691.

114. Field-Fote EC, Roach KE. Influence of a locomotor training approach on walking speed and distance in people with chronic spinal cord injury: a randomized clinical trial. *Phys Ther.* 2011;91:48-60.

115. Katalinic OM, Harvey LA, Herbert RD. Effectiveness of stretch for the treatment and prevention of contractures in people with neurological conditions: a systematic review. *Phys Ther.* 2011;91:11-24.

116. Morris SL, Dodd KJ, Morris ME. Outcomes of progressive resistance strength training following stroke: a systematic review. *Clin Rehabil.* 2004;18:27-39.

117. Ouellete MM, Le Brasseur NK, Bean JF, et al. High-intensity resistance training improves muscle strength, self-reported function, and disability in long-term stroke survivors. *Stroke.* 2004;35:1404-1409.

118. Rietberg MB, Brooks D, Uitedehaag BMJ, Kwakkel G. Exercise therapy for multiple sclerosis. *Cochrane Database Syst Rev.* 2004;3. CD003980. doi: 10.1002/14651858.CD003980.pub2.

119. Goodwin VA, Richards SH, Taylor RS, et al. The effectiveness of exercise interventions for people with Parkinson's disease: a systematic review and meta-analysis. *Mov Disord.* 2008;23:631-640.

120. Salbach NM, Mayo NE, Robichaud-Ekstrand S, et al. The effect of a task-oriented walking intervention on improving balance self-efficacy post-stroke: a randomized, controlled trial. *J Am Geriatr Soc.* 2005;53:576-582.

121. Allen NE, Sherrington C, Paul SS, et al. Balance and falls in Parkinson's disease: a meta-analysis of the effect of exercise and motor training. *Mov Disord.* 2011;26:1605-1615.

122. Gupta S, Rao B, Sd K. Effect of strength and balance training in children with Down's syndrome: a randomized controlled trial. *Clin Rehabil.* 2011;25:425-432.

123. Howe TE, Rochester OL, Neil F, et al. Exercise for improving balance in older people. *Cochrane Database Syst Rev.* 2011;11. CD004963. doi: 10.1002/14651858.CS0049563.pub3.

124. Schmidt RA, Lee TD. *Motor Control and Learning: A Behavioral Emphasis.* Champaign, IL: Human Kinetics; 2011.

125. Fitts PM, Posner MI. *Human Performance.* Belmont, CA: Brooks/Cole; 1967.

126. Winstein CJ. Knowledge of results and motor learning—implications for PT. *Phys Ther.* 1991;71:140-149.

127. Vander Linden DW, Cauraugh JH, Green TA. The effect of frequency of kinetic feedback on learning an isometric force production task in nondisabled subjects. *Phys Ther.* 1993;73:79-87.

128. Wright DL, Smith-Munyon VL, Sidaway B. How close is too close for precise knowledge of results? *Res Q Exerc Sport.* 1997;68:172-176.

129. Schmidt FA, Young DE, Swinnen S, et al. Summary of knowledge of results for skill acquisition: support for the guidance hypothesis. *J Exp Psy.* 1989; 14:352-359.

130. Schmidt RA, Lange C, Young DE. Optimizing summary knowledge of results for skill learning. *Human Mov Sci.* 1990;9:325-348.

131. Winstein CJ, Schmidt RA. Reduced frequency of knowledge of results enhances motor skill learning. *J Exp Psychol.* 1990;16:677-691.

132. Winstein CJ, Pohl PS, Lewthwaite R. Effects of physical guidance and knowledge of results on motor learning: support for the guidance hypothesis. *Res Q Exerc Sport.* 1994;65:316-323.

133. Swinnen SP, Schmidt RA, Nicholson DE, et al. Information feedback for skill acquisition: instantaneous knowledge of results degrades learning. *J Exp Psychol.* 1990;16:1706-1716.

134. Maslovat D, Brunke KM, Chua R, Franks IM. Feedback effects on learning a novel bimanual coordination pattern: support for the guidance hypothesis. *J Mot Behav.* 2009;41:45-54.

135. Park J-H, Shea CH, Wright DL. Reduced frequency concurrent and terminal feedback: a test of the guidance hypothesis. *J Mot Behav.* 2000;32:287-296.

136. Kleim, JA, Barbay S, Nudo RJ. Functional reorganization of the rat motor cortex following motor skill learning. *J Neurophysiol.* 1998; 80: 3321–3325.

137. Kleim JA. Principles of experience-dependent neural plasticity: implications for rehabilitation after brain damage. *J Speech Lang Hear Res.* 2008;51:S225-S239.

138. Kleim JA, Barbay S, Cooper NR, et al. Motor learning-dependent synaptogenesis is localized to functionally reorganized motor cortex. *Neurobiol Learn Mem.* 2002;77:63-77.

139. Shea JB, Morgan RL. Contextual interference effects on the acquisition, retention, and transfer of a motor skill. *J Exp Psychol Hum Learn Mem.* 1979;4:179-187.

140. Hanlon RE. Motor learning following unilateral stroke. *Arch Phys Med Rehabil.* 1996;77:811-815.

141. Shea CH, Lai Q, Black C, et al. Spacing practice sessions across days benefits the learning of motor skills. *Hum Move Sci.* 2000;19:737-760.

142. Carr J, Shepherd R. *Neurological Rehabilitation: Optimizing Motor Performance.* Oxford, UK: Butterworth Heinemann; 1998.

143. Carr J, Shepherd R. *Stroke Rehabilitation: Guidelines for Exercise and Training to Optimize Motor Skill.* Edinburgh, Scotland: Butterworth Heinemann; 2003.

144. Bass-Haugen J, Mathiowetz V, Flinn N. Optimizing motor behavior using the occupational therapy task-oriented approach. In: Trombly Latham CA, Radomski MV, eds. *Occupational Therapy for Physical Dysfunction.* 6th ed. Baltimore, MD: Williams & Wilkins; 2008.

145. Kwakkel G, Wagenaar RC, Twisk J, et al. Intensity of leg and arm training after primary middle-cerebral artery stroke: a randomized trial. *Lancet.* 1999;354:189-194.

146. Rossignol S. Locomotion and its recovery after spinal injury. *Curr Opin Neurobiol.* 2000;10:708-716.

147. Winstein CJ, Rose DK, Tan SM, et al. A randomized controlled comparison of upper-extremity rehabilitation strategies in acute stroke: a pilot study of immediate and long-term outcomes. *Arch Phys Med Rehabil.* 2004;85:620-628.

148. Boyd LA, Quaney BM, Pohl PS, et al. Learning implicitly: effects of task and severity after stroke. *Neurorehabil Neural Repair.* 2007;21:444-454.

149. Sullivan KJ, Knowlton BJ, Dobkin BH. Step training with body weight support: effect of treadmill speed and practice paradigms on poststroke locomotor recovery. *Arch Phys Med Rehabil.* 2002;83:683-691.

150. Field-Fote EC, Roach KE. Influence of a locomotor training approach on walking speed and distance in people with chronic spinal cord injury: a randomized clinical trial. *Phys Ther.* 2011;91:48-60.

151. Stevenson VL. Spasticity management. *Clin Rehabil.* 2010; 4:293-304.

152. Lieber RL, Steinman S, Barash IA, Chambers H. Structural and functional changes in spastic skeletal muscle. *Muscle Nerve.* 2004;29:615-627.

153. Katalinic OM, Harvey LA, Herbert RD. Effectiveness of stretch for the treatment and prevention of contractures in people with neurological conditions: a systematic review. *Phys Ther.* 2011;91:11-24.

154. Mortenson PA, Eng JJ. The use of cases in the management of joint mobility and hypertonia following brain injury in adults: a systematic review. *Phys Ther.* 2003;83:648-658.

155. Elbasiouny SM, Morok D, Bakr MM, et al. Management of spasticity after spinal cord injury: current techniques and future directions. *Neurorehabil Neural Repair.* 2010;24:23-33.

156. Yan T, Hui-Chan CW, Li LS. Functional electrical stimulation improves motor recovery of the lower extremity and walking ability of subjects with first acute stroke: a randomized placebo-controlled trial. *Stroke.* 2005;36:80-85.

157. Morris SL, Dodd KJ, Morris ME. Outcomes of progressive resistance strength training following stroke: a systematic review. *Clin Rehabil.* 2004;18:27-39.

158. Ouellete MM, Le Brasseur NK, Bean JF, et al. High-intensity resistance training improves muscle strength, self-reported function, and disability in long-term stroke survivors. *Stroke.* 2004;35:1404-1409.

159. Rietberg MB, Brooks D, Uitedehaag BMJ, Kwakkel G. Exercise therapy for multiple sclerosis. *Cochrane Database Syst Rev.* 2004;3. CD003980. doi: 10.1002/14651858.CD003980.pub2.

160. Goodwin VA, Richards SH, Taylor RS, et al. The effectiveness of exercise interventions for people with Parkinson's disease: a systematic review and meta-analysis. *Mov Disord.* 2008;23:631-640.

161. Dibble LE, Addison O, Pap E. The effects of exercise on balance in persons with Parkinson's Disease: as systematic review across the disability spectrum. *JNPT.* 2009;33:14-26.

162. Gordon NF, Gulanick M, Costa F, et al. Physical activity and exercise recommendations for stroke survivors: an American Heart Association scientific statement from the Council on Cardiology Subcommittee on Exercise, Cardiac Rehabilitation, and Prevention; the Council on Cardiovascular Nursing; the Council on Nutrition, Physical Activity and Metabolism; and the Stroke Council. *Circulation.* 2005;103:2031-2041.

163. Shumway-Cook A, Anson D, Haller S. Postural sway biofeedback for pretraining postural control following hemiplegia. *Arch Phys Med Rehabil.* 1988;69:395-400.

164. Winstein C, Gardner ER, McNeal DR, et al. Standing balance training: effect on balance and locomotion in hemiparetic adults. *Arch Phys Med Rehabil.* 1989;70:755-762.

165. Barclay-Goddard RE, Stevenson TJ, Poluha W, et al. Force platform feedback for standing balance training after stroke. *Cochrane Database Syst Rev.* 2004;4:D004129.

166. Salbach NM, Mayo NE, Robichaud-Ekstrand S, et al. The effect of a task-oriented walking intervention on improving balance self-efficacy poststroke: a randomized, controlled trial. *J Am Geriatr Soc.* 2005;53:576-582.

167. Allen NE, Sherrington C, Paul SS, et al. Balance and falls in Parkinson's Disease: a meta-analysis of the effect of exercise and motor training. *Mov Disord.* 2011;26:1605-1615.

168. Gupta S, Rao B, Sd K. Effect of strength and balance training in children with Down's syndrome: a randomized controlled trial. *Clin Rehabil.* 2011;25:425-432.

169. Howe TE, Rochester OL, Neil F, et al. Exercise for improving balance in older people. *Cochrane Database Syst Rev.* 2011;11. CD004963. doi: 10.1002/14651858.CS0049563.pub3.

170. Voss ED, Ionta MK, Myers BJ. *Proprioceptive Neuromuscular Facilitation: Patterns and Techniques.* 3rd ed. Philadelphia, PA: JB Lippincott; 1985.

171. Bohman I. *The Philosophy and Evolution of the NDT (Bobath) Approach.* Oak Park, IL: NDTA; 1984.

172. Bly L. A historical and current view of the basis of NDT. *Pediatr Phys Ther.* 1991;3:131-135.

173. Gordon J. Assumptions underlying physical therapy intervention: theoretical and historical perspectives. In: Carr J, Shepherd R, eds. *Movement Science: Foundations for PT Rehabilitation.* Gaithersburg, MD: Aspen; 2000.

174. Howle JM. *Neuro-Developmental Treatment Approach: Theoretical Foundations and Principles of Clinical Practice.* Laguna Beach, CA: NDTA; 2002.

175. Wade DT. Outcome measures for clinical rehabilitation trials: impairment, function, quality of life, or value? *Am J Phys Med Rehabil.* 2003;82(Suppl):S26-S31. doi: 10.1097/01. PHM.0000086996.89383.A1.

Chapter 18

PERSON FACTORS
Physiological

Sandra L. Rogers, PhD, OTR/L

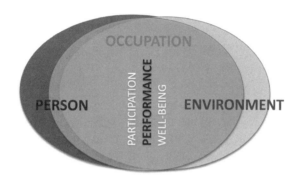

LEARNING OBJECTIVES

- Identify and define the primary physiological factors that influence performance and participation.
- Describe how constraints/barriers in physiological factors may affect a person's performance, participation, and well-being.
- Identify major health conditions or disabilities in which physiological factors influence performance, participation, and well-being.
- Identify established assessments that are evidence-based and measure capabilities and limitations related to occupational performance.
- Identify intervention principles to address physiological factors that are limiting occupational performance.
- Describe 3 to 5 intervention approaches that address limitations associated with physiological factors.
- Recognize the complexity of how physiological factors interact with other person and environment factors as it relates to performance in everyday life.

KEY WORDS

- Aerobic physical activity
- Body composition
- Body mass
- Bone-strengthening activity
- Cardiac endurance
- Flexibility
- General health
- Muscle endurance
- Nutritional status
- Physical fitness
- Skin integrity
- Sleep
- Stress

Christiansen CH, Baum CM, Bass JD, eds.
Occupational Therapy: Performance, Participation,
and Well-Being, Fourth Edition (pp 289-312).
© 2015 SLACK Incorporated.

INTRODUCTION

Adequate physiological functioning underlies the capacity of an individual to perform daily occupations. While individuals rarely consider physiological functioning as they go about their daily routines, it is pivotal in the ability of a person to function. Typically one only thinks of physiological functioning when something is not going well. For example, when a parent is not able to lift and carry a young child, an adult is not able to pass a physical examination for their work place, or an older adult is no longer able to do what they want to do.

Physiology is the study of biological function, how the body works, from cell to tissue, tissue to organ, organ to system. Physiology is the study of mechanisms, how things work, the study of function. Truly encompassing the function component of "body structure and function" in the ICF, physiology is a major player in the personal performance capabilities, as depicted in the PEOP Model. A study of physiology includes a study of all tissues, organs, and systems within the body and the functions associated with them.

As occupational therapy practitioners, we need to learn the basics of physiology and appreciate the ramifications of function within these systems because we must help our clients learn to manage the impact of illness on those physiologic functions we can observe. Practitioners often implicitly observe clients as they walk into a clinic or we walk into their home by observing any shortness of breath, breathing challenges, or alertness status, and we often assess the general conditioning of a client. We are, perhaps, most accustomed to dealing with the impact of disease on nervous, muscular, and skeletal systems. However, clinically we are also faced with the consequence of such things as spinal cord injury or typical aging on the integumentary system, as well as stress and illness on the endocrine, immune, and lymphatic systems.

It is useful to consider some of the primary aspects of healthy physiological functioning that influence an individuals' ability to participate in daily occupations without which a person may have difficulty participating.

PHYSICAL FITNESS

Physical fitness works well into our discussion of physiology because it represents overall wellness. Health-related physical fitness is of tremendous interest in health care because of its' potential to influence a variety of diseases. Additionally, many of these factors are under the partial control of an individual, at least to some extent. Research does not have a single method for determining physical fitness although it is defined most often defined as a combination of the following:

- Muscle strength
- Muscle endurance
- Flexibility
- Body composition
- Cardiorespiratory function

As such, it encompasses all systems described above in their healthy, functional state. These form the basis for human performance and are what a practitioner needs to consider in both wellness and disease or disability, because they are what will either prevent or allow participation in activities[1] and promote health. It is also an important consideration for clients faced with disability and disease.[2-7] Physical deconditioning can complicate the rehabilitation process.[7] For example a client may spend a considerable amount of time in bed while vital physiologic functions become stabilized. During this period of time their muscular and cardiorespiratory functions will have become compromised. As a result you will now not only be dealing with issues related to the primary health issue, you will be dealing with diminished heart and lung function, along with muscle weakness.

Muscle Strength

Muscle strength is the amount of force that can be exerted by one or a group of muscles in one voluntary maximum contraction. It is measured and developed using static (isometric) and dynamic (isotonic) means, but simply working on strength training is not generally the purview of an occupational therapy practitioner. However, it is important to know that static muscle strength is important in the development of posture and balance, while both forms of muscle strength play a role in all activities in which we engage, so the development of adequate muscle strength is a critical component of overall fitness. Additionally, it is an area critical to understanding typical and atypical muscle function and is addressed further in this text in Chapter 17.

Muscle Endurance

Muscle endurance is defined as the ability to repeat muscle contractions or maintain a single contraction as needed for a prolonged period of time. We need endurance in different ways in different muscles. Our postural control muscles must maintain posture against gravity for prolonged periods of time; our fine motor muscles, depending on what tasks we undertake, may need to repeatedly contract in the same way for prolonged periods of time. Our ability to perform such activities will depend on our muscular endurance. Muscle endurance is also tied to cardiorespiratory functions, as you might imagine.

Muscle endurance is typically evaluated by using a combination of the repetition maximum assessment, body-weight percentage, and calisthenics of push-ups and sit-ups. Metabolic equivalent (MET) levels are a reliable way to provide guidance as a measure of endurance. The MET of a task is a physiological measure expressing the energy cost of physical activities. It is defined as the ratio of metabolic rate (and therefore the rate of energy consumption) during a specific physical activity to a reference metabolic rate, set by convention as 1 kcal/kg/hour and roughly equivalent to the energy cost of sitting quietly. MET values of activities range from 0.9 (sleeping) to 18 (running at 17.5 km/h or a 5:31 mile pace). Different activities are assigned different MET levels depending on how much energy they take to do (see following section). The higher the MET level, the more energy the activity takes. A comprehensive table for many activities is available at https://sites.google.com/site/compendiumofphysicalactivities/.

Repetition Maximum and The Body-Weight Percentage are muscle endurance tests that allow a practitioner to analyze the muscle endurance capacity that a client demonstrates. They are highlighted in Table 18-1 and typically require more specialized testing situations. In a more typical clinical setting, calisthenics-type muscle endurance tests can be used more easily. Occupational therapy practitioners working with clients in wellness or promotion of physical fitness might use these techniques to establish a baseline to help the client identify progress and define success. The use of these measurement techniques in clients who have neurological impairment is limited; however, many clinicians use endurance as a way to measure progress in a variety of activities. For example, standing endurance during meal preparation following a stroke, or tolerance for completion of grocery shopping with clients who have chronic pain conditions.

Flexibility

Flexibility is defined as the range of motion at a joint, or at a sequence of joints. Flexibility will be influenced by the soft tissue around the joint(s), condition of the joint(s) themselves, and fat or excess muscle around the joint(s). Limited range of motion can clearly interfere with our ability to engage in many activities, including the very simple things such as combing the back of our hair or tying our shoes. Flexibility is measured in 2 ways: by simple measurement of degrees of movement to the ideal (range of motion measurement) and by functional testing.[1] Several resources are available to measure range of motion. Range of motion measures are useful to practitioners who seek to provide an indication of progression in therapeutic interventions but are not always indicative of

functional improvement and are most often used as in a comprehensive set of evaluations to measure progress.[11,12]

Functional evaluation includes measuring trunk, arms, and legs. There are several methods of measuring this flexibility. Some common examples are the sit and reach test, back scratch test, and the circumduction test. In the sit and reach test, which is a common measure of flexibility, the flexibility of the lower back and hamstring muscles are specifically measured. This test is important because tightness in this area is implicated in lumbar lordosis, forward pelvic tilt, and lower back pain. This test was first described by Wells and Dillon[13] and is now widely used as a general test of flexibility. The back scratch test measures how close the hands can be brought together behind the back; one then simply records the best score to the nearest centimeter or half inch.[14] This test is frequently used as an important test of general shoulder range of motion, particularly in seniors for driving evaluations and wellness.

Body Composition

Body composition refers to the fat and nonfat elements of the body. Both too little and too much body fat are thought to interfere with optimal body function, and either may interfere with our ability to engage in meaningful occupation.[15,16] Height and weight tables can give us some idea of ideal total body weight for people of the same sex and similar age and frame size. These tables tell us who is overweight or underweight with respect to the general population. However, these tables are not valid for determining an individual's lean to fat proportions. Body composition refers to the constituents of your body: lean mass, fat, and water. Scales weigh total body mass. Other measures are available for measuring whether weight is fat; lean mass including bone, ligaments, and muscle; or water.

In adults, overweight and obesity ranges are determined by using weight and height to calculate a number called the body mass index (BMI). BMI standard weight categories can easily be found on the web.[17] BMI is used because, for most people, it correlates with their amount of body fat. Calculating BMI is one of the best methods for population assessment of overweight and obesity.[18,19] Because calculation requires only height and weight, it is inexpensive and easy to use for clinicians and for the general public. The use of BMI allows people to compare their own weight status to that of the general population.[20]

Cardiorespiratory Function

The cardiovascular system is made up of the following:
- The heart, which provides the force for blood flow and maintains circulation
- The arterial system, which conducts oxygen-rich blood to tissues

Table 18-1. *Assessments for Cardiovascular and Muscle Endurance*

Assessment Name and Source	Type of Assessment	Description and Reference	Where It Can Be Obtained
Treadmill test	Cardiovascular assessments	Also called a stress test, it is the maximum effort attempted, beginning with walking and having the person produce as much effort until they have reached their tolerance. Routinely used in evaluation of cardiac fitness by physicians. Individual is connected to an ECG machine, and a blood pressure cuff is placed on one arm. Assessment is typically done by a technician in a laboratory setting.	Treadmill systems are available from many medical equipment companies.
Volume of Oxygen Measure (VO_2)		Calculates the volume of oxygen consumed for work per minute.	Oxygen and carbon dioxide analyzers, an ergometer on which workload may be modified, heart rate monitor, and a stopwatch. All equipment is available from a number of medical supply companies.
Relative Intensity		The level of effort required by a person to do an activity. When using relative intensity, people pay attention to how physical activity affects their heart rate and breathing, the so-called "talk test" is a simple way to measure relative intensity. As a rule of thumb, if a client is engaged in moderate-intensity activity she can talk (but not sing), during the activity. If you're doing vigorous-intensity activity, you will not be able to say more than a few words without pausing for a breath.	No specialized equipment needed.
Absolute Intensity is the amount of energy used by the body per minute of activity.		This establishes the intensity amount and is usually categorized according to light, moderate and vigorous. Absolute intensity can also be graded by using the speed at which an activity is performed, eg, running 6 mph.	Categorized according to light, moderate and vigorous.

(continued)

- The capillaries, which provide the medium for exchange between the blood and tissues
- The veins, which return blood to the heart and serve as an active blood reservoir

The amount of blood that the heart pumps in 1 minute is the cardiac output and is measured in milliliters per minute (mL/min). Cardiac output is the primary indicator of the ability of the heart to meet the demands of physical activity. Cardiac output is a product of the heart rate (beats

Table 18-1 (continued).   *Assessments for Cardiovascular and Muscle Endurance*

Assessment Name and Source	Type of Assessment	Description and Reference	Where It Can Be Obtained
Target heart rate	Cardiovascular assessments	To calculate this, a clinician first uses an age-predicted maximum heart rate and then obtains a resting heart rate. Then, using the Karvonnen formula, you determine the heart rate reserve by subtracting the resting heart rate (beats per minute) from the age predicted max heart rate. Heart rate reserve is the total number of heartbeats you have on reserve from rest to your maximum exercise effort.	Karvonnen Formula Target Heart Rate = ([max HR − resting HR] × % Intensity) + resting HR example
Borg Rating of Perceived Exertion (RPE)[8]		The most widely used physical exertion questionnaire. It is based on the physical sensations a person experiences during physical activity, including increased heart rate, increased respiration or breathing rate, increased sweating, and muscle fatigue.	(See Figure 18-1.) Public domain, reproduced in numerous publications.
A Physical Activity Readiness Questionnaire (PAR-Q)		PAR-Q is a brief 7-question questionnaire that will identify those persons who are: 1) at risk for beginning a moderate exercise program or 2) at-risk for undergoing an exercise test without prior medical examination. A very practical screening tool clinically as persons who are healthy enough to begin exercise without the expense of a medical examination or clinical exercise test or who need to be referred.[9]	Available at no cost: www. csep.ca/cmfiles/publications/parq/par-q.pdf (as long as it is used in its entirety).
Repetition maximum (RM)	Muscle endurance	RM is evaluated by having a client lift 40% to 60% of their estimated maximum weight using an exercise (eg, bench press) to lift weights 5 to 10 times. After a 2-minute rest, the load gets bumped up to 60% to 80% of the estimated maximum weight and lifted 3 to 5 times. Another rest period is added, then more weights are incrementally added. With 3- to 5-minute rest periods, this continues until the client has lifted as much as they can at least one time. That weight becomes the benchmark for muscle endurance. One then develops muscle strengthening routines that includes a client's maximum weight.	Technique is available to anyone.

(continued)

Table 18-1 (continued). *Assessments for Cardiovascular and Muscle Endurance*

Assessment Name and Source	Type of Assessment	Description and Reference	Where It Can Be Obtained
Body weight percentage[10]	Muscle endurance	This muscle endurance test utilizes a percentage of your total body weight and applies it to exercises that target specific muscle groups. A bench press repetition weight is derived from 66% of a man's body weight. For example if a man weighs 200 pounds, that amounts to 132 pounds. Thus, a 132-pound bench press would be repeated as many times as possible to find the muscle endurance for the pectorals. Using the same guidance, arm curls and leg curls are calculated at 33%, and leg extensions are figured at 50%. For women, lateral pull-downs, leg extensions and bench presses are calculated at 50%; leg curls, 33%; and arm curls, 25%.	No special equipment is required.
Calisthenics		These tests use basic exercises, such as push-ups and sit-ups. The sit-up test requires a rhythmical cadence of 50 beats per minute to measure the most sit-ups that can be performed without stopping or until the technique is lost. For example, for push-ups the chest must be lowered to the floor and raised back up, without buckling of the knees, as many times as possible without breaking technique.	No specialized equipment needed. Typically performed on a mat or carpeting for comfort.

per minute) and stroke volume (milliliters of blood ejected from the left ventricle with each stroke). The heart responds to a demand for increased blood flow with greater cardiac output by increasing both heart rate and stroke volume.

Cardiorespiratory fitness is defined as the ability to take in, transport, and use oxygen. As practitioners, it is important for us to be aware of the fact that this system is very sensitive to our needs and that the system works harder when the body is in different positions. The least stressful position for cardiorespiratory functions is supine, next is sitting, then standing. We ask more from our cardiorespiratory functions as we walk, run, etc. This seems quite logical, but needs to be kept forefront in our minds when we are dealing with a client who is not in good cardiorespiratory condition, especially when we begin to get

them into a sitting position from the supine position that they have maintained for several weeks at a time. It may take the cardiorespiratory functions a bit of catch-up time to function optimally, and we need to be cautious as practitioners to look for signs of overload to this system, which would be observed as shortness of breath, low blood pressure, or dizziness.

Screening will involve obtaining a health history and possibly a medical exam. The purpose of screening is to identify those individuals who may be at risk when beginning an exercise program and/or exercise testing. An exercise test may be recommended for those individuals who are deemed at a higher risk for exercise. Many of these types of exercise tests are medically supervised; focus is on cardiovascular risk and cardiopulmonary distress.[21] A physician performs a medical examination to determine

While doing physical activity, we want you to rate your perception of exertion. This feeling should reflect how heavy and strenuous the exercise feels to you, combining all sensations and feelings of physical stress, effort, and fatigue. Do not concern yourself with any one factor such as leg pain or shortness of breath, but try to focus on your total feeling of exertion. Look at the rating scale while you are engaging in an activity; it ranges from 6 to 20, where 6 means "no exertion at all" and 20 means "maximal exertion." Choose the number that best describes your level of exertion. This will give you a good idea of the intensity level of your activity, and you can use this information to speed up or slow down your movements to reach your desired range.

Try to appraise your feeling of exertion as honestly as possible, without thinking about what the actual physical load is. Your own feeling of effort and exertion is important, not how it compares to other people. Look at the scales and the expressions and then give a number.[22,23]

Borg Scale	Perceived Exertion	Modified Borg Scale
	Nothing at all	0.0
	Very, very weak	0.5
	Very weak	1.0
		1.5
	Weak	2.0
6		
7	Very, very light	
8		
9	Very light	
10		
11	Light	3
12		
13	Somewhat hard	4
14		
15	Hard (heavy)	5
16		6
17	Very hard	7
18		8
19	Extremely hard	9
20	Maximal exertion	10

Figure 18-1. Modified Borg Perceived Exertion Scale: Instructions for Borg Rating of Perceived Exertion (RPE) Scale.

any resting conditions that will need to be addressed before beginning participation in activities. Many of the risk factors for heart disease and special concerns for exercise may be identified on the health history. Clinical testing is warranted for those individuals who are at higher risk or already have a heart condition.[16] Clinical tests are highlighted in Table 18-1. More specific information can be located on the web by searching the National US Physical Activity Plan.

Other clinical measures include questionnaires that focus a client's attention on either his or her effort during physical exertion or on his or her readiness to participate in physical activity. The Borg Rating of Perceived Exertion (RPE) is the most widely used physical exertion questionnaire (Figure 18-1). Practitioners generally agree that perceived exertion ratings between 12 to 14 on the Borg Scale suggests that physical activity is being performed at a moderate level of intensity. Through experience of monitoring perceptions of how one's body feels, it becomes easier to help them modify intensity. For example, a walker who wants to engage in moderate-intensity activity

would aim for a Borg Scale level of "somewhat hard" (12 to 14). If he describes his muscle fatigue and breathing as "very light" (9 on the Borg Scale), he would want to increase his intensity. On the other hand, if he felt his exertion was "extremely hard" (19 on the Borg Scale), he would need to slow down his movements to achieve the moderate-intensity range. A high correlation exists between a person's perceived exertion rating times 10 and the actual heart rate during physical activity; so a person's exertion rating may provide a fairly good estimate of the actual heart rate during activity.[24] For example, if a person's rating of perceived exertion (RPE) is 12, then $12 \times 10 = 120$; so the heart rate should be approximately 120 beats per minute. The Borg Rating of Perceived Exertion is also the preferred method to assess intensity among those individuals who take medications that affect heart rate or pulse. Other commonly used questionnaires are highlighted in Table 18-1.

For older adults, a more comprehensive test of fitness, which includes a number of flexibility measures, endurance measures, and cardiovascular fitness, is available. The

Groningen Fitness Test for the Elderly[25] battery comprises tests of a range of fitness components. See Table 18-2 for the included tests. Alternatively, there is a fitness test for seniors based on common activities, ie, getting up from a chair, walking, lifting, bending, and stretching.[14,28]

INTERVENTION FOR FITNESS

Regular physical activity has overwhelming clear evidence associated with its' ability to help with weight control, stress reduction, lowering blood pressure, and lowering the chance of diabetes and heart disease.[29-31] While the evidence in favor of physical activity is clear, creating environments that support engagement are more challenging—as the near epidemic increases in obesity would suggest.[32] Evidence suggests that no one program works for any one individual, but that some guidelines may be helpful in starting a fitness program.[1,33,34] Initially, physical fitness goals and objectives, as well as assessing the 5 components of fitness, may be required. Then, a clinician might assist a client in choosing the exercise or activity that will achieve his or her goals. The exercise or activity programs for improving upper extremity strength, increasing low-back flexibility, or improving cardiovascular endurance will be different and specific. In collaboration with the client, an exercise program can be developed with specific recommendations for intensity, duration at each session, and frequency of the sessions. The intensity recommendations should be stated as ranges, with established upper level values that the client should not exceed and lower level, "insufficient load" values. In goal setting there needs to be a realistic determination for rate of change and amount of improvement to be achieved. Change is a function of various factors in each individual, including initial fitness levels, intensity of the training, type of training, age, general health, and psychosocial dimensions.[1]

A generic prescription for physical fitness might begin with a calculation of target heart rates and an administration of the PAR-Q. This is followed by development of a moderate physical activity program that is closely aligned to a client's routine and environment.[1,33] The Borg Exertion Scale would be used during physical exertion to monitor physical activity.[35] The MET levels would be used as a guide to help a client estimate the anticipation of physical exertion and choose activities that meet the level of fitness that is appropriate for them.[36] The success of a program for fitness is highly dependent on social, familial, personal preference; job and family responsibilities; and environment (eg, availability of exercise facilities and weather).[37-42] It's important for clients to schedule fitness for a time when there is little chance that they will have to cancel or interrupt it because of other demands. Additionally, fitness programs need to include all 4 aspects of physical fitness: flexibility, endurance, strength, and cardiorespiratory endurance. An example for a moderate-intensity program might include a warm up of walking for 5 to 10 minutes, a session of weight lifting followed by sit-ups and push-ups, 20 minutes of aerobic activity (brisk walking), stretching, and a 5- to 10-minute cool down (slow walking).

NUTRITION

More than one-third of adults and 17% of youth were classified as obese in 2009 and 2010. The rates for obesity have doubled for adults and tripled for children since 1980. While prevalence rates did not differ between men and women, the over-60 age group is more likely to be obese.[43] In the attempt to help stem the epidemic of obesity, nutrition guidelines have been established to help Americans make better choices. The Dietary Guidelines for Americans emphasize 3 major goals[44]:

1. Balance calories with physical activity to manage weight

2. Consume more of certain foods and nutrients, such as fruits, vegetables, whole grains, fat-free and low-fat dairy products, and seafood

3. Consume fewer foods with sodium (salt), saturated fats, trans fats, cholesterol, added sugars, and refined grains

The best diet is rich in fruits and vegetables, whole grains, and fat-free and low-fat dairy products for persons aged 2 years and older. The dietary and physical activity behaviors of children, adolescents, and adults are influenced by many sectors of society, including families, communities, schools, child care settings, medical care providers, faith-based institutions, government agencies, media, and the food and beverage industries and entertainment industries.[45] People who were obese had medical costs that were $1429 more than the cost for people of normal body weight.[43] Obesity also has been linked with reduced worker productivity and chronic work absence. Obviously practitioners need to grapple with issues related to obesity. It is clear that knowledge of a healthy diet alone is not enough to control weight.[46] Physical fitness, increasing engagement in a variety of non-sedentary activities, as well as changing habits to include more physical activity need to be addressed.[3,16,18,32,37,46-50]

When working with clients we can help clients choose a healthier balance of food when engaging in activities that include meal preparation, shopping, and eating. Like physical fitness no one strategy works for every individual.[18,46,48,50] Occupational considerations include the type of work, leisure activities, and how meals are consumed. In general, consumption of a healthier diet involves meal

Table 18-2. *The Groningen Fitness Test for the Elderly*[26,27]

Test	Method
Grip Strength Test: Upper body strength	Dynamometer
Leg Extension Test: Lower body strength	The participant sits on the table between the arm supports with their lower legs hanging down (knee angle 90 degrees). A shin guard attached to a resistance is fastened around the right lower leg of the participant, who must try to extend the right leg by raising the lower leg with maximum strength and then hold that position for 3 seconds. During the test, the participant may lean on the arm supports. Explosive movements should be avoided. The score is given in kilograms of force. After 1 practice trial, the best score of 3 trials is recorded. The resting period between trials is approximately 30 seconds.
Sit and Reach Flexibility: Hamstring and back flexibility	This test involves sitting on the floor with legs stretched out straight ahead. The soles of the feet are placed flat against the box. Both knees should be locked and pressed flat to the floor, the tester may assist by holding them down. With the palms facing downwards and the hands on top of each other or side by side, the subject reaches forward along the measuring line as far as possible. Ensure that the hands remain at the same level, not one reaching further forward than the other. After some practice reaches, the subject reaches out and holds that position for 1 to 2 seconds while the distance is recorded.
Circumduction: Shoulder flexibility	Using a cord that has a fixed handle on one end and a sliding handle on the other, the sliding handle is adjusted so that the length of the cord between the inside of the two handles is equivalent to the participant's shoulder width (from acromion to acromion). Then, holding the 2 handles of the cord, the participant passes the cord from in front of the body, over the head, and as far back as possible. This movement must be made with extended arms, and participants must try to keep their arms from fanning out more than is physically necessary to complete the movement. After a practice trial, the best score of 3 trials is recorded. Higher scores indicate better performance. The score is the angle of fanning out, in degrees, calculated with the following formula where S = how much the sliding handle shifted in centimeters during the movement and L = length of the arm in centimeters from acromion to the metacarpophalangeal joint of the middle linger.
Balance board (platform) test: Testing agility and balance	A wooden balance platform measures measuring 50 x 50 x 1.5 cm, with a small 2-cm-wide beam running lengthwise down the middle beneath it. Small stoppers are placed on the comers of the platform so that the board cannot tilt more than 18 degrees. Contacts connected to a timer are placed on the underside of the platform, exactly in the middle of the left and right halves. The participant is instructed to stand on the platform with toes pointed outward (15 degrees) and heels 15 cm apart. The participant must try to keep the platform balanced for a period of 30 seconds. The timer stops when the contacts touch the floor. After 1 practice trial, the best score of 3 trials is recorded. The score is the total time that neither contact touches the floor, expressed in counts (1 count = 0.3 seconds; 100 counts = 30 seconds). Thus the maximum score is 100 (for 30 seconds), and the higher scores indicate better performance.
Block transfer: A manual dexterity test or coordination test of fine motor abilities	In this test, 2 boards (56.5 x 23 x 2.4 cm), each punctuated with 40 holes (diameter, 4 cm; depth, 1.1 cm), and 40 blocks (diameter, 3.5 cm; height, 2.2 cm). The participant begins by sitting at a table with the 2 boards in front of them. Timing begins when the participant starts to move the 40 blocks from the first board to the second board, which is linked to the first board and farther away. The blocks must be moved in a prescribed sequence as quickly as possible using the preferred hand. The participant should practice with 5 blocks prior to the trial.

(continued)

Table 18-2 (continued).   *The Groningen Fitness Test for the Elderly*[26,27]

Test	Method
Reaction time test: A test of fine motor abilities	For this test a specially developed timer is used, which is connected to a hand-held module with a display light in the middle and a button on top, much like a stopwatch. The participant holds the module in the preferred hand and when the red light comes on must respond as quickly as possible by pushing the button. The reaction time (in milliseconds) is displayed on the timer. The time between the visual signals ranges between 4 and 9 seconds. After 3 practice trials, 15 trials are recorded. The score recorded is the median of the 15 trials.
Walking endurance test: Aerobic fitness test	This test uses a large flat non-slip area, tape recorder or CD player, a cassette tape or cd of the protocol, 3 yellow and 3 orange maker cones, and measuring tape. A rectangular course is marked out with the dimensions 16 2/3 x 8 1/3 meters, equaling a perimeter of 50 meters. Cones of alternating color are placed every 8 1/3 meters. The participants walk counterclockwise around the course, with the walking speed indicated by audible beeps. Between each 2 beeps the participant must walk 16 2/3 meters (one stage) from 1 cone to the next cone of the same color. The test starts off with a walking speed of 4 km/hr. Every third minute the pace is increased by 1 km/hr to a maximum of 7 km/hr. The test ends when the participant gives up or is unable to keep up the pace (eg, when they are more than 3 meters from a cone at 2 consecutive beeps) or successfully completes the last stage. The score is the number of 16 2/3 meter stages completed, the maximum possible score is 66. Higher scores indicate better performance.

preparation and this may require that an individual or family expend more energy and time planning meals, shopping, and cooking. Individuals or families that are heavily driven by a schedule (eg, have activities scheduled over and during meal times) will find this more difficult.[4,6,51] Environmental considerations are particularly important in nutrition, as it presents a barrier for individuals living in urban and lower socioeconomic areas who cannot readily access markets with fresh fruit and vegetables. A number of websites exist that help to present a balance of information regarding healthy nutrition that is evidence-based and directed to lay person's understanding of nutrition, for example: http://www.hsph.harvard.edu/nutritionsource/.

SLEEP

Sleep is typically defined as a period of rest for the body and mind, during which volition and consciousness are in partial or complete abeyance and the bodily functions are partially suspended. Sleep has also been described as a behavioral state marked by characteristic immobile posture, and diminished but readily reversible sensitivity to external stimuli.[52] Most theorists agree that sleep has value as a recuperative and adaptive function in the lives of humans. There are primarily 2 forms of sleep, both mea-surable on the basis of electroencephalographic (EEG) criteria and serve specific purposes in the resting cycle.[53]

Non-rapid eye movement (NREM) sleep, also called *orthodox* or *synchronized* (S) sleep, is the deep, dreamless period of sleep during which the brain waves are slow and of high voltage. Autonomic activities, such as heart rate and blood pressure, are low and regular. NREM sleep is subdivided into 4 stages. The EEG patterns of NREM sleep suggest that this is the kind of apparently restful state that supports the recuperative functions assigned to sleep. NREM sleep is increased after physical activity and has a relatively high priority among humans in the recovery sleep following extended periods of wakefulness.[53]

Rapid eye movement (REM) sleep, also called *paradoxical* or *desynchronized* (D) sleep, is the period of sleep during which the brain waves are fast and of low voltage. Autonomic activities, such as heart rate and respiration, are irregular. This type of sleep is associated with dreaming, mild involuntary muscle jerks, and REM. It usually occurs 3 to 4 times each night at intervals of 80 to 120 minutes, each occurrence lasting from 5 minutes to more than an hour. With each cycle, NREM sleep decreases and REM sleep increases, so that by the end of the night most of the sleep is REM sleep, which is when dreams occur. While everyone dreams every night, many do not remember dreaming; most people are aware, however, that they dream more just before rising.[52]

Patterns of Sleep Throughout Life

Factors affecting the total sleep pattern include age, state of physical health, psychological state, and certain drugs.[54] Newborns follow a pattern of several hours of sleep followed by a period of wakefulness. REM sleep occurs at the onset of sleep in infants; it rarely does in adults. As the child matures, there is an increasing tendency toward longer periods of nocturnal sleep. Elderly persons sometimes return to the shorter periods of sleep that are typical of infants. Although the average adult spends approximately 25% of total accumulated sleep in REM sleep and 75% in NREM sleep, the cyclic changes vary with individuals. The pattern of sleep, in addition to the REM and NREM states, also includes the periods of sleep and wakefulness within a 24-hour period.[55] Sleep requirements vary greatly among individuals. Infants usually require 16 to 20 hours of total sleep during a 24-hour period, and the amount decreases as the child matures. An adult usually requires 6 to 9 hours of total sleep, and requirements continue to decrease with aging.[54]

Relationship to Health

Sleep research consistently shows that sleeping too little can not only inhibit your productivity and ability to remember and consolidate information, but lack of sleep can also lead to serious health consequences and jeopardize safety for the individual and society.[19,56] For example, short sleep duration is linked with the following[57-62]:

- Increased risk of motor vehicle accidents
- Increase in BMI—a greater likelihood of obesity due to an increased appetite caused by sleep deprivation
- Increased risk of diabetes and heart problems
- Increased risk for psychiatric conditions including depression and substance abuse
- Decreased ability to pay attention, react to signals, or remember new information

A number of conditions are clearly linked to sleep pathology.[63] Most sleep disruption is temporary or can be linked to lifestyle routines that are more easily addressed by using a number of sleep patterning recommendations (see following interventions). Sleep pathologies on the other hand can stem from a number of neurological, physiological, psychological, and structural impairments that require more intensive intervention. Mental illness, drug addiction, dementia, and stroke are all associated with disregulations of sleep patterns and may benefit from intervention. Some impairments include:

- Insomnia
- Restless leg syndrome
- Sleep apnea
- Snoring
- Upper airway resistance syndrome (UARS)

These impairments would require a more intensive medical workup and may require that an individual participate in an overnight sleep study to evaluate the quality of sleep.

Sleep Assessments and Intervention

For an individual with a pattern of sleep insomnia or sleep apnea, a comprehensive and conclusive sleep assessment can only be done over a period of sleep with EEG monitoring. Consequently, sleep assessments are typically conducted with a questionnaire, for example the 11 questions featured on the Global Sleep Assessment Questionnaire (GSAQ) or Epworth Sleepiness Scale.[64,65] Two scales are free of charge to practitioners with a request for permission for use at these websites:

1. Epworth Sleepiness Scale: http://epworthsleepinessscale.com/
2. Pittsburgh Sleep Quality Index (PSQI): http://www.sleep.pitt.edu/content.asp?id=1484&subid=2316

These scales attempt to detail the extent of sleep pathology and determine if further more comprehensive assessment is required. While occupational therapy practitioners are not directly involved in the medical intervention for pathologies, they are often involved in helping clients to establish healthy sleep routines and may also be involved in helping clients to manage their medical issues.[66,67]

Other interventions include the use of tools that help to document healthy sleep patterns, including sleep diaries, documentation of pie of life, and establishment of routines and habits that support healthy sleep. The *Activity Card Sort* has been demonstrated to provide a reliable and valid tool to identify differences in competency among people on activities of daily living and assists the practitioner in documenting how a lack of sleep may inhibit participation in other occupations.[68-73] Additionally the Occupational Performance History Interview-II (OPHI-II) has been demonstrated to be sensitive to examining the impact that a lack of sleep is having on occupations.[74]

STRESS

The interaction of mind and body, while new to traditional medicine, has historically been implied as an important component of health in some areas of medicine, but was clearly articulated in occupational therapy. The implied relationship was that a reciprocal relationship existed between a healthy mind and a healthy body. As Mary Reilly so eloquently stated in her Eleanor Slagle Clark lecture, "Man, through the use of his hands, as they are energized by mind and will, can influence the state of his own health."[75]

While it is now widely accepted that the CNS interacts with the endocrine and immune system, and that these interactions are bi-directional, this research has largely been the work of the past 25 years. This knowledge of the bi-directional nature is extensively backed by both clinical and mechanistic evidence. The specifics of those relationships are beyond the scope of this chapter to discuss; however, the reader is encouraged to consult texts that focus on these topics.[76] As a brief review, it is helpful to note that 2 important aspects of these interactions include the production of stress hormones by the hypothalamic-pituitary-adrenal (HPA) axis and the sympathetic-adrenal-medullary (SAM) axis. Some of those components consist of cytokines that are products of the immune system activation and serve to alert the immune system and CNS that activation has taken place; hormones can modulate immune function by binding to their receptors, which are present on all immune cells.[77,78] It is important to note that stress has often been the focus of much research because stress (be it physiological or psychological) has been clearly shown to induce dysregulation across many aspects of both humoral (B-cell) and cellular (T-cell) responses.[79] The HPA axis and the autonomic nervous system provide 2 key pathways for immune system dysregulation: stressors can activate the sympathetic-adrenal-medullary (SAM) axis and the HPA axis, and thereby provoke the release of pituitary and adrenal hormones. For example, the catecholamines (adrenaline and noradrenaline), adrenocorticotropic hormone (ACTH), cortisol, growth hormone, and prolactin are all influenced by negative events and negative emotions, and each of these hormones can induce quantitative and qualitative changes in immune function. Furthermore, depression can substantially boost cortisol levels, and increases in cortisol levels can provoke multiple adverse immunological changes.[79]

Researchers have clearly demonstrated that stress, when it is coupled with lifestyle challenges or disease (ie, caregiving for those with dementia, HIV/AIDS, or psychopathology), will produce negative alterations in immune health.[78] Currently, it is unclear whether stress alone can create disease in otherwise healthy individuals or how well positive changes in lifestyle can buffer the potentially negative effects of stress.[76] Stress concepts can be broadly categorized as either resilience or cumulative burden/allostatic load. Cumulative burden (known as allostatic load) of adapting to environmental challenge can lead to physiological changes that result in compromise of the immune system (dysregulation) and can potentially lead to increased risk for disease and illness.[80-82] However, people vary in the extent to which life stress results in adverse consequences, giving rise to the concept of resilience.[83] The concept of resilience is critical, because maintaining a healthy immune system is central to good health and because research has shown that certain lifestyle characteristics may serve as buffers to stress. Accordingly, individuals with positive lifestyle patterns may experience fewer ill effects of stress.[84] A growing body of literature has examined these influences, including personal characteristics, coping styles, and social or lifestyle factors (ie, nutrition, smoking), which collectively point to great variation in individual responses to stressful life events.[78]

Assessment and Intervention

While stress has been clearly shown to have a negative impact on health, it is not clear that any one assessment or intervention can buffer one against stress. Clearly many of the lifestyle factors that have already been discussed (ie, body composition, nutrition, and physical fitness) may play an important role in controlling stress, but there is little evidence that simply adopting healthy lifestyles will be protective. Few studies measuring interventions have been completed to allow clinical utility. However, one important concept to consider for occupational therapy practitioners is the notion that engagement in meaningful activities and seeking a balance of activities could be seen as an intervention for reducing cumulative burden and providing a buffer to adverse consequences of stressful events.[85] It is unlikely that it is possible to lead a totally stress-free life, and many have promoted the idea of *eustress* (ie, humans benefit from some level of stress). It is unlikely to be the characteristics of the stressor that are of importance in determining hormonal alterations, but rather how the stressor is perceived by an individual and how well the individual is prepared to cope. Those 2 issues will then influence how the stress will alter the hormonal and immune milieu. Matuska and Christiansen suggest that the lifestyle configuration that may promote health and well-being is one that is quite dynamic and changes over time and over an individuals' circumstances.[86] This notion, and the beginning of evidence that this concept is accurate, gives practitioners some weight to their interest in an individual's engagement in personally satisfying tasks, and is worth investigating as part of an assessment. Some interventions investigated may show some promise to buffer the effects of stress, namely exercise, sleep, meditation, predictability and control over life events, social support, and spiritual support.[29,84,87-90]

In assessing stress, there are 2 categorizations of stress evaluation, *environmental* and *psychological*. Assessments that are more environmental include questionnaire and interview measures of major stressful life events, measures of chronic stress, as well as measures of daily events. The psychological measures include perceived stress and of negative affect. Examples of commonly used stress measures are listed in Table 18-3.

Table 18-3. *Commonly Used Measures of Stress*

Measure	Description	Primary Reference
Perceived Stress Scale (PSS)	The instrument used most often used. The PSS is a measure of the degree to which situations in one's life are appraised as stressful. Items were designed to tap how unpredictable, uncontrollable, and overloaded respondents find their lives. There are 3 versions of the scale, with 4 items, 10 items, or 14 items.	91,92
Hassle Scale	One rates a 53-item scale that includes both undesirable (hassles) and desirable (uplifts) events	93
Daily Stress Inventory (DSI)	Measures daily events; it is a 58-item questionnaire that asks about minor events occurring in the last 2 weeks	94
Positive Affect-Negative Affect Schedule (PANAS)	Measures negative affect A 60-item test that measures 11 specific affects: fear, sadness, guilt, hostility, shyness, fatigue, surprise, joviality, self-assurance, attentiveness, and serenity	95
Social Readjustment Rating Scale	An elaboration of this instrument developed by Holmes and Rahe. It is a rating scale of stressful life events that are believed to contribute to illness.	96

PAIN

Over one-third of the world's population reportedly suffers from persistent or recurrent pain, costing the American public alone approximately $100 billion each year in health care, compensation, and litigation.[97] Chronic pain is associated with conditions such as back injury, migraine headaches, arthritis, herpes zoster, diabetic neuropathy, temporomandibular joint syndrome, and cancer.[98] The International Association for the Study of Pain defines pain as "an unpleasant sensory and emotional experience associated with actual or potential tissue damage, or described in terms of such damage, or both."[99]

There are 3 primary underlying causes of pain:

- *Nociceptive pain* is from pain receptor stimulation. It may be somatic pain from activation of receptors in the musculoskeletal system or visceral pain that arises from receptors in the viscera.
- *Neuropathic pain* is pain due to changes in the peripheral or CNS.
- *Idiopathic pain* is pain without a known cause, and is not a diagnosis of psychogenic pain.

Additionally, pain can be classified as *acute* or *chronic*. Acute pain stems from a response to injury or illness is typically time-limited, is usually responsive to treatment, and inadequate treatment may result in delayed recovery. Chronic pain is a state in which pain persists beyond the usual course of an acute disease or healing of an injury, or that may or may not be associated with an acute or chronic pathologic process that causes continuous or intermittent pain over months or years.[97,98] Accurate assessment of the underlying cause and type of pain will allow more accurate selection of appropriate medications. However, chronic pain may be multifactorial and require multiple approaches to treatment. Chronic pain is the type of condition seen in a number of neurological (ie, stroke, headaches), orthopedic (ie, hand injuries, back injury), or ontological (ie, breast cancer) conditions.[100] The pain system may be grossly divided into the following components of *nociceptors*, the specialized receptors in the peripheral nervous system that detect noxious stimuli[101]:

- Primary nociceptive afferent fibers (normally Aδ and C fibers), which transmit information about noxious stimuli to the dorsal horn of the spinal cord
- Ascending nociceptive tracts, for example, the spinothalamic and spinohypothalamic tract (SHT), which convey nociceptive stimuli from the dorsal horn of the spinal cord to higher centers in the CNS
- Higher centers in the CNS that are involved in discrimination of pain, affective components of pain, memory components of pain, and motor control relate to the immediate aversive response to painful stimuli
- Descending systems that allow higher centers of the CNS to modify nociceptive information at multiple levels

Table 18-4. *Pain Intensity Scale*

Pain Numeric Rating Scale										
On a scale of 0 to 10, with 0 being no pain at all and 10 being the worst pain imaginable, how would you rate your pain RIGHT NOW?										
0	1	2	3	4	5	6	7	8	9	10
No Pain									*Worst Pain Imaginable*	
On the same scale, how would you rate your USUAL level of pain during the last week?										
0	1	2	3	4	5	6	7	8	9	10
No Pain									*Worst Pain Imaginable*	
On the same scale, how would you rate your USUAL level of pain during the last week?										
0	1	2	3	4	5	6	7	8	9	10
No Pain									*Worst Pain Imaginable*	
On the same scale, how would you rate your WORST level of pain during the last week?										
0	1	2	3	4	5	6	7	8	9	10
No Pain									*Worst Pain Imaginable*	

Mild pain is 1-3, Moderate pain is 4-6, Severe pain is 7-9.

Many of the currently available pain therapies for chronic pain are either inadequate or cause uncomfortable to deleterious side effects. Chronic pain results not just from the physical insult, but also from a combination of physical, emotional, psychological, and social abnormalities.[102,103] Because chronic pain persists after an insult is healed, the ongoing pain rather than the injury underlies the patient's disability. Untreated pain may become self-perpetuating, because pain has immunosuppressive effects that leave patients susceptible to subsequent diseases.[104] Chronic pain creates both physical and psychological problems that affect whether a person can engage in meaningful activities each day. Pain can decrease a person's strength, coordination, and independence, in addition to causing stress that may lead to depression.[97] It is now clear that if we can effectively treat the pain despite the underlying cause, it will be possible for patients to regain normal functioning.[98,102,103,105-111]

The management of pain is an important topic, and 9 states now require (5 states) or encourage (4 states) health care practitioners to obtain at least a portion of their annual continuing education credits in pain management.

Assessment and Intervention

The goals of pain assessment are to determine location, severity, and level of interference with ADL or QOL. The number of measures available to assess pain are numerous and broadly classified; they include intensity scales such as a visual analogue scale (VAS) or numeric rating scale (NRS) for assessment of pain intensity, pain drawings to identify location of the pain, observations of pain for those clients who are not capable of indicating pain (eg, dementia), and self-reports of pain which include intensity and time.[112-116] Because pain is a multidimensional sensory experience, it is unique to any one individual, consequently an important gauge of pain is the experience of the pain. As chronic pain may not be completely evaluated, it is important to use an assessment that is capable of monitoring progress.

The Numeric Rating Scale (NRS-11) (Table 18-4) is a widely used and clinically useful tool for measuring pain intensity in a variety of populations in many conditions, including children, elderly, cancer, and low back pain.[112-114,117] The McGill Pain Questionnaire can be used to monitor the pain over time and to determine the effectiveness of an intervention.[118] The questionnaire (available at many websites) is a widely-used method to evaluate a person experiencing significant pain.

Intervening to manage pain presents a challenge for practitioners due to the difficulties of or failure to properly assess pain, lack of pain relief standards, lack of accountability for effective pain relief, and poor reimbursement for pain care.[119] It has been reported that a common cause of unrelieved and unnecessary suffering stems from the failure of providers to fully or accurately assess pain, to accept a patient's subjective report of pain, and to perform actions to relieve the pain. It is recognized that pain assessment can be challenging in special populations such as neonates, children, and the cognitively or physically impaired. The additive effects of these pain treatment challenges have resulted in under-treatment and inappropriate treatment of a significant portion of patients suffering from acute or chronic pain.[97,98,100,103]

The goals of pain management should be to reduce pain, improve functioning, and improve the QOL. The results of a systematic review suggest that intervention techniques, such as mindfulness-based stress reduction programs and acceptance and commitment therapy, are not superior to CBT but can be good alternatives.[110] Compared with other non-disciplinary treatments, moderate evidence of higher effectiveness for multidisciplinary interventions was shown. In contrast to no treatment or standard medical treatment, strong evidence was detected in favor of multidisciplinary treatments. The evidence that comprehensive inpatient programs were more beneficial than outpatient programs was moderate.[110]

CBT is currently the most widely used psychological treatment for persistent pain. A critical review of the literature demonstrates some positive outcomes of cognitive-behavioral intervention, particularly when compared with no intervention. However, the evidence from this review is not conclusive.

SKIN INTEGRITY

The skin is a complex organ, the largest in the body, in which precisely regulated cellular and molecular interactions govern many crucial responses to our environment. Like other complex organs, the skin is composed of several interdependent cell types and structures that are functionally cooperative. The skin serves as a protective barrier, provides temperature control, conducts sensory information to the brain, synthesizes vitamin D (an essential vitamin for health), and provides communication and display (ie, blushing). The skin includes 3 primary layers: epidermis, dermis, and subcutaneous.[120]

Lack of skin integrity, or wounds, includes abrasions, punctures, bites, surgical wounds, diabetic ulcers, pressure ulcers, traumatic wounds, venous stasis ulcers, and arterial ulcers. Certain populations either exhibit or are at risk for wounds and from related complications. These populations include people with spinal cord injuries, cerebral palsy, hand injuries, diabetes, breast cancer, and burns, as well as those with sensory or mobility impairments. For example, more than 60% of non-traumatic lower-limb amputations occur among people with diabetes.[121]

Wounds and related conditions can affect a person's ability to participate in his or her daily life activities. There can be limitations with performing self-care or pursuing work, education, or other life roles. Sequelae of wounds can include depression, decreased social participation, and anxiety. Occupational therapy's perspective on working in this area combines an understanding of both physical disabilities and mental health, with a focus on supporting health and participation through engagement in daily life activities and occupations. Depending on the location and severity of the wound, a person may have difficulties with wound site management (applying wound treatments and promoting healing), clothing and footwear adaptations, and customizing and fitting pressure garments.[122]

Specialized training in wound care, debridement, splinting, active range of motion (AROM), and passive range of motion (PROM) associated with rehabilitation after a burn, traumatic hand injury, or hand or finger surgery can prevent adhesions and provide proper positioning for a client during wound healing. Wound care involves wrapping techniques with bandaging to maintain joint ROM and optimal functioning. It also can include direct wound care during therapy, whirlpool use, and client education on how to care for the wound. Making recommendations for support surfaces can include pressure relief surfaces for beds or wheelchairs. Adaptive equipment can allow a client to assist with or perform dressing changes. Training in use of equipment is necessary to complete basic ADL (eg, bathing, grooming, dressing, eating) and IADL (eg, assistive devices, special mattresses, special wheelchair cushions) that are pertinent to the individual. To promote sustained prevention, occupational therapy practitioners can help clients identify ways to incorporate recommended prevention measures into their ongoing daily routines. This can include selection and application of techniques to don and doff pressure garments to manage swelling and prevent upper-extremity lymphedema. Education in transfer techniques can minimize risk of skin tears.

Assessment and Intervention

The skin is easily accessible and therefore is more readily assessed. Occupational therapy practitioners help clients to examine their skin and ensure that skin is being properly cared for. Proper skin care is crucial to preventing skin breakdown. An initial skin assessment, which involves completion or assisting in the completion of skin assessment, could include assessing a wound in any area of the person's body that is affecting self-care. One frequently used skin assessment is the Braden Scale, available at the following website: http://www.bradenscale.com/faq.htm.

The following steps are basic to preserving skin integrity. Systematically inspect the skin at least once a day, paying particular attention to the skin over bony prominences. Cleanse the skin at frequent intervals with warm water and a mild, pH-balanced cleansing agent, then apply moisturizers and a barrier cream as indicated. During skin care, minimize the force applied to the skin. Avoid massaging over bony prominences and hyperemic areas, massage may destroy the underlying skin and damage blood vessels. Minimize skin exposure to moisture caused by incontinence, perspiration, or wound drainage. If the patient is incontinent, the skin should be cleansed at the time of soiling. When the source of moisture cannot be controlled, it is appropriate to use barrier creams or ointments to protect the skin. Absorbent products, such as briefs or pads, can be used to wick away the moisture. Minimize environmental factors, such as low humidity (less than 40%) and exposure to cold, which can lead to dry skin. Use proper positioning, transferring, and turning techniques to minimize skin injury caused by friction and shear forces.

To reduce friction injuries use lubricants (such as cornstarch and creams), protective films (such as transparent films and skin sealants), protective dressings (such as hydrocolloids), and protective padding. The topical skin care products used to prevent skin breakdown or to treat impaired skin integrity secondary to incontinence or wound drainage should be chosen according to the patient's skin type, product application and removal, cost, and desired outcome. Moisturizers, barrier creams, and cleansing agents all have different ingredients, and clinicians must take into account what is being applied to the patient's skin when developing a plan of care for prevention or intervention. Clinicians should also recognize the indications and contraindications of the products selected. This comprehensive understanding is often the best defense in maintaining skin integrity, controlling costs, and expediting the healing process.[122]

SUMMARY

There are many factors that affect performance other than physiologic variables. These other factors are discussed in depth elsewhere in this text. Physiological factors can affect an individual's observed performance during functional assessment in the clinical setting. They can influence actual individual daily activity levels, that in turn affect physical fitness. We must always remember that human performance is the product of physiologic and psychosocial variables that together influence individuals. Observable performance should never be assumed to be a clear indication of physiologic capacity.

Regular participation in adequate levels of physical activity is essential to health and physical fitness for everyone. Certain conditions and circumstances may limit an individual's ability to be active, and health and physical fitness decline. Diminished physical capacity as a result of inactivity or immobilization is an important, often overlooked, factor in disease-related impairment, functional limitation, and disability. The framework of physical fitness can be used in client evaluation and planning comprehensive treatment.

The physiologic basis of an individual's ability to perform tasks and engage in meaningful activities and occupational roles may be assessed, described, and changed within the organizational framework of physical fitness. It is essential to include fitness as an integral component of the rehabilitation process. Fitness information contributes to the understanding of disability and HRQOL. Physical fitness, as a measure of the physiologic basis of performance, must be assessed and addressed as a potentially modifying factor in the outcomes of disability and HRQOL.

What will you, the occupational therapy practitioner, do with this information on fitness? You will want to always consider the issues as they relate to wellness, because you should always be considering ways to incorporate concepts of wellness and the promotion of wellness into your intervention. From this perspective you can work with your clients to establish fitness goals once you understand fitness yourself, and then work with them on ways to increase the fitness complexity of activities they enjoy to meet their own fitness goals. You will also want to be aware of what to look for in your clients that would indicate compromised function in these fitness components. And there are times when your assessments and interventions will likely address aspects of fitness from an occupation/activity perspective, or occasionally from a component perspective, as they have been described here. Thus, you may be working with a client on muscle strengthening and endurance, but this could be incorporated into your client's functional activity of bread baking as your client works to knead and roll the dough. You will, of course, keep in mind that this task will challenge the cardiorespiratory functions for some of your clients, and you will need to keep an eye on them for signs of cardiorespiratory changes. The following tables identify a number of resources that will provide you with information to address the physiological factors highlighted in this chapter (Tables 18-5 to 18-7).

Table 18-5. *Evidence Table: Summary of Systematic Reviews Evaluating the Use of Exercise on a Variety of Populations*

Study Reference	Aim of Study	Methods and Studies Included	Results and Conclusions	Level of Evidence
Brazzelli, Saunders, Greig, and Mead[123]	Physical fitness training following a stroke	Systematic review included 32 trials involving 1414 participants that comprised cardiorespiratory, resistance, and mixed training. Two review authors independently selected trials, assessed quality, and extracted data. Data were analyzed using random-effects meta-analyses.	While there are limitations of the data, there is clear evidence that those in the post-stroke chronic phase (more than 1 month) benefit from physical fitness/exercise training as it is feasible and safe, and cardiorespiratory training improves measures of walking performance and reduces dependence during usual care. Training effects are retained at follow-up. The training effect may be greater when fitness training is specific or "task-related." There is insufficient data to conduct meaningful subgroup analyses to explore the effects of the type, "dose," and timing of training on outcome measures.	Systematic review Level I
Verschuren, Ketelaar, Takken, Helders, and Gorter[124]	Exercise programs focusing on muscle strength, cardiovascular fitness in children with CP	Systematic review included 20 studies of exercise including muscle strengthening, cardiovascular fitness, or a combination.	Exercise programs improve cardiovascular fitness and muscle strength, however outcome measures need to be expanded to include demonstration of performance in function.	Systematic review Level I
Bania, Dodd, and Taylor[125]	Increasing physical activity in people with CP	Systematic review included 3 RCTs and 2 qualitative studies, for a total of 21 participants.	Exercise programs can increase physical activity in people with cerebral palsy, but effects are not maintained when programs terminate. Outcomes measuring functional capacities were not included.	Systematic review Level I
Hayden, van Tulder, and Koes[126]	Effectiveness of individual exercise training on pain management and the improvement of functioning in chronic low back pain	Updated systematic review, included a meta-analysis of 43 RCTs on the utilization of exercise training odes and protocols effective in improving pain and function.	A wide variety of training protocols were effective in improving both function and lessening pain in individuals with chronic low back pain. Most effective were individually designed programs.	Systematic review Level I

(continued)

Table 18-5 (continued).   *Evidence Table: Summary of Systematic Reviews Evaluating the Use of Exercise on a Variety of Populations*

Study Reference	Aim of Study	Methods and Studies Included	Results and Conclusions	Level of Evidence
Shaw, Gennat, O'Rourke, and Del Mar[127]	To assess exercise as a means of achieving weight loss in people overweight or obese, using RCTs	Systematic review that included 43 studies and 3476 participants. Exercise was considered in combination with dieting or alone. Exercise was defined as differing in intensity demands of cardiovascular activity. Two authors independently assessed trial quality and extracted data.	The results of this review support the use of exercise as a weight loss intervention, particularly when combined with dietary change. Exercise is associated with improved cardiovascular disease risk factors, even if no weight is lost. Exercise combined with diet resulted in a greater weight reduction than diet alone. Increasing exercise intensity increased the magnitude of weight loss. Gains were made in lowered serum lipids, blood pressure, and fasting glucose.	Systematic review Level I
Waters, de Sliva-Sanigorski, and Hall[128]	This review updated the previous review of childhood obesity prevention research and determines the effectiveness of evaluated interventions, assessed by change in BMI. Additionally, it examines the characteristics of the programs and strategies to answer the question: "What works for whom, why, and for what cost?"	A systematic review of intervention studies for reducing obesity in children. This review includes 55 studies (an additional 36 studies were found for this update). The majority of studies targeted children aged 6 to 12. The meta-analysis included 37 studies of 27,946 children. Two review authors independently extracted data and assessed the risk of bias of included studies. Data was extracted on intervention implementation, cost, equity, and outcomes. Outcome measures were grouped according to whether they measured adiposity, physical activity-related behaviors, or diet-related behaviors. A meta-analysis was conducted using available BMI or standardized BMI (zBMI) score.	Review provides strong evidence to support beneficial effects of child obesity exercise programs on BMI, particularly for children aged 6 to 12. Demonstrated programs were effective at reducing adiposity, although not all individual interventions were effective and there was a high level of observed heterogeneity ($I2 = 82\%$). Interventions did not appear to increase health inequalities, although this was examined in fewer studies.	Systematic review Level I

(continued)

Table 18-5 (continued). *Evidence Table: Summary of Systematic Reviews Evaluating the Use of Exercise on a Variety of Populations*

Study Reference	Aim of Study	Methods and Studies Included	Results and Conclusions	Level of Evidence
Mead, Morley, Campbel, Greig, McMurdo, and Lawlor[129]	To determine the effectiveness of exercise in the treatment of depression	Systematic review that included 28 RCTs, of which 25 provided data for meta-analyses for a total of 907 participants. Effect sizes for each were calculated. All authors were involved in data extraction and analysis.	Exercise seems to improve depressive symptoms in people with a diagnosis of depression; but when only methodologically robust trials are included, the effect sizes are only moderate and not statistically significant. The effect of exercise was not significantly different from that of cognitive therapy. There was insufficient data to determine risks and costs.	Systematic review Level I
Scascighini, Toma, Dober-Spielmann, and Sprott[130]	To provide an overview of the effectiveness of multidisciplinary treatments of chronic pain and investigate about their differential effects on outcome in various pain conditions and of different multidisciplinary treatments, settings, or durations	A systematic review of all currently available RCTs in treatment of chronic pain by all 4 authors using a rating system to assess the strength of evidence with regard to the methodological quality of the trials.	Compared with other non-disciplinary treatments, moderate evidence of higher effectiveness for multidisciplinary interventions was shown. In contrast to no treatment or standard medical treatment, strong evidence was detected in favor of multidisciplinary treatments. The evidence that comprehensive inpatient programs were more beneficial than outpatient programs was moderate.	Systematic review Level I

Table 18-6. *Resources for Additional Information on Physiological Person Factors*

Organization	Description of Who They Serve	Web Address
The American Medical Society for Sports Medicine (AMSSM)	AMSSM is a multi-disciplinary organization of sports medicine physicians whose members are dedicated to education, research, advocacy, and the care of athletes of all ages. Founded in 1991, the AMSSM is now comprised of more than 2100 sports medicine physicians whose goal is to provide a link between the rapidly expanding core of knowledge related to sports medicine and its application to patients in a clinical setting.	http://www.amssm.org/
Center for Disease Control and Prevention (CDC)	A wealth of information including information for health professionals and families over a diversity of topics. Most relevant to this chapter include obesity and physical activity standards.	http://www.cdc.gov/nccdphp/dnpao/index.html
American Heart Association (AHA)	The AHA seeks to prevent heart disease and support both those with disease, their families, and health professionals.	http://www.heart.org/HEARTORG/
National Sleep Foundation (NSF)	NSF is dedicated to improving the QOL for Americans who suffer from sleep problems and disorders. They provide education to the public, support research, advocate for public policies that are based on sleep research, and outreach to health care providers for sleep research translation.	http://www.sleepfoundation.org/
Let's Move	Designed for families, schools, clinics, daycares, and wider communities to end childhood obesity. Focus is on physical activity and healthy food choices. There are strategies and initiatives for primary, secondary, and tertiary levels of involvement.	http://www.letsmove.gov/
National Heart, Lung, and Blood Institute Education Programs	Designed for health care professionals and for the general public providing tool kits for education about cardiovascular fitness, heart disease, obesity, and nutrition.	http://www.nhlbi.nih.gov/nhlbi/nhlbi.htm (general NHLBI site)
International Association for the Study of Pain (IASP)	IASP joins scientists, clinicians, health care providers, and policy makers to stimulate and support the study of pain and translate that knowledge into improved pain relief worldwide.	http://www.iasp-pain.org
Harvard School of Public Health: Nutrition Source	The Nutrition Source states as its' aims the provision of timely, evidence-based information on diet and nutrition for clinicians, allied health professionals, and the public. It serves to clarify information that is generated in public media and to provide the best evidence for nutrition practices	http://www.hsph.harvard.edu/nutritionsource/
National Physical Activity Plan	An initiative of companies and organizations begun in 2009 to encourage physical activity.	http://www.physicalactivityplan.org/healthcare.php
Physical Readiness Questionnaire	Canadian Public Health Ministry updated guidelines for physical activity and provides these guidelines, which are useful in gauging healthy living for children, youth, and adults	http://www.csep.ca/english/view.asp?x=804
CDC Physical Activity Guidelines and Plans	The CDC Control Guidelines and plans for physical activity in older adults.	http://www.cdc.gov/physicalactivity/everyone/guidelines/olderadults.html#Aerobic
National Center for Physical Activity and Disability	A CDC-sponsored initiative to support physical activity among persons with disabilities with useful readings and programs.	http://www.ncpad.org/

Table 18-7. *Organizations and Journals That Focus on Physiological Factors for Performance*

Organization or Journal	Description	Web Address
American Physiological Society	A nonprofit devoted to fostering education, scientific research, and dissemination of information in the physiological sciences.	http://www.the-aps.org/
Society for Neuroscience	A nonprofit membership organization of scientists and physicians who study the brain and nervous system.	http://www.sfn.org/
American Clinical Neurophysiology Society	Official journal of the Society for Neuroscience. Publishes papers on a broad range of topics of general interest to those working on the nervous system.	http://www.jneurosci.org/
Neural Plasticity	An international, interdisciplinary journal. Publishes articles related to all aspects of neural plasticity. Special emphasis placed on its functional significance as reflected in behavior and in psychopathology.	http://www.hindawi.com/journals/np/
Stroke Engine	A site for individuals who have experienced stroke, their families and health professionals who work in the field of stroke rehabilitation. Supports the use of evidence-based stroke rehabilitation in clinical practice.	http://stroke-ngine.ca/
Journal of Neurophysiology	Publishes original articles on the function of the nervous system. All levels of function are included, from the membrane and cell, to systems and behavior.	http://jn.physiology.org/
Physiology	Publishes peer review articles that highlight major advances in the broadly defined field of physiology.	http://physiologyonline.physiology.org/
Journal of Applied Physiology	Publishes original papers that deal with diverse areas of research in applied physiology that emphasize adaptive and integrative mechanisms.	http://jap.physiology.org/
Journal of Neuroscience	A peer-reviewed international journal that covers the structure, function, evolutionary history, development, genetics, biochemistry, physiology, pharmacology, informatics, computational neuroscience, and pathology of the nervous system.	http://www.jneurosci.org/

REFERENCES

1. Thompson WR, Gordon NF, Pescatello LS. *ACSM's Guidelines for Exercise Testing and Prescription*. Philadelphia, PA: Lippincott Williams & Wilkins; 2010.

2. Bean JF, Vora A, Frontera WR. Benefits of exercise for community-dwelling older adults. *Arch Phys Med Rehab*. 2004;85(7 Suppl 3):S31-42.

3. Gourlan MJ, Trouilloud DO, Sarrazin PG. Interventions promoting physical activity among obese populations: a meta-analysis considering global effect, long-term maintenance, physical activity indicators and dose characteristics. *Obes Rev*. 2011;12(7):e633-e645.

4. Katz DL, O'Connell M, Njike VY, Yeh MC, Nawaz H. Strategies for the prevention and control of obesity in the school setting: systematic review and meta-analysis. *Int J Obes (Lond)*. 2008;32(12):1780-1789.

5. Kutner NG, Barnhart H, Wolf SL, McNeely E, Xu T. Self-report benefits of Tai Chi practice by older adults. *J Gerontol Series B: Psychol Sci Soc Sci*. 1997;52(5):242-246.

6. Oude Luttikhuis H, Baur L, Jansen H, et al. Interventions for treating obesity in children. *Cochrane Database Syst Rev*. 2009;(1):CD001872.

7. Valentine RJ, Woods JA, McAuley E, Dantzer R, Evans EM. The associations of adiposity, physical activity and inflammation with fatigue in older adults. *Brain Behav Immun*. 2011;25(7):1482-1490.

8. Borg G. Perceived exertion as an indicator of somatic stress. *Scand J Rehab Med*. 1970;2(2):92-98.

9. Thomas S, Reading J, Shephard RJ. Revision of the Physical Activity Readiness Questionnaire (PAR-Q). *Can J Sports Sci*. 1992;17(4):338-345.

10. Heyward VH. *Advanced Fitness Assessment & Exercise Prescription*. 2nd ed. Champaign, IL: Human Kinetics; 2010.

11. Rybski M. *Kinesiology for Occupational Therapy.* Thorofare, NJ: SLACK Incorporated; 2011.

12. Houglum PA, Bertoti DB. *Brunnstrom's Clinical Kinesiology.* 6th ed. Philadelphia, PA: FA Davis; 2011.

13. Wells KF, Dillon EK. The sit and reach: a test of back and leg flexibility. *Res Q.* 1952;23:115-118.

14. Jones CJ, Rikli R. Senior fitness test manual. *J Aging Phys Act.* 2002;10(1):110-130.

15. Hoffman J. *Norms for Fitness, Performance, and Health.* Champaign, IL: Human Kinetics; 2006.

16. Nieman DC. *Exercise Testing and Prescription: A Health-Related Approach.* Boston, MA: McGraw-Hill; 2007.

17. World Health Organization. *Global Database on Body Mass Index: Classification.* World Health Organization; http://apps. who.int/bmi/index.jsp?introPage=intro_3.html.

18. Prentice A, Jebb S. Beyond body mass index. *Obes Rev.* 2001;2(3):141-147.

19. Wheaton A, Perry G, Chapman D, McKnight -EL, Presley-Cantrell L, Croft J. Relationship between body mass index and perceived insufficient sleep among US adults: an analysis of 2008 BRFSS data. *BMC Public Health.* 2011;11:295.

20. World Health Organization. *Global Database on Body Mass Index: Classification.* Geneva, Switzerland: World Health Organization; 2011.

21. Carpenito LJ. *Nursing Diagnosis: Application to Clinical Practice.* 12th ed. Philadelphia, PA: Lippincott Williams & Wilkins; 2007.

22. Borg G. Psychophysical bases of perceived exertion. *Med Sci Sports Exerc.* 1982;14(5):377-381.

23. Borg G. A category-ratio perceived exertion scale: relationship to blood and muscle lactates and heart rate. *Med Sci Sports Exerc.* 1983;15(6):523-528.

24. Borg G. *Borg's Perceived Exertion and Pain Scales.* Champaign, IL: Human Kinetics; 1998

25. Koen AP, Lemmink HK, Mathieu HGdG, Piet Rispens P, Stevens M. Reliability of the Groningen Fitness Test for the elderly. *J Aging Phys Act.* 2001;9:194-212.

26. Wells KF, Dillon EK. The sit and reach: a test of back and leg flexibility. *Res Q.* 1952;23(115-118).

27. Koen AP, Lemmink HK, Mathieu HGdG, Piet Rispens P, Stevens M. Reliability of the Groningen Fitness Test for the elderly. *J Aging Phys Act.* 2001;9:194-212.

28. Rikli RE, Jones CJ. Functional fitness normative scores for community-residing older adults, ages 60-94. *J Aging Phys Act.* 1999;7:162-181.

29. Fragala MS, Kraemer WJ, Denegar CR, Maresh CM, Mastro AM, Volek JS. Neuroendocrine-immune interactions and responses to exercise. *Sports Med.* 2011;41(8):621-639.

30. Shammas MA. Telomeres, lifestyle, cancer, and aging. *Curr Opin Clin Nutr Metab Care.* 2011;14(1):28-34.

31. Walsh R. Lifestyle and mental health. *Am Psychol.* 2011;66(7):579-592.

32. Centers for Disease Control and Prevention. Obesity: halting the epidemic by making health easier. In: *National Center for Chronic Disease Prevention and Health Promotion Division of Nutrition Physical Activity, and Obesity Report.* Washington, DC: Centers for Disease Control and Prevention; 2011.

33. Centers for Disease Control and Prevention. *Physical Activity Recommendations by Age Group.* Centers for Disease Control and Prevention. http://www.cdc.gov/physicalactivity/professionals/promotion/index.html. Published 2010. Accessed 2012.

34. Centers for Disease Control and Prevention. *Physical Activity Guidelines for Americans.* http://www.health.gov/paguidelines/guidelines/.

35. Borg G. A category-ratio perceived exertion scale: relationship to blood and muscle lactates and heart rate. *Med Sci Sports Exerc.* 1983;15(6):523-528.

36. Ainsworth BE, Haskell WL, Herrmann SD, et al. Compendium of physical activities: a second update of codes and MET values. *Med Sci Sports Exerc.* 2011;43(8):1575-1581.

37. Baker PR, Francis DP, Soares J, Weightman AL, Foster C. Community wide interventions for increasing physical activity. *Cochrane Database Syst Rev.* 2011;(4):CD008366.

38. Brown T, Summerbell C. Systematic review of school-based interventions that focus on changing dietary intake and physical activity levels to prevent childhood obesity: an update to the obesity guidance produced by the National Institute for Health and Clinical Excellence. *Obes Rev.* 2009;10(1):110-141.

39. Gillespie LD, Robertson MC, Gillespie WJ, et al. Interventions for preventing falls in older people living in the community. *Cochrane Database Syst Rev.* 2009;(2):CD007146.

40. Lee ACK, Maheswaran R. The health benefits of urban green spaces: a review of the evidence. *J Public Health (Oxf).* 2011;33(2):212-222.

41. Renalds A, Smith TH, Hale PJ. A systematic review of built environment and health. *Fam Community Health.* 2010;33(1):68-78.

42. Trost SG, Ward DS, Senso M. Effects of child care policy and environment on physical activity. *Med Sci Sports Exerc.* 2010;42(3):520-525.

43. Ogden CL, Carroll MD, Kit BK, Flegal KM. *Prevalence of Obesity in the United States, 2009-2010.* Hyattsville, MD: National Center for Health Statistics; 2012.

44. US Department of Agriculture, US Department of Health and Human Services. *Dietary Guidelines for Americans, 2010.* 7th ed. Washington, DC: US Government Printing Office; 2010.

45. Kushi L, Byers T, Doyle C, et al. American Cancer Society guidelines on nutrition and physical activity for cancer prevention: reducing the risk of cancer with healthy food choices and physical activity. *CA Cancer J Clin.* 2006;56:254-281.

46. Jensen M, Ryan D, Donato K, et al. Guidelines (2013) for managing overweight and obesity in adults. *Obesity.* 2014;22(S2):S1-S410.

47. Belanger-Gravel A, Godin G, Vezina-Im LA, Amireault S, Poirier P. The effect of theory-based interventions on physical activity participation among overweight/obese individuals: a systematic review. *Obes Rev.* 2011;12(6):430-439.

48. Shaw K, Gennat H, O'Rourke P, Del Mar C. Exercise for overweight or obesity. *Cochrane Database Syst Rev.* 2006;4:CD003817.

49. Tuah NA, Amiel C, Qureshi S, Car J, Kaur B, Majeed A. Transtheoretical model for dietary and physical exercise modification in weight loss management for overweight and obese adults. *Cochrane Database Syst Rev.* 2011;10:CD008066.

50. Verweij LM, Coffeng J, van Mechelen W, Proper KI. Meta-analyses of workplace physical activity and dietary behaviour interventions on weight outcomes. *Obes Rev.* 2011;12(6):406-429.

51. Reichert FF, Baptista Menezes AM, Wells JCK, Carvalho Dumith S, Hallal PC. Physical activity as a predictor of adolescent body fatness: a systematic review. *Sports Med.* 2009;39(4):279-294.

52. Chokroverty S. *Chokroverty: Sleep Disorders Medicine.* 3rd ed. Philadelphia, PA: WB Saunders; 2009.

53. Weilburg J, Stakes J, Roth T. Sleep physiology. In: Stern T, Rosenbaum J, Cobb S, et al, eds. Stern. *Massachusetts General Hospital Comprehensive Clinical Psychiatry.* 1st ed. Philadelphia, PA: Mosby Elsevier; 2008:285-301.

54. Wagner HL, Silber K. *Physiological Psychology.* New York, NY: BIOS Scientific Publishers: Taylor & Francis; 2004.

55. Lee, Ward TM. Critical components of a sleep assessment for clinical practice settings. *Issues Ment Health Nurs.* 2005;26(7):739-750.

56. National Highway Transportation Safety Administration. Traffic safety facts. In: National Highway Transportation Safety Administration. *Transportation.* Washington, DC: US Government; 2009.

57. Beccuti G, Pannain S. Sleep and obesity. *Curr Opin Clin Nutr Metab Care.* 2011;14(4):402-412.

58. Trotti LM. REM sleep behaviour disorder in older individuals: epidemiology, pathophysiology and management. *Drugs Aging.* 2010;27(6):457-470.

59. Romero-Corral A, Caples SM, Lopez-Jimenez F, Somers VK. Interactions between obesity and obstructive sleep apnea: implications for treatment. *Chest.* 2010;137(3):711-719.

60. Reed DA, Fletcher KE, Arora VM. Systematic review: association of shift length, protected sleep time, and night float with patient care, residents' health, and education. *Ann Intern Med.* 2010;153(12):829-842.

61. Chaput J-P, Klingenberg L, Sjodin A. Do all sedentary activities lead to weight gain: sleep does not. *Curr Opin Clin Nutr Metab Care.* 2010;13(6):601-607.

62. Cappuccio FP, D'Elia L, Strazzullo P, Miller MA. Quantity and quality of sleep and incidence of type 2 diabetes: a systematic review and meta-analysis. *Diabetes Care.* 2010;33(2):414-420.

63. Hauw J-J, Hausser-Hauw C, De Girolami U, Hasboun D, Seilhean D. Neuropathology of sleep disorders: a review. *J Neuropathol Exp Neurol.* 2011;70(4):243-252.

64. Johns MW. A new method for measuring daytime sleepiness: The Epworth Sleepiness Scale. *Sleep.* 1991;14(6):50-55.

65. Roth T, Zammit G, Kushida C, et al. A new questionnaire to detect sleep disorders. *Sleep Med.* 2002;3(2):99-108.

66. National Heart Lung and Blood Institute. Guide to Healthy Sleep. http://www.nhlbi.nih.gov/health/public/sleep/healthysleepfs.pdf.

67. National Heart Lung and Blood Institute. *At a Glance: Healthy Sleep.* http://www.nhlbi.nih.gov/health/public/sleep/healthysleepfs.pdf.

68. Albert SM, Bear-Lehman J, Burkhardt A. Lifestyle-adjusted function: variation beyond BADL and IADL competencies. *Gerontologist.* 2009;49(6):767-777.

69. Baum CM, Edwards DF. *Activity Card Sort.* 2nd ed. Bethesda, MD: AOTA Press; 2008.

70. Hartman-Maeir A, Eliad Y, Kizoni R, Nahaloni I, Kelberman H, Katz N. Evaluation of a long-term community based rehabilitation program for adult stroke survivors. *Neurorehabilitation.* 2007;22(4):295-301.

71. Hartman-Maeir A, Soroker N, Oman SD, Katz N. Awareness of disabilities in stroke rehabilitation—a clinical trial. *Disabil Rehabil.* 2003;25(1):35-44.

72. Hartman-Maeir A, Soroker N, Ring H, Avni N, Katz N. Activities, participation and satisfaction one-year post stroke. *Disabil Rehabil.* 2007;29(7):559-566.

73. Hildebrand M, Brewer M, Wolf T. The impact of mild stroke on participation in physical fitness activities. *Stroke Res Treat.* 2012:548-682.

74. Hamilton A, de Jonge D. The impact of becoming a father on other roles: an ethnographic study. *J Occup Sci.* 2010;17(1):40-46.

75. Reilly M. Occupational therapy can be one of the great ideas of 20th century medicine. *Am J Occup Ther.* 1962;16:1-9.

76. Rabin BS. *Stress, Immune Function and Health: The Connection.* New York, NY: Wiley-Liss; 1999.

77. Kiecolt-Glaser JK, McGuire L, Robles TF, Glaser R. Psychoneuroimmunology and psychosomatic medicine: back to the future. *Psychosom Med.* 2002;64(1):15-28.

78. Kiecolt-Glaser JK, McGuire L, Robles TF, Glaser R. Psychoneuroimmunology: psychological influences on immune function and health. *J Consult Clin Psychol.* 2002;70(3):537-547.

79. Glaser R, Kiecolt-Glaser JK. Stress-induced immune dysfunction: implications for health. *Nat Rev Immunol.* 2005;5:243-251.

80. Sapolsky RM. *Why Zebras Don't Get Ulcers: The Acclaimed Guide to Stress, Stress-Related Diseases, and Coping.* 3rd ed. New York, NY: Henry Holt & Company; 2004.

81. Sorrells SF, Caso JR, Munhoz CD, Sapolsky RM. The stressed CNS: when glucocorticoids aggravate inflammation. *Neuron.* 2009;64(1):33-39.

82. Calabrese EJ, Bachmann KA, Bailer AJ, et al. Biological stress response terminology: Integrating the concepts of adaptive response and preconditioning stress within a hormetic dose-response framework. *Toxicol Appl Pharmacol.* 2007;222(1):122-128.

83. Liston C, McEwen BS, Casey BJ. Psychosocial stress reversibly disrupts prefrontal processing and attentional control. *Proc Natl Acad Sci U S A.* 2009;106(3):912-917.

84. Seeman TE, McEwen BS, Rowe JW, Singer BH. Allostatic load as a marker of cumulative biological risk: MacArthur studies of successful aging. *Proc Natl Acad Sci U S A.* 2001;98(8):4770-4775.

85. Christiansen CH. Adolf Meyer revisited: connections between lifestyles, resilience and illness. *J Occup Sci.* 2007;14(2):63-76.

86. Matuska KM, Christiansen C, eds. *Life Balance.* Bethesda, MD: AOTA Press & SLACK Incorporated; 2009.

87. Kiecolt-Glaser JK, Christian L, Preston H, et al. Stress, inflammation, and yoga practice. *Psychosom Med.* 2010;72(2):113-121.

88. McEwen BS. Protective and damaging effects of stress mediators: central role of the brain. *Dialogues Clin Neurosci.* 2006;8(4):367-381.

89. Sapolsky RM. Stress and plasticity in the limbic system. *Neurochem Res.* 2003;28(11):1735-1742.

90. Zeitlin D, Keller S, Shiflett S, Schleifer S, Bartlett J. Immunological effects of massage therapy during academic stress. *Psychosom Med.* 2000;62:83-84.

91. Cohen S, Kamarck T, Mermelstein R. A global measure of perceived stress. *J Health Soc Behav.* 1983;24(4):385-396.

92. Cohen S, Williamson G. Perceived stress in a probability sample of the United States. In: Spacapan S, Oskamp S, eds. *The Social Psychology of Health.* Newbury Park, CA: Sage; 1988:31-67.

93. DeLongis A, Folkman S, Lazarus RS. The impact of daily stress on health and mood: psychological and social resources as mediators. *J Pers Soc Psychol.* 1988;54:486-495.

94. Brantley PJ, Jones GN. Daily stress and stress-related disorders. *Annals Behav Med.* 1993;15:17-25.

95. Watson D, Clark LA, Carey G. Positive and negative affectivity and their relation to anxiety and depressive disorders. *J Abnorm Psychol.* 1988;97:346-353.

96. Holmes T, Rahe R. The Social Readjustment Rating Scale. *J Psychosom Res.* 1967;11(2):213-218.

97. Loeser JD, Bonica JJ. *Bonica's Management of Pain.* Philadelphia, PA: Lippincott Williams & Wilkins; 2001.

98. Ballantyne J. *The Massachusetts General Hospital Handbook of Pain Management.* 2006. http://ovidsp.ovid.com/ovidweb.cgi?T=JS&NEWS=n&CSC=Y&PAGE=booktext&D=books&AN=00139962$&XPATH=/PG(0).

99. International Association for the Study of Pain. Definition 2012: official website for the society of pain. *International Association for the Study of Pain.* http://www.iasp-pain.org//AM/Template.cfm?Section=Home. Accessed June 2, 2012.

100. Veehof MM, Oskam M-J, Schreurs KMG, Bohlmeijer ET. Acceptance-based interventions for the treatment of chronic pain: a systematic review and meta-analysis. *Pain.* 2011;152(3):533-542.

101. Bear MF, Connors BW, Paradiso MA. *Neuroscience: Exploring the Brain*. Philadelphia, PA: Lippincott Williams & Wilkins; 2002.

102. Flor H, Turk DC. *Chronic Pain: An Integrated Biobehavioral Approach*. Seattle, WA: IASP Press; 2011.

103. McCracken LM. *Contextual Cognitive-Behavioral Therapy for Chronic Pain*. Seattle, WA: ASP Press; 2005.

104. Page GG, Shamgar B-E. The immune-suppressive nature of pain. *Semin Oncol Nurs*. 1997;13(1):10-15.

105. Carpenter L, Baker GA, Tyldesley B. The use of the Canadian Occupational Performance Measure as an outcome of a pain management program. *Can J Occup Ther*. 2001;68:16-22.

106. Hernandez-Reif M, Field TM, Krasnegor J, Theakston H. Lower back pain is reduced and range of motion increased after massage therapy. *Int J Neurosci*. 2001;106:131-145.

107. Ober KM. *Evaluation of the People with Arthritis Can Exercise Program (PACE) Using Three Approaches: Physiological, Clinical, and Subjective [Dissertation]*. Portland, OR: Nursing, University of Oregon; 1992.

108. Persson D, Andersson I, Eklund M. Defying aches and revaluating daily doing: occupational perspectives on adjusting to chronic pain. *Scand J Occup Ther*. 2011;18(3):188-197.

109. Robinson K, Kennedy N, Harmon D. Review of occupational therapy for people with chronic pain. *Aus Occup Ther J*. 2011;58(2):74-81.

110. Scascighini L, Toma V, Dober-Spielmann S, Sprott H. Multidisciplinary treatment for chronic pain: a systematic review of interventions and outcomes. *Rheumatology (Oxford)*. 2008;47(5):670-678.

111. Snodgrass J. Effective occupational therapy interventions in the rehabilitation of individuals with work-related low back injuries and illnesses: a systematic review. *Am J Occup Ther*. 2011;65(1):37-43.

112. von Baeyer C, Spagrud L, McCormick J, Choo E, Neville K, Connelly MA. Three new datasets supporting use of the Numerical Rating Scale (NRS-11) for children's self-reports of pain intensity. *Pain*. 2009;143(3):223-227.

113. Childs JD, Piva SR, Fritz JM. Responsiveness of the numeric pain rating scale in patients with low back pain. *Spine*. 2005;30(11):1331-1334.

114. Farrar JT, Young JP, LaMoreaux L, Werth J, Poole R. Clinical importance of changes in chronic pain intensity measured on an 11-point numerical pain rating scale. *Pain*. 2001;94(2):149-158.

115. Collins JJ, Byrnes ME, Dunkel IJ, et al. The measurement of symptoms in children with cancer. *J Pain Symp Manage*. 2000;19(5):363-377.

116. van Herk R, van Dijk M, Baar FPM, Tibboel D, de Wit R. Observation scales for pain assessment in older adults with cognitive impairments or communication difficulties. *Nurs Res*. 2007;56(1):34-43.

117. McCaffery M, Beebe A. *Pain: Clinical Manual for Nursing Practice*. Baltimore, MD: Mosby; 1993.

118. Melzack R. The McGill Pain Questionnaire: major properties and scoring methods. *Pain*. 1975;1(3):277-299.

119. Manchikanti L. Evidence-based medicine, systematic reviews, and guidelines in interventional pain management, part I: introduction and general considerations. *Pain Physician*. 2008;11(2):161-186.

120. Lazar AJF, Murphy GF. The skin. In: Kumar V, Abbas AK, Fausto N, Aster JC, eds. *Kumar: Robbins and Cotran Pathologic Basis of Disease*. 8th ed. Philadelphia, PA: Saunders Elsevier; 2010:1102-1119.

121. National Diabetes Information Clearinghouse. *Diabetes Numbers at a Glance*. National Diabetes Information Clearinghouse. http://ndep.nih.gov/publications/publication-detail.aspx?pubid=114. Published 2011. Accessed June 2, 2012.

122. Gardiner L, Lampshire S, Biggins A, et al. Evidence-based best practice in maintaining skin integrity. *Wound Practice and Research*. 2008;16(2):5-15.

123. Brazzelli M, Saunders DH, Greig CA, Mead GE. Physical fitness training for stroke patients. *Cochrane Database Syst Rev*. 2011;11:CD003316.

124. Verschuren O, Ketelaar M, Takken T, Helders PJM, Gorter JW. Exercise programs for children with cerebral palsy. *Am J Phys Med Rehabil*. 2008;87(5):404-417.

125. Bania T, Dodd KJ, Taylor N. Habitual physical activity can be increased in people with cerebral palsy: a systematic review. *Clin Rehabil*. 2011;25:303-315.

126. Hayden JA, van Tulder MW, Malmivaara A, Koes BW. Exercise therapy for treatment of non-specific low back pain. *Cochrane Database Syst Rev*. 2005;(3):CD000335.

127. Shaw K, Gennat H, O'Rourke P, Del Mar C. Exercise for overweight or obesity. *Cochrane Database Syst Rev*. 2006;4:CD003817.

128. Waters E, de Silva-Sanigorski A, Hall BJ, et al. Interventions for preventing obesity in children. *Cochrane Database Syst Rev*. 2011;12:CD001871.

129. Mead GE, Morley W, Campbell P, Greig CA, McMurdo M, Lawlor DA. Exercise for depression. *Cochrane Database Syst Rev*. 2009;3:CD004366.

130. Scascighini L, Toma V, Dober-Spielmann S, Sprott H. Multidisciplinary treatment for chronic pain: a systematic review of interventions and outcomes. *Rheumatology (Oxford)*. 2008;47(5):670-678.

PERSON FACTORS
Meaning, Sensemaking, and Spirituality

Aaron M. Eakman, PhD, OTR/L

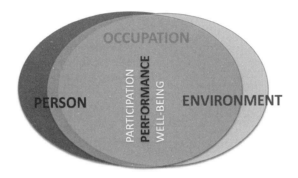

LEARNING OBJECTIVES

- Identify and define the primary factors that influence the personal narrative.
- Describe how constraints/barriers in meaning, sensemaking, and spirituality may affect a person's performance, participation, and well-being.
- Identify major health conditions or disabilities in which meaning, sensemaking, and spirituality have been seen as central to performance, participation, and/or well-being.
- Obtain an understanding of a personal narrative through interview.
- Identify established assessments that provide information about meaning, sensemaking, and spirituality.
- Identify principles and approaches that incorporate the personal narrative in intervention plans.
- Recognize the complexity of how the personal narrative interacts with other person and environment factors as it relates to performance in everyday life.

KEY WORDS

- Meaning
- Mind-body connections
- Motivation
- Personal life stories
- Personal well-being

INTRODUCTION

The PEOP Model represents a transactive approach that highlights intrinsic (personal) and extrinsic (physical, cultural and social) environmental influences on the performance of everyday occupations. Within this model, occupational performance involves the complex interactions between a person and his or her environment in which he or she carries out activities, tasks, and roles viewed as meaningful. This chapter will explore how to consider the idea of "meaningful" occupational

Christiansen CH, Baum CM, Bass JD, eds.
Occupational Therapy: Performance, Participation, and Well-Being, Fourth Edition (pp 313–331).
© 2015 SLACK Incorporated.

performance by drawing upon narrative meaning[1] or personal life stories as a principal means for accessing the inner subjective views of clients with whom occupational therapy practitioners interact. Models of human life span development, intrinsic motivation, meaning, and meaning making will be introduced as factors that influence personal life stories and meaning in day-to-day life. By gaining a deeper understanding of these factors, it will become evident how meaningful occupational performance influences health and well-being.

Critical information regarding personal motivations underlying occupational performance can be found by accessing and exploring meaning and the personal life stories of a client. The practitioner can come to understand how a client's past life experiences, values, and beliefs come to frame experience regarding their present situation as well as their goals for future occupational performance. The reader will be introduced to the importance of basic human needs (eg, control, autonomy, competence, belonging, and understanding) which appear to motivate and sustain occupational performance. Fulfillment of these needs through occupation is known to be linked to personal well-being, whereas occupational performance failing to meet these needs can lead to negative emotional reactions, stress, and ill-health.

Finally, meaning should be viewed as both a process embedded within ongoing occupational performance as well as an outcome arising from the PEOP Occupational Therapy Process.[2,3] The personal meaning that is associated with a given occupation is not necessarily a static thing. Models of meaning and meaning making indicate that meaning is constantly being developed and revised within occupational performance. Changes in personal beliefs, values, or goals, for example, influence both the motivations for engaging in tasks or activities and the experience of occupational performance. Furthermore, the experience of meaning we derive from our occupational performance can influence our sense of purpose and meaning in life, health, and well-being. Occupations that offer experiences of pleasure and joy connect us to those we care about and demonstrate competence in our valued social roles that ultimately make our lives worth living.

NARRATIVE AND BACKGROUND LITERATURE

I'm struggling with the disease. Part of me says I accept it and part of me refuses to accept it. I battle it—there's part of me that probably will never really accept it. I don't ever want to let go of my whole book of being able to do things that I've wanted to do. The hope has really been shattered. But part of my personality is I'm a fighter. I refuse to give up fighting. I'll fight the damned disease until they take my last breath. Or until something else gets me. Sometimes I feel like I'm winning and sometimes I feel like I'm losing.[4(p126)]

Boredom makes me look at myself. And I'm not an amazing person. And when you're bored, you don't want to look at yourself for that much time. But that's part of being bored, looking at yourself and your life… My life was pretty well boring… I was either getting high or I wasn't getting high, and that has been my life.[5(p113)]

Before I came here I was so lonely, I was afraid of going out of my mind. I'm not the type to sit around and watch TV and read magazines. That's why I came here. I like to mingle, to be around people, to have a roommate, to have company. It's what my disposition needs.[6(p153)]

A Brief Review of Meaning in Occupational Therapy

These 3 quotes offer a glimpse into how the personal narrative can be used to explore meaning in occupation. But how might we better understand the nature of meaning, its place in the day to day lives of our clients, and its role in the PEOP Occupational Therapy Process? What does "meaningful" occupation really mean? The term *meaningful* has often reflected valued, personally relevant, and subjectively positive experiences associated with activity or occupation. For example, in Kielhofner's[7] text *Health Through Occupation: Theory and Practice in Occupational Therapy*, contributors associated the experience of occupation with multiple perspectives on meaning, such as competence and mastery, valued goals, interests, self-efficacy, control, and creativity, which influence motivation to engage in occupation[8,9]; a sense of pleasure arising from personal competence which supports meaning in life[10]; whereas disruptions to valued activity due to illness and disability lead to a loss of life meaning.[11] To better understand the nature of personal meaning therefore requires insight into the personal and environmental factors that may serve to motivate and sustain occupational performance and knowledge regarding how personal experience arising from occupational performance influences future occupations and well-being.

There are a few definitions of meaning in occupation that help to frame this concept.[12] First, Keilhofner suggested the meaningfulness of activities is reflected in "an individual's disposition to find importance, security, worthiness, and purpose in particular occupations."[13(p505)] Second, Nelson indicated meaning or meaningfulness is related to an individual's interpretation of an occupational form such that "meaningfulness refers both to the perceptual sense it makes to the individual as well as to the cognitive associations elicited in the individual."[14](p635) Last, Christiansen and Baum defined meaning as "the personal significance of an event as interpreted by an individual."[15](p599)

Occupational therapy has wrestled with how best to conceptualize meaning in practice, most notably with respect to its role in supporting purposeful activity. This issue was relevant because purposeful activity defined as, "goal-directed behaviors or tasks… that the individual considers meaningful"[16](p865) was to serve as the basis of therapeutic occupation. Yet only limited agreement had been reached regarding the definitions of meaning and purpose and their roles in supporting occupational performance.[17,18] Present understanding, however, suggests meaning and purpose are intimately linked and one cannot be known without the other. For example, personal goals often underlie our purpose for action and inform both the narrative meaning we ascribe to our occupations and the experiences and feelings arising from engaging in those occupations.[19-21]

More recent perspectives in occupational therapy and occupational science have expanded how the concept of meaning may be understood. For instance, Crabtree[22] speculated that intrinsic motivation drives occupational performance, thereby imbuing activity with meaning. Jackson, Carlson, Mandel, Zemke, and Clark,[23] as well as Ikuigi,[24] support the importance of identifying personal values, interests, and life goals through narrative or interviewing, as well as assessing the experience of engaging in occupation to understand meaning. Further, Christiansen[25] proposed that competence, personal identity, and the social nature of a person's life serve to situate activity meaning within the life course, thereby contributing to life purpose and meaning. Finally, Johsson and Josephsson[26] suggest meaning in occupation is plastic and dynamic so the idea of change must be part of an understanding of meaning.

A Narrative Perspective on Meaning

The PEOP Model adopts narrative as the principal method for understanding a client's situation. Self-narratives refer to the personal stories persons tell about the events and experiences in their lives, and this narrative form offers an invaluable tool for considering meaning and occupation.[27] Our actions (past, present, and future) are inextricably linked with the passage of time, and our understanding of these actions require narrative to sift through and represent only the most relevant details from our experiences.[1] Self-narratives therefore have the potential to create coherence and meaning in everyday action and can imbue life itself with meaning and purpose.[25] Donald Polkinghorne has referred to "narrative meaning" and its functions as:

A scheme by means of which human beings give meaning to their experience of temporality and personal action. Narrative meaning functions to give form to the understanding of a purpose to life and to join everyday actions and events into episodic units. It provides a framework for understanding the past events of one's life and for planning for future actions. It is the primary scheme by means of which human existence is rendered meaningful.[28](p11)

Narrative has the capacity to bring order and coherence to our lives, though it is also concerned with desire, or shaping the will to act in the present towards some future goal or to realize a valued future self.[25,29] Our lives consist of past actions and experiences, yet we possess the uniquely human capacity to envision "hoped-for" goals for our future. Alternatively, a person's story can reflect a restricted future-self, or a regressive narrative, with limited aspirations, hopes, and dreams.[28] The onset of disability, unfortunately, plays havoc with a person's capacity to make sense of their present experiences. In turn, this incoherence may disconnect oneself from their idealized future self, resulting in significant emotional distress.[30] Narrative meaning within the PEOP Model, therefore, considers one's experience of their present occupational life as inexorably situated between one's known past and possible future.

Narrative also helps us to understand that the present-meaning found in occupation will be quite different depending on how one imagines their future. A person who is capable of connecting the relevance of their present activities and tasks to a future they wish to live builds a bridge of continuity and hope that inspires ongoing occupational pursuits.[31,32] Alternatively, if continuity between one's past, present, and future selves cannot be identified, if hope cannot be found, then the will to take risks and engage fully in occupational performance will be greatly diminished. Meaning in occupation is therefore dependent upon present beliefs, values, and goals that can serve to motivate action and propel an individual into a "hoped-for" future within an ongoing and larger life story.[1,25,32]

Finally, narrative offers both the person telling a story, and those listening (including the occupational therapy practitioner), access to the individual's salient life experiences, thoughts, and feelings. This, therefore, makes personal life stories a socially-situated event and affords great opportunities for new meanings to emerge.[29] Narrative in the PEOP Occupational Therapy Process involves the exchange of perspectives between both a client and a practitioner. A practitioner sensitive to a client's life experience can skillfully construct a therapeutic session that taps into a client's desires for the future. Well-constructed therapeutic occupations organize meaning by making the connection between the present and the "hoped-for" future explicit. The extent to which meaning in a therapeutic session is organized in this manner, by creating explicit therapeutic occupations and goals with clear relevance to a life one aspires to live, ultimately inspires purpose and motivation to the client's present actions.[32]

THE MODEL OF MEANING OF LIFE EXPERIENCES

King[2(p87-88)] has offered a model that may help to integrate the ideas surrounding narrative and meaning proposed in this chapter. Therefore, it will be important to introduce some of the more relevant aspects of this model. First, King proposes that personal meaning is acquired through 3 interrelated paths: *belonging* (the interconnections that a person has with others), *doing* (pursuing personal goals through participation in valued activities), and *understanding* (seeking to understand oneself and one's place in the world). Doing is central to this model, for without doing our potential for growth, development, and positive life experiences are thwarted.[33] The creation of meaning in our lives is therefore dependent upon the quality of our occupational performance. These paths to meaning, according to King, reflect human needs that are universal and fundamental to acquiring a sense of purpose and meaning in life. The model indicates that these 3 paths to meaning are intertwined and should be considered as mutually influencing.[34] For example, friendships provide a sense of belonging that can support an individual's belief in themselves as competent and provide access to others who offer assistance within preferred activities, tasks, and roles. To acquire and sustain meaning in life then requires the pursuit of personal needs for belonging, doing, and understanding. Notably, persons will differ with respect to which of these 3 paths to meaning are most relevant to their life. That is, though all 3 paths to meaning are needed, the relative emphasis for a given individual is determined by that person's needs and aspirations.[2]

Second, this model adopts a motivational and process approach to meaning in life experiences.[2] The motivational perspective reflects that the pursuit of occupations, and the nature in which occupational performance is perceived as meaningful, is related to the capacity of those occupations to satisfy the individual's basic needs. For example, the need for being with others may shape personal goals and motivate action as a person seeks out, develops, and maintains a satisfying personal relationship.[35] This perspective on needs does not define which occupations are pursued; rather, it suggests that needs can motivate occupation and leaves great room for variety in personal values and beliefs, and assumes a great multitude of occupations through which to pursue personally relevant goals.[36,37] The process perspective suggests that the

meaning we ascribe to our relationships, our occupations, and our understanding of ourselves is always open to change and revision. Personal meaning therefore is malleable and, often in the face of changing life circumstances, the meanings of our occupations can change.[26]

Lastly, the model of meaning in life experiences suggests that meaning (belonging, doing, and understanding) operates at 3 interacting levels within the individual.[2] At the foundational level, emotion, action, and cognition are implicated as the 3 fundamental ways in which a person processes and experiences his/her world. That is, for meaning to serve effectively in motivating action and imbuing our day-to-day occupations and our lives with meaning, we must consider the role of our emotional and cognitive processes. Emotional and cognitive processing offers instantaneous "felt meanings" of present-ongoing action[38]; a "here and now" sense of meaning that influences how we experience and understand our actions.[28] Our emotions (both positive and negative) are related to our interests and goals, values, and beliefs, and our experiences of meaning in occupations.[30,39-42] Access to our emotional and cognitive processing, our experience of our day-to-day occupations, and our sense of meaning in life may, in part, be gained through narrative.

A LIFESPAN THEORY OF CONTROL (PRIMARY AND SECONDARY CONTROL)

Perspectives on human development consistently indicate the central importance of control and mastery as persons pursue goals and engage in their day-to-day activities.[20,43-45] Occupational therapy has also recognized this aspect of human nature, and authors have suggested perceived control as one way to frame what we do as personally meaningful.[23,46,47] This idea of control can be understood as a fundamental human need and, therefore, it helps us understand how persons become motivated to engage in their everyday activities.[48] Alternatively, when persons lose control within their day-to-day lives and are not able to enact their will through occupation because of disease or disability, it can have significant negative implications for their personal well-being.[33,49]

The Motivational Theory of Life Span Development, which includes the ideas of primary and secondary control, is an ideal match with the PEOP Model because it is sensitive to both personal and environmental factors underlying occupational performance.[50,51] Primary control refers to the innate need of individuals to assert their will through action within their environment; or as "processes [that] are conceptualized as directed at changing the world to bring the environment into line with one's wishes."[48(p35)] Personal well-being and the meaning one imbues upon their daily activities are intimately affected by personal capacities and environmental affordances or barriers in support of valued activities and goals. One example of primary control may be seen in the actions of a toddler invested in play within a playground. This play may allow joy and exhilaration as the steps of a small slide are being mastered. Alternatively, when the child is not ready to end play, yet is led away by a parent, then it is likely that an immediate primary control need is being thwarted and emotional discomfort and crying ensues. As persons develop, they adopt valued personal goals and strivings[52-54] as extensions of primary control, and these goals serve in great part to organize the occupations of their day-to-day lives. Goal striving and our need for primary control remain constant throughout the life course and are a primary motivator for engagement in occupation; in part imbuing that participation with personal meaning.

When we consider the influences of primary and secondary control, we can better understand the nature of change in the meaningfulness of our day-to-day occupations. Secondary control interacts with primary control as a person matures and navigates the growing complexities of their day-to-day lives. Secondary control refers to cognitive and emotional processes aimed at modifying how one perceives and engages in the world or changing ones beliefs or values in the face of environmental challenges.[48] Despite our striving to maintain and assert primary control, our capacities for mastery and control can and will change throughout our lives. These changes may occur, for example, because of advancing age-related disability or because the environmental and activity demands exceed a person's abilities. For example, a young woman graduating from high school may have had a distinguished and enjoyable career playing volleyball for her team. However, as she transitions to a university, the competitive nature of team play may be above her skill level.

Secondary control strategies in this situation may lead the woman to one of a couple options that may alter the personal meaning she ascribes to volleyball. One secondary control strategy would entail enhancing commitment to a goal such that she places greater importance on "making the team," committing extra effort during team tryouts, and spending more time practicing. Secondary control may alternatively serve a role in disengaging from a goal and protecting oneself from the pain of failure.[55] From this perspective she may begin to either devalue the importance of "making the team," and/or increase her commitment to doing well in her classes, which would require additional study time that is currently taken up in tryouts and practice. In the latter case, this person is reestablishing a sense of primary control by increasing her focus on her academic success, which likely serves a critical role in enhancing her sense of well-being. In each of these scenarios, what should be clear is that the type and meaning of those occupations, whether in support of "making the team" or "academic success," will be quite different.

SELF-DETERMINATION THEORY (NEEDS FOR COMPETENCE, RELATEDNESS, AND AUTONOMY)

Need-based perspectives offer an important vantage point within the PEOP Model as a way to understand meaning and how socially-situated occupation may engender health and well-being. Examples of need-based perspectives in occupational therapy and occupational science have included occupational balance,[36] interventions for persons with mental illness,[56] and meaningful activity and meaning in life,[57] which have adopted the tenets of Self-Determination Theory (SDT).

SDT is at its core a modern theory of intrinsic (self-) motivation offering insights into why people do what they do.[37,58] Intrinsically motivated behavior or occupation refers to doing an activity for its own sake, for the satisfaction inherent in the doing. This may be contrasted with extrinsic motivation, which refers to engaging in an activity because of some imposed or socially dictated reason. Though in our lives certain occupations might lay at differing locations somewhere along this continuum, personal growth and well-being is maximized when our actions are perceived as being intrinsically motivated.

Within SDT persons are seen as having basic psychological needs that represent innate requirements or nutriments for well-being.[37] This theory is most compatible with the PEOP Model because it considers persons as agentic beings situated within social environments capable of either supporting or hindering these needs and, ultimately, supporting or hindering personal well-being. Further, through our being situated within social environments, the personal values, beliefs, and goal strivings that reflect the larger cultural miliieu may be adopted by an individual forming the basis of intrinsic motivation and supporting her/his basic psychological needs.

The 3 basic psychological needs referred to by SDT include competence, relatedness, and autonomy.[59] First, *competence* refers to feeling effective or skilled as one engages in occupations within their social environment. Second, *relatedness* refers to a feeling of being connected with, caring for, or being cared for by others within a community. Lastly, *autonomy* refers to an individual's perception that they are the source of their own occupational pursuits; that they have a say regarding the occupations in which they choose to engage. As an example, when people are autonomously motivated they experience volition and authorship over their actions. When the needs of competence and relatedness are supported through autonomous pursuit of valued life tasks, well-being is maximized[60,61] and motivation for future involvement is instilled.[62,63] Further, as well-being and motivation are impacted, there is an intimate association with finding meaning and value in the activities that support these needs.

Research has identified that the satisfaction of these basic psychological needs occurs on a day-to-day basis; these needs contribute to our perceptions of meaning in our daily occupations, and infuse our life with meaning. For example, persons reported greater levels of daily well-being when their activities were perceived as supporting their needs for competence, relatedness, and autonomy.[35] Alternately, well-being was consistently lower for these persons when their basic psychological needs were not being met within their daily occupations, signifying that the personal meaning of the activities was directly related to the support, or lack of support, of basic psychological needs. The needs of competence, relatedness, and autonomy have also been found to be related to both perceptions of meaningful activity and meaning in life; and there is evidence to suggest that meaningful activity may influence meaning in life directly, as well as indirectly, by supporting basic psychological needs.[57,64]

A MODEL OF MEANING MAKING (GLOBAL AND SITUATIONAL MEANING)

An important contribution to the meaning literature helps us to understand the nature of and change in meaning in response to stressful life events. Park and Folkman's[3,19] Integrated Model of Meaning Making draws from diverse psychological perspectives and frames meaning as both global meaning and situational meaning. *Global meaning* refers to the more generalized facet of a person's meaning system composed of 3 aspects of meaning:

1. Fundamental assumptions about the world (eg, one's overall sense of stability, control, and manageability of the world)
2. Personally valued goals and aspirations
3. A subjective sense of meaning and purpose in one's life

Situational meaning refers to meaning in the context of a particular event or situation within a person's life (eg, the onset of a disabling injury and the ensuing challenges found within day-to-day activities). In this model, well-being can be found when there is congruence between one's day-to-day activities and one's global meaning system, such that one perceives their occupations as enabling a sense of control and manageability where they achieve

their personal goals and maintain a strong sense of life purpose. However, when there is a discontinuity between global and situational meaning due to a traumatic event (ie, the presence of a spinal cord injury greatly disrupts ongoing occupations and compromises one's ability to achieve their personal goals), then stress ensues and well-being is greatly compromised.

This model informs how we might consider the role of meaning making as a process of coping with and hopefully surmounting difficult life circumstances. Central to the model are ongoing processes of personal appraisals (or evaluations) of perceived threats that a traumatic event poses in terms of achieving valued life goals.[65] The processes involved in appraisals (and meaning making) draw on both cognitive and emotional capacities as persons seek to understand their situation, and as they strive to bring their day to day occupations in line with their view of their life (eg, deeply held beliefs and goals).[19] For example, a person whose global meanings involve him being a good father, supportive partner, and contributing to his work and social communities will be faced with an agonizing reality following an appraisal of his very limited capacities to carry out even the most basic self-care activities after a traumatic spinal cord injury. In this example, there is a severe discrepancy between the person's global and situational meanings that creates great stress and emotional pain. The process of meaning making will likely require change in both the global and situational levels of meaning to again achieve their congruence and relative well-being.

Situational and global meaning maintain a transactive relationship such that situational meaning may change in response to a change in global meaning.[19] Ultimately, effective adaptation may be found when change in global beliefs permits realistic coping, perceived control and satisfaction with life.[3] A clinically oriented example may help to convey the ideas of global and situational meaning and their place in both the PEOP Model and in occupational therapy practice. Dubouloz et al[66] followed 5 persons with rheumatoid arthritis throughout the duration of their occupational therapy treatments and sought the personal narratives of their experiences. The authors initially identified a constellation of global meanings (referred to as *meaning perspectives)* held by the clients, including values and beliefs related to maintaining independence without help or limitation, staying active at all times, and helping others. Through the weekly treatment sessions that offered self-help strategies, these global meanings began to change. For example, the idea of independence gradually shifted to one of interdependence, because clients began to see the importance of caring for one's self and respecting pain and the physical limitations imposed by arthritis. The adoption of self-caring and self-respect beliefs was therefore required before persons could seek out or accept social supports or begin to effectively use self-pacing strategies within their daily occupations. Accepting assistance was eventually no longer viewed as a sign of dependence, which earlier in the process of treatment would have painfully challenged the global meaning of independence. Rather, newly adopted self-care and self-respect meanings served to engender a sense of control and satisfaction within the day-to-day lives of these clients. It appears the newly revised global meanings served as motivational resources for finding value and significance in the day-to-day activities these persons identified as helpful for realizing their goals, interests, and aspirations.

THE CENTRALITY OF EMOTIONS TO MEANING, HEALTH, AND WELL-BEING

Emotions and Meaning in Occupation

Elizabeth Yerxa, in her 1966 Eleanor Clarke Slagle Lecture,[67] argued that authentic occupational therapy requires that the emotions and will of the client are aroused and engaged; and further, an authentic therapeutic relationship requires acknowledging the emotional life of both the client and the practitioner. This suggests a central role for human emotions in the PEOP Occupational Therapy Process for how emotions are experienced within our daily lives, and the manner through which they shape occupational performance. Human emotion underlies much of what has been proposed within this chapter as defining the nature of and manner through which personal meaning may be experienced and understood. As well, emotions are relevant to the psychological, cognitive, sensory, motor, and physiological intrinsic factors within the PEOP Model. This section, therefore, will begin to highlight important ties between our emotions and how they enable us to construe meaning within our occupations and our lives. Further, this section will briefly address the role emotions are purported to serve with respect to stress, coping, and health.

Certain emotions have been characterized as basic and universal to human life, for example, anger, fear, disgust, sadness, surprise, and happiness. These "basic" emotions were identified because of the great consistency with which persons across all cultures shared similar patterns in facial expressions.[68] These basic emotional expressions are also related to personal subjective experiences which, with great consistency, underlie their physical expression[69]; for example, a person who appeared to be sad would indeed report that they were feeling sadness. Importantly, our emotional experiences reflect how we evaluate and appraise the events in our lives.[30] Our emotions are not blind, rather they have an intelligence which relies on past experiences, personal beliefs, and values regarding what should

or should not be.[70] Furthermore, our emotions underlie our personal goals and aspirations and motivate our actions, including our interactions with others as we are engaged in our daily lives.[71,72] For example, if one has an *interest* in achieving a certain goal, *cares* about a social cause, or *hopes* their actions can make a difference, then one has the motivating power of emotion supporting their occupations.

Emotions can be viewed as having an intelligence that informs our self-understanding and guides our actions, imbuing those actions with personally relevant meanings. One perspective on emotional intelligence suggests our cognitive and emotional capacities are intertwined and linked to 4 components of emotional processing.[73] First, emotional perception involves an individual's capacity to register, attend to, and make sense out of emotional messages. Accessing these emotional experiences is likely best achieved through the use of narrative and personal life stories.[28,74,75] Second, these emotional perceptions then serve as a reference for one to consider, appraise, and derive personal significance from a given situation or event. Awareness of one's anger, for example, reflects a personal judgment that some offense has been done to the person or to something with which the person identifies deeply.[70] Third, access to both emotional perception and awareness allows a person to understand and reason with their emotions. Emotional experience can reflect a complex blending of emotions (anger, frustration, and embarrassment), which when identified may help persons better understand their present experiences and navigate possible futures. Lastly, emotional management involves the capacity to reflect upon and modify one's emotions and the implications those emotions have with respect to personal goals, beliefs, values, and occupations. With personal reflection may come the awareness that a person has a responsibility for their emotions[70,76]; possibly leading to a reevaluation of their personal goals or values that in turn affects their emotional experience within occupational performance.[19,48]

Considering this model of emotional intelligence, there are indeed important connections with how the idea of meaning has been proposed earlier in this chapter. Emotions are not static, unitary, and fleeting experiences; rather they reflect a complex ongoing process of interpreting and experiencing meaning in our actions and in the actions of others. For as our emotional experiences change, so too do our meanings.[38] The salience of our emotions, whether powerful (such as anger and fear) or sublime (such as feeling at peace and belonging to a larger whole), speak to the broad range of experiences that imbue our present moments and our lives with meaning. Meaning, and by extension the notion of "meaningful," is therefore more complex than considering only emotions such as joy, love, hope, and happiness. Human lives, unfortunately, are also replete with emotions such as fear, anxiety, despair, and boredom. When personal goals, relationships with others, or a sense of one's self as a competent person have been thwarted, we would expect "meanings" that reflect fear, anger, loss, and sadness. Alternatively, occupational therapy practitioners may utilize therapeutic occupations that engage action and the experience of personal control and competence, thereby offering an emotional (and occupational) sign of hope for future recovery. Through authentic and emotionally intuitive occupational therapy practice,[77] clinicians can develop trusting therapeutic relationships that foster the desire and motivation within their clients to take risks towards an uncertain future.

Emotions, Stress, and Coping Through Meaning

Human emotions act as fundamental dynamic systems that guide personal adaptations within complex and changing social environments.[40] Further, our emotions serve to shape our personal goals and motivate our actions, thereby serving as a basis for experiencing purpose and meaning through occupation. Often, emotions (or affects) are construed more simply as being either positive (eg, interest, happiness, joy) or negative (eg, fear, worry, frustration) and act in parallel,[30,40,68,78,79] such that both positive and negative emotions may typically be experienced within our daily occupations. In short, good health and general well-being may be found in persons who are able to experience greater relative levels of positive vs negative emotions in their ongoing occupational lives. Negative emotions, however, may at times outweigh the positive in the face of substantial life stressors (eg, the onset of a traumatic injury or unsupported spousal caregiving to a person with dementia).

The persistence of relatively high levels of negative emotions in the face of life stressors is indeed predictive of poorer health outcomes and poses a greater risk for mortality. Quickly mounting evidence indicates that chronic negative emotions and stress are associated with depressed immune functioning[80,81]; decreased cognitive and physical functioning,[82] depression, arthritis, cardiovascular disease, Alzheimer's disease, frailty, and functional decline[81]; increased risk of infections, poorer wound healing, premature aging, and an increased risk of death.[81,83] Consistently, these studies have identified a mind/body connection that links the subjective experience of negative emotions and stress to physiological changes, and ultimately to poor health.

The burgeoning field of psychoneuroimmunology (PNI) plays a central role in advancing our understanding of this mind/body connection.[41,78,81,84] Briefly, research in PNI has primarily addressed the interactions amongst the CNS, the endocrine system, and the immune system

in response to stress. Components of this system include the hypothalamic-pituitary-adrenal (HPA) axis and the sympathetic-adrenal-medullary (SAM) axis, as well as an extremely vast array of associated antigens, antibodies, hormones, neuropeptides, neurotransmitters, and steroids.[83,84] Chronic stress and persistent negative affect in the face of day to day challenges leads to ongoing HPA and SAM activation, resulting in cumulative negative physiological effects and a diverse range of organ system breakdown and disease incidence.[83] In short, chronic stress and the concomitant negative emotions contribute to poorer health outcomes.

But what if we considered a different way to look at emotion and health? What if we asked, does the prolonged experience of positive emotions contribute to good health? This perspective on health adopts a "salutary" stance that aims to support and positively influence good health; as opposed to eliminate ill-health.[85,86] Indeed, evidence is mounting that positive emotions can support recovery, maximize health and well-being, and extend the number of years in which persons live a meaningful and engaged life. For example, positive emotions (eg, happiness, joy, and contentment) have been associated with greater immune functioning,[87] reduced cardiovascular disease risk and increased resistance to infection,[88] greater levels of both mental and physical health, and longevity.[89-92]

Furthermore, studies often report that positive emotions have a salutary effect, ie, a positive effect on health and well-being, which operates separately from negative emotions.[90,93,94] That is, the presence of negative emotions does not negate the important role that positive emotional experiences may play in coping with hardships or contributing to health and well-being. Coping can be fostered by establishing some semblance of control and competence within daily occupations or by engaging in tasks which bring pleasure or laughter, often through connecting with others, as well as reflecting on moments in which one felt joy, satisfaction, or contentment. These moments of positive emotions (ie, positive meaningful experiences in occupation) can bolster coping resources and offer a refuge from negative emotions when persons face the most difficult of life situations.[79]

Ryff and Singer[86,95] have extended this salutary perspective, making explicit links between a life well-lived, emotions, health, and well-being. Their model of human flourishing suggests engagement in occupations that satisfy our needs for positive relationships with others, mastery and control, positive self-regard, purpose in life, and personal growth are central to our physiological, mental, and physical health.[36] This model places human emotion at the nexus between the mind and body. For example, identifying that one's life has purpose has been associated with a lower incidence of Alzheimer's disease and mild cognitive impairment and a decreased risk for experiencing a heart attack.[96,97] Positive emotions, health, and well-being are therefore fostered when we pursue and make progress towards valued goals; have enduring satisfying relationships with others; and possess the resources to understand, cope with, and manage life's challenges.[85,86,98]

SPIRITUALITY AND MEANING

A significant focus on spirituality within occupational therapy occurred around the zenith of the 20th century. Some who advocated spirituality for the profession focused upon the inability of occupational therapy concepts, such as doing, performing, adaptation, and even meaning and purpose, to capture the rich and complex depths of human experiences found in occupation.[99,100] Spirituality was seen as a concept that could deepen the profession's understanding of occupational performance and participation beyond the person factors that had been identified at that time.[101,102] In the Canadian Model of Occupational Performance, for example, spirituality was identified as the essence of the person and was placed at the center of the model (nested between cognitive, physical, and affective performance factors) to emphasize the criticality of the concept.[102] Within the PEOP Model, spirituality is situated as a person factor along with psychological, cognitive, neurobehavioral, and physiological factors; and spirituality has been referred to as meanings that, "contribute to a greater sense of personal understanding about self and one's place in the world."[101(p248)]

Spirituality may be considered, as Christiansen had suggested, the quintessential element of humans.[100] It is in this idea that we find many connections between spirituality and other concepts central to meaning and occupation, such as living a meaningful and engaged life, or experiencing the sublime or extraordinary, as well as the moments of joy and contentment found in socially imbedded occupations. The notion of spirituality has been related to occupation directly, such that occupation offers a means for the expression of the inner self.[103] Therefore, spirituality may have much in common with concepts such as personal identity, creativity, personal beliefs, values and goals, as well as the process of self-understanding which arises out of occupation. Spirituality also offers a rich resource for reflecting upon how humans ultimately experience and engage with the world through occupation. Importantly, this opens up the likelihood that these facets of a person's life-world might be captured through personal narrative to inform therapeutic approaches within a clinical situation. As suggested by Kirsch, "reflection upon one's life, the path it has taken, and the road ahead is an important process in meaning making, and the basis for a narrative approach to addressing spirituality in occupational therapy."[104(p57)]

Spirituality can also be referred to with respect to sacred matters such as religion, inclusive of organized religion, its prevailing beliefs, and its related practices. In fact, this is a common understanding when the term spirituality is used.[105,106] This perspective clearly has significant implications for how persons experience meaning in their day-to-day occupations. Park[107] has suggested that religious aspects of a person's global meaning system involve the shaping of beliefs and the formation of related personal goals. These beliefs and goals may in turn afford opportunities for social support when engaged in religiously-based occupations; contribute to an individual's sense of life meaning; and bolster coping resources through offering a sense of control, understanding, and hope when persons are faced with difficult life situations. Though many occupational therapy practitioners see religiously-based spirituality as important, they may not be as comfortable with assessing this aspect of a person's life-world.[108] However, by making an effort to be open to a client's religiously-based beliefs and practices, practitioners may assist in guiding clients to identify and engage in valued occupations.

A BIT ON BOREDOM

The concept of boredom can be a useful perspective from which to consider meaning in occupation. Though there is not full agreement surrounding its definition, boredom has been characterized as an emotional experience that is uncomfortable and dissatisfying; awareness turns inward, time seems to slow, and complaints about a lack of "things to do" are common.[109-112] The presence of boredom seems to be related to an absence of meaningful occupation. Persons are more likely to experience boredom when engaged in occupations that are repetitious, lacking intrinsic value or worth, and do not have any clear purpose or end goal.[113] Within qualitative studies, boredom has been reported to occur when persons have limited commitments or concerns (ie, no purpose), an absence of personally fulfilling relationships, or lacked the skills to engage competently in occupation.[114] Further, the experience of boredom can also reflect negatively on one's sense of self and outlook on life as the following quote suggests: "I'm the source of whatever boredom is. It's not what's out here. It's me! And that just means I'm nowhere. Maybe that's what it is. Boredom is nowhere. I'm nowhere."[5(p117)]

Alternatively, boredom is least likely to occur when experiences of occupations are rich with positive personal meaning.[57] A key example is the concept of flow in which persons engage in occupations of interest to them, the skills of the person match the challenges of the task such that they experience competence and control, and there is consistent feedback reflecting the progress being made towards a valued goal.[115] Other factors that may decrease boredom are occupations that allow satisfying personal relationships, the experience of autonomy in work or leisure, and commitment to personally valued goals. Further, a full consideration of boredom requires understanding how the demands of the task, the affordances or barriers in an environment, as well as the capacities or limitations of the individual effect occupation. Alleviating boredom can therefore be addressed by creating a sense of belonging, offering choice and a sense of control, providing clear feedback on performance and structuring therapeutic occupations that interest a client and are matched to his or her skill level.[116] These therapeutic efforts, when embedded within the PEOP Occupational Therapy Process, can also lead to great benefits with respect to engagement in meaningful occupation.

Summary

To this point, the concept of meaning in occupation has been framed as being comprised of multiple ways to explore human motivation, action, and experience. The use of personal narrative allows us access to the beliefs, values, thoughts, and emotions of an individual as they strive to construe meaning upon past, present, and future occupations. Meaning found in life experiences requires we maintain this perspective, yet appreciate that human doing (occupation) is fundamental to the creation of meaning via our relationships with others and coming to understand ourselves and our place in a social world. The needs for control, autonomy, competence, and belonging, in part, underlie our personal beliefs and goals—offering us a perspective from which to understand a person's narrative and a resource for developing therapeutic occupations that motivate engagement. When a person perceives their occupations as failing to fulfill these fundamental human needs, ensuing negative emotions and stress may serve to compromise health and well-being. Alternatively, the experience of positive emotions that arise from our participation in fulfilling personal relationships and successfully striving towards and accomplishing valued goals ultimately serve to fill our occupations and our lives with meanings that foster health and well-being.

ASSESSMENTS AND EVALUATIONS: MEANING, SENSEMAKING, AND SPIRITUALITY

In the process of creating an effective therapeutic relationship between a client and practitioner, the use of a narrative approach to assessment is paramount. Assessing a person's perception of their present situation may be best achieved by eliciting personal stories related to valued occupations. King's Model of Meaning of Life Experiences offers a useful framework upon which to begin this process.[2] That is, the practitioner invites the client to share stories about those occupations they most like to do, as well as their present concerns and their hopes and dreams for the future. Open-ended questions can be used to determine a person's needs and goals related to doing, belonging, and understanding. Further, the practitioner should discover through interview what specific therapeutic goals a client has and why they are important to the client. King also indicates the importance of assessing a client's strengths and resources with respect to their family and social supports, their knowledge regarding their situation, as well as their abilities and skills with respect to doing, belonging, and understanding:

- Determine the client's degree of self-knowledge and self-efficacy (comfort level) in domains of interest
- Determine the client's strengths and competencies (and self-awareness with respect to these)
- Determine the client's knowledge of available recreational and vocational opportunities in the community
- Assess family factors such as financial resources and time availability
- Assess external supports such as existing friendships and other informal social supports

Theory development and research in occupational therapy and occupational science has recently led to instruments which validly assess meaningful experiences in occupation. The Value and Meaning in Occupations (ValMO) model describes 3 dimensions of value (or meaning) which can be found in the experience of occupation. These dimensions include self-reward value (eg, pleasure and relaxation), concrete value (eg, competent task completion), and symbolic value (eg, feeling close to others), which contribute to a sense of life meaning.[46] The Occupational Value Assessment with Predefined Items (OVal-pd) was developed from the ValMO model and validated in Sweden[117] and the US.[118] The Engagement in Meaningful Activities Survey (EMAS) is another instrument that validly assesses activity meaningfulness.[119] These self-report survey instruments offer occupational therapy practitioners the ability to quickly and easily measure the present level of meaning (or value) persons perceive in their daily occupations. Research employing the OVal-pd or the EMAS has demonstrated that meaningful occupation does indeed influence well-being. For example, greater levels of meaningful experiences in occupation have been associated with greater intrinsic motivation, life satisfaction, meaning and purpose in life, self-rated health, self-esteem, and QOL. Alternatively, lower levels of eaningful experiences in occupation have been associated with greater boredom, anxiety, stress, and depression.[47,57,120-125]

The instruments indicated in Table 19-1 offer a broad range of tools for assessing occupation and participation which practitioners might employ within the PEOP Occupational Therapy Process. Use of instruments such as the *Activity Card Sort*[126] or the COPM[127] offer opportunities to explore the presence and absences of occupations a client wants and needs to do. Further, these tools are useful for identifying occupationally focused goals as a basis for occupation-based interventions. Other assessments, such as the Children's Assessment of Participation and Enjoyment, Preferences for Activities for Children, or the Participation and Environment Measure for Children and Youth, assesses activity participation in younger populations with respect to frequency of activity participation across a range of activities, preferences for activity choices, as well as environments that support or hinder meaningful participation.[128,130]

INTERVENTIONS: MEANING, SENSEMAKING, AND SPIRITUALITY

Interventions in the PEOP Occupational Therapy Process require a client-centered perspective aimed at supporting engagement in meaningful occupations. As with assessment, intervention requires an ongoing narrative dialogue between the client and practitioner to assure progress towards valued goals are being achieved. Importantly, King's Model of Meaning of Life Experiences[2] supports the idea that effective goal setting and clinical interventions should be based upon doing or the use of therapeutic occupation. For example, by selecting tasks that are of interest to a client, the individual can best come to understand their present capacities. The competent experience found in a therapeutic occupation can also serve as a sign that the person is capable of achieving their personal goals, likely motivating future commitment to the therapeutic process. Choosing occupations that enable opportunities to connect with others and develop personal relationships weaves together the 3 pillars of King's model (doing, belonging, and understanding) and maximizes opportunities to infuse meaning in daily occupations and foster well-being.

By considering the importance of human needs, occupational therapy practitioners can also create meaning within the context of therapy. Therapeutic experiences that support the basic psychological needs of autonomy, competence, and belonging[131] infuse therapy with meaning. Working collaboratively with clients, goals can be developed that maximize opportunities for successfully meeting these basic needs through occupation.

Practitioners also must consider how the capacities of the individual, the characteristics of the environment, and the demands of a given task interact to support or thwart a person's experience of basic needs fulfillment. For example, the need to exert control over one's environment through occupation may be effectively met by marshaling social support that fosters increased opportunities and resources for achieving an individual's personal goals.[48] Further, the experience of control may be achieved in therapeutic occupations by creating that "just-right challenge" between a person's capacities and the demands of a given task and environment. The following examples offer some insights into how these aims may be understood and achieved in a therapeutic context.

The therapeutic encounter, an event in which client and practitioner are engaged as partners in creating healing and well-being, offers unique opportunities for crafting meaning. Within this context, the creation of meaning is realized not only within the actions and experience of the client, but relies on the ongoing interplay between the client and practitioner. Mattingly[29] presents a compelling analysis of a therapeutic encounter between a young child with motor performance difficulties and her adept occupational therapy practitioner. Within this event, typical therapeutic activities used to develop motor skills are transformed into a culturally shared narrative script, an "Olympic event" in which the child is momentarily transformed into an elite athlete. The child is encouraged to guide the session, which the practitioner skillfully shapes to enable and highlight personal competencies. This rich encounter affords the child motivating and meaningful experiences, such as feelings of social support and collaboration, autonomy, competence, joy, and excitement, which are too often absent within the child's day-to-day life. Through this encounter the routine and mundane qualities of therapy have been transformed to exercises worth performing, "making life, clinical life, more worth living."[29(p202)]

The meaning in this event can be envisioned from the multiple perspectives adopted within this chapter. First, the social nature of this encounter uses a shared cultural meaning, the Olympics, to situate therapy. Second, interwoven within the social exchange of action is the evident capacity of the practitioner to support the child's needs for autonomy and control by allowing her to direct the event, while the practitioner remarks on skilled and competent performances. Comments from the practitioner highlight the child's competence and validate the child's sense of efficacy and control. Third, through this socially embedded action, the child's motivation is supported and meaningful life experiences are realized, thereby creating a successful therapeutic encounter.

Table 19-1.   *Assessments of Participation in Meaningful Occupation*

Assessment	Construct Assessed	Description and Reference	Where It Can Be Obtained
Activity Card Sort, 2nd Edition	Participation and meaning	An assessment of activity participation for older and institutional adults that includes photographs of persons in activities to indicate length of time in activities, frequency of participation, and social interaction during participation.[126]	http://myaota.aota.org/shop_ aota/prodview.aspx? TYPE=D&PID=763&SKU=1247
COPM, 2nd Edition	Participation and meaning	An individualized assessment designed to detect change in a client's self-perception of occupational performance over time.[127]	www.caot.ca
Children's Assessment of Participation and Enjoyment (CAPE) and Preferences for Activities for Children (PAC)	Participation and meaning	The CAPE assesses an individual's day-to-day participation and the PAC assesses an individual's preference for activities; used for persons aged 6 to 21.[128]	www.pearson assessments.com
Engagement in Meaningful Activities Survey	Participation and meaning	A brief 12-item survey that assesses perceptions of meaningfulness in daily activities.[119,125]	Dr. Aaron Eakman, Department of Occupational Therapy, Colorado State University, Fort Collins, CO. Email: aaron.eakman@colo-state.edu
Meaningful Activity Participation Assessment	Participation and meaning	An assessment of the frequency and meaningfulness of 28 types of activities; used for older adults.[124]	http://digitallibrary.usc.edu/ cdm/compoundobject/collection/p15799coll127/id/514873/rec/6
Occupational Gap Questionnaire	Participation and meaning	A 28-item assessment which identifies a discrepancy (gap) between activities persons want to perform but are not performing or activities persons are performing but do not wish to be performing; used for adults with neurologically-related disabilities.[129]	Dr. Gunilla Eriksson, Division of Occupational Therapy, Karolinska Institutet, Huddinge, Sweden. Email: gunilla.eriksson@ki.se (Swedish version)
Occupational Value Instrument with Pre-Defined Items	Participation and meaning	A 28-item assessment of perceived value (concrete, self-reward, and symbolic) in daily occupations derived from the Value and Meaning in Occupation Model.[118]	Dr. Mona Eklund, Department of Health Sciences, Lund University, Sweden. Email: mona.eklund@med.lu.se (English version)
Paediatric Activity Card Sort	Participation and meaning	This instrument assesses occupational performance and engagement using pictures of children engaged in typical childhood occupations; for persons aged 5 to 14.	www.caot.ca

(continued)

Table 19-1 (continued).   *Assessments of Participation in Meaningful Occupation*

Assessment	Construct Assessed	Description and Reference	Where It Can Be Obtained
Participation and Environment Measure for Children and Youth	Participation and Meaning	This instrument assesses the frequency and extent of involvement and desire for change in typical home, school, and community environments, including supports and barriers to participation within each setting; for persons aged 5 to 17.[130]	Chia-Yu Lin Research Coordinator, CanChild Centre for Childhood Disability Research, McMaster University, Hamilton Ontario. Email: lin-chia@mcmaster.ca

The Motivational Theory of Life Span Development and its focus on primary and secondary control also provide insights for practitioners regarding meaning and change in meaning through occupation.[48] Importantly, the principal focus of therapy from this perspective is directed at maintaining primary control and supporting competence in striving toward client goals in valued occupations. Specific examples lie in a study of older adults with macular degeneration in which narrative data were used to determine how persons adapted to their disease.[132] Primary control was achieved through adopting compensatory strategies as these older adults endeavored to maintain satisfying occupational performance. One informant indicated, "I make contrast everywhere, I just bought new white mugs so I can see where the coffee is and I'm constantly figuring out contrast."[132(p28)] Compensations such as using vision aids (eg, a magnifying glass), seeking and accepting informal assistance in the community (eg, help reading a menu), and formal help (eg, help with reading labels during weekly visits to grocery store) helped persons assert their primary control needs through completing valued daily occupations. Occupational therapy practitioners may also focus on increasing primary control by encouraging sustained effort in tasks, developing needed occupational performance skills, or prioritizing valued occupations to support time management.

Secondary control strategies, in which persons actively strive to change their perception of their situation, also influenced how persons experienced and coped with their visual disability within occupations. By providing information regarding the disease process to a client, a person could attribute loss in capacities (a loss of primary control) to the disease and aging, thereby minimizing the likelihood of self-blame. Attempting to identify some benefits may also assist in coping with loss, such as developing new friendships with caregivers or deeper relationships with family. Also, persons may devalue goals to persist in occupations they no longer can competently perform, as one informant commented, "It's not life or death to give up playing tennis, it's just something I enjoyed and I now enjoy watching it. I try to watch as much as I can and appreciate it."[132(p28)] Therapy may therefore consist of assisting a client to identify alternative interests in occupations they are able to competently perform, and acknowledging their successes in that occupation. This effort can aid a person who has to "let go" of a valued occupation they can no longer do by focusing on tasks in which they are interested and competent.

Lastly, King's Model of Meaning of Life Experiences[2] directs practitioners to consider the variety of ways to support meaningful occupational engagement in areas of interest to the client. The use of narrative is central to this process, as the practitioner elicits the personal perspective of the client and matches intervention approaches to the client's most pressing concerns and goals:

- Promote belonging or social support (eg, support groups, clubs, drop-in programs)
- Promote competency and provide feedback about skill level (eg, involvement in sports and recreation programs; volunteer and paid employment)
- Promote self-awareness (eg, self-discovery programs, involvement in "values clarification" exercises and workshops)
- Provide instructions in the fundamental skills needed for belonging (eg, programs that assist the client in developing pro-social skills)
- Provide instructions in the fundamental skills needed for doing (eg, problem-solving and decision-making skills, skills needed to perform activities of daily living, vocational counseling)

OUTCOMES: MEANING, SENSEMAKING, AND SPIRITUALITY

Outcomes central to meaning will rest principally in a person's capacity to experience health and well-being through occupation. This proposition, however, considers the following factors. First, clients should hope to achieve the occupationally relevant goals that they have identified through the treatment process. This reflects the understanding that doing or engagement in occupation is an essential aspect of human existence and therefore a requisite concern within the goal setting process. Measures of occupational performance and participation outcomes are required, which can indicate that an increase in participation in preferred occupations has been demonstrated following the PEOP Occupational Therapy Process. Measures identified previously, and found in Table 19-1, may be used for this purpose. Second, experiences engendered through occupational performance and participation are crucial to well-being and are therefore key considerations in assessing occupational therapy outcomes. Therefore, valid measures of subjective experiences related to occupational performance and participation, also found in Table 19-1, should also be adopted within practice. Last, justifying occupational therapy practice continues to require that the outcomes of our services result in benefits that are important to our clients and to society. Participation in occupation is emerging as a concept that is gaining great appeal as such an outcome; however, occupational therapy practitioners should also consider assessing therapeutic outcomes with respect to measures of health-related quality, meaning and purpose in life, and well-being, such as those found in Table 19-2.

The study of meaning, personal well-being, sensemaking, and spirituality—though of great interest to occupational therapy practitioners—are gaining strength in medicine and community health. Table 19-3 was included to provide resources to help practitioners keep abreast of advances in these issues.

Table 19-2.   *Assessments of Well-Being and Related Constructs*

Assessment	Construct Assessed	Description and Reference	Where It Can Be Obtained
Basic Psychological Needs Scale—General	Well-Being	A 21-item assessment of the basic psychological needs for autonomy, competence, and relatedness.[57]	www.selfdetermination theory.org/ questionnaires/10-questionnaires/[53]
Boredom Proneness Scale (Short Form)	Boredom	A brief 12-item assessment of boredom proneness composed of 2 components: internal and external stimulation.[133]	133
COPE (complete and abbreviated versions)	Coping	Assesses a broad range of coping responses with either a 60-item version, or less burdensome 28-item version.[134]	www.psy.miami. edu/ faculty/cca-rver/CCscales.html
Swinburne University Emotional Intelligence Test	Emotional intelligence	A 64-item assessment of 5 forms of emotional intelligence including emotional recognition and expression, understanding emotions, emotional management, and emotional control.[135]	www.research-bank. swinburne.edu.au
Meaning in Life Questionnaire	Meaning in life	A 10-item assessment of the presence of meaning in life and the search for meaning in life.[136]	www.michaelfsteger. com/ ?page_id=13
Medical Outcome Health Survey Short Form (SF-36) Version 2	HRQOL	A 36-item survey which broadly assesses 2 aspects of HRQOL: physical and mental health.[137]	www.qualitymetric.com
Positive and Negative Affect Schedule	Emotion (affect)	A 20-item assessment of affect, including descriptors of positive (eg, interested, enthusiastic, inspired) and negative (eg, upset, scared, afraid) emotions.[138]	138
Purpose in Life Test	Meaning in life	A 20-item assessment reflecting Victor Frankl's conception of life purpose and meaning.[139]	139
Sense of Coherence Scale	Meaning in life	A 29-item assessment of personal resources for managing stress comprised of comprehensibility, manageability, and meaningfulness.[140]	140
Ryff Scales of Psychological Well-Being (long and medium forms)	Well-being	Assesses 6 dimensions of well-being with either 84 or 54 items, including self-acceptance, positive relations with others, autonomy, environmental mastery, purpose in life, and personal growth.[61]	www.liberalarts. wabash.edu/ ryff-scales
Satisfaction with Life Scale	Well-being	A short 5-item instrument designed to assess global cognitive judgments of satisfaction with one's life.[141]	http://internal. psychology.illinois. edu/~ediener/ SWLS.html
Ways of Coping Questionnaire	Coping	A 66-item questionnaire that assesses thoughts and actions that individuals use to cope with the stressful encounters of everyday living.[142]	www.mindgarden. com

Table 19-3.   *Organizations and Journals That Focus on Meaning, Sense Making, and Spirituality Factors for Performance*

Organization or Journal	Description	Web Address
Society for Emotional Well-Being Worldwide	Works to build a community of individuals and organizations dedicated to expanding access to mental healthcare, to promote exchange of knowledge and information on Global Mental Health (particularly in resource-poor settings), and to ultimately strengthen the emotional well-being of people in need by making mental health a reality for all.	http://seww.org/
Psychology of Well-Being	A peer-reviewed open access journal published under the brand SpringerOpen, devoted to understanding the biopsychosocial and behavioral factors leading to enhanced well-being, optimal emotional processing, and the prevention of psychological dysfunction.	http://www.springer.com/ psychology/ klinische+psychologie/ journal/13612
Journal of Spirituality in Mental Health	Interdisciplinary professional journal devoted to the scholarly study of spirituality as a resource for counseling and psychotherapeutic disciplines.	http://www.tandfonline. com/toc/wspi20/current
International Journal of Wellbeing	Journal that welcomes timely original high-quality scholarly articles of appropriate length on the topic of well-being; broadly construed.	http://www.internation-aljournalofwellbeing.org/ index.php/ijow
Journal of Religion, Disability and Health	Provides an interfaith, interdisciplinary forum that supports people with disabilities and their families through religious, spiritual, clinical, educational, and scientific perspectives.	http://www.tandfonline. com/toc/wrdh20/current#. U4aF9PldXrE

REFERENCES

1. Bruner J. *Acts of Meaning.* Cambridge, MA: Harvard University Press; 1990.
2. King GA. The meaning of life experiences: application of a meta-model to rehabilitation sciences and services. *American Journal of Orthopsychiatry.* 2004;74:72-88.
3. Park CL, Folkman S. Meaning in the context of stress and coping. *Review of General Psychology.* 1997;1:115-144.
4. Becker G. *Disrupted Lives: How People Create Meaning in a Chaotic World.* Berkeley, CA: University of California Press; 1997.
5. Corvinelli A. Boredom in recovery for adult substance users with HIV/AIDS attending an urban day treatment program. *Occupational Therapy in Mental Health.* 2010;26:99-130.
6. Kaufman ER. *The Ageless Self: Sources of Meaning in Late Life.* Madison, WI: University of Wisconsin Press; 1986.
7. Kielhofner G, ed. *Health Through Occupation: Theory and Practice in Occupational Therapy.* Philadelphia, PA: FA Davis; 1983.
8. Rogers JC. The study of human occupation. In: Kielhofner G, ed. *Health Through Occupation: Theory and Practice in Occupational Therapy.* Philadelphia, PA: FA Davis; 1983:93-124.
9. Fidler GS, Fidler JW. Doing and becoming: the occupational therapy experience. In: Kielhofner G, ed. *Health Through Occupation: Theory and Practice in Occupational Therapy.* Philadelphia, PA: FA Davis; 1983:267-280.
10. Engelhardt HT. Occupational therapists as technologists and custodians of meaning. In: Kielhofner G, ed. *Health Through Occupation: Theory and Practice in Occupational Therapy.* Philadelphia, PA: FA Davis; 1983:139-145.
11. Sharrott GW. Occupational therapy's role in the client's creation and affirmation of meaning. In: Kielhofner G, ed. *Health Through Occupation: Theory and Practice in Occupational Therapy.* Philadelphia, PA: FA Davis; 1983:213-233.
12. Reed KL. An annotated history of the concepts used in occupational therapy. In: Christiansen CH, Baum CM, Bass-Haugen J, eds. *Occupational Therapy: Performance, Participation, and Well-Being.* Thorofare, NJ: SLACK Incorporated; 2005:567-626.
13. Kielhofner G, ed. *A Model of Human Occupation.* Baltimore, MD: Williams & Wilkins; 1985.
14. Nelson DL. Occupation: form and performance. *American Journal of Occupational Therapy.* 1988;42:633-641.
15. Christiansen CH, Baum CM. Glossary. In: Christiansen CH, Baum CM, eds. *Occupational Therapy: Overcoming Human Performance Deficits.* Thorofare, NJ: SLACK Incorporated; 1997:591-606.

16. Hinojosa J, Kramer P. Fundamental concepts of occupational therapy: occupation, purposeful activity, and function. *American Journal of Occupational Therapy.* 1997;51:864-866.

17. Nelson DL. Therapeutic occupation: a definition. *American Journal of Occupational Therapy.* 1996;50:775-782.

18. Trombly CA. Occupation: purposefulness and meaningfulness as therapeutic mechanisms. *American Journal of Occupational Therapy.* 1995;49:960-972.

19. Park CL. Making sense of the meaning literature: an integrative review of meaning making and its effects on adjustment to stressful life events. *Psychological Bulletin.* 2010;136:257-301.

20. Carver CS, Scheier MF. *On the Self-Regulation of Behavior.* New York, NY: Cambridge University Press; 1998.

21. Little BR. Personal projects and free traits: personality and motivation reconsidered. *Social and Personality Psychology Compass.* 2008;2/3:1235-1254.

22. Crabtree JL. The end of occupational therapy. *American Journal of Occupational Therapy.* 1998;52:205-214.

23. Jackson J, Carlson M, Mandel D, Zemke R, Clark F. Occupation in lifestyle redesign: the well elderly study occupational therapy program. *American Journal of Occupational Therapy.* 1998;52:326-336.

24. Ikiugu MN. Meaningfulness of occupations as an occupational-life-trajectory attractor. *Journal of Occupational Science.* 2005;12:102-109.

25. Christiansen CH. Defining lives: occupation as identity: an essay on competence, coherence, and the creation of meaning. *American Journal of Occupational Therapy.* 1999;53:547-558.

26. Jonsson H, Josephsson S. Occupation and meaning. In: Christiansen CH, Baum CM, eds. *Occupational Therapy: Performance, Participation, and Well-Being.* Thorofare, NJ: SLACK Incorporated; 2005;116-132.

27. Kielhofner G. *Model of Human Occupation.* 4th ed. Baltimore, MD: Lippincott Williams & Wilkins; 2008.

28. Polkinghorne DE. *Narrative Knowing and the Human Sciences.* Albany, NY: State University of New York Press; 1988.

29. Mattingly C. Emergent narratives. In: Mattingly C, Garro LC, eds. *Narrative and the Cultural Construction of Illness and Healing.* Los Angeles, CA: University of California Press; 2000:181-211.

30. Lazarus RS. *Stress and Emotion: A New Synthesis.* New York, NY: Springer Publishing; 1999.

31. Clark F, Ennevor BL, Richardson PL. A grounded theory of techniques for occupational storytelling and occupational story making. In: Zemke R, Clark F, eds. *Occupational Science: The Evolving Discipline.* Philadelphia, PA: FA Davis Company; 1996:373-392.

32. Mattingly C. *Healing Dramas and Clinical Plots: The Narrative Structure of Experience.* Cambridge, UK: Cambridge University Press; 1998.

33. Wilcock AA. *An Occupational Perspective of Health.* 2nd ed. Thorofare, NJ: SLACK Incorporated; 2006.

34. King GA, Brown EG, Smith LK. *Resilience: Learning from People with Disabilities and the Turning Points in their Lives.* West Port, CT: Praeger; 2003.

35. Reis HT, Sheldon KM, Gable SL, Roscoe J, Ryan RM. Daily well-being: the role of autonomy, competence, and relatedness. *Personality and Social Psychology Bulletin.* 2000;26:419-435.

36. Matuska K, Christiansen CH. A proposed model of life balance. *Journal of Occupational Science.* 2008;15:9-19.

37. Ryan RM, Deci EL. Self-determination theory and the facilitation of intrinsic motivation, social development, and well-being. *American Psychologist.* 2000;55:68-78.

38. Gendlin E. *Experiencing and the Creation of Meaning: A Philosophical and Psychological Approach to the Subjective.* Evenston, IL: Northwestern University Press; 1962/1997.

39. Damasio A. *Looking for Spinoza: Joy, Sorrow, and the Feeling Brain.* New York, NY: Harcourt Books; 2003.

40. Zautra AJ. *Emotions, Stress, and Health.* New York, NY: Oxford University Press; 2003.

41. Kemeny ME, Shestyuk A. Emotions, the neuroendocrine and immune systems, and health. In: Lewis M, Haviland-Jones JM, Barrett LF, eds. *Handbook of Emotions.* 3rd ed. New York, NY: Guilford Press; 2008:661-675.

42. Eccles JS, Wigfield A. Motivational beliefs, values, and goals. *Annual Review of Psychology.* 2002;53:109-132.

43. Heckhausen J. *Developmental Regulation in Adulthood.* Cambridge, MA: Cambridge University Press; 1999.

44. Baltes BB, Baltes MM. *Successful Aging.* Cambridge, MA: Cambridge University Press; 1990.

45. Bandura A. *Self Efficacy: The Exercise of Control.* New York, NY: WH Freeman; 1997.

46. Persson D, Erlandsson L-K, Eklund M, Iwarsson S. Value dimensions, meaning, and complexity in human occupation—a tentative structure for analysis. *Scandinavian Journal of Occupational Therapy.* 2001;8:7-18.

47. Eakman AM, Carlson ME, Clark FA. Factor structure, reliability and convergent validity of the Engagement in Meaningful Activities Survey for older adults. *OTJR: Occupation, Participation and Health.* 2010;30:111-121.

48. Heckhausen J, Wrosch C, Schulz R. A motivational theory of life-span development. *Psychological Review.* 2010;117:32-60.

49. Carlson M, Clark F, Young B. Practical contributions of occupational science to the art of successful ageing: how to sculpt a meaningful life in older adulthood. *Journal of Occupational Science.* 1998;5:107-198.

50. Schultz R, Heckhausen J. A lifespan model of successful aging. *American Psychologist.* 1996;51:702-714.

51. Heckhausen J, Schultz R. A life-span theory of control. *Psychological Review.* 1995;102:284-304.

52. Brunstein JC, Schultheiss OC, Maier GW. The pursuit of personal goals: a motivational approach. In: Brandtstädter J, Lerner RM, eds. *Action and Self Development.* Thousand Oaks, CA: Sage; 1999:169-196.

53. Emmons RA. *The Psychology of Ultimate Concerns.* New York, NY: Guilford; 1999.

54. Little BR, Salmela-Aro K, Phillips SD, eds. *Personal Projects: Goals, Action, and Human Flourishing.* Mahwah, NJ: Lawrence Erlbaum Associates; 2007.

55. Rassmussen HN, Wrosch C, Scheier MF, Carver CS. Self-regulation processes and health: the importance of optimism and goal adjustment. *Journal of Personality.* 2006;74:1722-1748.

56. Wu C-Y, Chen S-P, Grossman J. Facilitating intrinsic motivation in clients with mental illness. *Occupational Therapy in Health Care.* 2000;16(1):1-14.

57. Eakman AM. Convergent validity of the Engagement in Meaningful Activities Survey in a college sample. *OTJR: Occupation, Participation and Health.* 2011;30:23-32.

58. Deci EL, Ryan RM, eds. *Handbook of Self-Determination Theory.* Rochester, NY: University of Rochester Press; 2002.

59. Ryan RM, Deci EL. Overview of self-determination theory: an organismic dialectical perspective. In: Deci EL, Ryan RM, eds. *Handbook of Self-Determination Research.* Rochester, NY: University of Rochester; 2002:3-33.

60. Cantor N, Sanderson CA. Life task participation and well-being: the importance of taking part in daily life. In: Kahneman D, Diener E, Schwarz N, eds. *Well-Being: The Foundations of Hedonic Psychology.* New York, NY: Sage; 1999.

61. Ryff CD, Keyes LM. The structure of psychological well-being revisited. *Journal of Personality and Social Psychology.* 1995;69:719-727.

62. Carlson M. The self-perpetuation of occupations. In: Zemke R, Clark F, eds. *Occupational Science: The Evolving Discipline.* Philadelphia, PA: FA Davis; 1996:143-157.

63. Kielhofner G. *A Model of Human Occupation: Theory and Application.* Baltimore, MD: Lippincott Williams & Wilkins; 2002.

64. Eakman AM. Relationships betwen meaningful activity, basic psychological needs, and meaning in life: test of the Meaningful Activity and Life Meaning Model. *OTJR: Occupation, Participation and Health.* 2013;33:100-109.

65. Lazarus RS, Folkman S. *Stress, Appraisal, and Coping.* New York, NY: Springer Publishing; 1984.

66. Dublouloz C-J, Laporte D, Hall M, Ashe B, Smith D. Transformation of meaning perspectives in clients with rheumatoid arthritis. *American Journal of Occupational Therapy.* 2004;58:398-407.

67. Yerxa EJ. Authentic occupational therapy. *American Journal of Occupational Therapy.* 1966;1:155-173.

68. Ekman P. An argument for basic emotions. *Cognition and Emotion.* 1992;6:169-200.

69. Matsumoto D, Keltner D, Shiota MN, O'Sullivan M, Frank M. Facial expression of emotions. In: Lewis M, Haviland-Jones JM, Barrett LF, eds. *Handbook of Emotions.* 3rd ed. New York, NY: Guilford Press; 2008:211-234.

70. Solomon R. *The Passions: Philosophy and the Intelligence of Emotions.* Chantilly, VA: The Teaching Company; 2006.

71. Klinger E. The search for meaning in evolutionary perspective and its clinical implications. In: Wong PTP, Fry PS, eds. *The Human Quest for Meaning: A Handbook of Psychological Research and Clinical Applications.* Mahwah, NJ: Lawrence Erlbaum Associates; 1998:27-50.

72. Klinger E. *Meaning & Void.* Minneapolis, MN: University of Minnesota; 1977.

73. Mayer JD, Salovey P, Caruso DR. Emotional intelligence as zeitgeist, as personality, and as a mental ability. In: Bar-On R, Parker JDA, eds. *The Handbook of Emotional Intelligence. Theory, Development, Assessment, and Application at Home, School, and in the Workplace.* San Francisco, CA: Jossey-Bass; 2000:92-117.

74. McAdams DP, Anyidoho NA, Brown C, Huang YT, Kaplan B, Machado MA. Traits and stories: links between dispositional and narrative features of personality. *Journal of Personality.* 2004;72:761-784.

75. Sarbin TR. Emotions as narrative employments. In: Packer MJ, Richard BA, eds. *Entering the Circle: Hermeneutic Investigation in Psychology.* Albany, NY: State University of New York Press; 1989:185-201.

76. Sarte JP. *Existensialism and Human Emotions.* Secaucus, NJ: Citadel Press; 1957.

77. Chaffey L, Unsworth CA, Fossey E. Relationship between intuition and emotional intelligence in occupational therapist in mental health practice. *American Journal of Occupational Therapy.* 2012;66:88-96.

78. Sapolsky RM. *Why Zebras Don't get Ulcers.* 3rd ed. New York, NY: Henry Holt and Company; 2004.

79. Folkman S, Moskowitz JT. Stress, positive emotion, and coping. *Current Directions in Psychological Science.* 2000;9(4):115-118.

80. Herbert TB, Chohen S. Stress and immunity in humans: a meta-analytic review. *Psychosomatic Medicine.* 1993;55:364-379.

81. Kiecolt-Glaser JK, McGuire L, Robles T, Glaser R. Emotions, morbidity, and mortality. *Annual Review of Psychology.* 2002;53:83-107.

82. Seeman T, Singer B, Rowe JW, Horwitz R, McEwan B. The price of adaptation: allostatic load and its health consequences. *Archives of Internal Medicine.* 1997;157:2259-2268.

83. Glaser R, Kiecolt-Glaser JK. Stress-induced immune dysfunction: implications for health. *Nature Review: Immunology.* 2005;5:243-251.

84. Pert CB. *Molecules of Emotion.* New York, NY: Touchstone; 1997.

85. Antonovsky A. *Unraveling the Mystery of Health.* San Francisco, CA: Jossey-Bass; 1987.

86. Ryff CD, Singer B. The contours of positive human health. *Psychological Inquiry.* 1998;9:1-28.

87. Marsland AL, Pressman S, Cohen S. Positive affect and immune function. In: Ader R, ed. *Psychoneuroimmunology 4.* San Diego, CA: Academic Press; 2007:761-779.

88. Steptoe A, Dockray S, Wardle J. Positive affect and psycho-biological processes relevant to health. *Journal of Personality.* 2009;77:1747-1776.

89. Diener E, Chan MY. Happy people live longer: subjective well-being contributes to health and longevity. *Applied Psychology: Health and Well-Being.* 2011;3:1-43.

90. Chida Y, Steptoe A. Positive psychological well-being and mortality: a quantitative review of prospective observational studies. *Psychosomatic Medicine.* 2008;70:741-756.

91. Xu J, Roberts RE. The power of positive emotions: it's a matter of life or death—subjective well-being and longevity over 28 years in a general population. *Health Psychology.* 2010;29:9-19.

92. Howell RT, Kern ML, Lyubomirsky S. Health benefits: meta-analytically determining the impact of well-being on objective health outcomes. *Health Psychology Review.* 2007;1:83-136.

93. Ong AD. Pathways linking positive emotion and health in later life. *Current Directions in Psychological Science.* 2010;19:358-362.

94. Folkman S. Positive psychological states and coping with severe stress. *Social Science and Medicine.* 1997;45:1207-1221.

95. Ryff CD, Singer B. Biopsychosocial challenges of the new millenium. *Psychotherapy and Psychosomatics.* 2000;69:170-177.

96. Boyle PA, Buchman AS, Barnes LL, Bennett DA. Effect of a purpose in life on rise of incident Alzheimer disease and mild cognitive impairment in community-dwelling older persons. *Archives of General Psychiatry.* 2010;67:304-310.

97. Kim ES, Sun JK, Park N, Kubzansky LD, Peterson C. Purpose in life and reduced risk of myocardial infarction among older U.S. adults with coronary heart disease: a two-year follow-up. *Journal of Behavioral Medicine.* 2012:1-10.

98. Baumeister RF. *Meanings of Life.* New York, NY: The Guilford Press; 1991.

99. Peloquin SM. The spiritual depth of occupation: making worlds and making lives. *American Journal of Occupational Therapy.* 1997;51:167-168.

100. Christiansen CH. Acknowledging a spiritual dimension in occupational therapy practice. *American Journal of Occupational Therapy.* 1997;51:169-172.

101. Christiansen CH, Baum CM, Bass-Haugen J, eds. *Occupational Therapy: Performance, Participation, and Well-Being.* 3rd ed. Thorofare, NJ: SLACK Incorporated; 2005.

102. Townsend EA, Polatjko H. *Enabling Occupation II: Advancing an Occupational Therapy Vision for Health, Well-Being and Justice Through Occupation.* Ottawa, ON: CAOT Publications ACE; 2007.

103. Hasselkus BR. *The Meaning of Everyday Occupation.* Thorofare, NJ: SLACK Incorporated; 2002.

104. Kirsch B. A narrative approach to addressing spirituality in occupational therapy: exploring personal meaning and purpose. *Canadian Journal of Occupational Therapy.* 1996;63(1):55-61.

105. Emmons RA, Palouttzian RE. The psychology of religion. *Annual Review of Psychology.* 2003;54:377-402.

106. World Health Organization. *International Classification of Functioning, Disability, and Health: ICF.* Geneva, Switzerland: World Health Organization; 2001.

107. Park CL. Religiousness/spirituality and health: a meaning systems perspective. *Journal of Behavioral Medicine.* 2007;30:319-328.

108. Enquist DE, Short-DeGraff M, Gliner J, Oltjenbruns K. Occupational therapists' beliefs and practices with regard to spirituality and therapy. *American Journal of Occupational Therapy.* 1997;51:172-180.

109. Farmer R, Sundberg ND. Boredom proneness: the development and correlates of a new scale. *Journal of Personality Assessment.* 1986;50(1):4-17.

110. Farnsworth L. Doing, being, and boredom. *Journal of Occupational Science.* 1998;5:140-146.

111. Mikulas WL, Vodonovich SJ. The essence of boredom. *Psychology and Behavioral Sciences.* 1993;43:3-12.

112. Stafford SP, Gregory WT. Heidegger's phenomenology of boredom, and the scientific investigation of conscious experience. *Phenomenology and the Cognitive Sciences.* 2006;5:155-196.

113. Bracke P, Bruynooghe K, Verhaeghe M. Boredom during day activity programs in rehabilitation centers. *Sociological Perspectives.* 2006;49:191-215.

114. Martin M, Sadlo G, Stew G. The phenomenon of boredom. *Qualitative Research in Psychology.* 2006;3:193-211.

115. Csikszentmihalyi M. *Flow: The Psychology of Optimal Experience.* New York, NY: Harper & Row; 1990.

116. Corvinelli A. Alleviating boredom in adult males recovering from substance use disorder. *Occupational Therapy in Mental Health.* 2005;21(2):1-11.

117. Eklund M, Erlandsson L-K, Persson D, Hagell D. Rasch analysis of an instrument for measuring occupational value: implications for theory and practice. *Scandinavian Journal of Occupational Therapy.* 2009;16:118-128.

118. Eakman AM, Eklund M. Reliability and structural validity of an assessment of occupational value. *Scandinavian Journal of Occupational Therapy.* 2011;18:231-240.

119. Eakman AM. Measurement characteristics of the Engagement in Meaningful Activities Survey in an age-diverse sample. *American Journal of Occupational Therapy.* 2012;66:e20-e29.

120. Eakman AM, Eklund M. The relative impact of personality traits, meaningful occupation and occupational value on meaning in life and life satisfaction. *Journal of Occupational Science.* 2012;iFirst:1-13.

121. Eklund M, Erlandsson L-K, Persson D. Occupational value among individuals with long-term mental illness. *Canadian Journal of Occupational Therapy.* 2003;70(5):276-284.

122. Eklund M, Leufstadius C. Relationships between occupational factors and health and well-being in individuals with persistent mental illness living in the community. *Canadian Journal of Occupational Therapy.* 2007;74:303-313.

123. Bigelius U, Eklund M, Erlandsson L-K. The value and meaning of an instrumental occupation performed in a clinical setting. *Scandinavian Journal of Occupational Therapy.* 2010;17:4-9.

124. Eakman AM, Carlson ME, Clark FA. The Meaningful Activity Participation Assessment: a measure of engagement in personally valued activities. *International Journal of Aging and Human Development.* 2010;70:299-317.

125. Goldberg B, Brintnell ES, Goldberg J. The relationship between engagement in meaningful activities and quality of life in persons disabled by mental illness. *Occupational Therapy in Mental Health.* 2002;18(2):17-44.

126. Baum, CM, Edwards, DF. *Activity Card Sort.* Bethesda, MD: AOTA Press; 2008.

127. Law M, Baptiste S, Carswell A, McColl MA, Polatjko H, Pollock N. *Canadian Occupational Performance Measure.* 2nd ed. Ottawa, ON: CAOT Publications ACE; 1994.

128. King GA. Measuring children's participation in recreation and leisure activities: construct validation of the CAPE and PAC. *Child Care Health and Development.* 2007;33:28-39.

129. Bergström AL, Guidetti S, Tistad M, et al. Perceived occupational gaps one year after stroke: an explorative study. *Journal of Rehabilitation Medicine.* 2012;44:36-42.

130. Coster W, Bedell G, Law M, et al. Psychometric evaluation of the Participation and Environment Measure for children and youth. *Developmental Medicine and Child Neurology.* 2011;53:1030-1037.

131. Deci EL, Ryan RM. The "what" and "why" of goal pursuits: human needs and the self-determination of behavior. *Psychological Inquiry.* 2000;11:227-268.

132. Boerner K, Brennan M, Horowitz A, Reinhardt JP. Tackling vision-related disability in old age: an application of the lifespan theory of control to narrative data. *Journal of Gerontology: Psychological Sciences.* 2010;65(B)(1):22-31.

133. Vodanovich SJ, Wallace JC, Kass SJ. A confirmatory approach to the factor structure of the boredom proneness scale: evidence for a two-factor short form. *Journal of Personality Assessment.* 2005;85:295-303.

134. Carver CS. You want to measure coping but your protocol's too long: consider the brief COPE. *International Journal of Behavioral Medicine.* 1997;4:92-100.

135. Palmer B, Stough C. *SUEIT: Swinburne University Emotional Intelligence Test: Interim Technical Manual.* Melbourne, Australia: Swinburne University Organisational Psychology Research Unit; 2001.

136. Steger MF, Frazier P, Oishi S, Kaler M. The meaning in life questionnaire: assessing the presence of and search for meaning in life. *Journal of Counseling Psychology.* 2006;53:80-93.

137. Ware JE, Kosinski M, Dewey JE. *How to Score Version 2 of the SF-36® Health Survey.* Lincoln, RI: Quality Metric Incorporated; 2000.

138. Watson D, Clark LA, Tellegen A. Development and validation of brief measures of positive and negative affect: the PANAS scales. *Journal of Personality and Social Psychology.* 1988;54:1063-1070.

139. Crumbaugh JC, Maholick LT. *Manual of Instruction for the Purpose in Life Test.* Munster, IN: Psychometric Affiliates; 1969.

140. Antonovsky A. The structure and properties of the sense of coherence scale. *Social Science Medicine.* 1993;36(6):725-733.

141. Diener E, Emmons RA, Larsen RJ, Griffin S. The satisfaction with life scale. *Journal of Personality Assessment.* 1985;49:71-75.

142. Folkman S, Lazarus RS. An analysis of coping in a middle-aged community sample. *Journal of Health and Social Behavior.* 1980;21:219-239.

ENVIRONMENT FACTORS THAT SUPPORT OCCUPATIONAL PERFORMANCE

PEOP: Enabling Everyday Living

THE NARRATIVE
The past, current and future perceptions, choices, interests, goals and needs that are unique to the Person, Organization, or Population

PERSON
- Cognition
- Psychological
- Physiological
- Sensory
- Motor
- Spirituality

OCCUPATION
- Activities
- Tasks
- Roles

ENVIRONMENT
- Culture
- Social Determinants
- Social Support and Social Capital
- Education and Policy
- Physical and Natural
- Assistive Technology

Personal Narrative
- Perception and Meaning
- Choices and Responsibilities
- Attitudes and Motivation
- Needs and Goals

Organizational Narrative
- Mission and History
- Focus and Priorities
- Stakeholders and Values
- Needs and Goals

Population Narrative
- Environments and Behaviors
- Demographics and Disparities
- Incidence and Prevalence
- Needs and Goals

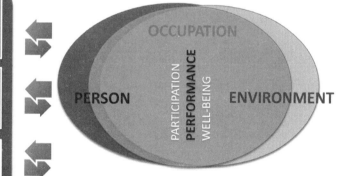

Section IV addresses the environment factors (the 'E' in the PEOP Model) that enable occupational performance. These factors have equal importance to person factors, and must be considered in all occupational therapy interventions. However, it is only in the last several decades that we have come to emphasize the various dimensions of the environment and their influences on occupational performance.

In this section, we examine 5 environmental factors: culture, social, physical and natural, policy, and technology. Thus, the environment includes more than just physical characteristics related to occupational performance; it also consists of societal factors as well. All of these environmental factors may support or limit performance, participation, and well-being.

The nature of occupational therapy evaluations and interventions for the environment will vary depending on the definition of the client (individual, organization, population) and the settings (home, public institution, community).

As you will see in this section, environment factors are just as important and complex as person factors. As you continue your learning, you will acquire specific knowledge about environmental interventions designed to improve the fit of person with environment and support occupational performance. Your skills will be valued as you contribute to improved personal and public environments for people with special needs.

Chapter	Title	FAQ
20	*Environment Factors: Culture* (Padilla)	• Why do individuals have multiple and overlapping cultural identities that must be considered, rather than a single cultural identity? • What value systems may be considered in developing occupational therapy interventions that support performance, participation, and well-being?
21	*Environment Factors: Social Determinants of Health, Social Capital, and Social Support* (Bass, Baum, Christiansen, Haugen)	• How do social determinants, social supports, and social capital influence occupational performance, participation, and well-being? • What opportunities are available for occupational therapy to support governmental, nonprofit, and international efforts to improve everyday life?
22	*Environment Factors: Physical and Natural Environment* (Stark, Sanford, Keglovits)	• How has our understanding of physical and natural environments that influence occupational performance evolved over time? • What aspects of the physical and natural environment should be considered in occupational therapy?
23	*Environment Factors: Health, Education, Social, and Public Policies* (Smith, Hudson)	• What key policies have supported occupational performance, participation, and well-being? • How are policies evaluated to determine whether they support individuals, organizations, and populations or communities?
24	*Environment Factors: Technology* (Polgar)	• What categories of assistive technology are considered in occupational performance? • How are technologies selected to support occupational performance, participation, and well-being?

Chapter 20

ENVIRONMENT FACTORS
Culture

René Padilla, PhD, OTR/L, FAOTA, LMHP

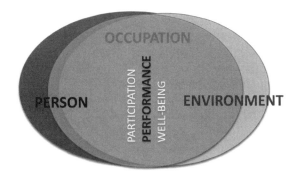

LEARNING OBJECTIVES

- Identify and define the primary cultural factors that influence performance, participation, and well-being.
- Discuss how cultural factors impact performance, participation, and well-being.
- Identify national and international efforts to address cultural factors that contribute to limitations in performance, participation, and well-being.
- Describe the influence of cultural factors on the practice of occupational therapy at the individual, organizational, and population/community level.
- Compare and contrast assessment and interventions regarding cultural factors in occupational therapy practice at the individual, organizational, and population/community level.
- Identify governmental, nonprofit, and international agencies that promote performance, participation, and well-being through work on cultural factors.

KEY WORDS

- Beliefs
- Customs
- Economic
- Individual vs population vs institution
- Organizational practice
- Policy
- Power/decision making
- Values

INTRODUCTION

Culture is a widely debated term that eludes a clear-cut definition. Perhaps the elusiveness in definition is due to its complexity and ubiquitous nature. One of the most famous definitions, proposed in 1871 by anthropologist E.B. Taylor, states that culture is "that complex whole

Christiansen CH, Baum CM, Bass JD, eds.
Occupational Therapy: Performance, Participation, and Well-Being, Fourth Edition (pp 335-358).
© 2015 SLACK Incorporated.

which includes knowledge, belief, art, morals, law, custom, and any other capabilities and habits acquired by man as a member of society."[1(p58)] Others proposed that culture is "a system of inherited conceptions expressed in symbolic forms by means of which people communicate, perpetuate, and develop their knowledge about and attitudes toward life"[2(p22)] or "an explanation of how the features of a particular population's behavioral repertoire are established, ie, by learning rather than by genetic processes."[3(p223)] Others add that "culture is a socially transmitted or socially constructed constellation consisting of such things as practices, competencies, ideas, schemas, symbols, values, norms, institutions, goals, constitutive rules, artifacts, and modifications of the physical environment."[4(p85)]

Scholars have attempted to identify cultural factors in order to guide research on their relationship with health behaviors. Some have described these factors as "the set of measurable characteristics that often are associated with a particular racial group, including religious influences, family practices, and beliefs about health care (such as experience of discrimination, perceived racism, medical mistrust)."[5(p441)] Research suggests that racial/ethnic health disparities are related to cultural factors,[6,7] and that such factors to some degree are determinants of education, economic status, and general social mobility.[8] The breadth of such definitions and implied factors can leave one wondering, "What is not culture?" Indeed, the notion of culture can be a "slippery concept, taking on a variety of definitions and meanings depending on how it has been socially situated and by whom."[9(p1)]

Many disciplines study culture, including anthropology, psychology, education, business, and the military, each subscribing to its own perspective of what the term encompasses. Consequently, there are literally hundreds of definitions. Constructs such as material culture (methods by which people share goods, services, technology), subjective culture (ideas and knowledge shared in a group), and social culture (shared rules of social behavior, institutions) have emerged,[10] and cultural continua, such as individualism-collectivism or independence-interdependence, have been described.[11] Many views of culture focus on what is inside the mind of people,[12] while others emphasize the collective (local and societal) and individual (public and intimate) levels of analysis.[13,14] Definitions are further complicated by an intense focus on geographic or ethnic variations, and a tendency to equate culture with country, which some scholars consider misguided.[15,16]

By virtue of attempting to reduce the notion of culture to an operational concept, definitions inherently have limitations. For example, the continuum of individualism-collectivism, often invoked to explain geographic or ethnic variation,[17-19] has been shown to be "neither as large nor as systematic as often perceived,"[20(p40)] to not account for

substantial internal variation within many groups,[21] and to produce research findings from limited samples that are likely not generalizable.[22] Some authors have proposed the idea of *cultural syndromes* to describe overlapping commonalities between groups of people living in a certain country, speaking a certain language, or during a particular historic period.[6(p409),20(p30)] Thus, a Native American student in Fremont, a Chinese-American grandmother in Lincoln, and a Jewish teacher in Omaha may share a language, a historic time period, and a geographic region and therefore all be considered "Nebraskans"; and at the same time not share their most important values, beliefs, norms, and attitudes. Likewise, an English-speaking Hispanic man in Omaha may share a similar cultural outlook with his long deceased Quechua-speaking great-grandmother in Ecuador and with a modern, Portuguese-speaking farmer in Brazil, yet not share language or even the same historic period. Perhaps they celebrate the same holidays, or have similar views about which foods may or may not be eaten, or about the nature and timing of sexual relationships. Yet, the Hispanic man may have more in common with the Brazilian farmer in some domains and in others with the Jewish teacher in Omaha. Consequently, any attempt to describe a particular cultural group must also acknowledge the multiple cultural variations that are likely to exist within it.

Wells and Black[23] offered a broad definition of culture that is particularly useful to occupational therapy, stating it is:

> The sum total of a way of living, including values, beliefs, standards, linguistic expression, patterns of thinking, behavioral norms, and styles of communication that influences the behavior(s) of a group of people that is transmitted from generation to generation. It includes demographic variables such as age, gender, and place of residence; status variables such as social, educational, and economic levels; and affiliation variables.[23(p270)]

While there are many definitions of culture, most have 3 characteristics in common that guide the content of this chapter. First, culture emerges in adaptive interactions between humans and environments; second, culture consists of shared elements between people; and third, culture is transmitted across time periods and generations.

The PEOP Model is consistent with this consensus in its recognition of the cultural environment as an extrinsic factor that influences, and in turn is influenced by, the occupational participation of people as individuals and as members of social groups, organizations, and populations.[24] The PEOP Model considers cultural factors to include values, customs, beliefs, power/decision making, organizational practices, and economic characteristics.[25]

NARRATIVE AND BACKGROUND LITERATURE

Culture can be described as a type of "lens" through which people perceive and understand the world they inhabit and in which they learn to live. A person is born into culture—culture is not present in his or her genetic makeup. This lens is learned over time through a process of enculturation. This understanding assumes that culture is constructed, shared, both objective and subjective, and both conscious and unconscious.

Unlike most animals, human beings are not born with the genetic programming that automatically prepares them to use the environment to find food and shelter—they need other people to care for them and teach them. Throughout life, humans must discover effective ways of interacting both with their environment and with each other. Through such interaction, we learn what is possible to do, what we are expected to do (and how we are to do it), and what we can count on the environment to provide for us. Culture encompasses this knowledge.

For example, if a child is born in a village high in the Andes of Perú, he is likely to not be permitted to crawl or creep extensively because homes have dirt floors. His parents might place him on a straw mat, and each time he crawls off of it they might move him back, gently chastising him verbally. Over time, the chastising may become harsher or even evolve into physical punishment until the child learns to accept the limits of the mat or is able to walk upright off the mat. Through this process the child enlarges his behavioral repertoire at the same time that the environment maintains boundaries on him. These boundaries signal the limits of what is permitted. The pleasure of movement within those boundaries reinforces the desire to creep or crawl, while the emotional pain from the verbal or physical chastising limits the exploration. In a very elementary way, the child learns to differentiate between "good" and "bad" through the boundaries placed on him. As his skills expand, so might also the boundaries; the discovery of additional freedoms give greater pleasure to movement and add meaning to his actions. This constant interaction with the human and physical environment shapes myriad skills and behavior options with their associated meanings, giving rise to all occupation.

At the same time that the environment sets boundaries on humans, we influence the world around us in many ways. In the previous example of the child born in an Andean village, it is easy to see that each time he crawls off the mat he is in turn shaping the behavior of his parents, who must react to his action and teach him the limits of his world. Their reaction will likely be quite different if his exploration is done while crying or loudly expressing his dissatisfaction over the boundaries, or if he does so by standing upright and holding on to furniture to aid his walking off the mat. In the first case the verbal reprimand may be harsher, while in the second situation he may be encouraged with clapping and words of admiration. The parents' actions are a response to the child's behavior, which in turn is shaped by the parents' encouragement. In this case, not only has the child learned to positively interact with the parents, he has also learned about the appropriate use of objects (ie, the furniture) in his environment.

While the physical environment may not offer verbal limits or reinforcements, it can shape the child's behavior in very powerful ways. To continue with this example, the presence of a mat on a dirt floor can provide freedoms of action to a child that he otherwise might not experience in a home that lacked the resources to fabricate or purchase a mat. Likewise, if there are objects the child can manipulate on the mat or in its close vicinity, he is likely to learn other behaviors and develop additional skills sooner than a child who lacks them in her environment. If a wooden stool is nearby, he might learn to hold on to it until he succeeds in standing. However, if the stool is not stable and tips over and injures him, he might avoid the stool in the future, or at least until he has developed many other skills that give him confidence over the stool. The child might eventually learn how to move the stool to another location while he holds on to it to stand. Thus, he has rearranged the environment to suit his curiosity, interests, or needs.

Some objects in the environment can be manipulated and changed, while others cannot. However, they all influence the person and, to some degree, the person can influence them as well. Their long-standing presence creates a sense of familiarity and predictability. The child in the Andean village may become very comfortable walking on steep paths, wearing thick clothes to guard against the cold weather, and feeling secure surrounded by high mountains. While he cannot change the weather or the mountains, he can build a fire to warm up or erect a fence that marks the land. He might not have been able to do this in an environment where people did not show him how to do certain things, where there was hot weather, or where the land was covered in jungle.

CULTURE IS CONSTRUCTED, SHARED, CONSCIOUS, AND UNCONSCIOUS

The previous examples illustrate how culture is not only constructed, but also how it is shared. As human beings interact with each other they come to share ideas, rules, and understandings as a group. Over time, the child comes to recognize the knowledge, attitudes and values of the various social groups he belongs to. In this way, cultural knowledge in the form of rules, values, attitudes, and preferences may be transmitted over generations. The smaller the group, the less variation there will be in this cultural knowledge, but each person brings to any group some level of individual variation of that cultural knowledge. The case of the child in the Andean village has already illustrated how parents can shape behavior. However, other social forces are at play at the same time. The family lives in the physical and social boundaries of the village, where parents are expected to behave in certain ways. There are likely parameters for parenting, and significant variation from those parameters may be dealt with by elders chastising young parents or removing the children if they are not cared for according to the group's standards. For example, if the infants are not clothed, elders may provide clothing for the child and angrily berate the parents for not meeting that responsibility. By choosing the clothing, elders also subtly indicate the type of clothes considered appropriate for the local tradition, physical environment demands, and so on. Because of these external reinforces, individuals acquire the cultural lens of the groups they inhabit in order to learn how to live in them. Without such shared perception, the continuity and cohesion of such groups would be unlikely.

Shared cultural knowledge and identification is transmitted from one generation to the next through formal and informal means. Formal means are those by which cultural knowledge is transmitted through direct instruction, as with schooling, religious training, and education into a trade or a profession. Informal means are those by which values and beliefs are transmitted indirectly or without formal instruction. Gender identification in Andean village culture, for example, is learned more by imitating the people in the village rather than through formal education. Whereas parents or the immediate family and social surroundings provided early or primary enculturation, organizations or institutions that are part of the group life that the individual inhabits provide secondary reinforcements.[26] Thus, schools, churches, clubs, and so on, which to some degree are sanctioned by the people who have primary influence over the individual, expand the experiences and repertoire of skills of the person within the context of a larger group. Television, movies, and so on (sometimes classified as tertiary or third level reinforcements)[26(p17)] may be diffuse, but nonetheless ubiquitous and powerful influences present in the social environment.[27]

The previous discussion illustrates why culture can also be described as objective and subjective, or conscious and unconscious. Objective elements of culture are the numerous visible and physical artifacts people create, including clothing, food, furniture and so on; subjective elements are the intangible aspects of people's lives, such as values, attitudes, beliefs, behavior norms, and hierarchy of roles.[14(p58),28] Conscious culture is the part of culture that we are aware of, can describe, and about which we can talk (and usually label as "culture"), while unconscious culture affects our behavior and thought without our awareness.[29] These dimensions of culture have been likened to an iceberg: what can be seen above the surface of the ocean (objective, conscious culture) is about 10% of the whole, whereas 90% of the iceberg lies beneath the surface (subjective, unconscious culture).[29] The hidden part of culture continually operates at the subconscious level, shaping our perceptions and responses to those perceptions. While this is likely the part of culture that is most meaningful to us, it also can be potentially the most dangerous, leading to numerous intercultural misunderstandings without us even knowing the source of the problem.[30]

Culture is very dynamic because it is socially constructed, objective and subjective, conscious and unconscious. Although a group may share some general cultural features in common, each individual in the group contributes uniquely to that shared meaning. Each individual in a society is in the process of "learning" culture and, consequently, is at a different point in the process. Shared and individual events in people's lives shape what the person learns and how he or she learns it. Further, individuals within a culture, and therefore cultures as a whole, are never static. For example, the mother of the child in the Andean village may have left when she was a teenager to work as a housekeeper in the city where she was taught to read and write. She may have experienced those skills as broadening her opportunities. Once she returned to the village and had her own family, she may have insisted on sending her oldest son to school in a nearby town, even if this was not the general practice in her own village. At the school, the son is in a new physical and social environment. There he is taught how to manipulate new objects, such as pencils and books; the appropriate way to act with his friends in the playground, such as taking turns; and how to speak in the presence of teachers or other people in authority, such as using words that identify the person's title. When he returns home in the afternoon he may re-enact some school experiences with his younger sister. In this way, the 2 children relate around the topic of school, but the context of their experience is quite unique.

Boundaries of culture, therefore, can be vague. It may seem superficially that people behave in the same way or hold the same values, but all persons are acting on the basis of their own perception of what they have learned as culture. We should always avoid using cultural generalizations to explain people's behavior, because no culture is homogeneous.[28(p26),31] Generalizations often lead to the development of stereotypes, cultural misunderstandings, prejudices, and, sadly, discrimination. Further, culture is never static because its members are constantly being influenced individually and collectively by other groups around them, or they themselves creatively generate new cultural expressions. A good example of this is how music evolves. Not all individuals of a region or country have the same preferences, yet local forms of music, ranging from traditional to contemporary, can be identified. Each new expression is likely the result of some external influences, but also the result of people seeking new forms of expression.

LEVELS OF CULTURE

There are multiple levels of cultural influence on occupation that could be contemplated, including global, societal, professional, and personal,[32] making this an even more complex topic. It may be most helpful to consider the contexts in which a person lives in order to identify dimensions of culture that may be significant in a person's life. Context "refers to a variety of interrelated conditions within and surrounding the [person] that influence [occupational] performance."[33(p613)] Cultural context, then, exists outside of us, but we internalize it to form part of our identities and as a way of regulating our relationships. Thus, cultural contexts in relation to occupation can be defined as,

> ... customs, beliefs, activity patterns, behavior standards, and expectations accepted by the society of which the individual is a member. Includes political aspects, such as laws that affect access to resources and affirm personal rights. Also includes opportunities for education, employment, and economic support.[33(p623)]

It is useful, therefore, to understand dimensions of occupation that are particularly related to cultural interpretation, while keeping in mind that culture is only one of many complex influences on health and participation in life. It is possible to overemphasize the importance of culture when trying to make sense of social problems or health conditions. Underlying physical and mental disorders may go untreated when professionals ascribe behaviors and symptoms to people's culture and fail to thoroughly analyze the situation.[34] Rather than being a catalogue or set of specific behaviors and artifacts, cultural contexts should be thought of as processes people use to guide their choices and actions.

Authors have classified contexts in various ways, mostly related to the types of social interactions that take place within them. For example, a scheme of 6 levels of culture (individual, team, functional, social identity group, organizational, and national) has been described within the context of business and commerce,[28(p27)] and 1 of 3 (playground, classroom, and institutional) for schools.[35] Hofstede[36] proposed a "Cultural Onion" Model, noting

that people's actions or practices occur more within a context of ideas or meanings, rather than of physical objects or spaces. Thus, he drew a series of concentric circles; at the center of which were values, with subsequent outer layers of rituals, heroes, and symbols. Others have used a similar onion model strategy to describe layers of social contexts that shape a person's values, meanings, and intentions.[31(p21)] This latter approach seems the most useful in understanding the culture learning process.[37] Krefting and Krefting[38] suggested viewing culture as a series of mutually influencing social levels that guide occupational choices. Within each level there are potentially many subgroups, each with their own concepts, rules, and social organizations. Although each of these subcultures developed from the larger culture and shares many of its concepts and values, each also has unique and distinctive features of its own. These levels include the individual, the family, the community, and the geographic region. Cultural norms and expectations vary greatly between these contexts across the world and influence the timing and availability of critical roles and responsibilities.[39]

One-to-one interactions, through which people learn and express their own perception of culture, take place at the individual level. This layer includes personal attributes, such as sense of humor, coping style, sense of personal space, and role choices. At the family level are the values and beliefs shared within the primary social group, such as gender roles and family structure. The earliest socialization takes place at this level. Secondary groups are at the community level, and include contexts such as school, work, profession, church, and neighborhood. Finally, at the regional level are the characteristics a person may share with people in a geographic area, such as language, holidays, mass communication media, and ethnicity. In most cultures, the family and immediate community levels have the greatest influence over the individual, and it is within those contexts that the person learns the pattern of behaviors that are expected or unacceptable at each level. Sometimes expectations at the various levels may contradict each other, at which times the person must make a choice about which level will take precedence. This often occurs with immigrant children who feel pulled between traditional values of the family and greater freedoms with school friends.[40] Thus, we can say that individuals have multiple and overlapping cultural identities, each representing a constellation of occupations, meanings, and participation associated with a social subgroup.[41]

The boundaries between these levels of culture can be clear-cut or hazy, or rigid or permeable, depending on the customs of the groups that inhabit the context. Every day we hear about how the world is becoming a "global village" with increasing integration of culture, economies, and borders. However, this does not dispel the fact that each

Figure 20-1. Sources of cultural identity acting on 4 levels of culture.

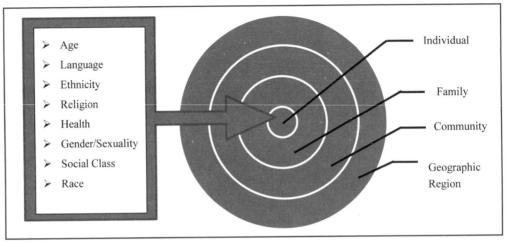

- ➤ Age
- ➤ Language
- ➤ Ethnicity
- ➤ Religion
- ➤ Health
- ➤ Gender/Sexuality
- ➤ Social Class
- ➤ Race

Individual

Family

Community

Geographic Region

nation of people has a distinct history of its own. Each country is unique in the way that its population is made up of a mosaic of cultures or people groups from all over the world, each group bringing a history of their own ancestry and culture. Tensions between groups may link back to historical processes and events from many different parts of the world (eg, tensions may exist between descendants from different Arab or Middle Eastern countries, depending on their religious background). On the other hand, certain problems may arise from the local cultural environment itself (eg, United States history has shown many conflicts between the government and Native American groups).

SOURCES OF CULTURAL IDENTITY

Levels of culture serve as primary lenses through which people learn about the surrounding cultural world and through which they form their cultural identities, usually expressed through the categorization of people. All societies have elaborate ways of moving people into and out of different categories, and also of confirming people to the categories into which they have been placed.[42] For example, wedding ceremonies constitute a process of moving people from the category of being single to married. Depending on the lens, such ceremony may be considered sacred and never to be undone, or temporary based on the partners' sense of self-actualization. In a sense, rehabilitation itself can be interpreted as a process of moving people from the category of disabled to able. Ultimately, the interactions between people and their social environments or contexts frame their cultural identities and direct their occupational meanings, choices, and participation. Some factors that influence cultural identity (depending on the importance placed on them in each context) include race, ethnicity, gender/sexuality, age, religion, language, social class, and health, among others (Figure 20-1).[43]

Race

The term *race* refers to a clustering of inherited biological or physical characteristics, sometimes referred to as "biological differences between populations."[44(p32)] While there has been some usefulness to the notion in health research, it has frequently been overvalued as a cultural categorization, with significant ethical consequences in society, and many scholars question its utility.[45] Different societies define different sets of physical characteristics when referring to the same race, and features that are considered significant in one society may be considered insignificant in others. Furthermore, the term has been used to refer to many characteristics that are not physical, as in the case of language (the "English speaking race"), religion (the "Jewish race"), or nationality (the "German race"). Therefore, race is best understood as a categorization of characteristics based on the particular values of a society. This is important not because of biology, but because of the cultural meaning the term may have in a particular society. For example, skin color and the shape of the lips or eyes are important differing criteria in the United States, while in many places in Latin America eye color and stature are more significant. Thus, someone classified as Black in Georgia or Michigan might be considered White in Perú or Bolivia.

Ethnicity

Ethnicity is defined culturally in a similar way to race. This term refers to the knowledge, beliefs, and behavioral patterns shared by a group of people with the same history and the same language.[46] Ethnicity is associated with a sense of "peoplehood" or loyalty to a "community of memory."[47] Ethnicity is also associated with a particular geographical region, although an ethnic group need no longer live in that region to feel a sense of belonging to it. For example, refugee groups in the United States, such as the Somali Bantu, have formed a tight community in several cities. Many continue to wear the traditional clothing and have learned to adapt traditional dishes to American foodstuffs, even though many of them were born in refugee camps in Kenya and have never been to Somalia.[48]

Another group of refugees, the Sudanese, are also an example of why ethnicity should not be confused with nationality. Nationality is a categorization based on citizenship of a country, and may not include shared ethnicity. Two large ethnicities are associated with Sudan—the northern group is traditionally Arabic in cultural practices, while the southern group is traditionally Christian. These identities have to do with the history of colonization of the region. When refugees began arriving in the United States from the country Sudan, they were often placed in group homes and apartment complexes together, expected to create small communities of support without consideration of their ethnic backgrounds. Although the northern and southern Sudanese may be biologically or genetically related by race and they may have the same nationality, they do not always identify with each other from the perspective of ethnicity, and old animosities have persisted in the United States.[49]

Gender

Gender is defined according to cultural meanings associated with male and female reproduction. These meanings are expressed through socially valued behaviors or roles that are assigned according to gender. These roles and behaviors may become so accepted that eventually they are thought to be naturally or biologically associated with the sex. However, gender is what it means to be male or female in a society, and roles, then, are those behaviors thought to be normal in the society when carried out by the assigned gender. As with race and ethnicity, particular behaviors considered naturally male or female vary greatly from society to society. Ultimately, any social or psychosocial trait can be "genderized" in favor of one sex or another.[2(p37),50,51] What in one society may be considered a typically female trait may be admired in males in another.[52] Despite growing evidence that sexual orientation is, in part, a function of innate biological characteristics,[53] persons that deviate from socially approved norms are often ostracized and even physically abused. The prevailing view in many societies is that sexuality is bimodal; only male and female are identified as possibilities.

Age

Age is culturally defined both by length of life and state of physical and mental development. Societies measure chronological age in different ways, such as a combination of calendar years, major social events, or natural cycles. For example, adulthood is legally recognized at age 21 in the United States, while a Jewish boy's Bar Mitzvah ceremony marks his transition to adulthood around the age of 13, and a male's entry into adulthood is marked by the first sexual experience amongst the Yekuana people in the Venezuelan rainforest regardless of chronological age.[54]

Religion

Religion and spirituality are based on shared ideas about the relationship between humans and a deity. These beliefs usually include a shared set of rules for living (moral values) that either enhance that relationship or with each other. Religious identity may include membership in a formalized religion (such as Islam, Christianity, or Buddhism) or loose affiliation with spiritualistic groups. Religious affiliation can engender community, pride in a shared history, and intense loyalty to the degree of extremism.[55] The cultural meaning of religion is often expressed through a sense of righteousness and virtue and, therefore, can be a powerful determinant of behavior.[56]

Language

Language is one of the most important sources of cultural learning.[57] Brain research has shown that humans are born with a predisposition for communication systems, whether vocal or gestural.[58] Language has meaning in its verbal (patterns of sound aggregated into words used to represent objects, people, and ideas) and nonverbal (gestures, norms regarding interpersonal space, and so on) properties and therefore can give us insight into another person's life[59] and to the cultural evolution of whole societies.[60]

Social Class

Virtually all societies have criteria for ranking its members in a stratified hierarchy.[61] Criteria to determine social class vary enormously between societies. For example, in the United States wealth is one of the most prevalent standards of social class, and other criteria (such as power, influence, and educational level) are strongly related to access to economic resources. Consequently, many experts consider social class the most significant culture-learning factor.[62] Class structure varies from society to society, and even within societies. In some societies the structure can be quite rigid, and people tend to remain for life in the class they were born into. For example, the caste system in regions of India is a social system where people are ranked into groups based on heredity. Because heredity cannot be changed, it is practically impossible to move out of that caste, although education and microeconomic loans are changing this slowly.[63,64] In contrast, in the United States it is almost a social expectation that individuals "move up" in social class as their education and careers progress, although growing evidence suggests this is becoming increasingly more difficult.[62(p63)]

Health Status

Finally, as with other sources of cultural identity discussed so far, health is also largely defined by a group's perception of what physical and mental states constitute being "healthy." In the Western world, the medical model has dominated the cultural definition of health. In this view, health has been defined as the absence of illness or disease, and in many instances become equated with "normalcy." The notions of ability and disability are closely related to the cultural construct of health. Ability is defined according to a society's view of what it means to be physically, mentally, and emotionally "able." Consequently, disabilities are sometimes deemed as states of ill health, when in fact it is possible to be a quite healthy person with blindness or developmental disabilities, for example. Obesity also is often considered a sign of poor health in the United States, largely because of the potential health problems it may bring and the associated costs in terms of loss of productivity and medical expenses. In other parts of the world, such as Mauritania, young girls and women are sometimes force-fed in order to make them fat as a sign of beauty.[65] Management of health in Western societies is largely biomedical. In this perspective, health practices considered mainstream in other countries, such as acupuncture, neuropathy, and faith healing, are deemed as "alternative." In most countries, however, health status is very much associated with socioeconomic level because illness and poor nutrition may result from poverty, unemployment, psychological stress, poor sanitation, alcohol abuse, inadequate housing, and lack of financial resources to pay for medical care.[66]

Value Systems

Of particular interest to understanding people's occupational choices are their value systems and their beliefs about the body, health, and healing. As noted earlier, every cultural context or level has a set of explicit and implicit values systems and assumptions to help its members differentiate between right and wrong, desirable and undesirable, or good and evil. These systems provide the basis upon which beliefs about the body, health, and healing are based. Cultural contexts affect people through their perceptions of what is consensually believed or, in other words, their perceptions of the views of people around them.[52(p583)] For example, American culture as a whole has been characterized as valuing individualism, materialism, privacy, and informality in social relationships.[67]

However, there are many value systems operating in any culture, and members of many Native American tribes would rather value community, shared resources, and formality in their relationships.[68] Value systems related to what is accepted as truth, how decisions should be made, what to do in the face of stress, issues of equality/inequality, and the use of time are some that have a clear influence on people's occupational choices and, therefore, on their health and participation in life.

What Is Considered Truth?

Cultural contexts teach people to arrive at a sense of truth in different ways, such as through fact, faith, or feeling.[41(p68)] Contexts that value fact expect people to examine objective evidence of the benefit of a choice before taking action. Contexts that value faith, on the other hand, use a value system derived from religious or political ideology to determine what is right and wrong, and evaluate action in comparison to the ideology. Finally, people in contexts that value feeling go with their "gut instinct" and choose actions based on intuition. Logic is used only to confirm the choice. The occupation of taking a vacation can exemplify these 3 value systems. People from a context that highly values facts will research options, list pros and cons, and compare costs and other factors before selecting their destination. On the other hand, people from contexts that value faith may select a destination where they can be involved in a service project for the poor, while people from contexts that value feeling might map out a vague destination and feel comfortable varying from it if an interesting option presents itself. While these 3 value systems can appear to be personality traits, they were learned in a context that supported them and, to some degree, expected these types of actions.

Individualism and Collectivism

The value systems of individualism or collectivism guide people in terms of the locus of decision making. Individualism is related to the degree to which a person first takes himself or herself into consideration when making decisions. Collectivism, in contrast, is related to the degree to which the person considers the group's consensus before taking action. Pure individualism or collectivism is actually rare. In most cultural contexts, people take into account the opinions of others when making decisions—otherwise it would be difficult for any sense of group identity to develop. In most cultures, persons can make individual choices. However, the cultural context will guide which decisions must particularly be guided by the predominant value. In addition, individualism tends to engender a high need for privacy and personal space, whereas collectivism reduces this need. This does not mean, however, that collectivist societies do not also highly value modesty. Individualism and collectivism are also related to belief systems of where people should turn when faced with stress. For example, when faced with inordinate stressors, people might turn to self-help types of resources in individualist contexts, and to interpersonal relationships in a collectivist culture. However, it is important to note again that it is unwise to generalize traits of any cultural context. The Japanese business culture illustrates this well. Japanese culture has many collectivist features in regards to identity, respect for hierarchy, and so on. Individual failure is perceived to bring shame and reflect poorly on the group, so stress is to be borne privately, giving rise to one of the highest suicide rates in the world.[69] Likewise, Russian business practices are described as "cut-throat-every-man-for-himself,"[70] yet tightly knit families and neighborhoods in some regions have been associated with lower rates of stress-related illnesses.[71]

Divisions of Power

Some form of division of power exists in all cultural contexts, whether explicit or implicit. Divisions of power can be based on financial resources, gender, race, age, or professional status. While divisions in power do not necessarily result in unfair advantages for some members of the group or disadvantages for others, most cultural contexts do seem to reinforce a hierarchy of leadership and responsibility.[72] The division of power will vary according to the predominant cultural identities, and can change based on individual member changes or collective changes. For example, although among the Yanomamo Indians in the Amazon basin tribal chiefdom is passed from males to males, decisions about daily life, including what to plant, where the men will hunt, and when to re-settle the village, are strictly matriarchal.[73] Formal and informal divisions of power and leadership, with their own unique rules and expectations, can be observed in nearly every context in which humans routinely meet, such as workplaces,[74] professions,[75] religious congregations,[76] and even school playgrounds.[77]

Use of Time

The use of time is a value system constructed uniquely in each cultural context as well. Time is used as a language, a way of handling priorities, and of revealing the way people feel about each other.[78,79] Anthropologist Edward Hall's[80] descriptions of monochromic and polychronic cultures are still are used today to guide research on how time is patterned in various contexts. People in monochronic cultural contexts tend to organize their lives with a "one-thing-at-a-time" mentality—time is a commodity that advances linearly and is lost if not used wisely and

intentionally. Consequently, punctuality, adherence to a pre-planned schedule, and efficiency are highly valued. In contrast, people from polychromic cultural contexts subordinate the use of time to social relationships rather than schedules. Thus, this context requires members of a group to stop and exchange social pleasantries even if late for an appointment, because the deference given to others is also expected for oneself.[81]

Beliefs About the Body, Health, and Healing

Culture-based beliefs about the body form another very important and complex influence over how people live their lives. In all societies, the body is the focus of many beliefs regarding its structure, function, and social and psychological significance.[82] Body image is acquired as part of growing up in a particular family, social group, and multiple cultural contexts. Three important aspects of this image that shape occupational participation are beliefs about the body's structure and function, beliefs about its optimal size, and beliefs about its boundaries.

For most people, the inner workings of the body are a matter of speculation.[42(p79)] Personal theorizing and experience, as well as inherited folklore, contribute to an "inside-the-body image," which is important to understand because it strongly influences people's perception and presentation of bodily symptoms and, consequently, their response to health interventions. People's knowledge of and cultural beliefs about the structure and function of the body vary greatly. For example, the belief that normal workings of the body depend on the harmonious balance between various forces (external, internal, or both) has different expressions around the world. In some regions of Latin America a "hot/cold theory of disease" supposes that health is strengthened or weakened by the effect of hot and cold temperatures on the body. Certain diseases are thought to be due to hot or cold temperatures in the environment. Therefore, they may shy away from ice cubes in a drink or from being outdoors in the early evening when the environmental temperature undergoes its biggest change, believing they may catch the flu *(resfrío)*. This theory is extended also to illnesses themselves—"hot illnesses" are treated by consuming "cold foods" and vice versa.[83] States of health themselves may be associated with a temperature. In certain regions of Central America and Mexico, pregnancy is considered a "hot" state, and people believe the mother's consumptions of too many "hot" foods will produce an ill-tempered baby.[84] The classification of which condition or food is hot and which is cold varies throughout the world, and what is considered hot in one subgroup may be considered cold in another. Further, how these elements work to balance each other is thought of differently.[85] These beliefs may ultimately lead people to consume a less nutritional diet and even become malnourished; not because of a lack of availability of needed foods, but because of the beliefs associated with them.[86]

Culture-based beliefs about how the body works are too numerous to discuss in detail here. Such beliefs can be part of a broad cosmology (such as in the case of Chinese or Tibetan traditional medicine) linking the individual to greater forces in the universe. "Maps" of the human body may bear little resemblance to Western anatomical textbooks, such as the body mapped by a crisscross of meridians along which the vital energy of chi flows.[87] Other beliefs about the body in the Western world seem borrowed from science and technology, such as imagining the body functioning in subdivisions as a combustion engine or the plumbing system in a house. Central to these models is the belief that health is maintained by the uninterrupted flow of various substances, and that individual parts of the body, like parts of a car or plumbing system, may stop working and sometimes need to be replaced. The essential reductionism of Western medicine with its advances in diagnostic technology has reinforced in many people the belief that the body is composed of many progressively smaller pieces, making a "medical body" another culturally-based explanation of how the body works. New ways of conceptualizing the human body (such as the composite body made up of transplanted parts, the cyborg body made up of mechanical parts that exist outside the body, and the virtual body that exists only in cyberspace) have appeared in the Western industrialized world.[42(p83)] What is important to note is that these various conjectures or cultural models lead people to participate in certain occupations and accept interventions that conform to their cultural beliefs and reject those that do not.[52(p591)]

Another important dimension of culture that may greatly influence occupational participation has to do with beliefs of what the body should look like and how it should be used. In almost every society the human body is viewed as having physical and social dimensions.[88] Social dimensions have to do with ideal size, shape, adornment, and interpersonal boundaries, to name a few. Culturally defined notions of beauty direct people to value certain features and engage in occupation to modify their bodies through such means as dieting, exercising, tattooing, piercing, and clothing. The tendency to link physical attractiveness to positive personal attributes has long been documented in multiple cultural contexts.[82(p22)] To conform to culturally defined standards of beauty, people use orthodontics to straighten their teeth, undergo plastic surgery, use wigs, paint their fingernails, and so on. All these modifications to the body ultimately are based on the symbolism groups of people share within a cultural context and, as with any other value system, can be at odds within a society. For example, older members of health professions in the United States tend to consider tattoos as signs of lack of education, while educated younger generations consider them admirable signs of individuality.[89] This latter example shows how the social body not only communicates culturally defined aesthetic values, it can also communicate status and power. Clothing is particularly important in this regard. Jewelry or certain color and design of clothing might be worn as a display of wealth. In Westernized societies, the white laboratory coat and starched uniforms that health workers wear serve not only the purpose of cleanliness, but many people also associate them with membership in a profession of high status. Clothing can also indicate transitions in status (ie, wedding dress to indicate transition from single to married or black clothing to indicate mourning over the death of a loved one).

Human beings' sense of identity extends beyond the border of the skin.[87(p33)] We are surrounded by a series of "symbolic skins" that represent boundaries of relationships. For example, Hall[90] identified 4 invisible layers or concentric circles of space that surround bodies of middle-class Americans. These include intimate distance (0 to 18 inches, entered by only people with whom the person has a very close relationship), personal distance (18 inches to 4 feet, entered by friends), social distance (4 to 12 feet, where impersonal business transactions take place), and public distance (12 to 25 feet or more, where no interaction is expected). Similar schemes have been documented for other cultural groups with variations in distance and who is permitted to enter such spaces. A person's sense of boundaries includes the verbal and nonverbal language used in social interactions.[91] In some groups, men greet by hugging and kissing on both cheeks or the lips even if meeting for the first time, whereas such behavior in other cultural contexts would be considered highly inappropriate. In other groups women and men are not allowed to have physical contact, so they do not greet by shaking hands. However, it appears that all cultural groups value some form of greeting and such greeting may be highly ritualized.[92]

These beliefs about body structure and function are closely related to beliefs about how the body maintains health or overcomes states of illness. Food in particular can be a central feature of a cultural group because of the broad range of symbolic meanings it occupies in each society.[93] In addition to the "hot/cold" theory discussed previously in which certain functions of the body are classified as fitting either of those categories and there is parallel classification of foods, other types of classification systems have been identified, including food vs non-food, sacred vs profane food, and medicinal and social foods.[94] These classification systems, which can coexist in single cultural contexts, are evidence that diet is often based on cultural criteria rather than nutritional value. Further, classification systems are usually based on historical associations, and some systems may be quite flexible, while others very rigid. What may be considered food to one group may not be to another, such as frog legs being considered a delicacy in France but not in Latin America, or guinea pigs a delicacy in Andean countries but not in the United States. Religious connotations limit foods that one may ingest or even come into contact. For example, some Catholics temporarily abstain from eating meat during Lent, while Orthodox Jews have a permanent prohibition against pork. Food classification systems often overlap (as in foods considered medicinal) or can be mutually exclusive (as in food considered sacred or medicinal in one cultural context and ordinary in another).

Finally, definitions of what constitutes health, illness, or disability vary between individuals, families, and cultural groups. Usually health is seen as more than the absence of unpleasant symptoms, it is explained as a balance of the relationship of people with nature, with each other, or with the supernatural world. Kleinman[95] coined the term *explanatory model* (EM) to refer to the ways patients and health practitioners "offer explanation of sickness and treatment to guide choices among available therapies and therapists and to cast personal and social meaning on the experiences of sickness."[95(p106)] A person's EM is assembled over time within the social, economic, and dominant ideology context within which the person lives. Given that each person experiences that context uniquely, people's EMs overlap significantly, but are never identical.[96] Examples of EMs in Latin America include *mal de ojo* (poor sleep, headaches, and sadness caused by a hex or a gaze from a more powerful or stronger person looking at a weaker one), *espanto* (anxiety caused by the soul leaving the body temporarily because of a sudden fright), and *empacho* (perceived stomach or intestinal blockage caused by altered eating habits or overeating).[97] Variations of these themes exist around the world, as in *koro* in China, *amok* in Malaysia, and the *tabanka* in Trinidad. EMs are also prevalent among some groups in industrialized countries like the United States, such as the moralistic ascription of AIDS as the punishment from God for drug use or homosexual behavior,[98] or blood diseases such as leukemia or sickle cell anemia caused by the intermarriage of races.[99] EMs often include an indication of what should be done to manage or counteract the illness. This may include self-help or assistance-seeking strategies that guide the establishment of new temporary or long-lasting daily routines.

Multiculturalism and Disparities

Although the coexistence of multiple cultural or ethnic groups within a social system (or "multiculturalism") raises the potential for many positive developments in society, it can also bring about the possibility of segregation and division.[100,101] In some cases, it creates a feeling of "otherness" by implying that people can be divided into "us" and "them" groups. "Us" often indicates the White dominant culture, while "they" are the "other" who do not belong wholly to the dominant culture for whatever reason (virtually all the sources of cultural identity mentioned previously can be used as markers of difference between people). This message is reinforced by unexamined use of concepts such as "tolerance," "accommodation," "sensitivity," "harmony," and "diversity."[102] Because the word "tolerance" implies accommodating something that is not entirely desired, emphasis on this and related concepts can suggest that one must accept and deal with "the other" within the dominant (superior) culture, without necessarily respecting or feeling equal with the different cultural groups. By not acknowledging underlying racism and xenophobia, the seemingly harmless beliefs that are nurtured through the use of words like "tolerance" and "diversity" are hidden. Although a country may be home to a large variety of cultural, ethnic, or racial groups, the underlying belief that there exists 2 groups consisting of "us" and "them" sometimes leads to tensions and bad feelings toward people in visible minority groups and/or people who recently immigrated to the country. The term *xenophobia* describes this phenomenon, whereby the dominant group of a country feels a fear of "foreigners," their customs, and culture.[103]

Racism and xenophobia can be expressed as subtly as through gestures or glances, or through more overt displays of prejudice. Statements such as "immigrants are stealing our jobs," or telling a person of color to "go back to where you came from" often contradict the reality that the jobs filled tend to be low-income with difficult working conditions. Furthermore, it may be that the person being told to "go back to where you came from" was born and raised in the United States. In these cases it is mostly fear and lack of information which are the culprits.

Racism and xenophobia may be manifested in many different ways, reaching from the everyday slurs and discrimination felt by people of minority groups, to systemic discrimination within an institution's or country's policies. For example, the history of United States immigration policy contains many instances where discriminatory practices were pervasive, such as minimum monetary requirements (known as head taxes) from only certain groups of immigrants (eg, the Chinese) or giving immigration officials the power in the early 1920s to prohibit admission to people if they were deemed undesirable due to their "peculiar customs, habits, modes of life, and methods of holding property and because of their probable inability to become readily assimilated."[104(p108)] Present-day policies may not be as overtly discriminatory as these examples, but often pose barriers for members of specific minority groups. A particularly illustrative example is the "points system," which determines whether or not an immigrant will be allowed admission to the United States. Points are awarded to potential immigrants on a scale that rates ability and potential in certain areas, such as education and work experience.[105] It can be argued that such a system inherently favors certain groups over others, especially for immigrants who have been schooled in English and were in a position to afford sufficient education. Institutional or organizational examples of subtle racism or xenophobia include production of printed materials in complex technical language, charging high processing fees, unequal pay for members of minority groups, or lack of access to needed medical procedures or health services for people who cannot pay for them.

Professions are also susceptible to subtle discriminatory practices.[106,107] Occupational therapy practitioners, just like members of any profession, are acculturated into the particular profession and encouraged to embrace its values found in core professional documents, such as our *Code of Ethics*.[108] Occupational therapy practitioners learn cherished beliefs and traditions that guide our work, such as the importance of occupation in the development of health, client-centered care, and holistic practice, to name a few. Traditional perspectives, such as the emphasis on independence and productivity, individualism, autonomy and self-direction, and Western European images of life roles, can belie subtle racist or xenophobic organizational attitudes and practices. Practitioners can easily assume that everyone shares these beliefs and viewpoints, thus indirectly communicating that other perspectives do not have value or are inferior. Such assumptions are strongly associated with privileged social groups and ethnocentrism, and can lead to "denial of equal access to institutional opportunities, political rights, economic rewards, and respect for human dignity."[109(p35)] Ultimately, the over-emphasis on individualist care can easily lead practitioners to overlook and contribute to population-specific differences in access to health care or health outcomes. Disparities in health, which most markedly exist among ethnic and racial-minority populations, have strongly been associated with discrimination, bias, and stereotyping in health care systems and legal and regulatory bodies.[66(p103)]

To provide excellent client-centered care, practitioners must also provide culturally competent care.[32(p12),110] Such care not only is sensitive to clients' unique aspirations and beliefs regarding health, but values those perspectives and collaboratively develops appropriate interventions that are meaningful to clients. Further, such care explores contributing causes of ill health beyond the individual and advocates for changes in organizations, agencies, institutions, and policies so that inequalities that perpetuate disparities may be corrected.[111,112]

ASSESSMENTS AND EVALUATIONS

Occupational therapy practitioners have an obligation to measure the need for service, design interventions based on knowledge gained from measurement, and evaluate the results of interventions. Culture can have a significant effect on therapy outcomes.[113] As noted in the preceding sections, culture affects performance of occupation in many ways. Culture prescribes norms for the use of time and space, influences beliefs regarding the importance of various tasks, and transmits attitudes and values regarding work and play, as well as what people are expected to do at different moments or phases of their lives. Therefore, cultural preferences must be considered and accommodated by occupational therapy practitioners as the need for intervention is being considered and strategies are planned and implemented. Culture may influence one's very perception of whether they need intervention, let alone the meaning, purpose, and importance they may associate with interventions.[113(p209)] It is important to note that culture refers not only to individuals or families, but also to organizations, including professions. The latter have patterns of shared assumptions, values, and beliefs practiced among its members, which permits them to understand acceptable and unacceptable behaviors. Thus, it is quite easy for a practitioner to unwittingly impose professional or organizational values that contradict the client's and potentially undermine desired intervention outcomes.

Practitioners should make a special effort to understand cultural dimensions from the perspective of their clients and adapt evaluation and intervention accordingly. Two of the most important strategies practitioners can use are *asking questions* and *observing behavior carefully*. The values and beliefs that encompass "culture" direct clients in their particular way of showing their symptoms, both verbally and non-verbally. In addition, these values and beliefs direct how clients perceive and interpret the behavior and communication of practitioners. Research has shown that patients or clients consider *respect* one of the most valued characteristics of culturally competent care on the part of health care practitioners.[114-117] Providing culturally responsive services to diverse clients therefore has the potential to improve access to care; quality of care; and, ultimately, health outcomes. Thus, the Office of Minority Health (OMH) of the US Department of Health and Human Services proposed enhanced national standards of culturally and linguistically appropriate service (CLAS) to "advance health equity, improve quality, and help eliminate health care disparities by establishing a blueprint for health and health care organizations."[118(p13)] Although the CLAS standards were primarily directed at health care organizations, individual practitioners were also encouraged to use the standards to make their practices more culturally and linguistically accessible. These standards,

Table 20-1. *Culturally and Linguistically Appropriate Services Standards*

CLAs Standards

Principle Standard

- *Standard 1.* Provide effective, equitable, understandable, and respectful quality care and services that are responsive to diverse cultural health beliefs and practices, preferred languages, health literacy, and other communication needs.

Standards Related to Governance, Leadership, and Workforce

- *Standard 2.* Advance and sustain organizational governance and leadership that promotes CLAS and health equity through policy, practices, and allocated resources.
- *Standard 3.* Recruit, promote, and support a culturally and linguistically diverse governance, leadership, and workforce that are responsive to the population in the service area.
- *Standard 4.* Educate and train governance, leadership, and workforce in culturally and linguistically appropriate policies and practices on an ongoing basis.

Standards Related to Communication and Language Assistance

- *Standard 5.* Offer language assistance to individuals who have limited English proficiency and/or other communication needs, at no cost to them, to facilitate timely access to all health care and services.
- *Standard 6.* Inform all individuals of the availability of language assistance services clearly and in their preferred language, both verbally and in writing.
- *Standard 7.* Ensure the competence of individuals providing language assistance, recognizing that the use of untrained individuals and/or minors as interpreters should be avoided.
- *Standard 8.* Provide easy-to-understand print and multimedia materials and signage in the languages commonly used by the populations in the service area.

Standards Related to Engagement, Continuous Improvement, and Accountability

- *Standard 9.* Establish culturally and linguistically appropriate goals, policies, and management accountability, and infuse them throughout the organization's planning and operations.
- *Standard 10.* Conduct ongoing assessments of the organization's CLAS-related activities and integrate CLAS-related measures into measurement and continuous quality improvement activities.
- *Standard 11.* Collect and maintain accurate and reliable demographic data to monitor and evaluate the impact of CLAS on health equity and outcomes and to inform service delivery.
- *Standard 12.* Conduct regular assessments of community health assets and needs and use the results to plan and implement services that respond to the cultural and linguistic diversity of populations in the service area.
- *Standard 13.* Partner with the community to design; implement; and evaluate policies, practices, and services to ensure cultural and linguistic appropriateness.
- *Standard 14.* Create conflict and grievance resolution processes that are culturally and linguistically appropriate to identify, prevent, and resolve conflicts or complaints.
- *Standard 15.* Communicate the organization's progress in implementing and sustaining CLAS to all stakeholders, constituents, and the general public.

US Department of Health and Human Services, Office of Minority Health, 2013.

listed in Table 20-1, were organized along a principal standard and 3-themed framework: governance, leadership, and workforce; communication and language assistance; and engagement, continuous improvement, and accountability. Practitioners should assure these standards are met and exceeded in their organizations. Some resources for practitioners to evaluate their own and/or their organization's cultural competence appear in Table 20-2.

Table 20-2. Assessment Tools to Measure Cultural Competence

Reference	Title of Assessment	Construct or Factor Assessed	Description
Suarez-Balcazar, Balcazar, Taylor-Ritzler, Protillo, Rodakowski, Gracia-Ramirez, and Willis[119]	Cultural Competence Assessment Instrument (CCAI-UIC)	Measures cultural awareness/knowledge, cultural skills, and organizational support	24-item scale; respondents rate the frequency with which they engage in certain behaviors or access resources
National Center for Cultural Competence[120]	Cultural Competence Health Practitioner Assessment (CCHPA)	Cultural knowledge in 6 categories: values and belief systems, cultural aspects of epidemiology, clinical decision-making, life cycle events, cross-cultural communication, empowerment/health management	Online self-assessment and self-directed learning recommendations for individuals working in health care; Likert scale format responses
Rooda[121]	Cultural Fitness Survey (CFS)	Measures attitudes toward and knowledge about 3 specific racial and ethnic groups: African American, Hispanic, and Asian American	Self-administered paper and pencil format
Bernal, Froman[122]	Cultural Self-Efficacy Scale (CSES)	Degree of confidence in caring for 3 distinct populations (Blacks, Puerto Ricans, and Southeast Asians)	30-item self-assessment Likert scale
Mendenhall, Stevens[123]	Global Competencies Inventory (GCI)	Assesses the likelihood to work effectively in an environment where there are cultural norms different from one's own. Report focuses on 3 aspects of intercultural adaptability: perception management, relationship management, and self-management.	150-item scale
Hammer, Bennett, Wiseman[124] Hammer[125]	Intercultural Development Inventory (IDI)	Measures capability for perceiving cultural differences and commonalities and modifying behavior to cultural context. Includes the following scales from ethnocentrism to ethnorelativity: denial/defense, minimization, acceptance, adaptation, integration.	50-item, theory-based, self-rating.
Portolla, Chen[126]	Intercultural Effectiveness Scale (IES)	The IES focuses on 3 dimensions of intercultural effectiveness: continuous learning (interest and curiosity about oneself), interpersonal engagement (interest and curiosity about others), and hardiness (effort to interact with people different from oneself).	76-items self-rating Likert scales

(continued)

Table 20-2 (continued).   *Assessment Tools to Measure Cultural Competence*

Reference	*Title of Assessment*	*Construct or Factor Assessed*	*Description*
Campinha-Bacote[127]	Inventory for Assessing the Process of Cultural Competence Among Health Care Professionals (IAPCC)	Cultural awareness, cultural knowledge, cultural skill, cultural encounters, and cultural desire	20-item self-assessment Likert scale
Sue, Bernier, Durran, Feinberg, Pedersen, Smith[128] Sodowsky, Taffe, Gutkin, Wise[129]	Multicultural Counseling Inventory (MCI)	Multicultural counseling skills, awareness, relationships, and multicultural counseling knowledge	Self-assessment
Mason[130]	Cultural Competence Self-Assessment Questionnaire (CCSAQ)	Knowledge of communities served; personal involvement with cultural groups, awareness of resources and linkages, representativeness in organization, reaching out to communities	79-item scale, measure designed to assist service agencies working with children with disabilities and their families in self-evaluation of their cross-cultural competence; used to identify an agency's cultural competence training needs

Occupation is everything that humans do in life, including actions, tasks, activities, thinking, and being. Engagement in occupation describes the interaction of the individual with his or her self-directed activities. Occupational performance is the doing of occupation in order to satisfy life needs.[131] It is essential that occupational therapy practice and assessment focus clearly on occupational performance, assisting clients to become actively engaged in their life activities. Assessment can and should be sensitive to and take place at multiple levels of culture in order to obtain important contextual information to support occupational engagement. It is very appropriate for a practitioner to consider not only the occupational performance issues of clients, but their past routines and habits (personal/individual level of culture) as well. Further, it would be important to have an understanding of the roles that clients and people close to them see them occupy (family and community levels of culture), and the traditions they find meaningful (community and geographic region levels of culture). These may vary substantially between clients. For example, 2 65-year-old women from Somalia who have had a stroke may require quite different interventions. While both may have hemiplegia and need similar assistance in dressing and other ADLs, what they each value as a therapeutic outcome may be quite dissimilar. One may wish to be completely independent in performing all ADLs, while the other may be comfortable retaining assistance with bathing and dressing (personal level of culture). One may feel relieved that she no longer has to be responsible for all food preparation for the family, while the other may be quite distressed about it because the responsibility has been shifted to someone else and she no longer sees herself as a provider (family level of culture). Likewise, one woman may welcome the care from extended family members and neighbors, while the other may not have people around her she trusts or they may not be able or willing to provide assistance (community level of culture). Finally, even though both are from Somalia and may value continuing to dress in the traditional gown or abaya, one may be comfortable covering her head with a simple scarf while the other may insist on continuing to wear the traditional Islamic two-piece hijab (regional level of culture). Therefore, practitioners should routinely make use of a variety of assessment strategies and, whenever possible, select assessment instruments that have been tested for cultural relevance and validity.[33(p651)] Table 20-3 provides some examples of such instruments.

Occupational therapy practitioners may serve organizations or populations in addition to individual clients.[33(p623)] Concerns over the contexts and environments that support or inhibit participation and engagement in desired occupations will be particularly critical at these levels. Institutionalized prejudices may perpetuate barriers that limit access to care and often go unrecognized. Attitudes, such as the assumption that people from diverse backgrounds are more primitive or deficient in genetic makeup and, therefore, inherently susceptible to more pathologies, or that members of ethnic minorities or of lower socioeconomic groups are somehow responsible for the health disparities or social inequities they experience, can pervade research and service delivery.[142-146]

The WHO developed the International Classification for Functioning Disability and Health,[8] often referred to as the ICF, in order "to provide a unified and standard language and framework for the description of health and health-related states."[147(p1)] It describes health domains and health-related domains from the perspective of the body, the individual, and society in 2 basic lists: (1) body functions and structures and (2) activities and participation. It also lists environmental factors that interact with all these factors. The ICF thus "mainstreams" the experience of disability and recognizes it as a universal human experience. The ICF can serve to organize description of what a person can do (function) and the restrictions the person may experience (disability). Such systematic description is intended to assure recognition of personal and societal influences that restrict or enable participation in order to address them. The *Occupational Therapy Practice Framework*[33] integrated aspects of the ICF into a guide for the profession. The PEOP Model is also very compatible with the ICF, particularly in its desire to address restrictions and enable participation of people with disabilities. Thus, the ICF can assist in identifying areas for specific assessment and intervention, as well as articulate desired outcomes of such intervention.

INTERVENTIONS

Culturally-sensitive intervention is essentially client-centered and contextually-driven.[9(p1),42(p186),88(p37),118(p7)] Practitioners must constantly orient their interventions to the contexts that clients find most important, because these interventions will be the most meaningful and be most likely to result in occupational participation.[148] Table 20-4 provides examples of national and international efforts to address cultural factors that contribute to limitations in performance, participation, and well-being. Occupational therapy intervention is intended to be health promoting.[33(p652)] Interventions vary depending on the client—person, organization, or population.[149] Interventions that focus on the person (or on a small group of people who support or care for the client, such as family members, caregivers, etc.) should address the interaction among intrinsic (person) and extrinsic (environment) factors and the activity demands of the occupations the person wishes to perform. Interventions should not only be client-centered and context driven, they should also be occupation-based.[150] Further, interventions should be evidence-based and dynamically interrelated with ongoing assessment. Cultural context will likely influence not only the expectations of the social groups the client belongs to, but also shape the demands of the activities themselves. For example, the 2 Somali women we referred to previously who had strokes may need intervention to increase their endurance. Both typically cooked family meals and wish to continue participating in that occupation. However, for one client making a sandwich may be a culturally acceptable intervention, for the other client it may not. The first client may value the practicality of accomplishing the task of feeding the family quickly, while the other may consider the meal insufficient to express care for loved ones and be a symbol of personal inadequacy.

Therefore, based on assessment results, intervention strategies should be adapted to the client's desires, goals, and cultural meanings. In other words, the occupational therapy professional must seek to learn what the clients' preferred occupations are and how he or she used to go about participating in them. Task analyses assist occupational therapy practitioners to assess the performance components of an activity that are not congruent with the client's ability at that time. This knowledge will provide the basis for adapting activities in order for the client to gradually participate in them once again. Considerations should be made over the social traditions, gender and age appropriateness, religious preference, language mastery, socioeconomic resources, and values related to communication, health, and body from the client's perspectives. Allowances should also be made to consider family members and close social relationships to the degree that they support the client's participation in occupation.

An important consideration should also be the degree to which a client wishes or needs to learn new culturally bounded behaviors. It would be wrong to assume that a person will only wish to maintain past or familiar occupational engagements. Just because people are facing temporary or long-standing disabilities does not mean that they

Table 20-3. *Examples of Assessment Instruments With Cultural Validity Used in Occupational Therapy*

Reference	Title of Assessment	Construct or Factor Assessed	Description
Baum, Edwards[132]	*Activity Card Sort,* 2nd edition (ACS)	Summarizes clients' occupational history for instrumental, leisure, and social activities.	Performed as a semi-structured interview that includes 3 setting versions and allows for documentation of percentage of activities retained.
Fisher, Bray-Jones[133,134]	Assessment of Motor and Process Skills (AMPS)	Observational assessment that is used to measure the quality of a person's activities of daily living (ADL).	The quality of the person's ADL performance is assessed by rating the effort, efficiency, safety, and independence of 16 ADL motor and 20 ADL process skill items while the person is doing chosen, familiar, and life-relevant ADL tasks.
Townsend, Stanton, Law, Polatajko, Baptiste, Thompson-Franson, Kramer, Swedlove, Brintnell, Campanile[135] Law, Baptiste, Carswell, McColl, Polatajko, Pollock[136]	Canadian Occupational Performance Measure (COPM)	Clients identify, prioritize, and evaluate important issues they encounter in occupational performance. Self-perception of actual performance and satisfaction with this performance over time.	Individualized, client-centered semi-structured interview designed for use by occupational therapy practitioners to detect change in a client's self-perception of occupational performance over time. Tool was developed to be used in conjunction with the COPM and Engagement.
King, Law, King, Hurley, Rosenbaum, Hanna, Kertoy, Young[137]	Children's Assessment of Participation and Enjoyment/Preference for Activities of Children (CAPE/PAC)	Participation in leisure activities is assessed.	Designed for children and young people with and without disabilities between the ages of 6 to 21 in several countries. The tool is designed to measure if and how children participate in 55 illustrated informal and formal activities that measure participation in 5 dimensions: diversity, frequency, with whom, where, and the enjoyment of activities (answers from 1 = not at all, to 5 = love it).
Loewenstein, Amigo, Duara, Guterman, Hurwitz, Berkowitz, et al[138] McDougall, Becker, Vaughan, Acee, Delville[139]	Direct Assessment of Functional Status-Revised (DAFS-R)	Time orientation, communication abilities, transportation knowledge, financial skills, shopping skills, eating skills, and dressing/grooming skills; is administered in outpatient settings	85-item scale, shown to have high inter-rater and test-rest reliability among patients identified as possibly having memory disorders and among normal controls

(continued)

Table 20-3 (continued). *Examples of Assessment Instruments With Cultural Validity Used in Occupational Therapy*

Reference	Title of Assessment	Construct or Factor Assessed	Description
Kielhofner, Mallinson, Forsyth, Lai[140]	Occupational Performance History Interview II (OPHI-II)	Activity/occupational choices, critical life events, daily routine, occupational roles, and occupational behavior settings	Semi-structured interview, scales for rating the information obtained in the interview, and a format for recording qualitative (ie, narrative) data. The interview is organized into thematic areas.
Haley, Coster, Ludlow, Haltiwanger, Andrellos[141]	Pediatric Evaluation of Disability Inventory (PEDI)	Detects whether a deficit or delay exists in children with regard to functional skill development and, if so, to describe the extent and content area of the delay or deficit.	Performed as a parental interview and provides outcome measures as both normative and scaled scores.

Table 20-4. *Examples of National and International Efforts to Address Cultural Factors That Contribute to Limitations in Performance, Participation, and Well-Being*

Organization	Purpose	Contact Information
American Association of People with Disabilities (AAPD)	Promotes equal opportunity, economic power, independent living, and political participation of people with disabilities.	http://www.aapd.com/
Disability Rights International	Organization dedicated to promoting the human rights and full participation in society of people with disabilities world-wide. Documents human rights abuses, publishes reports on human rights enforcement, and promotes international over-sight of the rights of people with mental disabilities.	http://www.disability-rightsintl.org/about/
Disabled Parents Network	International organization that aims to increase society's acceptance of disability in parenthood and provide support information and advice to disabled parents and their families.	http://disabledparentsnet-work.org.uk/
Disabled People's International	Network of national organizations or assemblies of disabled people established to promote human rights of disabled people through full participation and equalization of opportunity and development.	http://www.dpi.org/
Mobility International USA (MIUSA)	A cross-disability organization serving people with cognitive, hearing, learning, mental health, physical, systemic, vision, and other disabilities. Its mission is to empower people with disabilities to achieve their human rights through international exchange and international development.	http://www.miusa.org/

(continued)

Table 20-4 (continued).   *Examples of National and International Efforts to Address Cultural Factors That Contribute to Limitations in Performance, Participation, and Well-Being*

Organization	Purpose	Contact Information
National Council on Disability (NCD)	Independent federal agency charged with advising the President, Congress, and other federal agencies regarding policies, programs, practices, and procedures that affect people with disabilities.	http://www.ncd.gov/
National Organization on Disability NOD)	Private, nonprofit organization that promotes the full participation of America's 54 million people with disabilities in all aspects of life, but with an emphasis on employment.	http://www.nod.org/
Rehabilitation International	Worldwide network of people with disabilities, service providers, government agencies, academics, researchers, and advocates working to improve the quality of life of people with disabilities.	http://www.riglobal.org/
United Nations High Commission for Refugees (UNHCR)	Agency mandated to lead and coordinate international action to protect refugees and resolve refugee problems worldwide. Its primary purpose is to safeguard the rights and well-being of refugees. It strives to ensure that everyone can exercise the right to seek asylum and find safe refuge.	http://www.unhcr.org/ cgi-bin/texis/vtx/home
World Health Organization (WHO)	Specialized agency of the United Nations (UN) concerned with international public health. The WHO Task Force on Disability that ensures WHO programs and projects across the world are designed and implemented, taking into account people with disabilities. This task force spearheaded development of resources for community-based rehabilitation and ICF.	http://www.who.int/en/

will not be interested in learning new ways of being. Further, some clients may need to learn new behaviors in order to maintain desired autonomy. For example, the Somali women alluded to earlier will need to interact with health care provided in a potentially unfamiliar context for some time. Part of the occupational therapy intervention they need may be assistance with adapting to unfamiliar routines and expectations, particularly when materials needed for preferred occupations aren't readily available or they do not count on needed resources. Thus, an appropriate intervention may be to experiment replacing the traditional Somali *lahoh* (a pancake-like bread) with ready-made flour tortillas for breakfast meals. While tortillas may not be an exact match to the traditional food, this intervention may satisfy the desire to simplify meal preparation for the first woman, and for continuing to provide more traditional meals for her family for the second.

This latter example also illustrates why the dynamic interaction between client and community or social contexts should also be considered when providing intervention.[33(p628)] While one of the women may prefer

not to re-engage fully in the occupation of providing meals for her family, there may not be another alternative for that family because the children are too young or relatives and friends are not available to take on that responsibility. If the woman has the capacity, community needs may have to take precedence over personal preference.[151-153]

OUTCOMES

The ultimate purpose of occupational therapy intervention is to foster occupational engagement that results in participation.[33(p646)] Therefore, determination of success largely lies on whether the client has reached desired targeted outcomes and whether those outcomes result in greater participation in life.[147(p2)] Occupation-based outcomes are high-level outcomes because they relate to satisfactory role performance, identity and the realization of self, life satisfaction, well-being (happiness), and the creation of meaning.[154] Each of these outcomes will signify something unique in each cultural context. The constellation of life roles will vary from people group to people group, even if some activities or tasks associated with each role overlap. Occupational therapy outcome measurement, then, should include a determination of the client's level of satisfaction with role performance, sense of agency, adaptability in managing life situations, perception of confidence and self-esteem, QOL (quality of life), and personal fulfillment, among others. While any measure that can reliably and validly document change as a result of planned intervention can be a suitable measure of therapeutic outcome,[154(p525)] practitioners are encouraged to consult test manuals and published reviews of measures to determine their cultural suitability for use in measuring the attainment of specified client or program goals.

SUMMARY

Culture emerges in adaptive interactions between humans and environments, consists of shared elements between people, and is transmitted across time periods and generations. The PEOP Model recognizes the cultural environment as an extrinsic factor that influences, and in turn is influenced by, the occupational participation of people as individuals and as members of social groups, organizations, and populations.[24(p244)] Cultural factors include values, customs, beliefs, power/decision-making, organizational practices, and economic characteristics.[25] Culture is very dynamic because it is socially constructed, objective and subjective, conscious and unconscious. Cultural generalizations should not be used to explain people's behavior because no culture is homogeneous.[28(p25),32(p16)] Although a group may share some general cultural features in common, each individual in the group contributes uniquely to that shared meaning, is in a different point of learning culture, and acts based on his or her experiences and interpretations. Individuals have multiple and overlapping cultural identities, each representing a constellation of occupations, meanings, and participation associated with a social subgroup.[41(p62)] Culture is only one of many complex influences on health and participation in life. Race, ethnicity, age, gender, religion, language, social class, and health status all influence when, where, and how a person engages in occupation and participates in social life. Culturally-sensitive occupational therapy intervention is client-centered and contextually driven.[9(p1),42(p186),118(p7)] Value systems related to what is considered truth; individualism and collectivism; divisions of power; use of time; and beliefs about the body, health, and healing must be considered throughout the occupational therapy process to foster occupational engagement that results in participation.[33(p646)]

REFERENCES

1. Harris M. *The Rise of Anthropological Theory: A History of Theories of Culture*. Walnut Creek, CA: Altamira Press; 2001.
2. Geertz C. The Interpretation of Cultures. New York, NY: Basic Books; 1973.
3. Kroeber A, Kluchohn C. *Culture: A Critical Review of Concepts And Definitions*. Papers: Peabody Museum of Archeology & Ethnology, Harvard University. 1952;47(1):223.
4. Fiske AP. Using individualism and collectivism to compare cultures—a critique of the validity and measurement of the constructs: comment on Oyserman et al. *Psychol Bull*. 2002;128:78-88.
5. Myaskovsky L, Burkitt KH, Lichy AM, et al. The association of race, cultural factors, and health-related quality of life in persons with spinal cord injury. *Arch Phys Med Rehabil*. 2011;92:441-448.
6. Mays VM, Ponce NA, Washington DL, Cochran SD. Classification of race and ethnicity: implications for public health. *Ann Rev Public Health*. 2003;24:83-110.
7. Williams DR, Mohammed SA. Discrimination and racial disparities in health: evidence and needed research. *J Behav Med*. 2009;32:20-47.
8. Urban G. A method for measuring the motion of culture. *Am Anthropol*. 2010;112:122-139.
9. Iwama MK. Meaning and inclusion: revisiting culture in occupational therapy [guest editorial]. *Aust Occup Ther J*. 2004;51:1-2.
10. Chiu, CY, Hong YY. *Social Psychology of Culture*. New York, NY: Psychology Press; 2006.
11. Cohen AB. Many forms of culture. *Am Psychol*. 2009;64:194-204.
12. Kleinman A. *Writing at the Margin: Discourse between Anthropology and Medicine*. Berkeley, CA: University of California Press; 1995.
13. Nisbett RE. A psychological perspective: cultural psychology—past, present, and future. In: Kitayama S, Cohen D, eds. *Handbook of Cultural Psychology*. New York, NY: Guilford Press; 2007:837-844.
14. Triandis HC. Culture and psychology: a history of the study of their relationships. In: Kitayama S, Cohen D, eds. *Handbook of Cultural Psychology*. New York, NY: Guilford Press: 2007: 59-76.
15. Triandis HC. *Individualism and Collectivism*. Boulder, CO: Westview; 1995.
16. Triandis HC. The psychological measurement of cultural syndromes. *Am Psychol*. 1996;51:407-415.
17. Hui CH, Yee C. The shortened Individualism–Collectivism Scale: its relationship to demographic and work-related variables. *J Res Pers*. 1994;28:409-424.
18. Etgar M, Rachman-Moore D. The relationship between national cultural dimensions and retail format strategies. *J Retail Cons Serv*. 2011;18:397-404.
19. Özbilgin M, Tatli A. Mapping out the field of equality and diversity: rise of individualism and voluntarism. *Hum Relat*. 2011;64:1229-1253.
20. Oyserman D, Sorensen N. Understanding cultural syndrome effects on what and how we think: a situated cognition model. In: Wyer RS, Chiu C, Hong Y, eds. *Understanding Culture: Theory, Research, and Application*. New York, NY: Psychology Press; 2009:25-52.
21. Goldberg DT. Racial europeanization. *Ethn Racial Stud*. 2006;29:331-364.

22. Sharma P. Demystifying cultural differences in country-of-origin effects: exploring the moderating roles of product type, consumption context, and involvement. *J Int Cons Market.* 2011;23:344-364.

23. Wells SA, Black RM. *Cultural Competency for Health Professionals.* Bethesda, MD: American Occupational Therapy Association; 2000.

24. Baum C, Christiansen C. Person-environment-occupation-performance: an occupation-based framework for practice. In: Christiansen C, Baum C, Bass Haugen J, eds. *Occupational Therapy: Performance, Participation, and Well-Being.* 3rd ed. Thorofare, NJ: SLACK Incorporated; 2005:243-266.

25. Christiansen CH, Baum CM, Bass JD, eds. *Occupational Therapy: Performance, Participation, and Well-Being.* 4th ed. Thorofare, NJ: SLACK Incorporated; 2015.

26. Knudson DM, Cable TT, Beck L. *Interpretation of Cultural and Natural Resources.* 2nd ed. State College, PA: Venture Publishing; 2003.

27. Denzin NK. *Symbolic Interactionism and Cultural Studies: The Politics of Interpretation.* Hoboken, NJ: Wiley-Blackwell; 2007.

28. Fischer R. Where is culture in cross cultural research? An outline of a multilevel research process for measuring culture as a shared meaning system. *Int J Cross Cult Manage.* 2009;9:25-49.

29. Bardi A, Guerra V. Cultural values predict coping using culture as an individual difference variable in multicultural samples. *J Cross Cult Psychol.* 2011;42:908-927.

30. Good BJ, Del-Vechio MJ, Hyde ST, Pinto S. Postcolonial disorders: reflections on subjectivity in the contemporary world. In: Del-Vechio MJ, Hyde, ST, Pinto S, Good BJ, eds. *Postcolonial Disorders.* Berkeley, CA: University of California Press; 2008:1-42.

31. Gallardo ME, McNeill BW. *Intersections of Multiple Identities: A Casebook of Evidence-Based Practices with Diverse Populations.* New York, NY: Routledge; 2009.

32. Black RM, Wells SA. *Culture and Occupation: A Model of Empowerment in Occupational Therapy.* Bethesda, MD: AOTA Press; 2007.

33. American Occupational Therapy Association. Occupational therapy practice framework: domain and process. *Am J Occup Ther.* 2014;68(Suppl 1):S1-S48.

34. Charon R. *Narrative Medicine: Honoring the Stories of Illness.* Oxford, UK: Oxford University Press; 2006.

35. Schoen LT, Teddlie C. A new model of school culture: a response to a call for conceptual clarity. *School Effectiveness and School Improvement.* 2008;19:129-153.

36. Hofstede GH. *Cultures and Organizations: Intercultural Cooperation and its Importance for Survival.* New York, NY: McGraw-Hill; 2010.

37. Johnson AG. *Privilege, Power and Difference.* New York, NY: McGraw-Hill; 2005.

38. Krefting LH, Krefting DV. Cultural influences on performance. In: Christiansen C, Baum CM, eds. *Occupational Therapy: Overcoming Human Performance Deficits.* Thorofare, NJ: SLACK Incorporated; 1991:101-124.

39. Edwards D, Christiansen CH. Occupational development. In: Christiansen C, Baum C, Bass Haugen J, eds. *Occupational Therapy: Performance, Participation, and Well-Being.* 3rd ed. Thorofare, NJ: SLACK Incorporated; 2005:43-63.

40. Suarez-Orozco C, Hernandez MG. Immigrant family separations: the experience of separated, unaccompanied, and reunited youth and families. In: Garcia-Coll C, ed. *The Impact of Immigration on Children's Development.* Basel, Switzerland: S. Karger AG; 2011:122-148.

41. Holland D, Lachicotte W, Skinner D, Cain C. *Identity and Agency in Cultural Worlds.* Cambridge, MA: Harvard University Press; 2001.

42. Helman C. *Culture, Health and Illness.* 5th ed. New York, NY: Oxford University Press; 2007.

43. Rothman J. *Cultural Competence in Process and Practice: Building Bridges.* Boston, MA: Allyn & Bacon; 2007.

44. Omohundro JT. *Thinking like an Anthropologist: A Practical Introduction to Cultural Anthropology.* Boston, MA: McGraw-Hill; 2008.

45. Lorusso L. The justification of race in biological explanation. *J Med Ethics.* 2011;37:535-539.

46. Cornell SE, Hartmann D. *Ethnicity and Race: Making Identities in a Changing World.* 2nd ed. Thousand Oaks, CA: Sage Publications; 2007.

47. Bellah RN, Mardsden R, Sullivan WS, Swindler A, Tipton SM. *Habits of the Heart: Individualism and Commitment in American Life.* 3rd ed. Berkeley, CA: University of California Press; 2007.

48. Rutledge D. *The Somali Diaspora: A Journey Away.* Minneapolis, MN: University of Minnesota Press; 2008.

49. Abusharaf, RM. *Wanderings: Sudanese Migrants and Exiles in North America.* Ithaca, NY: Cornell University Press; 2002.

50. Benedict R. *Patterns of Culture.* Boston, MA: Houghton-Mifflin; 1989.

51. Fine C. *Delusions of Gender: How our Minds, Society, and Neurosexism Create Difference.* New York, NY: WW Norton; 2010.

52. Zou X, Tam KP, Morris MW, et al. Culture as common sense: perceived consensus versus personal beliefs as mechanisms of cultural influence. *J Pers Soc Psychol.* 2009;97:579-597.

53. Balthazart J. *The Biology of Homosexuality.* New York, NY: Oxford University Press; 2012.

54. Adiele F, Frosch M. *Coming of Age Around the World.* New York, NY: The New Press; 2007.

55. Azlan R. *Beyond Fundamentalism: Confronting Religious Extremism in the Age of Globalization.* New York, NY: Random House; 2010.

56. McCullough ME, Willoughby BL. Religion, self-regulation, and self-control: associations, explanations, and implications. *Psychol Bull.* 2009;135:69-93.

57. Romaine S. Language, culture, and identity across nations. In: Banks JA, ed. *The Routledge International Companion to Multicultural Education.* New York, NY: Routledge; 2009:373-384.

58. Thomas MS, Johnson MH. New advances in understanding sensitive periods in brain development. *Curr Dir Psychol Dev.* 2008;17:1-5.

59. Chomski N. *Language and Mind.* Cambridge, UK: Cambridge University Press; 2006.

60. Salzmann Z, Stanlaw J, Adachi N. *Language, Culture and Society: An Introduction.* 5th ed. Boulder, CO: Westview Press; 2011.

61. Grusky D. *Social Stratification: Class, Race, and Gender in Sociological Perspective.* 3rd ed. New York, NY: Westview Press; 2008.

62. Ornstein AC. *Class Counts: Education, Inequality, and the Shrinking Middle Class.* Lenham, MD: Rowman & Littlefield Publishers; 2007.

63. Jadhav N. *Untouchables: My Family's Triumphant Escape from India's Caste System.* Berkeley, CA: University of California Press; 2007.

64. Sachs J. *The End of Poverty: Economic Possibilities for Our Time.* New York, NY: Penguin; 2006.

65. Aaron GJ, Wilson SE, Brown KH. Bibliographic analysis of scientific research on selected topics in public health nutrition in West Africa: review of articles published from 1998 to 2008. *Glob Public Health.* 2010;5(suppl):S42-S57.

66. Barr DA. *Health Disparities in the United States: Social Class, Race, Ethnicity, and Health.* Baltimore, MD: The Johns Hopkins University Press; 2008.

67. Torelli CJ, Chiu, CY, Tam K, Au, AK, Keh HT. Exclusionary reactions to foreign cultures: effects of simultaneous exposure to cultures in globalized space. *J Soc Issues.* 2011;67:716-742.

68. Staurowsky EJ. American Indian imagery and the miseducation of America. In: King CR, ed. *The Native American Mascot Controversy: A Handbook.* Lanham, MD: Rowman & Littlefield; 2010:63-77.

69. Kaga M, Takeshima T, Matsumoto T. Suicide and its prevention in Japan. *Leg Med.* 2009;1(suppl):S18-S21.

70. Morrison T, Conway WA. *Kiss, Bow, or Shake Hands.* 2nd ed. Avon, MA: Adams Media; 2006.

71. King L, Hamm P, Stuckler D. Rapid large-scale privatization and death rates in ex-communist countries: an analysis of stress-related and health system mechanisms. *Int J Health Serv.* 2009;39(3):461-489.

72. Prince DW, Hoppe MH. *Communicating Across Cultures.* Greensboro, NC: Center for Creative Leadership; 2007.

73. Chagnon NA. *Yanomamo.* Belmont, CA: Wadsworth; 2012.

74. Wageman R, Gardner H, Mortensen M. The changing ecology of teams: new directions for teams research. *J Organ Behav.* 2012;33:301-315.

75. Noordegraaf M, Van Der Meulen M. Professional power play: organizing management in health care. *Public Adm.* 2008;86:1055-1069.

76. Kane MN, Jacobs RJ. Perceptions of humaneness of religious leaders among university students. *J Spiritual Ment Health.* 2012;14:59-81.

77. Martin B. *Children at Play: Learning Gender in the Early Years.* Oakhill, UK: Trentham Books, Ltd; 2011.

78. Allen JF. Towards a general theory of action and time. In: Mani I, Pustejovsky J, Gaizauskas R, eds. *The Language of Time.* Oxford, UK: Oxford University Press; 2005:251-276.

79. Muñiz C, Rodríguez P, Suárez M. The allocation of time to sports and cultural activities: an analysis of individual decisions. *International Journal of Sport Finance.* 2011;6:245-264.

80. Hall ET. *The Dance of Life: The Other Dimensions of Time.* New York, NY: Anchor Books; 1984.

81. Lindquist JD, Kaufman-Scarborough C. The polychromic-monochromic tendency model: PMTS scale development and validation. *Time & Society.* 2007;16:253-285.

82. Grogan S. *Body Image: Understanding Body Dissatisfaction in Men, Women and Children.* New York, NY: Routledge; 2008.

83. Lovera JR. *Food Culture in South America.* Westport, CT: Greenwood Publishing Group, Inc; 2005.

84. Cosminsky S. Maya midwives of Southern Mexico and Guatemala. In: Huber BR, Sandstrom, AR, eds. *Mesoamerican Healers.* Austin, TX: University of Texas Press; 2001:179-210.

85. Erikson PI. *Ethnomedicine.* Long Grove, IL: Waveland Press; 2007.

86. Tafur MM, Crowe TK, Torres E. A review of curanderismo and healing practices among Mexicans and Mexican Americans. *Occup Ther Int.* 2009;16:82-88.

87. Howson A. *The Body in Society: An Introduction.* Oxford, UK: Blackwell Publishing; 2004.

88. Womack M. *The Anthropology of Healing.* Plymouth, UK: AltaMira Press; 2010.

89. Favazza AR. *Bodies Under Siege: Self-Mutilation, Non-Suicidal Self-Injury, and Body Modification in Culture and Psychiatry.* 3rd ed. Baltimore, MD: The Johns Hopkins University Press; 2011.

90. Hall ET. Proxemics. In: Low SM, Lawrence-Zúñiga DD, eds. *The Anthropology of Space and Place: Locating Culture.* Malden, MA: Blackwell Publishers; 2003:51-73.

91. Knapp ML, Hall JA. *Nonverbal Communication in Human Interaction.* 7th ed. Boston, MA: Wadsworth; 2010.

92. Duranti A. Universal and culture-specific properties of greetings. In: Duranti A, ed. *Linguistic Anthropology: A Reader.* Malden, MA: Blackwell Publishing; 2009:188-213.

93. Nichter M. *Global Health: Why Cultural Perceptions, Social Representations, and Biopolitics Matter.* Tucson, AZ: The University of Arizona Press; 2008.

94. Barthes R. Toward a pshychosociology of contemporary food consumption. In: Counihan C, ed. *Food and Culture.* 2nd ed. New York, NY: Routledge; 2007:20-27.

95. Kleinman A. *Patients and Healers in the Context of Culture.* Berkeley, CA: University of California Press; 1980.

96. Ghane S, Kolk AM, Emmelkamp PM. Direct and indirect assessment of explanatory models of illness. *Transcult Psychiatry.* 2012;49:3-25.

97. Adato M, Roopnaraine T, Becker E. Understanding use of health services in conditional cash transfer programs: insights from qualitative research in Latin America and Turkey. *Soc Sci Med.* 2011;72:1921-1929.

98. Wald KD, Calhoun-Brown A. *Religion and Politics in the United States.* Lanham, MD: Rowman & Littlefield Publishers; 2011.

99. Telles EE, Sue CA. Race mixture: boundary crossing in comparative perspective. *Ann Rev Sociol.* 2009;34:129-146.

100. Lichter DT, Parisi D, Taquino MC, Grice SM. Residential segregation in new Hispanic destination: cities, suburbs, and rural communities compared. *Soc Sci Res.* 2010;39:215-230.

101. Pietila A. *Not in My Neighborhood: How Bigotry Shaped a Great American City.* Chicago, IL: Ivan R. Dee, Publisher; 2010.

102. Lentin A, Title G. *The Crises of Multiculturalism: Racism in a Neoliberal Age.* New York, NY: Zed Books; 2011.

103. Herrig C. Combating racism and xenophobia on both sides of the Atlantic. In: Herrig C, ed. *Combating Racism and Xenophobia: Transatlantic and International Perspectives.* Chicago, IL: Institute of Government & Public Affairs, University of Chicago; 2011.

104. Schrag P. *Not Fit for Our Society: Immigration and Nativism in America.* Berkeley, CA: University of California Press; 2010.

105. Bray I. *US Immigration Made Easy.* 15th ed. Berkeley, CA: NOLO; 2011.

106. Ayers I. *Pervasive Prejudice? Unconventional Evidence of Race and Gender Discrimination.* 2nd ed. Chicago, IL: the University of Chicago Press; 2010.

107. Wang, LI. *Discrimination by Default: How Racism Becomes Routine.* New York, NY: New York University Press; 2006.

108. American Occupational Therapy Association. Occupational therapy code of ethics. *Am J Occup Ther.* 2005;59:639-642.

109. Banakar R. *Rights in Context: Law and Justice in Late Modern Society.* Farnham, England: Ashgate Publishing Limited; 2010.

110. Benz JK, Espinoza O, Welsh V, Fontes A. Awareness of racial and ethnic health disparities had improved only modestly over a decade. *Health Aff.* 2011;30:1860-1867.

111. David R, Messer L. Reducing disparities: race, class and social determinants of health. *Matern Child Health J.* 2011;15(suppl):S1-S3.

112. Kosoko-Lasaki S, Cook CT. Cultural competency instrument: a description of a methodology, part II. In: Kosoko-Lasaki S, Cook CT, eds. *Cultural Proficiency in Addressing Health Disparities*. Sudbury, MA: Jones and Bartlett; 2008.

113. Owen J, Imel Z, Tao KW, Wampold B, Smith A, Rodolfa E. Cultural raptures in short-term therapy: working alliance as a mediator between clients' perceptions of microaggressions and therapy outcomes. *Counseling and Psychotherapy Research*. 2011;11:204-212.

114. Gazmarian JA, Ziemer DC, Barnes C. Perception of barriers to self-care management among diabetic patients. *Diabetes Educ*. 2009;35:778-788.

115. Lucas T, Lakey B, Arnetz J, Arnetz B. Do ratings of African-American cultural competency reflect characteristics of providers or perceivers? Initial demonstration of a generalizability theory approach. *Psychol Health Med*. 2010;15:445-453.

116. Paez KA, Allen JK, Beach MC, Carson KA, Cooper LA. Physician cultural competence and patient ratings on patient-physician relationship. *J Gen Intern Med*. 2011;24:495-498.

117. Starr SS, Wallace DC. Client perceptions of cultural competence of community-based nurses. *J Community Health Nurs*. 2011;28:57-69.

118. Office of Minority Health. *National Standards for Culturally and Linguistically Appropriate Services in Health Care: Final Report*. Washington, DC: US Department of Health and Human Services; 2001.

119. Suarez-Balcazar Y, Balcazar F, Taylor-Ritzler T, et al. Development and validation of a cultural competence assessment instrument. *J Rehabil*. 2011;77:4-13.

120. National Center for Cultural Competence. *Cultural Competence Health Practitioner Assessment (CCHPA)*. Georgetown University: Center for Child and Human Development: National Center for Cultural Competence. http://www11.georgetown.edu/research/gucchd/nccc/features/CCHPA.html. Accessed May 28, 2012.

121. Rooda LA. Knowledge and attitudes of nurses toward culturally different patients: implications for nursing education. *J Nurs Educ*. 1993;32:209-213.

122. Bernal H, Froman, R. The confidence of community health nurses in caring for ethnically diverse populations. *J Nurs Scholarship*. 1987;19:201-203.

123. Mendenhall ME, Stevens MJ, Burd A, Oddou GR. Specification for the content domain of the Global Competencies Inventory (GCI). *The Kozai Working Paper Series*. http://kozaigroup.com/inventories/the-global-competencies-inventory-gci/. Published 2008. Accessed May 28, 2012.

124. Hammer MR, Bennett MJ, Wiseman R. Measuring intercultural sensitivity: the Intercultural Development Inventory. *Int J Intercult Rel*. 2003;27:421-443.

125. Hammer MR. Additional cross-cultural validity testing of the Intercultural Development Inventory. *Int J Intercult Rel*. 2011;35:474-487.

126. Portolla T, Chen GM. *The Development and Validation of the Intercultural Effectiveness Scale*. Paper presented at: Annual Meeting of the International Association for Intercultural Communication Studies; 2009; Kumamoto, Japan.

127. Campinha-Bacote J. A model and instrument for addressing cultural competence in health care. *J Nurs Educ*. 1999;38:203-207.

128. Sue DW, Bernier JE, Durran A, Feinberg L, Pedersen P, Smith EJ. Position paper: cross-cultural counseling competencies. *Couns Psychol*. 1982;10:45-52.

129. Sodowsky GR, Taffe RC, Gutkin TB, Wise SL. Development of the Multicultural Counseling Inventory (MCI): a self-report measure of multicultural competencies. *J Couns Psychol*. 1994;41:137-148.

130. Mason JL. *Cultural Competence Self-Assessment Questionnaire: A Manual for Users*. Portland, OR: Portland State University, Research and Training Center on Family Support and Children's Mental Health; 1995.

131. Law M, Baum C, Dunn W. Occupational performance assessment. In: Christiansen C, Baum C, Bass Haugen J, eds. *Occupational Therapy: Performance, Participation, and Well-Being*. 3rd ed. Thorofare, NJ: SLACK Incorporated; 2005:339-372.

132. Baum CM, Edwards D. *Activity Card Sort*. 2nd ed. Bethesda, MD: AOTA Press; 2008.

133. Fisher AG, Bray-Jones K. Assessment of Motor and Process Skills. *Vol. 1: Development, Standardization, and Administration Manual*. 7th ed. Fort Collins, CO: Three Star Press; 2010.

134. Fisher AG, Bray-Jones K. *Assessment of Motor and Process Skills*. Vol. 2: User Manual 7th ed. Fort Collins, CO: Three Star Press; 2010.

135. Townsend E, Stanton S, Law M, et al. *Enabling Occupation: An Occupational Therapy Perspective*. Rev ed. Ottawa, ON: Canadian Association of Occupational Therapists; 2002.

136. Law M, Baptiste S, Carswell A, McColl MA, Polatajko H, Pollock N. *Canadian Occupational Performance Measure*. 4th ed. Toronto, ON: Canadian Association of Occupational Therapists; 2005.

137. King G, Law M, King S, et al. *Children's Assessment of Participation and Enjoyment and Preferences for Activities of Children*. San Antonio, TX: Harcourt Assessment Inc; 2004.

138. Loewenstein DA, Amigo E, Duara R, et al. A new scale for the assessment of functional status in Alzheimer's disease and related disorders. *J Gerontol*. 1989;44:114–121.

139. McDougall GJ, Becker H, Vaughan PW, Acee TW, Delville CL. The revised direct assessment of functional status for independent older adults. *Gerontologist*. 2009;50:363-370.

140. Kielhofner G, Mallinson T, Forsyth K, Lai JS. Psychometric properties of the second version of the Occupational Performance History Interview (OPHI-II). *Am J Occup Ther*. 2001;55:260-267.

141. Haley S, Coster W, Ludlow L, Haltiwanger J, Andrellos P. *Pediatric Evaluation of Disability Inventory (PEDI)*. Version 1.0. Boston, MA: New England Medical Center Hospitals; 1992.

142. Gryczynski J, Schwartz RP, Salkever DS, Mitchell SG, Jaffe JH. Patterns in admission delays to outpatient methadone treatment in the United States. *J Subst Abuse Treat*. 2011;41:431-439.

143. Harrington C, Kang T. Disparities in service utilization and expenditures for individuals with developmental disabilities. *Disabil Health J*. 2008;1:184-195.

144. Mendez DD, Hogan VK, Culhane J. Institutional racism and pregnancy health: using Home Mortgage Disclosure Act data to develop an index for mortgage discrimination at the community level. *Pub Health Rep*. 2011;126(suppl 3):102-104.

145. Saegert S, Fields D, Libman K. Mortgage foreclosures and health disparities: serial displacement as asset extraction in African American populations. *J Urban Health*. 2011;88:390-402.

146. Stone J, Moskowitz GB. Non-conscious bias in medical decision making: what can be done to reduce it? *Med Educ*. 2011;45:768-776.

147. World Health Organization. *International Classification of Functioning, Disability and Health: ICF*. Geneva, Switzerland: World Health Organization; 2001.

148. Fitzgerald MH. A dialogue on occupational therapy, culture and families. *Am J Occup Ther*. 2004;58:489-498.

149. Moyers PA, Dale LM. *The Guide to Occupational Therapy Practice*. 2nd ed. Bethesda, MD: AOTA Press; 2007.

150. Youngstrom MJ, Brown C. Categories and principles of intervention. In: Christiansen C, Baum C, Bass Haugen J, eds. *Occupational Therapy: Performance, Participation, and Well-Being.* 3rd ed. Thorofare, NJ: SLACK Incorporated; 2005:397-420.

151. Dawad S, Jobson G. Community-based rehabilitation programme as a model for task-shifting. *Disabil Rehabil.* 2011;33(21/22):1997-2005.

152. Maya T. Reflections on community-based rehabilitation. *Psychology in Developing Societies.* 2011;23:277-291.

153. Pollard N, Sakellariou D. Operationalizing community participation in community-based rehabilitation: exploring the factors. *Disabil Rehabil.* 2008;30:62-70.

154. Baum C, Christiansen C. Outcomes: the results of interventions in occupational therapy practice. In: Christiansen C, Baum C, Bass Haugen J, eds. *Occupational Therapy: Performance, Participation, and Well-Being.* 3rd ed. Thorofare, NJ: SLACK Incorporated; 2005:523-540.

Chapter 21

ENVIRONMENT FACTORS
Social Determinants of Health, Social Capital, and Social Support

Julie D. Bass, PhD, OTR/L, FAOTA; Carolyn M. Baum, PhD, OTR/L, FAOTA;
Charles H. Christiansen, EdD, OTR, FAOTA; and Kathryn Haugen, REHS/RS

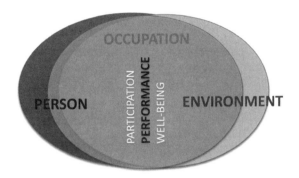

LEARNING OBJECTIVES

- Identify and define the primary social factors that influence performance, participation, and well-being.
- Discuss how social factors influence performance, participation, and well-being.
- Identify national and international efforts to address social factors that contribute to limitations in performance, participation, and well-being.
- Describe the influence of social factors on the practice of occupational therapy at the individual, organizational, and population/community level.
- Compare and contrast assessment and interventions regarding social factors in occupational therapy practice at the individual, organizational, and population/community level.
- Identify governmental, nonprofit, and international agencies that promote performance, participation, well-being through work on social factors.

KEY WORDS

- Health disparities
- Health equity
- Health inequalities
- Health inequities
- Social capital
- Social cohesion
- Social connectedness
- Social determinants of health
- Social support

INTRODUCTION

Social factors have long been recognized as contributing to individual, organization, and population health and well-being. There are multiple terms and models used to

Christiansen CH, Baum CM, Bass JD, eds.
*Occupational Therapy: Performance, Participation,
and Well-Being, Fourth Edition (pp 359-386).*
© 2015 SLACK Incorporated.

BOX 21-1

PERSON-CENTERED NARRATIVE: TAYLOR AND JORDAN

Taylor has lived with his spouse, Jordan, in the same urban neighborhood for over 35 years. Their daughter, a health professional, and his brother and sister-in-law live within an easy commute. Taylor retired about 7 years ago and greatly enjoyed the social activities that happened right outside their home as people walked by with their dogs and gathered informally to chat about weather, gardening, and politics. Taylor is often identified as the unofficial community organizer because of his genuine interest in others and helpful nature. Taylor and Jordan are especially close with their immediate neighbors; they have shared both happy and sad times over the years and looked out for each other.

Taylor was diagnosed with cancer 5 years ago and recently found out it had metastasized. Taylor and Jordan have been overwhelmed with the outpouring of support from family and neighbors. Neighbors have been taking care of the yard, dropping off cards, and doing errands. Taylor and Jordan believe it is the help, thoughts, and prayers of family and neighbors that are sustaining them and enabling them to participate in their community, even as Taylor nears the end of his life. Taylor's daughter and brother have just started taking turns staying at night to assist Taylor and provide relief to Jordan, but feel they will need information and equipment to provide this support in the days ahead. A neighbor who is an occupational therapist encourages them to ask their physician about hospice. Because of the poor prognosis, pain, fatigue, and increasing difficulty performing meaningful activities, Taylor and Jordan decide to obtain hospice services in the home.

Social Determinants of Health: Taylor and Jordan are grateful for their retirement pensions and supplemental health insurance plans, and describe their situation as "middle class." These resources have enabled them to enjoy many activities during Taylor's remissions from cancer, including travel, volunteering, and community classes.

Social Support: Taylor and Jordan describe strong social support from family, friends, neighbors, and health professionals. Their information about home care, assistance with chores, and just being there has made it possible for Taylor to stay at home most of the time.

Social Capital: Taylor and Jordan are proud of their neighborhood and the numerous connections among the families. This community has received several awards for their stewardship of the environment, beautification efforts, and social networks. Neighbors share news, have social gatherings, and volunteer to help families in need.

An occupational therapist visits with Taylor and Jordan in the home to learn about their needs and goals. Taylor has chosen not to receive any more cancer treatments. At times, he is in a lot of pain and states he is sleeping a lot. Taylor and Jordan have goals of:

- Managing fatigue and pain to enable spending some meaningful time together with a few family/friends

- Developing a care routine and obtaining equipment to make it possible for Taylor to be at home as long as possible and support Jordan and other caregivers

- Arranging for Jordan to learn some of Taylor's home responsibilities

---

describe the influence of social factors on health, including social determinants of health, social support, social capital, and social cohesion. These social factors are aspects of the environment in the PEOP Model that may serve as enablers or barriers to occupational performance, participation, and well-being.

Consider the social influences on performance, participation, and well-being in the PEOP Occupational Therapy Process Narrative for the following hypothetical scenarios:

- *Taylor and Jordan.* Taylor lives in a supportive urban neighborhood with his spouse, Jordan. Taylor has cancer that has metastasized and will be receiving hospice services (Box 21-1).

- *Jenny.* Jenny lives in the same mid-size city as her mother and 3 adult children. She has chronic mental illness and has had several different supported living environments in the last few years (Box 21-2).

- *Employees at Risk for Heart Disease and Stroke in a Governmental Organization.* In recent years, the human resources department has become concerned about health claims in a governmental division that suggest employees are at risk for heart disease and stroke (Box 21-3).

- *Children at Risk for Obesity and Related Conditions in a City.* A collaboration among governmental agencies, health care providers, churches, and schools has established a goal to pilot a public media campaign

---

BOX 21-2

PERSON-CENTERED NARRATIVE: JENNY

Jenny now lives in the same midsize city where she was born. She had a happy childhood, relatively carefree school years, and a promising future in college with her natural athletic ability and love of outdoor recreation and environmental science. But her mental health deteriorated when she was a young adult. Jenny returned to her hometown about 25 years ago to raise her 3 children after she was diagnosed with a severe mental illness and her husband left her. Over the years, she has had ongoing crises requiring hospitalization. Although some high school friends still live in the same community, she gradually lost contact with them after these episodes. Jenny's parents had to periodically step in and assume responsibility for raising her young children. This contributed to strain with some of her siblings, who believed Jenny was taking advantage of her parents' generosity. Jenny's children are now adults and have created lives of their own. The last few years have been especially hard for Jenny. She has moved from one living situation to another and been hospitalized several times after going off her medications; thus, she has no peer group or sense of community. Her father died a couple of years ago and her mother has become increasingly frail. Even though she is not stable enough to work, she would like to resume volunteering so she could meet new people, but it has been hard because of the side effects of her medication, limited motivation to maintain her hygiene, and lack of transportation. Jenny recently told her case worker that her mom and adult daughter are the only people left who will do anything with her on a regular basis.

Social Determinants of Health: Jenny is on a very limited disability income, but her state has some growing supports and programs for individuals with chronic mental illness. She describes the challenges of living with a chronic mental illness due to stigma, inadequate health services, few employment opportunities, and frequent changes in living environments. Jenny reports these circumstances have contributed to isolation and a tedious daily routine.

Social Support: Jenny states her mother is her primary support, but wonders what will happen when she is gone. Jenny's daughter is helpful when she has time, but she is busy with her job and young family. Jenny's sons check in once in awhile but they are still young men trying to figure out their own lives. Jenny enjoys her visits with a couple of high school friends once or twice a year when they return to visit their families, but she doesn't really feel like she can call them when she needs a friend or has a crisis.

Social Capital: Jenny has lived in 3 places during the last 5 years, including a low-income high-rise apartment, group home, and now in adult foster care. She states people keep to themselves in these settings and don't really help each other. Jenny has goals to:

- Create a weekly routine which gives her a purpose in life, a reason to get out of the house each day, and some hope of stopping the "revolving door"

- Take better care of herself—hygiene and grooming, eating better, exercise, clothing and laundry, medication

- Meet some people who she can do things with once in awhile and accept her for who she is

---

for the elementary school children in a metropolitan area with diverse socioeconomic and cultural communities (Box 21-4).

What are the social factors in each situation and how do these factors influence quality of life? These narratives highlighted the interactions of individuals, organizations, and populations/communities with their social environments and the effect of social factors on occupational performance, participation, and well-being. Occupational therapy has had a long-standing role in serving the occupational needs of individuals within a social context. There are now emerging opportunities to apply an occupational lens to local, national, and global health and societal issues that are influenced by social factors and identified as pri-

orities for governments and international organizations. A variety of concepts have been proposed as possible social factors at play, including social determinants of health, social support, social capital, social cohesion, and social connectedness.

SOCIAL DETERMINANTS OF HEALTH

The term social determinants of health is used to describe many of the complex person and environment factors that influence health along with performance, participation, and well-being. Consider an example of 2 equally capable high school students involved in

---

BOX 21-3

ORGANIZATION-CENTERED NARRATIVE: STATE AGENCY

In a governmental department, there have been alarming increases in the number of employees with serious cardiovascular health issues. After 4 heart attacks occurring in 2 months, the human resources manager decides to consult with an occupational therapist regarding workplace health and wellness programs. The occupational therapist meets with administrators and staff to gather information. From the administrators' perspective, this governmental organization is currently dealing with substantial challenges. Declining financial and staff resources force all departments to attempt to do more with less. Many employees have chronic health conditions (eg, obesity, heart disease, diabetes, stroke) that contribute to decreased productivity and increased absenteeism and long-term disability. Productivity has also been affected by overall low morale, high levels of stress, and negative attitudes, especially from "problem" employees. While most employees work hard to accomplish major tasks, there are inconsistent efforts day-to-day, leading to a difficulty in achieving division expectations.

Employees had a different take on many of the same issues. They indicated declining resources and sedentary jobs were significant sources of chronic stress. Inadequate staffing numbers, from multiple rounds of layoffs and attrition, led to increasing workloads and an inability to accomplish tasks. Accommodations, raises, and approved leaves of absence were rare. Workplace morale was low due to feelings of isolation, lack of support, powerlessness, and stagnation. Employees encounter barriers in time and access to regular physical activity and nutritious foods during the work day. Even though some employees participate in a lunch hour walking group, there are very few other indicators of healthy workplace initiatives.

The current physical environment does not support regular interaction, but a core group of employees indicate a commitment to getting through this difficult economic time together. Employees also reported a strong spiritual faith, a large social support network, and a high level of involvement and connection within their churches and communities.

Social Determinants of Health: This governmental organization has limited resources (eg, salaries, benefits, workplace programs) compared to its counterparts in other states. Recent economic trends have contributed to this inequity. Many employees have lifestyles and life circumstances (eg, nutrition, physical activity, responsibilities, chronic stress) that put them at risk for poor health.

Social Support: Employees describe strong social support outside of work, but report wide variation in levels of social support in the workplace. This variation may be related to the physical layout of offices, level of collaboration needed, organizational structure, and competition for resources.

Social Capital: Employees take pride in major accomplishments but they report little recognition by administration or general public. Employees demonstrate collective devotion to their work but report diminishing capacity to influence real change.

The occupational therapist collaborates with administrators and staff to identify organizational goals for improving cardiovascular health. This governmental organization has goals of:

- Improving overall physical health of employees to support improved retention and productivity
- Decreasing stress and improving morale of employees through cost-effective workplace initiatives
- Developing a model workplace program for other governmental organizations

---

educational occupations and preparing for college. What might be some social determinants that explain differences in their high school achievement and college entrance exam scores? Student A has computers and internet at home, a parent who has helped with homework, financial resources to pay for college exam preparation courses, academic enrichment summer camps during childhood, family financial resources to limit the need to work outside of school and provide opportunities for extracurricular activities, a nearby library, and social con-

nections to help navigate the college search process. Student A has substantial supports in place that make it easier to achieve high marks in most courses. Student B does not have any of these supports and spends a lot of time using public transportation to get to the library for computer access, working to save for college, taking care of younger siblings during the summer months, and using the resources in the counseling office after school to explore affordable options for college. Student B has the same capability as Student A, but not the same level of

---

BOX 21-4

POPULATION-CENTERED NARRATIVE: OBESITY

Childhood obesity is a major, global health issue, with over 42 million children under the age of 5 who are overweight or obese.[1] One major United States city has estimated that over 50% of its children are overweight or obese, and thus has decided to form a coalition of governmental agencies, health care providers, schools, and media outlets to identify and address the underlying issues of childhood obesity. An occupational therapist is asked to be a member of the coalition.

A number of environmental barriers contribute to high levels of childhood obesity in this city. The food sources in many neighborhoods are limited to fast food restaurants and corner stores that sell highly processed foods. Working parents often have limited time or resources to cook healthy foods for their children. Public transportation is available, but some neighborhoods have inconsistent service. There are very few safe parks and green spaces for children to play. Parents do not allow children to play outside or walk to nearby recreation centers due to the high levels of crime. Many elementary schools have discontinued physical education classes and recess due to budget constraints. Children have limited involvement in extracurricular sports and activities because of increased costs and time commitments. The regional culture is known for its rich traditional foods high in fat and sodium. Recreational activities in this area focus on music, attending sport events, and socializing.

The coalition has identified positive factors that will support efforts to reduce childhood obesity. Some nonprofit agencies have committed to funding programs and services for the city's most disadvantaged children. Professional athletes are considered role models, and thus many students desire to become involved in sports. Several local celebrities and athletes have agreed to become involved in campaigns advocating for increased levels of physical fitness. School marching bands, twirlers, and dance teams are an important element of the culture, and are popular in parades and local events. While there are currently few areas to walk or bike, the city has begun to incorporate bike lanes and paths into their long-term plan. There has been a gradual increase in the locations and hours for farmers markets.

Social Determinants of Health: This city has wide variation in family, community, and system factors including health care, schools, and services.

Social Support: There is strong social support from extended families and church communities. Some at-risk children live in families and neighborhoods without these supports.

Social Capital: Families maintain long-term connections with their schools and are strong supporters of youth activities and sports teams. Environmental barriers pose challenges to maintaining community connections and interest.

The occupational therapist contributes to this city's goals of:

- Establishing a culture of healthy living

- Developing a user-friendly guide for all community agencies that categorize activities from passive (reading) to active (flag football)

- Forming partnerships among schools, recreation centers, churches, businesses, and other organizations for youth activity and nutrition programs

- Using social media and celebrities to promote local events and build enthusiasm for healthy lifestyles

---

support/resources, so lower marks are earned in most courses. In a sense, many of the high marks for Student A may not be earned, but instead be artifacts of the social supports, socioeconomic status, and social capital of the family. This scenario may be repeated many times over for other individuals and groups—adults with health conditions and disabilities, children with special needs, and elders living in different communities.

There is strong agreement that social determinants of health influence performance, participation, and well-being, but there are different definitions of the concept by governmental agencies, international organizations, and individual researchers. The glossary provides definitions of social determinants of health and other terms that should be reviewed at the start of this chapter: social determinants of health, social support, social capital, social cohesion, health disparities, health inequalities, and health inequities (Table 21-1). The World Health Organization (WHO) and its recent Commission on the Social Determinants of Health along with governmental agencies have provided

Table 21-1. *Definitions of Social Factor Terminology*

Term	Definition	Reference
Social determinants of health	"The conditions in which people are born, grow, live, work and age, including the health system. These circumstances are shaped by the distribution of money, power and resources at global, national and local levels, which are themselves influenced by policy choices. The social determinants of health are mostly responsible for health inequities—the unfair and avoidable differences in health status seen within and between countries."[2(np)]	WHO[2(np)]
	"The complex, integrated, and overlapping social structures and economic systems that are responsible for most health inequities. These social structures and economic systems include the social environment, physical environment, health services, and structural and societal factors. Social determinants of health are shaped by the distribution of money, power, and resources throughout local communities, nations, and the world."[3(np)]	CSDH[3(np)]
Social cohesion	"A state of affairs concerning both the vertical and the horizontal interactions among members of society as characterized by a set of attitudes and norms that includes trust, a sense of belonging, and the willingness to participate and help, as well as their behavioural manifestations."[4(p290)]	Chan, To, Chan[4(p290)]
Social connectedness	"Refers to an individual's engagement in an interactive web of key relationships, within communities that have particular physical and social structures that are affected by broad economic and political forces."[5(p13)]	MN Department of Health[5(p13)]
Social support	"Social support is a general rubric that encompasses at least 3 distinct types of support: perceived support, enacted support and social integration...Perceived support (also known as functional support) is the subjective judgment that family and friends would provide quality assistance with future stressors. Enacted support reflects the same kinds of assistance just listed, but emphasizes specific supportive actions, whereas perceived support emphasizes the stressed person's judgment that such actions would be provided if needed. Social integration refers to the number or range of different types of social relations, such as marital status, siblings, and membership in organizations such as churches, mosques or temples."[6(np)]	Lakey (NIH)[6(np)]
Social capital	"Fabric of a community and the community pool of human resources available... individual and communal time and energy that is available for such things as community improvement, social networking, civic engagement, personal recreation, and other activities that create social bonds between individuals and groups."[69(np)]	CDC[7(np)]
	"The degree of social cohesion which exists in communities. It refers to the processes between people which establish networks, norms, and social trust, and facilitate coordination and cooperation for mutual benefit...Social capital is created from the myriad of everyday interactions between people, and is embodied in such structures as civic and religious groups; family membership; informal community networks; and in norms of voluntarism, altruism, and trust. The stronger these networks and bonds, the more likely it is that members of a community will cooperate for mutual benefit. In this way social capital creates health, and may enhance the benefits of investments for health."[8(p19)]	WHO[8(p19)]
Health equity	"Attainment of the highest level of health for all people. Achieving health equity requires valuing everyone equally with focused and ongoing societal efforts to address avoidable inequalities, historical and contemporary injustices, and the elimination of health and health care disparities."[9(np)]	DHHS, OMH[9(np)]

(continued)

Table 21-1 (continued). *Definitions of Social Factor Terminology*

Term	Definition	Reference
Health disparities	"A particular type of health difference that is closely linked with social or economic disadvantage. Health disparities adversely affect groups of people who have systematically experienced greater social and/or economic obstacles to health and/or a clean environment based on their racial or ethnic group; religion; socioeconomic status; gender; age; mental health; cognitive, sensory, or physical disability; sexual orientation; geographic location; or other characteristics historically linked to discrimination or exclusion."[9(np)] "Differences in health outcomes and their determinants between segments of the population, as defined by social, demographic, environmental, and geographic attributes."[10(p3)] "Systematic, potentially avoidable differences in health—or in the major socially determined influences on health—between groups of people who have different relative positions in social hierarchies according to wealth, power, or prestige."[11(p181)]	DHHS, OMH[9(np)] Truman et al[10(p3)] Braveman[11(p181)]
Health inequalities	"The huge and remedial differences in health between and within countries"[10(inside cover)] "where systematic differences in health are judged to be avoidable by reasonable action globally and within society they are, quite simply, unjust."[3(p26)] "Is sometimes used interchangeably with the term health disparities, is more often used in the scientific and economic literature to refer to summary measures of population health associated with individual- or group-specific attributes (eg, income, education, or race/ethnicity)."[10(p3)] "Difference in health status or in the distribution of health determinants between different population groups."[12]	Truman et al[10(p3)] CSDH[3(p26)] WHO[12]
Health inequities	"The huge and remedial differences in health between and within countries."[3] "Where systematic differences in health are judged to be avoidable by reasonable action globally and within society they are, quite simply, unjust."[3(p26)] "A subset of health inequalities that are modifiable, associated with social disadvantage, and considered ethically unfair."[10(p3)]	Truman et al[10(p3)] CSDH[3(p26)]

many of the most commonly used definitions of these terms.

Conceptual models and frameworks for the social determinants of health continue to evolve. In this chapter, an adaptation of the conceptual framework of social determinants of health as proposed by the WHO Commission on the Social Determinants of Health will be used (Box 21-5).[13(p5-7)] In this framework, social determinants of health and well-being include both structural determinants and intermediary determinants. The social and political context is the basis for these existing hierarchies. Structural and social determinants consist of the key institutions and systems within the socioeconomic and political context, as well as the structural indicators that are measures of individuals' position within society. These structural and social determinants have been proposed as

the main factors associated with health inequities.[1(p5-7)] Intermediary determinants of health are the individual and life circumstances that are distributed unequally in populations and thus, are also factors that contribute to health inequalities. In this framework, health care is also identified as an intermediary factor because of unequal access and services among some groups.[1(p5-7)] Thus, social determinants of health include not only specific social factors, but also other system and individual factors that occur unequally in populations. Some of these factors are discussed in other chapters of this text. Social support and social capital, 2 primary concepts discussed in this chapter, are represented in this framework. Social support is identified as an intermediary determinant of health, while social capital is placed along both the structural and intermediary dimensions.[13(p5-7)]

BOX 21-5

SOCIAL DETERMINANTS OF HEALTH

Structural and Social Determinants		Intermediary Determinants
Socioeconomic/Political Context	*Structural Indicators*	*Individual Context*
Social Policies	Social Capital	
Culture and Societal Values	Social Cohesion	
Public Policies	Socioeconomic	Social Support / Psychosocial Factors
Microeconomic Policies	Social class	Behaviors / Biological Factors
Governance	Gender / Ethnicity	Material Circumstances
	Education	Health System
	Occupation	
	Income	

Adapted from Solar O, Irwin A. *A Conceptual Framework for Action on the Social Determinants of Health: Social Determinants of Health Discussion Paper 2 (Policy and Practice)*. Geneva, Switzerland: World Health Organization Press; 2010.

Conceptual models differ in their explanation of the underlying factors that contribute to risk for disease.[14] Social determinants of health models propose that social inequalities (eg, unequal distribution of social and economic resources) explain the related factors that in turn influence health. Health disparity models suggest that there are a variety of related social and individual factors that interact and impact health. Multiple stressor models identify specific stressors at the individual and community level and explicitly examine race and discrimination as contributing to health disparities.

Different organizations have proposed concepts for social determinants of health that are used to summarize current knowledge, track trends in populations, and develop action plans for health improvement. *Healthy People 2020* provides the following examples of social determinants: "availability of resources to meet daily needs, such as educational and job opportunities; living wages, or healthful foods; social norms and attitudes, such as discrimination; exposure to crime, violence, and social disorder, such as the presence of trash; social support and social interactions; exposure to mass media and emerging technologies, such as the Internet or cell phones; socioeconomic conditions, such as concentrated poverty; quality schools; transportation options; public safety; and residential segregation."[15(np)] Health Canada proposes 4 foci for research on social determinants of health: community

health (eg, community capacity, resilience, efficiency), social capital, socioeconomic inequality (eg, income, social status), and social cohesion (eg, shared community values, challenges, opportunities).[16]

The Robert Wood Johnson Foundation has focused on social factors for vulnerable populations, particularly as it relates to social policy. It has identified critical social factors of early life experience, education, income, work, housing, community, race and ethnicity, and the economy as the main drivers of health for infant and child health, obesity, and adult chronic conditions. Specific social characteristics are embedded in each these factors.[17]

The social determinants of health are believed to contribute to health access and equalities (or conversely health disparities and health inequalities). Health disparities and health inequalities have been identified as priorities in both national and global health agendas. Three theoretical influences have guided the current thinking on social determinants of health as it relates to health inequalities: psychosocial factors (based on people's perceptions and experiences of their social status), social (production of disease/political and economy of health), and ecosocial (integration of social and biological factors).[13]

Specific social determinants have been identified as target areas related to health disparities and health inequalities. Bioethicists have proposed that justice in health care needs to be modified to include a social paradigm. A social paradigm considers not only the medical explanation related to differences in health but also the social factors that affect risk and may be remedied through social action.[18] For individuals with disabilities, limitations in function have been linked to social gradient or social class; in general, American adults from higher social classes have fewer functional limitations.[19] Marmot summarized the evidence on social determinants of health as related to social gradient, stress, early life, social exclusion, work, unemployment, social support, addiction, food, and transport.[20] For each social determinant of health, specific policy recommendations and target interventions have been proposed. For example, designing community facilities that promote social interaction may provide opportunities for individuals to develop relationships with others, which in turn may improve mental health and support feelings of personal worth.[20,21]

Goals are developed to address the social determinants of health and reduce health inequalities and health disparities. The Commission on Social Determinants of Health Final Report identified 3 principles for action as it relates to social determinants of health and health disparities[3(p2)]:

- Improve conditions of daily life—the circumstances in which people are born, grown, live, work, and age.
- Tackle the inequitable distribution of power, money, and resources—the structural drivers of those conditions of daily life—globally, nationally, and locally.
- Measure the problem, evaluate action, expand the knowledge base, develop a workforce that is trained in the social determinants of health, and raise public awareness about the social determinants of health.

Community action plans have been recommended as one strategy to address social factors that are barriers to performance, participation, and well-being; the tools that are included in these plans help communities identify and develop activities related to health goals and community needs. One such program is CHANGE (Community Health Assessment aNd Group Evaluation), an initiative by the Centers for Disease Control and Prevention, Healthy Communities Program.[22] The National Partnership for Action to End Health Disparities (DHHS) has identified 5 goals that should be adopted by professionals as part of any multifaceted plan: increase awareness (significance, impact, actions), enhance leadership at all levels, improve health care and health outcomes for targeted populations, improve health professionals' cultural and linguistic competency, and improve data collection and dissemination.[23(p4)]

There are beginning efforts to address social determinants of health within occupational therapy, but much more work is needed. Occupational therapy practitioners will want to become more familiar with the current evidence and goals related to social determinants of health and participate on interdisciplinary initiatives to improve health equalities. The AOTA issued a societal statement on health disparities[24] and commissioned a task force to summarize the issues related to health disparities.[25] However, there are still few studies in occupational therapy that examine relevant social factors and their influence on health disparities.[26] The Canadian Association of Occupational Therapy (CAOT) issued a response to the WHO Commission on Social Determinants of Health and stated CAOT "recommends that the Commission consider how occupational rights of individuals and groups—by way of participation in meaningful activity—may be highlighted within the discussion of social determinants of health."[27(p2)]

SOCIAL SUPPORT

Social support is central to individuals as they engage in the complexities of everyday life. Consider how social support makes you feel when a friend or even a stranger expresses comfort and caring—emotional support. There are 3 additional aspects to social support. Informational support is provided when advice and guidance on issues is needed; this support is necessary for recovery and adaptation. There is also tangible support; such support is the provision of material or service such as a loan, transportation, assistance with housing. The last type of social support is the support of belonging. Such support comes from being a part of something and produces a sense of belonging. This classification of social support can be attributed to Thoits[28] and has been written about by many, including Bowlby,[29] McColl and Rosenthal,[30] and Uchino.[31]

Bowlby described the stage theory of adjustment to loss to describe the support needed by people in a variety of situations including the onset of disabilities or chronic illness.[29] He suggested that in a crisis stage emotional support will be the most meaningful, but in the transactional phase informational support is necessary, and in the long-term the individual will need tangible support. Knowing how restricted the time for rehabilitation has become with decreased hospital and rehabilitation stays, occupational therapy practitioners recognize the role of social support in a person's recovery and address the need for emotional, informational, and tangible support in the rehabilitation process with both the client and the family.

The lack of social support contributes to "failure to thrive" in infants, limited social interaction and disrupted interpersonal relations in childhood and adulthood, and actual social isolation in older adulthood. Restricted social interaction causing high levels of social stress and anxiety appear to increase an individual's risk for development of schizophrenia spectrum disorders.[32,33] Recent reports indicate social exclusion causes changes in brain function and may lead to poor decision making and diminished learning ability.[34]

To be effective, social support must be perceived as positive, supportive, helpful, and satisfactory.[35] Studies of persons with stroke and spinal cord injury suggest that support is important to participation and satisfaction,[36,37] but little is known about the degree to which people are satisfied with their support systems.[38] It is acknowledged that cognitive capacity may play a role in determining how satisfied the person is with the social support that is available.[38] Studies show that as time passes, the availability of social support changes even when the condition requires ongoing support.[39]

Society is requiring health professionals to place more and more emphasis on participation. Social support plays a huge role in enabling participation in daily life performance. Community integration requires people to have tangible support such as services, transportation, and resources; information to access community resources and programs; emotional support to achieve personal and work satisfaction; and a sense of belonging in families, groups, and society.[35]

How does an occupational therapy practitioner determine a client's needs for social support? The practitioner elicits the narrative of the client in the PEOP Occupational Therapy Process to determine social supports and needs related to performance, participation, and well-being.

Social support is also central to the work of other health professionals, particularly social work. However, occupational therapy practitioners appreciate that social support is an important environmental factor that influences performance, participation, and well-being, and is an integral part of many of the occupations of individuals, families, organizations, and populations.

SOCIAL CAPITAL

In this section, social capital is discussed as one of the characteristics of communities that influence health and well-being. In so doing, we will start with a definition of the term, discuss explanations from social biology about how the behaviors underlying social capital evolved, and consider evidence that shows a relationship between this social indicator and health, with particular attention given for its relevance to the PEOP Model. We conclude the section with a short review of research on social capital and health, with special attention to the implications of this research for occupational therapy interventions with groups, organizations, communities, and populations.

What Is Social Capital?

Social capital is defined here as the extent to which members of a community or society cooperate and support one another in ways that provide benefits to all. The original concepts underlying social capital originate from the work of the French sociologist Emile Durkheim, who described attributes of social groups from the standpoint of integration, alienation, and anomie.[40] Durkheim's intent was to explain how an individual's ties to society helped to explain that person's mental state or pathological conditions. Modern sociologists, such as Pierre Bourdieu,[41] James Coleman,[42] and more recently Robert Putnam,[43] have resurrected current interest in this social phenomenon through examination of the societal implications of collective perceptions of trust and feelings of connectedness.

In his popular bestseller *Bowling Alone,* and its sequel *Better Together,* Putnam[43-45] described the collapse of the American community, suggesting that a return to the higher levels of social capital of a half century ago requires more emphasis on the value of cooperation, association, and social support within communities. Putnam's writings emphasized that the term *social capital,* which embodies the broader concepts inherent in the more common term *community,* implies a sense of trust, of reciprocal responsibility, and community connectedness and obligation. His thesis clearly asserts that various forms of civic engagement create social capital that becomes a tangible good that benefits both individuals and groups.

For example, when an occupational therapy practitioner volunteers to provide free (pro bono) services, her acts benefit the broader community by making services available to people who otherwise could not afford it. At the same time, her benevolence benefits the practitioner herself, by creating social contacts and helping to establish her reputation as a community-minded professional person. Her acts of goodwill toward the community also serve as an example for others. Research has shown that, when observed, positive social behaviors encourage similar behaviors by others.[46-48] Such altruistic behaviors confer status on those doing them, increasing the possibility of reciprocity or benefits from others in the group at some future point. Putnam asserts that investments in altruistic service and other forms of kindness create environments that are characterized by greater cooperation, mutual support, trust, and institutional effectiveness—collectively creating social capital.[43]

As a sociological concept, social capital has evolved out of the creation of interdependent communities. Although Americans take great pride in the ideas of self-reliance and independence, it is well known that societies, communities, and organizations exist not as a consequence of independence and individual autonomy, but rather as the result of the efficiency and effectiveness resulting from people working together to achieve mutual benefits. Cooperative and altruistic behaviors are more than nice social traditions that evolved with the advancement of modern civilization. Instead, they seem to be genetically encoded and neurally based adaptations of the human species that evolved over time because of their survival benefits.[49-52]

Altruism and Cooperation From the Perspective of Evolutionary Biology

A widely accepted theory of evolutionary psychology asserts that humans came to live in groups because of the survival advantages of doing so for protection and subsistence. Language is thought to have evolved from group living, especially social grooming.[53] The development of language, which evolved from close group interactions, fostered other cooperative behaviors as well as the ideas of trust, reputation, and standing.[52] Individuals exhibited altruistic behavior in support of group welfare.[54] Free riders, or group members who took advantage of altruism, evolved the need for group sanctions, such as loss of group membership or exclusion for those who were uncooperative.[55] Thus, it is readily understandable that today groups work best when there is trust, when there is a mutual or reciprocal sense of obligation, and when the threat of losing group acceptance works to create expectations for social behaviors that support the well-being of everyone.[49,52] These principles seem to apply whether we are describing families, organizations, or communities.

Social Capital of Communities

The creation of social capital comes directly from acts of civility and kindness sponsored not by governments, but by individuals within informal social networks in neighborhoods, communities, and organizations. Social capital results from perceived trust, civic-mindedness, and generosity, and this begins with individuals within their communities.[43] Social capital extends beyond the horizontal connections of bonding within homogenous groups and bridging with others outside one's customary social network, to vertical linking in ways that enable people to access and share power and influence within the established power hierarchies of organizations and political jurisdictions. Sociologist Amatai Etzioni has advocated what he refers to as *communitarian practices*.[56] Similar to other communitarian advocates, Etzioni proposes that a careful balance between an individual's rights and a community member's responsibilities to the greater good will foster greater social capital.[56] This concept underlies definitions of social capital as the reciprocal relationship between civic participation and interpersonal trust.[57(p1000)] The idea expressed in this definition is that an individual's participation with others in the community creates higher levels of trust, which then leads to an increased likelihood of further community participation. Thus, collective individual experiences of increasing trust contribute to the overall state of a community's (or a population's) social capital.[42,43]

Health and Social Capital

Among the beneficial consequences that are theorized to result from social capital are improved economic growth and development, as well as more effective political systems and governance; which presumably lead to safer communities, better educational and health systems, and other features that might strengthen social environments and contribute to a higher quality of life.[58] Naturally, investigators have also been interested in studying how social capital influences measures of physical and mental health.

Many studies of health and social capital have been published, and reviews of these efforts have consistently concluded that they are difficult to summarize. This difficulty stems from the lack of a consensus definition of social capital, which has led to different approaches to measuring the construct and thus a difficulty in grouping and comparing studies.[59] Also, because of the complexity of social capital, which can be viewed from multiple perspectives or levels ranging from the individual to the community, it is difficult to interpret observed associations among variables. For example, socioeconomic status tends to predict educational level in the same way that educational status predicts health status. Communities with higher levels of social capital tend to have better services for education and health care. So if one finds a relationship between social capital and health, is this due to the social networks that explain social capital or to the improved education and socioeconomic circumstances that also result from having higher levels of social capital? These questions are representative of the difficulties inherent in studying and understanding the influence of social capital on health status and outcomes. There are other challenges as well. Halpern[60] has criticized the methodology of some studies based on the probability of uncontrolled sampling biases, which under-represent community members in very poor physical or mental health who may either fail to participate in studies or provide skewed responses that are influenced by their emotional states.

While a number of studies have shown positive and significant associations between measures of social capital and measures of community or population health, there have been few studies that link specific individual behaviors associated with social capital (such as membership in civic organizations, social trust, volunteerism, and sense of belonging) to such measured outcomes. In a review of studies of social capital and self-rated health and mortality, Gilbert noted that studies of social capital are inconsistent in estimating effect sizes and that measures and levels of social capital are so varied that they create difficulties in summarizing results.[61] He concluded that despite these limitations, modest associations do seem to exist between social capital and health, recommending that future studies improve the clarity and consistency of both constructs and measures. Gilbert observed that social capital can be measured at either the individual or ecological (community level), or combine both levels using multi-level analysis.[61]

Various governmental authorities and governmental agencies have commissioned reviews and meta-analyses of studies of social capital and health. These studies are continuously building on previous work to improve the precision of measures, control confounding variables, and reduce sampling bias. However, it appears that when attention is given to improving the conditions that facilitate the participation of individuals in community groups (and when communities promote the creation of bonds, networks, and social support systems through attention to transportation, safe neighborhoods, and community meeting places) trust, volunteerism, reciprocal altruism, and an improved sense of community obligation result. These, in turn, lead to social mobility, civic involvement, improved educational systems, and the other characteristics that collectively define social capital, creating environments with conditions that enable people to thrive and flourish. Intuitively, one would expect such environments to lead to improved measures of population health and greater longevity. Early study findings suggest this is the case, but explaining the specific mechanisms through which this occurs will continue to be studied. The belief in the health promoting characteristics of social capital has resulted in widespread endorsement of the Ottawa Charter for Health Promotion,[62] leading to global efforts to promote healthy cities and communities. Three of the central tenets of the movement are squarely aligned with social capital, including health public policy, supportive environments, and strengthening community.

Implications of Social Capital for the Person-Environment-Occupation-Performance Model

The concept of social capital provides an ideal a way to describe environmental or community characteristics that both foster and enable participation and create conditions that influence health status. Just as the PEOP Model can be applied to individuals, groups, and populations, so too

can social capital be considered from multiple levels, ranging from individuals to organizations and larger communities. The characteristics that lead to higher levels of social capital in one group may be different than those that foster networks, civic participation, and closer bonds in another. Within the PEOP Model, some of the social factors that create social capital may also bear upon the resources that influence participation. Thus, social capital is an important environmental consideration when the PEOP Model is being applied. Further study is needed on how individual engagement and participation resulting from occupational performance provides explanatory power in models of social capital and health.

SOCIAL FACTORS AND THE PERSON-ENVIRONMENT-OCCUPATION-PERFORMANCE OCCUPATIONAL THERAPY PROCESS

Social factors are important in all stages of the PEOP Occupational Therapy Process.[63,64] Narratives, assessments/evaluations, interventions, and outcomes all have a social dimension that influence and are influenced by other person, environment, and occupation factors.

The narrative provides important contextual information and the client's perspective on social factors at play that influence performance, participation, and well-being. The narrative engages clients in thinking about the issues associated with social connectedness and social factors and identifies priorities that may be addressed in supportive environments to help transitions in home, family, and community life. The skilled occupational therapy practitioner's therapeutic use of self elicits a rich narrative that is the foundation for the PEOP Occupational Therapy Process.[63,64]

Obtaining clients' perspectives on social determinants of health, social support, and social capital is relevant, regardless of whether clients are individuals, organizations, or populations. The narrative is typically obtained through interviews, self-reports, and observations of clients. Evidence from qualitative research may also provide background for a narrative that informs the PEOP Occupational Therapy Process. In the 4 hypothetical scenarios introduced at the beginning of the chapter, identify the social factors (social determinants, social support, social capital) that were gathered by an occupational therapy practitioner at the narrative stage (see Boxes 21-1 to 21-4).

ASSESSMENTS AND EVALUATIONS

When the goals of the client (individual, community/population, organization) can be met by interventions within the scope of occupational therapy practice, the practitioner continues the PEOP Occupational Therapy Process by selecting assessments and completing an evaluation to document current capabilities/enablers and constraints/barriers for occupations, person, and environmental factors. The outcome of this stage informs intervention planning. Social factors are inherent in assessments of meaningful occupations, personal characteristics, and the environmental context. For example, the *Activity Card Sort* assessment may be helpful in identifying the lost social activities or occupations for a person who has multiple sclerosis.[65] At the individual, organization, or population level, the *Minimum Data Set* (MDS) assessment may help in the evaluation of preferences for customary routine and activities that are social in nature for residents in Medicare-certified and Medicaid-certified nursing homes.[66]

Assessments and evaluations help occupational therapy practitioners and their clients understand the social factors that influence specific aspects of occupational performance (personal care attendants who help with meal preparation), participation (employers who provide accommodations), and well-being (family/friends who bring joy to major life events). Assessments and evaluations also provide an important mechanism for monitoring differences in performance, participation, and well-being for some groups and documenting progress toward societal goals for eliminating health disparities and health inequalities.

When assessments and evaluation are used to examine health disparities and health inequalities, social factors are incorporated into measures of health and social position, and the evaluation process seeks to understand the relationship between these 2 factors.[11] A comprehensive, national surveillance of healthy equity includes measures of health inequities, health outcomes, and consequences of ill-health (including social consequences) as compared to determinants of health, which include daily living conditions, health behaviors, physical and social environment (including social capital), working conditions, health care, social protection (including coverage and generosity), gender, social inequities (including social exclusion), and sociopolitical context.[3(p182)] Additional dimensions may be considered when measuring social capital, including groups and networks, trust, collective action, social inclusion, and information and communication.[67]

In the PEOP Occupational Therapy Process, the evaluation is a summary of the findings from all of the selected occupation, person, and environment assessments. For occupational therapy practitioners who are still developing their clinical reasoning skills and for complex cases, graphic organizers along a continuum scale may help to visually represent the outcome of assessments used in evaluation; the factors that support and limit occupational performance; and the interplay between occupation, per-

son, and environment. For the hypothetical cases introduced at the beginning of the chapter, the outcome of assessments and evaluation are illustrated in Figures 21-1 to 21-4. After reviewing the figures, complete a written evaluation or give a verbal report to summarize the capabilities/enablers and barriers/constraints for each client.

There are a wide variety of assessments that examine social factors for individuals, populations, and organizations. Some assessments are more standardized and objective, while others are designed to elicit active involvement from diverse communities (eg, Photovoice, community observation/audits, concept mapping, health impact assessment, focus groups).[68] For social capital, measures of sense of community, trust, social support, and networks; organizational partnerships and memberships; and collective efficacy are obtained through surveys and questionnaires. Table 21-2 identifies some assessment tools occupational therapy practitioners may use to structure the collection of information in evaluation and guide the selection of interventions. Specific assessments of social determinants of health, social support, and social capital will be influenced by the conceptual framework for evaluation and clients' goals.

INTERVENTIONS

After the assessment/evaluation stage, the occupational therapy practitioner has information to select interventional approaches and help clients as they work on goals related to performance, participation, and well-being. Intervention approaches that address social determinants of health are more likely to target groups, communities, and populations. Intervention approaches that build social support are more likely to serve clients who are individuals, families, and groups. Intervention approaches to develop social capital may be directed at individuals or communities. For the hypothetical cases presented at the beginning of the chapter, sample intervention approaches are summarized in Figures 21-1 to 21-4.

Social Determinants of Health

Interventions that address social determinants of health often have an underlying goal of eliminating health disparities and health inequalities. Although occupational therapy is just beginning to engage in major public health and population health initiatives related to social determinants of health, there are numerous examples of occupational therapy practitioners from the past and today who have made it their personal mission to work with disadvantaged populations. The interventions used in population health and public health are selected to be cost-efficient, reach larger groups of people, and coordinated by

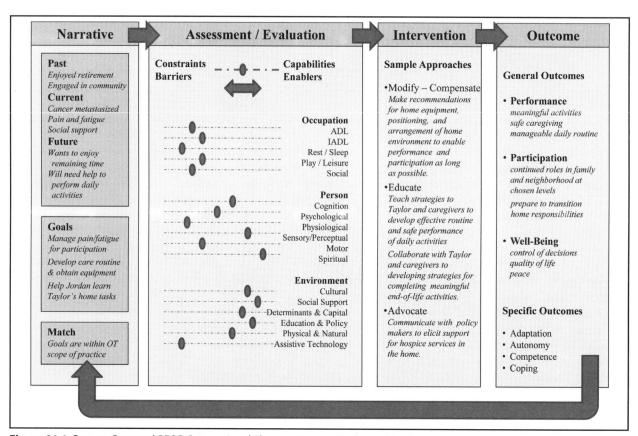

Figure 21-1. Person-Centered PEOP Occupational Therapy Process: Taylor and Jordan.

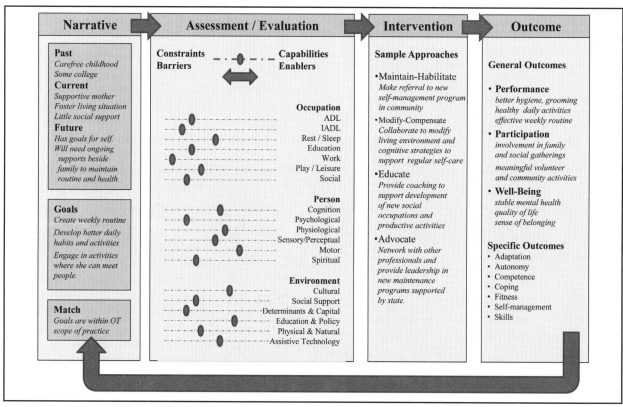

Figure 21-2. Person-Centered PEOP Occupational Therapy Process: Jenny.

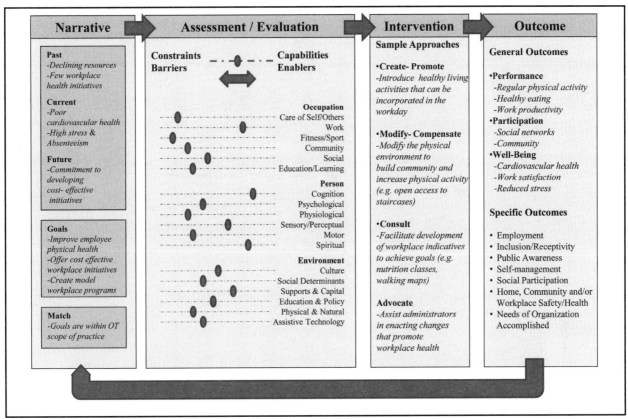

Figure 21-3. Organization-Centered PEOP Occupational Therapy Process: State Agency.

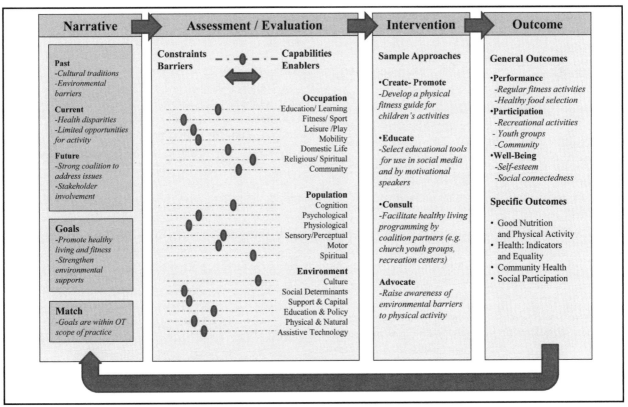

Figure 21-4. Population-Centered PEOP Occupational Therapy Process: Obesity.

Table 21-2. *Assessments for Social Factors*

Title of Assessment	Construct or Factor Assessed	Description	Reference/Source
Social Determinants of Health			
American Community Survey	Population: Basic, social, economic; Housing: Financial, physical, economic	Annual United States survey; sampling of about 1 in 38 United States households each year	http://www.census. gov/acs/www/[69]
Behavioral Risk Factor Surveillance System	Risk behaviors and events, chronic health conditions, use of preventive services (national and state level data)	Annual United States health-related interviews; sample of more than 400,000 adults	http://www.cdc. gov/brfss/[70]
ENACT, THRIVE (Prevention Institute)	Community-level characteristics that have been found to be important for strong communities	Community-level inventories of social determinants of health and related strategies to address barriers	http://prevention-institute.org/tools. html[71]
Kids Count Data Center (Annie E. Casey Foundation)	Well-being of children in the United States (national and state level data)	Provides population-based data for the United States and by state for demographics, economic well-being, education, family and community, health, safety, and risky behaviors	http://datacenter. kidscount.org/[72]
CHANGE: Community Health Assessment and Group Evaluation	Assets and limitations of community institutions/organizations, health care, schools, and work-site sectors as they relate to an assessment of community health at large.	Data may be collected using observation, survey, focus groups, walkability audits, and Photovoice	http://www.cdc. gov/healthycom-munitiesprogram/ tools/change/ downloads.htm[22]
Social Support			
Social Support Questionnaire (SSQ)	Availability and satisfaction with social support	27-item self-administered scale; 6-point rating scale; overall support score (SSQN) calculated; established criterion validity, inter-item correlation, internal consistency, test-retest reliability	Sarason et al[73,74]
Interpersonal Support Evaluation List (ISEL)	Perceived availability of potential social resources	20-item scale; 4 support subscales: tangible, belonging, self-esteem, appraisal	Cohen and Hoberman[75]
Social Relationship Scale	Extent of a network of social relationships and perceived helpfulness of these relationships on the life stresses and health	6 items representing work, monetary and finances, home and family, personal health, personal and social, and society in general	McFarlane et al[76]
Berkman-Syme Social Network Index (SNI)	Type, size, closeness, and frequency of contacts in the current social network	11 items; self-reported questionnaire; published predictive validity	Berkman and Syme[77]

(continued)

Table 21-2 (continued). *Assessments for Social Factors*

Title of Assessment	Construct or Factor Assessed	Description	Reference/Source
The Inventory of Socially Supportive Behaviors (ISSB)	Frequency of received social support in the last month	40 items; 5-point Likert scale	Barrera and Ainlay[78]
Social Capital			
Social Capital Assessment Tool (SOCAT)	Social capital data on households, communities, and organizations	Qualitative/quantitative; includes both structural and cognitive components at the household level	The World Bank Group[79]
Social Capital Integrated Questionnaire (SOCAP IQ)	Social capital for 6 dimensions: groups and networks, trust and solidarity, collective action and cooperation, information and communication, social cohesion and inclusion, empowerment and political action	Quantitative; part of a larger household survey; focused on developing countries	The World Bank Group[79]
Inequality			
Disability Adjusted Life Year (DALY)	Population measure of the burden of disease	DALY = YLL + YLD, where YLL is years of life lost due to premature death and YLD is years of life lost due to disability	WHO[80]
Gini Index	Individual or group measure of inequality (eg, income, premature mortality)	Relative difference in individuals or groups on a theoretical scale from 1 to 0 (1 = perfect or maximum inequality, 0 = perfect equality)	Truman et al (CDC)[10]
HALex	Individual measure of health-related QOL	Measures self-rated health and activity limitation in national surveys on a theoretical scale from 0 to 1 (1 = no activity limitation; excellent health, 0.10 = limited in activities and health)	Truman et al (CDC)[10]
Healthy days	Group measure of the number of healthy days (physical and mental health) in last 30 days	Estimated by the BRFSS; comparisons by state, income levels, and other population groups	Truman et al (CDC)[10]

interdisciplinary teams. Thus, prevention, education, consultation, and advocacy are intervention approaches that are commonly used to address social determinants of health. Specific examples of interventions for social determinants of health are summarized in Table 21-3 and include consciousness raising, community development, social action, health promotion, media advocacy, and policy and environmental change.[68] There are growing examples of evidence-based health and social interventions that may be applicable to occupational therapy and are designed to address social determinants of health.[68,81,82]

- *Health:* Free/accessible care, community health workers, home visits, professional-family partnership programs, health incentives

Table 21-3. Social Determinants of Health: Intervention Approaches

Specific Approach/ Occupational Therapy Approach	Definition	Uses/Applications	Professional Role
• Consciousness raising • Educate • Consult • Advocate	"A process through which people come together to discuss the relationship between individual or group experiences or concerns and the social or structural factors that influence them."68(p59)	Ensures "both "insiders" and "outsiders" develop a common understanding of issues and concerns, stimulating discussion and motivating partners to address the issues and concerns."68(p59) To help: • Group members understand how social and structural factors influence health. • Identify specific factors that influence current inequities and develop plans for change. • Partners frame issues to bring groups together for action	Professionals may facilitate discussion by: • Sharing experiences or responses to images of issue • Presenting hypothetical vignettes • Readings • Critical reflection: What is happening? Why is it happening?
• Community development or locality development • Consult • Educate	"A set of processes or efforts to create community change at the local level through strengthening social ties, increasing awareness of issues affecting the community, and enhancing community member participation in addressing these issues."68(p61)	To develop: • New partnerships or transition existing partnership to new initiative • Shared group identity • Motivation for action	Professionals may provide: • Community members with opportunities for leadership • Support to community leaders on conducting meetings, problem solving, consensus building/conflict resolution
• Social action • Consult • Educate	"An approach that focuses on altering social relationships or resources" and may include "activities that explicitly highlight an issue."68(p64)	To increase: • Awareness of issues • Community participation • Commitment at beginning of change initiative	Professionals may: • Provide information and data • Identify target audiences • Help frame the message

(continued)

Table 21-3 (continued). Social Determinants of Health: Intervention Approaches

Specific Approach/ Occupational Therapy Approach	Definition	Uses / Applications	Professional Role
• Health promotion • Prevent • Modify-compensate	"Activities designed to help people improve their health or prevent illness through changes in environments, lifestyle, and behavior."68(p65)	To develop initiatives that: • Address social determinants of health that support behavior change • Target social ties, physical/built environment, availability of resources, partner organizations, cultural competency, participatory approaches • Are promotional, informational, skill-based • Directed toward organizational, policy, or environmental changes	Professionals may: • Select interventions that address knowledge, skills, attitudes, behaviors • Address need for change at individual, social, organizational, community, and governmental levels
• Media advocacy • Educate • Advocate	"Strategic use of media coverage to encourage social, economic, or environmental change."68(p67)	To increase: • Public understanding of issues and their contributing social, economic, environmental conditions	Professionals may facilitate: • Development/review of mission and vision and related goals and objectives • Selection of audience and invitation of media representatives • Development of message • Selection of media outlet
• Policy and environmental change • Advocate • Consult • Modify-Compensate	"A plan or course of action intended to influence and determine decisions, actions, and rules or regulations that govern our collective daily life."68(p70)	To promote: • Creation or change in policies or environments to address social determinants of health	Professionals may: • Serve as researchers or active players in policy/environment work along with partners • Guide definition of the problem and unite concerned groups

Box 21-6

MESSAGES THAT EXPLAIN HOW SOCIAL DETERMINANTS OF HEALTH INFLUENCE PERFORMANCE, PARTICIPATION, AND WELL-BEING

- Health begins where we live, learn, work, and play.
- Health starts long before illness—in our homes, schools, and jobs.
- All Americans should have the opportunity to make the choices that allow them to live a long, healthy life, regardless of their income, education, or ethnic background.
- Your neighborhood or job shouldn't be hazardous to your health.
- Your opportunity for health starts long before you need medical care.
- The opportunity for health begins in our families, neighborhoods, schools, and jobs.

Copyright 2010 Robert Wood Johnson Foundation.

- *Community:* Services and resources, partnership building, environmental modification, participatory action research, activities, additional income, housing support, community treatments, neighborhood improvement projects
- *Education:* Health education, popular education, media campaigns, early childhood, academic enrichment, school-based programs
- *Political:* Workplace policies/practices, political action training, building common knowledge/language, policy recommendations, monitoring public agendas
- *Social Support:* Social support groups, story circles, work capacity building, case management

Many intervention approaches for social determinants of health are targeted for the community. The University of Kansas Community Tool Box provides a variety of resources for initiatives that promote community health and well-being.[83] For example, one section describes the importance of creating "good places for interaction" to promote social support, social capital, and equity. The characteristics of environments that support social interaction provide reasons to go there, reasons to stay there, safety and comfort, accessibility, and a welcoming feel.

Communication is an important principle, particularly for occupational therapy interventions that address social determinants of health. The terminology and language chosen for different clients is critical for achieving goals related to social factors. This is particularly true when working with clients representing different political persuasions and world views. The Robert Wood Johnson Foundation (RWJF) conducted seminal work on social determinants of health and how to talk about them with different groups.[84] In their research, they identified 7 lessons that guided development of the eventual messages describing beliefs about social determinants of health:

1. Academic phrases like social determinants of health or social factors do not resonate with most audiences
2. Messages should be framed in everyday, values-based, expressive language
3. Messages should consist of 1 key fact that is compelling
4. Potential solutions should communicated along with the problems
5. Personal responsibility to make healthy choices should be included in messages
6. Conservative and progressive values should be incorporated into messages
7. Focus primarily on how factors affect all individuals rather than specific groups

Through an iterative process, the RWJF proposed 6 messages that helped audiences understand issues related to social determinants of health (Box 21-6).

Social Support

In occupational therapy interventions, goals may be developed to help the client put social supports in place that will offer tangible, information, and emotional and belonging support that will be essential to achieve community participation. Social support is just one of the environmental factors that must be considered to improve a client's performance, participation, and well-being. It may be that a person will benefit from an attendant, such a person will provide tangible support that will allow the person to have assistance with their basic daily activities so they have time to spend in their other roles. If the client wants to explore what an attendant could offer, a first step may be to link the client with the local independent living center to learn how an attendant may help them achieve their goals. This process itself would classify as a social support strategy, as the occupational therapy practitioner is providing informational support.

Another form of social support is helping the client develop the skills to manage their health and conditions that may be secondary to their condition. Self-management programs are one example of an intervention that provides tangible, informational, and emotional support. An occupational therapy practitioner may offer social support by creating opportunities for the client to receive emotional support early in their recovery; such support will help the client gain a sense of belonging. Activities during a rehabilitation stay may be structured to involve friends and family. The goal would be to enable successful experiences that would re-engage clients with friends and their social network (eg, a sports team, a church group, or a bridge club). An activity as simple as preparing a meal, watching videos, or visiting with a pet may offer a sense of belonging. Some practitioners create opportunities for socialization that involves only the therapy staff. Although this may provide some level of support, professionals will not be there for clients once they go home—social events should involve clients' own social network to begin to reestablish relationships for when they do go home.

Social Capital

The creation of social capital comes directly from acts of civility and kindness sponsored not by governments or programs, but by individuals within informal social networks in neighborhoods, communities, and organizations. Social capital results from perceived trust, civic-mindedness, and generosity, and this begins with individuals within their communities. Nonetheless, many of the same intervention approaches designed to address social determinants of health and social support indirectly facilitate social capital. Strategies to increase social capital may be described as part of capacity building, community capacity building, or community development initiatives.

Communities develop a sense of commitment and emotional support in times of need as members generate shared beliefs, traditions, and goals through communal activities. Feeling safe and supported by a group engenders feelings of loyalty and attachment. McMillan and Chavis describe 4 ways in which group members generate a "psychological sense of community."[85] This occurs by creating a sense of belonging, through fulfillment of member needs,

by providing influence, and by offering shared connections.[85] These kinds of community-enhancing activities seem more likely to occur if a general climate of trust, friendliness, and goodwill is present.

Social capital is also created through community cooperation and interdependence. This is exemplified in collective efforts to build physical structures—either for the community at-large or for individuals, as occurs in well-known volunteer enterprises such as Habitat for Humanity.[86] In rural communities, social capital is developed through cooperative endeavors such as barn-raisings, furnishing meals for families undergoing adversity, or even through collective work efforts to plant or harvest crops for farm families experiencing adversity.

RESOURCES

Social factors are receiving increased attention as important components of many health initiatives. A variety of organizations have developed resources that may be used in learning activities and as part of public awareness campaigns to increase understanding of the influence of social factors on health. These resources are valuable to occupational therapy practitioners who want to address those social factors that support performance, participation, and well-being. Tables 21-4 and 21-5 provide information on readily available resources on social factors that influence health and evidence from recent research.

SUMMARY

This chapter introduced social determinants of health, social support, and social capital as important environmental factors in the PEOP Model. These factors have received increased emphasis in research and programs that target the health of communities and populations. Four case studies were used to illustrate how social factors are evaluated and addressed within the PEOP Occupational Therapy Process. Interdisciplinary assessments and interventions were identified and framed within an occupational therapy context. There are many opportunities to address social factors as a means to improve performance, participation, and well-being.

Table 21-4. *Organizations That Focus on Social Factors and Performance, Participation, and Well-Being*

Organization or Journal	Description	Web Address
Blue Cross Foundation	Social determinants are one of the priority areas for this foundation. The website provides information on research, resources, and community initiatives.	http://www.bcbs-mnfoundation.org/
Centers for Disease Control and Prevention	The CDC provides information on resources, publications, and definitions for professionals who are interested in the social determinants of health.	http://www.cdc.gov/socialdeterminants/
Healthy People 2020	Social determinants are one of the *Healthy People 2020* leading health indicator topics. The website provides an overview of social determinants, discusses determinants for different life stages, and summarizes latest tracking data.	http://www.healthy-people.gov/2020/LHI/socialDetermi-nants.aspx
Prevention Institute	Nonprofit organization focused on health and social equity, prevention, and community initiatives. Has developed assessments and interventions for the community level.	http://www.prevention institute.org/
Robert Wood Johnson Foundation	The Foundation has a mission to "improve the health and health care of all Americans." The website has a variety of resources related to social determinants of health.	http://www.rwjf.org/en.html
University College London	The Institute of Health Equity provides resources and research on a variety of programs that address social determinants of health, and other factors that contribute to health inequities.	http://www.institu-teofhealthequity.org/
UNICEF	Organization monitors maternal and child health and well-being through data collection and analysis, development of methods and indicators, and publications.	http://www.child-info.org/
Unnatural Causes	A 7-part documentary that introduces viewers to the "racial and socioeconomic inequalities in health." The website includes video clips, action toolkits, and resources related to social determinants of health.	http://www.unnatu-ralcauses.org/
The World Bank	Website provides information and resources on theories of social capital, measures, and a framework for implementing social capital into its operations. The website contains resources and publications.	http://go.worldbank.org/C0QTRW4QF0
The World Health Organization	Organization has targeted social determinants of health as one of its programs and provides information on evidence, actions, global commitments, publications, and learning opportunities.	http://www.who.int/social_determinants/en/

Table 21-5. Evidence Table of Studies Exploring the Relationships of Social Factors to Performance, Participation, or Well-Being

Ref	Aim of Study	Methods	Participants	Results and Outcomes	Conclusions and Implications	Level or Type of Evidence
87	Determine whether socioeconomic status is associated with treatment and mortality	Secondary analyses of treatment records, vital statistics data, and median neighborhood income by quintiles	38,945 stroke patients admitted to Ontario hospitals	There were differences in occupational therapy services by income level, with 36% of patients in lowest quintile and 47% of patients in highest quintile receiving therapy	There were differences in occupational therapy services by income even when occupational therapy was part of a universal health insurance system; additional research is needed	Cross-sectional
88	Examine relationships between social, productive, and physical activity in mortality	Sociodemographics; social, productive, and fitness activities; and health status were collected by structured interview	2761 individuals aged 65 and older; residents of CT. Data collected in annual telephone interviews	Survival rates were similar for social and productive activities as compared to fitness activities	Social and productive activities were as effective as fitness activities in decreasing risk of mortality; social activities may increase quality and length of life	Prospective cohort study
89	Determine effectiveness of health promotion interventions to address social isolation and loneliness in older people	30 studies were identified and classified by type of intervention (group activities, individual, service provision, community development); most were conducted in North America	16/30 were RCTs; participants were older adults who received intervention to prevent social isolation	9/10 effective interventions were group-based activities; 6/8 ineffective interventions were the other types of approaches	Health promotion group activities for older adults may be effective in addressing social isolation and loneliness	Systematic review
90	Define participation and meaning from perspective of individuals with disabilities	Focus groups	63 individuals with various disabilities; multi-site	Participation consisted of active and meaningful engagement; feeling part of, having choice, access, opportunity and control; entails responsibilities and impact, providing social support, social connectedness inclusion and membership	Definitions of participation from the perspectives of individuals with disabilities emphasizes the social factors that are inherent in participation; consideration of social factors should be considered in providing services to increase participation	Qualitative studies

(continued)

Table 21-5 (continued).   Evidence Table of Studies Exploring the Relationships of Social Factors to Performance, Participation, or Well-Being

Ref	Aim of Study	Methods	Participants	Results and Outcomes	Conclusions and Implications	Level or Type of Evidence
91	Examine relationship between social factors and well-being, health, and happiness	Secondary analyses of data from World Values Survey, US Benchmark Survey	Large national and international samples	Social capital and social support (family, friends, neighbors, colleagues, community members) are associated with health, happiness, life satisfaction, and well-being	Conclusions about causation are not possible with this research design; however, occupational opportunities that promote social connections may contribute to improved well-being.	Cross-sectional study
92	Examine the association between socioeconomic status, social network, competence, and subjective well-being for older adults	Meta-analysis of 286 correlational studies. Measures included: socioeconomic status (education, income), social network (quantitative/qualitative), subjective well-being (life satisfaction, happiness, self-esteem)	All studies included some participants who were 60+ years old	Older adults who report greater life satisfaction, self-esteem, and happiness tend to have greater socioeconomic status, social networks, and competence. There are age and gender differences in these trends.	Conclusions about causation are not possible with this research design. However, this study demonstrates relationships among subjective well-being, socioeconomic status, social factors, and competence that provide support for greater consideration of social factors in occupational therapy programs.	Meta-analysis
93	Examine whether chronic illness, social factors, and socioeconomic status predict quality of life	Secondary analysis of English longitudinal study of aging (ELSA); multiple regression of survey data	N = 11,234 older English adults who were non-institutionalized	All variables were statistically significant predictors of quality of life. Negative impact: poor finances, depression, performance limitations; positive impact: good neighborhood, trusting relationships, affluence	Prediction of quality of life for older adults requires consideration of social and contextual factors in addition to performance factors	Longitudinal descriptive study

(continued)

Table 21-5 (continued).   Evidence Table of Studies Exploring the Relationships of Social Factors to Performance, Participation, or Well-Being

Ref	Aim of Study	Methods	Participants	Results and Outcomes	Conclusions and Implications	Level or Type of Evidence
94	Examine the relationship between neighborhood characteristics and community and social engagement (ie, social capital)	Survey data; independent variable: walkability rating. Dependent measures of social capital: knowing neighbors, political participation, trust in other people, social participation Multivariate logit models	279 households living in 3 types of walkability (most to least) in neighborhoods in Ireland: city center, mixed use, suburban	The higher the neighborhood walkability, the higher all measures of social capital	Occupational therapists who recommend environmental modifications should consider neighborhood-level improvements that may increase social capital and social participation.	Cross-sectional survey
26	Examine how income/poverty status and race/ethnicity are associated with specific person-environment-occupation characteristics	Survey data available from US Census and National Center for Health Statistics. Variables: race/ethnicity, income levels, social, economic, housing, health and disability status, family, health care, community characteristics	United States citizens. Data from 2001 to 2006 available through governmental sources. Sample size varied by data source	There is evidence of health disparities for children and adults by income levels and race/ethnicity for "health and behavioral characteristics, activity profiles, home and work environments, experiences in health systems, and outcomes of health care services."	There are opportunities relevant for occupational therapy to address social determinants of health and other factors influencing health disparities.	Cross-sectional surveys
95	Identify significant predictors of community participation and social and home participation after rehabilitation	Personal interviews collected at baseline, 1, 6, 12 months post-discharge. Data collected on demographic variables, impairments, cognitive status, severity of illness, social support, persistence, activity, participation. Linear mixed model, latent growth model.	435 adults from 2 rehabilitation hospitals in the Boston, MA area. Participants had a diagnosis of neurologic disorder, lower extremity orthopedic trauma or other complex condition	Community participation: social support had a positive association at 6 and 12 months post-discharge Social and home participation: social support had a positive association at 1, 6, and 12 months post-discharge	Social support is an important domain in rehabilitation that is predictive of post-discharge community, social, and home participation. Occupational therapy should consider this person factor in the PEOP Occupational Therapy Process.	Longitudinal cohort design

REFERENCES

1. World Health Organization. *Global Strategy on Diet, Physical Activity, and Health: Childhood Overweight and Obesity.* World Health Organization. http://www.who.int/dietphysicalactivity/childhood/en/. Updated 2014. Accessed March 23, 2014.

2. WHO. *Social Determinants Of Health.* WHO. http://www.who.int/social_determinants/en/. Updated 2014. Accessed March 23, 2014.

3. Commission on Social Determinants of Health (CSDH). *Closing the Gap in a Generation: Health Equity through Action on the Social Determinants of Health: Final Report of the Commission on Social Determinants of Health.* Geneva, Switzerland: World Health Organization; 2008.

4. Chan J, To HP, Chan E. Reconsidering social cohesion: developing a definition and analytical framework for empirical research. *Social Indicators Research.* 2006;75(2):273-302.

5. Minnesota Department of Health: Community and Family Health Division: Office of Public Health Practice. *Social Connectedness Evaluating the Healthy People 2020 Framework: The Minnesota Project.* St. Paul, MN; Minnesota Department of Health; 2010. http://www.health.state.mn.us/divs/opi/resources/db/docs/1007socialconnectedness_report.pdf. Published July 2010. Accessed March 23, 2014.

6. Lakey, B. *Social support.* US National Institutes of Health: National Cancer Institute. http://dccps.cancer.gov/brp/constructs/social_support/index.html. Accessed March 23, 2014.

7. US Centers for Disease Control and Prevention. *Healthy Places: Social Capital.* US Centers for Disease Control and Prevention. http://www.cdc.gov/healthyplaces/healthtopics/social.htm. Updated February 14, 2013. Accessed March 23, 2014.

8. WHO. *Health Promotion Glossary.* Geneva, Switzerland: WHO; 1998. http://www.who.int/healthpromotion/about/HPR%20Glossary%201998.pdf?ua=1. Published 1998. Accessed March 31, 2014.

9. US Department of Health and Human Services: National Partnership to End Health Disparities. *Health Equity and Disparities.* US Department of Health and Human Services. http://www.minorityhealth.hhs.gov/npa/templates/browse.aspx?lvl=1&lvlid=34. Updated March 4, 2011. Accessed March 23, 2014.

10. Truman BI, Smith CK, Roy K, et al. Rationale for regular reporting on health disparities and inequalities—United States. *MMWR Surveillance Summaries.* 2011;60(Suppl):3-10.

11. Braveman P. Health disparities and health equity: concepts and measurement. *Annual Review of Public Health.* 2006;27:167-194.

12. World Health Organization. *Health Impact Assessment (HIA): Glossary of Terms Used.* World Health Organization. http://www.who.int/hia/about/glos/en/index1.html. Updated 2014. Accessed March 31, 2014.

13. Solar O, Irwin A. *A Conceptual Framework for Action on the Social Determinants of Health: Social Determinants of Health Discussion Paper 2 (Policy and Practice).* Geneva, Switzerland: World Health Organization Press; 2010.

14. Linder SH, Sexton K. Conceptual models for cumulative risk assessment. *American Journal of Public Health.* 2011;101(Suppl 1):S74-S84.

15. US Department of Health and Human Services. *HealthyPeople.gov.* HealthyPeople.gov. http://www.healthypeople.gov/2020/default.aspx. Updated August 28, 2013. Accessed March 23, 2014.

16. Health Canada. *Social Capital as a Health Determinant: How is it Defined?* Health Canada: Policy Research Communications Unit, Minister of Public Works, Government Services Canada; 2003. http://publications.gc.ca/collections/Collection/H13-5-02-7E.pdf. Published March 2003. Accessed March 23, 2014.

17. Robert Wood Johnson Foundation: Commission to Build a Healthier America. *What Drives Health.* Robert Wood Johnson Foundation. http://www.commissiononhealth.org/whatdriveshealth.aspx. Updated 2014. Accessed March 23, 2014.

18. Jecker NS. A broader view of justice. *American Journal of Bioethics.* 2008;8(10):2-10.

19. Minkler M, Fuller-Thomson E, Guralnik JM. Gradient of disability across the socioeconomic spectrum in the United States. *New England Journal of Medicine.* 2006;355 (7):695-703.

20. Marmot M. Social determinants of health inequalities. *Lancet.* 2005;365(9464):1099-1104.

21. Wilkinson RG, Marmot MG. *Social Determinants of Health: the Solid Facts.* Geneva, Switzerland: World Health Organization Press; 2003.

22. US Centers for Disease Control and Prevention. *Community Health Assessment and Group Evaluation (CHANGE) Action Guide: Building a Foundation of Knowledge to Prioritize Community Needs.* Atlanta, GA: US Department of Health and Human Services; 2010. http://www.cdc.gov/nccdphp/dch/programs/healthycommunitiesprogram/tools/change/pdf/changeactionguide.pdf. Published April 2010. Accessed March 23, 2014.

23. National Partnership for Action to End Health Disparities. *National Stakeholder Strategy for Achieving Health Equity.* Rockville, MD: US Department of Health & Human Services, Office of Minority Health; 2011.

24. Braveman B. AOTA's statement on health disparities. *American Journal of Occupational Therapy.* 2006;60(6):679.

25. Bass Haugen J, Blakeney A, Dunbar S, Opacich K, Abreu B, Jackson L. *AOTA Board Task Force on Health Disparities Report.* Bethesda, MD: AOTA; 2005.

26. Bass Haugen J. Health disparities: examination of evidence relevant for occupational therapy. *American Journal of Occupational Therapy.* 2009;63(1):24-34.

27. CAOT. *Response to the World Health Organization's Commission on Social Determinants of Health Final Report from the Canadian Association of Occupational Therapists.* CAOT. http://www.caot.ca/pdfs/CAOT_WHO_Response_EN.pdf.pdf. Published December, 31, 2008. Accessed on March 23, 2014.

28. Thoits PA. Conceptual, methodological, and theoretical problems in studying social support as a buffer against life stress. *Journal of Health and Social Behavior.* 1982;23:145-159.

29. Bowlby J. *Attachment and Loss: Loss, Sadness and Depression.* Vol. 3. New York, NY: Basic; 1980.

30. McColl MA, Rosenthal C. A model of resource needs of aging spinal cord injured men. *Spinal Cord.* 1994;32:261-270.

31. Uchino BN. *Social Support and Physical Health: Understanding the Health Consequences of our Relationships.* New Haven, CT: Yale University Press; 2004.

32. Thornicroft G, Norman S. The course and outcome of depression in different cultures: 10-year follow-up of the WHO Collaborative Study on the Assessment of Depressive Disorders. *Psychological Medicine.* 1993;23(4):1023-1032.

33. Verdoux H, Os JV. Psychotic symptoms in non-clinical populations and the continuum of psychosis. *Schizophrenia Research.* 2002;54(1):59-65.

34. D'Zurilla TJ, Nezu, AM Development and preliminary evaluation of the Social Problem-Solving Inventory. *Psychological Assessment: A Journal of Consulting and Clinical Psychology.* 1990;2(2):156-163.

35. McColl MA. Social support and occupational therapy. In: Christiansen C, Baum C, eds. *Occupational Therapy: Overcoming Human Performance Deficits.* Thorofare, NJ: SLACK Incorporated; 1997:411-425.

36. McColl MA, Friedland J. Development of a multidimensional index for assessing social support in rehabilitation. *Occupational Therapy Journal of Research.* 1989;9(4):218-234.

37. McColl MA, Skinner H. Assessing inter-and intrapersonal resources: social support and coping among adults with a disability. *Disability and Rehabilitation.* 1995;17(1):24-34.

38. Kinsella G, Ford B, Moran C. Survival of social relationships following head injury. *Disability and Rehabilitation.* 1989;11(1):9-14.

39. Cohen S, Syme S. *Social Support and Health.* San Diego, CA: Academic Press; 1985.

40. Durkheim, E. *Suicide: A Study in Sociology* (1897). Spaulding JA, Simpson G, trans. Glencoe, IL: Free Press; 1951.

41. Bourdieu P. The social space and the genesis of groups. *Theory and Society.* 1985;14(6):723-744.

42. Coleman JS. Social capital in the creation of human capital. *American Journal of Sociology.* 1988;94:95-120.

43. Putnam R. *Bowling Alone.* New York, NY: Simon and Schuster; 2000.

44. Putnam RD. Bowling alone: America's declining social capital. *Journal of Democracy.* 1995;6:65-78.

45. Putnam RD. *Better Together: Restoring the American Community.* New York, NY: Simon and Schuster; 2004.

46. George JM. State or trait: effects of positive mood on prosocial behaviors at work. *Journal of Applied Psychology.* 1991;76(2):299-307.

47. Phenice LA, Griffore RJ, Lee K. Altruism in public: holding open doors for those who follow. *European Journal of Social Sciences.* 2010;16(1):7-10.

48. Schwartz SH. Normative influences on altruism. *Advances in Experimental Social Psychology.* 1977;10:221-279.

49. Bateson P. The biological evolution of cooperation and trust. In: Gambetta D, ed. *Trust: Making and Breaking Cooperative Relations.* New York, NY: Basil Blackwell; 1988:14-30.

50. Fehr E, Rockenbach B. Human altruism: economic, neural, and evolutionary perspectives. *Current Opinion in Neurobiology.* 2004;14:784-790.

51. Rilling JK, Gutman DA, Zeh, TR, Pagnoni G, Berns, GS, Kilts, CD. A neural basis for social cooperation. *Neuron.* 2002;35:395-405.

52. Trivers RL. The evolution of reciprocal altruism. *Quarterly Review of Biology.* 1971;46:35-57.

53. Dawkins R. *The Selfish Gene.* 2nd ed. Oxford: Oxford University Press; 1989.

54. Hamilton WD. The evolution of altruistic behavior. *The American Naturalist.* 1963;97(896):354-356.

55. Kropotkin P. *Mutual Aid: A Factor in Evolution.* Montreal, QC: Black Rose Books; 1989.

56. Etzioni A. *The Spirit of Community: Rights, Responsibilities and the Communitarian Agenda.* New York, NY: Crown; 1993.

57. Brehm J, Rahn W. Individual-level evidence for the causes and consequences of social capital. *American Journal of Political Science.* 1997;41(3):999-1024.

58. Helliwell JF. How's life? Combining individual and national variables to explain subjective well-being. *Economic Modelling.* 2003;20(2):331-360.

59. Cullen M, Whiteford H. *The Interrelations of Social Capital with Health and Mental Health.* Canberra, Australia: Government of Australia; 2001.

60. Halpern D. *Social Capital.* Cambridge, MA: Polity Press; 2005.

61. Gilbert KL. *A Meta-analysis of Social Capital and Health. Unpublished Doctoral Dissertation.* Pittsburgh, PA: University of Pittsburgh; 2009.

62. World Health Organization, Health and Welfare Canada, Canadian Public Health Association. *Ottawa Charter for Health Promotion.* Ottawa, ON: World Health Organization; 1986.

63. Baum CM, Christiansen CH, Bass JD. The Person-Environment-Occupational-Performance (PEOP) Model. In: Christiansen CH, Baum CM, Bass JD, eds. *Occupational Therapy: Performance, Participation, and Well-Being.* 4th ed. Thorofare, NJ: SLACK Incorporated; 2015.

64. Bass JD, Baum CM, Christiansen CH. Interventions and Outcomes of OT: PEOP Occupational Therapy Process. In: Christiansen CH, Baum CM, Bass JD, eds. In: *Occupational Therapy: Performance, Participation, and Well-Being.* 4th ed. Thorofare: SLACK Incorporated; 2015.

65. Baum CM, Edwards D. *ACS: Activity Card Sort.* Bethesda, MD: AOTA Press; 2008.

66. US Department of Health and Human Services, Centers for Medicare and Medicaid Services. *Minimum Data Set 3.0 Public Reports.* CMS.gov: Centers for Medicare and Medicaid Services. http://www.cms.gov/Research-Statistics-Data-and-Systems/Computer-Data-and-Systems/Minimum-Data-Set-3-0-Public-Reports/index.html. Updated November 14, 2012. Accessed March 23, 2014.

67. The World Bank Group. *Measuring Social Capital.* The World Bank. http://go.worldbank.org/A77F30UIX0. Updated 2011. Accessed March 23, 2014.

68. Brennan Ramirez LK, Baker EA, Metzler M. *Promoting Health Equity: A Resource to Help Communities Address Social Determinants of Health.* Atlanta, GA: US Department of Health and Human Services, Centers for Disease Control and Prevention; 2008.

69. US Department of Commerce, US Census Bureau. *American Community Survey.* United States Census Bureau. http://www.census.gov/acs/www/. Published 2012. Updated March 6, 2014. Accessed March 23, 2014.

70. US Centers for Disease Control and Prevention. *Behavioral Risk Factor Surveillance System (BRFSS).* US Centers for Disease Control and Prevention. http://www.cdc.gov/brfss/. Updated December 24, 2013. Accessed March 23, 2014.

71. Prevention Institute. *Tools.* Prevention Institute. http://preventioninstitute.org/tools.html. Accessed March 23, 2014.

72. The Annie E. Casey Foundation. *KIDS COUNT Data Center.* KIDS COUNT Data Center. http://datacenter.kidscount.org/. Updated 2014. Accessed March 23, 2014.

73. Sarason A, Levine HM, Basham RB, Sarason BR. Assessing social support: the Social Support Questionnaire. *Journal of Personality and Social Psychology.* 1983;44:127-139.

74. Sarason IG, Sarason BR, Shearin EN, Pierce GR. A brief measure of social support: Practical and theoretical implications. *Journal of Social and Personal Relationships.* 1987;4(4):497-510.

75. Cohen S, Hoberman H. Positive events and social supports as buffers of life change stress. *Journal of Applied Social Psychology.* 1983;13:99-125.

76. McFarlane AH, Neale KA, Norman GR, Roy RG, Streiner DL. Methodological issues in developing a scale to measure social support. *Schizophrenia Bulletin.* 1981;7:90-100.

77. Berkman LF, Syme SL. Social networks, host resistance, and mortality: a nine-year follow-up of Alameda county residents. *American Journal of Epidemiology.* 1979;109:186-204.

78. Barrera M, Jr, Ainlay SL. The structure of social support: a conceptual and empirical analysis. *Journal of Community Psychology.* 1983;11:133-143.

79. The World Bank. *Social Capital: Measurement Tools*. The World Bank. http://go.worldbank.org/KO0QFVW770. Published 2011. Accessed June 15, 2013.

80. World Health Organization. *Metrics: Disability-Adjusted Life Year (DALY)*. World Health Organization. http://www.who.int/healthinfo/global_burden_disease/metrics_daly/en/. Updated 2014. Accessed March 23, 2014.

81. Williams DR, Costa MV, Oduntami AO, Mohammed S. Moving upstream: how interventions that address the social determinants of health can improve health and reduce disparities. *Journal of Public Health Management Practices*. 2008;14(Suppl):S8-S17.

82. Dobbins M, Tirilis D. *Social Determinants of Health: A Synthesis of Review Evidence*. Exchange Working Paper Series, PHIRN: University of Ottawa, Ottawa, Canada. 2011;S1(2):1-2. http://www.rrasp-phirn.ca/images/stories/docs/commissioned-reports/cps_summary_fall2011_en.pdf. Published 2011. Accessed March 30, 2014.

83. University of Kansas, Work Group for Community Health and Development. *Community Tool Box: Table of Contents*. Community Tool Box. http://ctb.ku.edu/en/tablecontents/index.aspx. Updated 2013. Accessed March 23, 2014.

84. Robert Wood Johnson Foundation, Carger E, Westen D. *A New Way to Talk About the Social Determinants of Health: Vulnerable Populations Portfolio*. Robert Wood Johnson Foundation. http://www.rwjf.org/en/research-publications/find-rwjf-research/2010/01/a-new-way-to-talk-about-the-social-determinants-of-health.html. Published January 1, 2010. Accessed March 23, 2014.

85. McMillan DW, Chavis DM. Sense of community: a definition and theory. *Journal of Community Psychology*. 1986;14(1):6-23.

86. Hays RA. Habitat for humanity: building social capital through faith based service. *Journal of Urban Affairs*. 2003;24(3):247-269.

87. Kapral MK, Wang H, Mamdani M, Tu JV. Effect of socioeconomic status on treatment and mortality after stroke. *Stroke*. 2002;33(1):268-275.

88. Glass TA, Mendes de Leon C, Marottoli RA, Berkman LF. Population based study of social and productive activities as predictors of survival among elderly Americans. *BMJ: British Medical Journal*. 1999;319(7208):478-483.

89. Cattan M, White M, Bond J, Learmouth A. Preventing social isolation and loneliness among older people: a systematic review of health promotion interventions. *Ageing and Society*. 2005;25:41-67.

90. Hammel J, Magasi S, Heinemann A, Whiteneck G, Bogner J, Rodriguez E. What does participation mean? An insider perspective from people with disabilities. *Disability and Rehabilitation*. 2008;30(19):1445-1460.

91. Helliwell JF, Robert D. Putnam RD. The social context of well-being. *Philosophical Transactions-Royal Society of London Series Biological Sciences*. 2004:1435-1446.

92. Pinquart M, Sörensen S. Influences of socioeconomic status, social network, and competence on subjective well-being in later life: a meta-analysis. *Psychology and Aging*. 2000;15(2):187.

93. Netuveli G, Wiggins RD, Hildon Z, Montgomery SM, Blane D. Quality of life at older ages: evidence from the English longitudinal study of aging (wave 1). *Journal of Epidemiology and Community Health*. 2006(4):357-363.

94. Leyden KM. Social capital and the built environment: the importance of walkable neighborhoods. *American Journal of Public Health*. 2003;93(9):1546-1551.

95. Jette AM, Keysor J, Coster W, Ni P, Haley S. Beyond function: predicting participation in a rehabilitation cohort. *Archives of Physical Medicine and Rehabilitation*. 2005;86(11):2087-2094.

ENVIRONMENT FACTORS
Physical and Natural Environment

Susan Stark, PhD, OTR/L; Jon Sanford, MArch; and Marian Keglovits, OTD, MSCI

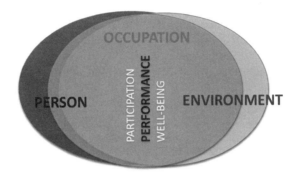

LEARNING OBJECTIVES

- Gain an understanding of the role of the environment in successful occupational performance.
- Understand the theoretical environment models that support the PEOP Model.
- Understand the strategies used to modify the physical environment.
- Understand the major environmental determinants that impact occupational performance.

KEY WORDS

- Built environment
- Natural environment
- Occupational performance
- Physical environment

OVERVIEW

This chapter introduces the important concepts and theories about environment and how the environment influences occupational performance. The discussion will include a historical review of environment in both occupational therapy and rehabilitation. Specific models of intervention will be described and applied to a case study to assist the reader in understanding how the environment can influence occupational performance.

INTRODUCTION

This chapter emphasizes the important role of the physical environment in occupational performance. Occupational performance is the result of complex interactions between intrinsic person factors and extrinsic factors of the environment and what people need and want to do. Environmental attributes interact with human capabilities

Christiansen CH, Baum CM, Bass JD, eds.
Occupational Therapy: Performance, Participation, and Well-Being, Fourth Edition (pp 387-420).
© 2015 SLACK Incorporated.

to enable performance, while others present barriers to an individual's attempts at meaningful interactions with his or her surroundings. In this chapter, we will explore this balance and the relationship between humans and the context within which they perform their occupations. Although the focus of this chapter is the physical environment, aspects of the social or policy environment are also addressed when appropriate given the inter-related nature of context.

Environment is the context that is external to the person and in which activity occurs.[1] Environments consist of physical elements, both built and natural (eg, doors, ramps, pathways) and social influences (eg, policy, culture, support and attitudes). As such, the environment is the context for people's performance and includes everything that a person encounters during participation as a human being in society. Environmental influences, depending on how they affect a person, can facilitate or hinder occupational performance. As a result, there is increasing recognition of the importance of environmental factors in contributing to occupational performance, particularly among more vulnerable populations (such as people with disabilities).[2-7] This view of the environment has not only greatly impacted the concept of disability, but also rehabilitation professionals' views of the disablement processes.

Typical medical models of health attribute the inability of individuals to perform their daily activities to the functional limitations caused by impairments. Environmentally or socially influenced models suggest that disability is a construct imposed by circumstances. Impairments do not become disabilities until they converge with the environment and the person cannot do what he or she needs or wants to do.

Conceptually, disability can be viewed as an expression of the misfit between person and environment. The outcomes of a person-environment match can be far reaching, beyond simply improving the performance of individuals with disabilities. As a result, modifying the environment has become an important intervention strategy to help manage chronic health care conditions; maintain or improve functioning, increase independence, ensure safety, ease of use, security, self-esteem, self-confidence; reduce the need to relocate to institutional facilities, and even reduce the costs of personal care services. A growing body of evidence has demonstrated these positive impacts. For example, Gitlin et al concluded that home modifications improved daily activity performance and reduced mortality.[8,9] Home modifications are effective in reducing falls when provided by occupational therapy practitioners.[10] Additionally, home modifications have been effective in reducing caregiver stress.[11] The physical environment is comprised of the built and natural environment.[12] We all live our lives interacting with the physical environment. Therefore, it is not surprising that the environment is conceptualized, studied, and written about by numerous disciplines, including architecture, environmental science, geography, psychology, policy, landscape and interior design, as well as occupational science. The body of knowledge that comprises many of these disciplines will be reviewed in this chapter to develop a better understanding of environmental contributions to occupational performance and provide the foundation to begin building interventions that support occupation.

Specifically, the first part of this chapter will focus on the historical view of the environment in occupational therapy practice and rehabilitation models. This discussion will be followed by an in-depth discussion of 5 models of person-environment interaction that can form the basis of a comprehensive understanding of the person-environment interaction for intervention. Each model represents a different perspective on this interaction, yet all are important in understanding environmental contributions to successful occupational performance, and each provides the foundation for environmental intervention. Having provided the foundation for environmental intervention, the third part of the chapter will present aspects of the physical environment that effect occupational performance. The fourth component of the chapter will describe intervention approaches to modification of the physical environment. The last part of this chapter will explore a case study using the PEOP Occupational Therapy Process that explores the environment factors that influence performance.

THE EVOLUTION OF ENVIRONMENT IN OCCUPATIONAL THERAPY AND REHABILITATIVE MODELS

Occupational Therapy Models

Historically, occupational therapy literature has recognized the importance of creating opportunities for meaningful interactions with the environment as the basis for promoting health through occupation.[13,14] Although these visionaries challenged the profession to address the environment, it was not until the 1970s and 1980s that occupational therapy practitioners began to talk about the environment as central to the experience of occupation. The first to do so was Dunning, who talked about space as important to consider in analyzing how an activity can be performed.[15] Kiernat conceptualized the environment as an occupational therapy modality that is purposely manipulated to either challenge or support the client's competencies.[16] In turn, the client's abilities expand in order to maintain a comfortable level of fit with the environment. Later Reed and Sanderson divided the environment into

3 constructs: physical, psychobiological, and societal.[17-19] They viewed the environment as interacting forces that shape the performance of individuals as they engage in occupation. The first occupational therapy model that focused on the environment was published in 1982. It was at that time that Howe and Briggs proposed the Ecological Systems Model.[20] They viewed the environment as composed of nested layers. The immediate settings were embedded in the social networks, and then both were in an ideological system. Beginning in 1985, more explicit models began to emerge and all have included the environment as critical elements in their models. In Table 22-1 you can see that there is beginning to be agreement that the environment influences the development and maintenance of the person; however, how the environment is conceptualized is somewhat model dependent.

The Evolution of Rehabilitation Models That Include the Environment

At the same time that concepts of the environment were emerging in occupational therapy, work was going on in the area of disability policy. Some of the changes to rehabilitation models were directly related to occupational therapy practitioners serving in the policy arena and working with other colleagues and consumers of rehabilitation services to shape new models. Prior to 1993, models of disability viewed pathology and disability interchangeably and excluded the consideration of the environment as a determinate of function. The models that view disability resulting from the interaction between the characteristics of the individual and the barriers in the environment are just beginning to emerge (Table 22-2).[34]

The National Medical Rehabilitation Research Center (NMRRC) report to the US Congress in 1993 introduced the idea of social participation and clearly articulated the role of the environment in both the definition of disability and societal limitations. In 1997, the Institute of Medicine (IOM) formed a panel in response to a request from Congress to prepare a report that would assess the current knowledge base in rehabilitation science and engineering. Their task was to evaluate the utility of current rehabilitation models, to describe and recommend mechanisms for the effective transfer and clinical translation of scientific findings to promote health and heath care for people with disabling conditions, and to critically evaluate the current federal programmatic efforts in rehabilitation science and engineering. A panel was constructed that included scientists from public health, sociology, rehabilitation, engineering, public policy, medicine, and both occupational and physical therapy.[34] This report proposed a new model, the Enabling-Disabling Process Model, in which the environment represents both physical space and social structures. It suggests that people with disabling conditions are dislocated from their prior integration in an environment. The model depicts the rehabilitation process as an attempt to rectify this displacement, by either restoring the individual's function or expanding access to the environment that removes barriers that limit performance (Figure 22-1).

Concurrent with the NCMRR and IOM reports to the US Congress, the WHO was initiating the revision of the ICIDH.[12] The ICIDH classification was developed in 1980 as a means of classifying the consequences of disease. With the revision of the ICD-10, which addresses functional states of health conditions, it was important to go beyond the functional status of the individual to guide and plan for the needs of people as they strive to return to active participation in meaningful lives. The ICIDH was revised during a 7-year process involving 65 countries and rigorous scientific examination of the document. The result of the revision process was approved by the WHO in 2001. The new publication, the ICF, has been accepted as the international standard to describe and measure health and disability (Figure 22-2).[12]

While traditional health indicators are based on the mortality (ie, death) rates of populations, the ICF shifts focus to "life" (ie, how people live with their health conditions and how these can be improved to achieve a productive, fulfilling life). The ICF takes into account the social aspects of disability and provides a mechanism to document the impact of the social and physical environment on a person's functioning.

The goal for the revision was to provide a unified and standard language and framework for the description of human functioning and disability as an important component of health. The classification evolved to cover disturbances in functional states associated with health conditions and the body, the individual and society level, and included 2 dimensions. The first dimension includes the functioning and disability factors and is divided into 2 sections. The body structure and function component includes the anatomical and physiological functions of the human body, while the activities and participation component covers the complete range of activities performed by an individual and describes areas of life in which an individual is involved. The second section includes the environmental and personal factors. The entire model is presented here (see Figure 22-2); however, the environmental aspects of the model will be discussed later in the chapter.

MODELS OF PERSON-ENVIRONMENT INTERACTION

Environmental theory has been developed, studied, and presented in the environment behavior studies (EBS) literature. These theories support the PEOP Model and

Table 22-1. *Occupational Therapy Models That Address Environment Factors*

Year	Authors	Model	Role of Environment in the Model
1983	Canadian Occupational Therapy Association[21]	Client-Centered Practice of Occupational Therapy	Introduced the environment as a critical element in supporting occupational performance.
1985, 1995, 2002	Kielhofner[22-24]	Model of Human Occupation	Environment includes objects, persons, and events with which the person interacts. The environment affords or presses occupational behavior.
1991, 1997; 2005; 2015	Christiansen and Baum[4,5]; Baum, Christiansen, and Bass-Haugen[25]; Baum, Christiansen, and Bass[26]	Person-Environment Occupation-Performance Model	The environment enables or acts as a barrier to occupational performance. The environment was described to include social support, social policies and attitudes, culture, and physical and natural attributes.
1992	Polatajko[27]	Occupational Competence Model	Occupational competence is the product of the dynamic interaction between the environmental demand and the individual's ability. The environmental dimensions include physical, social, and cultural.
1992	Stewart[28]	Model for the Practice of Occupational Therapy	The occupational therapy process involves interaction between client, practitioner, environment, and activities.
1992	Schkade and Schultz[29]	Occupational Adapation Model	Performance calls for an occupational environment to support the occupational response and includes the contest in which occupations occur (self- maintenance, play, and leisure).
1994	Dunn, Brown, and McGuigan[3]	Ecology of Human Performance Model	Environmental cues are used by a person to support the performance of tasks.
1995, 2000	Hagedorn[30,31]	Competent Occupational Performance in the Environment Model	Environmental demand is defined as the challenge presented by the environment that provides the press that supports occupational performance.
1995	Bass Haugen and Mathiowetz[32]	Contemporary Task-Oriented Approach Model	The environmental and performance context (physical, socioeconomic, and cultural), as well as personal characteristics, are important in determining occupational and role performance.
1996	Law, Cooper, Strong, Stewart, Rigby, and Letts[6]	Person-Environment-Occupation Model	The environment defined as those contexts and situation outside the individual (social, political, economic, institutional, and cultural) that elicit responses from the person.
1997	Canadian Association of Occupational Therapists[33]	Canadian Model of Occupational Performance	The environment includes the physical, institutional, cultural, and social factors. The environment forms the outer ring of a conceptual model that supports the person as he or she engages in occupation.

Table 22-2. The National Medical Rehabilitation Research Center Model[34]

Pathophysiology	Impairment	Functional Limitation	Disability	Societal Limitation
Interruption or interference of normal physiological and developmental processes or structures	Loss and/or abnormality of mental, emotional, physiological, or anatomical structure or function; includes all losses or abnormalities, not just those attributable to the initial pathophysiology, also includes pain.	Restriction or lack of ability to perform an action or activity in the manner or within the range considered normal that results from impairment or failure of an individual to return to the pre-existing level of function	Inability or limitation in performing socially defined activities and roles expected of individuals within a social and physical environment with external factors and their interplay	Societal policy, attitudes, and actions, or lack of, that creates physical, social, or financial barriers to access health care, housing, and vocational/avocational opportunities
Level of Reference				
Cells and tissues	Organs and organ systems	Organism—Action or activity performance (consistent with the purpose or function of the organ or organ system)	Individual—Task performance within the social and cultural context	Society

Adapted from work initially developed by the Institute of Medicine and published in *Disability in America,* 1991.

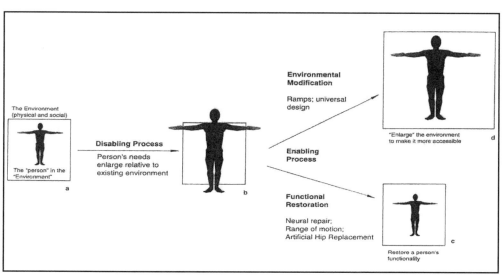

Figure 22-1. The Institute of Medicine Model.[21] (Reprinted with permission from *Enabling America: Assessing the Role of Rehabilitation Science and Engineering.* © 1997 by the National Academy of Sciences. Courtesy of the National Academies Press, Washington, DC.)

provide the operational definitions and theoretical assumptions necessary to understand how environment can influence behavior (or occupational performance). There is a rich history of important models that occupational therapy can explore and study. In this section we will introduce EBS theories, discuss their relevance to occupational therapy model and theory development using examples from the EBS literature, and review 4 theories that provide a basis for understanding aspects of the environment that effect occupational performance.

Figure 22-2. The International Classification of Function, Disability and Health (ICF): Interaction between the Components of ICF. (Reprinted with permission from the World Health Organization. *International Classification of Functioning, Disability and Health.* Geneva, Switzerland: World Health Organization; 2001. © 2001 WHO.)

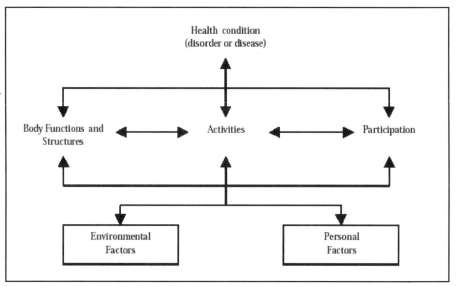

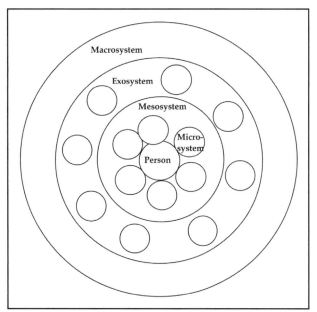

Figure 22-3. Broffenbrenner's model. (Reprinted with permission from Bronfenbrenner U. The ecology of cognitive development: research models and fugitive findings. In: Wozniak RH, Fischer KW, eds. *Development in Context: Acting and Thinking in Specific Environments.* New York, NY: Erlbaum; 1993:3-44. © 1993 Taylor & Francis Group LLC.)

Each of the models presented represents a transactional relationship between an individual's functional abilities and limitations and environmental factors, in general.[35,36] The models are presented from a broad to specific conception of the environment. The Bronfenbrenner model depicts the nested relationships of an individual within a community and society. The ICF Model is similarly broad in describing context and environment. The more specific transaction of an individual in their

context is described by Lawton and Nahemow's Ecological Model. Specific abilities in relation to context are predicted with the Enabler Model and, finally, Sanford and Connell's framework focuses directly on the impact of, specific characteristics and attributes of environments on occupational performance.

Bronfenbrenner

Urie Bronfenbrenner developed a model that is useful in understanding the influence of person-environment interactions that effect development.[37,38] Bronfenbrenner assumed that development occurred within an environmental context when he developed the ecological paradigm that he said captures the context-specific person-environment interaction that "emerges as the most likely to exert influence on the course and content of subsequent psychological developments in all spheres, including cognitive growth."[38(p10)]

Bronfenbrenner rejected the common assumption of most of his contemporaries in psychology that developmental attributes could be examined out of the context of an individual's life.[37,38] Instead, he identified individual spheres of environmental influence that influenced development and set out to explore development in context. Bronfenbrenner's ecological model consists of microsystems, mesosystems, exosystems, and macrosystems.[37,38] These environmental spheres of performance describe the nested networks of interactions that create an individual's ecology (Figure 22-3). Bronfenbrenner assumes that this ecological network changes over time as an individual develops.

Briefly, there are 4 major spheres of influence within Bronfenbrenner's ecological model.[37,38] The microsystem is a specific interaction that occurs between the developing person and one or more others. Parent child interactions or parent teacher interactions would occur within the microsystem. A mesosystem consists of interactions between and among 2 or more microsystems. An exosystem comprises an environment that has an impact on the developing individual, but does not contain him or her. The community represents such a system. Finally, the macrosystem contains a person's entire microsystem, mesosystem, and exosystem, and involves the entire realm of developmental possibilities for him or her. Macrosystems are temporally and culturally specific to that individual, and are dynamic rather than static. The macrosystem places the person in the context of his or her developmental ecology.[37,38]

The complex interactions within and between each system can inhibit or enhance development. For example, the possibility of developing an identity as a child with a disability is provided—or not provided—by the macrosystem of modern culture, but then an individual must also have microsystems, mesosystems, and exosystems that provide opportunities for that identity to develop.[37,38]

Environmental Features That Interact With Skills and Abilities: International Classification of Functioning, Disability and Health Classification

Understanding and describing the range of environmental factors that impact the performance of individuals is difficult given the vast number of environments and different features associated with each. Moreover, for each individual, occupations occur within a context that is unique to their circumstance. Each human lives in a life space that is built on a system of environments. The environments include a mix of physical and social elements. Physical elements can include the built environment, objects within the environment, and the geographical and climactic features of the natural environment. Social elements can include people, including their attitudes and cultural values, as well as social support offered by these people. Policies and services are also social elements in the environment that influence performance. The PEOP Model environment factors are made up of the physical dimensions of the environment, including the built environment; the natural environment; and the social dimensions of the environment such as the cultural, societal, social support and economic factors in an environment.

The PEOP Model works well with the WHO's classification of the environment that is part of the ICF.[12] Table 22-3 includes the ICF classification of environmental factors in terms of specific features and elements, including products and technology, natural and human made changes to the environment, support and relationships, attitudes and services, and systems and policies. This classification system is being developed in conjunction with a broader classification index of disability and the precursors to disability.[12] The development of the environmental classification index is still in its infancy; however, to date it is the most comprehensive description of environmental elements that contribute to the disablement process.

While the ICF classification provides a fairly complete list of all of the environmental features and elements that may influence performance, there is still no description of these features and elements from which a direct link between the environment and performance can be ascertained. For instance, a 30'-long, accessibility code-compliant, 1:12 (ie, 1" rise for every 12" of run) ramp at a building entrance might facilitate entry to that building for a young individual who uses a wheelchair, but an older wheelchair user who also has diminished upper body strength might not be able to push himself or herself up the same ramp. In contrast, the same older individual might be able to use a 1:16 ramp or one that was only 20 feet long.

For example, the ramp is an environmental feature that falls into the ICF model, and removing it entirely would not help the older individual get into the building. Moreover, it is unlikely that bodybuilding to improve upper body strength will be of much help. On the other hand, changing specific characteristics of the ramp, such as slope and length that place too high a demand on the older wheelchair user, would facilitate that individual's access to the building. The following model begins to illustrate how impairment and environmental characteristics affect occupational performance.

Person-Environment Fit: Environmental Press Model

Person-environment fit can be operationalized as the outcome of the transaction or interaction between the person and the environment.[35] Optimal fit occurs when an individual's capacities are consistent with the demands and the opportunities within his or her environment. Conversely, when the demands of the environment exceed an individual's abilities, there is person-environment misfit.

The extent to which the environment affects an individual's ability to perform an activity was initially defined as environmental press by Murray in 1938, and further explicated by Lawton and Nahemow's Ecological (Environmental Press) Model.[39] This model graphically illustrates the differential impact of the environment on behavior and performance as a function of an individual's competence. Most importantly for occupational therapy practitioners, the Environmental Press Model supports the process of determining the types of environmental

Table 22-3. *International Classification of Environment Factors*[12]

Environmental Factors	Examples
Products and technology	• Products or substances for personal consumption • Products and technology for personal use in daily living • Products and technology for personal indoor and outdoor mobility and transportation • Products and technology for communication • Products and technology for education • Products and technology for employment • Products and technology for culture, recreation, and sport • Products and technology for the practice of religion and spirituality • Design, construction, and building products and technology of buildings for public use • Design, construction, and building products and technology of buildings for private use • Products and technology of land development • Assets • Products and technology, other specified • Products and technology, unspecified
Natural environment and human-made changes to environment	• Physical geography • Population • Flora and fauna • Climate • Natural events • Human-caused events • Light • Time-related changes • Sound • Vibration • Air quality • Natural environment and human-made changes to environment, other specified • Natural environment and human-made changes to environment, unspecified
Support and relationships	• Immediate family • Extended family • Friends • Acquaintances, peers, colleagues, neighbors, and community members • People in positions of authority • People in subordinate positions • Personal care providers and personal assistants • Strangers • Domesticated animals

(continued)

Table 22-3 (continued). *International Classification of Environment Factors[12]*

Environmental Factors	Examples
Support and relationships (continued)	• Health professionals • Health-related professionals • Support and relationships, other specified • Support and relationships, unspecified
Attitudes	• Individual attitudes of immediate family members • Individual attitudes of extended family members • Individual attitudes of friends • Individual attitudes of acquaintances, peers, colleagues, neighbors, community members • Individual attitudes of people in positions of authority • Individual attitudes of people in subordinate positions • Individual attitudes of personal care providers and personal assistants • Individual attitudes of strangers • Individual attitudes of health professionals • Individual attitudes of health-related professionals • Societal attitudes • Social norms, practices, and ideologies • Attitudes, other specified • Attitudes, unspecified
Services, systems and policies	• Services, systems, and policies for the production of consumer goods • Architecture and construction services, systems, and policies • Open space planning services, systems, and policies • Housing services, systems, and policies • Utilities services, systems, and policies • Communication services, systems, and policies • Transportation services, systems, and policies • Civil protection services, systems, and policies • Legal services, systems, and policies • Associations and organizational services, systems, and policies • Media services, systems, and policies • Economic services, systems, and policies • Social security services, systems, and policies • General social support services, systems, and policies • Health services, systems, and policies • Education and training services, systems, and policies • Labor and employment services, systems, and policies • Political services, systems, and policies • Services, systems, and policies, other specified

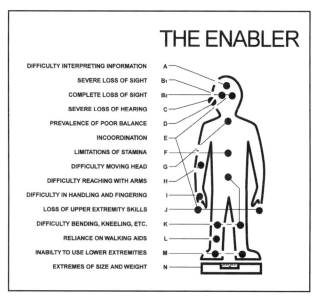

THE ENABLER

DIFFICULTY INTERPRETING INFORMATION — A
SEVERE LOSS OF SIGHT — B₁
COMPLETE LOSS OF SIGHT — B₂
SEVERE LOSS OF HEARING — C
PREVALENCE OF POOR BALANCE — D
INCOORDINATION — E
LIMITATIONS OF STAMINA — F
DIFFICULTY MOVING HEAD — G
DIFFICULTY REACHING WITH ARMS — H
DIFFICULTY IN HANDLING AND FINGERING — I
LOSS OF UPPER EXTREMITY SKILLS — J
DIFFICULTY BENDING, KNEELING, ETC. — K
RELIANCE ON WALKING AIDS — L
INABILTY TO USE LOWER EXTREMITIES — M
EXTREMES OF SIZE AND WEIGHT — N

Figure 22-4. The Enabler.[42-44]

changes that must be made to match the abilities of an individual, a critical component to the occupational therapy treatment process.

The level of an individual's competencies (eg, functional, cognitive, social, and behavioral skills and abilities) are represented on the Y axis of a graph and the amount of press resulting from demands are represented on the X axis. Competence ranges from low to high, and environmental press ranges from weak to strong. The outcome of a transaction is depicted on the graph at the intersection of an individual's skill level and the strength of environmental demand. The central diagonal line or adaptation level represents the "average" or baseline environmental press for that person. This is the point at which there is optimal person-environment fit. At this point, an individual does not need to adapt his or her behavior, skills, or environment.[39]

The ranges on either side of the baseline represent generally positive affect and successful performance of the person, as demands are in line with the skills of an individual. However, as an individual moves farther away from the baseline, performance outcomes decrease, either as a result of an environment that is too challenging (as represented by stronger demands) or one that is not sufficiently challenging (as represented by weaker demands). When demands are greater or less than an individual's skill level, negative outcomes or maladaptive behavior occurs, resulting in environmental interactions that are marked by poor occupational performance. For example, when a grab bar is located too far away (demand) for a frail older individual to reach (competency), he or she may lose balance, fall, or

experience fear of falling. As a consequence, the individual may require assistance in toileting, or may avoid the toilet altogether (maladaptive behavior).[39]

Two general principles/hypotheses derived from the Environmental Press Model are important in understanding the impact of the environment on people with diminished skills. First, the "Environmental Docility Hypothesis" proposes that persons with diminished physical, cognitive, or psychological capacity are at a greater risk for influence by the environment.[40,41] Thus, more-impaired individuals are likely to be more susceptible to environmental demands than less-impaired individuals. Second, excess disabilities occur when the environment is not responsive to an individual's capabilities. Thus, when there is a mismatch between environment and ability, observed levels of dependency would be greater than those expected given an individual's level of impairment.[40,41]

The Environmental Press Model provides an explicit understanding of the transactional relationship between person and environment and establishes the basis from which outcomes of a supportive environment can be measured. Whereas the model provides a basic understanding of the transactional nature of person environment fit, it does not identify specific environmental factors that can be targeted for intervention. Therefore, the next step is to break down the environment a little further and explore the specific environmental features that might impact the component skills and abilities of an individual.

Environmental Factors and Impairment: The Enabler Model

As the ramp example illustrates, environmental features can either support (ie, enablers) or hamper (ie, barriers) performance. Whether an environmental feature is supportive or not depends on both the skills and abilities of an individual (competence) and the characteristics of the environment (press). The Enabler Model begins to address these issues by linking competence defined by impairments to a limited set of press-producing environmental characteristics (Figure 22-4).[42-44]

As described in Section III, each person has abilities regardless of impairment diagnosis. Each measurable and objective ability exists on a continuum from personal capacity to disability. Within any environmental context, personal capacity can be viewed as the person's occupational performance potential, whereas disability can be viewed as diminished performance.[39]

Based on the work of Murray and Lewin, the Enabler Model captures the broad spectrum of abilities for individuals with a variety of limitations.[36,44] The Enabler explores the capacities of the person, including cognitive, sensory, internal body regulation, and motor capacities. The major contribution of this work to the current understanding of the person-environment interaction is the concept that a person with a disability is not simply "disabled," but has a unique set of abilities and limitations that are differentially impacted by various environmental factors.

The Enabler Model has specifically been used to assist in understanding accessibility in the physical environment and, more recently, to everyday occupations in the home.[42,43] To measure the impact of environmental factors on occupational tasks, Iwarsson has applied the Enabler Model to home activities as a method of evaluating environmental barriers to performance in the home. The evaluation tool is a helpful conceptualization of the home barriers. A list of 144 environmental barriers is provided (eg, narrow paths, irregular walking surfaces, and unstable walking surfaces) for the home environment. The list is coded by the types of impairments that may encounter barriers if this environmental attribute is present. Each barrier is rated by severity by impairment and a score as been assigned based on a 4-point system. The potential of the barriers can be rated as follows:

1. Potential problem
2. Problem
3. Severe problem
4. Impossibility

For example, if stairs are present in the home of an individual who depends on a wheelchair, a score of 4 will be tallied for that barrier.[42,43]

The Enabler Model clarifies, at the conceptual level, the relationship between impairment and a specific set of environmental factors. But how do we know that the set of environmental factors included in Iwarsson's model cover all of the possible environmental factors that impact performance? And just as importantly, how can we be sure that functional abilities imbedded in generic descriptions of impairment truly represent the skills and abilities of all individuals with those particular impairments? To answer these questions, we need to look at the conceptual framework suggested by the fourth model, which defines environmental characteristics by occupational tasks and links those characteristics to an individual's occupational performance, regardless of impairment.[42,43]

Linking Environmental Characteristics and Performance: A Framework for Home Modification

As noted earlier in this chapter, environmental features and elements, in and of themselves, do not exert demands on individuals. Rather, the characteristics of those features, such as the length and slope of a ramp, the height and location of a toilet, the number of family members available to provide assistance and support, or the types of transportation services available, create demands that impact occupational performance. Similarly, competence is defined by abilities and skills, such as range of motion; not by impairments, such as low vision or difficulty bending. The issue then is to construct a model that describes who (ie, ability and skill levels) is impacted by what (ie, environmental characteristics) and when (ie, occupational performance). To understand these relationships, a task analytic approach is useful. Such an approach relies on defining task-relevant environmental characteristics, rather than ones that are impairment-related. As a result, occupational performance can be linked to environmental characteristics irrespective of personal factors including impairment, skills, and abilities. Unlike the prospective approach of the first 3 models, this model is retrospective, based on actual performance of what an individual can or cannot do in a real environment.

One application of this approach is the conceptual framework to guide the process of developing home modification.[45,46] The conceptual framework (illustrated in Table 22-4) links occupational performance to the physical environment of the home and permits the assessment of occupational performance in the context of the environmental features and characteristics used in the conduct of each activity. Each activity is subdivided into its component and requisite tasks (eg, turning on the water, regulating water temperature, getting in the tub, grabbing the soap, etc). These tasks are linked to multiple characteristics of relevant environmental features. For example, bathing is dependent upon such task-related characteristics as the location of the tub relative to other fixtures in the bathroom, and the type and location of faucet handles.

Specifically, the framework describes the major environmental features of the home, including spaces, products, and hardware/controls, and the critical characteristics of these features that impact occupational performance for each task.[45,46] These are briefly discussed in the following sections.

Spaces

The physical characteristics of rooms and other spaces place demands on people that can determine successful performance or require excess effort to complete a task. For example, the layout of the tub and toilet in a bathroom can determine if a lateral wheelchair-to-toilet transfer is possible, and light levels can determine if an individual with low vision can read the label on a medicine bottle. Specific spatial characteristics that create demands include the following[45,46]:

- Size and spatial configuration/layout
- Entry dimensions (doorway width and threshold height)

Table 22-4. *Example of Physical Environment Characteristics That Impact Bathing Performance*

Space	Product	Controls/Hardware
Bathroom	**Tub/Shower**	**Faucet**

• Entry: doorway width, threshold height
• Size
• Layout
• Systems locations:
  ◦ Plumbing, electric
  ◦ Lighting, ventilation
• Floor materials/finishes
• Ambient conditions
	• Type (description)
	• Size/dimensions
	• Hardware configuration (location of hardware)
	• Lighting
	• Materials/finishes
		• Type (description)
		• Size
		• Approach: distance and angle
		• Force required
		• Operational characteristics
		  ◦ Direction, distance
		  ◦ Calibration
		• Materials/finishes

- Systems locations (location of switches, outlets, fixtures, and appliances)
- Floor materials/finishes
- Ambient conditions (illumination and noise)

Products

The design of products, including fixtures, appliances, and other off-the-shelf items, also creates demands that impact occupational performance. For example, the location of controls at the rear of an electric range requires an individual in a wheelchair to reach across the burners to operate the appliance; or the weight of a pot may be too much for an individual with limited strength to pick up. Product characteristics of interest include the following[45,46]:

- Type
- Size
- Force required to activate, engage, operate, lift, or move
- Materials/finishes (type, texture, and color contrast)
- Auditory/visual signals (intended to alert user to take some further action)

Controls and Hardware

Controls and hardware include a variety of user interfaces. They are either operable (such as a doorknob) or fixed (such as a drawer pull). Generally their function is to operate products, although occasionally inoperable hardware, such as grab bars, serves its own independent function. Controls and hardware typically create demands that require the user to manipulate the environment using fine motor control to grasp, twist, rotate, push, or pull an object,

although many interfaces also require the ability to attend to sensory feedback. For example, round doorknobs may be difficult for someone with arthritis to grasp, a black knob on a black appliance might not have sufficient color contrast for someone with a vision impairment to locate, or the sound of an oven control clicking into a heat setting may not be loud enough for an individual with a hearing impairment. Specific characteristics of controls and hardware that affect use include the following:

- Type of device (opener, dispenser, plumbing, lock, assist, receptacle, controls)
- Minimum approach distance and angle
- Hardware configuration
- Size
- Force of activation
- Operational characteristics (direction and distance to be moved, calibration, type of sensory feedback)
- Materials/finish (type, texture, and color contrast)

Although this conceptual framework was developed for linking physical characteristics to occupational performance in the home, it is relevant and adaptable to any setting. Moreover, using characteristics to describe environmental features is equally applicable to the social environment as it is to the physical environment.[45,46]

Summary of Theoretical Models

This set of theoretical models provides occupational therapy practitioners with a set of tools to guide clinical reasoning when developing compensatory interventions that involve changes to the physical environment. The models introduced here provide a basic understanding of the key environmental influences on occupational performance. Lawton and Nahemow's Ecological Model is often cited by occupational therapy literature to guide an understanding the balance between support and challenge that must be present in order for us to perform maximally our daily occupations.[39] The Enabler provides a matrix to guide clinical reasoning as we consider the various person factors that feel the influence of the environment.[43] The types of environmental features that impact performance are understood using the ICF *Classification Framework*.[12] Through this hierarchical organization of the environment from its broadest conceptualization as the context in which activity occurs to the link between specific characteristics and task performance, occupational performance can be understood, measured, and ultimately intervened upon by those interested in minimizing the impact of a disabling environment. The Bronfenbrenner model provides an important understanding of how the environment influences development and QOL.[37,38]

ASPECTS OF THE ENVIRONMENT THAT EFFECT OCCUPATIONAL PERFORMANCE

In this section, the features of the physical environment that influence performance will be introduced. Although not the focus of this chapter, social and political aspects of the environment as they influence physical interventions will be discussed. These features will be discussed in terms of their contribution to occupational performance and their potential to serve as supports or barriers. The physical and social features of the environment will be described in terms of how they can be modified to improve occupational performance. Physical interventions will be described in terms of adapted strategies, assistive technologies, adapted devices, and design changes. These intervention strategies will be followed by a discussion of the environmental characteristics that must be taken into consideration during intervention (ie, the natural environment, culture, economics, and social attitudes).

Strategies to improve occupational performance at the level of the physical environment may include changes to the person (eg, skill acquisition, adaptive strategies, prosthesis, or physical rehabilitation), occupation (eg, replacing one activity with another), or the environment (eg, assistive technologies, adaptive devices, design changes, caregiver support or personal attendant services). In most instances, a combination of strategies is needed to promote successful occupational performance. In this section we will focus on environmental modification strategies. Although strategies provided during occupational therapy are often focused on the home; the work, school, and community facilities are also potential areas where person-environment fit intervention strategies can help individuals with disabilities reach their occupational performance goals.

As noted in the previous section, the identification of environmental strategies is embedded in a detailed understanding of the specific environmental characteristics that affect occupational performance. However, a simple understanding of relevant characteristics does not ensure that a strategy will be successful. Rather, successful environmental modifications require matching the intervention to the situation. The PEOP Model—person-environment-occupation as it affects performance—defines the situation.

The Physical Environment and Its Effect on Occupational Performance

The physical environment can be organized into 3 categories using the domains of the ICF. These include the built (or human made environment), products and technology (appliances, fixtures, controls, and hardware—including [AT]), and the natural environment.[12] These 3 organizing factors will be used in the following discussion of the built environment.

Built Environment

There are 2 basic approaches to modifying the built environment. They include 1) re-structuring, reorganizing, or addition of a built environment; and 2) replacement, alteration, or addition of fixtures, appliances, or other environmental products and use of assistive technologies. Any or all of these approaches may be needed to accommodate a particular individual. Restructuring the built environment can be the most or least expensive approach. Building an addition to a home or community space, moving walls to reconfigure interior space, or changing the topography by grading to reconfigure the natural landscape can be expensive but necessary in some instances. On the other hand, re-arranging furniture in rooms, converting a downstairs study into a bedroom, and using the least demanding parts of the natural environment can be achieved at little or no cost. The second approach focuses on changing off-the-shelf products, such as a standard toilet with an elevated one or a bathtub with a curbless/roll-in shower. Alternatively, products can be used to provide information about environmental demands for users to make informed decisions about their ability to perform a task successfully.

Products and Technology

Another important method of changing the environment is the provision of products or AT. Products can include the addition of adaptive hardware or modification to environmental controls. AT is defined as any product or system that is used to improve the functional capacity of persons who have disabilities.[47] This technology is designed to make best use of an individual's abilities in order to overcome environmental barriers that may prevent the person from achieving maximal occupational performance.[48] There are numerous types of assistive devices and systems, including seating and mobility devices that can influence community access, computer access systems, augmentative communication devices, adapted driving devices, and environmental control units, as well as pieces of adaptive equipment that make it possible to accomplish tasks such as dressing. When providing AT, the costs must be considered, as much of AT available today is still costly and may not be funded by a health insurance program.[49] The possibility of disuse or "abandonment" of AT by individuals for various reasons, such as complexity of use or embarrassment related to using something different, may occur.[50] These factors may affect an individual's ability to maximize his or her independence.

Finally, changing hardware and controls might entail replacing an individual interface, such as a light switch, faucet, or door handle; adding a variety of electronic controls (eg, timers, photocells, or motion sensors) to automate tasks; or replacing an entire fixture, such as an oven, because the controls are too hard to reach or see.

Natural Environment

Often the natural environment presents features that cannot be modified. For example, the terrain in San Francisco presents hills, the climate in Montana will offer snow and ice, and the climate in Florida may offer extreme heat and humidity. These aspects of the natural environment including climate, atmospheric pressure, terrain, and even population density may impact the performance of individuals with disabilities. Although these features themselves can often not be changed, modifications can be made to address the elements present in the natural environment. For example, providing a covered drop off area in a driveway may allow someone who has a mobility impairment the time and protection they need from rain in the Seattle area. An older adult in Minnesota may benefit from a heated walkway that would melt snow and eliminate the need to shovel.

There may be policy or legal protections that are possible to improve occupational performance. For example, ensuring that accessible parking places, sidewalks, and curb cuts are free of snow or providing air conditioners for individuals at risk during extreme heat may make the difference between occupation and disablement. In some cases, natural terrain cannot be modified for individuals who have disabilities. For example, an accessible path from the top to the bottom of the Grand Canyon is not possible given the technology that is currently available. In this case, information may be the most important accommodation possible. A trail map that provides information about the terrain, rest areas, or alternative methods of accessing the trail (horseback) would be important information to allow an individual to choose which aspects of the trail they would like to experience.[51]

Support and Relationships and Their Effect on Occupational Performance

The use of social supports both formal (programs and services) and informal (family and friends) are common strategies to compensate for physical barriers. There are many definitions of social support. From a therapeutic perspective, social support for individuals with disabilities is often defined by determining whether they are cared for, loved and able to count on others should the need arise.[52,53] Social support can include practical support, informational support, and emotional support.[54] Practical support is generally considered tangible, physical support; assistance with transfers, preparation of meals, or driving one to a doctor's appointment are examples of practical support. This support can be informal (provided by a family member or loved one) or formal (provided by a paid caregiver or personal care attendant). Informational support is generally considered advice or guidance. For example, providing one with a list of tips for saving energy, identifying a support group in the community, or advising a client on the type of equipment to purchase for bathing may be considered advice or information. Often professionals or peers (individuals with the same or similar disability) provide this type of information, although family or friends can be a source of informational support. Emotional support is generally the provision of a sense of belonging or esteem. While professionals may provide this type of support, it is generally the role of family members and peer groups to provide everyday opportunities to be a member of a group or provide moral support during difficult times.[52-54]

Social supports can improve the match between the person and the environment in the same way that physical changes can improve performance. For example, the occupation of eating a meal may be disrupted in the life of a person who is temporarily using a wheelchair for mobility. The person may be unable to move about her kitchen due to the environmental barriers that include narrow space in the kitchen, no turning area, cabinets that are out of reach, and the inability to see what is cooking on the stove. One strategy may be to modify the space by increasing the clear floor space, moving furniture to make more room, moving cabinets, and installing an angled mirror above the stove, as seen in Figure 22-5. An alternative would include teaching the individual to use a microwave and providing one at a height that can be reached from a wheelchair.[55]

A third solution may be to engage a home-delivered meal service (practical support, formal). A fourth alternative would include engaging the individual's family or friends and asking them for help or assistance in preparing and providing meals (practical support, informal). Although problems can be solved by providing these approaches, the outcome results are often negative when practical support has been offered as a solution to environmental barriers, while informational support (for example, instruction in the use of a microwave) has been perceived as helpful when provided by professionals.[55-57] Emotional support has consistently been shown to demonstrate positive outcomes, pointing out the importance of providing interventions that allow caregivers the opportunity to provide more support and less instrumental (practical) assistance.[58] In some cases, the care of family members with disabilities in the home has been attributed to increased caregiver stress or burden.[59] In that case, the intervention plan that includes social support may be provided for the caregiver.[60] Often changes in the physical environment can influence lives of caregivers. For example, Calkins and Namazi found that caregivers often made effective physical changes that increased safety, security, or comfort for their loved ones with Alzheimer's disease.[61]

Socioeconomic and Political Aspects of the Environment That Influence Occupation

Other important factors that influence occupational performance include policies, economic factors, and attitudes toward people with disabilities. These factors may change slowly based on scientific outcome research, political or social pressure, or shifts in attitudes, but they are present and deserve consideration in their present state during any modification. They are also important considerations for occupational therapy practitioners who should consider their role in influencing policy, laws, and economics for people with disabilities, as well as understanding them. Culture, policy, laws, economics, and attitudes and beliefs, all features described in the ICF, will be discussed in light of the influence they have on the occupational performance of people with disabilities.

Culture

Culture includes the values, norms, customs, beliefs, behaviors, and perceptions that are shared by a group or society.[62] Culture can be relevant at the level of the individual, organization, community, and the societal level. Individually, culture can determine the level of independence that an individual desires. For example, it may be acceptable for an older adult to accept assistance during dressing from their spouse due to the cultural beliefs that the couple holds. Culture can also effect physical changes to

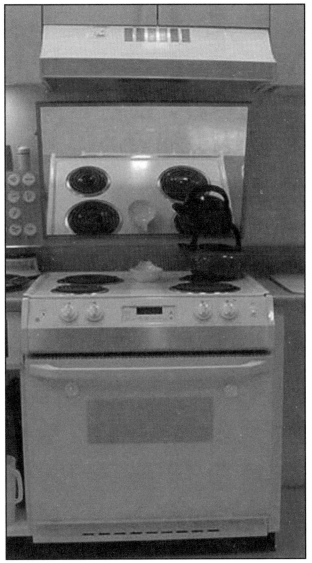

Figure 22-5. Modified stove.

the environment. For example, in Japan, an accepted cultural norm of removing one's shoes upon entering the home has shaped the design of houses. Typically, a landing that is higher than the floor surface inside the door is the area where the shoes are removed and stored until the wearer is ready to leave the home. This tradition makes wheelchair access more difficult to achieve, due to the lack of a level surface in the home and the important cultural meaning of the landing. Culture may be one of the most difficult aspects of the environment to understand, as often we do not realize what it is we do not know.[63] Rather, recognizing that cultural values may influence what an individual is willing to do in order to achieve his or her goals, and determining what those cultural values are, is an important consideration.

Policies and Laws Supporting the Built and Natural Environment

Policies that direct the funding of programs to benefit individuals with disabilities may play a role in whether there is funding or services available. There are few countries (ie, Sweden and Denmark) with policies that support home modifications for individuals with disabilities. Currently in the United States there is no federal program to provide home modifications for individuals who have disabilities.[64] Insurance programs will cover the cost of nursing home placement and home health aides, but will not fund the provision of simple environmental modifications that would increase the independence of individuals who have disabling conditions so they could stay at home. This requires that individuals rely on local services and programs for environmental modification assistance, while others fund the changes themselves. Often, individuals with disabilities do not have the resources to pay for costly home modifications, and thus rely on family or informal caregivers to support their daily activity performance. Caregiving has been associated with primary stressors, such as hardships and problems anchored directly in caregiving.[65] Physical environmental support may be necessary for increased independence for individuals with disabilities and also to relieve caregivers from the physical demands of care giving. Personal assistance provided to adults with disabilities amounts to 21.5 billion hours of help per year for informal, unpaid support; reducing the demands of caregiving is an high priority.[66]

Laws

To a great extent, many practical programs and policy changes that influence the built environment have been put in place as a result of legislation. As an example, a series of legislative acts have shaped the policies of the United States since the Vocational Rehabilitation Act of 1920 (Table 22-5).

Occupational therapy practitioners who intervene using the physical environment need to understand the legislative acts that can impact the physical environment. For example, legislation can influence funding and the types of modifications that may be possible. The Americans with Disabilities Act of 1990 (ADA), the Amendments to the Fair Housing Act in 1988, and the Individuals with Disabilities Education Act (IDEA, formerly called PL 94-142 or the Education for all Handicapped Children Act of 1975) are just a few of the laws that influence the physical environment.[68] These legislative acts reflect an interesting shift in public attitude toward people with disabilities. The recognition of the needs of individuals with disabilities has become more explicit with each successive legislative action. With the passage of the ADA, the focus of laws targeting people with disabilities has changed to a more comprehensive, broad-reaching approach focusing on protecting the civil rights of people who have disabilities.[69]

An Organizing Continuum for Understanding the Environmental Features That Influence Occupational Performance

Compensating for the physical environment can include changes to the physical or natural environment or social support to overcome physical barriers. These changes are made in a political, cultural, or economic context. How do we organize and think about the factors that determine how the changes will be made?

Individual characteristics, in addition to other environmental factors, must be considered when making decisions about environmental modification. One strategy to use when considering environmental issues is to envision the environment as hierarchically arranged, with those environments most frequently encountered in the center of a circle and those larger, more contextual environments surrounding the inner circle with progressively larger circles.[30,54] The environment can be conceptualized in a continuum from proximal to distal, with the most proximal environments consisting of those most personal places that one uses most frequently; and distal being the wider, more expanded layer of the environment that includes community.[37,70] Each of these layers of the environment contains physical and social attributes that affect how an individual performs.

Concurrent with the need to understand the impact of the environmental attribute on the performance of an individual, is the need to understand the impact of proximal versus distal environments. The personal environment is the environment most easily controlled by an individual. Thus, logically, the more personal or proximal an environment, the more likely it will support or inhibit performance.[37,70]

Figure 22-6 depicts an individual within his or her environment. A person can be viewed as the center of his or her own individual environment, with the layer that immediately surrounds him or her consisting of his or her own personal spaces. Personal spaces can include the home in which his or her lives or perhaps a place that his or her occupies and influences during their primary occupations. These places could also include a dorm room or a personal car. The closest personal relationships occur in these places; these are the spaces that are likely to have the greatest influence on the performance of an individual and are most likely to be influenced by an individual. Personal spaces are most likely to be adapted or customized for use by the occupants. Examples of these types of environments

Table 22-5. *Important Legislation That Affects Occupational Performance*[67]

Legislation	Summary and Effect
ADA, 1990	The ADA prohibits discrimination on the basis of disability in employment, state and local government, public accommodations, commercial facilities, transportation, and telecommunications. It also applies to the US Congress. To be protected by the ADA, one must have a disability or have a relationship or association with an individual with a disability. An individual with a disability is defined by the ADA as a person who has a physical or mental impairment that substantially limits one or more major life activities, a person who has a history or record of such impairment, or a person who is perceived by others as having such impairment. The ADA does not specifically name all of the impairments that are covered.
Fair Housing Act, 1988	The Fair Housing Act, as amended in 1988, prohibits housing discrimination on the basis of race, color, religion, sex, disability, familial status, and national origin. Its coverage includes private housing, housing that receives Federal financial assistance, and state and local government housing. It is unlawful to discriminate in any aspect of selling or renting housing or to deny a dwelling to a buyer or renter because of the disability of that individual, an individual associated with the buyer or renter, or an individual who intends to live in the residence. Other covered activities include, for example, financing, zoning practices, new construction design, and advertising.
	The Fair Housing Act requires owners of housing facilities to make reasonable exceptions in their policies and operations to afford people with disabilities equal housing opportunities. For example, a landlord with a "no pets" policy may be required to grant an exception to this rule and allow an individual who is blind to keep a guide dog in the residence. The Fair Housing Act also requires landlords to allow tenants with disabilities to make reasonable access-related modifications to their private living space, as well as to common use spaces. (The landlord is not required to pay for the changes.) The Act further requires that new multifamily housing with 4 or more units be designed and built to allow access for persons with disabilities. This includes accessible common use areas, doors that are wide enough for wheelchairs, kitchens and bathrooms that allow a person using a wheelchair to maneuver, and other adaptable features within the units.
Air Carrier Access Act	The Air Carrier Access Act prohibits discrimination in air transportation by air carriers against qualified individuals with physical or mental impairments. It applies only to air carriers that provide regularly scheduled services for hire to the public. Requirements address a wide range of issues including boarding assistance and certain accessibility features in newly built aircraft and new or altered airport facilities. People may enforce rights under the Air Carrier Access Act by filing a complaint with the US Department of Transportation, or by bringing a lawsuit in Federal court.
Civil Rights of Institution-alized Persons Act	The Civil Rights of Institutionalized Persons Act (CRIPA) authorizes the US Attorney General to investigate conditions of confinement at state and local government institutions, such as prisons, jails, pretrial detention centers, juvenile correctional facilities, publicly operated nursing homes, and institutions for people with psychiatric or developmental disabilities. Its purpose is to allow the Attorney General to uncover and correct widespread deficiencies that seriously jeopardize the health and safety of residents of institutions. The Attorney General does not have authority under CRIPA to investigate isolated incidents or to represent individual institutionalized persons.

(continued)

Table 22-5 (continued). *Important Legislation That Affects Occupational Performance*[67]

Legislation	Summary and Effect
Individuals with Disabilities Education Act	The Individuals with Disabilities Education Act (IDEA) (formerly called PL 94-142 or the Education for all Handicapped Children Act of 1975) requires public schools to make available to all eligible children with disabilities a free appropriate public education in the least restrictive environment appropriate to their individual needs. IDEA requires public school systems to develop appropriate Individualized Education Programs (IEPs) for each child. The specific special education and related services outlined in each IEP reflect the individualized needs of each student. IDEA also mandates that particular procedures be followed in the development of the IEP. Each student's IEP must be developed by a team of knowledgeable persons and must be at least reviewed annually. The team includes the child's teacher; the parents, subject to certain limited exceptions; the child, if determined appropriate; an agency representative who is qualified to provide or supervise the provision of special education; and other individuals at the parents' or agency's discretion.
Rehabilitation Act	The Rehabilitation Act prohibits discrimination on the basis of disability in programs conducted by federal agencies, in programs receiving federal financial assistance, in federal employment, and in the employment practices of federal contractors. The standards for determining employment discrimination under the Rehabilitation Act are the same as those used in Title I of the ADA.
Architectural Barriers Act (ABA)	The ABA requires that buildings and facilities designed, constructed, or altered with federal funds, or leased by a federal agency, comply with federal standards for physical accessibility. ABA requirements are limited to architectural standards in new and altered buildings and in newly leased facilities. They do not address the activities conducted in those buildings and facilities. The ABA covers facilities of the US Postal Service.

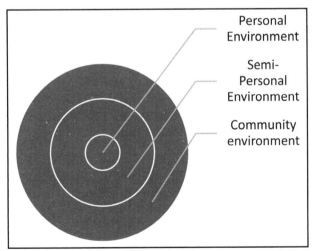

Figure 22-6. Proximal to distal layers of the environment.[37,70]

include one's home, workstation or office, and even one's car. For example, we can organize our toothbrush and toiletries in a manner that suits us best in our own homes, or we adjust the seat, mirrors, and items in our car that best facilitate our ability to drive.[37,70]

The second layer of the environment includes the semi-personal spaces encountered by individuals during their occupations. Semi-personal environments include those spaces frequented by individuals during their daily occupations. These spaces can include workspaces or "offices," local stores visited often, a favorite restaurant, a club, or religious facility. These spaces may or may not be customized to suit an individual's needs. Individuals are known and recognized in these environments. Occupations occur within these contexts and can be supported or impeded depending on the mix of social and physical influences. Semi-personal environments, or those public places that we pass through or experience frequently, typically surround proximal environments. Examples of public spaces can include a mall or a shopping center, library, or government building. These spaces may have adaptations that were made for the use of all individuals. These spaces may actually even have modifications made specifically for an individual. For example, a frequent patron of a coffee shop who uses a wheelchair may have influenced the proprietor to add an accessible bathroom, or the proprietor may allow the user to use his private bathroom because it is accessible. Generally, these spaces provide less accommodation than proximal or personal spaces.[37,70]

The third layer, or public sphere of performance, includes those spaces that an individual may or may not travel to on a frequent basis. These are community spaces used by many individuals in a society. They can include community-gathering places, such as arenas; public services, such as government facilities; and areas of public accommodation, such as stores or restaurants. The social and physical features are least likely to be customized to an individual's needs in this environment. The environment is typically designed to adhere to general anthropomorphic guidelines or governmental procedures. The outer layer of the environment is the public area. These spaces are the public or community spaces that may or may not be used by individuals, but they are part of the community within which the person operates.[37,70]

To better understand how the environment, made up of these physical and social influences, can have an effect on the performance of each individual, it is important to consider each element of the environment within the context that is relevant to that person. It is important to remember that while the elements can be explored individually, they continuously change and influence each other. While individuals are constantly changing throughout the developmental process, the environment is also constantly changing as a result of physical, social, and economic factors. In order to conceptualize the environment of an individual, it is helpful to consider the person within the context of the world in which they live (Table 22-6).

The layers of the environment do not exist in isolation, but are influenced by each other. For example, policy and services that are offered to individuals within a community may influence the type of housing that an individual can obtain. Thus, the public environment might greatly influence the personal environment of an individual.

These factors must be considered when determining modifications, as they may play a role in the success or failure of the person to do what he or she needs and wants to do. Does the client define independence by the level of assistance they need from another human? Does the individual's cultural beliefs or family system determine the amount of informal family support the person desires? Is the person interested in technology and interested in gadgets and physical support? Are they predisposed to using technology successfully or will they abandon the expensive equipment in favor of assistance from their spouse?[71,72]

INTERVENTION AT THE HOME AND COMMUNITY LEVEL

Home Modifications

The most common intervention provided by occupational therapy at the proximal level of the environment is modification to the home.[73] There is a large body of evidence supporting home modifications as an effective intervention for improving occupational performance. Home modifications can be used to improve the occupational performance of frail older adults, older adults with postoperative hip repair, adults and older adults with low vision, adults with schizophrenia, caregivers, and older adults with dementia.[74-80] Home modifications are also an important fall prevention strategy for older adults.[81] Although most of the literature has been developed for older adults, there is a growing body of evidence to support home modifications for caregivers or adults and children.

It is the role of the occupational therapy practitioner to determine the environmental factors that are influencing an individual's performance, consider the context of the occupations of the client and family, and identify a plan to resolve those barriers with the clients. Home modification interventions vary in intensity; they may include one visit using a checklist of standard home hazards, or a performance-based evaluation with follow-up and training. However, effective home modification interventions are a multi-step process including evaluation, development of an intervention plan, facilitation to implement recommendations, and training in the use of the modifications.[10]

Occupational therapy practitioners often work with a team to implement home modification interventions. Members of the team may include social workers, physical therapy practitioners, contractors, architects, representatives from funding sources, and family members. Training in the evaluation of the interaction between person and environment makes occupational therapy practitioners a key component to effective home modification interventions.[10,82] Home modification interventions are initiated and implemented across the continuum of care, with team members changing accordingly. For example, an inpatient occupational therapy practitioner recommends installation of a raised toilet seat and tub bench prior to discharge. Following discharge, the home health occupational therapy practitioner provides training to the client and family on the safe use of the new equipment and provides additional recommendations, such as rearranging furniture to increase accessibility.

Table 22-6. Examples of Environment Elements Found in Personal, Semi-Personal, and Public Environments

	Personal Environment	Semi-Personal Environment	Community
Built environment	• Home • Dorm room	• Places of employment • Neighborhood paces • Daycare	• Community spaces (sporting arenas, grocery stores, city hall)
Products and technology	• Assistive devices and technology designed or prescribed for and individual during self-care, or leisure or productive pursuits • Food, drugs • Clothing	• Assistive devices and technology designed or prescribed for an individual during education or employment outside the home, or during school such as augmentative communication devices, or specialized software	• Technology used in the community, such as motorized carts at the grocery store • Products used in the community, such as automatic teller machines
Transportation systems	• Personal car • Personal means of transportation (horse and buggy, bicycle)	• Transportation systems belonging to friends or family	• Public transportation including busses, cabs, airplanes
Natural environment	• Geography • Climate • Flora and fauna • Light, sound, and air quality	• Geography • Climate • Flora and fauna • Light, sound, and air quality	• Geography • Climate • Flora and fauna • Light, sound, and air quality
Cultural/societal factors	• Personal values • Tasks that must be accomplished by individual related to culture/religion	• Culture of workplace • Policy of organizations • Religious practices in group settings • Attitudes of a small group or individual toward disability	• Belief system of a society • Attitudes (of a society or group) toward disability • Public service systems and policies • Health care systems and policies
Social support	• Close friends • Family • Partner	• Casual friends • Work colleagues • Informational support • Emotional support	• Groups • Institutions • Professionals
Economic factors	• Personal resources	• Resources of community	• Community wealth (tax base)

The first step of the home modification process is evaluation. Important contextual information such as culture, important roles, and occupations or meaning of home are important and can be ascertained during the narrative and occupational profile interview.[83] Next, an evaluation of the person-environment fit and resulting occupational performance can be guided by one of the theoretical models presented in this chapter. The occupational therapy practitioner selects standardized assessments guided by the theoretical models, but customized to the treatment setting and health conditions. The evaluation should be conducted in the client's home (or use appropriate telerehab assessment approaches) to determine the baseline status of occupational performance and identify the unique environmental characteristics.[46,84] During evaluation, Connell's and Sanford's models can guide an environmentally focused task analysis to identify the influence of environmental barriers on occupational performance.[85,86] There are a number of standardized instruments available. For example, if fall prevention is the focus of the assessment, the HOME-FAST or the Westmead might be selected.[87,88] If accessibility of a potential apartment is the issue, and the person is not able to be assessed in the home, the Housing Enabler may be selected.[89] If a congregate living facility is being assessed, the Physical and Architectural Features Checklist of the Multiphasic Environmental Assessment Procedure (MEAP) may provide useful information.[90]

The next step is the development of an intervention plan. Taking an individual's unique personal and environmental factors into consideration, the occupational therapy practitioner identifies potential solutions and outcomes to meet the goals of the client(s). Availability and acceptability of personal assistance, ability to maintain equipment, and importance of aesthetics are examples of factors that may be considered when developing an intervention plan. Meetings with the home modification intervention team, as well as the client, to present potential home modifications and expected outcomes should be conducted to develop a final intervention plan. In order to increase the acceptability and usability of home modification strategies, it is necessary for the client to play an integral part in the decision making for the final intervention plan.

Which intervention is best? Once the practitioner has identified potential modifications, they should be reviewed with the client. Often there are multiple solutions that will address a single barrier. Environmental constraints, such as economic, architectural, and social barriers, might influence the choices of a home modification solution. For example, funding is often the most challenging obstacle for individuals with disabilities attempting to make home modifications. Building renovations are expensive, and funding currently is not available through most insurance companies for modifications to the home. People often rely on personal resources or social service agencies to fund the modifications. It is important to plan for modifications that will continue to meet the needs of the client (and their family members) over time. Aesthetic preferences can also influence the acceptability of a home modification for a client and their family. Clients should understand the range of solutions that could solve a barrier and the benefits and liabilities with each choice. Clients can then weigh costs in relation to their individual or family needs, priorities, aesthetic tastes, and values.

Once an intervention plan has been finalized, the occupational therapy practitioner may assist in obtaining and setting up equipment or AT and facilitate appropriate architectural modification. The occupational therapy practitioner may work directly with contractors or architects in order to ensure appropriate modifications occur to match the individual's personal abilities. Next, training on safe and appropriate use of the implemented strategies should be provided to the client and caregivers. Components of training include education, demonstrations, and activity training to ensure the client is able to achieve occupational goals. Although habits and routines are often disrupted by home modification strategies, during training the occupational therapy practitioner should try to incorporate them into the use of home modifications to increase adherence.

During training, it is possible the practitioner will identify modifications to the intervention plan to optimize occupational performance. These changes may be completed during activity training (ie, changing the way an individual completes an activity) or may require discussion with the team (ie, a need for an additional grab bar in the shower) before implementation. Furthermore, the occupational therapy practitioner should educate the client on any necessary maintenance, providing contact information for service providers and appropriate instruction manuals. For example, the practitioner should ensure a client who had a residential elevator installed has contact information for service companies readily available in case the elevator malfunctions.

Community Modifications

There is emerging evidence to support the role of occupational therapy practitioners in modifying the physical environment in communities. The community contains spaces such as government agencies, cultural venues, shopping complexes, and stores people visit on a less frequent basis than the home. Although people often spend less time in community spaces, they are important environments that serve as links between more private spaces, such as work and home, and they also contain critical goods and services necessary for successful participation in community life. Community spheres are important for socialization, recreation, and civic and social engagement. Environments with poor accessibility can negatively impact the participation of persons with disabilities.

The intervention approach is similar, the narrative and an occupational profile, a comprehensive assessment of community members and the physical environment, and a plan to reduce or remove barriers. There are a variety of reasons why occupational therapy practitioners address the physical environment in the community. In some cases the practitioner is working with an individual client, in other cases the intervention is directed to "public health" or an agency. A community assessment may be required as part of the process of understanding an individual client's abilities and limitations in different contexts or the general accessibility of a community space. The theoretical models support either of these intervention approaches, but the choice of assessment may change. Community assessments are presented in Table 22-7. An individually focused assessment might include the Craig Hospital Inventory of Environmental Factors (CHIEF) or the Home and Community Environment Assessment (HACE).[109-111] These types of assessment results can be helpful to occupational therapy practitioners to better understand the experiences of the individual client, and to set priorities with the client to enhance participation in occupational performance in the community. If the intervention is directed at the public health level, assessments such as the Community Health Environment Checklist (CHEC) may be used.[91]

Public places are not customized to meet individual needs. Rather, public spaces are typically designed to meet the needs of average individuals and are based on general guidelines, such as the ADA Accessibility Guidelines. Barriers to participation are highly prevalent in community spaces, including public transportation facilities.[112-115]

We can achieve greater accessibility by working directly with clients, by working with community property owners or consultants, and by working as advocates in the community. Occupational therapy practitioners can bring their knowledge of accessibility standards and theory to community agencies or organizations, or they can work directly with individual clients. Physical barrier removal may not always be possible in community settings. It is the role of the occupational therapy practitioner to understand current legislation and minimum standards and to help the client advocate for change. It is also possible to identify barriers through the assessment process to help clients make decisions about how they might access and use spaces using self-management strategies.

CASE EXAMPLE USING THE PERSON-ENVIRONMENT-OCCUPATION-PERFORMANCE MODEL

Modifying the environment has been a common strategy for supporting people who have limited capacities due to disabilities. It is the role of the occupational therapy practitioner to determine the environmental factors that are influencing an individual's performance, consider the context of the occupations of the client and family, and identify a plan to resolve those barriers with the clients. The following case provides an example of this intervention method. We will use Jen's story to illustrate how these theoretical constructs, intervention strategies, and the PEOP Model and person-centered PEOP Occupational Therapy Process support decisions to make environmental changes to improve the occupational performance of an individual with a disability.

Narrative

Jen is a 12-year-old girl who has cerebral palsy. Jen is active in her school, which promotes inclusion, and she is interested in pursuing social relationships of a typical adolescent. Her long-term goal is to graduate from high school and consider post-high school education options. She wants to eventually live in her own apartment. Jen currently lives in a single story home with her 15-year-old brother Frankie, her mother Rita, and her father Jim. Jim owns a small pest control business and Rita, previously a stay-at-home mom, has become an administrative assistant for a parent advocacy group. Jen is bright and outgoing. She has tremendous support from her family and is well liked by her peers and teachers. She is interested in supporting her school's athletic teams by attending their games and has recently considered becoming a cheerleader. She also has always enjoyed attending her friend's parties and "hanging out" with her peers. Jen has no cognitive limitations but has significant neuromotor and communication difficulties. Her speech is disarthric, it is difficult for anyone who does not know her well to understand her. She has some movement of her right arm and hand but experiences choreoathetoid movements and has trouble gripping items. She is unable to walk or transfer independently. She relies on a power wheelchair for mobility and her mom lifts her to the toilet, bathtub, and bed. Jen has self-concept scores that are lower than her non-disabled peers. She wishes that she could visit more of her friends and is beginning to feel left out of her group as her friends become more active in the community and begin to assert their independence.

Jen has become nearly 5 feet 10 inches tall, and would tower over her petite mother if she were standing. Rita has recently hurt her back and is having tremendous problems transferring Jen. She has become concerned that with her new job she will need to travel and will not be at home to accommodate Jen's needs. She is interested in finding a means to enable Jen to become more independent.

Currently, Jen has the enablers of a supportive family, economic resources, policy support from her state (programs to assist funding the changes her family may wish

Table 22-7. *Assessments of the Physical Environment*

Assessment	Physical Environment Construct	Description
Home		
Community Health Environment Checklist (CHEC)[91]	Receptivity of physical environment for participation	• Designed to be administered by community health professionals and community members using rule book and glossary • Focus on mobility impairments • Total destination and features scores
Canada Mortgage and Housing Corporation (CMHC)[92]	Barriers to occupational performance in the home	• Can be used by occupational therapy practitioners or other professions with experience in environmental adaptations • Translates well within a multidisciplinary team • Focus on individuals who are losing physical autonomy • Interview and observation • Identifies problematic activities, barriers in the home, and enabling adaptations
Comprehensive Assessment and Solution Process for Aging Residents (CASPAR)[93]	Environmental features impacting occupational performance	• Administration must be completed by practitioner or health care professional with training • Provides ratings of level of difficulty and use of mobility device for task completion • Problems are rated by urgency, along with client goals • Emphasis on mobility impairments • Assesses occupation and environment, does not document change in performance • Provides room-specific modifications
Enabler[94]	Physical barriers in the home	• Strong emphasis on person-environment interaction • Interview format • Individuals with functional limitations, with an emphasis on mobility issues • Identifies functional limitations, use of mobility devices, and physical barriers • Information used to create an accessibility score on 4-point ordinal scale
Home Environment Assessment Protocol (HEAP)[95]	Physical dimensions of safety in the home of persons with dementia	• Subscales include hazards, adaptations, clutter, and comfort • Addresses physical aspects, privacy, and meaning of objects • Measures change in hazards • Caregivers of persons with dementia • Professionals and nonprofessionals with training
Home-Fast[96]	Environmental hazards in the home	• Screening tool for fall risks in the homes of older adults • 25 items covering environmental and functional home safety concerns • Professionals and nonprofessionals can administer the assessment

(continued)

Table 22-7 (continued). *Assessments of the Physical Environment*

Assessment	Physical Environment Construct	Description
Home		
Home Observation for Measurement of the Environment (HOME)[97]	Quality and quantity of support and stimulation in the home environment	• Versions for ages 1 to 14, child care settings, and children with disabilities • Conducted in home with child and primary caregiver • Semi-structured interview and observation
In-Home Occupational Performance Evaluation (I-HOPE)[98]	Environmental barrier's influence on occupational performance	• Client identifies priority problematic activities • 4 subscales: activity participation, self-rating on performance, satisfaction with performance, and severity of environmental barriers (objective rating by practitioner) • Must be completed by an occupational therapy practitioner • Can be used to measure the impact of home modification interventions on occupational performance
Multiphasic Environmental Assessment Procedure (MEAP)[99]	Physical and social environments of residential settings for older adults	• Qualified clinicians, consultants, program evaluators, and researchers can use the MEAP • 5 instruments: resident and staff information, physical and architectural checklist, policy and program information, sheltered care environment scale, and rating scale (function) • Interviews, records, staff and administrator reports, and direct observation components

Safety Assessment of Function and the Environment for Rehabilitation (SAFER-Tool and SAFER-HOME)[100]	Safety concerns in the home	• SAFER-Tool
		  ◦ Identify safety concerns and guides intervention
		  ◦ Interview and in-home observation
		  ◦ Nominal score: no problem, problem
		• SAFER-HOME
		  ◦ Outcome measure of home modifications
		  ◦ Ordinal scale: no problem, mild problem, severe problem

Westmead Home Safety Assessment[101]	Physical and environmental fall hazards	• Completed by practitioner during home visit • Older adults • Interview, on-site observation, and performance-based components
Community		

ADA Checklist for Readily Achievable Barrier Removal[102]	Aspects of public areas that may be modified by removing barriers in existing facilities to meet ADA requirements	• A checklist that addresses 4 main barriers in public areas:
		  ◦ Approach and entrance
		  ◦ Goods and services
		  ◦ Public toilets
		  ◦ Other items: water fountains, public telephones

(continued)

Table 22-7 (continued). *Assessments of the Physical Environment*

Assessment	Physical Environment Construct	Description
Community		
Craig Hospital Inventory of Environmental Factors (CHIEF)[103]	Environmental influence on participation (adults-older adults)	• Client-perceived frequency and magnitude of environmental barriers • 5 subscales: policy, physical, work and school, attitudes and support, and services and assistance • People with disabilities aged 16 to 95 • Interview or self-report
Home and Community Environment Instrument (HACE)[104]	Physical aspects of the home and community environment influencing participation	• Interview and self-report • Adults and older adults with mobility impairments • Assesses 6 environmental domains: home mobility, community mobility, basic mobility devices, communication devices, transportation factors, and attitudes
Measure of Quality of the Environment (MQE)[105]	Environmental influence on participation	• Client provides self-ratings on the influence of environmental factors on participation • Addresses physical, social, and cultural influences on participation • Individuals with disabilities, self-administered
Workplace		
Work Environment Impact Scale (WEIS)[106]	Environmental characteristics that facilitate successful work-related occupations	• Semi-structured interview • Addresses individual perception of social and physical environments, supports, temporal demands, objects used, and job functions • 4-point rating scale measuring the overall impact of the work environment on the worker • Adults who have difficulty completing work tasks
Work Experience Survey[107]	Environmental barriers to access of job sites and productivity on the job	• Interview • Administration should be completed by a rehabilitation professional • Helps adults with disabilities identify barriers and direct accommodation planning • Assesses essential job functions, job mastery, and job satisfaction
School		
School Setting Interview (SSI)[108]	Identify aspects of the environment influencing function and participation across school settings including classroom, playground, gym, corridors, field trips	• Semi-structured interview • Students with physical disabilities age 10 years and older

to make to the environment), and a great belief in her abilities and success. Jen's parents have instilled a belief in her that she is a valuable person with contributions to make in life. Jen looks forward to making a contribution to society, to working, and having a satisfying life. Jen's family perceives these environmental modifications as an important learning opportunity for Jen. They want her to understand that the environment can be a support and that asking for modifications will be an important part of how she will be able to participate in society. Jen believes that she will achieve her goals and seeks the assistance of an occupational therapy practitioner to bridge her current situation to her goals by providing environmental support. The local school system has coordinated efforts with the family. For example, they have made sure that the equipment they provide for Jen to enhance her learning (computer) fit within the home context so that she can study. The family has also applied for and been granted tax credits to assist in paying for the changes to their home.

Jen has many roles as a pre-teen, daughter, friend, classmate, student, "included child," and person with a disability. Her mother, the primary caregiver to Jen (and also a client), has multiple roles as well. She is a mom, advocate for her daughter, and persons with disabilities spouse, and community leader, as well as a friend and caregiver.

Jen and her family face several environmental barriers. Most of them are in the built environment (her home, the context of this intervention). Her home has a small bathroom with a typical bathtub. She is currently unable to manipulate the handles of the bathroom faucet and is unable to see herself in the bathroom mirror because it is located at a height that she cannot use in a seated position (from her wheelchair). She is unable to transfer into the bathtub without maximum assistance from her mother. She is required to make a 3-point turn in order to get into the bathroom because of the narrow hallway and the configuration of the space. It is difficult to maneuver Jen's chair to the tub for transfers due to the limited space.

Since both Jen and Rita are involved, it is important to consider the goals of each client. Jen has immediate goals of being able to fix her own hair and wash her own hands. She would like to be able to get into the bathroom without bumping into everything. Rita is interested in transfers that are safer and cause less strain on her back.

Jen is interested in graduating and considering college or vocational opportunities. She is interested in being independent and living in and managing her own home someday; Rita has the same long-term goals.

Evaluation

First, using the PEOP Occupational Therapy Process and the Enabler Model to guide the organization of Jen's capabilities and constraints to her performance, the occu-

pational therapy practitioner would begin to think about the environment in terms of the capacity that Jen currently has, as well as the potential changes in her performance that may be expected given the prognosis of her diagnosis and her expected development.[116] Using the PEOP Occupational Therapy Process and Enabler as a guide, the practitioner begins to think about the assessment results and place them in the framework in order to consider the potential person and environment relationships that may be preventing Jen from reaching her desired goals. Jen has problems with mobility, reaching, grasping, and manipulating, and she uses a wheelchair for mobility. The practitioner identifies potential barriers in the home. These can then be verified by standardized measures that are based on observation of performance.

The evidence that has been presented thus far suggests that modification of the environment can increase the performance of individuals who have limited functional abilities. For example, as you recall from the beginning of this chapter, Connell and Sanford found that people with disabilities who modified their homes had little to moderate difficulty and dependence in the conduct of daily activities.[117] Gitlin et al concluded that home modifications slowed the rate of functional dependency and enhanced caregiver self-efficacy.[79] Mann et al reported that the rate of decline in independence of older adults and costs for personal assistance and health care were reduced through increased use of AT and environmental interventions.[118] These are critical pieces of evidence that, when coupled with the theories presented, suggest that environmental modifications are an appropriate intervention for Jen and her family.

Intervention

As a practitioner with a set of tools to provide environmental modification, the practitioner will continue to use the theory and models presented in this chapter to develop an intervention plan for Jen. When considering potential opportunities for modification, the practitioner can rely on the ICF environmental factors to organize his or her thinking about the potential environmental strategies that are possible. The framework by Connell and Sanford can guide the practitioner in his or her decisions about the characteristics of the environment that would support the occupational performance of the client.[117] So, in the present case, the plan was developed by the practitioner, the clients, and the contractor and included modification of the existing bathroom. The changes included enlarging the room by breaking through a wall into a spare bedroom to provide a larger area with a 6-foot circle of clear space in the middle of the room. This additional space accommodated Jen's power chair and a caregiver at the same time.

Jen and her mom also opted for an overhead lift system to make transfers to the bath or toilet easier for her mom and give Jen more independence. They chose the overhead lift system instead of the option of a roll in shower because Jen enjoyed relaxing in the bathtub. A special seating system was included in the tub so Jen could sit in the tub independently. The mirror over the sink was lowered to a height of 36 inches so Jen could easily check her appearance. The sink included a lever-type faucet and clear knee space so Jen could roll under.

Outcomes

Upon re-evaluation and observation of Jen in her bathroom, the short-term goals that Jen and her mom had for safer, easier transfers, and increased independence using a mirror and sink were achieved by using environmental modifications. Jen's mom reports decreased stress on her back, and Jen is delighted to see herself in the mirror. Her mom reports that Jen often rolls into the bathroom to check her appearance.

Although the intervention in Jen's case was in the home, there were other issues that the occupational therapy practitioner asked Jen about. The context of Jen's other occupations, the school she attends and the community in which she lives, were other potential places for environmental barriers. By revisiting Jen's goals and considering her new occupational performance priorities, Jen decided to address her desire to spend time with her friends. She was currently facing many problems accessing the community center and the movie theater.

Jen and her occupational therapy practitioner have developed an educational program that Jen presented to the Chamber of Commerce about living with disabilities. As a result of her presentation, several local businesses have been working with the local ADA Technical Assistance Center to improve the physical accessibility of the community. Jen and her family look forward to her development as a teenager, and feel that the control that Jen can exhibit over her environment truly helps her feel like a valued and important citizen.

SUMMARY

A fundamental shift in how disability is defined has occurred within the past decade. No longer is the individual "disabled" based on functional capacity, but rather that *he or she can become disabled by an environment that prevents optimum performance.* This new definition requires new intervention strategies by practitioners.

This chapter has provided some important concepts to use in understanding the role of the environment on the performance of occupations. We have summarized 5 important models that describe the person-environment-occupation-performance relationship that is inherent in the PEOP Model, including Lawton and Nahemow's Ecological Model, the ICF list by WHO, the Enabler Model by Steinfeld et al,[43] and the Conceptual Framework to Guide the Process of Developing Home Modification by Connell and Sanford,[117] and used them to explore the interventions possible in the physical and social environment. The environmental context where these changes occur was examined, and a discussion of the contextual features that need to be considered when making environmental modifications was presented (Table 22-8). Finally, a case study was presented to illustrate how the PEOP Model and the PEOP Occupational Therapy Process could be applied to a real case.

The occupational therapy process as defined by the PEOP Model explicitly defines the role of environmental modifications as improving the occupational performance of individuals who have limited capacity. The use of these theories and intervention strategies is central to the process of eliminating a "disabling" environment and maximizing occupational performance for the individual and society.

ACKNOWLEDGMENT

The authors wish to gratefully acknowledge the contribution of Carolyn Baum, PhD, to the discussion of the evolution of environment in occupational therapy and rehabilitative models. Dr. Baum personally influenced the IOM and WHO models, and her experience is appreciated in the development of this section.

Table 22-8.   Evidence Table: Interventions Addressing the Physical Environment for a Variety of Populations

Study Reference	Aim of Study	Methods	Results and Conclusions	Level of Evidence
Campbell, Robertson, La Grow, et al[119]	Efficacy of a multi-component intervention to reduce falls and fall injury (older adults with low vision)	Participants were randomized to 4 intervention groups: home safety and modifications, exercise, home modifications and exercise, or social visits. The home safety program used a checklist completed by a practitioner.	• The individuals who received home modifications reported 41% less falls than those that did not. There was no difference in falls occurring in the home or outside of the home. • The cost per fall prevented by the home safety program was $432.	RCT Level I
Clarke, Ailshire, Nieuwenhuijsen, and de Kleijn-de Vrankrijker[120]	Investigate environmental characteristics impacting participation for adults at risk for health-related impairments and activity limitations	Observational data was collected using systematic social observation on neighborhood characteristics.	• Adults with visual impairments living in heavy traffic areas demonstrated 20% lower odds of receiving preventative health care. • Odds of participating in regular interpersonal interaction were 45% higher for adults with mobility impairment living in areas with higher residential security. • Adults with mobility difficulties who live in areas with high proportion of poor condition streets have 60% lower odds of voting.	Cross-sectional Level IV
Close, Ellis, Hooper, Glucksman, Jackson, and Swift[121]	Effects of occupational therapy home modification intervention on falls over 12 months (older adults presenting to emergency department with a fall)	In-home evaluation including removal of home hazards, minor home repair, equipment, and referral for more extensive modifications. Safety education was also provided.	• Intervention group demonstrated lower risk and rate of falling compared to controls. Both experienced a decrease in ADL/IADL performance over time, but the intervention group exhibited less decline.	RCT Level I
Dooley and Hinojosa[122]	Effects of home modification intervention on QOL (individuals with Alzheimer's disease and caregivers)	Home modification assessment with treatment plan, environmental adaptations, and education; included caregiver strategies and referral to community-based services.	• The treatment group had a significant main effect for caregiver burden, positive affect, activity frequency, and self-care status.	RCT Level I

(continued)

Table 22-8 (continued). *Evidence Table: Interventions Addressing the Physical Environment for a Variety of Populations*

Study Reference	Aim of Study	Methods	Results and Conclusions	Level of Evidence
Gitlin, Corcoran, Winter, Boyce, and Hauck[123]	Short-term effects of home modification intervention (caregivers and dementia patients)	Multi-component intervention including the physical and social environmental modifications and education on the impact of the environment on dementia-related behaviors. In total, 75% of the recommendations were implemented.	• Intervention group caregivers reported less decline in the care recipient's IADL dependence than the controls. • Caregivers in the intervention group experienced reduced upset. • Different types of caregivers may respond differently to the home modification interventions: women had enhanced feelings of self-efficacy in managing behaviors, and women and minorities had enhanced feelings of self-efficacy managing functional dependence.	RCT Level I
Hammel, Jones, Gossett, and Morgan[124]	Identify community participation goals, barriers, and supports/strategies for individuals who have experienced a stroke	Observations and environmental audits with participants during participation in home and community environments.	• Physical barriers accounted for a significant amount of access barriers. • Adapting the environment was the primary way participants enabled participation. • Social barriers including supportive family and societal attitudes influenced participation.	Qualitative Level VI
Mann, Ottenbacher, Fraas, Tomita, and Granger[125]	Effects of home AT on occupational performance (frail older adults)	Functional and home assessment by an occupational therapy practitioner with recommendations, provision, and training in AT and environmental interventions.	• Individuals who received spent less on medical and other in-home assistance services and long-term nursing home costs.	RCT Level I

(continued)

Table 22-8 (continued). *Evidence Table: Interventions Addressing the Physical Environment for a Variety of Populations*

Study Reference	Aim of Study	Methods	Results and Conclusions	Level of Evidence
Ostensjo, Carlberg, and Vollestad[126]	Impact of assistive devices and environmental modifications on daily activities (young children with CP)	Survey and parent interview to describe the use of assistive devices and modifications and the benefits for function and caregiving.	• Use of assistive devices and modifications support daily activities for children with cerebral palsy. • Caregiver assistance was reduced substantially with use of assistive devices and modifications for mobility and eating. • Use of assistive devices is support by housing and transportation adaptions.	Cross-sectional Level IV
Petersson, Kottorp, Bergstrom, and Lilja[127]	Impact of home modifications on daily activities (adults aging with disabilities)	Occupational therapy practitioners interviewed participants before and after receiving home modifications through government grants. Intervention areas included bathrooms, entrances, elevators, and other areas of the home.	• The intervention group reported significantly less difficultly completing daily activities than the control group at 6 months. • Time waiting for home modifications was a confounding factor for difficulty completing activities.	Quasi-experimental pre-test/post-test Level II
Pighills, Torgerson, Drummond, Bland[128]	Efficacy of home modifications delivered by occupational therapy practitioners and trained assessors (older adults with a history of falls)	Home hazard assessment and removal completed by either an occupational therapy practitioner or a trained assessor.	• The occupational therapy practitioner group had a significantly higher number of home modification recommendations and adherence rates. • The occupational therapy practitioner group reported significantly fewer falls than the control group and no significant affect for the trained assessor group • There was no reported difference in ADL between groups. • There was no effect on fear of falling in either group.	RCT Level I

(continued)

Table 22-8 (continued).   *Evidence Table: Interventions Addressing the Physical Environment for a Variety of Populations*

Study Reference	Aim of Study	Methods	Results and Conclusions	Level of Evidence
Stark, Landsbaum, Palmer, Somerville, and Morris[129]	Effect of a home modification intervention on functional performance (older adults with functional limitations)	Participants received a structured in-home evaluation with home modifications, , education, and follow-up training. In total, 80% of recommended home modifications were followed.	• At 1 month, participants demonstrated a significant increase in functional independence, performance, and satisfaction with performance. Additionally, at 2 years post there was no change in functional performance.	Quasi-experimental design, pre- and post-prospective study Level III
Velligan, Diamond, Mueller, Li, Maples, Wang, and Miller[130]	Effects of cognitive adaptive training (CAT), generic environmental supports (GES), and treatment as usual (TAU) on function (adults with schizoaffective disorder)	Participants received CAT (individualized environmental supports), GES, or TAU.	• Participants in CAT used a higher proportion of supports than the GES group. • The CAT and GES group differed significantly in global functioning at 3 months post, compared to TAU. • Higher utilizers of environmental supports were more likely to improve target behaviors.	RCT Level I

REFERENCES

1. Carver V, Rodda M. *Disability and the Environment.* London, UK: Elek Books; 1978.
2. Barris R. Environmental interactions: an extension of the model of occupation. *American Journal of Occupational Therapy.* 1982;36(1):637-644.
3. Dunn W, Brown C, McGuigan A. The ecology of human performance: a framework for considering the effect of context. *American Journal of Occupational Therapy.* 1994;48(7):595-607.
4. Christiansen C, Baum C. *Occupational Therapy: Enabling Function and Well-Being.* 2nd ed. Thorofare, NJ: SLACK Incorporated; 1997.
5. Christiansen C, Baum C. *Occupational Therapy: Overcoming Human Performance Deficits.* Thorofare, NJ: SLACK Incorporated; 1991:847-860.
6. Law M, Cooper B, Strong S, et al. The person-environment-occupation model: a transactive approach to occupational performance. *Canadian Journal of Occupational Therapy.* 1996;63(1):9-23.
7. Law M. 1991 Muriel Driver lecture: the environment: a focus for occupational therapy. *Canadian Journal of Occupational Therapy.* 1991;58(4):171-180.
8. Gitlin LN, Winter L, Dennis MP, et al. A randomized trial of a multicomponent home intervention to reduce functional difficulties in older adults. *Journal of the American Geriatrics Society.* 2006;54(5):809-816.
9. Gitlin LN, Hauck WW, Winter L, Dennis MP, Schulz R. Effect of an in-home occupational and physical therapy intervention on reducing mortality in functionally vulnerable older people: preliminary findings. *Journal of the American Geriatrics Society.* 2006;54(6):950-955.
10. Clemson L, Mackenzie L, Ballinger C, Close JC, Cumming RG. Environmental interventions to prevent falls in community-dwelling older people: a meta-analysis of randomized trials. *Journal of Aging and Health.* 2008;20(8):954-971.
11. Gitlin LN, Winter L, Corcoran M, et al. Effects of the home environmental skill-building programf on the caregiver-care recipient dyad: 6-month outcomes from the Philadelphia REACH Initiative. *Gerontologist.* 2003;43(4):532-46.
12. WHO. *International Classification of Functioning, Disability and Health.* Geneva, Switzerland: World Health Organization; 2001.
13. Meyer A. The philosophy of occupation therapy. *Archives of Occupational Therapy.* 1922;1(1):1-10.
14. Reilly M. Occupational therapy can be one of the great ideas of 20th century medicine. *American Journal of Occupational Therapy.* 1962;16:300-308.
15. Dunning H. Environmental occupational therapy. *American Journal of Occupational Therapy.* 1972;26(6):292-298.
16. Kiernat JM. Promoting community awareness of architectural barriers. *American Journal of Occupational Therapy.* 1972;26(1):10-12.
17. Reed KL, Sanderson SR. *Concepts of Occupational Therapy.* Baltimore, MD: Williams & Wilkins; 1980.
18. Reed KL, Sanderson SR. *Concepts of Occupational Therapy.* 2nd ed. Baltimore, MD: Williams & Wilkins; 1983.
19. Reed KL, Sanderson SR. *Concepts of Occupational Therapy.* 3rd ed. Baltimore, MD: Williams & Wilkins; 1992.
20. Howe MC, Briggs AK. Ecological systems model for occupational therapy. *American Journal of Occupational Therapy.* 1982;36:322-327.

21. Department of National Health and Welfare, Canadian Association of Occupational Therapists. *Guidelines for the Client-Centred Practice of Occupational Therapy.* (H39-33/1983E). Ottawa, ON: Department of National Health and Welfare; 1983.

22. Kielhofner G. *A Model of Human Occupation: Theory and Application.* Baltimore, MD: Williams & Wilkins; 1985.

23. Kielhofner G. *A Model of Human Occupation: Theory and Application.* 2nd ed. Baltimore, MD: Williams & Wilkins; 1995.

24. Kielhofner G. *A Model of Human Occupation: Theory and Application.* 3nd ed. Baltimore, MD: Williams & Wilkins; 2002.

25. Christiansen C, Baum C, Bass Haugen J. Person-Environment-Occupation-Performance: an occupation-based framework for practice. In: Christiansen C, Baum C, Bass Haugen J, eds. *Occupational Therapy: Performance, Participation and Well-Being.* Thorofare, NJ: SLACK Incorporated; 2005:242-267.

26. Baum CM, Christiansen C, Bass JD. The person-environment-occupation-performance model. In: Christiansen CH, Baum CM, Bass JD, eds. *Occupational Therapy: Performance, Participation, and Well-being.* Thorofare, NJ: SLACK Incorporated; 2015.

27. Polatajko HJ. Naming and framing occupational therapy: a lecture dedicated to the life of Nancy B. *Canadian Journal of Occupational Therapy.* 1992;59(4):189-200.

28. Stewart AM. The Casson Memorial Lecture 1992: always a little further. *British Journal of Occupational Therapy.* 1992;55(8):296-302.

29. Schkade JK, Schultz S. Occupational adaptation: toward a holistic approach for contemporary practice, part 1. *American Journal of Occupational Therapy.* 1992;46(9):829-837.

30. Hagedorn R. *Tools for Practice in Occupational Therapy: A Structured Approach to Core Skills and Processes.* Edinburgh, Scotland: Churchill Livingstone; 2000.

31. Hagedorn R. *Occupational Therapy: Perspectives and Processes.* Edinburgh, Scotland: Churchill Livingstone; 1995.

32. Bass Haugen JB, Mathiowetz V. Contemporary task oriented approach. In: Trombly CA, ed. *Occupational Therapy for Physical Dysfunction.* 4th ed. Baltimore, MD: Williams & Wilkens; 1995: 510-527.

33. Canadian Association of Occupational Therapists. *Enabling Occupation: An Occupational Therapy Perspective.* Ottawa, ON: CAOT Publications; 1997.

34. Brandt EN, Pope AM. Executive summary. In: Brandt EN, Pope AM, eds. *Enabling America: Assessing the Role of Rehabilitation Science and Engineering.* Washington, DC: National Academy Press; 1997:1-23.

35. French JR, Rodgers W, Cobb S. Adjustment as person-environment fit. In: Coelho GV, Hamburg DA, Adams JE, eds. *Coping and Adaptation.* New York, NY: Basic Books, Inc; 1974:316-333.

36. Lewin K. *Field Theory in Social Science.* New York, NY: Harper; 1951.

37. Bronfenbrenner U. *The Ecology of Cognitive Development.* Cambridge, MA: Harvard University Press; 1979.

38. Bronfenbrenner U. The ecology of cognitive development: research models and fugitive findings. In: Wozniak RH, Fischer KW, eds. *Development in Context: Acting and Thinking in Specific Environments.* New York, NY: Erlbaum; 1993:3-44.

39. Lawton MP, Nahemow L. Ecology and the aging process. In: Eisdorfer C, Lawton MP, eds. *Psychology of Adult Development and Aging.* Washington, DC: American Psychological Association; 1973:619-674.

40. Lawton MP, Simon B. The ecology of social relationships in housing for the elderly. *Gerontologist.* 1968;8:108-115.

41. Lawton MP. Residential environment and self-directness among older people. *American Psychologist.* 1990;45(5):638-640.

42. Steinfeld E, Schroeder S, Duncan J, et al. *Access to the Built Environment: A Review of Literature.* Washington, DC: US Government Printing Office; 1979.

43. Iwarsson S, Isacsson Å. "The Enabler" applied to occupational therapy: reliability of a usability rating scale. In: Steinfeld E, Danford GS, eds. *Enabling Environments: Measuring the Impact of Environment on Disability and Rehabilitation.* New York, NY: Springer Science + Business Media, Kluwer Academic/Plenum Publishers; 1999:93-109.

44. Murray HA. *Explorations in Personality.* New York, NY: Oxford University Press; 1938.

45. Connell BR, Sanford J. Individualizing home modification recommendations to facilitate performance of routine activities. In: Laspry S, Hyde J, eds. *Staying Put, Adapting the Places to the People.* Amityville, NY: Baywood Publishing; 1997:113-147.

46. Sanford JA, Jones M, Daviou P, Grogg K, Butterfield T. Using telerehabilitation to identify home modification needs. *Assistive Technology.* 2004;16(1):43-53.

47. US Senate and House of Representative of the United States of America in the 100th Congress. *Public Law 100-407: The Technology-Related Assistance for Individuals with Disabilities Act of (1988).* Uscode.house.gov. http://uscode.house.gov/statutes/1988/1988-100-0407.pdf. Published August 19, 1988. Accessed January 1, 2014.

48. Seelman KD. Assistive technology policy: a road to independence for individuals with disabilities. *Journal of Social Issues.* 1993;49(2):115-136.

49. O'Day BL, Corcoran PJ. Assistive technology: problems and policy alternatives. *Archives of Physical Medicine and Rehabilitation.* 1994;75(10):1165-1169.

50. Gitlin LN, Corcoran M, Leinmiller-Eckhardt S. Understanding the family perspective: an ethnographic framework for providing occupational therapy in the home. *American Journal of Occupational Therapy.* 1995;49(8):802-809.

51. Axelson L. Development and use of the Swedish road weather information system. *Rwis.net: Sensor Integration Center: Swedish National Road Administration.* http://www.rwis.net/. Published 2000. Updated 2013. Accessed January 1, 2014.

52. McColl MA, Friedland J. Social support and occupational therapy. In: Christiansen C, Baum C, eds. *Occupational Therapy: Enabling Function and Well-Being.* 2nd ed. Thorofare, NJ: SLACK Incorporated; 1989:411-425.

53. McColl MA, Friedland J. Development of a multidimensional index for assessing social support in rehabilitation. *Occupational Therapy Journal of Research.* 1989;9(4):218-234.

54. McColl MA. Social support and occupational therapy. In: Christiansen C, Baum C, eds. *Occupational Therapy: Enabling Function and Well-Being.* 2nd ed. Thorofare, NJ: SLACK Incorporated; 1997:411-425.

55. Kondo T, Mann W, Tomita M, Ottenbacher K. The use of microwave ovens by elder persons with disabilities. *American Journal of Occupational Therapy.* 1997;51(9):739-747.

56. McColl MA, Rosenthal C. A model of resource needs of aging spinal cord injured men. *Paraplegia.* 1994;32:261-270.

57. Weinberger M, Tierney WM, Booher P, Hiner SC. Social support, stress and functional status in patients with osteoarthritis. *Social Science and Medicine.* 1990;30:503-508.

58. Holicky R, Charlifue S. Aging with a spinal cord injury: the impact of spousal support. *Disability and Rehabilitation.* 1999;21:250-257.

59. Zarit SH, Todd PA, Zarit JM. Subjective burden of husbands and wives as caregivers: a longitudinal study. *The Gerontologist.* 1986;26(3):260-266.

60. Gallo J. The effect of social support on depression in caregivers of the elderly. *Journal of Family Practice.* 1990;30:430-440.

61. Calkins M, Namazi K. Caregivers' perceptions of the effectiveness of home modifications for community living adults with dementia. *Journal of Alzheimer's Care and Related Disorder Research.* 1991;6(1):25-29.

62. Barris R, Keilhofner G, Levine R, Neville A. Occupation as an interaction with the environment. In: Kielhofner G, ed. *A Model of Human Occupation: Theory and Application.* Baltimore, MD: Williams & Wilkins; 1985:42-62.

63. Barney K. From Ellis Island to assisted living: meeting the needs of older adults from diverse cultures. *American Journal of Occupational Therapy.* 1991;45:586-593.

64. The Center for Universal Design. *A Blueprint for Action: A Resource for Promoting Home Modifications.* Raleigh, NC: North Carolina State University, School of Design; 1997.

65. Pearlin LI, Mullan JT, Semple SJ, Skaff MM. Caregiving and the stress process: an overview of concepts and their measures. *Gerontologist.* 1990;30(5):583-594.

66. LaPlante MP, Harrington C, Kang T. Estimating paid and unpaid hours of personal assistance services in activities of daily living provided to adults living at home. *Health Services Research.* 2002;37(2):397-415.

67. Federal Citizen Information Center (FCIC). *Publications.USA. gov: ACA.* Publications.USA.gov. http://www.pueblo.gsa.gov/cic_text/misc/disability/disrits.htm#ADA. Accessed April 2, 2014.

68. Peterson W. Public policy affecting universal design. *Assistive Technology.* 1998;10(1):13-20.

69. US Access Board. *ADA standards.* US Access Board. http://www.access-board.gov/guidelines-and-standards/buildings-and-sites/about-the-ada-standards/ada-standards. Published 2002. Updated 2012. Accessed January 1, 2014.

70. Lawton MP. *Environment and Aging.* Monterey, CA: Brooks-Cole; 1980.

71. Batavia AE, Hammer GS. Toward the development of consumer-based criteria for evaluation of assistive devices. *Journal of Rehabilitation Research and Development.* 1990;27(4):425-436.

72. Scherer MJ. *Living in a State of Stuck.* Cambridge, MA: Brookline Books; 1994.

73. Wahl HW, Fänge A, Oswald F, Gitlin LN, Iwarsson S. The home environment and disability-related outcomes in aging individuals: what is the empirical evidence? *Gerontologist.* 2009;49(3):355-367.

74. Mann WC, Ottenbacher KJ, Fraas L, Tomita M, Granger CV. Effectiveness of and environmental interventions in maintaining independence and reducing home care costs for the frail elderly: a randomized controlled trial. *Archives of Family Medicine.* 1999;8(3):210-217.

75. Hagsten B, Svensson O, Gardulf A. Early individualized postoperative occupational therapy training in 100 patients improves ADL after hip fracture: a randomized trial. *Acta Orthopaedica Scandinavica.* 2004;75(2):177-183.

76. Brunnstrom G, Sorensen S, Alsterstad K, Sjöstrand J. Quality of light and quality of life—the effect of lighting adaptation among people with low vision. *Ophthalmic and Physiological Optics.* 2004;24(4):274-80.

77. Velligan DI, Diamond PM, Maples NJ, et al. Comparing the efficacy of interventions that use environmental supports to improve outcomes in patients with schizophrenia. *Schizophrenia Research.* 2008;102(1-3):312-319.

78. Velligan DI, Diamond P, Mueller J, et al. The short-term impact of generic versus individualized environmental supports on functional outcomes and target behaviors in schizophrenia. *Psychiatry Research.* 2009;168(2):94-101.

79. Gitlin LN, Corcoran M, Winter L, Boyce A, Hauck WW. A randomized controlled trial of a home environmental intervention: effect of efficacy and use in caregivers and on daily function of persons with dementia. *Gerontologist.* 2001;41(1):4-14.

80. Graff MJ, Vernooij-Dassen MJ, Thijssen M, et al. Community based occupational therapy for patients with dementia and their care givers: randomized controlled trial. *BMJ (Clinical Research Edition).* 2006;333(7580):1196.

81. Chase CA, Mann K, Wasek S, Arbesman M. Systematic review of the effect of home modification and fall prevention programs on falls and the performance of community-dwelling older adults. *American Journal of Occupational Therapy.* 2012;66(3):284-291.

82. Pighills AC, Torgerson DJ, Sheldon TA, Drummond AE, Bland JM. Environmental assessment and modification to prevent falls in older people. *Journal of the American Geriatrics Society.* 2011;59(1):26-33.

83. Tanner B, Tilse C, De Jonge D. Restoring and sustaining home: the impact of home modifications on the meaning of home for older people. *Journal of Housing for the Elderly.* 2008;22(3):195-215.

84. Hoenig H, Sanford JA, Butterfield T, et al. Development of a teletechnology protocol for in-home rehabilitation. *Journal of Rehabilitation Research and Development.* 2006;43(2):287-298.

85. Watson DE, Wilson SA. *Task Analysis: An Occupational Performance Approach.* Bethesda, MD: AOTA Press; 2003.

86. Watson DE, Wilson SA. *Task Analysis: An Individual and Population Approach.* Bethesda, MD: AOTA Press; 2003

87. Mackenzie L, Byles J, Higginbotham N. Designing the home falls and accidents screening tool (HOME FAST): selecting the items. *British Journal of Occupational Therapy.* 2000;63(6):260-269.

88. Clemson L, Fitzgerald MH, Heard R. Content validity of an assessment tool to identify home fall hazards: the Westmead Home safety assessment. *British Journal of Occupational Therapy.* 1999;62(4):171-179.

89. Iwarsson S, Slaug B. *Housing Enabler: An Instrument for Assessing and Analyzing Accessibility Problems in Housing.* Nävlinge, Sweden: Veten & Skapen HB & Slaug Data Management; 2001.

90. Moos RH, Lemke S. *Evaluating Residential Facilities: The Multiphasic Environmental Assessment Procedure.* Thousand Oaks, CA: Sage Publications, Inc; 1996.

91. Stark S, Hollingsworth HH, Morgan KA, Gray DB. Community Health Environment Checklist. *Disability and Rehabilitation.* 2007;29(2):123-137.

92. Maltais D, Canada Mortgage and Housing Corporation. *Maintaining Seniors' Independence: A Guide to Home Adaptations.* Ottawa, ON: Public Affairs Centre, CMHC; 2012. http://www.cmhc.ca. Published 1989. Updated 2012. Accessed January 14, 2014.

93. Sanford JA, Pynoos J, Tejral A, Browne A. Development of a comprehensive assessment for delivery of home modifications. *Physical and Occupational Therapy in Geriatrics.* 2001;20(2):43-55.

94. Iwarsson S. *The Enabler: A Method for Analyzing Accessibility Problems in Housing.* Sweden: Lund University; 1997. http://www.enabler.nu/index.html. Updated December 9, 2009. Accessed April 2, 2014.

95. Gitlin LN, Schinfeld S, Winter L, Corcoran M, Boyce AA, Hauck,W. Evaluating home environments of persons with dementia: interrater reliability and validity of the Home Environmental Assessment Protocol (HEAP). *Disability and Rehabilitation.* 2002;24(1-3):59-71.

96. Mackenzie L, Byles J, Higginbotham N. Designing the Home Falls and Accidents Screening Tool (HOME FAST): selecting the items. *British Journal of Occupational Therapy.* 2000;63:260-269.

97. Bradley RH, Caldwell BM. The HOME inventory and family demographics. *Developmental Psychology.* 1984;20:315-320.

98. Stark SL, Somerville EK, Morris JC. In-Home Occupational Performance Evaluation (I-HOPE). *American Journal of Occupational Therapy.* 2010;64(4):580-589.

99. Moos RH, Lemke S. *Evaluating residential facilities: the multiphasic environmental assessment procedure.* Thousand Oaks, CA: Sage Publications; 1996.

100. Chui T, Oliver R, Oliver L, Oliver M, Letts L. *Safety Assessment of Function and the Environment for Rehabilitation Tool (SAFER).* Toronto, ON: Comprehensive Rehabilitation and Mental Health Services; 2001.

101. Clemson L. *Westmead Home Safety Assessment (WeSHA).* Sydney, Australia: Co-Ordinates Publications; 1997.

102. Institute for Human Centered Design. *ADA Checklist for Readily Achievable Barrier Removal.* New England ADA Center. www.ADAchecklist.org. Published 1995. Updated 2011. Accessed April 2, 2014.

103. Craig Hospital Research Department. *Craig Hospital Inventory of Environmental Factors (CHIEF) Manual.* Version 3.0. Englewood, CO: Craig Hospital; 2001. http://tbims.org/combi/chief/index.html. Published 2001. Updated 2012. Accessed April 2, 2014.

104. Keysor J, Jette A, Haley S. Development of the Home and Community Environment (HACE) instrument. *Journal of Rehabilitation Medicine.* 2005;37(1):37-44.

105. Fougeyrollas P, Noreau L, St-Michel G, Boschen K. *Measure of Quality of the Environment (MQE).* Version 2.0. Lac St-Charles, Quebec, Canada: International Network of the Disability Creation Process, Canadian Society of the International Classification of Impairments, Disabilities, and Handicaps: 1999.

106. Kielhofner G, Shei Lai J, Olson L, et al. Psychometric properties of the work environment impact scale: a cross-cultural study. *Work.* 1999;12(1):71-77.

107. Roessler RT, Gottcent J. The work experience survey: a reasonable accommodation/career development strategy. *Journal of Applied Rehabilitation Counseling.* 1994;25(3):16-21.

108. Hemmingsson H, Kottorp A, Bernspång B. Validity of the school setting interview: an assessment of the student-environment fit. *Scand J Occup Ther.* 2004;11:171-178.

109. Whiteneck GG, Harrison-Felix CL, Mellick, DC, et al. Quantifying environmental factors: a measure of physical, attitudinal, service, productivity, and policy barriers. *Archives of Physical Medicine and Rehabilitation.* 2004;85(8):1324-1335.

110. Whiteneck G, Meade MA, Dijkers M, et al. Environmental factors and their role in participation and life satisfaction after spinal cord injury. *Archives of Physical Medicine and Rehabilitation.* 2004;85(11):1793-1803.

111. Keysor J, Jette A, Haley S. Development of the home and community environment (HACE) instrument. *Journal of Rehabilitation Medicine.* 2005;37(1):37-44.

112. McClain L, Todd C. Food store accessibility. *American Journal of Occupational Therapy.* 1990;44(6):487-491.

113. McClain L, Cram A, Wood J, Taylor M. Wheelchair accessibility—living the experience: function in the community. *Occupational Therapy Journal of Research.* 1998;18(1):25-43.

114. Grabois EW, Nosek MA, Rossi D. Accessibility of primary care physicians' offices for people with disabilities. *Archives of Family Medicine.* 1999;8:44-51.

115. Iwarsson S, Ståhl A, Carlsson G. Accessible transportation–novel occupational therapy perspectives. In: Letts L, Rigby P, Stewart D, eds. *Using Environments to Enable Occupational Performance.* Thorofare, NJ: SLACK Incorporated; 2003.

116. Iwarsson S. *The Enabler: A Method for Analyzing Accessibility Problems for Housing.* Sweden: Lund University, Department of Community Health Services; 1997.

117. Connell BR, Sanford JA. Difficulty, dependence, and housing accessibility for people aging with a disability. *Journal of Architecture and Planning Research.* 2001;18(3):234-242.

118. Mann WC, Ottenbacher KJ, Fraas L, Tomita M, Granger CV. Effectiveness of and environmental interventions in maintaining independence and reducing home care costs for the frail elderly. A randomized controlled trial. *Archives of Family Medicine.* 1999;8(3):210-217.

119. Campbell AJ, Robertson MC, La Grow SJ, et al. Randomised controlled trial of prevention of falls in people aged ≥75 with severe visual impairment: the VIP trial. *BMJ.* 2005;331(7520):817-825.

120. Clarke PJ, Ailshire JA, Nieuwenhuijsen ER, de Kleijn-de Vrankrijker, MW. Participation among adults with disability: the role of the urban environment. *Social Science and Medicine.* 2011;72(10):1674-1684.

121. Close J, Ellis M, Hooper R, et al. Prevention of falls in the elderly trial (PROFET): a randomised controlled trial. *Lancet.* 1999;353(9147):93-97.

122. Dooley NR, Hinojosa J. Improving quality of life for persons with Alzheimer's disease and their family caregivers: brief occupational therapy intervention. *American Journal of Occupational Therapy.* 2004;58(5):561-569.

123. Gitlin LN, Corcoran M, Winter L, Boyce A, Hauck WW. A randomized controlled trial of a home environmental intervention: effect of efficacy and use in caregivers and on daily function of persons with dementia. *Gerontologist.* 2001;41(1):4-14.

124. Hammel J, Jones R, Gossett A, Morgan E. Examining barriers and supports to community living and participation after a stroke from a participatory action research approach. *Topics in Stroke Rehabilitation.* 2006;13(3):43-58.

125. Mann WC, Ottenbacher KJ, Fraas L, Tomita M, Granger CV. Effectiveness of and environmental interventions in maintaining independence and reducing home care costs for the frail elderly: a randomized controlled trial. *Archives of Family Medicine.* 1999;8(3):210-217.

126. Østensjø S, Carlberg EB, Vøllestad NK. The use and impact of assistive devices and other environmental modifications on everyday activities and care in young children with cerebral palsy. *Disability and Rehabilitation.* 2005;27(14):849-861.

127. Petersson I, Kottorp A, Bergström J, Lilja M. Longitudinal changes in everyday life after home modifications for people aging with disabilities. *Scandinavian Journal of Occupational Therapy.* 2009;16(2):78-87.

128. Pighills AC, Torgerson DJ, Sheldon TA, Drummond AE, Bland JM. Environmental assessment and modification to prevent falls in older people. *Journal of the American Geriatrics Society.* 2011;59(1):26-33.

129. Stark S, Landsbaum A, Palmer J, Somerville EK, Morris JC. Client-centered home modifications improve daily activity performance of older adults. *Canadian Journal of Occupational Therapy.* 2009;76:235-245.

130. Velligan DI, Diamond P, Mueller J, et al. The short-term impact of generic versus individualized environmental supports on functional outcomes and target behaviors in schizophrenia. *Psychiatry Research.* 2009;168(2):94-101.

ENVIRONMENT FACTORS
Health, Education, Social, and Public Policies

Diane L. Smith, PhD, OTR/L, FAOTA and Stan A. Hudson, MA

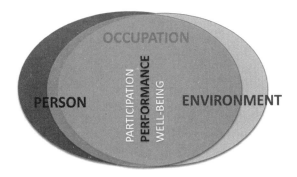

LEARNING OBJECTIVES

- Identify and define the primary health, education, social, and public policies that influence performance, participation, and well-being.
- Discuss how these policies impact performance, participation, and well-being.
- Identify national and international efforts to address health, education, social, and public policies that contribute to limitations in performance, participation, and well-being.
- Describe the influence of these policies on the practice of occupational therapy at the individual, organizational, and population/community level.
- Compare and contrast assessments and interventions regarding important health, education, social, and public policies in therapy practice at the individual, organizational, and population/community level.
- Identify governmental, nonprofit, and international agencies that promote performance, participation,

well-being through work on influential health, education, social, and public policies.

KEY WORDS

- Advocacy
- Agenda setting
- Committees
- Earmark
- Environment
- Equality
- Health care utilization
- Health promotion
- Health/public policy
- Occupational justice
- Scanning/awareness of social change
- Self-advocacy
- Social justice

Christiansen CH, Baum CM, Bass JD, eds.
Occupational Therapy: Performance, Participation, and Well-Being, Fourth Edition (pp 421-440).
© 2015 SLACK Incorporated.

INTRODUCTION

Case Study

Verna is an 85-year-old female who experienced a left-sided stroke approximately 2 months ago. Verna had acute care therapy services, but was not admitted to the rehabilitation unit as she could not tolerate 3 hours of therapy. She has been receiving outpatient rehabilitation (occupational, physical, and speech therapies) services at a local clinic and is showing improvement. However, because Verna broke her hip earlier this year and received occupational therapy and physical therapy, she is limited under the Medicare Therapy Cap and will be at her limit following the next visit. Verna has not achieved all of her goals and is a safety risk for living independently. She does not want to live in a nursing home.

Verna's case is not unique, in that occupational therapy intervention is frequently limited by health care policy. Therefore, it is imperative that occupational therapy practitioners be knowledgeable of the environmental influence of health care policy on practice. This chapter will discuss the role of policy in the PEOP Model, followed by a description of the policy process and its influence on access, reimbursement, and health. Strategies for how occupational therapy practitioners can assess and develop interventions to address and influence policy are presented.

Health and Public Policy in the Person-Environment-Occupation-Performance Model

As stated earlier in this text, the development of the PEOP Model was influenced by many emerging ideas and innovations in health care, disability, social policy, technology, rehabilitation, and public health. The PEOP Model further defines occupational performance as the complex interactions between the person and the environments in which he or she carries out activities, tasks, and roles that are meaningful or required of them. This chapter presents health policy as a significant environmental influence on occupational performance.

The PEOP Model views the client in context, including the environmental characteristics that provide support, whether those include places, people, policies, or technologies. Ultimately the comprehensive assessment of the policy environment clients inhabit will determine the interventions aimed at enabling the client to perform valued roles, activities, and tasks that are central to living, whether these pertain to management of self and others, or work or community engagement. The "top down"

approach considers the individual in context, identifying the client's roles, occupations, and goals. The model requires the occupational therapy practitioner to use this context to address the personal performance capabilities/constraints and the environmental performance enabler/barriers, such as those provided by health policies, that are central to the occupational performance of the individual (or client).

When considering the effect of policy, the "client" can be the health care consumer, health care practitioner, select groups (eg, older adults), or organizations (eg, outpatient rehabilitation facilities). *Environment* is defined as "the external physical and social environment that surrounds the client and in which the client's daily life occupations occur."[1(p19)] Policies provide an environmental context that can either be a barrier (eg, the therapy cap) or facilitator (eg, access to health insurance) to the client's ability to perform roles, activities, and tasks (eg, management of health) that are central to living.

Environmental factors in the PEOP Model central to occupational performance include cultural environment, social support, social determinants and social capital, health education and public policy, physical and natural environment, and assistive technology. Most relevant to this chapter are health education and public policy, which includes policy and access, funding, advocacy, and political infrastructure. However, cultural factors, which include values, customs, beliefs, policy, power/decision making, organizational practices, policies, and economic characteristic, must also be considered. Consideration of health policies also affects emerging areas of practice for occupational therapy, which addresses the occupational issues of communities and populations, such as health literacy. It is important for the occupational therapy practitioner to identify occupational therapy roles and areas of concern for the population and community, utilizing the occupational therapy practitioner's unique knowledge of factors that support or limit occupational performance (eg, policies).

NARRATIVE AND BACKGROUND LITERATURE

International Classification of Functioning, Disability and Health Areas Related to Policy

The ICF classifies health policies that occupational therapy practitioners need to be aware of under environmental factors. "Environmental factors make up the physical, social, and attitudinal environment in which people live and conduct their lives."[2(p171)]

Specific to this chapter, the environmental factors considered would fall under the category concerning services, systems, and policies, although these factors are not mutually exclusive of other environmental factors. The most relevant policies are the health policies and political policies, but other environmental policies mentioned affect receipt of health services, occupational performance, and participation. Table 23-1 outlines ICF-related areas that are specific to health policy affecting occupational therapy practice.

Public Policy Process

Politics is typically defined as the "art or science of government or governing, especially the governing of a political entity such as a nation, and the administration and control of its internal and external affairs."[3(np)] Policy is defined as "a plan or course of action, as of a government, political party, or business, intended to influence and determine decisions, actions and other matters."[3(np)] Kingdon suggests that politics affect policy in numerous ways:

> Those in power have the ability to shape laws or regulations, appoint those who will enact policies favorable to their points of view, allocate resources for enforcement or monitoring, and use their positions to advocate for policies.[4(p207)]

The role of occupational therapy practitioners is usually in the realm of influencing policy and not typically in politics.

According to Mason et al, policy "encompasses the choices that a society, segment of society, or organization makes regarding its goals and priorities and the ways it will allocate its resources."[5(p8)] However, policy is also a process in which views of the problem and possible solutions to it, ethical arguments, and political ideologies are continually being contested.[6] The policy process has been characterized as including problem definition, policy advocacy, agenda setting, policy analysis (including selection among alternative proposed solutions), policy implementation, and policy evaluation (Figure 23-1).[7,8] Passing a law or making a regulation does not by itself cause policy change; policy requires ongoing implementation activities, monitoring, and evaluation. For example, Title I of the ADA was passed in 1990 to prohibit discrimination against persons with disabilities in the workplace; however, there are no clear enforcement procedures and therefore little remarkable change in employment for persons with disabilities.[9,10]

> Public policies are authoritative decisions that are made in the legislative, executive, or judicial branches of the government. These decisions are intended to direct or influence the actions, behaviors, or deci-

sions of others. When public policies pertain to health or influence the pursuit of health, they become health policies.[7(p4)]

Malone states that policy has several distinctive aspects.[11] First, policy always has generality; that is, it is intended to address more than one person, and more than one individual set of circumstances. Therefore, although occupational therapy practitioners may encounter the effects of a policy on a single individual, such as having to adjust their treatment plans to fit within the allowable limits set by a patient's health insurance, understanding of the effect of policies on populations/communities is also necessary. Second, policy sets the norms. Policies formalize implicit and explicit normative judgments about what course of action is good or better than alternatives. It also determines the rules under which those alternatives will be weighed.[11] Third, policy has scale. Policies target different levels of social organization, and policies at one level can supersede or preempt those at "lower" levels. Another aspect of scale pertinent to policy is the level of specificity or scope involved. For example, some policies provide abstract principles on the basis of which individuals, groups, or governments are to take actions, whereas others proscribe, require, or restrict specific actions to be taken.[11] For example, the ADA has the intention of prohibiting discrimination against persons with disabilities in a broad and abstract way, whereas the Voting Accessibility for the Elderly and Handicapped Act was specific in mandating that polling places be accessible. Finally, policy is always decided by someone.[11] Knowing who is in a position to make policy decisions (eg, the Budget Committee) is a vital part of assessing the policy environment and of effecting implementation or change in a health policy that affects occupational therapy clients.[11]

Health, Health Policies, and the Environment

Although health is a universally important concept, its definition is far from universally agreed upon. However, the way in which health is conceptualized or defined by various cultures in a society is "important because it reflects society's values regarding health and how far society might be willing to go in aiding or supporting the pursuit of health and policies among its members."[7(p2)] Generally, negative and narrow conceptualizations of health lead to interventions that focus on correcting or reducing an undesirable state. Positive and broad conceptualizations of health stimulate proactive interventions aimed at many variables in the quest for health. Occupational therapy typically views health positively and broadly, similar to the WHO definition of health as the

Table 23-1. *ICF Areas Related to Health Policy*[2]

Number	Title	Description
e5802	Health policies	Legislation, regulations, and standards that govern the range of services provided to individuals for their physical, psychological, and social well-being. Occurs in a variety of settings including community, home-based, school and work settings, general hospitals, specialty hospitals, clinics, and residential and non-residential care facilities. Can include policies and standards that determine eligibility for services; provision of devices, AT, or other adaptive equipment; and legislation such as health acts that govern features of a health system such as accessibility, universality, portability, public funding, and comprehensiveness.
e5952	Political policies	Laws and policies formulated and enforced through political systems that govern the operation of the political system, such as policies governing election campaigns, registration of political parties, voting, and members in international political organizations (including treaties, constitutional, and other laws governing legislation and regulation).
e5152	Architecture and construction policies	Legislation, regulations, and standards that govern the planning, design, construction, and maintenance of residential, commercial, industrial, and public buildings, such as policies on building codes, construction standards, and fire and life safety standards.
e5202	Open space planning policies	Legislation, regulations, and standards that govern the planning, design, development, and maintenance of open space (including rural land, suburban land, urban land, parks, conservation areas, and wildlife reserves) such as local, regional, or national planning acts, design codes, heritage or conservation policies, and environmental planning policies.
e5252	Housing services policies	Legislation, regulations, and standards that govern housing or sheltering of people, such as legislation and policies for determination of eligibility for housing or shelter, policies concerning government involvement in developing and maintaining housing, and policies concerning how and where housing is developed.
e5352	Communication policies	Legislation, regulations, and standards that govern the transmission of information by a variety of methods (including telephone, fax, post office, electronic mail, and computer-based systems) such as eligibility for access to communication services, requirements for a postal address, and standards for provision of telecommunications.
e5402	Transportation policies	Legislation, regulations, and standards that govern the moving of persons or goods by road, paths, rail, air, or water, such as transportation planning acts and policies, policies for the provision, and access to public transportation.
e5552	Associations and organizational policies	Legislation, regulations, and standards that govern the relationships and activities of people coming together with common noncommercial interests, such as policies that govern the establishment and conduct of associations and organizations, including mutual aid organizations, recreational, and leisure organizations, cultural and religious associations, and nonprofit organizations.
e5702	Social security policies	Legislation, regulations, and standards that govern the programs and schemes that provide income support to people who, because of age, poverty, unemployment, health condition, or disability, require public assistance, such as legislation and regulations governing the eligibility for social assistance, welfare, unemployment insurance payments, disability, and related pensions and disability benefits.

(continued)

Table 23-1 (continued).   *ICF Areas Related to Health Policy*[2]

Number	Title	Description
e5852	Education and training policies	Legislation, regulations, and standards that govern the delivery of education programs such as policies and standards that determine eligibility for public or private education and special needs-based programs) and dictate the structure of local, regional, or national boards of education or other authoritative bodies that govern features of the education system, including curricula, size of classes, numbers of schools in a region, fees and subsidies, special meal programs, and after-school care.
e5902	Labor and employment policies	Legislation, regulations, and standards that govern the distribution of occupations and other forms of remunerative work in the economy, such as standards and policies for employment creation, employment security, designated and competitive employment, labor standards and law, and trade unions.

"state of complete physical, mental, and social well-being, and not merely the absence of disease or injury."[12(p1315)]

Generally health policies affect or influence groups or classes of individuals (eg, physicians, the poor, older adults or children) or types or categories of organizations (eg, medical schools, managed care organizations, employers). Health policies are established at federal, state, and local levels of government. Despite a substantive role for government in health affairs, most of the resources used in the pursuit of health in the United States are controlled and delivered by the private sector.[7] Even when government is directly involved in health care (eg, the Veteran's Administration), it focuses on ways to ensure broader access to those health services that are provided predominantly through the private sector and financed through a unique mix of both public and private payments for these services.

When considering the relationship between health policy and health, especially with regard to ways in which health policy can affect health, it is necessary to consider the role of health policy in environmental conditions, including physical, sociocultural, and economic environments under which people live.[7]

Physical Environment

Thompson points out that government has been involved in a variety of efforts to reduce environmental health hazards through public policies.[13] Examples of such federal policies include the Clean Air Act, the Occupational Health and Safety Act, the Consumer Product Safety Act (PL 92-573), and the Safe Drinking Water Act. More specific to occupational therapy practice, examples of federal policies directed at the physical environment, especially with regard to removal of barriers, include the Architectural Barriers Act, the Rehabilitation Act of 1973, the Voting Accessibility for the Elderly and

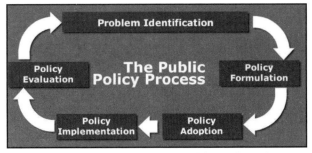

Figure 23-1. Policy process. (Reprinted from The policy process. ThisNation.com. http://www.thisnation.com/textbook/processes-policyprocess.html. Accessed September 2, 2013.)

Handicapped Act, the Americans with Disabilities Act of 1990, and the Americans with Disabilities Amendments Act of 2008. In the latter examples, by removing physical barriers persons with disabilities are provided with access to public and private facilities necessary for meaningful participation.[14]

Examples of similar international policies include the Equal Rights of Persons with Disabilities Law (Israel), the Disability and Equality Act of 2010 (United Kingdom), the Canadian Human Rights Law (Canada), and the Magna Carta for Disabled Persons (Philippines).

Sociocultural and Economic Environments

In addition to their physical environments, the sociocultural and economic environments in which people live also play important roles in their health. Issues of social injustice include chronic unemployment, the absence of a supportive family structure, poverty, homelessness, substance abuse, violence, and despair, which affect the health of people as much as harmful viruses or pollution.[1,7,15,16] These environmental barriers can prevent occupational therapy clients from achieving maximum performance and participation in society. Therefore, these are also issues in direct conflict with the notion of occupational justice.[1,17,18]

Health Care Affordability

Every society has limited health care resources and must ration care by some means. In universal and more socialistic systems, care is rationed by need. For example, there are long wait times for non-emergent surgeries (like hip replacements) in the UK and Canada.[19] In the United States we ration care by one's ability to pay for the service. American society does value emergency care and has policies requiring emergency rooms to see a patient regardless of their ability to pay, but by and large access to health care and good health status in the United States is proportional to one's income and form of employment. This is why people who live in poverty experience measurably worse health status than people who are more affluent.[20] Instead of receiving care that is coordinated, continuing, and comprehensive, the poor are far more likely to seek and receive fragmented services, provided by emergency rooms, public hospitals, or local health departments. The impact of economic conditions is especially dramatic for children. Impoverished children have double the rates of low birth weight and more than double the rates of conditions that limit school activity compared to other children.[21] These children are often those who require occupational therapy services. Reimbursement policies that provide health care (eg, Medicaid, CHIP) for these vulnerable populations can improve health and participation in the broadest sense.

Health Care Access

Another important determinant of health equality is the availability of and access to health services.[1] Health "services can be preventive, acute, chronic, restorative, or palliative in nature."[7(p16)] The production and distribution of health services require a vast set of resources, including money, people, and technology that health policies heavily influence. Passed in 2010, the Patient Protection and Affordable Care Act has several components that address access of vulnerable populations that can benefit from occupational therapy services such as guaranteed coverage for children.[22]

Living in an inner city or a rural setting often increases the challenge of finding health services because the availability of health providers is not adequate in many of these locations.[7] Lack of or inadequate information about health and health services is a significant disadvantage, one compounded by language barriers and functional illiteracy. Health policies that mitigate the negative influences of physical, sociocultural, and economic environments on

health or that take advantage of their positive potential for affecting health are important aspects of any society's ability to help its members achieve higher levels of health, occupational performance, and participation.

Health Care Costs

Economically, the implications of the level of health expenditures and their rate of increase over the past several decades, as well as projections of future increases, are significant.[23] The increasing health expenditures have reduced many people's access to health services by making it more difficult for them to purchase either the services or the insurance needed to cover those services. Because federal and state governments now pay for so much of health care, rising health expenditures have put substantial pressure on their budgets. These rising costs are unsustainable and are resulting in significant reforms to reimbursement policies. In some countries like Japan, there are specific policies limiting the cost, or how much may be charged for a service. The United States has very few direct policies focused on cost controls; rather, cost control is largely done indirectly through reimbursement policy. It is therefore imperative that occupational therapy practitioners be knowledgeable regarding health care utilization and policies that can benefit clients, as well as advocate for policies as decisions are made regarding resource allocation.[1] In addition, evidence of the cost-effectiveness of occupational therapy can assist in ensuring adequate coverage for services as changes to reimbursement are proposed and implemented.

Key Policies That Influence Performance, Participation, and Well-Being

It would be a daunting task to show all of the policies that affect occupational therapy practice at the individual (client or practitioner), organizational (facility), or population/community level. Table 23-2 discusses the evolution of policies that have affected and continue to affect the vulnerable populations served by occupational therapy practitioners. It is important to note in this evolution that as the changes occur in policy, the societal view of, for example, persons with disabilities also changes (eg, from support of the medical model to inclusion and civil rights). These policies address access (eg, Air Carriers Access Act), expand education (eg, IDEA), and prohibit discrimination (eg, ADA). Therefore, these policies are key components of the environmental influence considered in the PEOP Model that must be considered by occupational therapy practitioners in order to collaborate with clients for maximum occupational performance and participation.

Table 23-2. *Key Policies for Occupational Therapy Practice*

Year	Policy	Description
1918	Smith-Sears Veterans Rehabilitation Act	Provided for vocational rehabilitation and return to civil employment for disabled persons discharged from the US military
1921	Maternity and Infancy Act	Provided grants to states to plan maternal and child health services
1924	Veteran's Act of 1924	Codified and extended federal responsibility for health care services to veterans who receive aid if they are injured in the line of service
1935	Social Security Act	Established federally funded old age benefits and funds to states for assistance to blind individuals and disabled children
1943	LaFollette-Barden Vocational Rehabilitation Act	Added physical rehabilitation to the goals of federally funded vocational rehabilitation programs, and provided funding for certain health care services
1946	The Hill-Burton Act	Authorized federal grants to states for the construction of hospitals, public health centers, and health facilities for rehabilitation of people with disabilities
1950	Social Security Amendments	Established a federal-state program to aid permanently and totally disabled persons
1954	Vocational Rehabilitation Amendments	Authorized federal grants to expand programs available to people with disabilities
1956	Social Security Amendments	Created Social Security Disability Insurance (SSDI) for disabled workers ages 50 to 64
1958	Social Security Amendments	Extended SSDI benefits to dependents of disabled workers
1960	Social Security Amendments	Removed the age restriction from SSDI
1963	The Mental Retardation Facilities and Community Health Centers Construction Act	Authorized federal grants for the construction of public and private non-profit community mental health centers
1965	Social Security Amendments	Established Medicare and Medicaid
1965	Vocational Rehabilitation Amendments	Authorized federal funds for construction of rehabilitation centers, expansion of existing vocational rehabilitation programs, and creation of the National Commission of Architectural Barriers to Rehabilitation of the Handicapped
1968	Architectural Barriers Act	Prohibited architectural barriers in all federally owned or leased buildings
1970	Urban Mass-Transit Act	Required all new mass transit vehicles be equipped with wheelchair lifts; implementation was delayed for 20 years
1971	Fair Labor Standard Act	Amended to bring people with disabilities into the sheltered system
1972	Social Security Amendments	Created supplemental security income program, relieving families of the financial responsibility for caring for their adult disabled children
1973	Rehabilitation Act of 1973	Sections 501, 503, and 504 prohibited discrimination in federal programs and services and all other programs or services receiving federal funds
1973	Federal-Aid Highway Act	Authorized federal funds for construction of curb cuts
1975	Education of All Handicapped Children Act	Required free, appropriate public education in the least restrictive setting

(continued)

Table 23-2 (continued). *Key Policies for Occupational Therapy Practice*

Year	Policy	Description
1975	Developmentally Disabled and Bill of Rights Act	Provided federal funds to programs serving people with developmental disabilities and outlined rights for those who are institutionalized
1978	Rehabilitation Act Amendments	Established the first federal funding for consumer-controlled independent living centers
1980	Civil Rights of Institutionalized Persons Act	Authorized the US Justice Department to file civil suits on behalf of residents of institutions whose rights were being violated
1981	Telecommunications for the Disabled Act	Mandated telephone access for deaf and hard-of-hearing people in public places
1983	Rehabilitation Act Amendments	Provided for the Client Assistance Program, an advocacy program for consumers of rehabilitation and independent living services
1984	Voting Accessibility for the Elderly and Handicapped Act	Mandated that polling places be accessible
1985	Canadian Human Rights Act	Legislated that all individuals should have an opportunity equal with other individuals to make for themselves the lives that they are able and wish to have and to have their needs accommodated, without being hindered in or prevented from doing so by discriminatory practices based on race, national or ethnic origin, color, religion, age, sex, sexual orientation, marital status, family status, disability, or conviction for an offense for which a pardon has been granted
1985	Consolidated Omnibus Budget Reconciliation Act (COBRA)	Mandated that an insurance program give some employees the ability to continue health insurance coverage from their workplace after leaving the job; in addition, hospice care is made a permanent part of Medicare and extended to states for Medicaid
1985	Mental Illness Bill of Rights	Required states to provide protection and advocacy services for people with psychological disabilities
1986	Employment Opportunities for Disabled Americans Act	Allowed recipients of SSI and SSDI to retain benefits after they obtain work
1986	Protection and Advocacy for Mentally Ill Individuals Act	Set up protection and advocacy agencies for people who are inpatients or residents of mental health facilities
1988	Air Carriers Access Act	Prohibited airlines from refusing to serve people simply because they are disabled, and from charging people with disabilities more for airfare than nondisabled travelers
1988	Civil Rights Restoration Act	Clarified the original intention of the Rehabilitation Act; stating that discrimination in any program or service that receives federal funding, not just the part which actually receives the funding, is illegal
1988	Fair Housing Act Amendments	Prohibited housing discrimination against people with disabilities and families with children; also provided for architectural accessibility of certain new housing units, renovation of existing units, and accessibility modifications at the renter's expense

(continued)

Table 23-2 (continued). *Key Policies for Occupational Therapy Practice*

Year	Policy	Description
1990	Americans with Disabilities Act (ADA)	Provided comprehensive civil rights protection for people with disabilities; mandated that local, state, and federal governments and programs be accessible, that businesses with more than 15 employees make "reasonable accommodations" for disabled workers, and that public accommodations such as restaurants and stores make "reasonable accommodations" to ensure access for disabled members of the public; the act also mandated access in public transportation, communication, and in other areas of public life
1990	Education for All Handicapped Children Act Amendments	Amended and renamed the Individuals with Disabilities Education Act (IDEA)
1992	The Magna Carta for Disabled Persons (Philippines)	Mandated that the state shall give full support for the total well-being of disabled persons and their integration into society. It provides for the rights and privileges of disabled persons in employment, education, health social services, telecommunications, accessibility, political, and civil rights; prohibits discrimination
1996	Health Insurance Portability and Accountability Act (HIPAA)	Improved the continuity of health insurance coverage in group and individual markets for people who lose their job; also promotes medical savings accounts and improves access to long-term care services and coverage
1997	State Children's Health Insurance Program (SCHIP)	Helps provide medical care to children in low-income families that are not poor enough to qualify for Medicaid
1999	Equal Rights of Person with Disabilities Law (Israel)	To provide a basis for the right of a persons with a disability to equal and active participation in society in all spheres of life, and also a fitting response to his or her special needs in a manner that will enable him/her to life his or her life with maximum independence, privacy, and dignity
1999	Work Incentives Improvement Act (Ticket to Work)	Allowed those persons with disabilities who require health care benefits to work
2004	IDEA Amendments	Focused on student performance, emphasized coordination with No Child Left Behind Act, and strengthened provisions for disciplinary actions, IEPs, and due process services to children enrolled in private schools and transition services
2008	ADA Amendments	Clarified the original intention of ADA, broadened definition of disability
2009	SCHIP Amendments	Reduced barriers and improved access for pregnant women and low income children, now called Children's Health Insurance Program (CHIP)
2010	Patient Protection and Affordable Care Act	Provisions through 2014 to improve access to health care, provide relief for small businesses, extend coverage for young adults to age 26 under their parents' health plan, improve access to prescriptions for older adults and people with disabilities, prohibit denial of coverage for pre-existing conditions, increase accountability for insurance company spending, and improve preventive care
2010	Disability and Equality Act (UK)	Prevents discrimination by providing legal rights for people with disabilities in the areas of employment; education; access to good, services, and facilities—including private clubs and land-based transport services, buying and renting land or property, or functions of public bodies

ASSESSMENTS AND EVALUATIONS

A number of benefits derive from the effective analysis by occupational therapy practitioners of the health policy environment.[7] Such analyses help occupational therapy practitioners do the following:

- Classify and organize complex information about the public policy-making process and about health policies that can or might affect their profession and/or clients
- Identify and assess current health policies that do or will affect their profession and/or clients
- Formulate and advocate health policies or amendments to existing policies that affect their profession and/or clients
- Speculate in a systematic way about health policies that might emerge in the future and affect their profession
- Link information about health policies to the goals and strategies of their profession and, thus, to the resulting influence on occupational performance

Assessments are used to understand the capabilities and enablers, along with those factors that are current constraints or barriers to performance, participation, and well-being. When assessing and evaluating the influence of policy on occupational performance level, most factors will be environmental. For example, the lack of an accessible playground for children, inadequate public transportation to support older adult's community independence, and poor or confusing signage at the health center would each represent environmental factors. Assessing the policy environment is essential to adequately understand the issues in order to direct intervention and treatment.

Malone proposes a working framework that occupational therapy practitioners can use for assessing policy environments for individuals, organizations, or populations/communities.[11]

1. *What is the problem?* Seen from different disciplinary, theoretical, or practical perspectives, the same set of policy-relevant conditions can be defined very differently as a problem.[24,25] Each definition will call for a different policy solution. Our unique perspective as occupational therapy practitioners frames what we identify as problems and how we define them.

2. *Where is the process?* Kingdon suggests that policy agenda setting involves problems, politics, and visible participants.[4] Therefore, it is important to identify who has the power to influence health policy affecting occupational therapy clients. Kingdon also notes that policy consensus tends to result from bargaining and trading rather than persuasion. This means that effective participation in the politics of policy involves building organizations or coalitions that have the ability to trade their support on one issue for efforts on others that they espouse, or that have enough public support to give them bargaining power on their issue.[26] For example, reimbursement issues affecting all practitioners (occupational, physical, and speech-language pathology) can be addressed or supported by building a broader coalition of representatives from the AOTA, the American Physical Therapy Association (APTA), and the American Speech-Language-Hearing Association (ASHA).

3. *How many are affected?* Problems that affect only a small number of people are difficult to get addressed through policies, because the politics of policy-making tends to rely on building coalitions and leveraging power. Health issues that affect a small number may have a better chance of success if those affected or concerned are powerful individuals or groups, or if the issues can be reframed in such a way as to build ongoing public or media concern. For example, if an actor or other famous person has a sudden illness or condition (eg, Christopher Reeve and spinal cord injury) he or she may raise national awareness and support of the issue. Occupational therapy practitioners could frame issues around function instead of diagnosis to broaden defined problems and leverage support.

4. *What possible solutions could be proposed?* Before committing to any single solution to a policy problem, it is important to examine other options and determine the political viability and feasibility of the preferred solution. Alternatives need to be explored if the solution could be perceived as politically unpalatable, practically unworkable, or otherwise difficult to achieve. Which of these solutions is pursued depends on how the problem appears on the policy agenda. Therefore, it is important for occupational therapy practitioners to frame problems and solutions in a way that appeals to those in power.

5. *What are the ethical arguments involved?* Health policy decisions are always ethical decisions insofar as they involve making choices that will affect the lives of others. They often also involve allocation of resources and decisions about prioritizing these (eg, reimbursement decisions). Occupational therapy practitioners can utilize the *Code of Ethics* to understand the ethical concerns that are at stake for the key actors in the process and how another solution might address these ethical concerns most effectively, thus potentially removing an obstacle to compromise.[27]

6. *At what level is the problem most effectively addressed?* Deciding on what level may be appropriate is dependent on numerous factors, including the scope of the problem, the relevance to the policy agendas at different levels, where the problem is in the policy process, whether any particular regulatory agency has jurisdiction, and what kind of mobilization is possible. Occupational therapy practitioners must be knowledgeable about resources at the local, state, and federal levels in order to appropriately advocate for clients. Local resources could include city or county public agents or management and administration of local health care facilities.

7. *Who is in a position to make policy decisions?* As noted, some person or group of persons always makes policy decisions. Contacting one's governmental representative can be a quick way of learning the identity and contact information of decision makers on specific issues. Advocacy groups (eg, AOTPAC) working on the issue are also good sources for this kind of information. It is good to understand what motivates these policy-makers, as their interests are vital in structuring your positions and appeals in ways that align and connect to those interests.

8. *What are the obstacles to policy interventions?* Obstacles to policy intervention include lack of media attention, ideological opposition from those in decision-making positions, lack of sufficient monetary resources, advocacy leadership struggles, and efforts by those actively opposed to the policy. For example, with the ADA, strong opposition was expressed by the transportation industry and small business coalitions because it required them to invest in costly infrastructure improvements. Reimbursement for occupational therapy services may be opposed by politicians reacting to other issues and may be unaware of actual benefits of treatment. Therefore, evidence-based research and marketing remain important to reinforce the benefit of occupational therapy intervention.

9. *What resources are available?* Resources include information resources, advocacy resources, and economic resources. Information on a policy issue or set of concerns may be obtained from governmental agency websites, advocacy groups, professional organizations, policy researchers, media reports, and libraries. Advocacy resources include grassroots volunteer groups, advocacy organizations, professional organizations (eg, AOTA), political allies, and others. Economic resources include money raised from various resources such as political action groups or from fundraising.

Table 23-3 outlines selected assessments of health policy. At this point, there are no occupational therapy specific assessments of health policy. However these assessments are examples of assessments of the effects of policy prospectively (eg, Comprehensive Assessment of Reform Efforts) and retrospectively (eg, Health Impact Assessment, Policy Assessment Tool). Occupational therapy practitioners could incorporate these assessments with other health care and public health professionals in order to determine the effects of health policies on clients served. Once these assessments are made, strategies to address areas of concerns can be developed using the perspective of facilitation of enablers and removal of barriers that affect client's optimal participation.

INTERVENTIONS

Advocacy

Occupational therapy practitioners have a vested interest in understanding the health policy-making process. In addition, they must consistently be aware of social change affecting their clients.[1] Such an understanding is the first step in developing a high degree of political competence.[28] This, in turn, supports the ability to assess the impact of public policies on the profession's domain of interest or responsibility or the ability to exert influence in the public policy-making process.[29] Table 23-4 illustrates examples of how occupational therapy practitioners can provide interventions that affect health policy.

Kronenberg and Pollard describe the concept of political activities of daily living (pADL) that can help investigate "the political nature of everyday conflict and cooperation situations and offer a framework for the development of political competency."[31(p70)] Politically competent occupational therapy practitioners can become involved in the policy process at many points. For example, in the formulation phase of public policy-making, they might become involved in setting the policy agenda by helping to define the problems that policies might address, by participating in the development of possible solutions to the problems, or by helping to create the political circumstances necessary to turn ideas for solving problems into actual policies.[32] Remember that most policy-makers are not experts in the delivery of therapy and need assistance in understanding the issues and even in formulating effective policy. Politically competent occupational therapy practitioners also know how to participate effectively in the actual drafting of legislative proposals and in providing testimony at hearings in which legislation is developed. They can also influence health policy in the implementation phase of the process by focusing on rule-making that

Table 23-3. *Policy Assessments*

Assessment	Construct or Factor Assessed	Description and Reference (Source)
Health Impact Assessment (HIA) (Sponsor: Robert Wood Johnson Foundation)	A combination of procedures, methods, and tools that systematically judges the potential (sometimes unintended) effects of a policy, plan, program, or project on the health of a population, including the distribution of those effects within the population, and identifies appropriate actions to manage those effects.	An HIA follows a series of well-defined steps. The first steps focus on identifying whether a proposed policy or program is likely to have significant health effects, either overall or for particularly vulnerable subgroups, and also on assessing the scope and extent of those efforts. These findings provide the basis for recommending appropriate actions to be considered by community members, other stakeholders, and policy-makers. The final step focuses on evaluating whether the HIA has been effective, both in shaping the decision-making process and in improving relevant health outcomes. • http://www.healthimpactproject.org/hia
Comprehensive Assessment of Reform Efforts (Sponsor: Rand Corporation)	A micro-simulation model that projects how households and firms would respond to health care policy changes based on economic theory and existing evidence from similar scale changes (eg, changes in Medicaid eligibility).	The first step in using the micro-simulation is to compute the status quo—the way things now stand. The second step is using the model to simulate a policy option, done by altering the values of appropriate attributes (eg, health insurance premiums, regulatory requirements) and allowing the agents to respond to these changes and settle into a new equilibrium. The outcome of a policy option is then computed by comparing the new equilibrium with the status quo. The model not only predicts the effect of various health policy options on spending, coverage, and health outcomes, but it also predicts how specific design features influence the effects of a policy option. • http://www.rand.org/health/feature/compare.html
Policy Implementation Assessment Tool (Sponsor: US Agency for International Development)	Helps government and civil society advocates to "take the pulse" of policies in their countries. With this information, stakeholders can better understand policy dynamics and identify recommendations for translating health policies in to action.	Composed of 2 interview guides: one for policy-makers and one for implementers and stakeholders. The interview guides are designed to be flexible so that users can adapt them to their country context, the specific policy, topic area, and level of inquiry. The interview guides are organized around 7 dimensions that influence policy implementation: (1) the policy, its formulation, and dissemination; (2) social, political, and economic context; (3) leadership in policy implementation; (4) stakeholder involvement in policy implementation; (5) planning for implementation and resource mobilization; (6) operations and services; and (7) feedback on progress and results. The tool is applied through a step-by-step approach, which typically takes about 4 to 6 months: (1) select a policy, (2) form a core country team, (3) make decisions about study parameters, (4) adapt the interview guide, (5) identify interviewees and/or focus group participants, (6) conduct the interviews/ focus groups, (7) analyze data, and (8) share findings. • http://www.healthpolicyinitiative.com/policyimplementation

Table 23-4. *Policy Interventions*

Construct, Mechanism, or Factor	Intervention and Reference	How Policy Interventions Relate to PEOP Model
Advocacy-Political Competence	Occupational therapy practitioners can participate effectively in the actual drafting of legislative proposals or in providing testimony at hearings in which legislation is developed. They can also influence health policy in the implementation phase of the process by focusing on rule-making that helps guide the implementation of polices. Such involvement could include providing formal comment on proposed rules, or providing ideas and comments to task forces and commissions established by rule-making agencies as a means to obtain advice on their work.[27]	The PEOP Model defines occupational performance as the doing of meaningful activities, tasks, and roles through complex interactions between the person and environment. According to the PEOP, the client has the right and the practitioner has the responsibility to review and share available evidence on options for interventions that will support achievement of goals in the most effective and efficient manner. Occupational therapy interventions in the policy environment may advocate for change to remove societal barriers at the individual, organizational, or population/community level that limits occupational performance.
Advocacy-Clients	Occupational therapy practitioners can assess, identify, and advocate for (or on behalf of) political issues that affect client care; provide information to clients on options for impacting policy; and work to effect policy change through professional and advocacy organizations.	
Advocacy-Education	Occupational therapy faculty can work to develop policy skills and new policy roles for occupational therapy practitioners that complement and support the work of occupational therapy practitioners providing direct patient care, and researchers can conduct policy studies and explicate the policy implications of their work.	
Advocacy-Community	If an occupational therapy practitioners' work entails broad population/community initiatives and responsibilities (eg, public health, labor, legislative), he or she may work with others (individuals, organizations, or populations/communities) to implement advocacy strategies as part of an overall plan.	
Advocacy-Community Empowerment	Occupational therapy practitioners can empower consumer involvement to become self-advocates in policy, research, and practice that includes consumers' ideas or addresses their concerns; improved implementation of research findings; better care and better health.[1,28,29]	
Evidence-Based Policy-Making	Evidence-based policy-making requires sustained relationships and trust between researchers and policy makers. It also requires researchers to provide timely, locally relevant findings in multiple formats that are accessible and understandable to policy-makers and a broad range of other stakeholders, and support to build the capacity of policy-makers and media for using research findings. Evidence helps in policy-making to document the existence, extent, and correlates of problems; anticipate undesired or unintended consequences of policy decisions; identify options to address problems; and raise the quality of the health issues debate.[30]	

helps guide the implementation of polices. Such involvement could include providing formal comment on proposed rules or providing ideas and comments to task forces and commissions established by rule-making agencies as a means to obtain advice on their work.

According to the PEOP Model, the client has the right and the practitioner has the responsibility to review and share available evidence on options for interventions that will support achievement of goals in the most effective and efficient manner. Occupational therapy interventions in the policy environment may advocate for change to remove societal barriers at the individual, organizational, or population/community level that limit occupational performance.

Occupational therapy practitioners can assess, identify, and advocate for (or on behalf of) political issues that affect client care; provide information to clients on options for impacting policy; and work to effect policy change through professional and advocacy organizations. In addition, occupational therapy faculty can work to develop policy skills and new policy roles for occupational therapy practitioners that complement and support the work of occupational therapy practitioners providing direct patient care, and researchers can conduct policy studies and explicate the policy implications of their work.

If an occupational therapy practitioner's work entails broad population/community initiatives and responsibilities (eg, public health, labor, legislative), he or she may work with others (eg, individuals, organizations, populations or communities) to implement these strategies as part of an overall plan. At the organizational level, many of the factors will be environmental. Examples might include the lack of training of managers on how to make accommodations for workers who wish to return to work after an accident or injury, or facilities that do not consider ADA guidelines for accessibility. Occupational therapy practitioners can empower consumer involvement to become self-advocates in policy, research, and practice that includes consumers' ideas or addresses their concerns; improved implementation of research findings; better care and better health.[1,30,33] For example, the WHO *Declaration of Alma Ata* states that "the people have the right and duty to participate individually and collectively in the planning and implementation of their health care."[34(p1)] It is important to note that consumers may offer different and complementary perspectives to those of professionals. However, little research is available on the effect of consumer involvement in health policy.

Evidence-Based Policy

Health policies can be impacted by basic and clinical research findings, and research can be impacted by health policy.[35] Occupational therapy practitioners' involvement in informing health policy is a critical and powerful way of improving the health, occupational performance, and participation of the individuals and of populations we serve. Brown, among others, has identified several ways in which research can impact health-related policy making that can be incorporated by occupational therapy practitioners.[36] These include accurately and objectively documenting the existence, quantifying the extent, and demonstrating the correlates of the problem; analyzing the problem to identify the undesired and unintended consequences of policy decisions; suggesting or prescribing options to address the problem; and, perhaps most importantly, raising the quality of the debate about health issues to include scholarly evidence as well as anecdotes and biases.[37]

The effect is the promotion of *evidence-based policy-making* as a direct analogy to evidence-based clinical practice.[38] In one survey, almost 90% of policy makers and their staff valued researchers' thoughts on the policy implications of their work.[39] Table 23-5 highlights research focused on the development of evidence-based policy making. Although it is clear from the literature that evidence-based policy making is necessary, little research has been conducted looking at this relationship. The need for this input will continue to grow at the local, state, and federal levels, as new discoveries from translational efforts introduce new challenges for policy and regulation. Several actions have been proposed to maintain the relationship between researcher and policy maker.[41-46] These include, most importantly, building sustained relationships and trust between researcher and policy makers. Other activities promoting success including developing processes for providing timely, relevant information; synthesizing and disseminating findings into (multiple) formats that are accessible and understandable by policy makers and the broad range of other stakeholders; demonstrating the local applicability of results; and building the capacity of policy-makers and staff and media to better use research findings. An example of evidence-based policy making in occupational therapy is a report entitled *Occupational Therapy: Effective School-Based Practices within a Policy Context* in which "the authors were charged with the task of reviewing the research to identify evidence-based and effective practices for school-based occupational therapy, specifically for children serviced under Part B of IDEA."[40(p4)]

OUTCOMES

Policy Modification

In the policy process, without a modification phase policies would remain in their original version, despite the consequences of the policies.[7] In practice, however, the

Table 23-5. *Evidence Table*

Ref	Aim of Study	Methods	Partici-pants	Results and Outcomes	Conclusions and Implications	Level/ Type of Evidence
Swinth, Spencer, and Jackson[40]	• Evidence-based practice • Determine if there is evidence to support practice supported by the IDEA	Comprehensive literature review	None	Lack of high-level research-based evidence due to the few Level I and Level II studies available to guide school-based occupational therapy	School-based occupational therapy practice at times is based more on policy than research; need a stronger research agenda	V
Feder[37]	• Framing of research questions • How research questions are related to the policy agenda	Commentary	None	Research questions should be based on what *should* be on the policy agenda	Presently research questions are too influenced by the policy agenda in its current form	V
Hanft[41]	• Use of data for policy analysis • How can social science data be used effectively for policy analysis	Commentary	None	Major issues in using data for policy analysis include problems of assumption, use of data, inadequate data, the political process, and responsible research	Problems with data can affect its use in policy analysis; consideration of these problems must be made before its use in policy analysis	V
Cookson[38]	• Evidence-based policy-making • The importance of using evidence as a basis for policy making in health care	Commentary	None	The use of evidence is important in policy making in health care, as shown in large-scale policies of health reform in England	More evidence is needed to inform health policy making	V
Sorian and Baugh[39]	• Evidence-based policy-making • Determine how policy-makers are using data	Descriptive; survey	N = 292 Government policy-makers	Officials are overwhelmed by the volume of information, and prefer concise information relevant to current debates	Evidence to policy-makers should be relevant and scientific	IV

consequences, both anticipated and unintended, may cause some individuals, organizations, and populations/communities to seek modification of existing policies. At minimum, modification of policies that provide benefits to certain individuals, organizations, or interest groups may be sought by those who would benefit from a change. To the contrary, those affected by policies in a negative way will seek to modify them in order to minimize the negative consequences.

Policy Evaluation

To be most valuable as a source of information to guide policy modification, evaluation must be more than simply an activity that occurs after a policy has been implemented. Effective policy evaluation is part of a continuum of analytical activities that can begin in agenda setting and pervade and support the entire policy-making process. The continuum of these activities can be organized as "ex-ante policy analysis, policy maintenance, policy monitoring, and ex-post policy evaluation."[7(p234)]

Ex-Ante Policy Analysis

"This type of analysis, which is also called 'anticipatory' or 'prospective' policy analysis, has its utility mainly in influencing agenda setting, whether in the original formulation of a policy or its subsequent modification."[7(p234)] This analysis clarifies problems that decision makers may have to face, and evaluates the various potential solutions to those problems. It may also include cost-benefit analysis and consideration of costs of the various alternatives, to assist decision makers in determining the potential consequences of their decision.

Policy Maintenance

"This type of analysis is typically undertaken to help ensure that policies are implemented" as their formulators designed them and intended them to be implemented.[7(p234)] This analysis examines whether the original policy goals are being met, and identifies any unintended consequences that have resulted from implementation. This can assist in designing any modifications to a policy.

Policy Monitoring

This consists of the actual measurement and recording of the ongoing operations of a policy's implementation, and is sometimes the precursor to a more formal ex-post policy evaluation. Policy monitoring can "play a useful role in the exercise of appropriate managerial control and legislative oversight in the implementation phase, pointing out when and where modifications in rules and regulations or in operations might be needed."[7(p234)]

Ex-Post Policy Evaluation

"This is also called 'retrospective' evaluation, the process through which the real value of a policy is determined."[7(p234)] This can be a difficult process, depending on which outcomes of the policy are evaluated, the politics and motives of the evaluator, and any fiscal limitation. This type of evaluation looks at the contribution and cost-effectiveness of the policy on a program and policy level.

Evaluation Design

Evaluation of policies, especially in terms of their impacts and consequences, is a highly technical procedure that can be approached in a variety of ways, although typically one or more of a small number of basic approaches are used. These include "before-and-after comparisons, with-and-without comparisons, actual-versus-planned performance comparisons, experimental and quasi-experimental designs, and cost-oriented policy evaluation approaches."[7(p235)] Evaluations based on before-and-after comparisons involve comparing conditions or situations before a policy is implemented and after it has had the opportunity to make an impact and to produce consequences for the individuals, organizations, and groups who are affected.

A variation on this approach, known as with-and-without comparisons, involves assessing the consequences for individuals, organizations, or groups with the policy in place and comparing them to situations in which the policy does not exist (eg, state health policies). An example would be assessing the consequence of client social participation in a state that supports funding of personal assistants vs a state that does not fund personal assistants.

Another useful approach to policy evaluation (actual-vs-planned performance comparisons) involves comparing post-implementation policy objectives (eg, health status improvements) with actual post-implementation results. None of these approaches can show whether the policy was the cause of the change. Nevertheless, these approaches are widely used because they tend to be easy to implement and cost relatively little.

Experimental and quasi-experimental designs for policy evaluations can permit more meaningful conclusions, in that the results are based on a stronger research design and are evidence-based.[47] In policy evaluations that use experimental designs, individuals are randomly assigned to control or experimental groups so that the actual impact of the policy being evaluated can be better assessed. This important analysis clearly demonstrates the usefulness of the approach for policy evaluation, but the approach is very expensive and difficult to conduct. Quasi-experimental designs do not have the scientific rigor of randomized design, but they can serve a useful purpose in the conduct of policy evaluations, especially when a true experiment is too expensive or impractical for other reasons. Quasi-experimental designs can provide one of the most useful aspects of the policy evaluation: the ability to explore causality to a particular policy, although this is typically extremely difficult to do.

A final type of approach to policy evaluation is one based on cost-oriented evaluations. This approach can be especially important in the context of the search for policies that can provide value for public dollars. Cost-benefit analysis (CBA) and cost-effectiveness analysis (CEA) are the 2 most widely used forms of cost-oriented policy evaluation. In CBA, an evaluation is based on the relationship between the benefits and costs of a particular policy where all costs and benefits are expressed in monetary terms. Such analyses can help answer the fundamentally important evaluation question of whether the benefits of a policy are at least worth its costs.[48] CEA evaluation "is based on the desire to achieve certain policy objectives in the least costly way."[7(p236)] This form of analysis compares alternative policies that might be used to achieve the same or very similar objectives. Typically the results of CEA evaluations are expressed as "the net costs required to produce a certain unit of output measured in terms of health, eg, quality-adjusted years of life."[40(pJS2-JS3)]

Organizations and Agencies That Provide Resources for Policies

In order to appropriately advocate and provide resources for clients regarding policies that enable or act as a barrier for optimal performance, occupational therapy practi-

tioners must be aware of organizations at all levels that can provide resources, advocacy, and peer support (Table 23-6). Most of these organizations are nonprofit national organizations; some are specific to a disability (eg, blind, deaf) and some are broader (eg, National Organization on Disability). Several are support or advocacy organizations (eg, Disability Rights Education and Defense Fund), while others are focused on accessibility (eg, Institute for Human Centered Design). Again, these are selected organizations. Occupational therapy practitioners should, as a part of intervention planning, identify organizations specific to the needs of the client.

SUMMARY

This chapter discussed the important role of health policy as an environmental influence for the clients that occupational therapy practitioners serve, and for the profession itself. The policy process and the influences along the process were discussed in order to provide occupational therapy practitioners with the information they would need in order to advocate for clients, especially with regard to access and reimbursement. Assessments and interventions were discussed on a broad level, as no specific occupational therapy assessments or interventions regarding policy have been developed. Therefore, the need for more participation in evidence-based policy-making was stressed. Policy, especially health care policy, will continue to be a significant influence on occupational therapy practice and, more specifically, on the clients we serve.

Table 23-6. *Health Care and Disability-Related Organizations*

Organization	Description	Web Address
American Association of People with Disabilities	Largest, nonprofit, nonpartisan, cross-disability organization in the United States	http://www.aapd.com
American Council of the Blind	National organization advocating on behalf of persons who are blind or have low vision	http://www.acb.org
American Foundation for the Blind	National organization devoted to enabling people who are blind or visually impaired to achieve equality of access and opportunity to ensure freedom of choice in their lives	http://www.afb.org
The Arc	Country's largest voluntary organization committed to the welfare of all children and adults with mental retardation and their families	http://www.thearc.org
Designing Accessible Communities	Nonprofit organization providing information and education about accessibility to people with disabilities and to professionals in the fields of design, construction, code development, and enforcement	http://www.designingaccessiblecommunities.org
Disability.gov	One-stop inter-agency portal for information on federal programs, services, and resources for people with disabilities, their families, employers, service providers, and other community members	https://www.disability.gov
Disability Resources, Inc.	National nonprofit organization that provides information about resources for independent living.	http://www.dria-bilene.org
Disability Rights Education and Defense Fund	National law and policy center dedicated to protecting and advancing the civil rights of people with disabilities through legislation, litigation, advocacy, technical assistance, and education, as well as training of attorneys, advocates, persons with disabilities, and parents of children with disabilities.	http://www.dredf.org
Disability Statistics Center	Produces and disseminates statistical information on disability and the status of people with disabilities in American society, and establishes and monitors indicators of how conditions are changing over time to meet their health, housing, economic, and social needs	http://dsc.ucsf.edu
Disabled American Veterans	National organization advocating on behalf of veterans with disabilities	http://www.dav.org
Easter Seals	Serves children and adults with disabilities, their families, and communities through early intervention and child development services, vocational training and employment services, and physical medicine and rehabilitation	http://www.easterseals.com
Institute for Human Centered Design	Addresses environmental issues that confront people with disabilities and older adults through education, technical assistance, training, consulting, publications, and advocacy	http://www.humancentereddesign.org

(continued)

Table 23-6 (continued). *Health Care and Disability-Related Organizations*

Organization	Description	Web Address
Independent Living Centers	Typically they are nonresidential, private, nonprofit, consumer-controlled, community-based organizations providing services and advocacy by and for persons with all types of disabilities to assure physical and programmatic access to housing, employment, transportation, communities, recreational facilities, and health and social services	http://www.ilru.org
National Association of the Deaf	National consumer organization representing people who are deaf and hard of hearing	http://www.nad.org
National Disability Rights Network	Voluntary, national membership association of protection and advocacy systems and client assistance programs	http://www.napas.org
National Federation of the Blind	National organization advocating for people who are blind or have low vision	http://www.nfb.org
National Information Center for Children and Youth with Disabilities	Clearinghouse for information on disabilities and disability-related issues concerning children and youth (0 to 22)	http://www.icdri.org
National Organization on Disability	Promotes full and equal participation and contribution of people with disabilities in all aspects of life	http://www.nod.org
United Cerebral Palsy Association	Nonprofit organization that is dedicated to advancing the independence, productivity, and full citizenship of people with CP and other disabilities	http://www.ucp.org
United Spinal Association	Membership organization serving individuals with spinal cord injuries or disease	http://www.united-spinal.org
World Institute on Disability	International public policy center dedicated to carrying out research on disability issues and overcoming obstacles to independent living	http://www.wid.org

REFERENCES

1. Baum C, Barrows C, Bass Haugen JD, et al. Blueprint for Entry-Level Education. *Am J Occup Ther.* 2010;64(1):186-194.

2. World Health Organization. *ICF: International Classification of Functioning, Disability and Health.* Geneva, Switzerland: World Health Organization; 2001:171.

3. Politics. *The Free Dictionary by Farlex: American Heritage Dictionary of the English Language.* 4th ed. New York, NY: Houghton Mifflin Company; 2000. http://www.thefreediction-ary.com/politics. Published 2000. Updated 2009. Accessed May 1, 2011.

4. Kingdon, JW. *Agendas, Alternatives, and Public Policies.* Boston, MA: Little, Brown; 1984.

5. Mason, DJ, Leavitt, JK, Chaffee MW. Policy and politics: a framework for action. In: Mason DJ, Leavitt JK, Chafee MW, eds. *Policy and Politics in Nursing and Health Care.* 4th ed. St. Louis, MO: Saunders; 2002:1-18.

6. Malone RE. Policy as a product: morality and metaphor in health policy discourse. *Hastings Cent Rep.* 1999;29:16-22.

7. Longest BB. Health Policymaking in the United States. 2nd ed. Chicago, IL: Health Administration Press; 1998.

8. Mott J. *American Government and Politics.* Thisnation.com: American government and politics online. http://www.thisnation.com/. .

9. Smith DL. The employment status of women with disabilities from the behavioral risk factor surveillance system. *Work.* 2007;28:1-9.

10. Smith DL. The relationship of type of disability and employment status from the behavioral risk factor surveillance survey. *J Rehabil.* 2007;73:32-40.

11. Malone RE. Assessing the policy environment. *Policy Polit Nurs Practice.* 2005;6:135-143.

12. WHO. *Constitution of the World Health Organization. Basic Documents.* 15th ed. Geneva, Switzerland: WHO; 1948. http://apps.who.int/gb/bd/PDF/bd47/EN/constitution-en.pdf. Published 1948. Updated 2013. Accessed September 2, 2013.

13. Thompson FJ. *Health Policy and the Bureaucracy: Politics and Implementation*. Cambridge, MA: Institute of Technology Press; 1981.

14. US Department of Justice: Civil Rights Division. *Information and Technical Assistance on the Americans with Disabilities Act*. ADA.gov: US Department of Justice: Civil Rights Division. http://www.ada.gov/. Accessed April 18, 2012.

15. Commission on Social Justice. *Social Justice: Strategies for National Renewal*. The Report of the Commission on Social Justice. London, UK: Vintage/Ebury; 1994.

16. Wilcock AA. *An Occupational Perspective of Health*. 2nd ed. Thorofare, NJ: SLACK Incorporated; 2006:344.

17. Christiansen CH, Townsend EA, eds. *Introduction to Occupation: The Art and Science of Living*. Upper Saddle River, NJ: Prentice Hall; 2004:278.

18. Townsend EA, Wilcock AA. Occupational justice. In: Christiansen CH, Townsend EA, eds. *Introduction to Occupation: The Art and Science of Living*. Upper Saddle River, NJ: Prentice Hall; 2004:243-273.

19. The Commonwealth Fund. *2011 Commonwealth Fund International Health Policy Survey*. The Commonwealth Fund. http://www.commonwealthfund.org/Surveys/2011/Nov/2011-International-Survey.aspx. Updated 2013. Accessed September 2, 2013.

20. Klerman LV. Nonfinancial barriers to the receipt of medical care. *Future Child*. 1992;2:171-185.

21. Starfield B. Child and adolescent health status measures. *Future Child*. 1992;2:25-39.

22. US Department of Labor. *Affordable Care Act*. US Department of Labor. http://www.dol.gov/ebsa/healthreform/. Accessed April 18, 2012.

23. Schieber GJ, Poullier JP, Greenwald LM. US health expenditures performance: an international comparison and data update. *Health Care Fin Rev*. 1992;13:1-87.

24. Linder SH. On cogency, professional bias, and public policy: an assessment of four views of the injury problem. *Milbank Q*. 1987;65:276-301.

25. Malone RE. Heavy users of emergency services: social construction of a policy problem. *Soc Sci Med*. 1995;40:469-477.

26. Dodd CJ. Can meaningful health policy be developed in a political system? In: Harrington C, Estes, CL, eds. *Health policy and Nursing: Crisis Reform in the US Health Care Delivery System*. 2nd ed. Sudbury, MA: Jones and Bartlett; 1997:416-428.

27. AOTA. *Occupational Therapy Code of Ethics and Ethics Standards*. AOTA. http://www.aota.org/~/media/Corporate/Files/AboutOT/Ethics/Code%20and%20Ethics%20Standards%202010.ashx. Published 2010. Accessed September 2, 2013.

28. Goodman-Lavey M, Dunbar S. Federal legislative advocacy. In: McCormack G, Jaffe E, Goodman-Lavey M, eds. *The Occupational Therapy Manager*. 4th ed. Bethesda, MD: AOTA Press; 2003:421-438.

29. Longest BB. *Seeking Strategic Advantage Through Health Policy Analysis*. Chicago, IL: Health Administration Press; 1997.

30. WHO. *The Ottawa Charter for Health Promotion: First International Conference on Health Promotion, Ottawa, 21 November 1986*. WHO. http://www.who.int/healthpromotion/conferences/previous/ottawa/en/print.html. Published November 21, 1986. Updated 2013. Accessed September 2, 2013.

31. Kronenberg F, Pollard N. Overcoming occupational apartheid: a preliminary exploration of the political nature of occupational therapy. In: Kronenberg F, Simó Algado S, Pollard N, eds. *Occupational Therapy without Borders: Learning from the Spirit of Survivors*. Oxford, UK: Elsevier-Churchill Livingstone; 2005:58-86.

32. Kingdon JW. *Agendas, Alternatives, and Public Policies*. 2nd ed. New York, NY: HarperCollins College Publishers; 1995.

33. Dawson J. *Self-Advocacy: A Valuable Skill for Your Teenager With LD*. GreatSchools. http://www.greatschools.org/special-education/health/797-self-advocacy-teenager-with-ld.gs. Published 2007. Updated 2013. Accessed September 2, 2013.

34. World Health Organization. *Declaration of Alma Ata: Report of the International Conference on Primary Health Care*. Geneva, Switzerland: World Health Organization; 1978.

35. Mirvis DM. From research to public policy: an essential extension of the translation research agenda. *Clin Translational Sci*. 2009;2:379-381.

36. Brown L. Knowledge is power: health services research as a political resource. In: Ginzburg E, ed. *Health Services Research*. Cambridge, MA: Harvard University Press; 1991.

37. Feder J. Why truth matters: research versus propaganda in the policy debate. *Health Serv Res*. 2003;38:783-787.

38. Cookson R. Evidence-based policy making in health: what it is and what it is not. *J Health Serv Res Policy*. 2005;10:118-121.

39. Sorian R, Baugh T. Power of information: closing the gap between research and policy. *Health Aff*. 2002; 21: 264-273.

40. Swinth Y, Spencer KC, Jackson LL. *Occupational Therapy: Effective School-based Practices within a Policy Context (COPSSE Document Number OP-3)*. Gainesville, Florida: University of Florida, Center on Personnel Studies in Special Education; 2007.

41. Canadian Health Services Research Foundation. *The Theory and Practice of Knowledge Brokering in Canada's Health System*. Ottawa, ON: Canadian Health Services Research Foundation; 2003.

42. Hanft RS. Use of social science data for policy analysis and policy-making. *Milbank Q*. 1981;59:596-603.

43. Institute of Health Economics. *Effective Dissemination of Findings from Research*. Alberta, Canada: Institute of Health Economics; 2008.

44. Lomas J. *Improving Research Dissemination and Uptake in the Health Sector: Beyond the Sound of One Hand Clapping*. Hamilton, ON: McMaster University Centre for Health Economics and Policy; 1997.

45. Lomas J. Using "linkage and exchange" to move research into policy at a Canadian foundation. *Health Aff*. 2000;19:236-240.

46. Mitton C, Adair CE, McKenzie E, Patten SB, Perry BW. Knowledge transfer and exchange review and synthesis from the literature. *Millbank Q*. 2007;85:729-768.

47. Cook TP, Campbell DT. *Quasi-Experimentation: Design and Analysis Issues for Field Settings*. Chicago, IL: Rand McNally; 1979.

48. Elixhauser A, Luce BR, Taylor WR, Reblando J. Health care CBA/CEA: an update on the growth and composition of the literature. *Med Care*. 1993;31(Suppl):JS1-JS11.

Chapter 24

ENVIRONMENT FACTORS
Technology

Jan Miller Polgar, PhD, OTReg(Ont), FCAOT

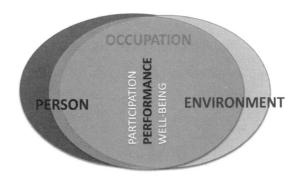

LEARNING OBJECTIVES

- Identify and define the primary technology factors that influence performance, participation, and well-being.
- Discuss how technology factors impact performance, participation, and well-being.
- Identify national and international efforts to address technology factors that contribute to limitations in performance, participation, and well-being.
- Describe the influence of technology factors on the practice of occupational therapy at the individual, organizational, and population/community level.
- Identify governmental, nonprofit, and international agencies that promote performance, participation, and well-being through work on technology factors.
- Describe how technology applies to the PEOP Model and enables performance, participation, and well-being.

- Define assistive technology from conceptual and regulatory perspectives.
- Discuss the issues that affect the recommendation and use of technology, including personal, occupational, and contextual factors.
- Apply a PEOP Occupational Therapy Process for intervention with assistive technology.
- Discuss future implications to technology use in daily occupations, including ethical considerations.

KEY WORDS

- Accessible design
- Assistive technology
- Context
- Device discontinuance
- Digital technology
- Ergonomics

Christiansen CH, Baum CM, Bass JD, eds.
*Occupational Therapy: Performance, Participation,
and Well-Being, Fourth Edition* (pp 441-464).
© 2015 SLACK Incorporated.

- Expert user
- Extrinsic enabler
- Human factors
- Human technology interface
- Novice
- Outcome evaluation
- Persuasive computing
- Robotics
- Usability
- Virtual technology

INTRODUCTION

Technology is a pervasive part of our daily occupations. It has the capacity to simplify occupation through enhancing or replacing personal, physical, sensory, or cognitive capacities. Think about how much further and faster you can move in your community when using a bicycle or private or public transportation vs walking or running. The technology augments your physical ability to move. This chapter will explore a specific classification of technology: assistive technology (AT) as it relates to the PEOP Model.

SITUATING ASSISTIVE TECHNOLOGY WITHIN THE PERSON-ENVIRONMENT-OCCUPATION-PERFORMANCE MODEL

AT is a component of the environment in the PEOP Model, congruent with the placement of AT in the WHO ICF.[1] This component of the model includes AT, ergonomics, accessible and universal design, and virtual and digital technology. While both the PEOP Model and ICF situate AT in the environment, it is conceptually different from other environmental elements in that it is more intimate to the person. Sanford[2(p55)] suggests that AT is "more individualized and usually follows the person." It is not a feature of a particular environment. Commonly, we think of the environment as structures (physical, social, institutional) that exist within a context (eg, ramps at a building entrance, policies that guide practice in a business environment). AT comes with the person to a situation, affecting how they perform their occupations within the environment. For example, a wheelchair does not typically exist in the environment separate from the user. It comes with the person who has a mobility limitation, enabling movement in the environment; it is not shared with others in the environment, having been recommended for that person based on his or her own unique configuration of needs, experiences, and goals.

This chapter explores AT as an intervention, as something that enables occupational performance through augmentation or replacement of functional abilities. The process of determining appropriate AT is framed in the PEOP Occupational Therapy Process and supplemented by the Human Activity Assistive Technology (HAAT) Model,[3] which is specific to AT.

Assistive Technology as an Enabler of Occupational Performance, Participation, and Well-Being

AT has the potential to affect occupational performance through augmentation or replacement of physical, sensory, and/or cognitive abilities. At the performance level, AT enables the completion of occupations by supporting these abilities. On a physical level, it can enhance or replace the client's strength, endurance, balance, coordination, or range of motion. At the sensory level, it can enhance information from the environment and convert it into a form the client is able to use. Cognitive technologies support numerous cognitive functions, such as memory, task sequencing, organization, and attention. AT ranges in complexity from something as simple as a sock aid or built-up handle on an eating utensil, to complex systems that allow a client to remotely control objects within their environment or that monitor[4] and cue the client's occupational performance.[5] AT that is congruent with the client's goals and life situation has the potential to enable occupational participation in many different contexts. Studies of the use of wheeled mobility have demonstrated that clients travel further and participate in more community activities following the acquisition of either a manual or powered wheelchair.[6,7]

Technologies that support communication are instrumental in assisting users to engage in many occupations. For example, the ability to communicate through the use of augmentative and alternative communication devices facilitated the participation of children with speech impairments in a community theater program.[8] The client's well-being, conceptualized as their satisfaction, has been demonstrated across the use of many different types of AT, including powered mobility,[9] electronic aids to daily living,[10,11] and closed-circuit televisions (CCTV).[12]

NARRATIVE AND BACKGROUND LITERATURE

Definition of Assistive Technology

It is important to clarify what we mean by AT, as there are numerous categories of technology that the

Table 24-1. *Additional Classifications of Assistive Technology[3]*

Classification	Description
Low vs high	Low technology is relatively easy to make or obtain; devices that are more expensive, require expertise to make, and may require a recommendation from a professional are considered high technology.
Hard vs soft	Hard technologies include tangible items, such as a wheelchair, computer, software, or ADL devices. Soft technologies are the supports for the training and ongoing use of AT, these include print or electronic materials that support use, clinician reasoning, and education of an AT team member in the selection, set-up, and ongoing use.
Minimal to maximal	This categorization is actually a continuum. On one end are those technologies that augment function; in specific circumstances extending the client's own abilities. The other end of the continuum includes those devices that replace a significant proportion of the client's abilities.
General vs specific	General technologies have a wide range of application, while specific technologies have one unique application.
Commercial to custom	This category is also represented by a continuum. On one end are technologies that are available commercially, either those designed for the general public or for persons with disabilities, and can be used "right out of the box." The other end includes those technologies that are custom made for one specific user.

occupational therapy practitioner may encounter. A common definition is from US PL 108-364, The Assistive Technology Act of 1998, as amended in 2004: "Any item, piece of equipment or product system whether acquired commercially off the shelf, modified, or customized that is used to increase, maintain, or improve functional capabilities of individuals with disabilities."[13]

The WHO ICF defines assistive products and technology as "any product, instrument, equipment or technology adapted or specially designed for improving the functioning of a disabled person."[1] These definitions both refer to enablement of function by products that are specifically designed for individuals with disabilities and/or those that are mass-produced for the general population.

Locating Assistive Technology Within the International Classification of Functioning, Disability and Health

AT is specifically mentioned in the Products and Technology chapter of the Environmental Factors component of the WHO ICF.[1] Technology that is designed for persons with a disability is found in many different environmental factors, including products and technology for daily living, education, employment, culture, recreation and sport, religion and spirituality, indoor/outdoor mobility and transportation, and communication.[1] Some of the classifications, such as indoor/outdoor mobility and trans-

portation, communication, and education (defined as acquisition of knowledge), are most closely linked to ICF activities. The remaining WHO categories that include AT refer to broader types of occupations, ie, employment, community and civic life, recreation, and daily activities, for which many different categories of AT are useful and are more closely linked to the participation category.

Categories of Assistive Technology

This chapter includes those devices that are intended to assist someone to complete his or her daily activities. It does not include technology that is used primarily in a rehabilitation setting as part of therapy, parallel bars for example. Major categories of technology will be reviewed, including technology that augments or replaces mobility, communication, sensory, cognitive, and/or manipulation function. Table 24-1 shows additional ways to classify AT.

Seating and Mobility

Seating and mobility products assist the client to achieve and maintain a functional seated position and/or move from one location to another safely and efficiently. They include specialized seating, wheelchairs, canes, walkers, and scooters. Seating products (mainly seat cushions and backs) are recommended for 3 main purposes:

1. Assist the user to maintain an optimal position for function
2. Minimize the likelihood of developing a pressure ulcer
3. Comfort

Wheelchairs form the major group of mobility products recommended by occupational therapy practitioners. They include both manual and power products. Manual wheelchairs are propelled either by the user or by a caregiver. A power wheelchair has a motor that drives the wheels, requiring the user to control the speed, direction, and to start and stop the chair. Common options include the ability to change the seat so that it is either tilted or reclined, which provides greater comfort and pressure relief. Some wheelchairs have a mechanism that moves the seat so that the user may be in a reclining or standing position.

Augmentative and Alternative Communication

Augmentative and alternative communication (AAC) devices enable communication for individuals for whom oral expression is challenging.[14] These devices range from simple communication boards that display pictures or words required by the user, to electronic devices that transform keystrokes or text to speech.[3] They are portable, mounted on a wheelchair to be available as needed.

Computers and Computer Access Technology

Information and communication technology (ICT) (eg, computers, smart phones, and tablets) provide a tremendous opportunity for us all, including individuals with disabilities. The combined functions of the software and hardware enable occupational performance across many settings (eg, home, work, and school) for individuals with cognitive and physical disabilities. ICT is an excellent example of technology that is mass-produced for the general population and is readily used by individuals with a wide range of abilities, often with little or no modification. Most of these devices have some form of accessibility options as part of their operating system that allow the user to modify the device input or output.[3]

Access technology includes joystick controls, various switches, head arrays (switches that are embedded into a wheelchair headrest), and sip-n-puff switches that are operated through breath control.[3] These technologies are paired with input to computers, powered wheelchairs, and electronic aids to daily living, making it possible for a client with limited movement to use these devices.

Assistive Technology for Manipulation

Technology that augments or replaces manipulation ranges from very simple devices (eg, a simple reacher) to complex electronic aids to daily living that control other devices in the home.[3,4] These devices support manipulation for self-care, educational, employment, community

involvement, or leisure occupations. This category is one in which AT has crossed over to more commercially available devices. For example, many commercially available tools have enlarged handles, which were originally only available from rehabilitation suppliers. Robotics is an emerging area of technology with promise for the future. Most of the robotic systems that support manipulation are used primarily in a laboratory or clinical settings at this time. These systems often include some form of arm that the user controls. Typically, these devices remain fixed to a table or desk top, limiting the location in which they can be used.

Cognitive Technologies

Cognitive technologies support learning and memory or daily occupations by reducing cognitive demand. These devices include smart phones, specialized memory devices, watches, electronic calendars with large video display, and sensor technology.[3] These devices augment cognitive function of memory, time management, concept organization, and language.

Vision Technologies

Vision technologies support 2 primary functions: movement in the environment and reading. The long cane is the main technology used for the first function. Reading is supported by magnifying lenses, screen readers, CCTV, and optical character recognition (with which text can be scanned into a computer and then converted to speech).[3]

Hearing Technologies

Although hearing aids are the most common form of hearing technologies, they are not included in this chapter as their provision is not part of the occupational therapy practitioner's scope of practice or expertise. Other devices that support hearing include personal amplification systems, closed captions, visual displays, and alerting devices (such as an alarm clock that vibrates and emits light to awaken the user).

Pervasive Computing Technologies

Another emerging area of AT is pervasive computing technologies, which involves 3 components:[5]

1. *Ubiquitous computing:* integration of computer power with sensors into a broad range of objects
2. *Ubiquitous communication:* anytime, anywhere between person and/or object
3. *Intelligent-user-friendly interfaces* that enable flexible and natural control of the environment

These technologies monitor the behavior of a client, typically in their home environment. Examples include movement sensors to detect falls, telecommunication technology that allows interaction across geographical locations, and sensors that detect when an appliance has been left on.

Table 24-2. *Assistive Technology Organizations and Resources*

Name of Organization or Resource	Brief Description of Inter-Professional Resources	Web Address or Publisher
RESNA	International organization that promotes research and knowledge translation in the area of AT. Sets standards of practice and code of ethics for practitioners and manages professional designation (AT Provider)	www.resna.org
International Association for Augmentative and Alternative Communication	International organization that promotes advancement, research, and professional development for clients and clinicians using AAC	www.isaac-online.org
DAISY (Digital Accessible Information System) Consortium	Organization that develops, maintains, and promotes international standards for access to digital information	www.daisy.org
International Seating Symposium	Annual conference held in North America on matters concerning seating and mobility; proceedings are available online	www.iss.pitt.edu www.interprofessional. ubc.ca
European Seating Symposium incorporating AT	Annual conference, usually held in Ireland, for seating and mobility, with some AT	www.seating.ie
CSUN	International conference on technology, primarily digital technologies and vision aids	www.csun.edu/cod/conf/ index.html
Closing the Gap	International conference on AT and disability	www.closingthegap.com
Alternative and Augmentative Communication	Official journal of ISAAC; publishes scientific articles concerning AAC assessment, intervention, theory, and technology	http://informahealthcare. com
Assistive Technology	Journal published by RESNA	www.resna.org
Disability and Rehabilitation: Assistive Technology	Journal publishes a broad range of content about technological developments that have the potential to enhance rehabilitation and client outcomes; one of the primary journals advancing rehabilitation science	http://www.informa-healthcare.com
Journal of Rehabilitation Research and Development	Official journal of Rehabilitation Research and Development Service, US Department of Veterans Affairs	www.rehab.research. va.gov/jrrd

Assistive Technology Team Members

A number of different individuals participate on the AT service delivery team. The client, his or her family, and/or caregiver are primary participants on the team. Research suggests that better outcomes of device use are achieved when the client perceives that he or she was included actively in the assessment and decision-making process.[3] Health care professionals include physicians, occupational and physical therapy practitioners, speech-language pathologists, audiologists, optometrists, kinesi-ologists or ergonomists, and rehabilitation aides. Rehabilitation engineers or technicians and AT vendors or distributors may also be involved. In some jurisdictions, the designation of Assistive Technology Provider (ATP) is awarded to individuals who have completed a specialization process and examination. If the technology is used in the educational system, a teacher, learning resource specialist, and/or educational assistant may also be involved in service delivery. Table 24-2 lists a number of organizations and resources that support these team members.

Table 24-3. *Characteristics of Devices That Predict Use*[3,15]

Characteristic	Definition
Efficiency	Device assists the user to complete the desired occupation in a reasonable amount of time without undue fatigue, frustration, or dissatisfaction
Learnability	Device is easy to learn how to use
Ease of use	Device is easy to use on an on-going basis
Memorability	Degree to which the operation of a device can be remembered and the ease with which it can be used after a prolonged period of nonuse
Errors	Operator errors are detected by the device, transmitted to the user, and have a minimal impact on the performance of the device
Satisfaction	The sense of satisfaction the user has with the device
Portability	The ability to move the device from one location to another with ease
Maintenance/ongoing support	The device is easy to maintain, either by the client and family or through access to customer support; on-going support for the use of the device is accessible
Cost/benefit	The benefit achieved from device use is at least equal to the cost of obtaining and maintaining it

Device Use and Discontinuance

AT that is not used has significant functional and financial cost to the client and their family, and a financial cost to the funder and society at large if devices are funded through a health care program. Studies of device use suggest rates of discontinuance ranging from 8% to 75%.[3] These rates and the associated costs make device discontinuance a significant factor of AT service provision and emphasize the need for an evidence-based device selection and delivery system.

Multiple reasons for discontinuance of devices, including personal, device, and environmental factors, are described in the literature. Only key ones will be identified here.[3,15] Personal reasons for discontinuance include the client no longer needing the device due to improvement or decline in function, and/or the client never saw the need for the device. Environment reasons include accessibility issues and stigma associated with using AT in a public location. Device issues include the device is not reliable, difficult to use, and/or has high costs. Table 24-3 shows additional device characteristics that affect use. The first 2 groups of reasons may be minimized through a systematic assessment process, which will be described later. A design process that includes the user and health care professionals minimizes the device issues.

Human factors are the study of the interaction of the user with a device, with a focus on how the design of the device affects its use and operation. Devices that require a complex set of steps for successful operation; those that are difficult to see, hear, or manipulate; and those that do not provide sufficient feedback to detect or repair an error are often left unused.

Norman discusses design principles that affect the usability of a device, ie, the efficiency, effectiveness of and satisfaction with device use.[16] His principles include the following:

- Visibility—the relevant operation features are seen easily
- The conceptual model of how the device works is conveyed through the design

The latter principle is achieved through careful mapping of the user's actions to the device response, providing cues about the device operation and constraints that limit unsafe or incorrect operation and giving feedback.

Principles of Selecting Assistive Technology to Enhance Performance, Participation, and Well-Being

The client drives the selection process; the AT does not. The client, including family and other relevant stakeholders, are an active part of the selection process. His or her needs and goals are primary; the technology is selected to match the client's situation.

An evidence-based process guides the clinical reasoning that results in AT recommendation. The clinician uses a systematic process to identify and assess the client's needs, relevant components of client performance and perception, and the environment; make AT recommendations;

implement; and then evaluate the outcome of the recommendations.

A minimalist approach is used for equipment selection. Only the equipment and options that a client needs or is likely to use should be recommended.

The professional follows a code of ethics in the selection process, balancing the needs of the individual with those of society. The clinician balances client needs with public resources that fund AT provision. Further, enhancement of client safety, such as with sensors that monitor client activity, is balanced with the client's right to risk-taking and self-determination.[17]

The Human Activity Assistive Technology Model

The HAAT Model[3] has many elements that are consistent with the PEOP Model, with one difference; it specifically considers the contribution of AT to occupational performance. In short, the HAAT Model considers someone doing something within a context (environment) using AT. The model is depicted in Figure 24-1. The HAAT Model, consistent with the PEOP Model, considers the influence of the person, the environment, and the AT on occupational performance. A premise of the model is that the outcome of assessment of the activity, human, and context elements drives the selection of the AT.

Activity

The *activity* parallels the *occupation* in the PEOP Model. Because the HAAT Model was designed for use in the AT field by professionals (who include, but are not exclusively, occupational therapy practitioners), the word activity is used rather than occupation. The activity includes all that an individual does in their daily activities. In addition, it includes factors such as time, location, and manner in which the activity is completed (independently or with assistance).[3]

The Human

The *human* element includes the client's physical, cognitive, and affective abilities and how they affect the ability to engage in desired occupations (ie, person factors in the PEOP Model). Further, it includes whether he or she is a novice or expert in the use of AT and the meaning that the occupation and technology use holds for him or her.[3]

Context

The HAAT Model refers to environmental influences as the context. This aspect identifies different influences of the context in which the client performs the activity, including physical, social, cultural, and institutional factors. The *physical context* includes the built and natural environment, including accessibility, light, sound, temper-

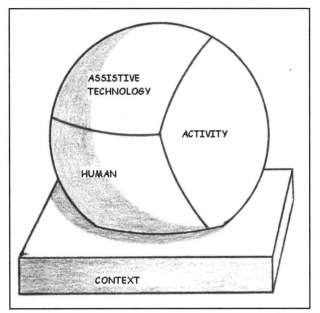

Figure 24-1. The Human Activity Assistive Technology (HAAT) Model. (Reprinted with permission from Cook AM, Polgar J. *Cook and Hussey's Principles of Assistive Technology.* 3rd ed. St. Louis, MO: Elsevier; 2008.)

ature, and transportation of the device. The *social context* includes other individuals with whom the client interacts: familiar, unfamiliar, and strangers. The influence of these groups is seen in their familiarity with the client, their needs and routines, expectations of the client, and their acceptance of the use of AT.[3] The *cultural context* includes beliefs, practices, rituals, and stories shared among a group of people.[18] Culture may influence the perception of disability, the willingness to accept assistance, attitudes toward contributions to the community or society, and rights and responsibilities of members of the culture.[3] The *institutional context* includes legislation, policies, and procedures that affect AT procurement, use, and service provision. It includes all levels of government, as well as policies of organizations such as schools and corporations. Table 24-4 lists some of the relevant pieces of legislation.

Assistive Technology

AT is labeled an extrinsic enabler, since it is something external to the person that enables his or her occupational performance.[3] It includes the human-technology-interface (HTI), a processor, an activity output, and an environmental interface, although not all devices have all of these elements. The HTI is the point of interaction between the client and the device, including a computer keyboard or mouse; an access switch; remote controllers; and wheelchair seat cushions, backs, and push rims.[3]

The processor is the component of the technology that receives input from the HTI or the environment and

Table 24-4. *Examples of Legislation Relevant to Assistive Technology*

Country	Name of Legislation	Purpose	Reference
United States	Rehabilitation Act of 1973, as amended	Mandates reasonable accommodation in all programs that are federally funded; includes right of access to AT	Rehabilitation Act of 1973, as amended, 29 U.S.C. §791,793,794,794d.
United States	IDEA Amendments of 1997 and 2004	Establishes the right of all children to an education that is free and provided in the least restrictive environment; includes the access to AT	IDEA 20 U.S.C. §1400 et seq.
United States	Assistive Technology Act of 1998, amended in 2004	Regulates the expansion of AT devices and services, mandates a consumer-driven approach to AT service provision and expands funding opportunities	Assistive Technology Act of 1998, as amended, PL 108-364, §§ 3, 118 stat 1707 (2004).
United States	ADA of 1990	Prohibits discrimination on basis of disability; mandates access to services and products that are provided in specific sectors	ADA of 1990, 42 U.S.C. §§ 12010 et seq.
Canada (relevant legislation is at the provincial level)	Accessibility for Ontarians with Disabilities, 2005	Legislates the development, implementation, and enforcement of accessibility standards across employment, buildings, structures and facilities, goods and services, and other accommodations	http://www.e-laws. gov.on.ca/html/stat-utes/english/elaws_statutes_05a11_e.htm
Australia	Disability Discrimination Act, 135 of 1992, as amended	Seeks to eliminate discrimination of persons with disabilities in employment and education, accommodate access to premises, and the provision of goods and services	http://www.comlaw.gov. au/Details/C2011C00747/ Html/Text#_Toc303846990
UK	Disabilities Discrimination Act	Legislation to eliminate discrimination against persons with disabilities in the provision of goods and services, and in education and employment	http://www.legislation.gov. uk/ukpga/2005/13/pdfs/ ukpga_20050013_en.pdf

transforms that input into some form of activity output. The processor is commonly a mechanical link or electronic component.[3] The activity output describes the function of the device, including communication, manipulation, mobility, sensory, and cognitive functions.[3] The environmental interface captures sensory input and augments or alters it in some usable form. Examples include lenses that magnify visual information, microphones that amplify auditory input, and haptic sensors that enhance external forces.

ASSESSMENT AND EVALUATION

The PEOP Model situates consideration of AT in the *assessment* aspect of the PEOP Occupational Therapy Process, congruent with the idea that the person performing occupations in context drives the selection of AT. The following

application of the PEOP Occupational Therapy Process integrates considerations specific to AT in the narrative.

THE NARRATIVE: CLIENT INFORMATION

The Occupational History

Consideration of the person engaged in occupation is one element of the narrative. Typically, the term *client* includes both the person with the occupational performance issue and significant others such as parents, spouses, or children who engage in co-occupations with that person and whose own situation affects whether and how AT will be used.

Identification of the occupations in which the client wants or needs to engage is informed by the perceptions and meanings the client has of these occupations. The dynamic link between person and occupation influences whether AT will be integrated into daily life. Understanding this dynamic for the client in the following areas forms a part of the occupational history: the meaning ascribed to or the motivation for different occupations, and the client's sense of agency influencing his or her choices regarding how an occupation is performed.

How the person views an occupation and his or her skill level influence whether AT will be accepted or not. An occupation that is highly meaningful for the person, one that he or she is highly motivated to continue, is one for which AT use is welcomed. In contrast, AT may not be used for occupations holding less meaning or for which a prior level of performance cannot be regained, eg, high performance athletics where re-engagement at a perceived lower performance level is not acceptable.

Understanding the client's experience of agency in performing his or her occupations aids the process of determining whether AT is an appropriate intervention. A dialogue will uncover the situations in which the person will accept assistance from another and/or use technology, and those in which he or she wants to perform independently. Here it is necessary to appreciate the client's self-perception, which will affect if, and, or when AT will be integrated into daily life.

Client's Description of Current Situation

Whether the client is a novice or expert user of AT will affect their perception of the current situation. A client whose ability to engage in occupations has changed suddenly and recently may feel quite bewildered by their current situation, with little sense of how to re-engage in desired occupations and often with little or no knowledge of AT.[1] In contrast, clients who have used AT over a long period (ie, expert users) have a different appreciation of their own abilities and the utility of AT. Their knowledge of AT may be quite extensive, defining their choices of specific products.

Gaining an appreciation of the client's understanding of the current situation also requires dialogue about the context in which the client performs occupations. More details on this aspect will be described in the following section; however, at this point the practitioner should elicit the client's perception of physical, social, cultural, and institutional contexts that might affect AT use.

Occupation

Relevant occupations are identified from the occupational history. Table 24-5 identifies assessments that are useful for this identification. Building on the history, the practitioner asks about how frequently these occupations

are completed, where they occur, and how the client chooses to complete them. An activity analysis is a useful to determine the components of the activity that can be replaced or augmented by the use of technology.

Person

A thorough evaluation of key physical, sensory, and cognitive skills and functional abilities is completed. Table 24-6 lists the components in each of these areas to be evaluated. Further, the clinician identifies any conditions that might affect function over time, such as growth or expected recovery or decline of function. Anticipated change in function affects the type of AT recommended. Because a device is only of benefit if the client uses it, the clinician needs to gain an understanding of the meaning that the technology holds for the client. Use of some devices may signify vulnerability or disability to the person (a wheelchair is a common symbol of disability). Use of devices viewed in this way may be resisted. A device that is viewed as a tool—something of utility—has a greater chance of being integrated in the client's daily occupations.[27]

Environment

Assessment of the physical context considers the interaction between the AT and the physical elements of the environment. It includes the natural and built environments; accessibility within and across environments; and the effect of physical elements of light, temperature and sound on the function and use of the technology.[3] Terrain, light, and temperature of the natural environment affect device operation and function outdoors. Consider how the client will move outdoors and identify the aspects of the outdoor environment that enable or hinder mobility. In the built environment, determine whether the client can get into and out of buildings, travel through a building to key locations (eg, a classroom), and access facilities (eg, washrooms and elevators). Physical elements of the indoor environment, such as light and ambient sounds, affect device use. If the AT is portable, identify how the device will be transported and who will be responsible for its care during transportation.[3]

Evaluation of the social environment includes interaction with and influence of others in the locations where the AT will be used. Determine who is present in the environment, the role they have in supporting AT use, their attitude toward AT use, and their knowledge of how to use it if they have responsibility for set-up, maintenance, and repair. It is also important to understand how the attitudes of unfamiliar others affect device use.[1]

Cultural beliefs about independence vs interdependence, disability, occupational, social justice, and the right

Table 24-5. *Assistive Technology Assessment for Intervention and Outcome Evaluations*

Assessment	Construct or Factor Assessed	Description and Reference	Where It Can Be Obtained
General Assistive Technology Intervention Measures			
Survey of Technology Use	Past/current experience with technology	Checklist designed to determine an adult client's previous experience with various types of technology	www.matchingpersonandtechnology.com
AT Device Predisposition Assessment	Match between client, general context, and technology	Checklists for adult clients and AT providers that identifies relevant aspects of the person, their environment, and the device to guide the AT selection process	www.matchingpersonandtechnology.com
Educational Technology Predisposition Assessment	Match between client and technology in educational context	Checklists for client and AT provider that identifies relevant aspects of the person, their environment, and the device to guide the AT selection process in the educational setting	www.matchingpersonandtechnology.com
Workplace Technology Predisposition Assessment	Match between client and technology in work context	Checklists for adult clients and AT providers that identifies relevant aspects of the person, their environment and the device to guide the AT selection process in the workplace	www.matchingpersonandtechnology.com
Health Care Technology Predisposition Assessment	Provider attitude toward technology	Checklist that helps a health care provider determine his or her attitude toward technology use	www.matchingpersonandtechnology.com
Matching AT and Children	Match between child, parents, context, and technology	Assessment that involves parents, health care, and educational providers to identify appropriate AT for a child	www.matchingpersonandtechnology.com
General Assistive Technology Outcome Measures			
Family Impact of Assistive Technology Scale (FIATS)	Impact of AT use on family	Measurement of the perceptions of parents about the aspects of their daily lives that are affected by AT use	Available from first author Ryan, Campbell, and Rigby[19]
Psychosocial Impact of Assistive Devices Scale (PIADS)	Psychosocial outcome (competence, self-esteem, and adaptability) of AT use	Measures the impact of AT on quality of life conceptualized with 3 factors: competence, self-esteem, and adaptability	Jutai and Day[20]
Quebec User Evaluation of Satisfaction with Assistive Technology (QUEST 2.0)	User satisfaction with AT	Evaluates user's satisfaction with a wide range of AT and with AT service provision	www.matchingpersonandtechnology.com Demers, Weiss-Lambrou, and Ska[21]

(continued)

Table 24-5 (continued). *Assistive Technology Assessment for Intervention and Outcome Evaluations*

Assessment	Construct or Factor Assessed	Description and Reference	Where It Can Be Obtained
Device Specific Outcome Measures			
AT Outcomes Profile—Mobility	Activity and participation	Measures the impact of mobility devices on activity and participation	www.atoutcomes.com Bode, Jutai, Heinemann, and Fuhrer[22]
Functioning Everyday in a Wheelchair Seating—Mobility Outcomes Measure	Activity and participation	Provides a profile of function, as perceived by the user of a wheelchair or scooter	www.Few.Pitt.edu Holm, Mills, Schmeler, and Trefler[23]
Wheelchair Outcome Measures (WhOM)	Body structures and function, activity, and participation	A user-centered measure of the functional and physical outcomes of wheelchair service delivery	Available from: WC Miller (author), Mortenson, Miller, and Polgar[24]
Wheelchair Skills Test	Wheelchair skills	Measure of basic and advanced skills required to use a power or manual wheelchair	www.wheelchairskillsprogram.ca
COMPASS	Computer skills	Provides a systematic evaluation of computer input skills, including keyboarding, use of a pointing device, text entry, and use of alternative input methods such as switches	Available from author Koester[25]
Language Activity Monitor	Verbal communication	Automated data logger that captures the utterances from an AAC device	www.aacinstitute.org Hill and Romich[26]

to choice and control over occupational engagement also influence technology selection and use. Views about personal space may influence the acceptance of technology, such as a wheelchair or some electronic aids to daily living that place a physical barrier between the client and others in their environment.

The final environmental component is the institutional environment. Here, the practitioner needs to consider the legislation and policies that affect AT provision in his or her jurisdiction, safety standards, and policies for use and ownership of technology in institutions, such as supported nursing facilities and funding requirements. Relevant legislation and accompanying policies have different functions. They may:

- Define what constitutes AT and what is excluded
- Identify the conditions under which AT must be provided
- Define eligibility for acquisition of AT

- Specify responsibilities for device recommendation/prescription, provision, and funding

The practitioner is responsible for learning about the legislation in his or her jurisdiction in order to comply with it. Funding is a very important element of the institutional environment. Policies governing funding change over time; it is the ethical responsibility of a clinician to remain current on the policies that affect his or her practice. The clinician must comply with the following aspects of funding policies:

- Determination of eligible products
- Assessment of clients to ensure that they are eligible for the equipment to be recommended
- Provision of required documentation to support equipment recommendation
- Repair and replacement schedules
- Determination of who (ie, which professional) is responsible for completing each aspect of the AT provision and funding process

Table 24-6. *Human Elements Assessed in the Assistive Technology Selection Process*

Human Element	Element Components
Physical	• Range of motion • Strength • Balance • Gross motor skills • Fine motor manipulation • Endurance • Postural control • Reflexes • Muscle tone • Presence of contractures—fixed/flexible • Involuntary movements and reactions • Motor planning
Tactile sensation	• Proprioception • Light touch • Deep pressure • Temperature perception • Pain
Vision (in conjunction with eye care specialist)	• Visual acuity • Depth perception • Visual field • Light sensitivity • Contrast sensitivity • Color discrimination
Hearing (information received from audiologist)	• Sound detection • Sound discrimination • Localization of sound • Speech discrimination • Vestibular function
Cognitive	• Attention • Memory • Perceptual functions • Spatial awareness • Abstraction • Organization and planning • Time management • Insight • Judgment • Problem solving
Affective	• Regulation of emotions • Range of emotions • Presence of diagnosis that will affect AT use

INTERVENTION

Intervention to Obtain Assistive Technology

Assistive technology modifies occupational performance through augmentation or replacement of body functions. Cook and Polgar describe 3 activity outputs that AT augments and replaces: manipulation, communication, and mobility.[3] In addition, they describe AT to support cognitive, visual, and auditory function. Table 24-7 lists these constructs and related AT interventions. The synthesis of information from the narrative, assessment, and evaluation phases influences the selection of AT. This synthesis is compared with the functionality of the AT in order to determine the most appropriate fit.[3,29] The following aspects of the device are considered:

- *Device function:* What does the device do? Does it have a single or multiple purpose(s)? Can it be used across multiple environments, as needed?
- *Ease of use:* Are there device functions that the client can use immediately? How much training is necessary to develop competence in use of the device?
- *Support the device provides to the client:* Does it provide the appropriate amount of support to the client, allowing him or her to use his or her own abilities without placing unreasonable demands on the client?
- What are the physical, cognitive, sensory, and affective requirements for *successful device use?*
- *Device esthetics:* Is the look of the device acceptable to the client?

Once specific AT is identified, best practice involves a trial period in which the client can use the AT in various contexts, over an appropriate time, for desired occupations, and with anticipated assistance in order to evaluate the match between the person and the technology.[29]

Acquisition of the Technology

The clinician's role at the time the client receives the device is to ensure proper fit, set-up, and facilitate training in use of the device. When a substantial length of time occurs between device recommendation and acquisition, re-evaluation may be necessary to determine if the equipment still meets the client's needs. Set-up of the equipment by positioning the client and/or the equipment ensures optimal use by the client. Programming may be necessary for some devices, such as the controller of a powered wheelchair or electronic aid to daily living. Biomechanical and ergonomic considerations ensure optimal positioning for occupational performance supported by the device.

Table 24-7. *Assistive Technology Intervention*

Construct, Mechanism, or Factor	Intervention and Reference	How It Relates to PEOP
Communication	• AAC[3,8,14] • Communication Boards • Speech Synthesis • Electronic communication devices • Computer Access[3,14] • Voice recognition • Alternate access • Word prediction/word completion software • Speech to text • Software to support alternate selection methods • Smart phone technology[3,5]	• Intervention for communication is relevant to the sensory and motor aspect of the person component of PEOP. • It facilitates occupation in all areas of activities, tasks, and roles within a number of different environments. • Aspects of the cultural and social environment influence the client's ability to use communication devices.
Cognition	• Memory aids[3,4] • Electronic organizers[3,4] • Computer apps[5] • Pill organizers[3] • Pervasive computing technology[4,5] • Sensors • Systems that cue occupational performance • Telehealth, telerehabilitation	• Cognitive technologies are pertinent to cognitive and perceptual functions of the person. • They influence occupational performance of most activities, across all environments. • Social and cultural contexts are influential.
Manipulation	• Simple[3] • Reachers • Built-up handles • Dressing and self-care aids • Aids for eating and meal preparation • Electronic aids to daily living[3,4,5,10,11] • Remote control of appliances and electronics • Remote control of living environment, including lights, temperature, window covering, doors • Telephone access • Robotics[4]	• Manipulation aids augment or replace physical function of the person, including strength, ROM, endurance, and coordination. • They support manipulative aspects of occupational performance. • Aspects of the physical, social, and cultural environments influence their use.
Hearing	• Alerting devices[3] • Assistive listening devices[3] • Close-captioned displays[3] • Computer access[3]	• Hearing devices support the sensory and perceptual aspects of audition for the person. • These are used to support hearing across all occupations. • They are influenced by social, cultural, and physical environments.

(continued)

Table 24-7 (continued).   *Assistive Technology Intervention*

Construct, Mechanism, or Factor	Intervention and Reference	How It Relates to PEOP
Mobility	• Canes[3] • Walkers[3] • Scooters[3] • Manual wheelchairs[3,28] • Powered wheelchairs[3,6,7,9,27,28] • Seating products[3,27] • Cushions • Backs • Headrests • Pelvic positioning devices • Driving aids[3]	• Mobility devices support physical function involving movement within and across multiple environments. Positioning devices support optimal position for function across occupations. • They support occupation by enabling a person to get from one place to another, and to achieve and maintain a stable position for occupational performance. • The natural, built, social, and cultural environments are influential.
Vision	• Magnification aids[3,12] • Optical • Non-optical • Electronic • Automatic readers[3,12] • Synthetic speech output[3,12] • Mobility aids[3,12]	• Vision aids support the sensory and perceptual aspects of vision. • They support the visual aspects of occupational performance across most occupations. • Physical aspects of the environment, such as noise and light, influence their use as well as social and cultural aspects.

Training/Education

The complexity of the device will determine the level of support required for the client to gain proficiency in its use. When a high level of skill is needed, a systematic training program is of benefit. Cook and Polgar suggest the following training strategies[30]:

- Familiarize with the basic functions of the device
- Start with simple operations and build to complex
- Start with occupations important to the client
- Build in success
- Engage the client and caregivers
- Evaluate throughout the training

Commonly, training involves use of the device in relevant environments. Virtual technology is an emerging training method that is showing promise.[28]

Advocacy

There are many opportunities for the practitioner to advocate on behalf of the client during intervention that includes AT. Technology is expensive, so the first opportunity often involves advocating for funding to support acquisition of AT. The practitioner provides the necessary justification for funding of the device (following policies established in his or her jurisdiction) and assists the client with the funding and procurement processes. The opportunity to receive necessary education on device use is limited in some jurisdictions. The occupational therapy practitioner advocates for funding and time to support a training program, particularly for clients who receive an unfamiliar device while living in the community. The practitioner may also advocate for contextual changes (eg, policy, social, and physical) that enable device use across relevant environments.

OUTCOMES

Outcome Evaluation

Evaluation of the outcome of AT provision, both at the client and the system level, provides important information for many stakeholders, including the client and family, the professional team, organizational service providers, funders, and policy-makers. The importance of efficacious AT outcomes was recently recognized with calls for a user-centered outcome model encompassing AT use, usability, and QOL,[31] as well as a framework that includes the interaction of device-specific characteristics, the user, and the environment.[32] Best practice suggests that follow up occurs at regular intervals over a longer period (eg, 3, 6, 12, or 24 months). Changes in the person, his or her occupations and roles, the context in which he or she engages in occupation, and available technology are considered.

Outcome evaluation can be achieved through informal or formal evaluations. Cook and Polgar suggest that an informal evaluation of AT includes use of AT and the human technology interface.[30] The use of AT is determined through observation or interview including occupational performance, amount of use, satisfaction, and assistance needed. Evaluation of the human AT interface includes device and client positioning; visual, auditory and manipulative aspects of device use; error detection and repair; and source of errors. Formal evaluation uses standardized tests with demonstrated psychometric properties for a defined use, which allow the practitioner to compare the client's performance with others or to quantify change in some aspect of client performance. Table 24-5 provides information about different standardized assessments specific to AT intervention and outcome evaluation.

Evidence Base of Assistive Technology Interventions

The range of AT products and interventions is vast, so this section will discuss some of the areas in which evidence exists and some of the challenges for establishing the evidence base for AT intervention. Table 24-8 shows some of the evidence supporting the effect of wheeled mobility on participation of adults, as an example of the evidence that exists.

Evidence supporting outcomes of AT includes effect on different populations (eg, children, adults, seniors, or diagnostic categories), across different environments (eg, home, school, work, community), across different categories of devices (as identified earlier in this chapter), and across different outcomes (eg, body structures and function, activity, and participation). Device categories such as AAC, computer access, and seating and mobility have been available for many years, with the result that many different bodies of research are available to support their use. Other categories, such as pervasive computer technology and robotics, exist primarily in a laboratory setting, so the evidence to support the effect of their use on occupational performance, well-being, and participation in a naturalistic setting is extremely limited.

Isolating the effect of AT use from other aspects of the client's function is a challenge to developing evidence. AT is often used in combination with assistance from others and environmental modifications, requiring research methods that account for confounding factors that influence occupational performance. The heterogeneity of the clients who use these devices makes it difficult to generalize across research findings. As Table 24-8 demonstrates, the range of research methods, dependent variables, outcome measures, and research protocols challenge the ability to generalize and build strong evidence supporting interventions.

The range of devices within a specific category and the amount of customization possible further complicate establishment of an evidence base. For example, pressure relief through the use of a wheelchair cushion is the subject of many research projects. Pressure relief cushions vary in terms of materials (eg, foam, air, or gel), construction, and configuration, which challenges the ability to make conclusions about any particular cushion and its effect on minimizing pressure ulcer incidence. Novel and rigorous research methods are needed to account for these multiple variables in order to demonstrate efficacy of AT intervention.

SUMMARY

Let's draw together some of the key ideas of this chapter in conclusion. Technology is only useful if it meets the client's needs and functions as expected. Technology that is poorly designed and clumsy to use is often put away, unused. Equally important is the meaning the technology has for the client. The client is more likely to integrate technology that evokes a sense of confidence in and satisfaction with his or her daily occupations. A client-centered, evidence-based evaluation and appropriate follow up are part of best practice to ensure effective device use. Ethical issues are more prominent in AT service provision, with the development of devices that can monitor a client's behavior. Best practice here suggests that the practitioner carefully considers the balance between enabling independence to live in the community with the limitations imposed by these technologies in the service delivery process. Finally, more attention needs to be directed to equitable and sustainable access to AT globally. The WHO *World Report on Disability* calls for increased use

Table 24-8. Evidence Table for Assistive Technology Intervention (Using Example of Effect of Powered Mobility on Participation)

Study	Aim of Study	Methods	Participants	Results and Outcome(s)	Conclusion(s) and Implications	Level or Type of Evidence
Baker et al[33]	Explore the lived experience of older adults using a wheelchair in the home and community.	Semi-structured interview asking about changes in lifestyle, activities, and self-perception since receiving wheelchair. Inductive data analysis involving 2 researchers. Member check with 2 participants, involving review of summary of themes and follow-up telephone interview.	N = 10. Inclusion criteria: older than 65 years, used wheeled mobility for at least 12 months, required assistance with activities of daily living (ADL), lived in community, lived in study area, could participate in interview in English. 80% male. Mean age = 75.5 years.	All participants expressed perception that wheelchair enabled occupation. Themes labeled using International Classification of Functioning, Disability and Health (ICF) framework and included (1) body structure and impairment elements related to urinary function and mobility; (2) activity and participation themes of dependence on others, especially outdoors, and relationship with caregiver; (3) environmental factors, including physical accessibility, caregiver health, and stigma; and (4) contextual factors of psychosocial benefits, lifestyle habits, comorbidities, and past experiences.	Understanding the past experiences and lifestyle choices of client informs both wheelchair selection and training aspects. Client training in wheelchair skills is necessary to reduce effort of use of chair. Understanding the abilities and needs of the caregiver is an important consideration of wheelchair selection.	Credibility: Moderate—team of researchers involved in data collection, framework, and theoretical foundation predetermined; single data collection time and method used. Transferability: Moderate—quantitative information provided on numerous key demographic factors; limited information on severity of impairment and functional level. Dependability: Moderate—process described well; data analysis congruent with ICF, which was foundational to work. Confirmability: Weak—limited confirmation of findings with participants; predetermined framework and theory used; no external peer review; 2 researchers involved in data analysis.

(continued)

Table 24-8 (continued). Evidence Table for Assistive Technology Intervention (Using Example of Effect of Powered Mobility on Participation)

Study	Aim of Study	Methods	Participants	Results and Outcome(s)	Conclusion(s) and Implications	Level or Type of Evidence
Brandt et al[34]	Investigate outcomes of powered wheelchairs by older adults and identify the risk factors of negative outcomes.	Cross-sectional study involving interviews. Study-specific questionnaire used, including questions about person, assistive technology (AT), activity, environment, and outcomes of wheelchair use. 12 Danish municipalities randomly selected to represent small-, medium- and large-sized communities. Participants recruited using municipal records of wheelchair users older than 65 years. Chi-square test used to determine male/female and summer/winter differences. Wilcoxon signed rank test used to determine difference in summer/winter frequency. Odds ratio (OR) calculated between negative outcome and personal characteristic.	111 powered wheelchair users interviewed. Mean age = 77 years. 56% male. Powered scooter users = 84; powered wheelchair users = 27. Mean time of wheelchair use = 4.5 years.	Majority of users felt wheelchair was important and used it outdoors for shopping, visiting, and going for a ride. Few used powered wheelchair on some form of vehicle. Males and females participated in most activities on equal basis. Odds ratio analysis identified age (>76 years), being female for prioritized activities, inability to transfer without assistance, and visual function as factors heightening risk of negative outcomes.	All older adult participants used the chair, and most felt it was of value and enabled them to participate in valued activities and social life. Transportation was a limiting factor. Risk factors identified may assist clinicians to understand what might limit the older adult's use of a powered wheelchair.	Level IV

(continued)

Table 24-8 (continued).   Evidence Table for Assistive Technology Intervention (Using Example of Effect of Powered Mobility on Participation)

Study	Aim of Study	Methods	Participants	Results and Outcome(s)	Conclusion(s) and Implications	Level or Type of Evidence
Cooper et al[35]	To determine the correlation between wheelchair activity recorded with a data logger and community participation.	Wheelchair activity recorded over 3-week period, including during participation at weeklong sporting event and 2 weeks at home using data logger attached to wheelchair. Major life activities at home and in community measured with the Participation Mobility Survey (PARTS/M). PARTS/M data reduced to provide a single score (range, 0-19). Data logger information included distance traveled, speed, number of stops, and drive time over 2-week home period.	N = 16. 15 males. Mean age = 49.13 years. 9 had tetraplegia; 7 had paraplegia. 7 manual wheelchair users; 9 powered wheelchair users.	Mean distance traveled per day = 3374.07 meters. Mean drive time per day = 68.65 minutes. Community participation score range (N = 14), 6.5-16.0 (mean, 11.98). Significant positive correlation between average speed and community participation areas of transportation and socialization. No significant differences between distance traveled and community participation.	Speed of travel significantly correlated with community participation for manual chair users only. Users capable of propelling chair at higher speeds may have higher functioning. Lack of a significant correlation between powered wheelchair and community mobility may be artifact of PARTS/M questions.	Level IV

(continued)

Table 24-8 (continued). Evidence Table for Assistive Technology Intervention (Using Example of Effect of Powered Mobility on Participation)

Study	Aim of Study	Methods	Participants	Results and Outcome(s)	Conclusion(s) and Implications	Level or Type of Evidence
Frank et al[36]	Explore the effects of powered wheelchairs on users, families, and caregivers.	Descriptive study using telephone-administered questionnaire and interview. Interview asked about effect of wheelchair use on family and caregivers. Authors describe work as "qualitative research approach."(p328) Inductive data analysis involved initial coding and analysis by 2 researchers and reanalysis by a third.	N = 64. 50% male. Range of conditions. Mean age = 41.7 years (range 10–81 years). Participants described as having severe disability. 18 participants received some form of assistance during interview, including reading, repetition of response when speech was difficult to understand, and assistance to hold phone. Used powered wheelchair for at least 10 months.	Main theme identified the reduced burden for caregivers when powered wheelchair was obtained, mainly from cessation of need to push wheelchair. Powered wheelchair also afforded more opportunities for community participation. Increased difficulties for caregivers involved lifting requirements when transferring chairs, challenges with transportation, and lack of curb cuts in community. Safety issues related to battery charge and appearance of vulnerability were identified.	Provision of powered mobility device affects more than mobility; it affords freedom and independence for user and their family and/or caregivers. Environmental aspects of transportation and accessibility seen as limiting factors of participation.	Credibility: Weak—data were collected at single point in time with single method; multiple researchers engaged in data analysis and confirmation; no recorded reflection of perceptions and values. Transferability: Moderate—significant amount of information provided about participants, although limited information on what is meant by "severe" disability. Dependability: Moderate—methods are well described; key quotes provided to support each theme. Confirmability: Moderate—data analysis done in 2 steps, with third researcher completing independent analysis following initial analysis by 2 other researchers; interviews conducted by researcher not connected with service provider; no apparent reflection on prior values and perceptions.

(continued)

Table 24-8 (continued). Evidence Table for Assistive Technology Intervention (Using Example of Effect of Powered Mobility on Participation)

Study	Aim of Study	Methods	Participants	Results and Outcome(s)	Conclusion(s) and Implications	Level or Type of Evidence
Hoenig et al[37]	To determine patterns of wheelchair use in different locations and compare use across locations.	Longitudinal cohort study. Participants interviewed 2-3 weeks after receipt of wheelchair. Outcome variables included self-reported wheelchair use in different life-spaces (in home, near home, at a distance). Independent variables included personal characteristics, characteristics related to wheelchair (mode of propulsion, transfers, met/unmet needs), and environment characteristics (steps, accessibility features, transportation). Kappa statistic used to compare wheelchair use across life-spaces. Bivariate regression used to compare wheelchair use with independent variables. Stepwise logistical regression used for final multivariate models.	N = 153. Mean age = 64.8 years. 92% male. Inclusion criteria: received manual or powered wheelchair, older than 21 years, lived within 65-mile radius of study site, had Short Portable Mental Status Questionnaire score of >6 of 10. Exclusion criteria: receiving identical wheelchair to one being replaced.	Stepwise regression showed number of impairments, home accessibility, and dependence on another for propulsion were significant predictors of wheelchair use in bathroom and kitchen. Accessibility of home was predictor of wheelchair use near home. Older age was negatively associated with wheelchair use distant to home. Independent propulsion, poverty, and accessible home were predictors of wheelchair use across all life-spaces.	Wheelchair use inconsistent across life-spaces and participants. Participants selectively determine where and for what purpose they will use their chairs. Wheelchair provision needs to consider various contexts in which wheelchair might be used. AT use is not simply use vs nonuse; multiple factors need to be considered regarding its use.	Level IV

(continued)

Table 24-8 (continued). Evidence Table for Assistive Technology Intervention (Using Example of Effect of Powered Mobility on Participation)

Study	Aim of Study	Methods	Participants	Results and Outcome(s)	Conclusion(s) and Implications	Level or Type of Evidence
Löfqvist et al[38]	Investigate outcomes of powered mobility use (wheelchair and scooter), including need for assistance, frequency, ease of mobility, and types of participation.	Prospective cohort study. Participants interviewed prior to receiving their first powered wheelchair or scooter (baseline) and then at 4 and 12 months. Nordic Mobility-related Participation Outcome Evaluation of Assistive Device Interventions (NOMO 1.0) used for data collection.	N = 47 (baseline), 42 (at 4 months) and 34 (at 12 months). Inclusion criteria: age 20 years or older, first-time wheelchair/scooter acquisition, cognitive capacity and verbal skills enabling participation in interview. 11% women. Mean age = 69 years.	By 4 months, 50% of participants were independent in use of device. No significant changes in number of activities in which participants engaged. Shopping, going for walk/ride, and spending time with family/friends increased between baseline and 4 months. This result remained stable at 1 year.	Changes in participation occur within first 4 months. Participants became independent with mobility after receiving powered mobility device.	Level III
Pettersson et al[39]	To gain perspective of persons who had a stroke on the effect of powered mobility on activity and participation.	Participants interviewed prior to and then 3-5 months after acquisition of powered wheelchair. Instruments included study-specific questionnaire, checklist of life events, Individually Prioritized Problem Assessment, and World Health Organization Disability Assessment Schedule II. Data analysis included within-group effect for IPPA and WHODAS II. Wilcoxon signed rank test used to determine significant differences between baseline and follow-up.	N = 32. 69% male. Mean age = 67 years (range, 45-85 years). Median age of onset of stroke = 24 months.	118 activity limitations identified at baseline. Of these, 41% were eliminated and 40% were reduced at follow-up. Community and civic life (ICF) was domain with greatest limitation. Limitations existed in areas related to environmental accessibility. Large effect size found for pre- and post-acquisition differences for community, social, and civic life and for getting around and self-care.	Powered wheelchair, used outdoors, can support greater participation in community activities, including leisure. Wheelchair perceived as an enabler of occupation in many areas by all participants.	Level III

(continued)

Table 24-8 (continued).   Evidence Table for Assistive Technology Intervention (Using Example of Effect of Powered Mobility on Participation)

Study	Aim of Study	Methods	Participants	Results and Outcome(s)	Conclusion(s) and Implications	Level or Type of Evidence
Rosseau-Harrison et al[40]	To document perceived impact of participants' first power or manual wheelchair on ADL and social participation.	Phenomenological study using semi-structured interviews. Based on the Disability Creation Process (DCP) model. Meaning associated with life habits and changes in life habits identified. Analysis modeled on methods used in phenomenological approach.	10 adults who used services of a specific seating and mobility program in Montreal, Canada, whose first wheelchair was received between July and December 2008. Range of disabling conditions. Able to participate in interview in French. Mean age = 64.3 years. 60% female. Mean time between wheelchair acquisition and interview = 315 days. 80% had progressive condition.	Participants indicated expectations were met in self-care and nutrition areas, with less perceived change in body condition and housing. Expectations for outdoor mobility were not met. Effect on social roles perceived as positive and strong; less effect on responsibilities and community life. Both positive and negative emotional responses identified.	In addition to changes in mobility, participants experienced emotional and social effects of wheelchair acquisition.	Credibility: Strengths include description of the DCP that guided the interview and conceptualization of the project and use of multiple participants in the analysis process. Limits to credibility include a single data collection point and means of data collection. Transferability: Participants thoroughly described; less information provided on setting. Dependability: moderate—more information on questions asked in interview and data analysis process would be helpful. Confirmability: Strengths include inclusion of DCP information and use of team for data collection; limitations include lack of indication that analysis was externally reviewed.

and affordability of AT.[27] It recommends that the AT be congruent with the circumstances of the local environment, and that sustainable and affordable AT provision includes devices that are produced locally from local materials. This idea is the next challenge for AT service provision.

ACKNOWLEDGEMENT

I want to acknowledge the substantial work of Albert M. Cook and Susan Hussey on the development of the initial HAAT Model, and Albert M. Cook for his efforts on the revised model that is presented here.

REFERENCES

1. WHO. *International Classification of Functioning, Disability and Health*. Geneva, Switzerland: WHO; 2001.

2. Sandord JA. *Universal Design as a Rehabilitation Strategy*. New York, NY: Springer Publishing Company; 2012.

3. Cook AM, Polgar J. *Cook and Hussey's Principles of Assistive Technology*. 3rd ed. St. Louis, MO: Elsevier; 2008.

4. Mann W, Milton B. Home automation and smart homes to support independence. In: Mann WC, ed. *Smart Technology for Aging, Disability and Independence*. Hoboken, NJ: Wiley-Interscience; 2005:33-66.

5. Bardram J, Mihalidis A, Wan D. *Pervasive Computing in Healthcare*. London, UK: CRC Press; 2007.

6. Auger C, Demers L, Gelinas I, Miller W, Jutai J, Noreau L. Life-space mobility of middle-aged and older adults at various stages of usage of power mobility devices. *Arch Phys Med Rehabil*. 2010;91:765-773.

7. Sonenblum S, Sprigle S, Harris F, Maurer C. Characterization of power wheelchair use in the home and community. *Arch Phys Med Rehabil*. 2008;98:486-491.

8. Batorowicz B, McDougall S, Shepherd T. AAC and communication partnerships: the participation path to community inclusion. *Augment Altern Comm*. 2006;22:178-195.

9. Buning ME, Angelo J, Schmeler M. Occupational performance and transition to powered mobility: a pilot study. *Am J Occup Ther*. 2001;55:339-344.

10. Jutai J, Rigby P, Ryan S, Stickel S. Psychosocial impact of electronic aids to daily living. *Assist Technol*. 2000;12:123-131.

11. Ripat J. Function and impact of electronic aids to daily living for experienced users. *Technol Disabil*. 2006;18:79-87.

12. Huber J, Jutai J, Strong G, Plotkin A. Psychosocial impact of closed-circuit television on persons with age-related macular degeneration. *J Vis Impair Blind*. 2008;102:690-701.

13. US Government Printing Office, 108th Congress. *Assistive Technology Act of 1998, as amended, PL 108-364, §§ 3, 118 stat 1707*. http://www.gpo.gov/fdsys/pkg/PLAW-108publ364/html/PLAW-108publ364.htm. Published 1998. Amended October 25, 2004. Accessed September 2, 2013.

14. Blackstone SW. Evaluating, selecting, and using communication devices. In: Galvin JC, Scherer MJ, eds. *Evaluation, Selecting, and Using Appropriate Assistive Technology*. Gaithersburg, MD: Aspen; 1996:97-124.

15. Fisk AD, Rogers WA, Charness N, Czaja SJ, Sharit J. *Designing for Older Adults: Principles and Creative Human Factors*. 2nd ed. London, UK: CRC Press; 2009.

16. Norman D. *Design of Everyday Things*. New York, NY: Basic Books (Perseus); 2002.

17. Blanchard J. Ethical considerations of home monitoring technology. In: Mann WC, Helal A, eds. *Promoting Independence for Older Persons with Disabilities*. Amsterdam, The Netherlands: IOS Press; 2006:121-126.

18. Davis W. *The Wayfinders*. Toronto, ON: Anansi Press; 2009.

19. Ryan S, Campbell K, Rigby P. Reliability of the Family Impact of Assistive Technology Scale for families of young children with cerebral palsy. *Arch Phys Med Rehabil*. 2007;88:1436-1440.

20. Jutai J, Day H. Psychosocial Impact of Assistive Devices Scale (PIADS). *Technol Disabil*. 2002;14:107-111.

21. Demers L, Weiss-Lambrou R, Ska B. The Quebec User Evaluation of Satisfaction with Assistive Technology (QUEST 2.0). *Technol Disabil*. 2002;14:101-105.

22. Bode R, Jutai J, Heinemann A, Fuhrer M. The Assistive Technology Outcomes Profile-Mobility (ATOP/M): development of activity limitations and participation restrictions. *Arch Phys Med Rehabil*. 2010;9:10.

23. Holm M, Mills T, Schmeler M, Trefler E. *The Functioning Everyday with a Wheelchair (FEW) Seating-Mobility Outcomes Measure*. FEW: University of Pittsburgh. http://www.few.pitt.edu/. Published 2003. Accessed September 2, 2013.

24. Mortenson B, Miller W, Polgar J. Measuring wheelchair intervention: development of the Wheelchair Outcome Measure (WhOM). *Disabil Rehabil: Assist Technol*. 2007;2:275-285.

25. Koester HH, LoPresti E, Ashlock G, McMillan W, Moore P, Simpson R. *Compass: Software for Computer Skills Assessment*. Paper presented at: CSUN 2003 International Conference on Technology and Persons with Disabilities; Los Angeles, CA; 2005.

26. Hill K, Romich B. A rate index for alternative and augmentative communication. *Int J Speech Technol*. 2002;5:57-64.

27. WHO. *World Report on Disability*. Geneva, Switzerland: WHO; 2011.

28. Archambault P, Tremblay S, Cachercho S, Routhier F, Boissey P. Driving performance in a power wheelchair simulator. *Disabil Rehabil: Assist Technol*. 2012;7(3):226-233.

29. Scherer M. The impact of assistive technology on the lives of people with disabilities. In: Gray DB, Quantrano LA, Lieberman ML, eds. *Designing and Using Assistive Technology: The Human Perspective*. Baltimore, MD: Paul H. Brookes; 1998:99-116.

30. Cook AM, Polgar J. *Essentials of Assistive Technology*. St. Louis, MO: Elsevier; 2012.

31. Lenker J, Paquet V. A new conceptual model for assistive technology outcomes research and practice. *Assist Technol*. 2004;16:1-10.

32. Fuhrer M, Jutai J, Scherer M, DeRuyter F. A framework for the conceptual modeling of assistive technology device outcomes. *Disabil Rehabil*. 2003;25:1243-1251.

33. Baker D, Reid D, Cott C. The experience of senior stroke survivors: factors in community participation among wheelchair users. *Can J Occup Ther*. 2006;73(1):18-25.

34. Brandt Å, Iwarsson S, Ståhle A. Older people's use of powered wheelchair for activity and participation. *J Rehabil Med*. 2004;36:70-77.

35. Cooper RA, Ferretti E, Oyster M, Kelleher A, Cooper R. The relationship between wheelchair mobility patterns and community participation among individuals with spinal cord injury. *Assist Technol*. 2011;23:177-183.

36. Frank A, Neophytou C, Frank J, De Souza L. Electric-powered indoor/outdoor wheelchairs (EPIOCs): user's view of influence on family, friends and careers. *Disabil Rehabil: Assist Technol*. 2010;5(5):327-338.

37. Hoenig H, Pieper C, Zolkewitz M, Schenkman M, Branch L. Wheelchair users are not necessarily wheelchair bound. *J Am Geriat Soc.* 2002;50:645-654.

38. Löfqvist C, Pettersson C, Iwarsson S, Brandt A. Mobility and mobility-related participation outcomes of powered wheelchair and scooter interventions after 4-months and 1-year use. *Disabil Rehabil: Assist Technol.* 2012;7(3):211-218.

39. Pettersson I, Törnquist K, Ahlström G. The effect of an outdoor powered wheelchair on activity and participation in users with stroke. *Disabil Rehabil: Assist Technol.* 2006;1(4):235-243.

40. Rosseau-Harrison K, Rochette A, Routhier F, et al. Perceived impacts of a first wheelchair on social participation. *Disabil Rehabil: Assist Technol.* 2012;7(1):37-44.

INTERVENTIONS
Principles and Emerging Approaches

PEOP: Enabling Everyday Living

THE NARRATIVE
The past, current and future perceptions, choices, interests, goals and needs that are unique to the Person, Organization, or Population

PERSON
• Cognition
• Psychological
• Physiological
• Sensory
• Motor
• Spirituality

OCCUPATION
• Activities
• Tasks
• Roles

ENVIRONMENT
• Culture
• Social Determinants
• Social Support and Social Capital
• Education and Policy
• Physical and Natural
• Assistive Technology

Personal Narrative
• Perception and Meaning
• Choices and Responsibilities
• Attitudes and Motivation
• Needs and Goals

Organizational Narrative
• Mission and History
• Focus and Priorities
• Stakeholders and Values
• Needs and Goals

Population Narrative
• Environments and Behaviors
• Demographics and Disparities
• Incidence and Prevalence
• Needs and Goals

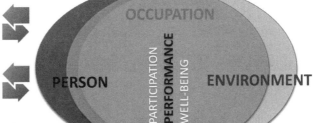

OCCUPATION

PERSON

PARTICIPATION PERFORMANCE WELL-BEING

ENVIRONMENT

Section V addresses the principles of professionalism and emerging approaches for occupational therapy interventions.

Developing a professional identity is just as important as the specific knowledge and skills for assessments and interventions you will acquire. Professional ideals and ethical principles are important to retain throughout your career. Your work toward the greater good of the profession and the people you serve are the rewards that come from being an occupational therapy practitioner.

In Section V, you are introduced to 4 intervention areas that are shaping the future of occupational therapy: learning strategies, self-management, educational and techno-logical strategies, and public and community health. There are 2 main themes that transcend the intervention priorities of the past and present with the opportunities of the future. First, we want our clients to be able to perform the occupations that are important and meaningful in their life. Engagement in these occupations supports their participation in society and defines their life. Second, we strongly believe that occupational performance supports overall health and well-being. If clients are supported to realize their occupational goals, we believe they will also experience improved physical, emotional, and mental health.

Chapter	Title	FAQ
25	*Principles Supporting Intervention and Professionalism* (Fleming, Moyers Cleveland)	• How do ethics, teaming, documentation of service delivery, advocacy, and continuing competence support professionalism? • What current and emerging competencies are recommended for health care professionals?
26	*A Person-Centered Strategy: Using Learning Strategies to Enable Performance, Participation, and Well-Being* (Wolf, Josman)	• How is "learning" an inherent part of occupational therapy? • How does an understanding of learning theories, enablers, and barriers help develop effective interventions?
27	*An Organization-Centered Strategy: Self-Management—An Evolving Approach to Support Performance, Participation, and Well-Being* (Hammel, Finlayson, Lee)	• How do self-management approaches support performance, participation, and well-being? • What person, environment, and occupation factors are addressed in self-management programs?
28	*Educational and Digital Technology Strategies* (Hamilton, Hamilton)	• How are education and educational technologies used in occupational therapy interventions? • How do educational/technology concepts and theories support occupational therapy interventions?
29	*A Population-Centered Strategy: Public and Community Health* (Stone)	• What terms and concepts from public and community health are essential to know for occupational therapy practitioners who work in this area? • How are public and community health assessments and interventions used in occupational therapy?

Chapter 25

Principles Supporting Intervention and Professionalism

John D. Fleming, EdD, OTR/L and Penelope A. Moyers Cleveland, EdD, OT/L, FAOTA

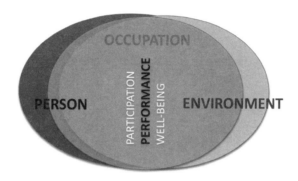

Learning Objectives

- Understand the principles necessary to support intervention and professionalism.
- Use ethical principles and codes of ethics in professional decision making.
- Understand the skills for professional interactions and communications.
- Know how to construct and use a professional portfolio incorporating principles for professional lifelong development.

Key Words

- Advocacy
- Attitudes
- Certification
- Code of Ethics
- Competencies
- Continuing competence
- Documentation
- Dynamic teaming
- Electronic health record
- Implementation science
- Interprofessional teams
- Knowledge
- Licensure
- Peer review
- Professional development
- Skills
- Values

Christiansen CH, Baum CM, Bass JD, eds.
Occupational Therapy: Performance, Participation, and Well-Being, Fourth Edition (pp 467-483).
© 2015 SLACK Incorporated.

INTRODUCTION

There are increased demands for flexibility and change in the world of health care today, impacting the practitioner's values and skills that underlie ethical health care practice, interprofessional communication, and lifelong learning. A major stimulus for these changes in health care comes from the Pew Health Professions Commission in their report, *Recreating Health Professionals Practice for a New Century.*[1] This report presents some major recommendations, including the demand for a change in the content of educational programs. There is a push for consistency in which professional programs meet emerging health care needs through the creation of a workforce that is competent and can practice with other health care disciplines rather than separately; and one that is engaged in public service as part of professional practice.

The Commission goes on to identify 21 competencies for the individual practitioner to develop to meet these recommendations in order to practice in a changing health care environment. These competencies include practicing in an ethical manner and developing a personal ethic of responsibility and service, partnering with communities in health care decisions and working in interdisciplinary teams, using effective communication technologies, and engaging in ongoing learning individually and with others. These competencies are directly stated in the PEOP Model as principles of intervention with individuals, organizations, and populations. Developing these skills and awareness about the need and benefits of these considerations will help the occupational therapy practitioner to create a more effective, ethical, and integrated practice serving the needs of clients and the advancement of the discipline of occupational therapy. This chapter will explain and explore ethics, professional communication interprofessional teams, and continuing competence for the occupational therapy practitioner.

Ethics

Using Ethical Principles to Support Intervention in the Person-Environment-Occupation-Performance Model

Ethics can be defined as a system of moral principles or a code of conduct.[2] These rules of conduct, or systems, are often related to a particular culture or profession, such as occupational therapy. Ethics can be differentiated from morals, in that morals are broader and generally reflect people's values and what they consider they believe to be right and good. Morals reflect what people feel they ought to do.[3] Ethics takes morals and critically examines these beliefs to form a set of criteria that particularly relate to

that culture or professional group. While not specifically becoming a law in a legal sense, ethical beliefs may have laws associated with them.

Ethical principles are fundamental laws or truths that have been developed over the history of civilization in order to provide guidance when situations arise that cause conflicts in ethics or morals. Table 25-1 defines and provides an application of selected ethical principles to health care practice.[4] Practitioners use ethical principles to guide a response to an ethical problem or dilemma, but these need to be used in a thoughtful way. These principles may conflict with each other, and in some cases application of 2 different principles may call for 2 different courses of action. What is good for the individual is not necessarily good for the organization or the population as a whole. The PEOP Model uses ethics and ethical reasoning as part of occupational therapy approaches and outcomes to allow individuals, organizations, and populations to perform occupation with the greatest quality of participation and well-being in our society. In order to try to come to grips with these dilemmas, researchers and those who study ethics have devised ethical models to help guide the practitioner through these difficult situations.

Ethical Decision Making

Several authors have developed models to guide a practitioner through decisions about ethical dilemmas. Table 25-2 provides a generalized view of basic steps in ethical decision making, adapted from several sources in the literature.[5,6] Information and knowledge of possible courses of action are critical to making a reasoned decision. As a practical matter, it is advisable for the practitioner to be thinking of these options for action on a regular basis, as time or circumstances may not allow for a prolonged debate in a situation. Communication with other health care professionals and team members may help one to determine the best course of action. Using evidence-based practice to know the possible practical options is also an important and ongoing professional activity for the practitioner to help expand his or her wealth of knowledge.

Assessing Outcomes of Ethical Decision Making

Assessment and evaluation is an ongoing part of ethical decision making as the practitioner decides on appropriate knowledge to gather, selects applicable ethical concepts, and chooses appropriate courses of action. Assessment also occurs when the practitioner looks at the effectiveness of their chosen course of action. Assessing outcomes may be difficult, as all outcomes of action are not generally known right away, and issues like the principle of double effect (ie, potential for an action to have both a planned good effect and an unknown, possibly evil or harmful effect) may play a part in long-term outcomes.

Table 25-1. *Selected Ethical Principles*[4]

Principle	Description	Related Health Care Issues/Examples
Common good	Actions that secure the best opportunity for individuals are also related to the best for society as a whole.	Allowing the individual client to reach his or her maximal potential allows him or her to contribute more effectively for the good of society.
Distributive justice	Society's ability to balance resources, individual needs, and the good of the whole society for appropriate health care outcomes.	Equitable access to health care, the person's basic right to health care.
Double effect	Potential for an action to have both a planned good effect and an unknown, possible evil or harmful effect.	Situations where health care policies are created to address one issue, but complicate or deprive others who have a related issue.
Respect for persons	Protection of individual autonomy and decision making.	Client-centered care and the ability to participate or decline treatment options and engagement as a research subject.
Stewardship	The obligation to maintain scarce resources and preserve human life and the natural environment.	Maintaining clinical supplies and resources; obligation to teach the next generation of practitioners about occupational therapy.
Ordinary vs extraordinary means	The determination of the intensity or length of medical treatment (means) versus the possible benefit or outcome of that treatment.	Health care directives, Do Not Resuscitate/ Intubate orders (DNR/I), decisions about hospice care, euthanasia.

Assessment of outcomes in ethical decision making can be viewed within 2 major schools of ethical thought. On one hand, there is the *deontologic approach* to outcomes. This approach states that ethical criteria are met when the practitioner acts according to the duties and rights of those involved. Duties are responsibilities one has to fulfill because of moral or legal obligations; for example, the legal duty to respect an individual's Do Not Resuscitate order would be a type of duty. The other school of thought is the *utilitarian approach,* which states that you are acting ethically if you are bringing out the best balance between benefits of the decision over its burdens. This school of thought is embodied in ethical principles of doing the most benefit for the most people or doing the greatest good. These 2 schools of thought may, and do, often clash. Consequently, practitioners have to decide what position they will take when considering potential legal liability and legal consequences.

American Occupational Therapy Association Code of Ethics

Occupational therapy has been guided by a concern for ethical practice since the first days of the profession. The current version of the *Code of Ethics* is a revision based on

a 2005 version, and can be traced back to the *Principles of Occupational Therapy Ethics* in 1977. The most recent versions of the *Code of Ethics* are also based on the identification and development of 7 core ethical principles. These principles were introduced in 1993's *Core Values and Attitudes of Occupational Therapy Practice.* The 7 values identified in this document included the ability to put the other person first (altruism), fairness with others (equity), allowing others to make choices for themselves (freedom), respecting laws (justice), the individual's value and self-worth (dignity), presenting accurate information (truth), and acting in a thoughtful way using appropriate clinical judgment (prudence).[6]

Overview

Table 25-3 identifies the 7 guiding beliefs of the *Code of Ethics Standards,* a definition of the related principle as stated in the document, and some examples of how the practitioner can demonstrate these principles in daily work as an occupational therapy practitioner. The examples are not meant to be exhaustive, but reflect some of the basic actions practitioners will come across in their practice. For a complete listing of the behaviors expected of

Table 25-2. *Generalized Ethical Decision-Making Process*[5,6]

Step	Pertinent Questions	Supporting Actions
Identify the problem	• What kind of problem is it? • How am I involved in this problem?	Check legal liability and supporting laws as applicable.
Gather information relevant to the problem	• What are the clinical indicators in this situation? • What are concerns/beliefs of the individual and the family? • What are the appropriate cultural/organizational/environmental factors? • Who is involved in this situation? (stakeholders)	Check with other stakeholders as needed. Research information about conditions, environmental and organizational factors. Use evidence-based practice findings as appropriate.
Identify ethical and moral concerns	• What values are involved here? • What ethical principles apply? • Are there any value conflicts, biases, or conflicts of interest involved?	Review the *AOTA Code of Ethics* and other ethical documents as needed.
Identify possible courses of action and their consequences	• What are ethical, moral, legal, financial, and practical alternatives to this issue?	Brainstorming, develop lists of possible practical, moral, ethical, financial, legal, and political consequences for actions.
Select a course of action	• Which possible course of action meets the greatest good of those involved? • Which course of action meets the needs that are determined to be most ethically good and beneficial?	Prepare materials and communication approaches to implement the course of action.
Implement the course of action	• How might this course of action best be implemented?	Use materials and communication skills to implement the decision.
Evaluate the course of action	• Did my action meet the demands of the ethical issue and at least some of the stakeholders involved? • What have I learned from this situation?	Self-reflection about situation and how it might be addressed in the future ; you may not be able to evaluate the situation fully right away.

occupational therapy personnel, please refer to the original document.[7]

Application to Practice

Ethical issues are a frequent and regular part of practitioners' daily lives. Practitioners must balance professionalism and the client relationship with situations, such as discontinuing treatment, choosing treatment with consideration of reimbursement issues, and possible cultural differences in health and ideas of well-being. In addition to discipline specific documents on ethics and ethical practice, practitioners may have guidelines from their health care organization in the form of organizational mission or philosophy statements, as well as in policies and procedures.

Dige identified 4 advantages for the use of written ethical interpretations described in policies guiding clinical practice. First, these interpretations within organizational guidelines can add precision and understanding to the practitioner's use of ethical principles.[8] Second, these organizational guidelines contribute to building and maintaining a shared professional identity. Third, these organizational guidelines put emphasis on client-centered evaluation and intervention. Finally, guidelines provide a useful framework for the ethical behavior of interprofessional teams.[8] Ethical codes and the use of ethical guidelines can

Table 25-3. *American Occupational Therapy Code of Ethics Standards*

Guiding Belief	Principle	Examples of Applications to Practice
Beneficence	Working to improve and maintain the health and happiness of occupational therapy consumers	Providing appropriate and timely services; considering and applying personal, social, and cultural contexts to provide the most effective interventions; discontinuing services when there is no need; making appropriate referrals to other services; practicing within the scope of one's own expertise
Nonmaleficence	Avoiding injury or harm to occupational therapy consumers	Avoiding injuring occupational therapy consumers in any way; practicing and maintaining appropriate professional boundaries; engaging in research that does not injure or put subjects at risk
Autonomy and confidentiality	Allowing the individual the right to make his/her own health care decisions and keeping medical information private	Establishing intervention plans using client-centered practice; getting informed consent of research subjects and informing them of their ability to voluntarily withdraw from treatment or research; maintaining integrity and confidentiality of all health care information, including electronic information
Social justice	Just, equitable, and appropriate distribution of occupational therapy services	Upholding the benefit of occupational therapy in health care and the larger society; educating others about the value of occupational therapy; working for the best health care for others
Procedural justice	Following and upholding current laws and rules regulating health care services	Applying the Code of Ethics, Occupational Therapy Standards of Practice, and other laws affecting treatment and reimbursement of health care services; appropriately supervising other occupational therapy staff and students; maintaining continuing competence and licensure in occupational therapy
Veracity	Being truthful and honest in any dealings as an occupational therapy practitioner	Avoiding fraud; reporting occupational therapy services rendered to clients accurately and on time; avoiding plagiarism and crediting others; avoiding false marketing of occupational therapy services
Fidelity	Maintaining collegial and respectful relationships within and without occupational therapy	Honoring occupational therapy and other professions and their competencies and traditions; respecting and protecting the private information of other colleagues; avoiding insider knowledge or conflict-of-interest situations; working to resolve interpersonal and organizational issues in an effective manner

Adapted from AOTA. Occupational Therapy Code of Ethics and Ethics Standards (2010). *American Journal of Occupational Therapy.* 2010; 64: S17-S26.

therefore help practitioners be more confident in their work and able to explain the value of occupational therapy to others outside the profession.

An emerging area in which practitioners need ethical understanding is within research. Needing to understand and apply research ethical principles is becoming increasingly frequent, as practitioners look to increase occupational therapy's understanding of effective clinical practice. Efforts by practitioners to complete and evaluate clinical research studies bring with it specialized concerns, such as ensuring research participants understand what they are doing in the research project and agree with the procedures (informed consent), have the opportunity to withdraw from the research project as they wish, and remain anonymous by keeping their personal information and involvement in a project private (confidentiality).

Organizations that review and evaluate these ethical issues in research projects have been created in institutions that obtain funding and carry out research. These organizations, called Institutional Review Boards (IRBs), are made up of community experts and clinical professionals with experience in research and research design to examine and monitor these research projects. Review by IRBs is mandated by the federal government for research involving human subjects, and has been in place since 1981. The purpose of IRBs is to protect the rights and well-being of research subjects, researchers, and the organizations involved in research from ethical and legal injury.[9] A major component of this ethical review is an analysis of the benefits of the research, balanced by the risks to research participants. Those practitioners doing research will need to create appropriate documents and go through IRB review of their projects. They may also take part in IRBs as reviewers of research.

Relationship to Licensure and Certification

While ethical dilemmas can often arise during everyday practitioner-client interactions, ethical principles and codes are also reflected in the laws and regulations that affect a practitioner's actions. The most obvious application to this is the laws and regulations that affect documentation and third-party payment for health care services. Occupational therapy personnel must provide services in a clear manner that demonstrates the connection of intervention to current practice guidelines and the best available evidence to address the health care issues. They also must report it in such a way that is accurate, truthful, and demonstrates the need and benefits for the intervention. Failure to practice in this fashion or abide by laws governing health care practice may lead to fines, criminal and civil suits, and/or the inability to practice.

Several levels of oversight are present in the American health care system to monitor and measure the appropriateness and quality of health care interventions and reimbursement practices. These include procedures to get care approved prior to giving occupational therapy interventions (prior authorization), review of documentation and care plans by other professionals after care is given (peer review), and reports made to agencies that grant funds for research. Included in this oversight may be the opportunity for clients and practitioners to appeal denial of services once it happens.

Occupational therapy practitioners and occupational therapy assistants have professional certification or licensure that indicates they are competent to deliver occupational therapy interventions to clients. This certification or licensure happens at the national and state levels. Students must pass a national certification exam to become a practicing occupational therapy practitioner or occupational therapy assistant. The National Board for Certification of Occupational Therapy (NBCOT) administers the certification exam and maintains continuing certification of occupational therapy practitioners nationwide. Most states also now have licensure or certification boards, and may even have a licensing board separate from other disciplines. Passing the national certification exam and paying the appropriate licensing fee is generally needed to obtain a state license. Practitioners and students should check with individual states to determine the specific procedures they need to take for obtaining a state certification or license to practice.

Occupational therapy practitioners have a professional responsibility to maintain competence and licensure/certification by participating in continuing education and professional activities. Ongoing competence must be demonstrated in a cyclical way by presenting evidence of the professional activities in which the individual has participated. Currently NBCOT requires certification every 3 years with 36 professional development units (PDUs). While attending workshops is one common way to accrue PDUs, individuals may do many other things to demonstrate ongoing competence, including supervising students, making professional presentations, mentoring others, or publishing material about occupational therapy.[10] State licensure or certification boards often count similar kinds of activities, but may have a different time period to complete these activities. It is practitioners' responsibility to know their cycles for certification or licensure, have their documentation available for employers or regulating agencies, and to keep a record of professional activities that they can use to meet the requirements.

Certification and professional membership organizations also play a role in situations where ethical principles or professional competency resulting in harm to the public occurs. These organizations all have a reporting process for situations of ethical or legal violation of professional practice. Each organization has a jurisdiction in terms of how it takes action in regards to the practitioner's credentials.[11,12] State licensing boards look to the NBCOT licensing examination to determine the occupational therapy practitioner's initial competency to enter practice after graduating from an accredited occupational therapy education program. State licensing boards make decisions on an ongoing basis affecting the practitioner's ability to provide occupational therapy services to clients in a particular state. AOTA and state occupational therapy associations have decision-making power about how a practitioner may participate in these professional associations.

Penalties for improper behavior may include fines; restriction in the ability to practice, including probation or outright revoking of licenses; and public reprimands and censure. All organizations have methods to let the health care and occupational therapy communities know of their decisions in such matters, making it difficult or impossible for practitioners to move their practice to another locality in order to continue to practice.

Other Ethical Codes Related to Population and Organizational Intervention

While the *Occupational Therapy Code of Ethics Standards* is a major guideline for occupational therapy practice, other ethical codes exist, and have historically come in use, that affect ethical decision making in occupational therapy. Table 25-4 describes these other major ethical codes in use. Together they form the basis for ethical practice in clinical and research settings. Many of them affect health care and research throughout the world, while other documents, such as the Health Insurance Portability and Accountability Act (HIPAA), relate only to the United States. Knowledge of these codes is important for the practitioner to gain a full understanding of ethical thinking and decision making.

Professional Interactions and Communication

Interprofessional Teams

The Pew Health Commission report[1] emphasizes the need for "interdisciplinary competence" amongst all professions, embodied in the use of interprofessional teams. The benefits of interprofessional teams are stated as the time use of resources without duplication of services, and the coalition of multiple areas of professional expertise in an environment where problem solving and creative solutions are often needed to bring about effective health care outcomes to clients.[21,22] While the idea of teaming in health care is not new, the health care environment has changed to create new demands for the practitioner as they work in teams.

Relationship to Emerging Practice

Health care literature has talked about teaming for research and clinical interventions for many years, starting in the 1980s. However, progress toward comprehensive and collaborative use of teams has been slow. Part of the challenge in developing widespread use of teams has been the multiple terms used for interprofessional teaming. Choi and Pak identified 3 terms for teaming in the literature: *interdisciplinary, multidisciplinary,* and *transdisciplinary.*[9,23] Although there is not a clear and consistent definition of these terms, *interdisciplinary* teams generally work jointly toward a common problem from their own discipline specific base; *multidisciplinary* teams work sequentially or in parallel toward a specific problem; and *transdisciplinary* teams work in a more holistic way, with shared skills and goals to solve a common problem. Teaming is becoming more important as occupational therapy personnel work outside of traditional medical settings, such as hospitals, and move to community and transitional models of care.

Dynamic Teaming

The directives of the Pew Report[1] emphasize the need for more work done in the transdiciplinary fashion, with true collaboration and emphasis on client outcomes, than teams that stick to individual disciplinary concerns and parallel interventions. An example of this new emphasis on teams is found in the concept of dynamic teaming, developed by Charles Savage.[10,24] Dynamic teaming emphases possibilities rather than problems and combines individual team member's talents and skills to learn, share, re-team, and create—rather than compete or posture. Savage calls this knowledge *networking,* as a way of providing opportunities for individual contribution of skills, learning from others, and leveraging knowledge rather than physical assets. Dynamic teaming also has greater potential to engage individual practitioners in the work, as they have a chance to personally contribute to the learning of their colleagues.

Characteristics of Effective Teams and Team Success

Increased research on the nature of teams and the qualities of effective teaming has generated conclusions about the factors that lead to successful teaming or create barriers that prevent effective teaming. Choi and Pak completed a meta-analysis of health care literature from 1982 to 2007 on health care teams in research, education, and policy work.[25] Table 25-5 summarizes their findings on factors promoting team success and those factors creating barriers to team success. While institutional and environmental factors can help or hinder effective teamwork, the makeup of the team and its communication skills can exert a great influence. Pearson et al provided support for this emphasis in a systematic review of literature on effective nursing teams in clinical practice.[26] Factors leading to successful nursing teams included shared accountability amongst members, commitment of team members toward the goals of the team, open communication amongst team members, enthusiasm for the work, and motivation by team members to participate in team activities and care.[26]

Team Communication

The discussion of factors affecting team success point out that many of them relate to basic communication

Table 25-4. *Primary Ethical Codes and Laws Related to Occupational Therapy*

Name of Document	Date Developed	Key Ethical Concepts and/or Protections
Hippocratic Oath[13]	Late 5th century BC	Created by Hippocrates, known as the father of Western medicine, or by one of his students. Lays out basic principles of sharing scientific knowledge, prevention of disease, respecting the privacy of individuals, and calling others in for consultation as necessary.
Nuremburg Codes[14]	1947	Developed at the end of World War II in response to human medical atrocities in concentration camps. Forms the basis for ethical research with human beings emphasizing voluntary consent of subjects, the necessity of doing the research, elimination of physical or other suffering in research, proper preparation of equipment and the qualifications of the researchers, and the ability to terminate the experiment by either subject or researcher if there is increased potential for injury or inability of the subject to continue.
Geneva Convention[15]	1864 to 1949	Set of 3 agreements tied together with a final accord in 1949. They deal with the treatment and protection of individuals, both civilian and military, during wartime. Ratified by over 190 countries at this time.
Ethical Code of the American Medical Association[16]	1957, latest revision 2001	Code affecting American physicians with 9 principles, including practicing competent care, upholding the law and medical standards, respecting individual rights and providing appropriate care, supporting medical intervention for all, the physician's independence in choosing whom to serve (except in emergencies), pursuing medical education and informing individuals medical information, and participating in activities that increase community health
Declaration of Helsinki[17]	1964, latest revision 2008	Developed by the World Medical Association to look at research ethics. The right of subjects for self-determination and making informed decisions. Also attends to the needs of vulnerable subjects, such as minors, and the use of research protocols with independent ethical review by a properly convened committee.
Belmont Report[18]	1978	Described 3 basic principles in the conduct of human subjects research, including: • Respect for persons—autonomous participation of subjects, courtesy, and informed consent • Beneficence—philosophy of doing no harm and balancing maximum benefits for the research while minimizing risks to the human subjects • Justice—equality and fairness in research procedures including recruitment procedures and fair distribution of costs and benefits to the research subjects
Health Insurance Portability and Accountability Act (HIPAA)[19]	1996	Federal law designed to allow individuals to move insurance (portability), limiting denial of coverage due to pre-existing conditions, and reform insurance fraud. It also protects an individual's medical information (Protected Health Information, PHI) and medical payment information in all forms, print or electronic. Health providers and organizations are charged to keep this information secure and confidential.

(continued)

Table 25-4 (continued). *Primary Ethical Codes and Laws Related to Occupational Therapy*

Name of Document	Date Developed	Key Ethical Concepts and/or Protections
Patient's Bill of Rights (as part of the Patient Protection and Affordable Care Act [PPACA])[20]	2001 to 2010	First proposed in 2001, but not passed in legislation at this time. Some of the basic principles are included in the PPACA, including several rights, eg, insurance coverage for pre-existing conditions, the ability to choose your doctor, keeping young adults covered, ending lifetime limits on insurance coverage, and ending a person's insurance coverage without warning or cause. It also provides review and information about any premium increases, barriers to emergency coverage, annual limits on health care benefits, preventive care, and the patient's right to appeal.

Table 25-5. *Factors Promoting Success and Creating Barriers in Interdisciplinary Teams*

Factors Promoting Success	Factors Creating Barriers
Good selection of team members	Poor selection of the disciplines of team members
Having good team members	Poor process of team functioning
Having mature and flexible team members	Lack of proper measures to evaluate interdisciplinary work
Having personally committed team members	Lack of guidelines for multiple authorship in research publications
Physical proximity of team members to each other	Language differences and understandings between disciplines
Access of the internet and email for support	Insufficient time for the project
Personal and organizational incentives	Insufficient funding for the project
Institutional support and changes which support teamwork	Institutional/organizational constraints
A common goal and shared vision	Discipline conflicts
Clarity and rotation of team roles	Team conflicts
Open and positive communication among team members	Lack of communication among disciplines
Constructive comments and feedback among members	Unequal power among disciplines

Adapted from Choi BC, Pak AW. Multidisciplinarity, interdisciplinarity, and transdisciplinarity in health research, services, education and policy: 2. promoters, barriers, and strategies of enhancement. *Clin Invest Med.* 2007;30(6):E224-E232.

skills. Errors in written and oral communication are a leading cause of death or serious injury to clients in health care facilities *(sentinel event)*. The Joint Commission Association of Healthcare Organizations, the major health care accrediting organization in the United States, identified communication issues as the third most commonly reported root cause of sentinel events in accredited health care facilities in 2011.[27]

An effective technique for team communication is the SBAR method. The team member communicates by describing the situation or what is going on (S), the clinical background or context (B), their assessment of the situation (A), and their recommendation (R). This approach to communication lets other team members know what is going on, as well as the speaker's view of the situation. Other communication methods that improve team communication include briefings, either leading up to or after an event, and meeting agendas and meeting minutes with action assigned to one or more team members.[28]

Assessment of Team Performance and Peer Review

The assessment of interdisciplinary teams can take many forms. Outcome measures have been used to investigate interdisciplinary team performance in health care.[29] Measures that can be used for continuous quality improvement projects (CQI), such as length of stay, patient satisfaction surveys, reduction in health care costs, and greater frequency of patient discharges back to their homes, can be used as a way to gauge the effectiveness of the team. It is important for the team to develop goals and objectives prior to interventions with clients to help determine the most appropriate outcome measures to use in the assessment process.

In addition to outcome measures, it is useful to have assessment performed within the team itself to determine the level of communication and teamwork present for the team. This could take place in several ways, including self-evaluation by team members and peer review of the work done by the team. These reviews may be centered on team communication skills and participation, or rating of team members around an agreed list of competencies and skills needed to produce the desired outcomes. Good team-building practice, such as joint agreement about roles, responsibilities, and expectations (norms) of teammate's behavior prior to starting the work of the team, may help increase effectiveness and lessen the chances of dysfunctional team behavior as the work continues.

Principles of Documentation for Individuals, Populations, and Organizations

Purposes of Documentation

With the emphasis on creating effective client outcomes and demonstrating the links between practice and available research, the documentation practitioners complete about their interventions is even more important. A practitioner's documentation serves several important purposes. At the most basic level, documentation of services provides a chronological record of occupational therapy interventions with a client. Documentation also facilitates communication about occupational therapy among professionals, clients, professionals, and their families. Documentation can be used to assess clinical outcomes and the quality of care. Documentation is used to meet reimbursement requirements and reflect the practitioner's clinical reasoning and thought process about client evaluation and intervention processes. Finally, documentation can also provide legal protection for the practitioner and the health care organization.[30]

The quality of the documentation a practitioner writes can affect how well these purposes are met. Effective documentation should be thorough and should be completed in a timely fashion. Documentation should also be accurate and indicate what has been done in collaboration with the client. Documentation should reflect the best practice as indicated by the evidence for the identified problem. What is documented should be relevant to the needs of the client and the anticipated therapeutic outcome the practitioner and client desires.

The Electronic Health Record and Use of Technology

The development of the electronic health record (EHR) or electronic medical record (EMR) is a major change in the way occupational therapy personnel document about client interventions. The idea of an EHR originated in the 1960s, and gained momentum in the 1980s and 1990s with advances in computer technology and the internet. Much of the current structure of EHRs in the United States came from HIPAA legislation in 2006 and the Health Information Technology for Economic and Clinical Health Act (HITECH) in 2009. This legislation mandates "meaningful use" of electronic records to achieve meaningful outcomes in care, as well as maintaining the integrity and privacy of individual's personal health information. The laws require physicians and medical systems to use EHRs by 2015, or suffer penalties for Medicare reimbursement.[31] Use of the EHR will become a reality for practitioners moving forward.

While research is still mixed about the advantages and disadvantages of the EHR, several factors have been identified. Advantages include ease of accessing records in multiple locations and ability of many professionals to view the record at the same time. Professionals can work more as a team, and records can go from one health care setting to another. EHRs can eliminate redundant testing conducted by multiple providers as a result of the patient's history being viewed in its entirety.

A major challenge and possible disadvantage to EHRs can be the challenge of maintaining record privacy and security, as the record can be exposed to hacking and piracy risks—as might any electronic data. Incompatibility between EHRs may also limit the portability advantage of the record. Training professional staff may be time consuming and affect costs and productivity. Small health care systems may also have cost issues in purchasing hardware and software to initiate EHRs. EHRs are still evolving, and further research is needed to determine if these advantages and disadvantages are accurate, and if advantages outweigh disadvantages.

Types of Written Reports

Whether they are written electronically or on paper, practitioners will need to compile several types of written reports in their professional careers. Many of these include reports about client care involving evaluation reports, progress notes, and discontinuation notes. In addition, practitioners may write business memos and email messages, formal business letters, proposals for grants or professional presentations, and business plans and reports as an entrepreneur or practitioner in private practice.

Types of Oral Reports

The importance of verbal communication has been noted earlier in this chapter. Oral reporting may be done informally, as in a communication with another team member as the need arises, or formally at a department or team meeting. Oral reports may also be given to individuals' families, over the phone for reimbursement purposes, or to other professionals or family members. While maintaining patient privacy and confidentiality is a critical ethical consideration in professional health care communication, it is especially important in verbal communication. Care must be taken to communicate orally in appropriate places and to not be in situations where one can be overheard.

Client and Professional Advocacy

Dimensions of Advocacy

Engaging in activities to bring about health care change has become an activity for all health care professions, including occupational therapy. Competencies around advocacy included in the Pew Report[1] include improving access to health care for those with unmet health needs, partnering with communities in health care decisions, and advocating for public policy that promotes and protects the health of the public. Advocacy is an ongoing and challenging responsibility for any practitioner as ethical dilemmas and the shifting nature of health care often create conflicts in the course of actions any one person might take. Advocacy can take place at any level from the individual client to national and population levels.

Advocacy for others has been an accepted role of practitioners in occupational therapy literature, but little research has been done to investigate why and how practitioners engage in advocacy. Dhillon et al explored the meaning of advocacy for occupational therapy practitioners and their experiences with advocacy.[32] Ten Canadian occupational therapy practitioners were interviewed about advocacy and their advocacy experiences, and grounded theory methods were used to analyze and identify findings. Six major reasons for advocating were identified and categorized according to practitioner effects, patient effects, and patient/practitioner effects. Practitioner-related reasons for advocating included personal satisfaction or fulfillment and using practitioner-related power and influence to affect change. Joint practitioner/patient reasons included engaging in occupation or allowing expanded opportunities for occupation and a commitment to client-centered practice. Reasons for advocacy related to the client included meeting human rights and basic needs and improving the client's quality of life.[32]

Occupational therapy practitioners learned about advocacy in their educational programs as well as through experiences on the job. Job-related skills in advocacy were developed when the situation arose, rather than through planned skill building or a strategic plan. Practitioners did have to learn skills of facing adversity and using diplomacy. The occupational therapy practitioners reported experiencing resistance to advocacy, and therefore had to learn how to challenge systems or beliefs of others in the environment that were not friendly toward what the practitioner was advocating.[32]

Practitioners may advocate for individuals and their families, a group having a certain diagnosis or social issue, or the profession of occupational therapy itself. Ethical issues are present at all of these levels of advocacy, but the nature of the ethical dilemma may change. For example, with individuals and their families, ethical values such as autonomy, beneficence, or nonmaleficence may take center stage.[33] When advocating for their clients, occupational therapy practitioners have to determine what is best for the client, particularly determining whether the client can make his or her own decisions about advocacy strategies. An example of autonomy clashing with beneficence during advocacy is wondering: "How does a chronic illness such as Alzheimer's dementia affect the well-being of the individual as well as those trying to take care of him or her? What care should the individual be given medically vs what services are covered by insurance or third party payers?" Any of these questions are complex and create a challenge in advocacy for the practitioner as they provide client-centered care.

At the population level, practitioners may advocate for policy change and health care practices that include prevention, health promotion, and evidence-based outcomes across a broader scale. This advocacy may include actions such as communicating with elected representatives about health care policy issues; educational and marketing efforts to alert others about the benefits and contributions of occupational therapy; and partnering with other health care professions to advance health care concerns locally, nationally, and internationally.[34]

Advocacy at the population level brings about other ethical concerns in addition to those ethical values mentioned previously in individual care situations. These ethical concerns include concepts of the common good, social and procedural justice, veracity, and fidelity. Edwards et al phrased these concerns as one of moral agency: the belief in the ability, either individually or in groups, to act morally and advocate for change.[35] Moral agency happens with the individual practitioner as well as in the broader social context, nationally and internationally.[36] This broader social context is an important arena for national and professional associations to make a contribution.

Structures to Help Practitioners Engage in Advocacy

Occupational therapy practitioners have many opportunities to engage in advocacy and receive support. Foundational to these efforts is activity and membership in state, national, and international occupational therapy associations, such as AOTA. These associations expend major resources to educate practitioners about policy issues that affect occupational therapy and the clients served, creating marketing and educational resources to allow practitioners to educate others about occupational therapy, and engaging professional advocates to bring occupational therapy-related concerns to elected officials and governmental agencies. AOTPAC is an occupational therapy organization federally recognized in the United States to raise and donate money to the political campaigns of those politicians having positions favorable to occupational therapy and its clients. AOTF (American Occupational Therapy Foundation) advances and supports scientific endeavors, including research, to spread knowledge about occupation and occupational therapy. Membership, volunteering, and making monetary contributions are ways an individual practitioner can become involved in advocating for the health care needs of clients.

International and interdisciplinary associations are additional avenues for advocacy in occupational therapy. WFOT (World Federation of Occupational Therapists) provides networking opportunities and a platform to engage in occupational therapy concerns outside the United States. Conferences are held every 4 years around the world and individual practitioners may attend, present research, and network with other professionals. Networking opportunities are also present in national and state asso-

ciations, and practitioners may also partner with agencies that address health care needs locally through United Way agencies and community boards. Other professional associations address priorities at the population level (eg, American Public Health Association) or provide forums for interdisciplinary care and specific health issues (eg, Brain Injury Association of America). Therefore, participating in these advocacy opportunities may significantly expand the work occupational therapy practitioners may do to benefit individuals in need.

Continuing Competence and Professional Development

All occupational therapy personnel and their leaders have the responsibility to establish a culture that values and supports their own active learning as an aspect of client-centered care that is evidence-based and of high quality. Creating a learning culture that integrates the practice change efforts of interprofessional teams, that include occupational therapy, produces high levels of competence beyond what can be accomplished when focusing professional development efforts primarily on the learning of individual practitioners.[37] In such learning cultures, practice is never static because occupational therapy practitioners and their colleagues from other disciplines understand that each client encounter is a learning opportunity for how to improve services and the outcomes of intervention.

Learning cultures are necessary because of the exploding knowledge base in health care delivery. As a result, there are widening gaps in the length of time to transfer knowledge from research to practice. Therefore, continuing competence only partially rests with each individual practitioner, and ultimately needs a system that forms learning communities where knowledge is used to continuously revise practice. Learning environments are supported through a well-coordinated, multi-pronged approach that addresses the multiplicity of factors essential for practice-based learning, offers guidance around the collection and analysis of relevant information that fosters learning, and includes initiatives to establish and build the learning infrastructure.

Hallmarks of a Learning Culture

Changing practice patterns or behaviors is a complex undertaking and is best accomplished through a leadership approach that targets entire teams of employees.[38] Leadership is needed to promote agreement among practitioners on the nature of the change and how it is to be enacted within the organization. Leadership prepares staff to facilitate the learning of others, plan and appropriately delegate workloads to allow for learning time, enhance communication of new knowledge, create opportunities for staff to receive feedback about their practice change, and recognize the importance of positive interactions as a foundation for sharing knowledge. Leadership needs to examine the flexibility of institutional policies in order to remove barriers to change. There should be organizational investment in feedback mechanisms to provide the data needed to assess change efforts.[39] Financial incentives, such as merit pay and bonuses, and promotions are important ways to motivate interest in making practice change.[40]

A learning culture promotes the partnering of occupational therapy staff members; not only with each other, but with staff throughout the organization in order to access the interprofessional knowledge needed to enhance service delivery. Clients take a central role in teaching providers about the expectations for services in terms of how they want their health care and occupational needs met, giving feedback about the intervention process itself regarding any gaps related to expectations. Occupational therapy practitioners in organizations with a learning culture are expected to serve as learning role models, encourage scholarly dialogue about occupational therapy practice and client-centered care, and provide constructive feedback to their peers in a variety of disciplines throughout the organization about ways to improve services. It is important to involve academic partners in this organizational learning in order to shape the educational experience of not only occupational therapy students, but of other health profession students. Academic partners also bring a distinctive perspective to the learning, given that they are situated in a different organizational experience than the service providers and may therefore bring "fresh eyes" to the situation. These academic partners are important in terms of the learning resources and supports they can offer to a service delivery organization. Faculty then can take their learning and integrate it back into their research and teaching.

Factors Affecting Learning and Development of Competence

In order to examine the factors affecting the development of competence, a good place to start is to clearly identify what the occupational therapy practitioners and their colleagues in other disciplines are to learn. Competencies are explicit statements that define specific areas of expertise and are related to effective or superior performance in a job.[41] A competency might state that "the occupational therapy practitioner integrates understanding of the client's context and occupational needs when administering and interpreting occupational performance assessments." To successfully enact this competency statement, the occupational therapy practitioner has to have knowledge of occupational performance assessments and their proper use; as well as knowledge about occupational performance and its underlying factors, client occu-

pational needs, and contexts. In addition, the occupational therapy practitioner has to have the skills to perform the assessments and the interpersonal skills to engage the client in the evaluation process. Additionally, the occupational therapy practitioner uses clinical and ethical reasoning to properly interpret the results.[42] Employers of occupational therapy practitioners can use the *Standards for Continuing Competence* as a framework for analyzing the learning needs implied in each competency statement.[43] In this way, there is clearer direction regarding whether learning is designed to target knowledge or skills, and their application to practice.

Addressing the knowledge gaps apparent in the competency statement is often where typical continuing education may focus. Depending upon the type of knowledge developed, knowledge gains pre-education and post-education can be measured through questionnaires and paper and pencil tests. This is true primarily for propositional knowledge emerging from ideas and concepts, expressed as informational statements.[44] However, practitioners who are learning together in cooperative inquiry examine their own experience and action in collaboration with others. In fact, cooperative inquiry results in using other kinds of knowing. For instance, experiential knowing is internalized, difficult to explain, and is derived from face-to-face interactions with people, places, and things. Presentational knowledge is expressed through imagery, such as storytelling or the arts. Practical knowledge results in a skill or competence. When these ways of knowing are congruent with each other, the knowledge base of practitioners is deeper, richer, and more valid.

Using competencies to understand how learning programs are developed to meet the needs of occupational therapy practitioners; however, remains a difficult process, especially when the target is to ultimately improve client outcomes and experiences. Employers may assume that knowledge alone will translate to improvement in the skills of their employees and thus client outcomes will change. Research has indicated that the learning of the practitioner does not necessarily produce an immediate corresponding improvement in practice performance.[45] In fact, learning is not necessarily a good initial predictor of practice performance quality. After an intensive learning episode, there may be no improvement in practice performance or there may even be periods of slight performance decline. Then, these periods of no change may be followed by sudden jumps in performance quality.[45] Learning about practice is a cognitively complex task, not only requiring cognitive reorganization, but also involving abandonment of previously held principles and ideas. Consequently, the impact of learning on practice appears to occur in sudden leaps, rather than through continuous and gradual change as commonly believed.

Given that practice learning is cognitively complex, the cognitive ability of the occupational therapy practitioner is a key determinant to successful performance. Cognitive ability means occupational therapy practitioners have to recognize their own gaps in knowledge and skills, as well as manage their time and relationships. In addition, an occupational therapy practitioner's ability to meet the criterion set for a competency may depend on other factors, such as motivation to change performance, tendency to act in a consistent manner, positive self-concept or self-image, or certain attitudes and values.[46] These continuing competence dimensions of cognitive ability and motivation respond poorly to continuing education and may require employers to examine their screening approaches used during the hiring process of occupational therapy practitioners.

Learning Infrastructure

When developing a learning infrastructure in an organization, principles from implementation science, which involve using evidence-based strategies to implement a practice change, should be considered.[47] For instance, implementation science outlines the common success factors of practice change as involving the knowledge, cognitions, attitudes, and routines of practitioners. In addition, the resources and the social influences of the organization are strong determinants of whether a practice change will occur. It is useful for occupational therapy practitioners to examine persisting ineffective practices in their service delivery in order to more aggressively focus on the development of implementation science in occupational therapy. Along with their organizational leaders and colleagues in other disciplines, occupational therapy practitioners should facilitate analysis of the relevant determinants for successful implementation of practice changes. Overlooking or "short-cutting" this analytic step can be tempting when facing pressures of cost reduction and of taking quick action to solve problems of poor quality outcomes. Leaders and occupational therapy practitioners have to resist these pressures to skip analysis, because using ineffective implementation strategies ultimately leads to expensive and unsuccessful results. Effective practice change results when consideration is given to the full range of alternative implementation strategies. Systematic reviews of previous implementation studies are helpful in considering strategies with known effectiveness. Well-chosen practice change strategies are ones that match determinants of the specific innovation, target group, and context.

This implementation science research indicates that singular approaches to learning, such as a workshop, are ineffective in translating knowledge, skills, and attitudes to practice.[48] Interactive learning approaches are needed and have been shown to increase translation, including role-playing, case discussions, and opportunities to practice skills. Knowledge deficits for instance, not only should be addressed by active learning strategies, but need to incorporate advanced organizers in study materials. Advanced organizers are graphic models that clarify the text structure of the assigned reading. In other words, these organizers improve understanding through identification of key topics within the text as well as the relationships among topics.[49]

In general, educational interventions supporting a practice change should be designed according to the goal of the learning. For example, role-playing and video feedback might be more effective when the learning is facilitating the development of interpersonal skills. In contrast, knowledge acquisition may occur with readings and case studies.[50] Critical and ethical reasoning development may require mentoring, reflective writing, simulations, educational outreach visits, collaborative learning groups, and peer teaching.[51] Performance skill development may require practitioners to demonstrate a skill to an expert who uses specific criteria to judge the performance. Finally, learning that is infrequent is also ineffective; instead, learning must occur in an ongoing manner that is consistently timed to occur prior to, during, and following a practice change.[52] Educational booster sessions may be needed to sustain a practice change given that all intervention processes degrade over time.

Currently, organizational infrastructure for learning to change practice is overly focused on each discipline's separate actions, rather than on interprofessional actions. This approach to supporting practice change is certainly being challenged, as client outcomes are dependent upon teams of health care professionals working carefully together to streamline and coordinate care. Examples of implementation strategies focused on interprofessional teams include norm-setting strategies, use of role models, social influence strategies, and leadership strategies.[53] Using norm-setting strategies to change attitudes of practitioners toward a practice change includes using 2 such strategies involving shifting the perspective of practitioners and stimulating practitioners to experience anticipated regret. For instance, practitioners may claim that a new method of practice may take too much time, and as a result they may not realize they have assumed a caregiver rather than a client-centered perspective. A shifting perspective strategy would involve asking practitioners to think of the client as someone in their family, and then to rethink whether they would consider lack of time as an acceptable excuse for insufficient implementation of a practice innovation. As an alternative strategy, anticipated regret attempts to trigger feelings of regret using hypothetical situations. Occupational therapy practitioners who claim asking the client about their occupational needs is too time consuming, could be asked, "How would you feel if the client goes home and is unable to engage in his or her meaningful activities and develops significant depression after you did not comply with the occupational therapy process, that begins with determining occupational needs?"

Even when implementation strategies for a practice change are focused on groups of professionals, as opposed to individuals in single disciplines, many of these learning strategies are voluntary in nature in terms of whether the staff actually participates. Grol and Grimshaw found that education alone resulted in mixed effects in facilitating a practice change when used in health care workers at large.[54] Mixed effects were also found for the commonly used strategy of giving staff feedback on performance. Therefore, other strategies from implementation science, such as reminders, decision support, and use of information and communication technology, may be more effective in encouraging implementation of innovations in practice. These alternative learning infrastructure supports are more likely to address the complexity, time needed, costs, and risks related to practice innovation. Facilitators of change should include ways to enhance the fit of the practice change with current practice. Such proposed changes should incorporate ways to adjust the innovation to the user's needs and insights. Furthermore, combined strategies from implementation science are identified as more effective than using single strategies alone, such as primarily using education approaches.

Actually, organizational learning infrastructure underuses strategies focused on extrinsic motivation of the practitioner and overuses intrinsic motivation strategies for individual practitioners and groups. For instance, clients are rarely involved in the implementation of innovations. However, Entwistle expressed ethical concerns about how a client-triggered practice change might send an implicit signal that clients cannot rely on basic elements of good care when they are at their most vulnerable.[55] Implementation science provides an alternative focus by describing what individuals themselves could do to enhance well-being. In the area of pressure ulcer prevention, individuals are often unaware of the risks until they actually develop a pressure ulcer. A client-directed practice change strategy could be to provide risk information and suggest how individuals themselves could avoid pressure ulcers. In this way, the clients of occupational therapy can be the extrinsic motivators for practice changes in occupational therapy because they already are engaging in healthy strategies themselves. Therefore, expectations for further care are raised.

Implementation science of practice change has examined the effectiveness of communicating injunctive rather than descriptive norms about practice. Descriptive norms describe actual practice (eg, "compliance of staff with hand hygiene policy is only at 50%"). In contrast, injunctive norms describe what we think the situation should be (eg,

"we believe noncompliance with hand hygiene prescriptions is not acceptable, as it threatens patient safety"). Van Achterberg, Schoonhoven, and Grol found that descriptive norms are counterproductive because they tend to create an acceptable norm for an unacceptable practice.[47] Achieving 80% implementation of a practice change might inadvertently be considered acceptable, even though 20% of the time clients may not be receiving the service most effective in producing a desired outcome.

A major challenge of creating learning infrastructure is to move beyond working on one practice innovation at a time, such as this year the organization will focus on fall prevention. Obviously there are risks to an organization that holds a "single project at a time" philosophy, because the organization is communicating to its employees there is lack of capability to handle complexity. In addition, the organization has not analyzed whether the sequence of projects could be inefficient. There is failure to recognize that many practice improvement projects may include similar processes. In contrast, the organization may reap multiple benefits in the maximization of cost control when examining how guidelines for preventing pressure ulcers, urinary tract infections, and falls may have related educational strategies and infrastructures.[47] It is clear that the development of implementation science in occupational therapy needs more research, including evaluation of actual strategy delivery vs the intended delivery and of implementation success in meeting preset targets, time, and costs.

Conclusions Regarding Continuing Competence

Lifelong learning is the cornerstone of continuing professional development, and continuing competence focusing on a broad array of knowledge, skills, and attitudes. And while the delivery of formal, continuing education activities should continue to be an important component in continuing competence, the current role of these formal structures in facilitating practice change is limited. As a result, while individual practitioners are likely to continue to improve practice through these mechanisms, components of learning are missing when other disciplines are not involved and when organizations fail to support learning. Therefore, limited learning strategies may cause practice change to occur sub-optimally. Practitioners may be subject to practice drift, where the intended practice change is poorly maintained due to lack of system supports in decision making and in facilitating the work flow involved in task completion. If organizational leaders are to have an important role in maintaining the competence of their practitioners, these leaders must understand and accept the limits of human abilities and propensities to self-identify and redress areas of weaknesses, and to voluntarily engage in appropriately designed learning activities.

By shifting perspective from educational activities being the primary focus of making a practice change, organizational leaders will be able to direct additional efforts at understanding how professional learning not only arises from practice, but actually occurs in and is informed by practice. By focusing implementation science research efforts on further understanding and developing methods to change practice, educational approaches may have a chance to become substantially more relevant to the continuing competence of practitioners.

SUMMARY

This chapter focused on ethics, teaming, documentation of service delivery, advocacy, and continuing competence. Each of these issues in practice is incorporated into the PEOP Model as principles forming the foundation for intervention with individuals, organizations, and populations. Developing skills in these foundational areas help the occupational therapy practitioner create a more effective, ethical, and integrated practice serving the needs of clients in ways they expect and find helpful in meeting their occupational needs.

REFERENCES

1. O'Neil EH, Pew Health Professions Commission. *Recreating Health Professional Practice for a New Century: The Fourth Report of the Pew Health Professions Commission.* San Francisco, CA: Pew Health Professions Commission; 1998. http://futurehealth.ucsf.edu/Content/29/1998-12_Recreating_Health_Professional_Practice_for_a_New_Century_The_Fourth_Report_of_the_Pew_Health_Professions_Commission.pdf. Published December 1998. Accessed July 19, 2013.

2. Dictionary.com. *Definition of Ethics.* Dictionary.com. http://dictionary.reference.com/browse/ethics. Updated 2013. Accessed July 19, 2013.

3. Fletcher J. Morality. In: Lewis MA, Tamparo CD, Tatro BM, eds. *Medical Law, Ethics, and Bioethics for the Health Professions.* 7th ed. Philadelphia, PA: FA Davis; 2012.

4. Purtilo R. *Ethical Dimensions in the Health Professions.* 4th ed. Philadelphia, PA: Elsevier Saunders; 2005.

5. Ryerson University. *The Ethics Network: Sample Ethical Decision Making Models.* Ryerson University. http://www.ryerson.ca/ethicsnetwork/resources/index.html. Accessed July 19, 2013.

6. AOTA. Core values and attitudes of occupational therapy practice. *American Journal of Occupational Therapy.* 1993;47(12):1085-1086.

7. AOTA. Occupational therapy code of ethics standards. *American Journal of Occupational Therapy.* 2010;64(6):S18-S26.

8. Dige M. Occupational therapy, professional development, and ethics. *Scandinavian Journal of Occupational Therapy.* 2009;16:88-98.

9. US Department of Health and Human Services. *Code of Federal Regulations: Title 45 Public Welfare: Part 46 Protection of Human Subjects: 46.102 Definitions.* US Department of Health and Human Services: code of federal regulations. http://www.hhs.gov/ohrp/humansubjects/guidance/45cfr46.html#46.102. Published July 14, 2009. Updated January 15, 2009. Accessed July 19, 2013.

10. National Board for the Certification of Occupational Therapists. *NBCOT Professional Development Units (PDU) Activity Chart.* National Board for the Certification of Occupational Therapists. http://www.nbcot.org/pdf/renewal/pdu_chart.pdf. Updated December 31, 2013. Accessed July 19, 2013.

11. US Department of Health, Education, and Welfare. *Credentialing Health Manpower (pub. No. OS-77-50057).* Bethesda, MD: US Department of Health, Education, and Welfare; 1977.

12. Willmarth C. State regulation of occupational therapists and occupational therapy assistants. In: Jacobs K, McCormack GL, eds. *The Occupational Therapy Manager.* 5th ed. Bethesda, MD: AOTA Press; 2011:455-457.

13. Tyson P. *The Hippocratic Oath Today.* Public Broadcasting System: NOVA. http://www.pbs.org/wgbh/nova/body/hippocratic-oath-today.html. Published March 27, 2001. Updated 2013. Accessed July 27, 2013.

14. *Nuremberg Code.* Princeton University. http://www.princeton.edu/~achaney/tmve/wiki100k/docs/Nuremberg_Code.html. Accessed July 27, 2013.

15. International Committee of the Red Cross. *The Geneva Conventions of 1949 and their Additional Protocols.* ICRC: International Committee of the Red Cross. http://www.icrc.org/eng/war-and-law/treaties-customary-law/geneva-conventions/index.jsp. Updated July 23, 2013. Accessed July 27, 2013.

16. American Medical Association. *AMA's Code of Medical Ethics.* American Medical Association. http://www.ama-assn.org/ama/pub/physician-resources/medical-ethics/code-medical-ethics.page. Published 2013. Accessed July 27, 2013.

17. World Medical Association (WMA). *WMA Declaration of Helsinki—Ethical Principles for Medical Research Involving Human Subjects.* World Medical Association. http://www.wma.net/en/30publications/10policies/b3/. Published June, 1964. Updated October, 2008. Accessed July 27, 2013.

18. US Department of Health and Human Services. *The Belmont Report.* HHS.gov: US Department of Health and Human Services. http://www.hhs.gov/ohrp/humansubjects/guidance/belmont.html. Published April 18, 1979. Accessed July 27, 2013.

19. US Department of Health and Human Services. *Health Information Privacy.* HHS.gov: US Department of Health and Human Services. http://www.hhs.gov/ocr/privacy/. Accessed July 27, 2013.

20. Centers for Medicare and Medicaid Services. *The Center for Consumer Information and Insurance Oversight: Patient Bill of Rights.* CMS.gov: Centers for Medicare and Medicaid Services. http://www.cms.gov/CCIIO/Programs-and-Initiatives/Health-Insurance-Market-Reforms/Patients-Bill-of-Rights.html. Accessed July 27, 2013.

21. Atwal A, Caldwell K. Do all health and social care professionals interact equally: a study of interactions in multidisciplinary teams in the United Kingdom. *Scandinavian Journal of Caring Sciences.* 2005;19:268-273.

22. Reeves S, Freeth D, McCrorie P, Perry D. 'It teaches you what to expect in future…': inter-professional learning on a training ward for medical, nursing, occupational therapy and physiotherapy students. *Medical Education.* 2002;36:337-344.

23. Choi BCK, Pak AWP. Multidisciplinarity, interdisciplinarity and transdisciplinarity in health research, services, education and policy: 1. definitions, objectives, and evidence of effectiveness. *Clin Invest Med.* 2006;29:351-364.

24. Savage C. *The Dynamic Teaming Handbook: World Café.* KEE International. http://www.kee-inc.com/downloads/Dynamic%20Teaming%20Handbook%20Rev.%203.4.pdf. Published 2004. Updated January 14, 2004. Accessed July 19, 2013.

25. Choi BCK, Pak AWP. Multidisciplinarity, interdisciplinarity, and transdisciplinarity in health research, services, education and policy: 2. promoters, barriers, and strategies of enhancement. *Clinical and Investigative Medicine.* 2007;30(6):E224-E232.

26. Pearson A, Porritt KA, Doran D, et al. A comprehensive systematic review of evidence on the structure, process, characteristics, and composition of a nursing team that fosters a healthy work environment. *International Journal of Evidence-Based Healthcare.* 2006;4:118-159.

27. The Joint Commission. *Sentinel Event Data: Root Causes by Event Type 2004-2011.* The Joint Commission: sentinel-event statistics. http://www.jointcommission.org/assets/1/18/Root_Causes_Event_Type_2004-2011.pdf. Accessed 2012.

28. Leornard M, Graham S, Bonacum D. The human factor: the critical importance of effective teamwork and communication in providing safe care. *Quality and Safety in Health Care.* 2004;13(1):185-190.

29. Fox R, Sampalli T, Fox J. Measuring health outcomes of a multidisciplinary care approach in individuals with chronic environmental conditions using an abbreviated symptoms questionnaire. *Journal of Multidisciplinary Healthcare.* 2008;1:97-104.

30. Sames K. *Documenting Occupational Therapy Practice.* 2nd ed. Upper Saddle River, NJ: Prentice Hall; 2010.

31. US Department of Health and Human Services. *HITECH Act Enforcement Interim Final Rule.* US Department of Health and Human Services. http://www.hhs.gov/ocr/privacy/hipaa/administrative/enforcementrule/hitechenforcementifr.html. Updated 2009. Accessed July 19, 2013.

32. Dhillon SK, Wilkins S, Law MC, Stewart DA, Tremblay M. Advocacy in occupational therapy: exploring clinicians' reasons and experiences of advocacy. *Canadian Journal of Occupational Therapy.* 2010;77(4):241-248.

33. Brewer BC. Do not abandon, do not resuscitate: a patient advocacy position. *Journal of Nursing Law.* 2008;12(2):78-84.

34. Lamb A, Meier M, Metzler C. Federal legislative advocacy. In: Jacobs K, McCormack GL, eds. *The Occupational Therapy Manager.* 5th ed. Bethesda, MD: AOTA Press; 2011:441- 454.

35. Edwards I, Delany CM, Townsend A, Swisher LL. Moral Agency as enacted justice: a clinical and ethical decision-making framework for responding to health inequities and social justice. *Physical Therapy.* 2011;91(11):1653-1663.

36. Galheigo SM. What needs to be done? Occupational therapy responsibilities and challenges regarding human rights. *Australian Occupational Therapy Journal.* 2011;58(2):60-66.

37. McWilliam CL. Continuing education at the cutting edge: promoting transformative knowledge translation. *Journal of Continuing Education in the Health Professions.* 2007;27(2):72-79.

38. Sebrant, U. The impact of emotion and power relations on workplace learning. *Studies in the Education of Adults.* 2008;40:192-206.

39. Townsend E, Sheffield SL, Stadnyk R, Beagan B. Effects of workplace policy on continuing professional development: the case of occupational therapy in Nova Scotia, Canada. *Canadian Journal of Occupational Therapy.* 2006;73:96-108.

40. Nelson JM, Cook PF. Evaluation of a career ladder program in an ambulatory care environment. *Nursing Economics.* 2008;26:353-360.

41. Spencer LM, Spencer SM. *Competence at Work.* New York, NY: Wiley; 1993.

42. Cleveland Moyers P, Hinojosa J. Continuing competence and competency. In: Jacobs K, McCormack GL, eds. *The Occupational Therapy Manager.* 5th ed. Bethesda, MD: AOTA Press; 2011:485-501.

43. AOTA. Standards for continuing competence. *American Journal of Occupational Therapy.* 2010;64:S103-S105.

44. Heron J, Reason P. *A Layperson's Guide to Cooperative Inquiry.* Bath, UK: Centre for Action Research in Professional Practice; 2004.

45. Handfield-Jones RS, Mann KV, Challis ME, et al. Linking assessment to learning: a new route to quality assurance in medical practice. *Medical Education.* 2002;36:949-958.

46. Epstein RM, Hundert EM. Defining and assessing professional competence. *Journal of the American Medical Association.* 2002;287:226-235.

47. van Achterberg T, Schoonhoven L, Grol R. Nursing implementation science: how evidence-based nursing requires evidence-based implementation. *Journal of Nursing Scholarship.* 2008;40:302-310.

48. Forsetlund L, Bjorndal A, Rashidian A, et al. Continuing education meetings and workshops: effects on professional practice and health care outcomes (Art. No. CD003030). *Cochrane Datebase of Systematic Reviews.* 2009;2(2).

49. Kools M, Ruiter RA, van de Wiel MW, Kok G. Testing the usability of access structures in a health education brochure. *British Journal of Health Psychology.* 2007;12(4):525-541.

50. Hugenholtz NIR, de Croon EM, Smits PB, van Dijk FJH, Nieuwenhuijsen K. Effectiveness of e-learning in continuing medical education for occupational physicians. *Occupational Medicine.* 2008;58:370-372.

51. Kowlowitz V, Davenport CS, Palmer MH. Development and dissemination of web-based clinical simulation for continuing geriatric nursing education. *Journal of Gerontological Nursing.* 2009;35:37-43.

52. Cleland JA, Fritz JM, Brennan GP, Magel J. Does continuing education improve physical therapists' effectiveness in treating neck pain? A randomized clinical trial. *Physical Therapy.* 2009;89:38-47.

53. Larson EL, Early E, Cloonan P, Sugrue S, Parides M. An organizational climate intervention associated with increased handwashing and decreased nosocomial infections. *Behavioral Medicine.* 2000;26:14–22.

54. Grol R, Grimshaw J. From best evidence to best practice: effective implementation of change in patients' care. *Lancet.* 2003;362(9391):1225-1230.

55. Entwistle VA. Differing perspectives on involvement inpatient safety. *Quality and Safety in Health Care.* 2007;16:82-83.

Chapter 26

A PERSON-CENTERED STRATEGY
Using Learning Strategies to Enable Performance, Participation, and Well-Being

Timothy J. Wolf, OTD, MSCI, OTR/L and Naomi Josman, PhD, OT(I)

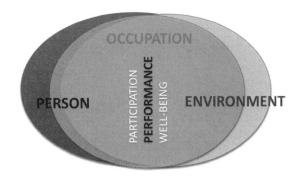

LEARNING OBJECTIVES

- Give context to therapy as learning.
- Compare and contrast the difference between cognitive learning and behavioral learning.
- Define and describe learning principles as they are used in the therapeutic process.
- Describe how behavioral and cognitive learning applies to different occupational therapy settings.
- Understand and identify how to adapt the learning strategies to meet the needs of different populations.
- Identify personal and environmental barriers that may influence the learning process for individuals.
- Identify appropriate interpretation of standardized and performance-based cognitive assessments to determine if an individual is capable of cognitive learning.
- Describe behavioral and cognitive learning theory principles and their application in several frames of reference.

KEY WORDS

- Automaticity
- Chaining
- Classical conditioning
- Cognition
- Declarative knowledge
- Domain-specific strategies
- Errorless learning
- Generalization
- Global strategy
- Goal
- Metacognition
- Operant conditioning
- Procedural knowledge
- Scaffolding
- Self-monitoring
- Transfer

Christiansen CH, Baum CM, Bass JD, eds.
Occupational Therapy: Performance, Participation, and Well-Being, Fourth Edition (pp 485-497).
© 2015 SLACK Incorporated.

INTRODUCTION

Joe is a 47-year-old accountant who works for a large firm in a metropolitan area. Joe's firm recently purchased new iPads (Apple Inc) for all of the accountants in order to allow them to work while traveling to and from home. Joe has never used an iPad before; however, he has a lot of experience using computers and other related technology. In order to learn how to use the iPad, Joe applies what he knows from working with computers to figure out how to turn it on and off, open and close applications, save files, use email, and all the other functions of the iPad. He applies strategies he has used with other devices to remember how certain applications work. In order to accomplish this, Joe has to use his cognitive abilities, such as executive function and memory, to plan and organize his behavior and respond to the novelty of learning a new activity. A few weeks later, Joe purchases an iPhone (Apple Inc). He is then able to apply the knowledge he has gained from learning how to use the iPad to working the iPhone. This pattern of behavior continues through all the activities humans do in everyday life; humans respond to learning novel activities by applying previous knowledge and strategies and adapting them as necessary to be successful.

This example of Joe is a simplified view of how people learn a new behavior. In the case of Joe, he was using cognitive learning that relied on his cognitive abilities (eg, memory, executive function) to learn how to work the iPad. In the case of some people with disabilities, they may have impairment in these functions and have to rely on other processes to learn a new behavior. Individuals who receive interventions from occupational therapy practitioners have to learn how to complete everyday life activities, use new AT devices, instruct their caregivers, and navigate in the home/community with a disability. Occupational therapy practitioners need to understand how people learn, the different ways people learn, and how best to facilitate learning with the interventions provided to clients. This chapter will review learning strategies and how they can be applied in a rehabilitation setting. Specifically, the chapter will compare and contrast these 2 theories of learning, discuss how to decide which approach is appropriate for a client, and identify strategies to implement with clients.

BACKGROUND LITERATURE

Learning can be defined as a relatively permanent change in behavior or capability of responding, as a result of acquiring skills or knowledge.[1] In its simplest terms, occupational therapy services can be thought of as learning activities to teach clients new ways of doing activities. Many factors play into an individual's ability to complete meaningful tasks and occupations. Occupational therapy practitioners are trained to be holistic and to evaluate every aspect of a person's ability to function in everyday life. Occupational therapy practitioners teach activities for several reasons, including, but not limited to, helping clients relearn skills after injury/illness, helping clients develop new or alternative strategies to perform occupations and/or roles, and helping caregivers learn how to support participation for persons with disabilities.[2] In order to teach activities in a beneficial way, occupational therapy practitioners must identify meaningful activities to the client, choose an instructional mode compatible with the client's current cognitive level, structure the learning environment, provide reinforcement and grading of activities as appropriate, and structure feedback and practice.[2] Teaching and learning are complex skills; but they are important because they increase the effectiveness of the services occupational therapy practitioners provide. To begin to address this topic, it is necessary to discuss 2 of the main schools of thought related to how people learn: *behavioral learning* and *cognitive learning* (Table 26-1).

Overview of Behavioral Learning Theory Principles for Therapeutic Application

Behaviorism is a school of thought in psychology that explains human reactions in terms of learned behaviors.[3] A central tenant behind behaviorism is that only observable behaviors are worthy of being researched, believing that cognitive processes like abstraction, mood, or thought are too subjective.[4] Behaviorists believe that everything people do, including thinking, feeling, and acting, should be regarded simply as behaviors and nothing more. Pathological behaviors can be treated by altering the environment or changing it through behavioral modification techniques.

John B. Watson (1878-1958) was the first psychologist to study how learning affects human behavior. His research formed the school of thought known as behaviorism. Watson believed that psychology in the behaviorist view is purely objective; the goal of which is to predict and control behavior, and only observable behaviors are worthy of being studied.[5] Ivan Pavlov (1849-1936) building on the work of Watson discovered the principle of classical conditioning—a process of behavior modification by which a subject comes to respond in a desired manner to a previously neutral stimulus that has been repeatedly presented along with an unconditioned stimulus that elicits the desired response.[3] In this work, Pavlov discovered the basis of the basic behavioral stimulus-response bond.[6] Even this basic concept of classical conditioning can be applied to occupational therapy interventions. For example, occupational therapy practitioners assist clients with memory difficulties through the use of external aids to

Table 26-1. *Comparison of Behavioral and Cognitive Learning Theories*

Characteristic	Behavioral Learning Theories	Cognitive Learning Theories
Primary theorists	John Watson, Ivan Pavlov, BF Skinner	Edward Tolman, Jean Piaget, Lev Vygotsky
Historical time	Early 20th century	Mid-20th century
Basic premise	Modifying observable behaviors; "*Learning to*"	Learning the cognitive processes behind observed behaviors; "*Learning that*"
Experimental method	Analyze observable behavior	Observe behaviors as indications for the mental processes responsible for the behaviors
Use of stimuli	Identify relationships between paired stimuli and observed behaviors	Describe how stimuli are processed, encoded, and retrieved
Teaching strategies	Provide rewards and punishments to modify behavior	Use past knowledge and individual motivation to strengthen encoding through schemes and mastery; enhance self-esteem through scaffolding
Learning strategies	Positive and negative reinforcements modify behaviors	Rehearse information, modify existing schemata, and organize information in a meaningful manner
Influence of consciousness	Consequences influence behavior without conscious awareness	Conscious awareness is responsible for the selected behavior due to past experiences
Cognitive processes	Are thought to be too abstract or subjective and not necessary to modify behavior	Are responsible for observed behaviors and improvement/changes in cognitive processes lead to behavior change

trigger reminders. Specifically, an alarm on a cellular phone can be used to cue a client to take medications. The alarm, a neutral stimulus, becomes a conditioned stimulus that produces a conditioned response of taking medications on time. BF Skinner (1904-1990) continued to build on the behavioral learning principles of Watson and Pavlov through the development of his own theories on operant conditioning. Operant conditioning is a process of behavior modification in which the likelihood of a specific behavior is increased or decreased through positive or negative reinforcement each time the behavior is exhibited, so that the subject comes to associate the pleasure or displeasure of the reinforcement with the behavior.[7] The principles of operant conditioning are very applicable to everyday learning. For example, if a parent is trying to teach her child to keep his room clean, the parent might reward the child when the room is kept clean all day by providing the child with a piece of candy. This would be an example of positive reinforcement for a good behavior, therefore increasing the likelihood that the behavior (the child keeping his room clean) will be repeated. If the child does not keep his room clean, then the parent might provide punishment by placing the child in time-out, there-

fore decreasing the likelihood that the negative behavior (the child not cleaning his room) will be repeated. The concept of reinforcement has become central to behavioral theories of learning.

The concepts of behavioral learning may seem overly simple and are probably something most occupational therapy practitioners are familiar with from their own life experience; however, in the appropriate situation with the appropriate clients, the proper application of these principles can help our clients become more independent with a specific behavior that they would otherwise require a higher level of assistance to complete. The major limitations with behavioral learning techniques are that they are time consuming and every behavior needs to be individually conditioned. Therefore, these techniques are most appropriate for individuals with a higher level of neurological impairment who are limited in their ability to learn cognitively.

Overview of Cognitive Learning Theory Principles for Therapeutic Application

Cognition is defined as a person's capacity to acquire and use information to adapt to environmental demands.[8,9]

This definition encompasses information-processing skills, learning, and generalization. The capacity to acquire information involves information-processing skills, or the ability to input, organize, assimilate, and integrate new information with previous experiences. Adaptation involves using previously acquired information to plan and structure behavior towards goal attainment. Thus, the ability to apply learning to a variety of situations is inherent within the concept of cognition.[9] Descriptions of specific components of cognition related to learning (eg, attention, memory, metacognition/awareness, executive function) can be found in Chapter 15.

Cognitive theory views learning as an (1) active process for processing and storing information that involves development and reorganization of cognitive structures, and (2) the learner as an active participant in the process of knowledge acquisition and integration.[10-12] Cognitive theory describes knowledge acquisition as a mental activity involving internal coding and structuring by the learner,[13,14] and suggests that learning is optimal under conditions that are aligned with human cognitive architecture.[15] Cognitivists typically concentrate their inquiry into what learners know and how they acquired their knowledge, rather than on what learners do. Therefore, the cognitive approach has focused on how to generate knowledge as a meaningful entity and on how to assist learners in structuring, organizing, and relating new information to knowledge stored in memory.[16] While cognitive learning concepts are more complex and abstract than behavioral concepts; just like behavioral learning principles, the proper application of cognitive learning principles to the appropriate clients in the appropriate context may help improve independence with everyday life activities.

Most intervention approaches incorporate both cognitive and behavioral components to support optimal learning. It is rare when a purely cognitive or behavioral approach is best suited for a specific client, and therefore specific components/techniques can be selected based on the client's skills and abilities. Cognitive-behavioral learning theory is based on the notion that thoughts change behaviors. According to this theory, it can be effective to use behavioral techniques (ie, chaining, reinforcement) while also helping the client learn new thinking patterns that can support their desired behaviors.[17]

Core Concepts of Learning

There are core concepts associated with learning, in terms of the type of knowledge gained from the learning experience and how that knowledge is to be used, that need to be considered when structuring a learning experience for a client. Behavioral, cognitive, and combinations of these 3 approaches can all lead to skill acquisition; however, the ability to use that skill in different contexts and/or apply principles associated with that skill can be different depending on how the learning experience is structured and the cognitive capacity of the client. These concepts need to be considered when selecting specific intervention activities, depending on the goals and expectations of the client (narrative) and occupational therapy practitioner.

Procedural and Declarative Knowledge

Procedural knowledge (memory) simply refers to knowing how to do something. It can be defined as the sequences, habits, and routines used to perform motor tasks.[18] An anecdotal description of procedural knowledge is when people say "just like riding a bike." This type of knowledge is also considered implicit or automatic, meaning that it is associated with behaviors that may not be consciously recalled and can be accomplished with little cognitive processing. For example, when a child is learning how to tie her shoelaces, she is explicitly told how to perform the task. As she practices, she gradually needs less and less cueing and/or cognitive processing to accomplish the task, and no longer has to think of each explicit step to perform the task. Eventually, she is able to tie her shoe without any cueing and without a lot of conscious thought. This can be accomplished through both behavioral and cognitive learning approaches. In a behavioral approach, chaining techniques could be employed to help the child learn one step at a time, and reinforcement is provided for correct performance. In a cognitive approach, a mnemonic may be taught to the child (eg, bunny ears) that the child rehearses, learns, and recalls when attempting to tie his or her shoes. It may also be more effective to combine these approaches and use aspects of behavioral learning (ie, chaining, reinforcement) with cognitive learning (ie, use of mnemonic) to learn that activity, depending on the skills and/or abilities of the child. While the skill of tying a shoe can be considered a procedural memory once learned, the ability to recall the steps or the specific events related to learning how to tie a shoe is a different form of knowledge.

Declarative knowledge is contrasted with procedural knowledge (memory). Where procedural knowledge is the knowing "how," declarative knowledge is considered knowing "that." Declarative knowledge is knowledge about information or facts (semantic) and events (episodic).[1] This type of knowledge is considered explicit, in that it is associated with memory that can be consciously recalled. Remembering the name of your first grade teacher, the first time you went on a trip, etc are considered examples of declarative knowledge. In rehabilitation, declarative knowledge allows clients to recall previous therapeutic interactions, remember previously learned strategies/concepts, and apply them to current activities. For example, if yesterday the occupational therapy practitioner worked with a client in the kitchen on learning energy conservation techniques, the practitioner would rely on the client's declarative knowledge from that event (episodic) and the principles of energy conservation he or she taught him (semantic) to be recalled and applied at today's therapy session, and hopefully when the client goes home. In contrast to procedural memory, which takes practice/time to acquire, declarative knowledge can be acquired in as little as a single exposure.[19] Most Americans can recall where they were and what they were doing the instant they heard about the planes hitting the World Trade Center on September 11, 2001. This was a single exposure that created long-term declarative knowledge. Declarative knowledge is typically more associated with cognitive learning as it is necessary for successful transfer of activities learned in therapy to different contexts. Clients can learn new skills (procedural knowledge) through behavioral learning approaches even without intact ability to learn new declarative knowledge.

Transfer and Generalization

Transfer of information relates to the way in which prior learning affects new learning. It is considered successful when an individual performs a learned task in a new environment.[1] Transfer should be considered in terms of the similarity of the new environment to the old environment where the original learning occurred, which is referred to as *similarity* or *distance of transfer*.[20] According to Toglia, treatment progresses along a horizontal continuum that gradually increases demands of transfer and generalization of strategies. Very similar activities that share surface or physical characteristics are considered "near-transfer." Somewhat similar activities are considered "intermediate-transfer," and activities physically different to the original activity are considered to be "far-transfers."[21] An example of near-transfer would be applying skills learned for making a cup of coffee in the clinic to making a cup of coffee using a different kettle or mug or coffee jar in the same clinical environment. Intermediate-transfer would be making a sandwich in the therapeutic kitchen and transferring the skills to making the same sandwich in the kitchen at home. Far-transfer would entail applying skills of light meal preparation in the clinic to loading and starting the dishwasher. Transfer is ultimately the goal of cognitive learning approaches and is typically not expected in behavioral approaches, as it requires the client to rely on executive function to perform activities in novel environments. The farther the transfer, the more cognitive processing is typically required. Practitioners can also assist with enhancing transfer by allowing the client to practice in a variety of environments to promote recognition of environmental cues for the desired behavior.[1] The distance of transfer is graded by the practitioner

according to the client's ability to use the same strategy across a variety of situations.[21] Transfer is also contrasted with generalization of learning.

Generalization of learning or "very-far transfer" occurs when an individual is able to transfer learned strategies in intervention to everyday context of functioning.[21] For example, during interventions, an individual may learn to make a bed and will transfer the strategies used to write a shopping list at home. The practitioner should vary the task to be learned on a regular basis to allow the individual the ability to generalize information learned when presented the opportunity. The varied tasks should be graded gradually according to the individual's present skill level and the client's problem areas.[1]

Characteristics That Support and/or Hinder Learning

In the PEOP Occupational Therapy Process, assessment/evaluation helps to identify the capabilities/enablers and barriers/constraints for person factors, environmental factors, and occupational performance. An understanding of these characteristics helps the occupational therapy practitioner develop learning experiences.

Person Characteristics

The following person characteristics, factors intrinsic to the person, can either support or hinder learning depending on the client's skills, abilities, and health conditions. Each of these factors can exist in a 2-way relationship with learning. While impairment in certain person factors (ie, cognition) or presence of other negative factors (ie, stress) can negatively impact learning, learning can also potentially help clients to compensate (ie, learning cognitive strategies to compensate for cognitive loss) or overcome (ie, learning progressive relaxation techniques to help mitigate stress) these limitations. It is important to examine these factors in the PEOP Occupational Therapy Process and determine whether they are supporting and/or hindering a client's ability to learn; this, in turn, helps identify interventions to promote learning and overcome limitations related to occupational performance.

Cognitive

The first section of this chapter addressed learning in terms of the cognitive capacity of the client. The selection of a learning approach hinges on the cognitive capacity of the client. For example, if a client has a neurological injury that limits his or her ability to attend to stimuli and encode, store, and recall memories, than a cognitive-based approach may not be appropriate to help the client achieve occupational performance goals. An expectation of generalization and transfer of what is learned may not be realistic either, given that in order to generalize and transfer, the client has to be able to use executive function to monitor the incoming sensory information and use previously obtained knowledge/skills to form a plan, organize behavior, and sequence activity to accomplish the task. Thus, it is necessary to evaluate the client's cognitive abilities and limitations before developing learning goals and beginning any intervention.

Physiological

There are several physiological factors that can affect learning, but for the purposes of this chapter only a few will be discussed. It is important to have an understanding of a client's health condition and prognosis of the physiological changes that are expected and need to be monitored before beginning any intervention. The following physiological factors are extremely common across health conditions.

Stress can potentially have both positive and negative effects on learning.[22] Stress may positively affect learning when the stressor is conceptually related to the information and considered important.[23] Good stress, or *eustress*, can motivate clients to want to do more while in therapy. More often than not though, stress is a hindrance to learning. Chronic exposure to stress hormones, specifically after injury or illness, can cause negative effects on the brain structures involved in cognition; specifically, stress is known to cause memory impairments.[24,25] Also, chronic stress can exacerbate pathophysiology of body systems (ie, nervous, immune, cardiovascular, and metabolic systems).[26] Following injury and/or illness, stress is extremely common across health conditions.

There is little evidence to show that pain supports learning in any capacity; however, there are studies that show that a person's level of acceptance of chronic pain may impact learning. A greater acceptance of pain has been shown to be related to lower reports of perceived pain intensity, less depression, less anxiety, less physical and psychosocial disability, and better work outcomes.[27] These positive outcomes can support learning. However, pain also forces an individual to attend to the pain source and this, in turn, may make it difficult to focus attention on other stimuli. Chronic pain has been shown to negatively affect cognition, especially attention and memory.[28] It is important to not only monitor pain that a client is experiencing, but also initially target an intervention at helping a client control pain as much as possible in order for other interventions to be effective.

Psychological

There are many psychological factors associated with learning; however, only a few concepts that are common across populations will be addressed here. Anxiety may have positive and negative effects on learning. A healthy amount of anxiety about something can be important (eg, feeling a little anxious before taking an exam can raise your level of awareness) and may motivate an individual to be prepared; however, too much anxiety can consume our cognitive resources and have a negative effect on learning/performance.[29] It may not be obvious how much anxiety a client is experiencing or how it is influencing his or her performance; thus, it is important to be aware of this tendency and monitor it appropriately.

Depression is characterized by changes in capacities to engage in goal-directed use of time, energy, interest, and attention.[30] Depression never facilitates learning; in fact, it is probably the most pervasive and strongest hindrance to learning in rehabilitation. It is common across almost all health conditions and may cause fatigue, lack of interest in activities previously enjoyed, antisocial behaviors, and social isolation. For individuals with depression, the ability to learn is negatively impacted.[31] However, learning new skills has also been shown to combat depression.[32] A core principle of occupational therapy is that engagement in activity can influence the state of one's health,[33] which is consistent with current knowledge about depression.

Motivation to perform a task increases if the task is meaningful to the individual.[34] Motivation is related to the *expectancy-value appraisal* of situations. If it is expected that a certain experience will be valuable, a person is more likely to learn/engage in that behavior.[35] Motivation may be intrinsic (ie, within the individual) or come from extrinsic sources (eg, family, practitioner, external reward). On the other hand, a lack of motivation may hinder learning if an individual is not engaged in activity. This idea supports the notion of finding the "just right" challenge for clients to help increase motivation and self-efficacy. Self-efficacy is defined as the belief that one can achieve a desired outcome by successfully performing certain behaviors.[36] That is, belief in one's ability to successfully accomplish a goal or outcome plays a large role in motivation. High levels of self-efficacy and goal attainment lead to an individual setting more challenging goals and learning new skills[37]; however, excessive feelings of self-efficacy or limited awareness about one's abilities may lead to negative or maladaptive behaviors (eg, setting goals/expectations too high or too low). Motivation and self-efficacy are critical components in learning and in recovery as they are necessary components for occupational engagement.

Spiritual

Spirituality is a central component of a person's meaning and motivation in life.[38] While spirituality is very individualized, it is necessary to understand the role it plays in a client's life and how the client derives meaning from activities. If an activity is not meaningful or purposeful, it can hinder performance and motivation for performance.[38] Spirituality influences occupational engagement both on a conscious and subconscious level. Though religion and spirituality are often regarded as synonymous, the term *spirituality* can be seen as an umbrella term under which one finds religion.[39] While some people have a religious affiliation, spirituality is applicable to all individuals.[40] Thus defined, spirituality has a tacit omnipresence that is entwined with meaning and motivation.[38]

Empirical investigation of the relationship between spirituality and learning is limited. In the field of adult learning, scholars have examined spirituality's role in learning, and its potential to enhance learning in academic settings.[41,42] Some scholars contend spirituality is always present in the learning environment.[43] They emphasize spirituality's co-existence with cognition in the learning process, rather than as a separate component.[41,42] Spirituality is inextricably linked to diverse outcomes and learning, meaning, and engagement in everyday life.[38,39,44,45] Thus, the spirituality domain is important in occupational therapy.[46-48]

Environment Characteristics

In the PEOP Occupational Therapy Process, it is important to consider the environmental aspects of learning. The social and physical environments where learning occurs can greatly impact the ability of the learner to process and obtain information. The occupational therapy practitioner considers the environment where learning is taking place and structures it according to the learner's goals and needs. The practitioner also considers the behavioral or cognitive approach when structuring the environment. In a behavioral approach, the environment is the most important aspect of the individual's desired responses. In a cognitive approach, the environment supports or hinders an individual's abilities to learn information. The individual's ability to learn information should also be considered when structuring the environment in a cognitive approach. The 2 factors are considered dynamically to reach optimal performance for the client.

The social environment includes the practitioner as an instructor. The practitioner makes the learner feel comfortable, safe, and respected in order to achieve optimal learning outcomes.[1] The practitioner also is aware of the individual's cultural influences and support systems as part of the social environment. Cultural environments may impact the way the learner understands information. Support systems, such as family members and friends, may enhance or hinder learning. Practitioners, family members, and friends may serve as positive role models for the learner.[49] On the other hand, a family member who provides too much assistance for a learner may hinder the learner's ability to achieve goals independently. The practitioner may have to consider encouraging new social environments for the learner when the social environment appears to be non-conducive to learning. For example, a learner involved in a gang may be unable to learn information because he is worried about his safety. The practitioner encourages the individual to remove himself from the social situation, so he can focus on learning new information.[1]

The physical environment for learning should also considered by the practitioner. In order to understand the influences of a person's capabilities and the environmental demands, Lawton and Nahemow[50] proposed an Ecological (Environmental Press) Model (Figure 26-1), which may be used to select behavioral or cognitive learning approaches in a given situation. The individual's competencies are listed on the Y axis from low to high. The environmental press is listed on the X axis from weak to strong. The interaction between an individual's competence and the environmental press is located at the intersection of the individual's abilities and environmental demand.[51] Ideally, occupational therapy practitioners should place an individual in an environment that best suits their abilities to reach the zone of maximal performance potential.[50]

For example, a noisy and loud environment, such as a therapy gym, may not be the ideal environment for teaching someone with a TBI. This environment provides many distractions that, as viewed by a cognitive learning approach, may remove the learner's attention from the information to be learned. It is recommended that the practitioner provide learning opportunities for this individual in a quiet, private room to enhance retention of information.[52] Cognitive learning approaches assume that an increase in an individual's competency is possible (and desired). This can be explained by Lawton's Ecological Model, as increases in the learner's competency allows for an increase in environmental press to reach the zone of maximal performance potential. Therefore, the practitioner can gradually increase the amount of distractions as the learner recovers to simulate real-world experiences.

Occupation Characteristics

Knowing the occupation that the client wishes to engage in helps to select an appropriate intervention approach and set realistic goals. As the complexity of an occupation or task increases, the amount of time to learn new skills and strategies to accomplish the task also increases. Use of behavioral approaches inherently takes more time than cognitive approaches. As previously discussed, cognitive approaches rely on the ability of the client to quickly gain new declarative knowledge and use that knowledge to improve future performance. Behavioral approaches require the use of stimulus-response mechanisms that rely on feedback/reinforcement, shaping, chaining, or other techniques that can require a considerable amount of time and may not be possible for extremely complex tasks (ie, managing a household budget). These

Figure 26-1. Environmental Press Model. (Reprinted with permission from Lawton MP, Nahemow L. Ecological theory of adaptation and aging. In: Preiser W, ed. *Environmental Design Research.* Stroudsburg, PA: Dowden, Hutchinson & Ross; 1973:24-32.)

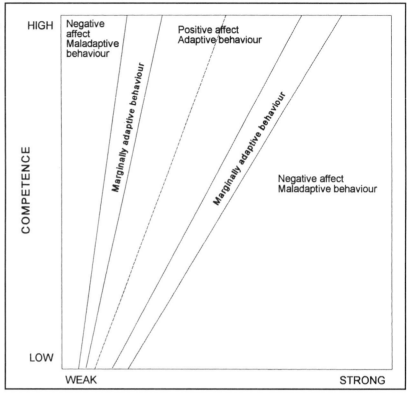

factors (the complexity of the activity, the clients' skills and abilities, the environment, the time the client will be in therapy, etc) need to be taken into account when structuring the learning activities and developing goals with the client.

ASSESSMENT

Since cognitive learning approaches are generally more effective for transfer and generalization of learned skills, it is preferred that a cognitive approach is used if appropriate for a client. Cognitive learning approaches are recommended for individuals who do not have any suspected neurological impairment, eg, physical disabilities; when a neurological impairment is indicated, the cognitive status of the client is evaluated to determine the approach that would be the most appropriate to facilitate learning. Standardized assessments are used in the PEOP Occupational Therapy Process to measure a client's baseline abilities so that therapy activities can be structured around improving those domains that are identified as problems on a given assessment (see Chapter 15). Standardized assessments are used as one tool to evaluate clients' cognitive status, but they may not always capture true functional abilities in everyday life.[53] Thus, occupational therapy practitioners should always interpret performance on standardized assessments in combination with

clinical observations and the client/family report in making the final determination of cognitive status.

If the practitioner determines that a client does not have sufficient capacity to learn a new activity, the practitioner should consider a behavioral approach for that client. A behavioral approach is recommended for individuals who are cognitively compromised, in order to enhance safety and intervention outcomes. Assessment of cognitive status is an iterative process using the PEOP Occupational Therapy Process and should be reconsidered as the client improves. For example, individuals with TBI or stroke may initially require a behavioral approach; however, as they recover it may be appropriate to shift from a behavioral to a cognitive approach.

For individuals with degenerative neurological impairments such as dementia, Parkinson's disease, Alzheimer's disease, Huntington's disease, and Amyotrophic Lateral Sclerosis (ALS), it may be appropriate to initially use a cognitive learning approach; however, as their condition progresses, they may require a shift to a behavioral learning approach. This also can further be explained using Lawton's Ecological (Environmental Press) Model.[50] If the client's competencies are improving due to recovery, a cognitive approach may be used to enhance the learner's abilities. If a learner's condition progresses to a point where their competencies have decreased and are not likely to improve, a behavioral approach is considered. Additionally, for clients with low baseline or current competencies, a behavioral approach is most appropriate; the environmental alterations made by the practitioner will enable them to perform at their optimal level.

The client's capabilities/enablers and constraints/barriers should be considered by the practitioner to select the appropriate learning approach for a client. A variety of diagnoses and conditions may contribute to low cognitive competencies. Standardized assessments may assist with determining if an individual is appropriate for cognitive vs behavioral learning. Formal and/or informal evaluations of additional person and environmental factors discussed earlier in this chapter will assist in selecting the appropriate intervention strategies, as well as help with structuring individuals' intervention sessions.

INTERVENTION

All intervention approaches discussed in this chapter have one core principle behind their development: they are focused on occupational performance. The PEOP Occupational Therapy Process emphasizes client-centered approaches that address goals related to occupational performance. Selecting a specific intervention approach is based upon the skills/abilities and prognosis of the client (person factors), the environment in which they will be performing their selected occupations (environment), and the occupation itself.

Behavioral Approaches

Behavioral learning strategies are used to elicit a specific behavior through the pairing of a stimulus and response and/or through the use of reinforcement; they rely on training an observable behavior without regard to whether or not cognitive processes are involved or not. (Cognitive strategies rely on training cognitive processes that can then be elicited and used to perform an activity.) For example, an alarm may be used as a stimulus to train someone with a TBI to take medications. Or a positive reinforcement may be given to a child with autism when he or she appropriately greets the neighbor. Some difficulties in using a behavioral approach lie in controlling the stimulus response pairing and the appropriate application of reinforcement. Behavioral learning strategies may be incorporated in a variety of rehabilitation intervention approaches. Specific principles that are central to behavioral learning are defined and discussed in the context of the following approaches.

Motor Learning

Motor learning theory is based on the principle of neural plasticity—the ability of the nervous system to repair or

rewire itself following injury. It assumes that the client has intact short-term memory in order to learn new movements, and also has long-term memory in order to both save and retrieve the information to make a lasting change. It is often used with clients who have had a stroke or brain injury with resultant motor performance deficits such as ataxia, apraxia, hemiparesis, or general muscle weakness. First, a functional problem must be identified and the motor components of the actions for a task are analyzed. (For example, if a client has difficulty picking up a glass of water, the practitioner break the task down into parts: flexing the shoulder to reach for glass, extending at the elbow, composite finger extension to open fingers around glass, maintaining the wrist in neutral, composite finger flexion to grasp glass, and elbow flexion to bring glass to mouth.) Next, the problem areas of the task are identified and those parts are practiced in isolation through visual, verbal, and manual guidance.[54] Once the problem areas are mastered, the task is practiced as a whole and all the parts are integrated into one task.

Mass repetition and practice are necessary for the acquisition of motor learning following nervous system injury.[55] For a client with apraxia, it may be more beneficial to schedule frequent short sessions rather than less frequent long sessions. The practitioner may also attempt to maximize the number of repetitions or practice trials per session. This can be accomplished by quickly reinforcing behaviors (either positively or negatively) and using activities that are functional and meaningful to the client. The mass practice should also be organized and structured so that environmental distractions are minimized. For clients with severe motor planning impairments, keeping the target number of repetitions or movements relatively small at first allows for enough massed practice to result in improved motor performance and facilitate motor learning and generalization. The types of schedules of feedback and reinforcements can also be structured by the practitioner to facilitate motor performance.[56] For example, in the beginning stages of therapy, immediate feedback might be more beneficial to the client so that errorless learning can occur; however, as the client improves and is able to accomplish the task on his or her own, the practitioner should attempt to provide less immediate and frequent feedback so that the client can problem solve independently and generalization can occur.[57]

Neurofunctional Approach

The neurofunctional approach is used with clients who have moderate to severe neurological impairments from injuries such as TBI, anoxia, and stroke. Using this approach there is little to no expectation of generalization or transfer to novel activities because of the low cognitive abilities of the client. It is a client-centered behavioral approach that targets function/behavior rather than impairment.[58] This approach often involves mass practice, cueing, reinforcement, chaining, scaffolding, and task-specific training.[58] Chaining can be either forward or backward. Forward chaining is used to teach multiple-step tasks. The practitioner demonstrates the first step on the first trial, then completes the first and second steps on the second trial. This is repeated until all the steps of the activity have been completed and the client can remember the entire sequence.[59] Backward chaining is also used to teach multiple-step tasks. The practitioner demonstrates all steps of the task on the first trial and then demonstrates all but the last step on the second trial and prompts the client to perform the missing step. With each trial, prompts and cues are minimized and this process is repeated until all the steps have been learned and the client is able to perform the whole task.[59] Another technique used in this approach is scaffolding. Scaffolding refers to tailoring the material to enhance optimal learning.[60]

The neurofunctional approach is also based in the concept of *errorless learning*. Errorless learning does not allow an individual to make a mistake when learning a new skill. The practitioner or family member interferes before a mistake is made.[1] This technique is based on the idea that once an individual with severe cognitive impairments makes a mistake, it is difficult for them to identify the mistake and correct it.[61] It employs many of the same principles as classical conditioning, in that a behavior is repeated to the point of automaticity—where a behavior can be accomplished with little to no conscious thought.[62] For example, a practitioner treating a client with a severe TBI may use a cueing system to assist the client with taking a shower safely. The client may need reminders to correctly sequence the steps of the task and also for safety. The goal would be for the client to safely take a shower in his or her own bathroom, with no expectation that the skill would transfer to other environments.

Cognitive Approaches

There are many intervention approaches that use cognitive-based learning in addressing occupational performance; however, only a few will be discussed in this section. Once an individual has a firm understanding of learning principles, he or she will be able to evaluate/learn a new intervention approach, understand the type of learning that is expected, and determine if a client is capable of that type of learning. A common theme in cognitive-based approaches is that clients are expected to have intact *metacognition*. Metacognition represents a learner's awareness of his own knowledge and ability to understand, control, and regulate his cognitive processes. The concept of metacognition includes 2 subcomponents: *metacognitive knowledge* and *metacognitive process*. Flavell

referred to metacognitive knowledge as declarative knowledge concerning the self, task, and strategy characteristics, whereas the metacognitive process refers to a set of skills and strategies geared to regulating/monitoring learning and problem solving.[63,64] The following examples of intervention approaches discuss the use of metacognitive abilities to learn new skills to improve occupational performance.

The Cognitive Orientation to Daily Occupational Performance

The Cognitive Orientation to daily Occupational Performance (CO-OP) approach was originally developed for use with children and has 3 main objectives: skill acquisition, development of cognitive strategies, and transfer and generalization of learning.[65] It uses a "goal-plan-do-check" method by which the practitioner assists the individual with guided discovery, encouraging the individual to develop problem-solving solutions when encountering issues with performance on their goals rather than giving explicit directions.[17] CO-OP uses the individual to promote learning, operating under the assumption that the individual is more likely to use and understand a solution to occupational performance issues if they discover the solution themselves.[65]

Individuals are taught the global strategy of "goal-plan-do-check" as a cognitive strategy for achieving personal goals. Global strategies may be used in a variety of situations and for long periods of time. The "goal-plan-do-check" global cognitive strategy is used as a general method for developing an individual's own approach to everyday tasks and activities.[66] A goal is set by the individual for a performance area and a plan is then designed to achieve successful performance. The plan is executed in the "do" stage. The individual then "checks" success through self-monitoring. If successful performance is achieved, the individual will continue to use the designed plan for future performance. If the performance was unsuccessful, the individual would then design a new plan, execute the plan, and check success until the desired performance was achieved.[66]

Other domain-specific strategies are used to support a specific part of a task. Domain-specific strategies are intended for a short period of use and may also vary by individual. For example, one child may remember to ride a bike by telling herself to pedal in a circle, where another child may tell himself to pedal like a clock. Another domain-specific task for riding a bike may be a child reminding himself to hold the handlebars like a motorcycle rider. Domain-specific strategies are incorporated within a global strategy and may emerge in the "plan" stage. They may also emerge in the "check" stage as an individual critiques performance.[66]

Learning is measured by development of cognitive plans that lead to skill acquisition and generalization/transfer of learning to other contexts and tasks.[65] The practitioner provides learning opportunities for the client through guided discovery. Guided discovery requires the practitioner to provide cues, model appropriate performance, and give feedback rather than explicitly stating a solution to a performance problem.[66]

This approach is appropriate for children with developmental coordination disorder (DCD), acquired brain injury, pervasive developmental disorder, higher-functioning austim, and cerebral palsy.[66-68] It has also been found to be an effective treatment approach for adults with TBI and stroke.[69,70] This evidence suggests that CO-OP may be an effective treatment strategy for a variety of adult and children diagnoses.[66] The approach is not appropriate for individuals who refuse to develop solutions, do not meet prerequisite cognitive abilities, or use unsafe or problematic self-guided discovery without appropriate supervision.

Dynamic Interactional Model

Toglia[71-73] developed the Dynamic Interactional Model (DIM) for cognitive rehabilitation, emphasizing metacognition and self-awareness, and the use of strategies in relation to performance for adults with brain injury. The DIM addresses the learning potential of the person and his or her ability to transfer learning to daily activities. It provides a framework for addressing cognitive impairments by changing the person's strategies or awareness, the activity, or the environment. The ability to transfer skills learned in one situation to another is monitored and worked on within a specific difficulty level of task. The client is asked to apply the targeted strategy within a variety of situations.

The DIM cognition constitutes a broad framework for integrating a range of treatment approaches.[21] Performance may be facilitated in a number of ways: by changing a client's self-awareness and use of strategy, manipulating activity and environment demands, or a combination of strategies. The DIM serves as a platform for a multi-context treatment approach that concentrates on altering a client's strategy and self-awareness. This multi-context approach guides strategies across a broad spectrum of meaningful occupations.[74-76] For example, a client who displays deficient planning, skips steps, or is inattentive when shopping or running errands may benefit from using a checklist or self-instructional procedure to remember items to be purchased or errands to be run.

This model has been proposed for people with brain injury and schizophrenia,[77] and suggested for other populations, including children with learning disabilities. There is preliminary support for its effectiveness with children with handwriting difficulties[78] and in improving grapho-motor abilities, self-care, and mobility in the rehabilitation of adolescents with TBI.[79]

Evidence suggests DIM may be an effective treatment strategy for a variety of adult and children populations.[21] The specific assessments and treatment techniques of this approach rely heavily on verbal mediation. Therefore, clients with major language impairment may not be capable of responding to mediation and verbal cues. The approach is also not appropriate for individuals who do not meet prerequisite cognitive abilities.

SUMMARY

Rehabilitation is a learning process. The occupational therapy practitioner designs the appropriate learning environment and selects the strategies for his or her clients. An understanding of the theories of learning, in addition to the facilitators and barriers to learning, inform intervention planning designed to maximize occupational performance.

ACKNOWLEDGMENTS

The authors would like to thank our students who graciously assisting the production of this chapter: Colleen Fowler, OTD/S and Morgan Rognstad, OTD/S at Washington University in St. Louis, MO; and Sonya Meyer, MSc/S at University of Haifa in Haifa, Israel.

REFERENCES

1. Berkeland R, Flinn N. Therapy as learning. In: Christiansen CH, Baum CM, Bass Haugen J, eds. *Occupational Therapy: Performance, Participation and Well-Being.* 3rd ed. Thorofare, NJ: SLACK Incorporated; 2005:421-448.

2. Richardson P. Teaching activities in occupational therapy. In: Pendleton H, Schultz-Krohn W, eds. *Pedretti's Occupational Therapy Practice Skills for Physical Dysfunction.* 6th ed. St. Louis, MO: Mosby Elsevier; 2006:101-109.

3. Gray P. *Psychology.* 4th ed. New York, NY: Worth Publishers; 2002.

4. Byrne JH. *Learning and Memory.* 2nd ed. New York, NY: Macmillan Reference USA; 2003.

5. Watson JB. Psychology as the behaviourist views it. *Psychological Review.* 1913;20(2):158-177.

6. Gardner RA, Gardner BT. *The Structure of Learning: From Sign Stimuli to Sign Language.* Mahwah, NJ: Lawrence Erlbaum Associates, Inc; 1998.

7. Nye RD. *The Legacy of B.F. Skinner: Concepts and Perspectives, Controversies and Misunderstandings.* New York, NY: Brooks/Cole Publishing Company; 1992.

8. Haywood HC, Lidz CS. *Dynamic Assessment in Practice: Clinical and Educational Applications.* New York, NY: Cambridge University Press; 2007.

9. Lidz CS, ed. *Dynamic Assessment: An Interactional Approach to Evaluating Learning Potential*. New York, NY: Guilford Press; 1987.

10. Good TL, Brophy JE. *Educational Psychology: A Realistic Approach*. 4th ed. White Plains, NY: Longman; 1990.

11. Merriam SB, Caffarella RS. *Learning in Adulthood: A Comprehensive Guide*. 2nd ed. San Francisco, CA: Jossey-Bass; 1999.

12. Simon HA. Learning to research about learning. In: Carver SM, Klahr D, eds. *Cognition and Instruction*. Mahwah, NJ: Lawrence Erlbaum; 2001:205-226.

13. Derry SJ. Cognitive schema theory in the constructivist debate. *Educational Psychologist*. 1996;31(3-4):163-174.

14. Spiro RJ, Feltovich PJ, Jacobson MJ, Coulson RL. Cognitive flexibility, constructivism, and hypertext: random access instruction for advanced knowledge acquisition in ill-structured domains. In: Steffe LP, Gale J, eds. *Constructivism in Education*. Hillsdale, NY: Lawrence Erlbaum Associates; 1992.

15. Sobel CP. *The Cognitive Sciences: An Interdisciplinary Approach*. Mountain View, CA: Mayfield; 2001.

16. Ertmer PA, Newby TJ. Behaviorism, cognitivism, constructivism: comparing critical features from an instructional design perspective. *Performance Improvement Quarterly*. 1993;6(4):50-72.

17. Meichenbaum DH, Goodman J. Training impulsive children to talk to themselves: a means of developing self-control. *Journal of Abnormal Psychology*. 1971;77(2):115-126.

18. Youngstrom MJ, Brown C. Categories and principles of interventions. In: Christiansen C, Baum C, Bass Haugen J, eds. *Occupational Therapy: Performance, Participation, and Well-Being*. 3rd ed. Thorofare, NJ: SLACK Incorporated; 2005.

19. Medin D, Ross B, Markman A. *Cognitive Psychology*. 4th ed. Hoboken, NJ: John Wiley & Sons, Inc; 2005.

20. Butterfield EC, Nelson GD. Theory and practice of teaching for transfer. *Educational Technology Research and Development*. 1989;37(3):5-38.

21. Toglia JP. The Dynamic Interactional Model of cognition in cognitive rehabilitation. In: Katz N, ed. *Cognition, Occupation, and Participation Across the Life Span: Neuroscience, Neurorehabilitation, and Models of Intervention in Occupational Therapy*. Bethesda, MD: AOTA Press; 2011:161-201.

22. Schwabe L, Bohringer A, Chatterjee M, Schachinger H. Effects of pre-learning stress on memory for neutral, positive and negative words: different roles of cortisol and autonomic arousal. *Neurobiology of Learning and Memory*. 2008;90(1):44-53.

23. Smeets T, Wolf OT, Giesbrecht T, Sijstermans K, Telgen S, Joëls M. Stress selectively and lastingly promotes learning of context-related high arousing information. *Psychoneuroendocrinology*. 2009;34(8):1152-1161.

24. Lupien SJ, McEwen BS, Gunnar MR, Heim C. Effects of stress throughout the lifespan on the brain, behaviour and cognition. *Nature Reviews: Neuroscience*. 2009;10(6):434-445.

25. Kim JJ, Yoon KS. Stress: metaplastic effects in the hippocampus. *Trends in Neurosciences*. 1998; 21(12): 505-509.

26. McEwen BS. Central effects of stress hormones in health and disease: understanding the protective and damaging effects of stress and stress mediators. *European Journal of Pharmacology*. 2008;583(2-3):174-185.

27. McCracken LM. Learning to live with the pain: acceptance of pain predicts adjustment in persons with chronic pain. *Pain*. 1998;74(1):21-27.

28. Dick BD, Rashiq S. Disruption of attention and working memory traces in individuals with chronic pain. *Anesthesia and Analgesia*. 2007;104(5):1223-1229.

29. Eysenck MW. Anxiety and cognitive-task performance. *Personality and Individual Differences*. 1985;6(5):579-586.

30. Devereaux E, Carlson M. The role of occupational therapy in the management of depression. *American Journal of Occupational Therapy*. 1992;46(2):175-180.

31. Naismith S, Hickie I, Ward P, Scott E, Little C. Impaired implicit sequence learning in depression: a probe for frontostriatal dysfunction? *Psychological Medicine*. 2006;36(03):313-323.

32. Custer VL, Wassink KE. Occupational therapy intervention for an adult with depression and suicidal tendencies. *American Journal of Occupational Therapy*. 1991;45(9):845-848.

33. Reilly M. The 1961 Eleanor Clarke Slagle lecture: occupational therapy can be one of the great ideas of 20th century medicine. *American Journal of Occupational Therapy*. 1962;16:1-9.

34. Kircher MA. Motivation as a factor of perceived exertion in purposeful versus nonpurposeful activity. *American Journal of Occupational Therapy*. 1984;38(3):165-170.

35. Bass Haugen J. Personal and environmental influences on occupations. In: Christiansen C, Baum C, Bass-Haugen J, eds. *Occupational Therapy: Performance, Participation, and Well-Being*. 3rd ed. Thorofare, NJ: SLACK Incorporated; 2005.

36. Bandura A. Self-efficacy: toward a unifying theory of behavioral change. *Psychological Review*. 1977;84(2):191-215.

37. Schunk DH. Goal setting and self-efficacy during self-regulated learning. *Educational Psychologist*. 1990;25(1):71-86.

38. Howard BS, Howard JR. Occupation as spiritual activity. *American Journal of Occupational Therapy*. 1997;51(3):181-185.

39. Kaye J, Raghavan SK. Spirituality in disability and illness. *Journal of Religion and Health*. 2002;41(3):231-242.

40. Johnstone B, Glass BA, Oliver RE. Religion and disability: clinical, research and training considerations for rehabilitation professionals. *Disability and Rehabilitation*. 2007;29(15):1153-1163.

41. English LM. Spiritual dimensions of informal learning. *New Directions for Adult and Continuing Education*. 2000;2000(85):29-38.

42. Love PG. Comparing spiritual development and cognitive development. *Journal of College Student Development*. 2002;43(3):357-373.

43. Tisdell EJ. *Exploring Spirituality and Culture in Adult and Higher Education*. San Francisco, CA: Jossey-Bass; 2003.

44. Greenstreet W. From spirituality to coping strategy: making sense of chronic illness. *British Journal of Nursing*. 2006;15(17):938-942.

45. Griffith J, Caron CD, Desrosiers J, Thibeault R. Defining spirituality and giving meaning to occupation: the perspective of community-dwelling older adults with autonomy loss. *Canadian Journal of Occupational Therapy*. 2007;74(2):78-90.

46. Christiansen C. Nationally speaking—acknowledging a spiritual dimension in occupational therapy practice. *American Journal of Occupational Therapy*. 1997;51(3):169-172.

47. Peloquin SM. The spiritual depth of occupation: making worlds and making lives. *American Journal of Occupational Therapy*. 1997;51(3):167-168.

48. Wilding C. Where angels fear to tread: is spirituality relevant to occupational therapy practice? *Australian Occupational Therapy Journal*. 2002;49(1):44-47.

49. Bandura A. Social-learning theory of identificatory processes. In: Goslin DA, ed. *Handbook of Socialization Theory and Research*. Chicago, IL: Rand McNally; 1969.

50. Lawton MP, Nahemow L. Ecological theory of adaptation and aging. In: Preiser W, ed. *Environmental Design Research*. Stroudsburg, PA: Dowden, Hutchinson & Ross; 1973:24-32.

51. Stark SL, Sanford JA. Environmental enablers and their impact on occupational performance. In: Christiansen CH, Baum CM, Bass Haugen J, eds. *Occupational Therapy: Performance, Participation and Well-Being*. 3rd ed. Thorofare, NJ: SLACK Incorporated; 2005.

52. Glang A, Ylvisaker M, Stein M, Ehlhardt L, Todis B, Tyler J. Validated instructional practices: application to students with traumatic brain injury. *Journal of Head Trauma Rehabilitation*. 2008;23(4):243-251.

53. Baum C, Morrison T, Hahn M, Edwards D. *Executive Function Performance Test: Test Protocol Booklet*. St. Louis, MO: Program in Occupational Therapy Washington University School of Medicine; 2003.

54. Wolf TJ, Birkenmeier R. Intervention to increase performance and participation following stroke. In: Christiansen CH, Matuska KM, eds. *Ways of Living: Intervention Strategies to Enable Participation*. 4th ed. Bethesda, MD: AOTA Press; 2011:281-298.

55. Guadagnoli MA, Lee TD. Challenge point: a framework for conceptualizing the effects of various practice conditions in motor learning. *Journal of Motor Behavior*. 2004;36(2):212-224.

56. Krakauer JW. Motor learning: its relevance to stroke recovery and neurorehabilitation. *Current Opinion in Neurology*. 2006;19(1):84-90.

57. Eiriksdottir E, Catrambone R. Procedural instructions, principles, and examples. *Human Factors: The Journal of the Human Factors and Ergonomics Society*. 2011;53(6):749-770.

58. Giles GM. A neurofunctional approach to rehabilitation after brain injury. In: Katz N, ed. *Cognition, Occupation, and Participation Across the Life Span: Neuroscience, Neurorehabilitation, and Models of Intervention in Occupational Therapy*. 3rd ed. Bethesda, MD: AOTA Press; 2011.

59. Gillen G. Managing memory deficits to optimize function. In: Gillen G, ed. *Cognitive and Perceptual Rehabilitation: Optimizing Function*. St. Louis, MO: Mosby Elsevier; 2009.

60. Vygotsky LS. *Mind and Society*. Cambridge, MA: Harvard University Press; 1978.

61. Squires EJ, Hunkin NM, Parkin AJ. Errorless learning of novel associations in amnesia. *Neuropsychologia*. 1997;35(8):1103-1111.

62. Medin DL, Ross BH, Markman AB. Attention. In: Medin DL, Ross BH, Markman AB, eds. *Cognitive Psychology*. 4th ed. Hoboken, NJ: John Wiley & Sons, Inc; 2005.

63. Flavell JH. *Cognitive Development*. Englewood Cliffs, NJ: Prentice Hall; 1985.

64. Veenman MVJ, Van Hout-Wolters BHAM, Afflerbach P. Metacognition and learning: conceptual and methodological considerations. *Metacognition and Learning*. 2006;1(1):3-14.

65. Polatajko HJ, Mandich A. *Enabling Occupation in Children: The Cognitive Orientation to Daily Occupational Performance (CO-OP) Approach*. Ottawa, ON: CAOT Publications ACE; 2004.

66. Polatajko HJ, Mandich A, McEwen SE. Cognitive orientation to daily occupational performance (CO-OP): a cognitive-based intervention for children and adults. In: Katz N, ed. *Cognition, Occupation, and Participation Across the Life Span*. 3rd ed. Bethesda, MD: AOTA; 2011.

67. Miller LT, Polatajko HJ, Missiuna C, Mandich AD, Macnab JJ. A pilot trial of a cognitive treatment for children with developmental coordination disorder. *Human Movement Science*. 2001;20(1-2):183-210.

68. Rodger S, Springfield E, Polatajko HJ. Cognitive orientation for daily occupational performance approach for children with asperger's syndrome. *Physical and Occupational Therapy in Pediatrics*. 2007;27(4):7-22.

69. Dawson DR, Gaya A, Hunt A, et al. Using the cognitive orientation to occupational performance (CO-OP) with adults with executive dysfunction following traumatic brain injury. *Canadian Journal of Occupational Therapy*. 2009;76(2):115-127.

70. McEwen SE, Polatajko HJ, Huijbregts MPJ, Ryan JD. Exploring a cognitive-based treatment approach to improve motor-based skill performance in chronic stroke: results of three single case experiments. *Brain Injury*. 2009;23(13-14):1041-1053.

71. Toglia JP. A dynamic interactional approach to cognitive rehabilitation. In: Katz N, ed. *Cognitive Rehabilitation: Models for Intervention in Occupational Therapy*. Boston, MA: Andover Medical; 1992:104-143.

72. Toglia JP. A dynamic interactional model to cognitive rehabilitation. In: Katz N, ed. *Cognition and Occupation in Rehabilitation*. Bethesda, MD: AOTA; 1998:5-50.

73. Toglia J. A dynamic interactional approach to cognitive rehabilitation. In: Katz N, ed. *Cognition and Occupation Across the Life Span*. 2nd ed. Bethesda, MD: AOTA; 2005:29-72.

74. Toglia J, Johnston MV, Goverover Y, Dain B. A multicontext approach to promoting transfer of strategy use and self regulation after brain injury: an exploratory study. *Brain Injury*. 2010;24(4):664-677.

75. Toglia JP. A dynamic interactional approach to cognitive rehabilitation. In: Katz N, ed. *Cognitive Rehabilitation: Models for Interventions in Occupational Therapy*. Stoneham, MA: Butterworth-Heinemann; 1992.

76. Toglia JP. The multicontext approach. In: Crepau EB, Cohen ES, Schell BAB, eds. *Willard and Spackman's Occupational Therapy*. 10th ed. Philadelphia, PA: Lippincott Williams & Wilkins; 2003:264-267.

77. Josman N. Reliability and validity of the Toglia Category Assessment test. *Canadian Journal of Occupational Therapy*. 1999;66(1):33-42.

78. Josman N, Schein A, Sachs D. Use of the dynamic interactional model for handwriting intervention in children: explanatory case studies. *Israeli Journal of Occupational Therapy*. 2011;20(1):E3-E27.

79. Zlotnik S, Sachs D, Rosenblum S, Shpasser R, Josman N. Use of the dynamic interactional model in self-care and motor intervention after traumatic brain injury: explanatory case studies. *American Journal of Occupational Therapy*. 2009;63(5):549-558.

AN ORGANIZATION-CENTERED STRATEGY

Self-Management—An Evolving Approach to Support Performance, Participation, and Well-Being

Joy Hammel, PhD, OTR/L, FAOTA; Marcia Finlayson, PhD, OTReg(Ont), OTR; and Danbi Lee, OTD, OTR/L

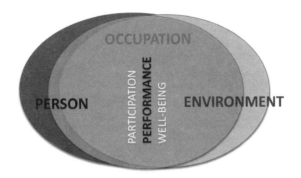

LEARNING OBJECTIVES

- Identify the broader context in which the principles of self-management have been developing.
- Discuss the different ways that the term *self-management* is used.
- Discuss similarities and differences between patient education and self-management.
- Identify key theories that can inform self-management program development and delivery.
- Examine the theoretical and practical links between self-management principles and occupational therapy.
- Apply self-management principles to enhance occupational therapy practice.

KEY WORDS

- Action planning
- Acute illness/disease
- Chronic care model
- Chronic illness/disease
- Consumer direction
- Decision making
- Decisional autonomy
- Developing partnerships
- Environmental management
- Goal setting
- Participation

Christiansen CH, Baum CM, Bass JD, eds.
Occupational Therapy: Performance, Participation, and Well-Being, Fourth Edition (pp 499-511).
© 2015 SLACK Incorporated.

Figure 27-1. Expanded Chronic Care Model. (Reprinted with permission from Barr VJ, Robinson S, Marin-Link B, et al. The expanded Chronic Care Model: an integration of concepts and strategies from population health promotion and the Chronic Care Model. *Hospital Quarterly.* 2003;7:73-82. © 2003 Longwoods Publishing.)

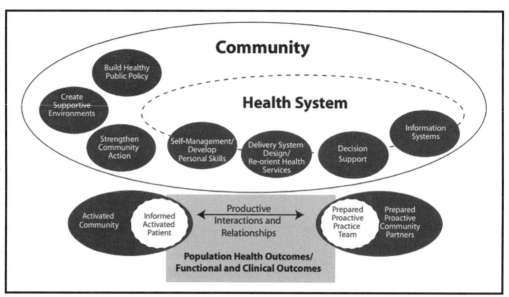

- Patient/client activation
- Patient education
- Problem solving
- Role management
- Self-efficacy
- Self-management
- Self-management support
- Social cognitive theory
- Social learning theory

INTRODUCTION

A primary aim of occupational therapy is to enable and support occupational engagement and full participation in society. In this chapter, occupations are conceptualized as "the ordinary and familiar things that people do every day."[1(p1015)] A growing emphasis and mandate in health care has been meeting the health and participation needs of people living with long-term disabilities and chronic illnesses. Research has shown that having a chronic illness involves constant management of everyday life. Chronic illness management also represents a significant portion of health care utilization and spending; changes in health care delivery systems are needed to improve services related to the everyday management of these conditions. The Expanded Chronic Care Model proposes a systems change framework for making these improvements, specifically citing self-management as an integral component that is theoretically informed and evidenced-based (Figure 27-1).[2]

Self-management is informed by social cognitive and self-efficacy theories, and focuses on "living life well" with a chronic illness and confidently managing everyday life. This approach involves a systematic process of problem identification, goal setting, and action planning. Thus, self-management philosophy and its associated intervention strategies fit nicely with those of occupational therapy.

To date, the focus in self-management has been on symptom and health management. Evidence supports the positive and important impact of building individuals' self-efficacy in order to be an effective self-manager. Increasingly, self-management interventions are being integrated with occupational therapy theory and interventions to also include the management of everyday participation and life roles in the home, community, school/workplace, and society. This innovative practice and area of research is focused on enhancing outcomes related to occupational engagement and participation in context, and examining the outcomes on long-term health, wellness, QOL, and health service utilization. This chapter provides information on chronic illness and implications for health care delivery; self-management approaches, theory and evidence base; and key intersection between self-management and occupational therapy, including the implications for occupational therapy practice.

THE BROADER CONTEXT FOR SELF-MANAGEMENT

Self-management may seem like an emerging trend in health care, but the reality is that it has been discussed in the medical, nursing, and general health care literature for at least 30 years.[3] The growing interest in and emphasis on self-management in health care and rehabilitation can be attributed to several factors:

- The growing personal, social, and financial burden of chronic, non-communicable (eg, depression, cardiovascular) and lifestyle-related and behavior-related (eg, smoking, physical inactivity) conditions.[4]

- The continuing mismatch between the health needs of people living with chronic conditions and the acute-care orientation of current health care systems.[2,5,6]

- The recognition that people who are living with chronic conditions must make day-to-day decisions about their health independent from their health care providers, and need the knowledge and skills to do so with confidence.[7]

- The increasing focus on client/patient-centered care, system-minded care, and shared decision making throughout health care systems to serve all people better.[8,9]

The PEOP Model enables occupational therapy practitioners to consider the potential challenges a person with a chronic condition (eg, diabetes, chronic obstructive pulmonary disease, cardiovascular disease) or a long-term disability (eg, stroke, cerebral palsy, intellectual disability) may face. Box 27-1 summarizes examples of some of these challenges.

When these challenges are ineffectively or only partially managed, people with chronic conditions or long-term disabilities can experience serious restrictions in their occupational performance, participation, well-being, and quality of life. In addition, these individuals tend to incur greater health care costs and experience more frequent or severe exacerbations of their condition, new symptoms, or the emergence of secondary conditions.[5]

For all of these reasons, there is a high level of recognition that health care systems worldwide are not well designed to serve people with chronic conditions.[2,8,12] These systems were designed at a point in time when acute and infectious diseases predominated and people could be diagnosed, treated, cured, and then sent home to continue on as before. This situation is no longer the case—even in developing countries.[12] Now, worldwide estimates suggest that 2 out of 3 deaths each year are attributable to chronic conditions.[13] In addition, estimates suggest that up to 75% of health care encounters in the United States are related to chronic conditions.[14] For the people with these conditions, the return home after these encounters still means having to find ways to perform daily tasks and pursue those activities that give meaning and pleasure to their lives. The Expanded Chronic Care Model is widely utilized as a framework for including people with chronic illness within health care delivery, pointing to self-management programming as a strategy to do so (see Figure 27-1).[2]

BOX 27-1

EXAMPLES OF CHALLENGES OF LIVING WITH A CHRONIC CONDITION[5,10,11]

- Knowing that the condition cannot be cured
- Experiencing an unknown prognosis
- Worrying about the potential for progression over time
- Knowing that treatment options are limited, unclear, or may be only partially effective or satisfactory
- Having to make and maintain behavioral/lifestyle and environmental changes to support participation and well-being
- Finding ways to build skills and resources to facilitate decision making related to health, health care, and future planning
- Needing to be vigilant and monitor the condition regularly to reduce risk of complications or declines

---

While occupational therapy practitioners often work extensively with their clients for several weeks or months at a time, the reality is that—for the most part—we move into and out of people's lives at critical junctures only; for example, when a significant new functional problem has emerged. Rarely do we have opportunities to maintain long-term relationships with our clients across the full continuum of their health and functioning, over time, or across settings. As a result, we have an obligation to understand the self-management process and support the development of self-management skills among our clients. By doing so, we can enable our clients to achieve important outcomes and assist them to maximize their abilities and achieve their goals when we are no longer actively involved in their care. With our focus on occupational performance, participation, well-being, and quality of life, occupational therapy practitioners are well-positioned to actively contribute to processes that support self-management skill development and related outcomes.

Efforts to change systems and better support people with chronic conditions or long-term disability have resulted in the development and evaluation of health care service delivery models, such as the Chronic Care Model[15] and the Expanded Chronic Care Model.[2] To varying degrees, these models do the following:

- Target function, prevention of complications, health promotion and participation as key outcomes of effective service delivery

- Focus on developing strong and effective partnerships and collaborations between informed consumers and proactive providers
- Value evidence-based approaches and the provision of decision supports for both consumers and health care providers
- Recognize that care occurs on a continuum, so self-management support must occur in both institutional and community settings
- Recognize the critical role of supportive environments, accessible communities, and healthy public policy to support consumers' efforts to fully participate in everyday life

WHAT IS SELF-MANAGEMENT?

There are many definitions and explanations of self-management, which can be confusing. Part of the problem is that the term *self-management* is used to describe a set of behaviors and skills, the process of building and maintaining those behaviors and skills, and a set of outcomes that can be expected if the actual use of the behaviors and skills is effective.[16]

Self-Management: Behaviors and Skills

One of the first descriptions of the behaviors necessary for self-management was published in the book *Unending Work and Care.*[17] Nursing researchers conducted in-depth interviews of 60 couples who were managing chronic illness at home. In some cases, only one partner had a condition, but in other cases both did. Their analysis indicated that the management of chronic conditions required engagement in 3 groups of tasks and activities (what occupational therapy practitioners would call occupations), all of which are focused on reducing impact of the condition on daily life.

The first group of self-management occupations revolve around *medical management,* which involves monitoring symptoms, responding to exacerbations, and following through on treatments that have been selected collaboratively with health care providers (eg, doing exercises, taking medications, using equipment as instructed). The second group focuses on *role management,* which involves examining personal values; deciding what activities are most important and meaningful; and making adjustments in habits, routines, and roles to ensure that one is spending time on the activities that are most important. The final one is *emotional management,* which involves finding ways to cope effectively with the emotional consequences of having a chronic condition; for example, fear of progression, uncertainty about consequences of new symptoms,

frustration at the lack of effective treatments, and all of the associated stresses of medical and role management.

Later, Lorig and Holman summarized a set of core skills that people with chronic conditions need to have to successfully engage in medical, role, and emotional management.[3] These skills included self-monitoring, problem solving, decision making, goal setting (also called action planning), finding and using resources, and building partnerships with health care providers and other caregivers. Other authors have suggested a much broader and more specific array of self-management skills, some of which include using medications correctly, managing medical emergencies, eating a healthy diet, staying physically active, reducing stress, adjusting to physical limits, soliciting support from family or friends, handling finances and benefits, managing pain, improving sleep, developing hobbies or leisure activities, and taking care of spiritual or religious needs.[18] What has not been discussed in the self-management literature to any great extent is management of the environment beyond social relationships, particularly physical, cultural, and institutional environments. This is one area to which occupational therapy practitioners could make important contributions.

Ultimately, the skills needed to self-manage a chronic condition or long-term disability will depend on the interaction among person's condition and associated restrictions, his or her occupational and role demands, and the characteristics of the environments in which he or she must function. The case presented in Box 27-2 illustrates the application of some of the behaviors and skills that have just been discussed.

Self-Management: Process

Building self-management skills and integrating them into daily habits and routines can be challenging for a person with a chronic condition; it is a process that requires behavior changes and confidence to maintain these changes over time. Health care providers cannot engage in this process on behalf of clients, but they can support its initiation and maintenance through a variety of strategies that are collectively referred to as self-management support.[19] Specifically, "self-management support is the care and encouragement provided to people with chronic conditions and their families to help them understand their central role in managing their illness, make informed decisions about care, and engage in healthy behaviors."[19]

According to Bodenheimer, MacGregor, and Shafiri, self-management support is a set of tools that providers can share to enable clients to make informed choices about their health as well as a collaborative relationship that aids and inspires clients to become informed and active participants in their care.[20] The essential elements of self-management support include giving information, teaching condition-specific skills, negotiating behavior changes, providing training for problem solving and emotional coping, providing regular follow-up, and engaging the client in the care process.[21]

How these elements are enacted varies across settings (ie, primary care, acute care, rehabilitation), disciplines, payment mechanisms, and countries. In a review of approaches used in Australia to support self-management, Lawn and Schoo found that the most commonly used approaches included group-based programs (eg, Chronic Disease Self-Management Program [CDSM]), care planning (eg, the Flinder's Model), brief primary care techniques (eg, 5A model), motivational interviewing, and health coaching.[22] Core features of these approaches are summarized in Table 27-1.

On the surface, some of these approaches, notably the group-based programs, may be confused with traditional patient education even though they are quite different in their guiding principles, facilitator and client roles, and expected outcomes.[7] Traditional patient education is based on the belief that greater knowledge will change a person's behavior. Therefore, these programs tend to be disease-specific, focus on technical skills related to symptoms or treatments, and be planned and directed by a professional with expertise in the area.[7] The expected outcome of patient education is adherence or compliance with a prescribed treatment regime which, in turn, is expected to result in improved health and functioning. Life skills groups and stress management groups are examples of patient education groups that occupational therapy practitioners may lead.

In comparison, group-based self-management programs are based on the belief that greater confidence in one's own skills and abilities will change behavior.[7] To build confidence, self-management groups address the problems raised by the clients rather than the professional. Both clients and professionals are recognized as having their own expertise, which is complementary and mutually informing. Rather than addressing knowledge and technical, disease-specific skills, self-management focuses on building skills to act on problems (eg, problem solving, decision making, goal setting, etc). Improved confidence is viewed as the proximal outcome that then supports improved health and functioning in the long-term.

In addition to the 5 common approaches to self-management support summarized in Table 27-1, several other strategies should also be noted. Examples include shared decision making and patient decision aids.[9,23] Since shared decision making is a critical component of client-centered care, occupational therapy practitioners are well-positioned to apply it to self-management support.[23] What the profession lacks at this point are decision aids

---

BOX 27-2

CASE: THE APPLICATION OF SELF-MANAGEMENT TASKS AND SKILLS

Mary has relapsing remitting multiple sclerosis (MS). For the most part, her symptoms are mild. Her most common symptoms are fatigue (particularly in the late morning), numbness in her lower legs, and a slight foot drop on her right side. As a result of her symptoms, she has adjusted her work schedule and requested accommodations (role management). She has also participated in some workshops through the MS Society and the MS Clinic to learn more about the disease and what she can expect (medical management). Although she worries about her future, she has elicited the support of friends and has taken up meditation to help herself stay grounded on what is important in her life (emotional management). One morning when she got up, she realized that she could not feel her right foot at all (self-monitoring). Rather than ignoring it, she reflected back on what she learned in her workshops (problem solving) and reviewed some of the materials she had received (using resources). She concluded that this symptom could be the early signs of a new exacerbation (problem solving), and contacted the MS Clinic (decision making) for an appointment. Before going to the clinic, Mary wrote down her observations and questions (medical management, action planning). During the visit, she explained what had happened and worked with the members of the MS care team to make a decision about how to proceed (building partnerships).

---

that provide clients with accurate, up-to-date, and comprehensive information, including risks and benefits of the occupational therapy interventions being offered.

Self-Management: Outcomes

At this point, self-management has been described as a set of behaviors and skills, and the process of building and maintaining those behaviors and skills over time. The key question is do these processes, behaviors, and skills produce meaningful outcomes? Evidence is growing to support an affirmative response to this question across a range of self-management support approaches, chronic conditions, settings, and disciplines.

Some of the strongest evidence to date comes from the work of Dr. Kate Lorig from Stanford University and the

Table 27-1.　Common Approaches for Self-Management Support, Programs, and Resources

Approach	Core Features	For More Information
CDSM	• Structured group program co-facilitated by a health care professional and a lay leader • Develops core self-management skills: problem-solving, decision-making, action planning, finding and using resources, developing partnerships with providers • Requires licensing fee and 1 week training to become a facilitator	http://patienteducation.stanford.edu/programs/cdsmp.html
Flinder's Program	• One-to-one care planning process that includes a client self-assessment of his or her self-management capacity, a "cue and response" interview, client identification of goals, and the development of a self-management plan • Incorporates elements of motivational interviewing and cognitive behavioral therapy • Requires certification to use	http://www.flinders.edu.au/medicine/sites/fhbhru/self-management.cfm
5 A's	• Originally developed to offer guidance to primary care physicians when encouraging health behavior change (eg, quitting smoking, getting more exercise) • The 5 A's reflect the steps that the provider takes with the client: (1) assess the situation by asking about the behavior; (2) advise and encourage behavior change; (3) agree on behavior change goals; (4) assist the client to acquire the necessary knowledge, skills, confidence, and supports; and (5) arrange follow up, referrals, and other necessary supports	http://www.ahrq.gov/professionals/clinicians-providers/guidelines-recommendations/tobacco/5steps.html
Motivational Interviewing	• Originally developed to support behavior change in people with a drinking problem • A counseling approach that explores and resolves ambivalence and supports motivation for behavior change • Focuses on client's own values, beliefs, and preferences to build motivation to change • Multiple levels of training are available	http://www.motivationalinterview.org/
Health Coaching	• One-to-one interaction that incorporates motivational interviewing, cognitive behavioral therapy, and other psychological principles to support a person's active engagement in self-management • Training and certification is available	http://www.nshcoa.com

work that she and her colleagues have done on the Chronic Disease Self-Management Program.[24-27] The success of this program has led to several derivatives, including a lay-lead version in the UK.[28] A recent systematic review of the most common outcomes evaluated for self-management programs found that they included[29]:

• Improved self-efficacy

• Changes in health behaviors (eg, activity engagement, self-monitoring)

• Improved health status (eg, self-rated health, symptoms, functional limitations)

• Health care utilization (eg, physician visits, hospital admissions)

• Quality of life

- Psychological indicators (eg, depression, anxiety, helplessness)

An earlier systematic review examined 145 self-management programs.[30] Despite methodological variability, there was a:

> growing body of evidence to show that, when compared to no intervention (ie, standard care), self-management approaches can provide benefits for participants particularly in terms of knowledge, performance of self-management behaviors, self-efficacy and aspects of health status.[30(p181)]

There was also some evidence for fewer emergency visits and fewer in-patient hospital stays—and therefore lower health care costs—as a consequence of self-management interventions. Ultimately, self-management encompasses all of the following[31,32]:

- Enabling consumers to live well despite the challenges of having a chronic condition
- Building skills that can be self-tailored to individual health situations and priorities
- Ensuring consumer participation, choice and control
- Building partnerships and collaborations between consumers and providers

Theoretical Underpinnings of Self-Management

Self-management interventions are broadly based upon social cognitive theory, and specifically on self-efficacy, problem solving, goal setting and patient activation, and social learning theories.[33] Social cognitive theories focus on the dynamic transactions of personal, behavioral, and environmental factors upon human agency, or the capacity to exercise control over life.[33,34] This agency includes direct personal agency (the ability to self-organize, plan ahead, self-reflect, and self-regulate), and collective agency (shared belief of a social group that they have the power to effect change and produce results together). Thus, social cognitive interventions focus on developing individual and collective (ie, social group) agency, power, and control.

Within social cognitive approaches, self-efficacy theory represents the most commonly cited and studied theory guiding self-management interventions. According to Bandura, self-efficacy is "the belief in one's capabilities to organize and execute courses of action required to manage prospective situations."[34(p18)] People with strong self-efficacy view their problems as challenging tasks to be mastered, develop deep motivation and commitment to actively engage in solving these issues, and recover quickly from setbacks or threats to this engagement. People with weak self-efficacy tend to avoid challenging tasks, believe that issues are outside of their control, focus on the nega-

tive, predict poor outcomes, and lose confidence in the face of setbacks or threats. Self-management focuses on developing positive expectations, performance, self-reflection, and self-monitoring skills specific to health management.

Self-efficacy is developed via mastery experiences (directly performing and problem solving), social modeling (watching similar people engage and problem solve), social persuasion (receiving positive feedback and encouragement from others or giving that feedback to others), and psychological responses (learning how to minimize stress and elevate mood to face difficult issues).

Self-management interventions use a combination of personal and social learning activities to promote self-efficacy, which helps to build positive, strong, and resilient engagement and problem solving over time, particularly in the face of difficult situations. In many cases, self-management interventions also use social learning theory to inform the specific delivery approach; that is, situating learning within real life scenarios through which individuals learn with and from other people with similar interests and issues.[33,35,36] As an example, the Stanford CDSM program has people with chronic conditions come together as a group to problem solve how to confidently manage a range of relevant issues.[37] These include health symptoms (eg, depression, fatigue, medication side effects); interactions with the health system and providers (eg, communications with health care providers); and the pursuit of important life goals through the use of strategies such as relaxation, communication, resource acquisition, and general health promotion. The group learns with and from each other, receiving and giving positive feedback and encouragement to pursue and meet life goals. The group is often co-facilitated by a lay or peer mentor who has experienced these issues and learned how to use self-management strategies and enable others to do so as well. Social learning theory shows that learners are more likely to establish rapport and trust with someone with similar issues and needs, seeing these people as social role models, coaches, and mentors.[3,33,34,38] Participants also actively learn and engage in concrete goal setting, problem solving, and action planning to increase their self-efficacy and support each other as a group. The Stanford Patient Education Research Center website and other resources provide information on programming and participant manuals and forms.[37,39]

Social problem solving, goal setting, and patient activation are additional practice frameworks that include processes and learning activities to support self-efficacy and develop confidence and resilience for engagement and life management. Social problem solving is a prescriptive model and process focused on effective problem management and proactive coping in times of stress.[40] The evidence-based problem-solving therapy approach is used by trained psychologists and focuses on developing 2 aspects

Figure 27-2. Goal-setting and action-planning practice framework for self-management. (Reprinted with permission from Scobbie L, Dixon D, Wyke S. Goal setting and action planning in the rehabilitation setting: development of a theoretically informed practice framework. *Clin Rehabil.* 2011;25[5]:468-482. © 2011 by SAGE.)

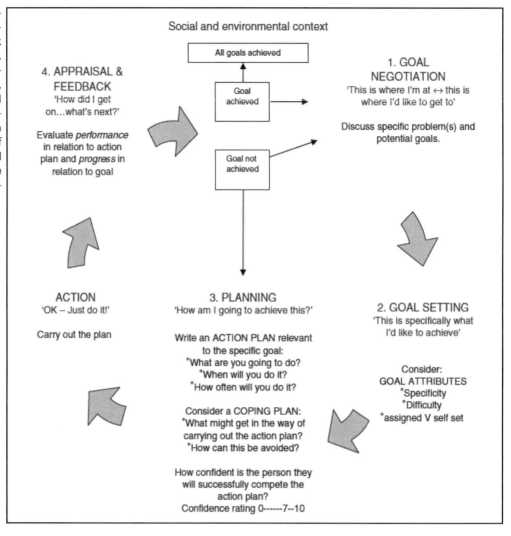

of social problem solving: problem orientation and specific problem-solving skills.[41] Problem orientation involves building a positive, strength-based approach to problem recognition, attribution, appraisal, perceived control, and time/effort commitment. Problem-solving skills focus on learning a process and skill set related to defining and formulating the problem, generating alternative solutions, making decisions, and implementing and verifying solutions. Social problem solving provides a tool kit of strategies that can be tailored to different styles (rational, impulsive, avoidant), as well as assessment tools such as the Social Problem Solving Inventory[42] and specific intervention protocols (for individual and group delivery).

Goal setting, consumer/patient activation, and health action and change are additional intervention approaches related to self-management of health and chronic conditions, and becoming an informed and effective self-manager. The goal setting and action planning practice framework is similar to the PEOP Occupational Therapy Process, in that it uses individuals' goals to establish a plan and measure outcomes, as seen in Figure 27-2.[43] The Patient Activation Measure (PAM) was created to assess a person's stage of activation or readiness to change and then to tailor interventions to fit the individual's needs and capacities.[43] There is a growing body of evidence supporting delivery of tailored self-management interventions that target specific consumer needs and styles vs delivery of a preset, fixed intervention. Tailoring also fits with occupational therapy's focus on client-centered practice and individualized occupational profiles and trajectories.

These approaches are evidence-based and provide support for integrating self-management ideas and interventions into occupational therapy. They also provide examples of assessment tools, intervention protocols, and strategies that may be applied with individuals with chronic conditions and long-term disabilities and delivered individually or within a social group context.

Self-Management and Occupational Therapy

Self-management approaches are compatible with the PEOP Model and PEOP Occupational Therapy Process. An individual's narrative (which includes perspectives and goals) guides the nature of the interaction between the client and the practitioner and the intervention process. Outcomes of self-management approaches are related to changes in performance, participation, and well-being. Specific issues that are addressed in self-management approaches and are relevant to occupational therapy include occupations of chronic illness and disability, role and role management, participation, environment and environment management, and client-centered goals.

Occupations of Chronic Illness and Disability

Occupational therapy practitioners conceptualize occupations as the "ordinary and familiar things that people do every day."[1(p1015)] Although self-management is not explicitly identified as an occupation in many occupational therapy models and the practice framework, the self-management literature repeatedly proposes that the management of chronic illness and long-term disability are major life occupations on a daily basis, over time, and across the lifespan.[17,45] If the management of chronic illness and disability is an everyday occupation, it is also likely that self-management contributes to personal identity. Occupational transitions occur across the lifespan, and chronic illness and disability may be particularly challenging during transition points, such as starting school, moving into a first apartment, finding work, starting a family, and selling a home. Occupational management of chronic illness and disability is particularly important for older adults, given the increased probability of experiencing multiple chronic illnesses during this life stage. Transitions may also correspond to times during which people with disabilities may not have occupational therapy consultation or services. Thus, occupational therapy practitioners may want to prepare clients for self-management of occupational transitions and provide information on long-term management supports.

Roles and Role Management: Becoming a Self-Manager

In the PEOP Model, roles are a central component of occupations; roles represent important indicators of personal identity and the ways identity is realized, coordinated with specific tasks and contexts, and performed. Major role changes and social isolation are common among people with chronic illness and long-term disabilities, affecting their sense of self and identity.[46-49] Identity and role disruption is a frequent result of having a chronic condition, as the physical or psychological difficulties, social attitudes, and expectations influence role participation. Gaining control over what one chooses to be and do—and how one then accomplishes this—involves redefining, prioritizing, and managing life roles.

Role management is also a core task of self-management.[3] It involves maintaining, changing, and creating meaningful life roles. Roles may be redefined through meaningful occupations; occupational therapy practitioners have a critical role in renewing clients' lives by supporting their process of role adaptation.[50,51]

Using the PEOP Occupational Therapy Process, an outcome of occupational therapy interventions could help clients become confident, effective self-managers. Occupational therapy practitioners may use narrative, assessment and evaluation, interventions, and outcomes as they guide a client to self-evaluate personal capacity and difficulties, set achievable short-term and long-term goals, perform and reflect on their goals, modify the environment to support goal achievement, and identify and utilize available resources and services needed to make goals possible. The process of gaining occupational competence and self-efficacy in a new role of self-manager may be facilitated by the tools self-management programming provides.[37] Increased self-efficacy in role management enables people to face daily issues and life challenges in a proactive, positive way; rather than a negative, reactive response or crisis management.

Participation and Self-Management

Self-management focuses on living life well with chronic illness or disability, which also corresponds to the PEOP Model and ICF focus on participation for everyday life situations.[37,52] The focus is not on remediation of impairments or independent performance (performing activities by self without supports), but rather on supporting long-term, meaningful, desired engagement in areas of participation (home, community, work/school/productive, social) of greatest importance to the person and the social world in which they operate. In occupational therapy, this will require practitioners to place more emphasis on participation in context, to respond to the long-term needs and desires of people with disabilities and chronic illness.

Environment and Environmental Management

Full participation occurs in a context, and the environmental context can either serve as an enabler or barrier to participation. A critical aspect of living life well with a disability or chronic illness, then, is on environmental management. Achieving participation goals may involve learning how to find and put into place environmental supports and information resources to address environmental barriers. Environmental management strategies may address many areas, for example:

- Physical (built and natural environment, community livability, AT, home modifications and safety, transportation access)
- Social (assertive communication with family and friends, asking for help without feeling dependent, dealing with overprotectiveness or lack of respect, hiring and managing personal attendants)
- Societal (strategizing supports for community living, navigating social service and health systems, troubleshooting economic and financial issues, advocating for rights and systems changes, changing attitudes, and building and being a part of disability community and culture)

Environmental problem solving and management is a key component of occupational therapy services related to self-management.

Client-Centered Practice

The goal of self-management is to create empowered, competent, informed consumers and self-managers (see Figure 27-1). Self-management approaches assert that individual self-efficacy, confidence, and autonomy drive activation of motivation and engagement. Thus, facilitating client-centered and consumer-directed approaches are critical to activation related to goal setting, problem solving, and action planning. When individuals actively lead engagement, they are more likely to realize goals, manage their health, and live life well. When engagement is done collectively with other people with similar interests and issues (eg, social learning), benefits are not only seen by the individuals, but also by people with disabilities as a social group; this encourages further engagement to change and build participation opportunities in society for the group.[33] Self-management offers a strong theoretical, programmatic, and evidence base for client-centered and social learning-based services and interventions that is aligned with the philosophy of occupational therapy.

Examples of Self-Management Principles to Enhance Occupational Therapy Practice

Self-management approaches and interventions may be used at many different times in the rehabilitation process, across the continuum of health care delivery services, and in both group and individual formats. The Flinders Program is a one-to-one collaboration between an individual with a chronic condition and a health professional; the aims of the program are to develop a strong client/health professional partnership, collaboratively identify problems and possible solutions, motivate the client for sustained changes in behaviors, measure changes over time, and improve outcomes.[52] The Flinders Program has been used in hospital settings and was shown to be effective with different client groups, including people with type-2 diabetes, mental illness, and diverse chronic illness.[52-56] Strategies such as motivational interviewing, client activation, and goal setting also can be used individually, and thus can also be integrated into rehabilitation settings. Studies have utilized these strategies to empower people with chronic illness and to improve their health outcomes.[57-61]

The Stanford CDSM program has extensive evidence of its impact on self-efficacy and health-related outcomes in community-based settings.[24,25,27] Programs have been developed to support people with chronic illness, offering specific modules for diabetes, arthritis, cancer, asthma, AIDS, and other chronic illnesses. Emerging evidence is also pointing to the need for and potential benefit of community-based self-management programs designed for people with stroke and brain injury—groups that have not been included in traditional chronic care models and self-management programs.[62,63] These community-based group programs also have much potential to be offered in outpatient settings as an alternative group intervention.

Recently, attention has been given to alternative delivery methods, such as internet and teleconferencing, to increase accessibility to clients with limited or poor access to traditional health care services. Research shows that these methods can provide viable and effective intervention delivery to people with different chronic illnesses.[27,64-66]

Most of the self-management interventions have not focused beyond symptom and health management. A growing body of research involves designing and evaluating self-management interventions that focus on managing everyday home, community, work, and social life and participation for people living with long-term disabilities and caregivers.[67-69] Strategies for building self-efficacy, such as goal setting, client activation, and action planning, are also being integrated into occupational therapy practice and interventions.[70-73] These trends highlight the importance of becoming more knowledgeable and proficient in delivering and evaluating self-management in occupational therapy practice. There are many resources and advanced training opportunities available to occupational therapy practitioners to gain skills to effectively implement self-management programs and to use self-management and self-efficacy strategies in their practice (see Table 27-1).

DIRECTIONS FOR THE FUTURE

There are many indicators that self-management approaches will continue to grow in their availability and demand, particularly given the international recognition and adoption of the Chronic Care Model.[2] Several jurisdictions, including Australia, Sweden, Canada, and the UK, have adopted self-management programming as an integral part of their health care system. In the United States, the Affordable Care Act proposes to implement new self and chronic disease/illness management services and demonstrations programs, utilizing a community-based, consumer-directed approach. Many self-management programs, such as the Stanford CDSM program, have already been adopted by federal and state agencies (such as the Administration of Aging and Area Agencies on Aging) and are provided free of cost within local communities; however, the focus is primarily on health and symptom management.[39] There are opportunities for occupational therapy to develop and evaluate self-management programs related to occupational engagement and participation in the home, community, school/workplace, and society.

Another future area of development for self-management and occupational therapy involves informed risk management or risk contracting, an approach that[74-76]:

1. Acknowledges the civil right of people with disabilities to fully participate and live in a restrictive setting of choice, including the right to take risks with dignity

2. Collaboratively assesses risks involved in this full participation so consumers, providers, and funders are aware of them

3. Establishes a comprehensive plan to realistically manage risks and provide needed environmental supports

4. Proactively monitors risks over time so supports can be tailored to meeting changing needs and issues

5. Evaluates the impact of supports on full participation, health and wellness, and service utilization to guide future resource allocation and changes in systems

Given occupational therapy's focus on occupational engagement and participation in context, an informed risk management approach could be part of formal occupational therapy services to shift the focus from evaluations of safety to interventions that make individuals as safe as possible, while still realizing their rights and desires.

SUMMARY

This chapter introduced self-management approaches for individuals with chronic conditions and the opportunities for occupational therapy to contribute to interventions that improve performance, participation, and well-being. The characteristics of and available resources for evidence-based self-management approaches were summarized. The PEOP Model and PEOP Occupational Therapy Process provide a framework for occupational therapy involvement in self-management programs at the individual, organization, and population level.

REFERENCES

1. Christiansen C, Clark F, Kielhofner G, Rogers J. Position paper: occupation. *American Journal of Occupational Therapy.* 1995;49(10):1015-1018.

2. Barr VJ, Robinson S, Marin-Link B, et al. The expanded Chronic Care Model: an integration of concepts and strategies from population health promotion and the Chronic Care Model. *Hospital Quarterly.* 2003;7:73-82.

3. Lorig KR, Holman H. Self-management education: history, definition, outcomes, and mechanisms. *Annals of Behavioral Medicine.* 2003;26:1-7.

4. Meetoo D. Chronic diseases: the silent global epidemic. *British Journal of Nursing.* 2008;17(21):1320-1325.

5. Holman H, Lorig K. Patient self-management: a key to effectiveness and efficiency in care of chronic disease. *Public Health Reports.* 2004;119:239-243.

6. Wagner EH, Austin BT, Michael VK. Organizing care for patients with chronic illness. *The Milbank Quarterly.* 1996;74:511-544.

7. Bodenheimer T, Lorig K, Holman H, Grumbach K. Patient self-management of chronic disease in primary care. *JAMA.* 2002;288:2469-2475.

8. Berwick DM. A user's manual for the IOM's 'quality chasm' report. Health Affairs. 2002;21(30):80-90.

9. Coulter A, Collins A. *Making Shared Decision-Making a Reality: No Decision About Me, Without Me.* London, UK: The King's Fund; 2011.

10. Jerant AF, von Friederichs-Fitzwater MM, Moore M. Patients' perceived barriers to active self-management of chronic conditions. *Patient Education and Counseling.* 2005;57(3):300-307.

11. Thorne S, Paterson B, Russell C. The structure of everyday self-care decision making in chronic illness. *Qualitative Health Research.* 2003;13:1337-1352.

12. WHO. *Noncommunicable Diseases Country Profiles 2011.* World Health Organization: WHO publications. http://whqlibdoc.who.int/publications/2011/9789241502283_eng.pdf. Published 2011. Accessed July 4, 2013.

13. Beaglehole R, Bonita R, Horton R, et al. Priority actions for the non-communicable disease crisis. *Lancet.* 2011;377(9775):1438-1447.

14. US Centers for Disease Control and Prevention. *Chronic Diseases: The Power to Prevent, the Call to Control.* US Centers for Disease Control and Prevention. http://www.cdc.gov/chronicdisease/resources/publications/aag/pdf/chronic.pdf. Published 2009. Accessed August 2, 2013.

15. Wagner EH, Davis C, Schaefer J, Von Korff M, Austin B. A survey of leading chronic disease management programs: are they consistent with the literature? *Managed Care Quarterly.* 1998;7(3):56-66.

16. McGowan, P. *Self-Management: A Background Paper.* University of Victoria: Centre on Aging. http://www.selfmanagementbc. ca/uploads/Support%20for%20Health%20Professionals/Self-Management%20support%20a%20background%20paper%20 2005.pdf. Published 2005. Accessed August 2, 2013.

17. Corbin JM, Strauss A. *Unending Work and Care: Managing Chronic Illness at Home.* San Francisco, CA: Jossey Bass Publishers; 1988.

18. Noël PH, Parchman ML, Williams JW, et al. The challenges of multimorbidity from the patient perspective. *Journal of General Internal Medicine.* 2007;22(3):419-424.

19. MacColl Center for Health Care Innovation. *Partnering in Self-Management Support: A Toolkit for Clinicians.* Improving chronic illness care. Seattle, WA: MacColl Center. http://www. improvingchroniccare.org/downloads/selfmanagement_support_toolkit_for_clinicians_2012_update.pdf. Published May 2009. Updated 2012. Accessed August 2, 2013.

20. Bodenheimer T, MacGregor K, Shafiri C. *Helping Patients Manage Their Chronic Conditions.* California Healthcare Foundation. http://www.chcf.org/publications/2005/06/helping-patients-manage-their-chronic-conditions#ixzz1jXzlWyDK. Published June 2005. Accessed August 2, 2013.

21. Bodenheimer T, Abramowitz S. *Helping Patients Help Themselves: How to Implement Self-Management Support.* California Healthcare Foundation. http://www. chcf.org/publications/2010/12/helping-patients-help-themselves#ixzz1jYBoR3B9. Published December 2010. Accessed August 2, 2013.

22. Lawn S, Schoo A. Supporting self-management of chronic health conditions: common approaches. *Patient Education and Counseling.* 2010;80:205-211.

23. Salzburg: Global Seminar. Salzburg statement on shared decision making. *BMJ (Clinical Research Ed.).* 2010;342(2011):d1745.

24. Lorig KR, Sobel DS, Stewart AL, et al. Evidence suggesting that a chronic disease self-management program can improve health status while reducing hospitalization: a randomized trial. *Medical Care.* 1999;37(1):5-14.

25. Lorig KR, Ritter P, Stewart AL, et al. Chronic disease self-management program: 2-year health status and health care utilization outcomes. *Medical Care.* 2001;39(110):1217-1223.

26. Lorig KR, Hurwicz ML, Sobel D, Hobbs M, Ritter PL. A national dissemination of an evidence-based self-management program: a process evaluation study. *Patient Education and Counseling.* 2005;59(1):69-79.

27. Lorig KR, Ritter P, Laurent DD, Plant K. Internet-based chronic disease self-management: a randomized trial. *Medical Care.* 2006;44(11):964-971.

28. Barlow JH, Wright CC, Turner AP, Bancroft GV. A 12-month follow-up study of self-management training for people with chronic disease: are changes maintained over time? *British Journal of Health Psychology.* 2005;10(4):589-599.

29. Du S, Yuan C. Evaluation of patient self-management outcomes in health care: a systematic review. *International Nursing Review.* 2010;57:159-167.

30. Barlow J, Wright C, Sheasby J, Turner A, Hainsworth J. Self-management approaches for people with chronic conditions: a review. *Patient Education and Counseling.* 2002;48:177-187.

31. Ryan P, Sawin KJ. The individual and family self-management theory: background and perspectives on context, process, and outcomes. *Nursing Outlook.* 2009;57(4):217-225.

32. Wilkinson A, Whitehead L. Evolution of the concept of self-care and implications for nurses: a literature review. *International Journal of Nursing Studies.* 2009;46(8):1143-1147.

33. Bandura A. Social cognitive theory: an agentic perspective. *Annual Review of Psychology.* 2001;52:1-26.

34. Bandura A. *Social Foundations of Thought and Action: A Social Cognitive Theory.* Englewood Cliffs, NJ: Prentice Hall; 1986.

35. Vygotsky LS. *Mind and Society: The Development of Higher Mental Processes.* Cambridge, MA: Harvard University Press; 1978.

36. Lave J, Wenger E. *Communities of Practice: Learning, Meaning, and Identity.* Cambridge, MA: Cambridge University Press; 1998.

37. Lorig KR, Holman H, Sobel D, Laurent D, González V, Minor M. *Living a Healthy Life With Chronic Conditions: Self-Management of Heart Disease, Arthritis, Diabetes, Depression, Asthma, Bronchitis, Emphysema and Other Physical and Mental Health Conditions.* 4th ed. Boulder, CO: Bull Publishing; 2012.

38. Bandura A. *Self-Efficacy: The Exercise of Control.* New York, NY: Freeman; 1997.

39. Stanford Patient Education Research Center. *Stanford Small-Group Self-Management Programs in English.* Stanford School of Medicine: patient education in the department of medicine. http://patienteducation.stanford.edu/programs/. Published 2013. Accessed on July 6, 2013.

40. D'Zurilla TJ, Nezu AM. *Problem-Solving Therapy: A Social Competence Approach to Clinical Intervention.* 2nd ed. New York, NY: Springer; 1999.

41. D'Zurilla TJ, Nezu AM. *Problem-Solving Therapy: A Positive Approach to Clinical Intervention.* 3rd ed. New York, NY: Springer Publishing Company; 2007.

42. D'Zurillo TJ, Nezu AM, Maydeu-Olivares A. *Manual for the Social Problem Solving Inventory—Revised.* 3rd ed. North Tonawanda, NY: Mental-Health Systems; 2002.

43. Scobbie L, Dixon D, Wyke S. Goal setting and action planning in the rehabilitation setting: development of a theoretically informed practice framework. *Clin Rehabil.* 2011;25:468-482.

44. Hibbard JH, Stockard J, Mahoney ER, Tusler M. Development of the Patient Activation Measure (PAM): conceptualizing and measuring activation in patients and consumers. *Health Service Research.* 2004;39:1005-1026.

45. Finlayson M. Concerns about the future among older adults with multiple sclerosis. *American Journal of Occupational Therapy.* 2004;58(1):54-63.

46. Christiansen CH. Defining lives: occupation as identity: an essay on competence, coherence, and the creation of meaning. *American Journal of Occupational Therapy.* 1999;53(6):547-558.

47. Asbring P. Chronic illness—a disruption in life: identity-transformation among women with chronic fatigue syndrome and fibromyalgia. *Journal of Advanced Nursing.* 2001;34(3):312-319.

48. Bury M. The sociology of chronic illness: a review of research and prospects. *Sociology of Health and Illness.* 1991;13(4):451-468.

49. Clarke P, Black SE. Quality of life following stroke: negotiating disability, identity and resources. *Journal of Applied Gerontology.* 2005;24:319-336.

50. AOTA. Occupational therapy practice framework: domain and process. 2nd ed. *American Journal of Occupational Therapy.* 2008;62:625-683.

51. Hoogerdijk B, Runge U, Haugboelle J. The adaptation process after traumatic brain injury: an individual and ongoing occupational struggle to gain a new identity. *Scandinavian Journal of Occupational Therapy.* 2011;18(2):122-132.

52. WHO. *International Classification of Functioning, Disability and Health.* Geneva, Switzerland: World Health Organization; 2001.

53. The Flinders Program. Flinders University. http://www.flinders.edu.au/medicine/sites/fhbhru/self-management.cfm. Updated July 23, 2013. Accessed July 6, 2013.

54. Lawn S, Lawton K. Chronic condition self-management support within a respiratory nursing service. *Journal of Nursing and Healthcare of Chronic Illness.* 2011;3:372-380.

55. Lawn S, Battersby MW, Pols RG, et al. The mental health expert patient: findings from a pilot study of a generic chronic condition self-management programme for people with mental illness. *International Journal of Social Psychiatry.* 2007;53:63-74.

56. Roy D, Mahony F, Horsburgh M, Bycroft J. Partnering in primary care in New Zealand: clients' and nurses' experience of the Flinders Program in the management of long-term conditions. *Journal of Nursing and Healthcare of Chronic Illnesses.* 2011;3(2):140-149.

57. Alegria M, Polo A, Gao S, et al. Evaluation of a patient activation and empowerment intervention in mental health care. *Medical Care.* 2008;46(3):247-256.

58. Britt E, Hudson SM, Blampied NM. Motivational interviewing in health settings: a review. *Patient Education and Counseling.* 2004;53(2):147-155.

59. Hibbard JH, Mahoney ER, Stock R, Tusler M. Do increases in patient activation result in improved self-management behaviors? *Health Services Research.* 2007;42:1443-1463.

60. Rosewilliam S, Roskell CA, Pandyan AD. A systematic review and synthesis of the quantitative and qualitative evidence behind patient-centered goal setting in stroke rehabilitation. *Clinical Rehabilitation.* 2011;25:501-514.

61. Stott NCH, Rees M, Rollnick S, Pill RM, Hackett P. Professional responses to innovation in clinical method: diabetes care and negotiating skills. *Patient Education and Counseling.* 1996;29:67-73.

62. Cadilhac DA, Hoffman S, Kilkenny, M. A phase II multicentered, single-blind, randomized controlled trial of the stroke self-management program. *Stroke.* 2011;42:1673-1679.

63. Huijbregts MPJ, Myers AM, Streiner D, Teasell R. Implementation, process, and preliminary outcome evaluation of two community programs for persons with stroke and their care partners. *Topics in Stroke Rehabilitation.* 2008;15(5):503-520.

64. Finlayson M, Preissner K, Cho C, Plow M. Randomized trial of a teleconference-delivered fatigue management program for people with multiple sclerosis. *Multiple Sclerosis Journal.* 2011;17(9):1130-1140.

65. Lorig K, Ritter P, Laurent D. Online diabetes self-management program: a randomized study. *Diabetes Care.* 2010;33(6):1275-1281.

66. Taylor DM, Cameron JI, Walsh L. Exploring the feasibility of videoconference delivery of a self-management program to rural participants with stroke. *Telemedicine and e-Health.* 2009;15(7):646-654.

67. Hammel J, Baum C, Wolf T, Lee D. *The Stroke Self-Management Program: Facilitators Manual.* Chicago, IL: University of Illinois; 2010.

68. Hammel J, Lee D, Fogg L, Baum C, Wolf T. *Evaluating a Self-Management Intervention for Home, Community and Work Participation After a Stroke: A Pilot Study.* Manuscript in preparation. 2013.

69. Finlayson M, Garcia JD, Preissner K. Development of an educational programme for caregivers of people aging with multiple sclerosis. *Occupational Therapy International.* 2008;15:4-17.

70. Bower K, Gustafsson L, Hoffmann T, Barker R. Self-management of upper limb recovery after stroke: how effectively do occupational therapists and physiotherapists train clients and carers? *British Journal of Occupational Therapy.* 2012;75(4):180-210.

71. Doig E, Fleming J, Cornwell P, Kuipers P. Qualitative exploration of a client-centered, goal-directed approach to community-based occupational therapy for adults with traumatic brain injury. *American Journal of Occupational Therapy.* 2009;63(5):559-568.

72. McEwen SE, Polatajko HJ, Davis JA, Huijbregts M, Ryan JD. 'There's a real plan here, and I am responsible for that plan': participant experiences with a novel cognitive-based treatment approach for adults living with chronic stroke. *Disability and Rehabilitation.* 2010;32(7):541-550.

73. Polatajko HJ, Mandich AD, Miller LT, Macnab JJ. Cognitive Orientation to Daily Occupational Performance (CO-OP) part II: the evidence. *Physical and Occupational Therapy in Pediatrics.* 2001;20(2-3):83-106.

74. Kane RA, Levin CA. Who's safe? Who's sorry? The duty to protect the safety of clients in home- and community-based care. *Generations.* 1998;22(3):76-81.

75. Duval N, Moseley C. *Negotiated Risk Agreements in Long-term Support Services.* Durham, NH: National Program Office on Self-Determination; 2001.

76. Galantowicz S, Selig B. *Risk Management and Quality in HCBS: Individual Risk Planning and Prevention, System-wide Quality Improvements.* Cambridge, MA: Thomson Medstat; 2005.

Chapter 28

EDUCATIONAL AND DIGITAL TECHNOLOGY STRATEGIES

Anita L. Hamilton, BAppSc(OT), MOccThy, Grad Cert(Higher Ed), PhD(Cand) and
Alec I. Hamilton, BEd(Sci), Grad Dip App Child Psych, MAnaly Psych, MCouns(Psych)

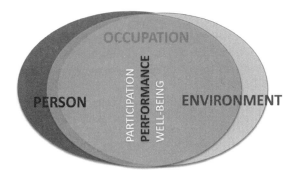

LEARNING OBJECTIVES

- Give context to *educate* as a fundamental enabling skill in occupational therapy.
- Review education and learning theory as it applies to occupational therapy practice.
- Describe how education is central in the PEOP Occupational Therapy Process.
- Define and describe how digital technologies can facilitate educational outcomes.
- Describe a practice exemplar where an occupational therapy practitioner created an education program for a specific population, integrating digital technology where appropriate.

KEY WORDS

- Digital inclusion
- Digital literacy
- Digital technology
- Educating
- Information literacy
- Learning
- Virtual

OVERVIEW

"Occupational therapy is a client-centered health profession concerned with promoting health and well-being through occupation. The primary goal of occupational therapy is to enable people to participate successfully in the activities of everyday life. Occupational therapy practitioners achieve this outcome by enabling people to do things that will enhance their ability to live meaningful lives or by modifying the environment to better support participation."[1(np)]

Christiansen CH, Baum CM, Bass JD, eds.
*Occupational Therapy: Performance, Participation,
and Well-Being, Fourth Edition (pp 513-525).*
© 2015 SLACK Incorporated.

This chapter focuses on the role of education and the use of education technology in interventions for individuals, groups, and communities. First, education and learning theories relevant to occupational therapy practice and an application model that exemplifies how education theory can be applied in occupational therapy will be introduced. Then, the role of digital technology in providing education to clients will be discussed. Finally, a practice exemplar will describe an occupational therapy practitioner working in an organization/community setting using education and digital technology as a tool of enablement. The practice exemplar will be described through the lens of the PEOP Occupational Therapy Process. Throughout this chapter the term *client* will mean individuals, groups, and/or whole communities.

INTRODUCTION

Occupational therapy practitioners often use education approaches to achieve occupational performance goals of clients[2,3] and promote learning, "the enduring ability of an individual to comprehend and/or competently respond to changes in information from the environment and/or from within the self."[4(p547)] Facilitation of learning is a core clinical competency in occupational therapy[5,6] that "aims to facilitate mastery of tasks and activities viewed as pivotal in a client's goal attainment."[3(p187)]

Education plays a role in all areas of occupational therapy practice. Education may be used to restore function or remediate or compensate for lost function. For example, a person undergoing total hip replacement surgery is given education about management of their affected limb to ensure they minimize the risk of dislocation, maximize stability, and return to full mobility. Education can be used in health promotion, injury, and illness prevention and to enable individuals or groups to self-manage their condition. Education may also be used in advocacy through community-wide education and campaigns aimed at removing barriers to occupational performance; an example is increasing public awareness about depression to reduce stigma through understanding of the complex issues surrounding the development and management of depression. Reducing stigma through education enables people with depression engage in meaningful activities.

EDUCATION AS A TOOL OF ENABLEMENT

Education is one of many tools of enablement that occupational therapy practitioners use as a therapeutic intervention. Therefore it is important that occupational therapy practitioners have foundational knowledge and skills in education theory to inform the design and development of the educational activities and materials that can meet the needs of individuals, families, groups, and communities with whom we work.[7] When occupational therapy practitioners educate they enable; that is, they "demonstrate, enlighten, instruct, inform, facilitate learning through doing, notify, present just-right challenge, prompt learning of skills, prompt rote and repetitive learning, prompt transformative learning, simulate, teach, train, tutor."[7(p114)]

Education and Learning Theory

In order to develop effective education interventions, it is important to understand the theory behind the approaches. School systems, including universities and colleges, have at their hearts a number of theoretical systems that drive their approach to learning. On the road to becoming therapy practitioners, school and university or college experiences have acculturated practitioners through theoretical approaches for education and learning; however, learners are often unaware of these theories and their background. This is not inherently problematic in the university setting, but it becomes an issue when occupational therapy practitioners unconsciously act within a particular paradigm from habit and not by design in practice. To work effectively with others, it is important to be consciously aware of the theories, models, and frames of reference that ultimately shape practice.

The primary education theories that influence occupational therapy practice are behaviorist, constructivist, developmental, and transformative theories.[8] Each has strengths and limitations; the key is to know the theory that is driving a specific intervention. Each theory has embedded within it specific assumptions. These assumptions determine the actions taken, the timing, and also how those actions are evaluated. The following section summarizes some of the predominant theoretical approaches to education and learning and the beliefs systems that are captured within their formulation.[8]

Behaviorist Theory

Behaviorist theories have dominated early educational approaches and continue to have a major impact on education today. Approaches to managing behavior, like Positive Behavioral Support (PBS) or Applied Behavioral Analysis (ABA), have their origins in the early ideas of behaviorism. In its simplest form, behaviorist theory sees the individual predominantly as an unknowable system; that is, a system only understandable via direct observation of the behavior the individual produces. Within this context, behavior is anything that is observable and captures the skills, physical abilities, and actions of individuals. Behavior does not include or describe the thoughts or feelings an individual may hold, as these are not observable and therefore not open to outside evaluation. Furthermore, and perhaps the key to this theory's approach to intervention, is that behaviors can be modified via reward and/or punishment. For example, university grading systems stem from this theory; they reward those who do well with points, credits, or some other extrinsically valued unit. In simple terms, some academic behavior (poor academic performance) can be negatively reinforced with low grades, while other academic behaviors can be positively reinforced with high grades. This is the essence of the behavioral approach. It is based on the fundamental belief that a positive behavior that is valued by a person will be repeated when the behavior is paired with a positive. Conversely, when external responses to undesired behaviors are negative or neutral, then the behavior is less likely to occur again. According to behaviorist theory it is these environmental responses that drive learning.[8]

Constructivist Learning Theory

Another central theory of learning is the constructivist approach, sometimes referred to as the social-constructivist approach and/or educational constructivism. While there are subtle differences between each of these, they are combined for the purposes of this general discussion. The basic premise of constructivism is that reality is constructed through language and social interaction. Human beings construct meaning out of their social interactions and the language used to describe and make meaning of the information around them. Within this theory there is no "true" reality, only the reality that is constructed.[8]

In the relationship between a more knowledgeable or experienced individual and the learner, social interaction occurs and meaning is created. Knowledge, skills, and abilities are developed through social interactions in contexts that hold value for the "teacher" and the "learner." This mode of guided learning requires a gradual movement from teacher dependence to learner independence. As time and learning progress, the learner develops understandings, knowledge, and skills that eventually do not require the support of the teacher. This evolution requires teacher and learner to continually renegotiate their roles and the power balance between them.[8]

Within the context of occupational therapy, constructivist theory requires practitioners to have knowledge or experience of their practice areas, and an understanding of how the client's experience might be enhanced. By combining the client's needs with the practitioner's knowledge, it is possible to collaboratively develop educational interventions that build client's skills, knowledge, or abilities.

The practitioner creates a "just-right" challenge at each stage of the education process.[8]

Developmental Learning Theories

Developmental theories propose that learning is like climbing a series of stairs, each step requiring a range of skills and abilities that are developed and honed at a particular time in an individual's life. Once the skills and/or tasks of the stage of life are accomplished, the individual moves forward up the staircase to the next step where a new set of skills and abilities are developed and accomplished. Life's journey is therefore a series of incremental steps or age and stage developmental tasks leading to some higher skill and ability. Developmental theories place the focus within the client, and any interventions on clients' level of age, ability, and/or skill. The assumption is an individual is unable to move forward until he or she has completed the necessary aspect of the relevant stage.[8]

An example of developmental theory guiding the education approach is teaching remedial handwriting skills to school-aged children. The occupational therapy practitioner works with the child and the teacher to facilitate appropriate body posture, pencil grip, and concentration while also paying close attention to selection of appropriate writing tools and writing activities. The intervention is carefully designed to align with the child's developmental stage and expectations of the school setting.[8]

Occupational Therapy Models

Over the past 30 years, occupational therapy scholars have articulated theoretical frameworks and developed models that have defined broader understanding of the concepts relating to occupation.[9] The current PEOP Model and PEOP Occupational Therapy Process have proposed that principles guiding occupational therapy interventions include client-centered, evidence-based, ethics, client advocacy, effective communication, cultural sensitivity, professional lifelong development, and current business fundamentals.[10,11] As knowledge regarding these principles develops, the ability of occupational therapy practitioners to provide interventions through education also evolves.

LEARNING

It is perhaps wise to pause here and discuss what is meant by the term *learn*. In the action of education there is an implied outcome; an outcome described as learning. Learning occurs when there is change in the individual, group, or community. This can be a simple change, like an increase in knowledge or an understanding of the way to

Table 28-1. *A Program to Address Life Balance[14] Aligned With Education Approaches*

Education Activity	Occupational Therapy	Technology	Education Approaches
Learning about life balance	OT gives explicit instruction/ explanation about dimensions of lifestyle balance[14,15]	Create a website, use a blog or wiki with links, cite references	Behaviorist Developmental
Learning how to monitor life balance	OT prompts monitoring of lifestyle balance in each of the essential domains	Use online survey or app to monitor lifestyle balance (eg, Life Balance Inventory[16])	Behaviorist Developmental Authentic
Learning how improve life balance	Client uses education, support, cues, and prompts to implement changes in lifestyle	Apps for recording management of domains of concern (eg, relaxation techniques, diet, finances, activities)	Constructivist Transformative Authentic
Learning how to manage on-going life balance	Client self-monitors, self-questions, and solves problems with lifestyle balance	Create or join an online support group about life balance (use an online discussion forum or attend a group in Second Life, a multi-user virtual world)	Transformative Authentic

act in certain circumstances. However, the work of occupational therapy practitioners goes beyond simple learning to relevant and important changes for the client, group or community, ie, authentic and transformative learning.

Authentic Learning

Authentic or learner-centered learning has principles common to constructivist education.[12] When an intervention is based within the authentic learning model, the focus is primarily on the client's capacity within context: the environment in which the learning occurs (eg, home, community, work) and the relationship between the client and the educator, education materials, and the teaching strategies used by the occupational therapy practitioner.[13] Authentic learning focuses on the ability of the learner without constraint of developmental theory (ie, the age or stage of development is not the primary focus). In other words, the learner's needs are the primary focus and not their developmental stage. By understanding what is important to the client (referred to as *the narrative* in the PEOP Occupational Therapy Process) and through the assessment and evaluation of the client's needs, the occupational therapy practitioner is able to understand the client's occupational performance goals and current capacity to achieve them. The occupational therapy practitioner can then develop and implement an educational intervention that includes functional learning tasks; works toward the client's goals; and takes into consideration the demands

of the client's skills, abilities, and environment. An example is using a program developed to address life balance (Table 28-1), illustrating how an intervention, theory, and practice connect.[14]

A related learning model is the Four-Quadrant Model of Facilitated Learning (4QM), developed by Greber et al.[3,17,18] The 4QM depicts the teaching–learning approach used in occupational therapy practice.[3] This model illustrates the range of approaches an occupational therapy practitioner might use in practice. "It uses the integration of two continua—(i) directness of the strategy; and (ii) source of initiation of prompting—to group learning strategies into clusters based on the learner needs they serve."[3(p187)]

Transformative Learning

Transformative learning involves a deep shift in consciousness that alters thoughts, feelings, and actions. Often these changes emerge from exploration and understanding of the self; power relations in society; concepts of race, gender, and class; and social justice. As a result, this may help to envision a new way to interact at work, with family, and in society that expands capacity for tolerance, acceptance, understanding, and compassion.[19]

As a field of study, transformative learning has grown to include multiple and diverse areas of educational concern. It also ranges across a wide diversity of practice settings, including adult and continuing professional education, higher education, workplace learning, and education for social change. Transformative learning approaches in occupational therapy can be evident in the following ways.

In the role of educator the occupational therapy practitioner will:

- Establish an environment that builds trust and facilitates development of sensitive relationships.[20]
- View clients as a "community of knowers," individuals who are "united in a shared experience of trying to make meaning of their life experience."[21(p320)]
- Serve as a role model and demonstrate willingness to learn by expanding and deepening understanding of subject matter and teaching approaches.[22]

Therefore, an occupational therapy practitioner using a transformative learning approach will[23]:

- Provide a just-right challenge in learning tasks and environments
- Be interested in the learners and the knowledge they bring
- Avoid taking the role of being the font of all knowledge
- Be a provocateur and enable discourse
- Facilitate deep learning
- Be self-reflective

PREPARING FOR THE ROLE OF EDUCATOR

Mortiboys[13] suggested there are 3 key components to being an effective educator: having subject expertise, using effective learning and teaching methods, and having emotional intelligence. In occupational therapy, subject expertise is developed through knowledge relevant to the individuals, groups, and communities in practice, as well as being informed and guided by strong professional theory. The needs of clients are more likely to be met when theory and effective learning and teaching methods are used. Subject expertise related to practice in occupational therapy is discussed in detail throughout this text. The following section will focus on being aware of and encouraging emotional states that are conducive to learning and various educational tools that are available.

Learning-Style Theory

This is a good point to once again pause and reflect. Do you know how you like to learn? Can you be flexible in how you learn? Can you take your knowledge about how you learn and adapt this to your role as an educator? A key notion in constructivist approaches to education is the importance of matching teaching style to the client's learning style.[12] Therefore, to be an effective educator, occupational therapy practitioners need to understand learning-style theory and how clients learn.

When we become aware of our own learning preferences, we may notice that this preferred learning style is also our preferred approach to providing education for clients. Understanding our own learning style can preempt the tendency to develop education strategies exclusively in our dominant style (eg, a visual learner may always choose charts, pictures, or diagrams to explain concepts). Once we understand our own learning style(s), we are in a better position to reflect on clients' learning styles and design approaches that fit their needs.

Learning-style theory suggests that individuals have a preference for how they filter or take in information, and for the way that information is communicated to others. Some people like to learn something new via pictures, diagrams, or mind maps; others may like facts and more concrete things like dates, times, or statistics. Those who like learning via pictures will often draw a picture to communicate, and those that feel comfortable with facts and concrete items will give tangible examples to make their point. Of the many learning style assessment tools available in mainstream use, 2 of the most commonly referred to are VARK[24] and Kolb's Learning Style theory.[25] Many learning style assessments are available online; they offer a good start to a conversation about learning styles and can be an excellent foundation for discussion about the education approaches to meeting a client's needs.[26-28]

Emotional Intelligence

Emotional intelligence is defined as the ability to recognize, process, and respond to one's own emotions as well as others' emotions.[13] The concept of emotional intelligence was first developed by Mayer and Salovey, but it was the work of Goleman in the 1990s[13] that brought the concept into the public domain. Mayer and Salovey then expanded on the definition by suggesting that emotional intelligence consists of 5 domains: "knowing one's emotions, managing emotions, motivating oneself, recognizing emotions in others, and handling relationships."[29(p43)] Goleman recently summarized this, suggesting individuals need to develop and exercise 20 emotional intelligent competencies nested within the following 4 domains[30]:

1. The ability to recognize emotions
2. The ability to regulate emotions
3. The need to be competent in achieving both of these within our selves
4. The need to be competent in achieving both of these with others

Occupational therapy practitioners may recognize the impact of emotional intelligence as they reflect on professional practice and themselves in the role of educator.[20] Occupational therapy practitioners need to be caring and establish an environment where clients feel respected, safe, and fairly treated.[20] Practitioners need to interact in a socially competent manner, be enthusiastic and positive about learning, and hold a positive view of clients and the therapeutic relationship. A constructive, emotionally intelligent and professional relationship must be formed between an occupational therapy practitioner and clients.

DIGITAL TECHNOLOGY AS A TOOL FOR EDUCATION

Over the past 15 years, digital technology has transitioned from Web 1.0 (which was primarily a place to search and download information), to Web 2.0 (which provides tools that people can use to interact with each other to collaborate and build communities around shared interests).[31] The key difference between Web 1.0 and Web 2.0 has been the development of interactive or social media tools, such as wikis, blogs, podcasts, social networks, and discussion forums. Because individuals can interact with each other, these tools can harness the collective intelligence of the users.[32]

There is a plethora of health-related organized activities and information online, enabling clients to obtain professional opinions as well as authentic information and support from others managing similar issues.[31] Pew Internet research indicates that 83% of Internet users living with chronic conditions seek health information online, and Wardell et al found that over 80% of the people with multiple sclerosis (MS) who responded to their survey stated that they were interested in using digital technology to access education and supports for their MS.[33,34]

Health care professionals are also discovering, exploring, and using the freely available digital technology tools such as podcasts, blogs, and Twitter to provide health care information.[35] Digital technology offers a fast and inexpensive method of communication that may have a deeper level of connection and personalization.[33] Through social media, health care professionals are able to reach a larger and more diverse audience, and consumers can be active participants by producing and distributing information through collaborative writing and sharing of information.[33]

Five categories of digital technology that are central to education are proposed in this chapter. The categories depict a specific role in education; however, many digital technologies may fit more than one category. A summary of the categories and digital technology tools are outlined in Table 28-2.

Content Management

Content management systems facilitate the storage and retrieval of data. They allow a large number of people to share and contribute to creating or using stored data. In this context, the term *data* refers to documents, images, texts, music, articles, etc. In most systems, the creator of the content management system can control the role of the users and what they can view, edit, and publish. This technology simplifies communication and can streamline activities, such as shared report writing. Examples of content management programs include Google Drive and Joomla. See Table 28-2 for further examples.

Content Publishing

Also called content sharing, this category of programs enables users to present information to others in an organized and professional way. Both blogs and wikis can be used to publish on the Internet, often in the form of a website. Other programs, such as virtual pinboards, online curation services, and presentation programs, enable occupational therapy practitioners to publicly share content with others. These programs are described in Table 28-2.

Communication

Digital technology has changed how people communicate with each other. Programs such as Skype and Google Hangout enable Internet users to have live conversations with each other, usually using audio and video. Also called voice over Internet protocol (VoIP), this technology is usually cheap and easy to use, as long as a reliable Internet connection is available. Health care practitioners use this type of technology for remote consultations with clients and to attend free online professional development activities, such as the occupational therapy 24-hour exchange (OT24Vx) held on World Occupational Therapy Day.[41,42]

Networking

Health care professionals use networking as an important means of advancing knowledge and skills.[43] Over the past 15 years, our capacity to network with colleagues has rapidly expanded due to improved access to digital technology. One of the biggest areas of growth in the online world has been through social networking sites such as Facebook and LinkedIn. Firewalls are in place at many workplaces to protect sensitive information held on the computing system, which means that access to social networks is usually prevented or limited. Many health care practitioners are working around this by using personal mobile technology or accessing the sites from home.

Table 28-2. *Application of Digital Technology in Occupational Therapy Practice*

Tools	Description	Application
Content Management		
Collaborative writing (eg, Google Drive, ZohoWriter)	An online program that stores documents created by one or more people in a cloud drive. Facilitates editing and reviewing of a document by multiple individuals, either synchronously or asynchronously.	Write collaboratively with colleagues or clients. See example: https://www.zoho.com/docs/zoho-docs-tour.html
Personalized home page for web browsing (eg, Netvibes)	An online page that uses widgets and gadgets to assemble social networks, email, calendar, videos, and blogs, etc on one customizable home page. RSS feeds (programs that push information to your computer) enable automatic updates.	Create a personalized home page for a client with memory loss.
Scholarly databases (eg, Pubmed, Google Scholar)	A freely accessible Web search engine that indexes the full text of scholarly literature across an array of publishing formats and disciplines.	Research evidence to develop a program you are planning.
Bookmarking: Social bookmarking (eg, Diigo, Delicious)	A tool to bookmark (save) Web URLs in a virtual/online environment rather than on an individual computer. The user's account can be public, semi-public, or private. You can store a range of useful websites, comment on them, categorize them using tags, and share.	Save and tag websites under topic headings and share with colleagues and clients with similar interests. See example: http://www.diigo.com
Content Publishing		
Blog/Weblog (eg, Blogger, Wordpress)	A website where items are posted on a regular basis, with the most recent posts at the top. Usually a blog is about a single topic or theme, they can be reflective and/or educational.	Create site about your area of occupational therapy expertise as a knowledge translation tool. See example: http://healthskills.wordpress.com
Wiki (eg, Wikipedia, Ask Dr. Wiki)	A wiki is an interactive Web page designed to enable anyone who is allowed access the ability to contribute or modify content.	Create a resource for clients about a specific topic. See example: http://udltechtoolkit.wikispaces.com
Microblog (eg, Twitter)	An online program where users can submit text, hyperlinks, video, or pictures. Text entries are restricted to 140 characters.	Create a professional Twitter account and share news stories about occupational therapy. Search: #OT #OTResearch #Occhat or #OTalk for conversations about OT.
Curation services (eg, Storify, Scoopit, PaperLi)	Curation services are programs that collect and organize topics of interest. They facilitate creation of theme-based digital publications (eg, newsletters) and "makes the noisy web sensible."[36,37]	Create a digital newsletter with your client group using a program like paper.li or Storify. See example: http://tinyurl.com/otdaily
Virtual pinboard (eg, Pinterest)	A content sharing service that allows members to "pin" images, videos and other objects to their online/virtual pinboard.	Create a pinboard about a topic of shared interest and teach others how to contribute. See example: http://tinyurl.com/otpinterest

(continued)

Table 28-2 (continued).   *Application of Digital Technology in Occupational Therapy Practice*

Tools	Description	Application
Content Publishing		
Virtual presentation (eg, Slideshare, Prezi)	A platform for business documents, videos, and presentations. Anyone can share presentations and video, and both allow for users to find relevant content and connect with other members who share similar interests.	Create a series of informative presentations for your client group. See example: http://www.slideshare.net/BekiDellow/the-kawa-model-reflective-practice
Podcast/ Video cast (eg, YouTube, iTunes)	A series of audio or video digital media files that is distributed over the Internet by syndicated download (RSS), through Web feeds, to portable media players and personal computers. Users can download or upload to YouTube, iTunes, etc.	Create an educational video or podcast about occupational therapy. See example: http://tinyurl.com/aboutot
Communication		
VoIP (eg, Skype, Elluminate)	Enable users to talk in real time using the Internet. Can be audio, video, or both. Can be recorded and replayed using supplemental computer programs.	Having access to this technology can enable clients to remain socially connected and interact with health care professionals remotely.
Survey tools (eg, SurveyMonkey, Fluidsurveys)	An online survey system to deliver surveys and collect and analyze results all through one central system. Many also include interpretive graphics and charts.	Having access to this technology can enable clients to remain socially connected and interact with health care professionals remotely.
Networking		
Social network sites (eg, Facebook, LinkedIn)	Online communities of people who share interests and activities or who are interested in exploring the interests and activities of others.	Join or create a Facebook discussion group about your area of practice to help you connect with other occupational therapy practitioners around the globe. See example: https://www.facebook.com/groups/MH4OT
Discussion forums (eg, phpBB)	An online discussion space for people to interact with others who share a specific interest. Unlike online chats in which participants communicate synchronously, most discussion forums are asynchronous.	Find or create a discussion forum for your client population to discuss topics of shared interest. Note, occupational therapy practitioners should visit the site and check the reliability of the information before recommending a client uses it for support. See example: http://www.healthboards.com
Multi-User virtual world (eg, Second Life)	A virtual world where the user is represented by an avatar in a 3D virtual environment. Users can interact with each other. Information can be presented using text, audio, and video.[38]	Facilitate a client to join a virtual support group. See example: Occupational Therapy Center at Thomas Jefferson University, Philadelphia, PA; http://tinyurl.com/otsecondlife

(continued)

Table 28-2 (continued). *Application of Digital Technology in Occupational Therapy Practice*

Tools	Description	Application
Gaming		
Cognitive (eg, memory games, SPARX[38,39]) Physical (eg, Nintendo Wii) Social (eg, Farmville)	Gaming as an educational tool and to improve cognitive, physical, and social functioning is a growth area of research and practice in occupational therapy. Watch "7 ways games reward the brain"[39,40] for more information about the role of gaming.	Before recommending a game the occupational therapist needs to identify clear objectives and trial the game to see if it meets these educational or therapeutic objectives. See examples: http://memoryimprovementtips.com http://youtu.be/8HbbBT32Dll

Gaming

Gaming has been used in formal education for over 75 years and was introduced by Dewey and the Gestalt theorists (Barnett); there is evidence that gaming has been used as a teaching strategy as far back as 3500 BC.[44] The use of gaming such as World of Warcraft (Blizzard Entertainment, Inc), Words With Friends (Zynga, Inc), and Farmville (Zynga, Inc), has risen in prominence recently due to the rapid development of digital technology.

Using games in education offers clear advantages over more traditional didactic methods.[45] As a learning methodology, gaming can facilitate learning in cognitive, affective, and psychomotor domains[33]; build enthusiasm[46]; and enrich the effectiveness of educational interventions with diverse groups of learners.[36] Games can provide a way to link theory to reality and provide a forum for immediate feedback for the learners[45]; they can motivate participants to learn by doing, solve problems, experience failure in a safe environment without serious consequences; and learn from experience.[44]

Enhancing Trust in the Online Environment

All consumers of online health care information need to consider the source of information they plan to use.[31] It is important that health care practitioners understand the factors that contribute to *online trust* and promote confidence in using digital technologies. A model of online trust was developed by Corritore, Kracher, and Wiedenbeck[47]; it suggests trust is the outcome of an interaction between external factors with the perception of credibility, ease of use, and risk of using the online technology. External factors are aspects of the environment, both physical and psychological, surrounding the user of

the online technology[47] and including the personal characteristics of the individual, such as their "general propensity to trust"[35(p750)] and prior experience with using digital technologies.

Credibility includes "honesty, expertise, predictability, and reputation."[35(p750)] The credibility of an online resource, such as a website, can be enhanced by the overall appearance of the site, verification logos (such as HONCode),[48] sponsorship by a recognized government body or reputable organization, provision of a list of references, and information that is regularly updated and reviewed. When occupational therapy practitioners create online resources, they need to ensure that the site contains credible information and is easy to understand. Professionals develop the content and control most of these factors, but information technology support can be helpful in making the site easy to access and navigate and have a professional appearance.

Ease of use is an essential component in selecting technology for use in an educational intervention with a client or group. Occupational therapy practitioners need to have a good understanding of the range of technology tools available and how they can be applied in education; they need to be able to understand the relationship between an intervention and learning styles[49] that enable learning to take place, and carefully select the right tools to meet the goals of the education. *Universal design* is another principle that is central to ease of use. It is very important that sites are universally accessible so that the broadest range of people can access the site.[50]

Risk in providing online technologies requires consideration of exploitation, vulnerabilities, and the controls given to the user.[47] Occupational therapy practitioners can and should be using online technologies to create educational resources for clients. However, with this opportunity comes the responsibility to protect vulnerable clients. Occupational therapy practitioners often work with people who are seen as vulnerable, for example an individual with a TBI. It is essential that occupational therapy practitioners address online privacy, password protection, and overall security when educating clients about the risks associated with using online technologies.

EDUCATIONAL INTERVENTIONS USING THE PERSON-ENVIRONMENT-OCCUPATION-PERFORMANCE OCCUPATIONAL THERAPY PROCESS

Developing Educational Interventions

A growing area of practice for occupational therapy is to address the occupational concerns of a population. In this section, a case example of a population-based intervention is used to illustrate the process. (Please refer to the PEOP Occupational Therapy Process for a description of each stage of the process.) The intervention was planned using sound education theory and applying digital technology where appropriate to meet the needs of a group of people with a shared concern. The intervention was the development of an evidence-based educational program for caregivers who were caring for a family member who had survived an acquired brain injury (ABI). The focus of the intervention was on facilitating caregivers to teach skills retraining in the home, focusing on skills that are important to the individual with ABI and the caregiver.

Narrative

The first stage of the PEOP Occupational Therapy Process is to understand narrative. The narrative is the past, current, and future perceptions; choices; interests; goals and needs that are important to the person, organization, or population. The process guides the occupational therapy practitioner to use this context to address the personal performance capabilities/constraints and the environmental performance enabler/barriers that are central to occupational performance. The occupational therapy practitioner that developed the caregiver education program noticed that sometimes when her clients came to her life skills program they had lost confidence or skills between sessions. When she investigated this further, one client mentioned that when she asked for help at home her son would just do it for her. The son had no way of knowing that taking over was negatively reinforcing the skills being learned in class and undermining the confidence the mother was slowly developing. The occupational therapy practitioner realized she had unintentionally contributed to this outcome because she had not

offered education sessions for caregivers. She needed to inform caregivers about the aims of the life skills program and how breaking the teaching and learning into small steps needed to be positively reinforced at home to support the new skills being developed. The occupational therapy practitioner decided she needed to understand the needs of the caregivers who were taking on the specific education and supporting roles. She started this process by researching the literature using online databases and reviewed the agency's digital newsletter. The practitioner then developed a list of common concerns. Using digital technologies, such as online databases and newsletters, increased her understanding of the caregivers' narrative.

Assessment and Evaluation

The second stage of the PEOP Occupational Therapy Process is to assess and evaluate to reveal the constraints/barriers preventing achievement of occupational performance goals, and the capabilities/enablers that support occupational performance. The practitioner uses evidence and expertise to help the client understand what is possible and the challenges involved in achieving identified goals.

The occupational therapy practitioner developed an online survey to assess the needs of the caregivers using the data she had collected in the narrative. Online surveys can provide a feeling of greater anonymity, are time and cost efficient, and (if designed well) are easy to interpret. The data obtained through the survey revealed that caregivers had concerns about their level of competence and confidence in supporting individuals with ABI to learn new skills.[51] The survey also revealed that the caregivers had difficulty balancing roles and managing relationships; some experienced financial strain, and others reported difficulty trusting the individual with ABI to be safe when learning a new task. A perceived lack of community-based support was also a major concern for the caregivers.[51]

The occupational therapy practitioner reported the findings of the survey to the key stakeholders at the agency: the Executive Director, the staff member running a caregiver support group, another occupational therapy practitioner, and a caregiver representative. The group discussed the findings in the context of the agency's vision and mission, funding, and other programs already offered and considered options for a future intervention that would meet the needs of these caregivers.

Intervention

Developing an intervention to overcome the limitations and barriers to work toward achieving the agreed goals is the third stage of the PEOP Occupational Therapy Process. The model highlights the importance of the client, practitioner, and caregivers all working collaboratively to implement interventions that will assist the client to achieve goals. The intervention must be based on the best available evidence and actively involve the client in the decision-making process. Identifying and communicating the evidence for a given intervention not only promotes sound reasoning, it also reflects the highest principles of ethical practice. This is also consistent with a constructivist approach to intervention.

The occupational therapy practitioner and caregivers collaborated to develop an education program with 3 components.[52] The first component was designed to teach caregivers about brain injury and recovery and how to manage the physical, cognitive, emotional, and behavioral issues of the individual with ABI. The second component was designed to assist the caregiver to understand the reasons why occupational therapy used a step-by-step educational process in the life skills program. Finally, each caregiver was given an opportunity to focus on one particular life skill that was needed to assist in working with the individual with ABI at home.

Outcome

The final stage of the PEOP Occupational Therapy Process is to identify the outcome of the intervention. To measure the outcome of the intervention, the occupational therapy practitioner designed a pre-program and post-program assessment. Pre-program and post-program assessments are important as they provide the practitioner with an understanding of the baseline, the starting point, and the finishing point of the participants. The information is used to illustrate the growth, development, and learning that occurred during the program. Including pre-assessments and post-assessments are particularly important for reporting tangible outcomes of the program, as it helps identify areas that worked well and areas for improvement for the next program. These findings may be reported at conferences and in journals so that others may benefit, when the learning was part of a research study that included approval from an institutional review board. (Of course, to conclude that the intervention had an effect on the outcome, it is important to have random assignment to an intervention and a control/comparison group and other characteristics of strong research designs to make definitive conclusions.) Information from pre- and post-assessments may also be used as evidence of efficacy and efficiency to support applications for funding of future programs.

In our example, the practitioner developed an online survey based on the needs assessment undertaken in the evaluation stage mentioned previously. The caregivers were also asked to complete an independent online assessment tool that examined the caregiver's level of "strain."[53]

Caregiver strain is a commonly found phenomenon in those who care for a family member. Utilizing an independent, online, simple assessment tool like the Modified Caregiver Strain Index (MCSI) provided the occupational therapy practitioner with further reliable and valid information. Following completion of the program, caregivers felt they were able to engage more effectively in their caregiver role and protect themselves against burnout. The outcome survey revealed that at times caregivers needed additional support between sessions and outside business hours. It was proposed that the agency could look into developing an online support service that would be run by the agency's staff and trained volunteers. At this point the practitioner returned to the first stage of the PEOP Occupational Therapy Process. In this scenario, the new narrative was providing ad-hoc support to caregivers who were actively engaged in ongoing rehabilitation in the home and who needed additional support outside business hours.

SUMMARY

The PEOP Occupational Therapy Process maps out the process of occupational therapy when working toward achieving improved occupational performance with individuals, groups, or populations. Education is a key approach to enabling occupation, therefore occupational therapy practitioners need to understand and apply education and learning theories in the context of their practice. Digital technology has emerged as a central tool to facilitate education. Therefore occupational therapy practitioners need to use and apply digital technologies in therapeutic and educational interventions.

REFERENCES

1. WFOT. Definition of Occupational Therapy. WFOT: About Occupational Therapy. http://www.wfot.org/aboutus/aboutoccupationaltherapy/definitionofoccupationaltherapy.aspx Published 2012. Accessed August 4, 2013.
2. Greber C, Ziviani J, Rodger S. Clinical utility of the four-quadrant model of facilitated learning: perspectives of experienced occupational therapists. *Australian Occupational Therapy Journal.* 2011;58(3):187-194.
3. Berkeland R, Flinn N. Therapy as learning. In: Christiansen C, Baum CM, Bass Haugen J, eds. *Occupational Therapy: Performance, Participation and Well-Being.* 3rd ed. Thorofare, NJ: SLACK Incorporated; 2005:421-448.
4. Christiansen C, Baum CM, Bass Haugen J. *Occupational Therapy: Performance, Participation, and Well-Being.* Thorofare, NJ: SLACK Incorporated; 2005.
5. McEneany J, McKenna K, Summerville P. Australian occupational therapists working in adult physical dysfunction settings: what treatment media do they use? *Australian Occupational Therapy Journal.* 2002;49(3):115-127.

6. Rodger S, Brown GT, Brown A. Profile of paediatric occupational therapy practice in Australia. *Australian Occupational Therapy Journal.* 2005;52(4):311-325.

7. Townsend E, Beagan B, Zofia K-T, et al. Enabling: occupational therapy's core competency. In: Townsend EA, Polatajko HJ, eds. *Enabling Occupation II: Advancing an Occupational Therapy Vision for Health, Well-Being and Justice Through Occupation.* Ottawa, ON: Canadian Association of Occupational Therapists; 2007:87-132.

8. Illeris K. *Contemporary Theories of Learning: Learning Theorists—In Their Own Words.* New York, NY: Routledge; 2009.

9. Hooper B. Epistemological transformation in occupational therapy: educational implications and challenges. *OTJR: Occupation, Participation and Health.* 2006;26(1):15-24.

10. Baum CM, Christiansen CH, Bass JD. The Person-Environment-Occupational-Performance (PEOP) Model. In: Christiansen CH, Baum CM, Bass JD, eds. *Occupational Therapy: Performance, Participation, and Well-Being.* 4th ed. Thorofare, NJ: SLACK Incorporated; 2015.

11. Bass JD, Baum CM, Christiansen CH. Interventions and Outcomes of OT: PEOP Occupational Therapy Process. In: Christiansen CH, Baum CM, Bass JD, eds. In: *Occupational Therapy: Performance, Participation, and Well-Being.* 4th ed. Thorofare, NJ: SLACK Incorporated; 2015.

12. Matthews WJ. Constructivism in the classroom: epistemology, history, and empirical evidence. *Teacher Education Quarterly.* 2003;30(3):51-64.

13. Mortiboys A. *Teaching with Emotional Intelligence: A Step-by-Step Guide for Higher and Further Education Professionals.* New York NY: Taylor & Francis; 2005.

14. Matuska KM, Christiansen CH. A proposed model of lifestyle balance. *Journal of Occupational Science.* 2008;15(1):9-19.

15. Wagman P, Håkansson C, Matuska KM, Björklund A, Falkmer T. Validating the model of lifestyle balance on a working Swedish population. *Journal of Occupational Science.* 2012;19(2):106-114.

16. Matuska KM. *Life Balance Inventory.* St. Catherine University: life balance inventory. http://minerva.stkate.edu/LBI.nsf. Published 2009. Accessed June 5, 2012.

17. Greber C, Ziviani J, Rodger S. The Four-Quadrant Model of Facilitated Learning (part 1): using teaching-learning approaches in occupational therapy. *Australian Occupational Therapy Journal.* 2007;54:S31-S39.

18. Greber C, Ziviani J, Rodger S. The Four-Quadrant Model of Facilitated Learning (part 2): strategies and applications. *Australian Occupational Therapy Journal.* 2007;54:S40-S48.

19. Mezirow J. *Learning as Transformation: Critical Perspectives on a Theory in Progress.* San Francisco, CA: Jossey-Bass; 2000.

20. Taylor RR, Lee SW, Kielhofner G, Ketkar M. Therapeutic use of self: a nationwide survey of practitioners' attitudes and experiences. *American Journal of Occupational Therapy.* 2009;63(2):198-207.

21. Loughlin KA. *Women's Perceptions of Transformative Learning Experiences Within Consciousness-Raising.* San Francisco, CA: Mellen Research University Press; 1993.

22. Cranton P. *Understanding and Promoting Transformative Learning: A Guide for Educators of Adults.* San Francisco, CA: Jossey-Bass; 1994.

23. Hamilton A, Burwash S. *Professional and Educational Conceptual Framework: Curriculum Philosophy.* Edmonton, AB: University of Alberta; 2008.

24. Leite WL, Svinicki M, Shi Y. Attempted validation of the scores of the VARK: learning styles inventory with multitrait-multimethod confirmatory factor analysis models. *Educational and Psychological Measurement.* 2009;70(2):323-339.

25. Kayes DC. Internal validity and reliability of Kolb's Learning Style Inventory. Version 3 (1999). *Journal of Business and Psychology.* 2005;20(2):249-257.

26. Clark D. *Learning Style Survey.* Big dog's & little dog's performance juxtaposition: learning style survey. http://www.nwlink.com/~donclark/hrd/styles/learn_style_survey.html. Published 2000. Accessed June 5, 2012.

27. Hay Group. Kolb Learning Style Inventory (KLSI). Version 4 Online. Hay Group. http://www.haygroup.com/leadershipandtalentondemand/ourproducts/item_details.aspx?itemid=118&type=2. Published 2012. Accessed June 5, 2012.

28. Fleming N. The VARK Questionnaire. VARK: a guide to learning styles. http://www.vark-learn.com/english/page.asp?p=questionnaire. Published 2010. Accessed June 5, 2012.

29. Goleman D. *Emotional Intelligence.* 10th anniversary ed. New York, NY: Random House Digital; 2012.

30. Goleman D. An EI-based theory of performance. In: Goleman D, Cherniss C, eds. *The Emotionally Intelligent Workplace: How to Select for, Measure, and Improve Emotional Intelligence in Individuals, Groups, and Organizations.* San Francisco, CA: Jossey-Bass; 2000:27-44.

31. Hamilton A. Diffusion of innovation: web 2.0. *Occupational Therapy Now.* 2010;12(1):18-21.

32. O'Reilly T. What is web 2.0: design patterns and business models for the next generation of software. *Communications and Strategies.* 2007;1:17.

33. Yarrow L. Becoming social media savvy: using web 2.0 to enhance education. *Topics in Clinical Nutrition.* 2012;27(1):34-40.

34. Wardell L, Hum S, Laizner A, Lapierre Y. Multiple sclerosis patients' interest in and likelihood of using online health-care services. *International Journal of MS Care.* 2009;11(2):79-89.

35. Hamilton A. Diffusion of innovation web 2.0. *Occupational Therapy Now.* 2010;12(1):18-21.

36. Gary R, Marrone S, Boyles C. The use of gaming strategies in a transcultural setting. *Journal of Continuing Education in Nursing.* 1998;29(5):221-227.

37. Rosenbaum S. Curate the cloud. *EContent.* 2011;34(10):28-29.

38. Lee M. How can 3D virtual worlds be used to support collaborative learning? An analysis of cases from the literature. *Journal of e-Learning and Knowledge Society—English Version.* 2009;5(1):149-158.

39. Merry SN, Stasiak K, Shepherd M, et al. The effectiveness of SPARX, a computerised self help intervention for adolescents seeking help for depression: randomised controlled non-inferiority trial. *BMJ.* 2012;344:e2598-e2598.

40. Chatfield T. *Tom Chatfield: 7 Ways Games Reward the Brain.* TED.com: ideas worth spreading. http://www.ted.com/talks/tom_chatfield_7_ways_games_reward_the_brain.html. Accessed June 12, 2012.

41. McMullen E. Use of audiovisual equipment (SKYPE) for the treatment of hand injuries for remote consultations. *Hand Therapy.* 2012;17(2):42-46.

42. OT4OT. Online technology 4 occupational therapy: using online technology to advance occupational therapy. *Online Technology 4 Occupational Therapy.* http://ot4ot.com/. Updated 2012. Accessed June 12, 2012.

43. Kashani R, Burwash S, Hamilton A. To be or not to be on Facebook: that is the question. *Occupational Therapy Now.* 2010;12(6):19-22. http://www.caot.ca/otnow/Nov10ENG/Facebook.pdf. Published 2010. Accessed August 4, 2013.

44. Henry JM. Gaming: a teaching strategy to enhance adult learning. *Journal of Continuing Education in Nursing.* 1997;28(5):231-234.

45. Barnett DJ, Everly Jr GS, Parker CL, Links JM. Applying educational gaming to public health workforce emergency preparedness. *American Journal of Preventive Medicine.* 2005;28(4):390-395. http://www.sciencedirect.com/science/article/pii/S0749379705000024. Published 2005. Accessed June 6, 2012.

46. Pennington J, Hawley P. Use of educational gaming to enhance theory learning. *Journal of the New York State Nurses' Association.* 1995;26(3):4-6.

47. Corritore CL, Kracher B, Wiedenbeck S. On-line trust: concepts, evolving themes, a model. *International Journal of Human-Computer Studies.* 2003;58(6):737-758.

48. Anon. *Health On the Net (HON): Health On the Net Code of Conduct (HONcode).* http://www.hon.ch/HONcode/. Accessed June 12, 2012.

49. Kirschner PA. Can we support CCSL?: educational, social and technological affordances. In: Three worlds of CSCL: can we support CSCL? Open Universiteit Nederland. http://dspace.ou.nl/bitstream/1820/1618/1/Three%20worlds%20of%20CSCL%20Can%20we%20support%20CSCL.pdf. Accessed September 21, 2014.

50. Horton S. *Universal Usability: A Universal Design Approach to Web Usability.* http://universalusability.com/. Accessed June 12, 2012.

51. Tang R. *Survey: Exploring Caregiver Education and Support Needs of Families Caring for a Person with an Acquired Brain Injury* (unpublished manuscript). Edmonton, AB: University of Alberta, Faculty of Rehabilitative Medicine, Department of Occupational Therapy; 2012.

52. Fong M. *Use of Logic Modelling and Knowledge Translation to Facilitate Skill Retraining in Acquired Brain Injury Survivors and Reduce Strain in their Caregivers* (unpublished manuscript). Edmonton, AB: University of Alberta, Faculty of Rehabilitative Medicine, Department of Occupational Therapy; 2012.

53. Onega LL. Helping those who help others: the modified caregiver strain index. *American Journal of Nursing.* 2008;108(9):62-69.

Chapter 29

A POPULATION-CENTERED STRATEGY
Public and Community Health

Gretchen V. M. Stone, PhD, OTR, FAOTA

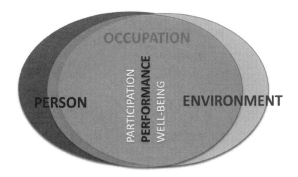

LEARNING OBJECTIVES

- Describe how the PEOP Model frames interventions focused on population-centered and community-centered outcomes, while retaining the occupational performance of a particular person as the ultimate desired outcome.
- Analyze how the health of a community is affected when barriers or enablers in one domain of the PEOP Model creates barriers or enablers in the other domains.
- Adopt language and terminology used in population health to describe how occupational therapy services contribute to the welfare of a community.
- Explain why it is important for occupational therapy practitioners to be knowledgeable about the goals of organizations and stakeholders they serve.
- On the basis of a case example, analyze how occupation-based assessment and intervention address priority population-based health concerns at the local, state, and national level.
- Compare and contrast population-centered intervention strategies that target disease management, health promotion, and delivery of health services.
- Explain how the PEOP Occupational Therapy Process may facilitate successful intervention outcomes.
- Identify ways that occupational therapy practitioners can learn more about public health.

KEY WORDS

- Community health assessment
- Comorbidity
- Consumer-directed care
- Disability-adjusted life year (DALY)
- Disease burden

Christiansen CH, Baum CM, Bass JD, eds.
Occupational Therapy: Performance, Participation, and Well-Being, Fourth Edition (pp 527-546).
© 2015 SLACK Incorporated.

- Epidemiology
- Health care utilization
- Health disparities
- Health promotion
- Health/public policy
- Home and community care services
- Integrated care
- Mission statement
- Morbidity rate
- Mortality rate
- Nongovernmental organization
- Participatory action research
- Patient-Reported Outcomes Measurement Information System (PROMIS) Global health measure
- Public-private partnership (PPP)

OVERVIEW

This chapter broadens occupational therapy practice to include public and community health. Public and community health encompasses prevention of avoidable diseases and conditions, promotion of desirable health-related behavior, and a broad spectrum of population-based intervention strategies designed to reduce the effects of progressive or chronic diseases and conditions.

- *Why are occupational therapy practitioners uniquely positioned to advance public and community health?*

Occupational therapy practitioners examine relationships among factors that influence health by drawing upon their foundation in science and theory to explain and influence how, why, and when people engage in some health-related activities and not others. Practitioners who adopt the PEOP Model examine how people use their time (their occupations), where and with whom they engage in occupations (their environment), strengths and challenges (unique to them as a person), and how they manage daily life activities (performance.) Each of these components in the model is critical to sustaining health, and therefore each of these components is incorporated either directly or indirectly into public and community health initiatives.

- *What obstacles are occupational therapy practitioners likely to face in public and community health settings?*

Occupational therapy practitioners must learn to adopt a population-based perspective as well as a person-centered perspective. Adopting a population-based perspective means learning new terminology and new ways of conceptualizing and measuring outcomes. People who embrace population-based perspectives formulate goals and design interventions based on targeted outcomes that are aligned with public policy and driven by available funding, rather than the needs of one person. Occupational therapy practitioners working in public health settings typically offer services within primary care and prevention models of health care, rather than models of health care focused on rehabilitation. They learn to work in an organizational structure with an interdisciplinary team perspective that is different from a more traditional medical model. People on the team include local elected officials, activists and advocates working outside the framework of government, health department employees, community health workers (CHWs), and many other people who are joined by common concerns. People working in population and community health settings may not be aware of what occupational therapy practitioners can offer, and don't know what to expect. It is critical for occupational therapy practitioners who are nested within communities to communicate effectively to a broad audience, note unmet needs, and offer strategies for addressing unresolved challenges and problems. The PEOP Model offers a working guide for occupational therapy practitioners as they identify problems and propose interventions for populations of people living within specific communities.

- *How are assumptions that guide population and community health different than assumptions that guide person-centered practice?*

Perspectives that guide population health are informed by knowledge of the collective strengths and challenges known to a group of people with a common condition or experience, rather than the needs and preferences of one person with an impairment or handicapping condition. Assessment and intervention is population-centered, in that needs and plans are calculated on the basis of large data sets representing factors that are known to determine health outcomes. Thus, the health of populations is defined in terms of determinants that describe characteristics of groups of people. Social determinants include a number of characteristics (eg, income, social status, social support, education, employment) and have been described in a variety of ways. Occupational therapy practitioners committed to population health are focused on the ability of a population of people to circumvent, change, or adapt to situations that affect their health so that they are able to participate in society

- *What knowledge and skills do occupational therapy practitioners have to inform public policy?*

The nature of services that enable populations of people with chronic and/or progressive conditions to engage in the same activities as other people and to live at home is of increasing interest to those who have the authority to formulate health policy and allocate funding for health care. Participation in society is a health outcome. Achieving this outcome requires careful examination of relationships among multiple factors. For example, exercise may be a health-promoting behavior among people with diabetes, but understanding why people with diabetes who live in a particular geographical area (a population) do not exercise on a regular basis begs investigation of multiple interacting factors. These interacting factors include how populations of people spend their time (their occupations), where and with whom they engage in occupations (their environment), their common strengths and challenges, and how they manage daily life activities (performance.) Analysis of interacting factors helps to clarify the relative impact of different determinants of health. This type of analysis is critical to inform health policy. Occupational therapy practitioners who choose careers in public and community health have the potential to implement change at the societal level.

INTRODUCTION

The profession of occupational therapy was founded in response to population-based needs, particularly the occupational needs of a population of people with mental illness living in a particular situation. Today, occupational therapy practitioners are expanding awareness of the value of human occupation in their own communities, across their native lands, and across the globe. The profession is claiming its rightful role in prevention of avoidable diseases and conditions and promotion of desirable health-related behavior by formulating occupation-based intervention strategies that reduce the effects of progressive or chronic diseases and conditions. Occupation-based intervention strategies based on the PEOP Model are population-specific and community-specific because the model adopts a systems perspective. Components of the model influence and are influenced by one another; that is, components of the model represent phenomena that are dynamic. The phenomena examined within each component of the PEOP Model are revealed in new ways when circumstances change. Systematic application of the PEOP Model and the PEOP Occupational Therapy Process influence the nature of occupation-based interventions critical for the health and well-being of populations living in different cultures and geographical regions and under different socioeconomic conditions.

Each section of this chapter adopts a similar format. Population and community health concerns are framed as questions informed by the literature, by evidence, and by official documents. An illustrative case describes how people worked together to develop low-cost strategies to address the unmet needs of an under-served population. This case is an example of the PEOP Model and PEOP Occupational Therapy Process for planning population-centered interventions. A state legislature, several universi-

ties, a community, and a group of dedicated health professions' students worked together to address the "burden of disease" by implementing strategies to meet the needs of people living with diabetes in a specific geographical region of Texas. The case will highlight a population of people living with or at-risk for diabetes in Texas, a specific community (colonia); and the organizations that work in this community; and one person in the colonia, Mrs. C., who has diabetes and other personal and environmental characteristics that are not uncommon in the colonia.

PUBLIC AND COMMUNITY HEALTH NARRATIVES

How Does a Case Illustrate the Narratives of the Population, Community, and Person?

The PEOP Occupational Therapy Process emphasizes the narrative as a starting point for planning occupational therapy interventions. This case is about a population of people with diabetes in Texas living in a poor community known as a colonia and a person, Mrs. C., who has diabetes and is a community member. Read and reflect on the narratives of the population, community, and person in this case to set the stage for learning about public and community health narratives (Box 29-1).

How Do People Across the World Work Together to Further the Goal of Public and Community Health?

Collective action is needed to establish the conditions that enable people to live healthy lives. The World Health Organization (WHO) was created as a means of:

> ... directing and coordinating authority for health within the United Nations system. It is responsible for providing leadership on global health matters, shaping the health research agenda, setting norms and standards, articulating evidence-based policy options, providing technical support to countries and monitoring and assessing health trends.[9(np)]

Promoting health involves processes that support people in assuming responsibility for their health.[10] Implicit in the WHO's definition of health and health promotion is the idea that health is influenced by the actions people take, the beliefs people hold, and the ability of people to access what they want and need to take care of themselves.

Cognitive Behavioral Therapies (CBTs) propose that what people know and think affects how they act.

BOX 29-1

THE NARRATIVE FOR A POPULATION, COMMUNITY, AND PERSON IN TEXAS

Population

Diabetes is a serious public health problem in Texas. In 2007, there were an estimated 1.8 million adults with diabetes and an additional 460,040 adults with undiagnosed diabetes. Prevalence is slightly higher in females (10.8%), Hispanics (12.3%), and non-Hispanic Blacks (12.9%), as compared to males (9.9%) and non-Hispanic Whites (8.5%). Diabetes is the sixth leading cause of death in Texas. In 2005, 5593 deaths were directly attributed to diabetes, for a mortality rate of 30 deaths per 100,000 persons. The mortality rates for Hispanics (52 per 100,000) and non-Hispanic Blacks (55 per 100,000) are more than double that of non-Hispanic Whites (21 per 100,000). In 2006, the financial costs of diabetes exceeded $12 billion in Texas. Hospitalization is a major contributor to the overall cost of diabetes in Texas; in 2003, 204,242 hospital admissions cost $3.6 million. The burden of diabetes and its complications are expected to increase in the coming years; it is estimated the total number of diabetes cases in Texas will increase by 59% in the next 30 years, from 1.8 million in 2007 to almost 2.9 million in 2040.[1] The burden of diabetes (ie, mortality and morbidity rates) are calculated from population data and has been linked with other medical conditions (eg, cancers, diabetic retinopathy, decline in mental function). Local government emphasizes the burden of diabetes care, because health services are provided by agencies within home communities and diabetes can be a complex medical condition.[2] People with diabetes may require multiple medications and need follow-up visits. Diabetes care for complex needs cannot be addressed within the 10- to 15-minute appointments typically scheduled with primary care providers. Thus, many agencies are unable to provide recommended national guidelines.[2(p1613)]

Community

The community in which Mrs. C. lives is known as a *colonia*. There are over 100 similar colonias throughout the region. This particular colonia consists of small mobile homes or wooden structures situated on ranch land that was divided into small plots nearly 40 years ago and sold to people who dreamed of owning their own homes. The land is not viable for growing home gardens due to drainage problems, poor soil, and insecticides from nearby crop fields.[3] A mountain-shaped toxic dump lies within several miles of the colonia, and is surrounded by a tall barbed wire fence, illuminated by flood lights, and kept under surveillance.[4] The community is non-incorporated, meaning there is no governmental responsibility for potable water, sewage, roads, or drainage. There is a small grocery store and a Catholic church within walking distance. The nearest community with high schools, medical clinics, or retail stores is more than 30 miles away. With a few exceptions, citizens are legal residents. Most men work as laborers on surrounding ranch land and many older men served in the military. Women have traditionally remained at home to care for their families; widows depend on their families for income or work as housekeepers some distance away. The population of children is dwindling as young adults seek employment in neighboring towns or enlist in the military. Houses are rarely sold and bought; family or other community members either remain in the same house for years or rotate among several different homes. Multigenerational families are the rule, rather than the exception. The prevalence of diabetes in the colonias is proportionately higher as compared with that in the county or larger region.[5] Type 1 diabetes is common among family members. This region reports the highest rate of amputations due to diabetes per square mile of any other region in the country. People in this community seek medical attention from a public health clinic in the neighboring town, or travel an hour to a hospital emergency room in the closest city. The cost of hospital re-admits incurred by people living in colonias, both in terms of Medicare and Medicaid, has become unsustainable. To address this problem, the state legislature awarded a 3-year grant for university–community partnerships to develop strategies for containing costs. The intent is to implement an integrated care model characterized by alignment and collaboration within and between the medical intervention and care at the level of organizations and providers.[6]

Person

Mrs. C. is a 54-year-old Hispanic woman diagnosed with hypertension, diabetes, obesity, and depression. She reports she has a bulging disc in her cervical spine and pain in her wrist, neck, and back. Mrs. C. uses a borrowed straight leg cane on her right side and wears a brace on her left wrist to alleviate pain. Her daughter, who lives

(continued)

BOX 29-1 (CONTINUED)

THE NARRATIVE FOR A POPULATION, COMMUNITY, AND PERSON IN TEXAS

nearby, purchased the brace from a drug store. Mrs. C. was a housekeeper most of her life, but is no longer able to work due to her physical status. Her daily routine includes doing dishes and laundry. Until recently, she was able to shop for groceries by using an electric cart provided by a small local store down the road. Now she is unable to walk the distance without falling, as the road is unpaved and lacks a drainage system. Mrs. C. has a car and is able to drive, but does not have money to pay for gas or car insurance, so is dependent upon her daughter, who lives nearby, to buy groceries and complete "bigger tasks." Although she is a legal resident of the United States, Mrs. C. has not contributed to social security and has no means of supporting herself. Her husband, a farm laborer, passed away 10 years ago of cancer. She lives alone in one of the colonia's mobile homes at the end of a dirt road, outside of an established health district.[7] Although Mrs. C. is eligible for county health services,[5] she chooses not to go there because of previous unpleasant experiences.[8] Her primary source of health care is the hospital emergency room approximately 30 miles away.

Perceptions, motivations, skills, and social environment are key influences on behavior. CBTs that stress awareness of thoughts and behaviors include the Health Belief Model, Transtheoretical Model (or Stages of Change), Theory of Planned Behavior (TPB), and Precaution Adoption Process Model (PAPM). Other theories have a social change focus on the level of society, including Social Cognitive Theory, Community Organization and Other Participatory Models, Diffusion of Innovations Theory, and Communication Theory.

How Do Communities Plan, Conduct, and Evaluate Health Promotion and Disease Prevention Programs?

Models for planning, conducting, and evaluating health promotion and disease prevention programs are typically created by governmental agencies or organizations (eg, US Centers for Disease Control and Prevention [CDC]) in partnership with state and local health departments, community groups, or by researchers in academic settings who partner with community health agencies and receive grant funding to cover their costs. University and community partnerships are tasked with developing models that are supported by evidence. Funding for these types of grants is available from the federal government or from nongovernmental agencies (NGOs), eg, the Robert Wood Johnson Foundation. One example of a project funded by the Robert Wood Johnson Foundation is Mobilizing Action Toward Community Health (MATCH): Metrics, Incentives, and Partnerships for Population Health.[11] MATCH was developed at the University of Wisconsin—Madison Population Health Institute. This model is designed to address 2 primary questions, "How are we doing, and how can we do better?" The model uses a logic

model to represent how goals, activities, metrics, and outcomes are related to one another. Logic models show how interventions or incentives can be used to improve population health and reduce health disparities. For example, the principal activities included in the MATCH logic model are

... 1) producing county health rankings in all 50 states, 2) examining partnerships and organizational models to increase involvement and accountability for population health improvement, and 3) developing incentive models to encourage and reward communities that implement evidence-based programs and policies that improve population health.[11(np)]

Other models have also been used to guide public health programs. Mobilizing for Action through Planning and Partnerships (MAPP), the Planned Approach to Community Health (PATCH), and the PRECEDE-PROCEED model (PRECEDE = Predisposing, Reinforcing, and Enabling Constructs in Educational/Ecological Diagnosis and Evaluation; and PROCEED = Policy, Regulatory, and Organizational Constructs in Educational and Environmental Development) are based on evidence and stresses collection of data to inform evidence-based public health practice.[12] Theories and models may seem abstract, but they are critical for communities who want to know how to plan, conduct, and evaluate health promotion and disease prevention programs. The US Department of Health and Human Services published a guide for health promotion practice that distinguishes the place of theories vs models in health promotion. According to this guide, *Theory at a Glance: A Guide for Health Promotion Practice*, theories are based on principles and they seek to explain processes.[13] Models do not attempt to explain, but offer a guide for applying theory by providing a plan to investigate a phenomenon.[13]

What Health Issues Take the Highest Priority, and How Are These Determined?

The US Department of Health and Human Services publicizes 10-year goals and objectives for health promotion and disease prevention under the title Healthy People 2020.[14] One significant change in Healthy People 2020 is a set of high-priority heath issues that represent significant threats to the public's health. There are 26 Leading Health Indicators (LHIs) organized under 12 topic areas. The LHIs address determinants of health that promote QOL (quality of life), healthy behaviors, and health development across all life stages.[14] Setting public health priorities is a process that focuses on improving the health of the population as distinct from focusing on the health of individuals, and leads to a more integrated approach to health care. Public health programs consider contextual influences (such as public policies, culture, and the natural environment) and community influences (such as material resources, collective lifestyles and health practices, social interactions, the built environment, health services, and biological characteristics).

PUBLIC AND COMMUNITY HEALTH ASSESSMENTS

How Does a Case Illustrate an Assessment of the Population, Community, and Person?

The PEOP Occupational Therapy Process emphasizes assessment/evaluation as an important next step for planning occupational therapy interventions. Continue your learning about the case and this population of people with diabetes in Texas living in a poor community known as a colonia and a person, Mrs. C., who has diabetes and is a community member. Read and reflect on the description of population, community, and person assessments (Box 29-2) and the graphic organizer figures for the community (Figure 29-1) and for Mrs. C. (Figure 29-2) to set the stage for learning about public and community health assessments.

How Are Public and Community Health Assessed?

Priority health issues are informed by observing and tracking the health of a population and health statistics.

Public health policies and practices also monitor societal conditions that people need to keep healthy. Although the primary goal of public health is prevention, it falls to public health to measure and monitor health-related concerns when people are not healthy. Epidemiology is the science that informs these functions and is the branch of medicine that deals with the incidence, distribution, and control of diseases. Epidemiological studies provide prevalence and risk factor data, mortality data, complication-specific data, and strategies for controlling complications from specific diseases. These studies also enable public health initiatives to target medical conditions or health-related impairments by providing information about health indicators such as geographic region, availability of local resources, socioeconomic status, occupational hazards, and vulnerability due to natural and man-made disasters. Epidemiology provides the data to calculate the *burden* of specific diseases and impairments; society strives to address the burden.

How Is the Cost of Poor Health Calculated?

From a population perspective, poor health is calculated in terms of *burden of disease*. There is no common definition for this phrase, although it represents a means of calculating the cost of providing medical intervention for a specific disease and associated lost productivity to society. In 2000, the WHO adopted a strategy for measuring overall disease burden.[31] This measure, known as the disability-adjusted life year, or DALY, is the number of years lost due to ill-health, disability, or early death. The DALY is based on the idea that time is the most appropriate measure of the effects of chronic illness, both time lost due to premature death and time spent disabled by disease. According the WHO website, DALYs are calculated by taking the sum of 2 components: (expected or average number of) Years of Life Lost (YLL) and Years Lived with Disability (YLD). One DALY, therefore, is equal to 1 year of healthy life lost.[31] Looking at the burden of diseases via DALYs is one indication of a population's health. When the prevalence of a disease increases, the cost of providing care for people living with that disease increases. Epidemiological studies in the US are largely under the purview of the CDC. One mission of the CDC is to identify national health priorities on the basis of available data. The CDC website includes links for Diseases and Conditions as well as Data and Statistics. This enables public health officials to secure data and trends for specific geographical regions. The CDC generates many different public reports about health, including those most central to the practice of occupational therapy, such as

BOX 29-2

ASSESSMENT AND EVALUATION FOR A POPULATION, COMMUNITY, AND PERSON IN TEXAS

Population

The Texas Department of State Health Services *Diabetes Data: Surveillance and Evaluation*[15] uses population data to evaluate diabetes prevention and control programs. Diabetes incidence, prevalence, morbidity, and mortality rates are tracked using several data sources and monitored especially for high-risk populations. The Texas Behavioral Risk Factor Surveillance System, Health Plan Employer Data and Information Set (HEDIS), and TMF Health Quality Institute provide reliable data for diabetes burden reports and planning and implementing programs.[15] The occupational therapy practitioner in this case example wanted to learn more about the cost of hospitalization and prevalent comorbidity of conditions related to the care of diabetes. She knew this would be a priority concern of officials in the area she serves, because her clients go to the emergency room when they feel ill rather than a personal physician. Sometimes they wait so long to seek help that it becomes necessary for them to be hospitalized. The burden of diabetes in terms of hospital costs is reflected in Diagnosis-Related Group data (DRGs) data. DRGs are part of a system created to classify hospital cases into groups. DRGs pay hospitals at a predetermined set rate based on the patient's diagnosis. This system was designed to replace cost-based reimbursement and determines how much Medicare and Medicaid will pay; the CMS[16] is one source of information. The occupational therapy practitioner commits to learning more about public health and decreasing the burden of diabetes on society, and so she joins national and state public health associations.

Community

After acquiring an understanding of the community's narrative, the occupational therapy practitioner may partner with organizations to meet the needs of individuals with diabetes in the community. The assessment focuses on people, occupations, and the environment to understand how interaction among these elements affects performance in common daily activities. Identifying underlying problems involves focusing on the near and far effects of physical and social environments, similar to the actions of a camera lens. A telescopic lens captures a close-up view, and a wide-angle lens captures a panoramic view of the same situation. However, neither view is enough to fully capture the situation. The problem may lie somewhere in the middle. For example, an assessment may determine a person is able to plan a menu, drive a car, find her way to the grocery store, purchase items on her list, and prepare food. But if the assessment doesn't find that individuals in the community have no money for gas and food, the PEOP Occupational Therapy Process falls short in identifying all barriers to meal preparation. In this example, the occupational therapy practitioner uses assessment to understand what people in the community needed to participate in daily life. A "windshield" survey provided a data source on the health status of a population of people with diabetes, and the actions and conditions that protect and improve their health.[17] These data were collected by CHWs and occupational therapy students as they drove vans down each street in the colonia and around the perimeter. The CHWs identified special buildings, markers, and houses and shared stories and history about the colonia. Students counted the number of houses, whether streets were paved, where the church was located, and noted resources in the built environment as well as geographical features. They learned the land is typically dry and barren, but several times a year a storm reaches the area, causing extensive flooding. People struggle to keep water from leaking through the roof or coming into the house from the ground. It can take 1 month for things to dry out. Mold and mildew are prevalent, especially on ceilings and around window frames. Dirt roads become difficult to navigate and shoes sink into the red, thick clay that surrounds every home. People stay at home during these periods. The months of July, August, and September can be nearly unbearable, as homes are not air conditioned.

The colonia offers a rich social environment; people know the names of their neighbors and are informed when people move away or change homes. They are not concerned about crime and, although they don't like to ask for help, they know most people would offer assistance if needed. The Catholic church is a common meeting place for worship and fellowship. Catholic Charities is an organization based in a nearby city that works in concert with the local church to provide resources for people with significant unmet needs. The itinerant priest at the church learns what people need and passes this information along to a social worker employed by Catholic Charities. The social worker arranges for a group of volunteers to construct ramps in households with the greatest need. She

(continued)

BOX 29-2 (CONTINUED)

ASSESSMENT AND EVALUATION FOR A POPULATION, COMMUNITY, AND PERSON IN TEXAS

also has a contact at the Jewish Federation who seems to be a ready source of used, good equipment, including wheelchairs, walkers, shower benches, and other assistive devices for people with disabilities. These community-based strengths are paired with associated challenges. People are reluctant to invite people they don't know into their homes. Some ramps don't have the correct incline or safety features. Donated equipment may not be suited for specific needs of recipients.

In addition to evaluating the broader environment, home visits were conducted to collect objective and self-report data regarding additional enablers and barriers. Students wrote descriptions of each person's performance capabilities and limitations during valued activities. Supplemental assessments included measures of "person factors," such as functional range of motion and strength during engagement in typical daily activity and cognitive functioning. Since the CHWs are part of the community, students interviewed all 6 CHWs and asked them to[18]:

- Identify the primary needs of people they visited in their homes

- Think about what needs to change and how things would be different if changes were implemented

- Reflect on what they observed occupational therapy and nursing students doing

- Report what they would like to learn how to do

- Consider what they think students should learn about

- Generate ideas for how students and CHWs could learn from one another

Priority concerns identified by CHWs during interviews were centered on the physical environment, such as public access to streets, open pools of sewage, lack of transportation, polluted water, mildew, and unsustainable living conditions, and were relayed to public officials. At the end of a year, the assessment was also shared with the Catholic Charities director and the county health department physician.

Person

The foundational principle of the PEOP Model is that performance of occupation (doing) enables the participation (engagement) in everyday life that contributes to a sense of well-being (satisfaction). Clearly, Mrs. C. is not engaging in daily life activities she finds satisfying. An assessment during a home visit revealed constraints/barriers and capacities/enablers. A CHW became aware of Mrs. C.'s falling in her bathroom from the neighbor who had given Mrs. C. the cane. The CHW contacted a social worker at Catholic Charities who obtained a walker from the Jewish Federation in a nearby city and arranged for one of the university's inter-professional teams to evaluate her at home and to deliver the walker.[19] Team members included clinical laboratory clinical science (CLS), nursing, and occupational therapy students, as well as nursing and occupational therapy faculty members.

During the home visit, the CLS student tested her Glycosylated haemoglobin A1c (HbA1) level. Then the nursing student checked her glucose level and vital signs, paying special attention to her blood pressure[20] and the inventory of insulin on hand.[21] She also checked to see if Mrs. C. was taking the medication properly, asked her about her diet, stressed the importance of good nutrition and water intake, and discussed foods to eat and avoid. The occupational therapy practitioner checked for possible hazards and supports in the environment for daily activities. She documented that the outside steps were constructed from 2-x-4 strips of lumber with a 4" gap between them and stagnant pools of water covered the ground. The inside walls were made from materials that could not support grab bars, the doorways were narrow, the linoleum flooring was peeling, and there were scatter rugs throughout the house. Other hazards included no lighting in the narrow hallway, mold growing along the bathroom ceiling, and a leak in the kitchen ceiling.[22] Piles of papers, boxes, and clothing were stacked in nearly every corner. The occupational therapy practitioner addressed some of these concerns, but most issues required follow up from the CHW.[23,24] The occupational therapy practitioner asked Mrs. C. about the brightly colored doilies carefully arranged across the back of the couch. Mrs. C. described how she had learned to crochet from her grandmother and how it saddened her that her daughter had not learned. The practitioner noted framed photographs and learned some of them were of Mrs. C.'s sons who had served in the military and died in Afghanistan. Mrs. C. was glad that she still had the steps constructed by her oldest son. They reminded her of how devoted he was to her. The occupational therapy practitioner concluded it would be a mistake to suggest removal of the steps even

(continued)

Box 29-2 (continued)

Assessment and Evaluation for a Population, Community, and Person in Texas

though they were dangerous; instead she would recommend that a ramp be added to the side of the porch. Mrs. C. reported her daughter helped with basic needs, but seemed resentful and rushed during infrequent visits. Mrs. C. disliked that her daughter only wanted to eat out at fast food restaurants and lived with a man who had 3 children. During the conversation it became apparent that episodes of depression, weight gain, and poor eating habits first emerged during her husband's prolonged illness and increased following the deaths of her sons. Mrs. C. had stopped going to church even though she missed the sense of community, the peace she gained through worship, and the fellowship of Wednesday night suppers and Ladies Circle meetings. Mrs. C. didn't want to ask other people for a ride and her daughter no longer attended church.

As was her habit, Mrs. C. made oatmeal for breakfast. She fumbled as she tried to grasp and hold a cup containing 4 cups of water. She poured water from a gallon container into the pot by tipping it to one side. When asked why she didn't draw water from the faucet, Mrs. C. turned the knob to show a rusty colored discharge.[25] Several tasks from the Kitchen Task Assessment indicated some minimal cognitive impairment.[26] Mrs. C. spends most of the day watching TV. She sits on a straight-backed kitchen chair because the couch is low and she cannot stand up without assistance. The falls she sustained occurred while getting in and out of the bath tub.[27] Mrs. C. explained her left leg is weak, so she uses the cane in her right hand to stabilize herself, steps over the ledge with her right leg, and then lifts her left leg to get into the tub. She was aware this was unsafe, but didn't want to bathe herself using the sink because there was no way to close the drain and she didn't feel as clean. Mrs. C. also reported she had pain and fatigue while standing to dress. In functional strength and range of motion, Mrs. C. had limitations in shoulder flexion to 90 degrees and internal and external rotation. This restricted her ability to don a bra and any garments that required her to put in one arm at a time. Before leaving, the occupational therapy practitioner commented on a photograph of Mrs. C. in which she had long braids wrapped around her head. When Mrs. C. was asked how she manages her hair now, she became distressed. Mrs. C.'s hair had been cut to shoulder length by her daughter when she couldn't raise her arms high enough to manage it herself. The CHW told Mrs. C. she would return on Monday.[28,29]

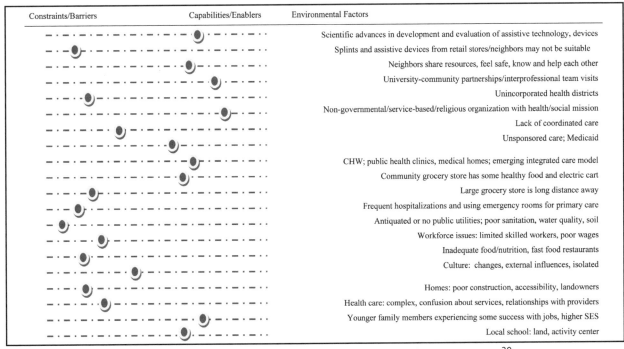

Figure 29-1. Assessment and evaluation of specific environmental factors for the colonia community.[30]

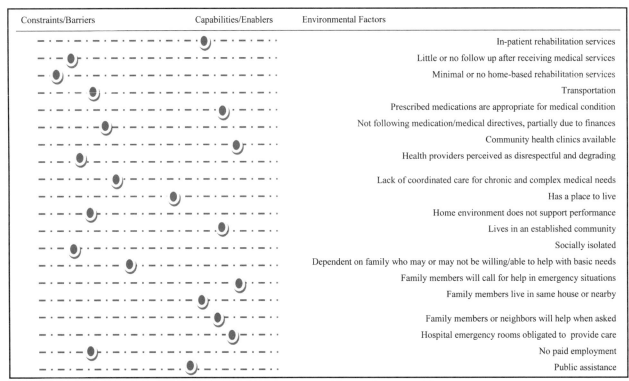

Constraints/Barriers	Capabilities/Enablers	Environmental Factors

In-patient rehabilitation services
Little or no follow up after receiving medical services
Minimal or no home-based rehabilitation services
Transportation
Prescribed medications are appropriate for medical condition
Not following medication/medical directives, partially due to finances
Community health clinics available
Health providers perceived as disrespectful and degrading

Lack of coordinated care for chronic and complex medical needs
Has a place to live
Home environment does not support performance
Lives in an established community
Socially isolated
Dependent on family who may or may not be willing/able to help with basic needs
Family members will call for help in emergency situations
Family members live in same house or nearby

Family members or neighbors will help when asked
Hospital emergency rooms obligated to provide care
No paid employment
Public assistance

Figure 29-2. Assessment and evaluation of specific environmental factors for Mrs. C.[30]

functional status, physical function, and percent of people in different age groups who need help with ADL.

Are Determinants of Health Included in Community Assessment Strategies?

Epidemiologists maintain and analyze public health data sets to link social determinants to health outcomes.[32,33] What skills and knowledge do occupational therapy practitioners have to inform population-based assessment? Population health data includes functional status and physical function, in addition to disease categories and conditions. Occupational therapy practitioners contribute to population health by developing and expanding the use of occupation-based, functional assessments that capture health outcomes in new ways; this requires specialized knowledge and advanced training in psychometrics.

What Is the Impact of Burden of Disease on Local Communities?

The burden of diabetes in terms of hospital costs is reflected in Diagnosis-Related Group data (DRGs). DRGs are part of a system created to classify hospital cases into groups. DRGs pay hospitals at a pre-determined set rate based on the patient's diagnosis. This system was designed to replace "cost-based" reimbursement, and determines how much public assistance programs, such as Medicare and Medicaid, will pay. One source of information about Medicare and Medicaid is the Centers for Medicare and Medicaid Services (CMS).[16]

By convention, the same terminology is used to describe and measure population health at the international, national, and state level. Local government officials are interested in population health because most health services are provided by agencies and organizations within home communities. However, rather than thinking in terms of the burden of a particular disease, which refers to disease-related morbidity and mortality issues, local concerns center on the burden of care.[2] The Agency for Health Research and Quality (AHRQ), is a resource for learning about a disease process, nutritional management, physical activity, medications, monitoring, acute complications, risk reduction, goal setting and problem solving, psychosocial adjustment, and other management issues. Occupational therapy practitioners have knowledge in several of these areas, thus they can make a significant contribution to inter-professional teams dedicated to disease care and prevention.

What Tools Are Used to Assess Population/Public Health?

The Association of Community Health Improvement (ACHI) Community Health Assessment Toolkit is a guide for:

> ... planning, leading, and using community health needs assessments to better understand—and ultimately improve—the health of communities. It presents a suggested assessment framework of 6 steps, and provides practical guidance drawn from experienced professionals and a variety of effective tools.[34(np)]

In the past, many hospitals have assessed health needs as part of their service to the community and as a way of gathering data to determine needs and plan for future services. Under the Patient Protection and Affordable Care Act of 2010, Community Health Needs Assessments (CHNAs) are now required of tax-exempt hospitals.[35]

A Public Health Assessment is not the same thing as a medical exam or a community health study. It can sometimes lead to those things, as well as to other public health activities. In a Public Health Assessment, representatives of an agency talk with people living or working in an area, local leaders, and health professionals (among other community members) about what they know about their area and health concerns. Community health concerns are addressed in every Public Health Assessment for every site. Before the Public Health Assessment is finished, it is available in the community during the Public Comment Period through communication channels, such as contact with local community groups, political leaders, health professionals, and articles in local newspapers and stories on television and radio. The Public Comment Period lets the community tell the agency how well the Public Health Assessment addressed their concerns. The agency then responds to the public's comments in the final Public Health Assessment, such as concerns about toxic substances.[36]

How Is the Community Involved in a Public Health Assessment?

The community plays a key role in a Public Health Assessment, and any activity that follows. Community Health Assessment (CHA) is a fundamental tool of public health practice. Its aim is to describe the health of the community by presenting information on health status, community health needs, resources, and epidemiologic and other studies of current local health problems. It seeks to identify target populations that may be at increased risk of poor health outcomes and to gain an understanding of their needs, as well as assess the larger community environment and how it relates to the health of individuals. It also identifies those areas where better information is needed, especially information on health disparities among different sub-populations, quality of health care, and the occurrence and severity of disabilities in the population. The CHA is the basis for all local public health planning, giving the local health unit the opportunity to identify and interact with key community leaders, organizations, and interested residents about health priorities and concerns. This information forms the basis of improving the health status of the community through a strategic plan.

Typically, CHA are used every 2 years to evaluate the health of a community.[37] The 1999 CHA's recommendation for local departments includes the following:

- Use data to plan for future public health services
- Develop local priorities and monitor progress toward meaningful outcomes
- Scan the environment continuously for changes in conditions and new health issues
- Assume a leadership role in community health assessment and involve other local groups
- Evaluate the local department's capacity for community health assessment

CHAs are used to develop initiatives that are carried out by the local public health department alone or in partnership with other organizations (eg, schools, universities, employers, health care, government, nonprofit organizations).[37]

PUBLIC AND COMMUNITY HEALTH INTERVENTIONS

How Does a Case Illustrate Interventions for a Population, Community, and Person?

The PEOP Occupational Therapy Process identifies interventions as the next step. Continue your learning about the case and this population of people with diabetes in Texas living in a poor community known as a colonia and a person, Mrs. C., who has diabetes and is a community member. Read and reflect on the description of population, community, and person interventions (Box 29-3) and the examples of occupational therapy interventions to set the stage for learning about public and community health interventions (Table 29-1).

BOX 29-3

INTERVENTIONS FOR A POPULATION, COMMUNITY, AND PERSON IN TEXAS

Population

In this case, a university and a community entered into a partnership to design and implement an intervention to contain the costs of health care. The desired outcome was to eliminate emergency room visits by people with diabetes and cut readmissions to the hospital by 50%. Funding from the university–community partnership paid the salaries for 6 CHWs and travel expenses for inter-professional health care teams of university students. Each team included a CHW, a nursing student, and an occupational therapy student. Sometimes a CLS also traveled with the team. Nursing and occupational therapy faculty members supervised all team members. Once a month the teams traveled in vans to colonias, arriving on Friday night and staying through Sunday evening. As prevention and monitoring were the primary goals of the teams, CHWs and students with experience on prior trips conducted follow-up visits while keeping in touch with faculty via smart phones with the capability of sending photos and videos. Faculty members supervised students traveling with the team for the first time and teams accompanied by faculty visited all new referrals. A community health nurse funded by Catholic Charities maintained medical records and was the primary source of referrals. Teams visited the homes of the most vulnerable people living with diabetes. Occupational therapy practitioners serving on the teams defined problems and solutions in new ways. They found unidentified needs and barriers to disease management and health promotion, ie social isolation and lack of participation in community activities. Intervention was developed in collaboration with consumers and lay providers and included delivery of health services in homes (or close to homes) and used available resources. The occupational therapy practitioner searched for a systematic review to identify characteristics of interventions effective for the population of people with diabetes. She found culturally appropriate health education interventions were well-supported, and drew upon this evidence to shape an educational intervention for the population she served. She knew she did not have the medical background to develop an intervention on her own, and the health education materials she found on her regional public health website were not well-suited to the population she was serving. She decided to work with an inter-professional health care team to create a multimedia instructional module. This module featured a person with diabetes and a practitioner organizing the person's daily routine around checking blood sugar and taking insulin. The module also included examples of what to do and what not to do when using glucose testing materials. These instructional materials were easily accessible to CHWs and people with diabetes. Developing and using materials in this way is an example of a population-centered intervention that evolved from the PEOP Occupational Therapy Process and focused on a population, the environments in which they lived and worked, and the occupations in which they engaged. This process generated new ways of thinking about health promotion. Another example of a population-based health promotion strategy was to initiate a TV campaign showing family members working together and enjoying one another as they prepared a meal of traditional, nutritious foods. The intent of this occupation centered strategy was to change attitudes. A "healthy foods" Wednesday night supper organized by the local church changed behaviors; school children published a cookbook with healthy recipes to make at home changed knowledge, behaviors, and attitudes. These population-based interventions emerged through the PEOP Occupational Therapy Process and involved active engagement in activities. In this situation an intervention specific to the population with diabetes focused on 2 primary goals: prevent obesity and promote self-management of the disease process.

Community

According to the PEOP Model, when intervention is designed for a person, the person is involved in setting goals and it is the client who ultimately determines desired outcomes. It follows that if intervention is designed for the community, it is the community that is involved in setting goals and it is the community that ultimately determines desired outcomes. Occupational therapy practitioners who serve communities begin by investing time and energy to learn about priority goals for the community and the current status of the community relative to those goals. Following is an example of a community that 1) described current reality and goals, 2) enacted steps to reach the goals, and 3) created their vision of an integrated care plan.[38]

CHWs, students, and people from the community systematically took time to ACT-LOOK-THINK. This approach, known as participatory action research (PAR) integrated assessment and intervention, processes into an iterative

(continued)

BOX 29-3 (CONTINUED)

INTERVENTIONS FOR A POPULATION, COMMUNITY, AND PERSON IN TEXAS

cycle.[39] The PEOP Model served as a framework for how to act, what to look for, and what to think about. The first ACTion occurred when the inter-professional team visited people referred to them by Catholic Charities. The team took the opportunity to LOOK at the reaction of neighbors. After THINKing about the fact that the community was not accustomed to outside visitors, team members decided to ACT by attending church services the next Sunday morning. At the start of the church service, the priest introduced them to the congregation. After LOOKing at the reaction of the congregation they realized (THINK) it would be a good idea for the priest to introduce them at all future services (ACT). Team members told the congregation they could self-refer by notifying a CHW they wanted a home visit from the team. The CHWs LOOKed at how many people asked for visits, took time to THINK about how to schedule them, and visited as many people as time allowed (ACT). Similarly, team members ACTed by contacting the ramp builders, LOOKed at the needs of people who still needed ramps, and took time to THINK about how to improve the process and develop a solution. Community volunteers built ramps to specifications drawn by occupational therapy students. The PAR process also generated a solution to a different problem. To ensure that people only received donated equipment they could actually use, 2 identical notebooks of numbered photos and pictures of equipment were made. The occupational therapy practitioner kept one scrapbook and the CHW kept the identical copy. Thereafter equipment was "prescribed" by referring to the assigned number for a piece of equipment that would be best the best fit for a particular person. This strategy enabled CHWs to carry a visual representation of the exact item needed as they scouted around for donated equipment.[39]

Person

The occupational therapy practitioner wondered if Mrs. C. could get into the tub another way. Perhaps Mrs. C. would be willing to sit on a chair near the edge of the tub. Mrs. C. liked this idea so the occupational therapy practitioner brought a plastic lawn chair from the front yard. When the chair was placed near the tub faucet, Mrs. C. could bathe herself and even extend her legs and dangle her feet in the water streaming from the faucet. After Mrs. C. had washed herself using a long-handled brush, the occupational therapy practitioner gave her a package of white cotton socks and recommended that Mrs. C. wear them with her shoes. The practitioner also gave Mrs. C. a long-handled mirror so that she could check the bottom of her feet and each of her toes. The therapy practitioner advised against using bedroom slippers. The occupational therapy practitioner taught Mrs. C. how to sit on the edge of her bed to help save energy and reduce pain while dressing, and how to safely ambulate with the new walker. After the occupational therapy practitioner assembled the donated walker, it became clear that it would not fit through the narrow doorways so, with Mrs. C.'s permission, the occupational therapy practitioner removed the molding from the door frames at the level of the walker and below, and secured the rough edges with duct tape. Mrs. C. learned to navigate through the doorways and to turn the walker in her bathroom. Then, the occupational therapy practitioner showed Mrs. C. how to wrap her hair into a pony tail and secure it to her head by placing her head on the kitchen table and using her hands together.[40]

Mrs. C. purchased water in gallon jugs because water from the faucet was not fit to drink (the environment). She and her daughter have been eating regularly at a fast food chain restaurant. Mrs. C. wanted to be able to prepare meals for herself and her daughter (occupation), but peripheral neuropathy limited the sensation in her hands (person). She compensated by asking her daughter to pour water into small containers so she could manage more easily (enhanced occupational performance). When she began preparing meals that her daughter enjoyed, they ate nutritious food at home more often. Eating at home rekindled the mother-daughter relationship (social environment). When she consistently ate good food, Mrs. C. felt healthier. Subsequently she expanded her range of health-sustaining occupations. Mrs. C. was less dependent on her daughter and she and her daughter enjoyed being together. Due to the mediating effects of occupation, improved health was an outcome even when poverty was a social determinant. The effects were far reaching, because the reclaimed occupation of cooking corn, beans, and rice at home had the potential to lower the incidence of intergenerational diabetes associated with restaurant chain food. This example of one woman in her own home generalized to interventions with the larger population.[27] Other people in this same population had similar strengths and challenges, therefore interventions for the entire population were likely to be effective.

Table 29-1. *Occupational Therapy Interventions and Outcomes for a Population: Obesity and Diabetes*

Intervention Approach	Outcome
Prevent Obesity	
Educate the population through TV campaign that promotes preparation of nutritious food at home, cost comparisons of healthy vs unhealthy food, church night suppers with healthy menus, classroom cook-books to educate children about healthy food	Enhanced occupational performance supports healthy eating
Prevent obesity through awareness of the benefits of exercise	Enhanced function with increased stamina and endurance during daily activities
Promote awareness of a problem and commitment among many people to address a major health concern through social media, advertising, talk shows	Interdependence among all citizens results in ownership of a shared problem
Self-Management	
Modify/compensate for lack of clean water by stocking stores with gallons of water	Increased consumption of (potable) water
Educate and employ CHWs	Competent workforce sensitive to the traditions and practices of the people needing services
Consult with inter-professional team members who specialize in home-based chronic disease management	Coordination in care and improved health outcomes
Restore ability of people with limited mobility to participate in community activities	Increased strength, range of motion, and endurance for community activities

What Is the Purpose of Population-Centered Intervention?

Population-centered intervention strategies address both disease management and health promotion. One readily available guide to health promotion priorities at the national level is Healthy People 2020.[6] Disease management is a population-based approach to health care that identifies patients at risk, interventions with specific programs of care, and related outcome measures. A multi-disciplinary approach to care for chronic disease coordinates comprehensive care along a disease continuum across health care delivery systems; health care delivery systems are expanding to include lay workers. CHWs effectively offer population-based interventions because they understand population-based needs within the communities in which they live and work. Occupational therapy practitioners can teach and support CHWs to optimize their skills. Optimizing the skill set of lay community workers reduces costs and provides services to more people. Increasing the number of skilled health providers available to meet the needs of people with diabetes is a systems-based disease management intervention strategy.

What Are Characteristics of Population-Centered Interventions?

Some population-based intervention strategies focus on participation in society, while others are customized to address specific educational needs of the population for disease management. Instructional strategies offer a variety of formats to increase knowledge, develop skills, and change attitudes so people will take needed actions to monitor their own health.[41] Experts in diabetes care argue that the correct systems are not in place to care for the population of individuals with diabetes.[2(p1613)]

What Is the Position of the American Occupational Therapy Association on Public and Community Health Intervention?

In 2008 the AOTA published a position statement on occupational therapy in the *Promotion of Health and the Prevention of Disease and Disability*,[42] and summarized

Table 29-2. Description of Current Reality and Desired State in Colonia and Steps to Achieve Goals

Current Reality	Desired State	Steps to Achieve Goals
County has 2 primary care clinic sites	Develop 3 county sites: north, mid, and south	County medical society convened a work group (for the second time in a decade) to deal with the issue of indigent health care
Obstetrical (OB) services were lost in parts of county	Restore OB services throughout the county	Community access coalition came together to submit a community access program grant
Secondary and tertiary care is covered at 21% federal poverty level	Cover secondary and tertiary care at 100% federal poverty level or greater.	University hosted an expert to speak on the impact of indigent health care on health policy
Funding for indigent health care is limited, uncertain	Identify sustained funding for indigent health care	County commissioners' court responded to the medical society's request by charging a public task force on indigent health care to study the issue and to formulate solutions
Secondary and tertiary care are episodic, lack of medical homes	Provide continuity of care and assure all individuals have medical home	Task force (composed of over 40 people) formed study groups on issues of government, health plan composition, financing, and education. Issue gained the support from media, and, movement of community cooperation and change developed

common definitions for prevention at 3 levels: primary, secondary, and tertiary.

> Primary prevention is defined as education or health promotion strategies designed to help people avoid the onset and reduce the incidence of unhealthy conditions, diseases, or injuries. Primary prevention attempts to identify and eliminate risk factors for disease, injury, and disability. Secondary prevention includes early detection and intervention after disease has occurred and is designed to prevent or disrupt the disabling process. Tertiary prevention refers to treatment and services designed to arrest the progression of a condition, prevent further disability, and promote social opportunity.[42(p 695),43]

Contemporary conceptions of occupation are expanding to capture the experiences of people from marginalized populations.[44] They may include descriptions of disconnectedness and isolation termed *occupational alienation*.[45] Other concepts refer to occupational deprivation and occupational justice; preclusion from engagement in activities available to others due to lack of control or opportunity.[46,47] The term *occupational rights* emphasizes the importance of engagement in meaningful occupations to support individual and community health and well-being.[47]

PUBLIC AND COMMUNITY HEALTH OUTCOMES

How Does a Case Illustrate Outcomes for a Population, Community, and Person?

The PEOP Occupational Therapy Process uses narratives, assessment and evaluations, and interventions to work toward outcomes that are important at the population, community, and person level. Continue your learning about the case and this population of people with diabetes in Texas living in a poor community known as a colonia and a person, Mrs. C. who has diabetes and is a community member. Read and reflect on the description of community's reality, desired state, and steps (Table 29-2) and a summary of the population, community, and person PEOP Occupational Therapy Process (Table 29-3). This case illustrated the challenges and rewards that an occupational therapy practitioner may experience when working in public and community health roles.

Table 29-3. A Community-Based Intervention Informed by Participatory Action Research and Facilitated by Occupational Therapy Practitioners

Narrative Goals	Assessment and Evaluation	Intervention Strategies	Outcomes Anticipated and Realized
People Living in Colonia			

• Improve sewage and drainage and contain environmental hazards	• Assets/Capabilities/Enablers
	  ◦ 40-year history of shared dreams
	  ◦ Multigenerational families live in homes or close proximity
	  ◦ Local grocery store
	  ◦ People know their neighbors, feel safe
	  ◦ Priest is well-known and liked
	  ◦ Living conditions now less crowded
	  ◦ Willingness to change diet
	  ◦ Occupational therapy students, friends, others willing to donate craft supplies
	  ◦ Empty wing of the elementary school
		• Environment
		  ◦ CHWs take environmental concerns to local authorities
		  ◦ Expose in local newspaper about environmental concerns
		• Garden
		  ◦ Activities center with cooking classes, garden
		• Grocery
		  ◦ CHWs meet with store owner to discuss needs for healthier foods
		• Community building
			• Environment
			  ◦ Local authorities develop and implement plan for colonia
			• Garden
			  ◦ Established a community garden
			• Grocery
			  ◦ Local grocery store expands offerings, and posts nutrition posters and cost comparisons of healthy/unhealthy foods
			• Community building

• Raise fruits and vegetables in home gardens			
• Expand local grocery store to include more healthy foods			

• Keep younger generation in the community	• Barriers
	  ◦ Next generation moving away
	  ◦ Prevalence of diabetes
	  ◦ Remote, unincorporated
	  ◦ People accept help but don't like to ask
	  ◦ Local grocery has few perishable items
	  ◦ People with mobility issues become socially isolated, don't attend church or activities
	  ◦ Difficulty getting fresh food
	  ◦ Fewer multigenerational families living under the same roof; older people are lonely and receive less support
	  ◦ People with mobility limitations alone during day spend time watching TV
	  ◦ Available wing of school needs paint
		◦ CHWs teach and learn low-cost crafts during home visits (eg, crocheting)
		  ◦ Activities center offers cooking classes, garden
		• Health care
		  ◦ Room in local school now has an outreach office
		  ◦ CHWs post phone numbers on refrigerator of people who will provide help when needed
		  ◦ CHWs inform priest when someone needs a ride to church/church events
		  ◦ Community center offers senior exercise classes
		  ◦ CHWs show women with diabetes how to add exercise routines into household chores
			◦ Bus route expanded to colonia
			  ◦ Expanded social networks among neighbors; eg, crochet group at the church on Wednesdays
			  ◦ People in the community open their homes to inter-professional teams
			• Health care
			  ◦ Regularly scheduled visits from inter-professional teams
			  ◦ Formalized communication networks in the homes of people who are vulnerable and live alone
			  ◦ Effective ride sharing program
			  ◦ People refer neighbors to CHW

• Access health care			

(continued)

Table 29-3 (continued). A Community-Based Intervention Informed by Participatory Action Research and Facilitated by Occupational Therapy Practitioners

Narrative Goals	Assessment and Evaluation	Intervention Strategies	Outcomes Anticipated and Realized
State and Local Government			
• Reduce incidence of obesity • Reduce hospitalization of people with diabetes • Reduce visits to the hospital emergency room	• Assets 　◦ All team members monitor meds • Barriers 　◦ Low Medicaid reimbursement rate 　◦ Medicare doesn't cover cost of care 　◦ Subject to changes in funding	• Increase public interest • Offer aerobics classes in refurbished activity centers • Conduct wide-spread public awareness campaign • Fund community/university partnerships	• Lost distinction of "fattest city in America" • Reduced hospitalizations for people with diabetes >50% • Reduced visits to the hospital emergency room >50% • Medicaid payment rate dropped
Nongovernmental Agencies			
• Catholic Diocese, mission is "spreading the gospel of Jesus Christ, administering its sacraments, and exercising charity"	• Assets 　◦ Predominantly Catholic population 　◦ Supported at multiple levels • Barriers 　◦ Youth leave area, don't attend church	• Provide an itinerant priest, a church building with regular services, a welcoming environment	• Church has an active role in referring parishioners with needs and supporting health team members in building relationships with parishioners
• Catholic Charities, mission "provide service to people in need, to advocate for justice in social structures, and to call the entire church and other people of good will to do the same."	• Assets 　◦ Committed donors and volunteers 　◦ Supported at the national and local level • Barriers 　◦ National economic downturn, contributions down	• Hire, train, supervise CHWs; maintain health records, serve as referral source, manage accounts, collect data, evaluate outcomes	• Established "Healthy Living" Center, social worker employed to serve people with diabetes

(continued)

Table 29-3 (continued).   *A Community-Based Intervention Informed by Participatory Action Research and Facilitated by Occupational Therapy Practitioners*

Narrative Goals	Assessment and Evaluation	Intervention Strategies	Outcomes Anticipated and Realized
Nongovernmental Agencies			
• Combined Jewish Appeal, Mission to "distribute funds"	• Assets ◇ Committed donors and volunteers ◇ Supported at the national and local level • Barriers ◇ Matching requests with funding priorities	• Secure equipment specific to individual needs, serve as a collection site for donated equipment	• Individuals have needed equipment
• Local food bank, mission "to serve the body, mind, and spirit of those in need through food distribution and nutrition education"	• Assets ◇ Committed donors and volunteers • Barriers ◇ Supported at the local and state level ◇ Donations unable to meet increased need	• Provide food boxes	• Individuals have access to nutritional food and information
• State university, mission "to provide scholarly teaching, innovative scientific investigation, and state-of-the-art patient care in a learning environment to better the health of society"	• Assets ◇ Informed and committed students/faculty, willing to take risks, develop new programs • Barriers ◇ Added to regular workload, extended time ◇ Unknown roles, requires trial and error	• Visit all people referred to team • Assess and provide intervention for all people referred • Retain representation on all inter-professional teams • Have experienced students mentor novice students	• Interventions provided • Occupational therapy is an important team member on teams • Experiences support student and faculty learning • Disseminated at occupational therapy conferences

SUMMARY

Occupational therapy practitioners who serve at-risk populations and communities offer evidence-based interventions that are sensitive to the needs of people of different races and ethnic groups.[23,48] By generating new possibilities for addressing health priorities, practitioners offer solutions for not only what could be done to promote health and well-being, but also what should be done given available choices and resources.[49] Health services research is one of the research priorities identified by the AOTF-AOTA Research Agenda.[44,50] Consistent with this priority, occupational therapy practitioners who design population-based and community-based intervention are positioned to evaluate performance outcomes for diagnostic groups based on type of occupational therapy intervention, site of service delivery, professional training, and/or team composition.

REFERENCES

1. Texas Diabetes Council. *Diabetes: A Comprehensive Approach: a Plan to Prevent and Control Diabetes in Texas.* Texas Department of State Health Services. www.dshs.state.tx.us/diabetes/PDF/TDC-State-Plan-1011.pdf. Published 2010. Accessed August 11, 2013.
2. Hirsch IB. The burden of diabetes (care). *Diabetes Care.* 2003;26(5):1613-1614.
3. US Food and Drug Administration. Protecting and Promoting Your Health. US Department of Health & Human Services: US Food and Drug Administration. http://www.fda.gov/default.htm. Updated August 16, 2013. Accessed August 18, 2013.
4. US Environmental Protection Agency. *Wastes—Hazardous Waste.* US Environmental Protection Agency. http://www.epa.gov/osw/hazard/. Updated April 8, 2013. Accessed August 12, 2013.
5. SNAP food benefits. Texas Health and Human Services Commission. http://yourtexasbenefits.hhsc.state.tx.us/programs/snap/. Accessed August 18, 2013.
6. Low L, Yap M, Brodaty H. A systematic review of different models of home and community care services for older persons. *Biomedical Central Health Services Research.* 2011;11(93):1-15. doi:10.1186/1472-6963-11-93.
7. Texas Secretary of State. *Colonias FAQs (Frequently Asked Questions).* Texas Secretary of State: John Steen: Texas border & Mexican affairs. http://www.sos.state.tx.us/border/colonias/faqs.shtml. Accessed August 18, 2013.
8. Lewin S, Skea Z, Entwistle VA, Zwarenstein M, Dick J. Interventions for providers to promote a patient-centred approach in clinical consultations. *Cochrane Database of Systematic Reviews.* 2001;4(10):CD003267.
9. WHO. About WHO. World Health Organization. http://www.who.int/about/en/. Updated 2013. Accessed August 6, 2013.
10. Health Promotion. Public Health Agency of Canada. http://www.phac-aspc.gc.ca/index-eng.php. Updated August 2, 2013. Accessed August 6, 2013.
11. Kindig DA, Booske BC, Remington PL. Mobilizing Action Toward Community Health (MATCH): metrics, incentives, and partnerships for population health. *Preventing Chronic Disease.* 2010;7(4):A68. http://www.cdc.gov/pcd/issues/2010/jul/10_0019.htm. Published 2010. Updated March 22, 2013. Accessed August 6, 2013.
12. MacDonald G. Evidence-based public health. *Preventing Chronic Disease.* 2004;1(2):1-2. http://www.cdc.gov/pcd/issues/2004/apr/04_0012.htm. Published April 2004. Updated March 22, 2013. Accessed August 6, 2013.
13. Rimer BK, Glanz K. *Theory at a Glance: A Guide for Health Promotion Practice.* 2nd ed. Washington, DC: US Department of Health and Human Services; 2005.
14. US Department of Health and Human Services: OASH Press Office. HHS Announces the Nation's New Health Promotion and Disease Prevention Agenda. HHS news. http://www.healthypeople.gov/2020/about/DefaultPressRelease.pdf. Published December 2, 2010. Accessed August 11, 2013.
15. Texas Department of State Health Services, Texas Diabetes Council. *Diabetes Data: Surveillance and Evaluation.* Texas Department of State Health Services. http://www.dshs.state.tx.us/diabetes/tdcdata.shtm. Updated April 26, 2013. Accessed August 18, 2013.
16. Centers for Medicare and Medicaid Services. Acute Inpatient PPS. Centers for Medicare and Medicaid Services. http://www.cms.gov/Medicare/Medicare-Fee-for-Service-Payment/AcuteInpatientPPS/index.html?redirect=/acuteinpatientpps/. Updated April 10, 2013. Accessed August 7, 2013.
17. National Network of Libraries of Medicine. *Guide 1: Set the Direction with a Community Assessment.* National Network of Libraries of Medicine. http://nnlm.gov/outreach/community/planning.html. Updated January 9, 2008. Accessed August 19, 2013.
18. CARE: community Alliance For Research and Engagement. Yale School of Public Health. http://www.care.yale.edu/index.aspx. Updated 2013. Accessed August 19, 2013.
19. Campus-Community Partnerships for Health. *Service-Learning.* Campus-Community Partnerships for Health: promoting health equity & social justice. http://depts.washington.edu/ccph/servicelearningres.html. Updated 2013. Accessed August 19, 2013.
20. American Diabetes Association. *American Diabetes Association.* American Diabetes Association. http://www.diabetes.org/. Updated 2013. Accessed August 19, 2013.
21. Ryan R, Santesso N, Hill S, et al. Consumer-oriented interventions for evidence-based prescribing and medicines use: an overview of systematic reviews. *Cochrane Database of Systematic Reviews.* 2011;5:CD007768.
22. Housing Assistance Council. *Housing for Persons With Disabilities in Rural Areas.* Housing Assistance Council: building rural communities. http://ruralhome.org/. Accessed August 19, 2013.
23. Bass Haugen JD. Health disparities: examination of evidence relevant for occupational therapy. *American Journal of Occupational Therapy.* 2009;63:24-34.
24. AOTA. AOTA's societal statement on health disparities. *American Journal of Occupational Therapy.* 2011;65:S76-S77.
25. Blakeney AB, Marshall A. Water quality, health, and human occupations. *American Journal of Occupational Therapy.* 2009;63:46-57.
26. Baum C, Edwards D. Cognitive performance in senile dementia of the Alzheimer's type: the kitchen task assessment. *American Journal of Occupational Therapy.* 1993;47(5):431-436.

27. Clarke IP, George LK. The role of the built environment in the disablement process. *American Journal of Public Health.* 2005;95(11):1933-1939.

28. Joyce K, Pabayo R, Critchley JA, Bambra C. Flexible working conditions and their effects on employee health and well-being. *Cochrane Database of Systematic Reviews.* 2010;2:CD008009.

29. Bosch-Capblanch X, Liaqat S, Garner P. Managerial supervision to improve primary health care in low- and middle-income countries. *Cochrane Database of Systematic Reviews.* 2011;9:CD006413.

30. Bass JD, Baum CM, Christiansen CH. Interventions and outcomes of occupational therapy: PEOP Occupational Therapy Process. In: Christiansen CH, Baum CM, Bass JD, eds. *Occupational Therapy: Performance, Participation, and Well-Being.* 4th ed. Thorofare, NJ: SLACK Incorporated; 2015.

31. WHO. Health Statistics and Health Information Systems: Metrics: Disability-Adjusted Life Year (DALY). World Health Organization. http://www.who.int/healthinfo/global_burden_disease/metrics_daly/en/. Updated 2013. Accessed August 7, 2013.

32. Johnson TD. Nation's overall health not improving, assessment finds: obesity, diabetes stalling US progress. *The Nation's Health.* 2012; 42(1): 1-18.

33. US Department of Health and Human Services: Office of Minority Health. Health Topics: Infant Health: Articles. US Department of Health and Human Services: Office of Minority Health. http://minorityhealth.hhs.gov/templates/browse.aspx?lvl=3&lvlid=326. Accessed August 7, 2013.

34. Association for Community Health Improvement, Health Research and Educational Trust. *ACHI Community Health Assessment Toolkit: A Practical Guide to Planning, Leading, and Using Community Health Assessments.* Hospitalconnect. com. http://www.assesstoolkit.org/. Updated 2007. Accessed August 11, 2013.

35. Internal Revenue Service. Community Health Needs Assessments for Charitable Hospitals. 78 FR 20523 (April 5, 2013).

36. US Centers for Disease Control and Prevention: Agency for Toxic Substances and Disease Registry. *Public Health Assessments.* Agency for Toxic Substances and Disease Registry: community matters. http://www.atsdr.cdc.gov/com/pha.html/. Updated April 16, 2003. Accessed August 11, 2013.

37. The Municipal Public Health Services Plan: Community Health Assessment: Guidance and Format. New York State Department of Health. http://www.health.ny.gov/statistics/chac/docs/chaguide.pdf. Updated October 1, 1998. Accessed August 11, 2013.

38. Raimer B, Tiernan K. *Texas Pioneers: Eliminating Disparities to Launch Health Care Reform.* Paper presented at: Communities Joined in Action National Conference; 2011; Washington, DC.

39. Baum F, MacDougall C, Smith D. Participatory action research. *Journal of Epidemiology and Community Health.* 2006;60(10):854-857.

40. Baum CM, Law M. Occupational therapy practice: focusing on occupational performance. *American Journal of Occupational Therapy.* 1997;51:277-287.

41. Smith D, Gutman, S. Health literacy in occupational therapy practice and research. *American Journal of Occupational Therapy.* 2011;65(4):368.

42. Scaffa M, VanSlyke N, Brownson CA. Occupational therapy in the promotion of health and the prevention of disease and disability. *American Journal of Occupational Therapy.* 2008;62(6):694-703.

43. Patrick DL, Richardson M, Starks HE, Rose MA, Kinne S. Rethinking prevention for people with disabilities part II: a framework for designing interventions. *American Journal of Health Promotion.* 1997;11:261-263.

44. Braveman B, Bass Haugen JD. From the desks of the guest editors—social justice and health disparities: an evolving discourse in occupational therapy research and intervention. *American Journal of Occupational Therapy.* 2009;63:7-12.

45. Wilcock AA. *An Occupational Perspective of Health.* 2nd ed. Thorofare, NJ: SLACK Incoporated; 2006.

46. Townsend E, Wilcock AA. Occupational justice and client-centered practice: a dialogue in progress. *Canadian Journal of Occupational Therapy.* 2004;71:75-87.

47. Whalley-Hammel K. Reflections on well-being and occupational rights. *Canadian Journal of Occupational Therapy.* 2008;75:61-64.

48. Breland HL, Ellis C Jr. The issue is—is reporting race and ethnicity essential to occupational therapy evidence? *American Journal of Occupational Therapy.* 2012;66:115-119.

49. Rogers JC. Clinical reasoning: the ethics, science, and art. *American Journal of Occupational Therapy.* 1983;37:601-616.

50. AOTA, AOTF. Occupational therapy research agenda. *American Journal of Occupational Therapy.* 2011;65(6 Suppl.):S4-S7.

FOUNDATIONAL KNOWLEDGE AND RESOURCES

PEOP: Enabling Everyday Living

THE NARRATIVE
The past, current and future perceptions, choices, interests, goals and needs that are unique to the Person, Organization, or Population

PERSON
•Cognition
•Psychological
•Physiological
•Sensory
•Motor
•Spirituality

OCCUPATION
•Activities
•Tasks
•Roles

ENVIRONMENT
•Culture
•Social Determinants
•Social Support and Social Capital
•Education and Policy
•Physical and Natural
•Assistive Technology

Personal Narrative
• Perception and Meaning
• Choices and Responsibilities
• Attitudes and Motivation
• Needs and Goals

Organizational Narrative
• Mission and History
• Focus and Priorities
• Stakeholders and Values
• Needs and Goals

Population Narrative
• Environments and Behaviors
• Demographics and Disparities
• Incidence and Prevalence
• Needs and Goals

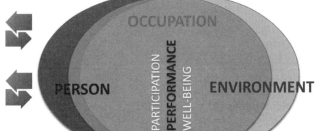

OCCUPATION

PERSON

ENVIRONMENT

PARTICIPATION

PERFORMANCE

WELL-BEING

Section VI provides an ending to this text, but also an important beginning for occupational therapy practice, education, and research.

A firm understanding of business principles is essential to be successful in a complex and changing health care environment. Occupational therapy and related concepts are similar to the language of other disciplines; sometimes we make assumptions about the underlying meaning and appropriate use of terminology in our profession or ignore how concepts have evolved over time to reflect new knowledge. Both of these chapters are intended to be used along with other sections of the text in integrative learning activities.

Chapter	Title	FAQ
30	*Enabling Successful Practice Through Application of Business Fundamentals* (Nellis)	• Why is knowledge of business fundamentals essential for occupational therapy practice and the profession? • What are the primary skills needed to be successful in the business of health care?
31	*Key Occupational Therapy Concepts in the Person-Occupation-Environment-Performance Model: Their Origin and Historical Use in the Occupational Therapy Literature* (Reed)	• Why is it important to examine the definitions and evolution of core concepts in occupational therapy? • What are some examples of concepts that have had different meanings over time or context?

Chapter 30

ENABLING SUCCESSFUL PRACTICE THROUGH APPLICATION OF BUSINESS FUNDAMENTALS

Patricia Nellis, MBA, OTR/L

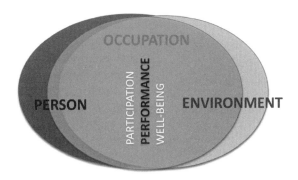

LEARNING OBJECTIVES

- Understand business principles as applied to occupational therapy.
- Understand how to use the PEOP Model to scan the environment in order to identify and analyze occupational therapy business opportunities.
- Understand legal business structures, and the implications of each on occupational therapy business ventures.
- Develop effective mission/vision/value statements that promote alignment and support future marketing efforts for occupational therapy services.
- Describe the key components of a marketing plan and how they relate to a business plan and successful implementation of a business concept aimed at improving the lives of others through participation.
- Describe the structure and purpose of a business plan to realize your practice objectives.

- Understand key financial components and metrics to measure and communicate success within your management structure/stakeholders.
- Understand reimbursement mechanisms in health care, school, and community settings.

KEY WORDS

- Corporation
- CPT (Current Procedural Terminology) codes
- Creating mission statements
- Creating vision statements
- Development of business plans
- Development of marking plans
- Individualized Education Program (IEP)
- Organizations
- Outcome measurements
- Outcomes

Christiansen CH, Baum CM, Bass JD, eds.
Occupational Therapy: Performance, Participation, and Well-Being, Fourth Edition (pp 549-563).
© 2015 SLACK Incorporated.

- Partnership
- Sole proprietorship
- Values

INTRODUCTION

The business of health care in the United States and abroad continues to grow and evolve. It was not until World War II that the US government began to embark on a mission to address health care for its citizens. Initial efforts included enacting legislation to fund the building of hospitals and to assure that certain health care services were available to the population at large.[1] Subsequent initiatives ushered in legislation to address the labor needs of health care providers, including occupational therapy practitioners, in the form of developing training programs and support.[1(p39)] Services at this time were geared toward episodic treatment of illnesses or related conditions, and were provided by a fragmented set of providers.

By the 1970s, the federal government began to appreciate the need to contain costs within an industry that was showing growth at an unsustainable rate. Imposing changes in reimbursement would support the need to contain costs and force providers to assess the services they delivered in order to streamline care, create standard practices, and eliminate waste. These activities, in theory, would eventually improve quality and lead to better outcomes. The first major change in reimbursement came in the form of how hospitals were paid. The formula shifted from cost-based (reimbursement based on itemized services delivered) to a "bundled" payment that was all inclusive.[2] This change was the beginning of a shift in payment methodology for all levels of care.

Between the mid-1980s to 1990s, various legislative acts continued to expand and mandate health-related services (eg, school age children; rehabilitation in nursing homes, home health), all the while continuing the practice of "bundling" services and reducing reimbursement to contain costs. With these acts came additional requirements for documentation, such as the Resident Assessment Instrument (RAI), the Patient Assessment Instrument (PAI), and the Outcomes Assessment Information Set (OASIS), all designed to move toward "standardizing" care, improving quality, and ultimately improving outcomes.[3] Changes during this period led to increases in the volume of therapy services delivered in practice areas such as schools, home health, outpatient, private practice, inpatient rehabilitation, and skilled nursing facilities.[1(p47)]

As the new millennium began, renewed efforts at reforming health care in the United States continued, with the primary focus being on cost containment, followed closely by concerns about access and quality. The delivery system remained fragmented and highly variable, with performance that is individualized but not standardized, and with a focus on volume, not value.[4] Today, due to continued legislation, cost pressures, and demographic changes, health care in the United States is slowly shifting from a focus on episodic treatment of illnesses in a fragmented delivery structure to a more coordinated, integrated system focused on prevention and population health, underpinned by the use of standards, guidelines, and outcome measures that support and guide quality.

Today, new trends have created many new opportunities for occupational therapy. Key drivers of change include changes in population demographics, such as aging and longevity, health care efforts to contain costs and reimbursement, changes in lifestyle choices and values, advances in science and technologies, and the kinds of health care services required, as well as where they are delivered.[5] These changes have led to broadened areas of practice that reach more settings, touch more populations, and address more concerns in an effort to promote healthful occupations in the changing world around us. From our humble beginnings of engaging disabled soldiers in purposeful activities, to addressing the psychosocial needs of children and promoting accessibility and QOL through the science of occupation, the world is now the market in which we operate and our "business" is enabling performance, participation, and well-being to individuals, organizations, and populations. Because the skills necessary for creating and managing businesses successfully are often not emphasized in formal occupational therapy education, practitioners may fail to see their relevance to effective practice or may overlook opportunities to deliver their services through creation of their own businesses.

ALIGNMENT OF OCCUPATIONAL THERAPY TRAINING/EDUCATION WITH USING THE PERSON-ENVIRONMENT-OCCUPATION-PERFORMANCE MODEL

The skills required for developing and managing a successful business are really very similar to the skills employed by an occupational therapy practitioner. A recent analysis suggests that out of 195 core skills and competencies identified in several pieces of literature, both practitioner and manager actively used 73% of all the skills listed.[1(p18)] This supports the proposition that practitioners are well aligned by way of education and training to be successful in the business of health care. Application of the PEOP Model through the systematic process of identifying and analyzing information and developing goals that align with needs and fit with the environment, along with sound planning, communication, and implementation skills, will lead to success in any setting, whether the results are an intervention for an individual, a new department program initiative, or a community-based program improving the health of a population.

Definition of Business

A business is an organization that is engaged in the "trade of goods, services, or both to an identified consumer or group of consumers."[6(np)] The word *business* is derived from the word *busyness*, a state of "purposeful activity"[7(np)] or occupation, which is a foundational concept in occupational therapy. The driving concept behind the trade or exchange of goods or services is the assumption that there is a good or service geared at filling a need or want and that it is perceived to be of value to a consumer who is willing to pay for it. An additional caveat of "value" is that it makes a difference in the life of a customer, either by way of increased skills, comfort, success, sense of well-being, or some other outcome. In providing health care services, standardized practices based on scientific evidence/best practice, meaningful measures to assess outcomes, and transparency/reporting performance toward these measures to the public are considered "value" added elements of care.[8] Accountability, adaptability, collaboration, teamwork, and the use of the Six Sigma or Lean Philosophy to eliminate waste, duplication, and organize processes are common skills and tools used to add value when meeting the needs of consumers.[9]

Business Structures

There are several legal forms of businesses (Table 30-1) that are subject to varying state/local jurisdictions, and there are typically certain "features" of these structures that distinguish one from another. Common features include taxation, liability, risk, decision-making control, continuity of existence, transferability of ownership, and expense/formality of setting up the business.[10] In many new businesses, liability, risk, and control are significant issues, thus most of our discussion here will be to compare the most common forms of business structures with these issues. The most common forms include sole proprietorships, partnerships, and corporations. Please note that this list is not all-inclusive, as there are variations between geographic jurisdictions, representing regions, and localities (eg, states and cities). In setting up any business, it is imperative to know the state and local requirements and investigate which would be the best fit for the type and level of business. Any business venture, even a new program proposal in an existing organization, is a *team sport*—meaning that you will need to seek assistance from professionals with expertise, eg, attorneys, financial planners, human resource professionals, tax advisors, accountants, etc.

A *sole proprietorship* is a type of business that is owned by one person; there is no legal distinction between the business and the owner. The owner/business is responsible for any debt incurred by the business, and the owner has full control over any and all decisions made regarding the business. Since the owner and business are one and the same, the owner is also at risk for any negligence, damage, or legal suit brought against them from a customer. This type of business is usually very small in size due to its inherent level of risk and liability, and is relatively easy to set up. Many clinicians choose not to permanently operate under this form due to liability and risk concerns.

A business owned by 2 or more people is a *partnership*. There are 3 typical classifications of partnerships: general partnerships where the partners share management control, property, profits, and financial liability in pre-determined proportions; limited partnerships where one or more partners has "limited" control and liability and is not considered a "general partner"; and limited liability partnerships (LLP) where one partner is not responsible for another partner's liability brought on by negligence or misconduct. LLPs are quite common among groups of professionals and are relatively less formal to set up.

A more recent business structure is that of a *limited liability company*, or LLC. This structure has both characteristics of a partnership or sole proprietorship and a corporation. An LLC is often referred to as a "corporation," but this reference is incorrect. Details of the requirements vary by state and country. An LLC may have one or more owners; the liability of this business structure is limited to what the owners have invested. In a legal suit, the plaintiffs pursue the company and not the owners or investors. Another benefit of an LLC is the pass-through taxation. Income or loss is reported as such on the owner's taxes in the United States and many of the state regulations provide further freedoms for taxation, allowing the company to choose to file as an LLC, S-Corporation, or C-Corporation. The requirements for setting up and maintaining an LLC are less complicated, and the company has greater flexibility in determining how the company is governed.

A *corporation* is a business that is a separate "entity," meaning it is legally separate from the members and the members are not liable for any debts incurred by the corporation. They are the most formal and complex to set up, and are by far the most common forms in large organizations. Corporations can be either owned by a government or individuals, and can organize as for-profit or nonprofit. A privately-owned, for-profit corporation is owned by shareholders who elect a board of directors to direct the corporation and hire its managerial staff. Nonprofit corporations are not owned by shareholders, and individuals do not receive a portion of any profits or excess revenue over expenses. Instead, any excess funds are put back into the

Table 30-1. *Comparing Forms of Business**

	Sole Proprietorship	General Partnership	Limited Liability Partnership	Limited Liability Company
Definition	A business owned and operated by one person for profit.	2 or more people who jointly own or operate a business for profit.	A form of partnership often used by professionals. The partner or investor's liability is limited to the amount he or she has invested in the company.	One or more partners have limited liability and no rights of management.
Ease of Formation	Easiest form of business to set up. If necessary, acquire licenses and permits, register name, and obtain taxpayer identification.	Easy to set up and operate; a written partnership agreement is recommended. Must acquire an Employer ID number and register company name.	File articles of organization with the state; adopt operating agreement, and file necessary reports. The name must show it is limited liability company.	Requires filing a Certificate of Limited Partnership. Name must show that business is a limited partnership. Must have written agreement, and must keep certain records.
Period of Existence	Terminates at will or on the death of the owner.	Terminates by agreement, or by death or withdrawal of partner, unless there is a partnership agreement to the contrary.		May terminate by agreement, or withdrawal of a member, depending upon operating agreement.
Liability	The owner's personal assets are at risk.	Each partner's personal assets are at risk.	Similar to rules for corporations	General partners' personal assets are at risk. A limited partner is liable only to the extent of his or her investment.
Dissolution	Easiest form of business to dissolve. Pay debts, taxes, and claims against business.	Pay debts, taxes, and claims against business; settle partnership accounts.	Pay debts, taxes, and claims against business. Distribute remaining assets to members. File articles of dissolution with the state.	Pay debts, taxes, and claims against business. Settle partnership accounts. File cancellation of certificate with the state.

*C and S Corporations are not depicted on this chart because individuals or small groups forming companies typically do not consider them.

program. Nonprofits also have a board that serves to provide guidance to the corporation.

EFFECTIVE SKILLS FOR BUSINESS SUCCESS

Business success is the end result of a process that includes gathering information, analyzing, and comparing it to some desired or future state; developing goals, interventions, and outcome measures; and implementing, re-evaluating, or modifying the plan as time goes on in order to achieve the desired goals. Key competencies and skills transcend the different types of services delivered, whether they are geared at traditional health care for individuals, for school age children, or for wellness and prevention programs at the community level. In addition to a professional responsibility of being a lifelong learner, there are 3 major categories of skills that impact effectiveness and success: communication, evaluation and planning, and implementation skills.

Communication Skills

Communication skills include all aspects of communication from verbal, nonverbal, or written on a one-to-one basis; to the same within organizations, markets, or industries. Examples of specific communication-based activities include advocacy and consultation; education, collaboration, leading, or motivating others; facilitating groups or teams; communicating with clients, insurance companies, community boards, and public organizations; and marketing. These activities are not all inclusive, and even though occupational therapy is an autonomous profession, the ability to collaborate is perhaps the most critical.[11]

Evaluation/Assessment and Planning Skills

Assessment and planning skills include the ability to collect data in an organized, focused manner and analyze it for decision making. These skills are fundamental to the implementation of interventions and services. Examples include collecting relevant financial data and analyzing it for efficiency, cost containment, or goal achievement; collection of performance or quality improvement measures; and analyses of job duties for staffing needs or additional resources. Planning based on the results of data gathering and analyses, and developing appropriate goals, interventions, and strategies creates the foundation for the next implementation, including managing and sustaining change.

Implementation Skills

Implementation skills include all aspects of putting plans in motion. Successful implementation often includes a plan that outlines the various steps one must take and activities one must complete to fully launch the plan that has been written. Effective skills in this area often require navigating and managing multiple processes simultaneously. Evaluation and assessment skills are foundational for developing an implementation plan, and communication skills are critical for the actual execution.[12] Examples of specific activities include deployment of specific interventions; developing and implementing team training initiatives, policies, or performance improvement activities; or integrating practice changes into an existing setting based on new evidence.

REIMBURSEMENT IN HEALTH CARE AND INFLUENCE ON OCCUPATIONAL THERAPY SERVICES/BUSINESS DEVELOPMENT

For many individuals in the United States, traditional health care services are funded either through public sources, such as Medicare or Medicaid; or through private sources, such as employer-based insurance programs or those purchased by individuals or groups from private insurance companies. In other countries, provisions for funding health care vary. However, in most developed countries a single government-funded health insurance scheme is typically the norm, sometimes supplemented at an individual's discretion by private insurance plans. Each of these insurance sources has a set of defined rules/regulations and specifications of what is covered and under which circumstances. Not all such plans may include coverage for occupational therapy services, and many do include either a deductible or set amount of money that must be paid by the insured before the insurer pays their part, as well as an additional co-pay amount for individual visits. The aim of this section will be to orient the practitioner to a basic understanding of the major reimbursement models and associated documentation needs.

Medicare is one of the largest payers in the United States, thus the policies, rules, and processes of this program also influence many other insurance organizations. Medicare provides health care services for people older than 65 years of age, for those with disabilities and/or end-stage renal disease. Medicare is comprised of the Hospital Insurance Program (Part A), the Medical Insurance Program (Part B), Medicare Advantage (managed care referred or Part C), and the Prescription Drug Program (Part D). Here, we will briefly examine the major components of the Part A and B programs, since both provide significant coverage for occupational therapy services.[13] Readers not based in the United States should consult applicable provisions of coverage for services, typically available on web-based resources identified by the specific funding agency. Although policies for Medicare are uniform across the 50 United States, in some countries, such as Canada, (provincial) health authorities may have specific policies governing coverage that vary by governing jurisdiction.

Medicare Part A Reimbursement and Documentation

US Medicare, Hospital Insurance, or Part A program includes acute hospital stays, inpatient rehabilitation, skilled nursing, home health, and services for end-stage renal disease. In acute hospitals, individuals are admitted either for a medical condition, testing that requires multiple services, or for certain procedures (eg, orthopedic surgery) that can only be provided on an inpatient basis. The specific occupational therapy assessment used may be chosen by the hospital, along with the style and contents of notes. Many hospitals include similar content such as past history, prior level of function, current functional status, goals, and a plan of care. Often, notes are entered upon the conclusion of each visit and the occupational therapy practitioner plays a role in helping to determine discharge needs for post-hospital care and follow-up services.

Individuals admitted to inpatient rehabilitation facilities (IRF) are deemed to need a higher level of intensive rehabilitation that includes occupational therapy, physical therapy, speech-language pathology, or prosthetic/orthotic training. The assessment tool in the IRF setting is the Patient Assessment Instrument (PAI), which captures certain patient characteristics along with their functional status in select areas of ADL.[14] This assessment occurs upon admission and again at discharge, and results in a "score" that translates into a case mix group that determines the reimbursement rate for the facility. The practitioner typically documents small contact notes on a daily basis and a longer, more comprehensive assessment note summarizing treatment on a weekly basis (at least). The content of the notes relates directly to the ADL areas on the PAI, such as eating, grooming, bathing, dressing, and transfers, and serves to support the coding of the patient's level of function on the PAI.

Skilled nursing facilities (SNF) Part A programs are "distinct" geographical areas that have a set number of their beds dedicated to the Part A program. The SNF Part A program requires that individuals must need skilled nursing and/or rehabilitation at least 5 days per week. The assessment used in this setting is the Resident Assessment Instrument (RAI), of which the Minimum Data Set (MDS) is a subset. The MDS contains screening components for conditions such as depression, as well as ratings for specific performance and support needs in physical functioning and ADL areas. The number of minutes of therapy is recorded on the MDS for a pre-determined assessment period. This total number of minutes, combined with select ADL scores, serves to place the individual into a resource utilization group (RUG).[3] The actual reimbursement for the SNF is based on the specific RUG group into which the individual falls, so close tracking of minutes of occupational therapy delivered is critical, along with supportive documentation. Documentation at the SNF level involves an initial assessment; brief daily contact notes, including minutes of therapy; and a longer, more in-depth weekly note summarizing progress.

Home Health Agencies (HHA) provide services to those who are homebound and in need of intermittent skilled nursing, physical therapy, or speech therapy. Occupational therapy is a covered service, but an individual cannot qualify solely on a need for occupational therapy until the need for nursing, physical therapy, or speech therapy has been established. Once occupational therapy has been determined as a need, services can be continued even when the other disciplines have been discontinued. Individuals receiving home health services need additional interventions aimed at improving performance, assuring safety, and preventing future problems. The Outcome and Assessment Information Set (OASIS) is the tool used by the HHA to assess and classify the individual receiving services. It is very comprehensive and covers many subjects including environmental support, health, and functional status and use of health services. The individual occupational therapy assessment must include information about ADL and IADL, and formal progress reports must be completed by a licensed occupational therapy practitioner on or before the 13th and 19th visits.[15] The report must summarize using objective measures, the individual's functional status compared against the initial, and any changes in the plan of care. Typically, less comprehensive treatment notes are completed on each visit.

Medicare Part B

The Medical Insurance Program (Part B) covers many different kinds of services, including occupational therapy. It provides reimbursement for services delivered in outpatient settings, and is the major insurance coverage in the section of a nursing home where residents live on a permanent basis. Reimbursement for services is based on Current Procedural Terminology (CPT) codes and descriptions. Medicare pays 80% of the stated reimbursed amount, with the remaining 20% either being paid by some type of co-insurance or by the individual. Currently, there are dollar limitations on the total reimbursement possible in a given year, and this practice has led to closer scrutiny by providers to assure that services are necessary and effective.

The assessment used at this level can be the choice of the provider, but must contain certain information including the individual's prior level of function, current level, specific problems, goals, interventions, and a plan of care. The plan of care must include the diagnosis, long-term goals, type, amount, duration, and frequency of treatment. Objective assessments where information is obtained systematically and consistently, including interpretation of the results, are required. The plan must be certified by a physician within 30 days and must be re-certified every 90 days. Required documentation includes an evaluation and plan of care, physician certification, progress reports, and treatment notes.[13] The progress report is a more extensive summary that must be completed by a licensed occupational therapy practitioner at a minimum of once every 10 visits. The treatment notes are brief, completed per visit, and must include details such as the time in/out and specific services provided, including a listing of timed/untimed CPT codes that will serve to support the bill for that session.

Schools

In the United States, school-based services are required by federal legislation. School-based services and reimbursement vary tremendously by state and individual districts. In some cases, the practitioner may be required to document and charge for public or private insurance if the model is such that the schools are billing for services. In other cases, the practitioner may be required to document progress against goals in the IEP. The practitioner may be employed by the district or serving the district through a contractual arrangement. The practitioner may provide services directly, within or outside of the classroom, or they may serve as a consultant working with/through teachers, paraprofessionals, or aides.[16]

Community Programs

Community-based programs vary broadly by purpose and populations served. Reimbursement for community-based programs may range from insurance (private and public), to public funding from other government sources, to general funding from private foundations or grants.[17] Documentation for community-based programs varies with the purpose, but mirrors the stated goals and objectives of each program. For those receiving grant funding, keeping detailed records of expenses and making sure they are aligned with the mission and objectives is critical. Documentation supporting effectiveness of the program is also critical in order to keep or obtain future funding. That process involves using tools for assessment when the individuals enter and exit the program to be able to measure the impact the program has had on addressing the needs of the population served.[17(p265)]

ASSESSMENTS AND EVALUATIONS

Assessment, evaluation, and analysis are the beginning points to any business planning venture. This process typically begins with a market analysis that leads to the identification of a smaller target market. A market consists of all potential consumers who are willing to pay for a service. A target market is simply a smaller group of consumers who have certain characteristics in common, such

as needs, economic resources, demographic characteristics, etc.[1(p128)] In occupational therapy, some examples of a target market would include seniors wishing to stay in their home, school-age children with developmental concerns, or community dwelling young adults with mental health challenges. The goal of a market analysis is to discover trends, assess needs/demands, and identify a viable target market (including competitors) in order to develop or improve upon a service. There are 2 major subsections to a market analysis, an environmental assessment and organizational assessment.[1(p132)]

Environmental Assessment

The environmental assessment considers all factors that are external to a business or organization that may have an impact on or influence how the business may function in the identified market. Common areas assessed include: demographics, economics, political climate, regulations, physical accessibility, use or availability of technologies, and social/cultural characteristics. Much of this information can be obtained from various national databases. In the United States, these would include the US Census, CDC, US Department of Education, Agency for Healthcare Research and Quality, or the US Department of Health and Human Services. Other information is best obtained by touring the geographical area to assess for community infrastructure such as schools, hospitals, churches, and other services, as well as investigating community service organizations and other local businesses.

Organizational Assessment

The goal of the organizational assessment is to identify factors, both internal and external to the organization, that may influence the ability of the business to be able to deliver the service in the selected target market. Many organizations use a SWOT analysis to meet this need, as it systematically assesses both internal and external factors. The "S" and "W" stand for strengths and weaknesses. These are internal to the organization and are accepted as factors being within the control of the business or individuals within the business. Examples could be knowledge, skills, or resources, some of which may include staffing, time, equipment, relationships, or money. The "O" and "T" stand for opportunities and threats, and are external factors to an individual or organization and thus out of the realm of direct control. However, they are expected to influence the outcomes of a business concept. Examples may include the number of competitors (or lack thereof) or the resources available in the environment, such as physical space, accessibility, laws, reimbursement practices, etc. Thus, whether a given factor is a threat or an opportunity depends upon its nature and characteristics within the environment under consideration. Some factors have the potential to be either threats or opportunities, while others remain only in one category regardless of circumstances. For example, a rapidly growing target population can be an opportunity. But fast growth can also overwhelm the ability to deliver quality services, and this factor then becomes a threat. On the other hand, rising liability insurance costs are always a threat to a business, as are legal actions.

It is important to elaborate on the process of completing a SWOT analysis at this point and to caution that it is not simply a "listing" of factors. Once the factors have been listed, there needs to be a step during which the factors are prioritized in order of importance or influence. For strengths and weaknesses, it is recommended to look at each individual item and determine the importance of each, based on how much the strength will help fulfill the business concept and how much the weakness will impact or prevent the concept from coming to life. The other necessary comparison is to determine how much the identified strengths can provide in terms of support to offset, or mitigate, the negative effects of the weaknesses listed. The same process applies to the analyses of the opportunities and threats. Table 30-2 provides a description of a rating process and summary table that illustrates a comparative process using priorities and weighting.

Identifying and Defining the Business Concept

In most cases, occupational therapy practitioners provide services in the form of defined interventions to individuals, organizations, or communities. Typical service models include prevention, wellness, educational, or niche specialty programs.[18] Once you have identified your target market and completed the organizational analysis, you can begin to develop the details of the services. This includes a clear description of the actual service(s), how often, when, and how they will be provided and all the resources needed to deliver the service such as people, technology, physical space, billing systems and marketing. It also includes a projection of anticipated income from the business; as well as legal fees, start-up costs, and other start-up expenses. Once completed, you'll begin the process of analyzing the feasibility of pursuing your concept.

Assessing Feasibility

The goal at this stage is to determine whether or not your business concept will be realistic and sustainable. Influencing factors include knowledge about the trends identified in your target market, namely the number of consumers or clients who will use your services, referral sources, availability, location, payment, funding, laws and regulations, competitors, potential labor market availability, and other considerations. Three specific areas of feasibility assessment include operational, technical, and economic.[19] Operational feasibility considers whether or not you have sufficient human resources, skills, knowledge, and processes to be effective. Technical feasibility looks at all the technological components, including equipment, computers, phones, software programs for billing, documentation, and technologies. Economic feasibility, perhaps the most critical, refers to whether or not you will have sufficient demand for your services that will produce enough revenue to cover costs, sustain, and eventually grow the business. Anticipating that beginning months will incur costs greater than revenues is an important part of considering economic feasibility. All combined, the results of an effective feasibility assessment will yield a determination that the plan is feasible, feasible with changes, or not feasible at all.

INTERVENTION

Mission, Vision, and Value Statements

Mission statements describe the purpose of your business, or what you do. This statement typically has 3 components: who you are, the services or products you provide, and how you deliver or provide that service or product.[18(p18)] Mission statements can vary from long narratives to very brief descriptions and, given the fact that they are often used in marketing efforts, it is advisable to target a version that is easily recognized and recalled. Vision statements are perhaps the most critical. They are the statements of dreams and desires. Vision statements are inspiring and grab the reader. They are easily recalled and resonate with consumers and others. They are dynamic, in that they inspire the mission to come to life and point the direction to the future. Vision statements often contain words such as *premier, leader, number one, best,* or *preferred;* all pave the way to being great or the only choice. Values statements are descriptions of the beliefs that serve to drive the purpose or mission and fuel the vision to become a living concept. They "guide" the behaviors and decisions of the individual or organization by defining what is important. It is important to carefully craft these statements and assure that they reflect what you provide, believe, and where you want to be in the future, because they will serve as the foundation for developing strategies, managing growth, and navigating changes in the business landscape.

Table 30-2. *Organizational Assessment SWOT Analysis Summary Matrix*

	Weight	Rating	Weighted Score	Comments
Factors: Strengths/Weaknesses				
S—Knowledgeable/dedicated providers	2.5	6	15	5 advanced clinicians
S—Software/systems capable	1	6	6	Billing and health records
W—Limited access to large amounts of capital	2	6	12	Not positioned to grow quickly
Factors: Opportunities/Threats				
O—Target market has few providers	2	6	12	Weak competitors
T—Limited physical location availability	1.5	6	9	Building is old, outdated, expensive to retrofit
O—Business climate incentives	1	6	6	Tax breaks
Total Score	10	36	6*	

(S=Strength, W=Weakness, O=Opportunity, T=Threat)
*Total column score divided by 10
Explanation: To create a SWOT Summary Matrix as shown in this example, select the 2 to 3 most important strengths/weaknesses and the 2 to 3 most important opportunities/threats. Assign a weight to each: 10 = most important; 0 = not important. The total for all MUST not exceed 10. Rate each factor based on the following scale. The rating compares how well-equipped the business is to manage the factor, or how well it is currently managed.
10 = Outstanding
9 = Above average and strengthening
8 = Above average and holding steady
7 = Above average, having difficulty sustaining
6 = Average and strengthening
5 = Average and holding steady
4 = Average, having difficulty sustaining
3 = Below average but strengthening
2 = Below average holding steady
1 = Below average, having difficulty sustaining
0 = Poor/incapable
Multiply weight times rating; then add weighted scores and divide by 10. You will get a number between 1 to 10. This will tell you which factors to utilize in determining goals/plans and how well the business is positioned to move forward.

Effective Business Planning

The objectives for writing a business plan are to describe the business concept in detail and to provide a financial picture or projection of what will be necessary to implement the plan.[20] Many choose to undertake writing a shorter business proposal, illustrating the basic concept before developing a full plan. Typical business plans can be anywhere from 20 to 30 pages long. There is no set format, but one should include at least the following basic sections[21]:

- *Executive Summary:* This should be the last section written and is a summary of every part of the plan. It should include a description of the mission, vision, values, names of owners, number of employees, description of services, and summary of the target market. It is the first section that is read, and must be concisely written to inspire and persuade others.

Table 30-3. *Key Components of a Marketing Plan*

Component	Description
Market research	• Description of market • Dynamics • Needs identified/scope of needs
Target market	• Description of who, where, and statistics • Specific needs • Describe any barriers to reaching the target market and strategies • Describe facilitators • Results of SWOT and strategies
Product/service	• Description of what will be offered • When, where, by whom • Description of how the service will fill the need • Referral sources/collaborators
Competitors	• List competitors and related information: location, strength of competition, brand, etc. • Describe how your service will be different from others providing the same/similar
Mission/vision statements/goals/objectives	• Describe statements • Identify details of goals/objectives

Market strategies	• Describe specific activities, below are a few ideas:
	  ◦ Networking?
	  ◦ Direct marketing: brochures, flyers?
	  ◦ Advertising: print, radio, web?
	  ◦ Increase awareness/expertise: write column, serve on board, train lay persons, volunteer activities
	  ◦ Personal sales: to whom?
	  ◦ Press releases

Marketing budget	• How much is set aside for each specific activity?
Measures and process	• Identify specific measures to assure you are focused • Describe how measurement process will work: what you will use, how often measures will be reviewed, etc.

- *Company/Business Description:* The detailed description should include goals and objectives that support the mission, vision, and values. Alignment of the goals, objectives, and measures assures that the practices, programs, and decisions are directly related to the mission or the reason the business exists, and to the vision or future direction.[22,23] This section also includes a description about the services, supporting evidence, and how they will be delivered. Lastly, this section should include a contingency, or exit plan, that details when and what will happen should the business fail to thrive.

- *Organization and Management:* This section includes details of the organizational structure in terms of who does what, number of employees, salaries, benefits, ownership, advisory board members, and roles, as well as a description of how the department or organization functions.

- *Marketing Plan:* The marketing plan is perhaps the most dynamic and action-oriented (Table 30-3). The marketing process systematically identifies and describes techniques and activities taken to attract and grow users of the services. This section also includes referral sources, collaborators, or community partners, as well as a description of the nature and scope of any competitors. Any environmental barriers or facilitators in the market that may impact your efforts should be described, along with the strategies you plan to implement to grow and sustain the business. Many market planning guides refer to a series of "P's" which include: Product (the service or product), Price (the cost, charge, reimbursement), Place (where the service is provided/offered), Promotion (the plan for promoting, growing), Position (the kind of service or position in market —niche, better quality, less costly, substitute for another service/product), Packaging (how your product/service appears, confidence of people delivering the service, types of assessments/interventions you offer), and People (EVERYONE in your business).[1(p128),24]

- *Funding Requests:* This section includes any funding needed, the amount, and what will be done with the funds. Some funding needs may include start-up costs, such as market research, legal, accounting, or contract fees.

- *Financial Projections:* This section includes projections of income, cash flow, and capital purchases. Typically, the projections are developed for a 5-year period. The first year should be broken down monthly, and years 2 to 5 can be quarterly. For any business/program that may have a "seasonal" component (eg, school-based services), it is advisable to extend monthly projections through the second year. It is advisable to seek the assistance of a qualified professional to assure projections are realistic and accurate. Pictures and graphs may be useful in this section.

- *Appendix:* This section contains all supporting information used in the narrative sections. It should include resumes, references, evidence tables/articles, legal documents, lists of consultants, attorneys, accountants, and any raw data.[21]

Implementing the Business Plan and Managing Change

Effective and successful implementation begins with the formulation of the plan, including clear goals, objectives, and measures. In an established system or organization, it also includes the management of change, since it is a change in practice and processes. In either scenario, managing the environment in terms of "marketing" the services to potential clients or "selling" the idea to stakeholders who will be impacted by the change is a key process, involving use of different communication strategies.[25] In marketing a new business, communicating the service provided and the value that it brings is a beginning

point, since the goal for a new start-up is to build the client base. In selling a new proposal in an existing organization, soliciting the input from key stakeholders in the initial development phases, along with communicating the value of the program and the "what's in it for me" to those who will be impacted by the change, is a key beginning point, since the goal is to gain support for the proposal. In either case, developing an implementation plan that includes specific activities, timelines, and measures of success is foundational.

OUTCOMES

Delivering services, measuring against identified goals and objectives, and changing interventions or strategies is a dynamic process. This need for change is a response to evolving person-environment factors. Tracking and analyzing measures is important, because it promotes a sustained focus on goals and objectives, supports effectiveness and efficacy, and helps to identify gaps in performance. Effective management of various measures may also lead to the discovery of new problems or issues or point to needed changes in strategies or processes.[25-27] Many measures fall into the 2 broad categories of financial and quality. Quality often includes subsets of measures focused on operations, processes, and outcomes.

Financial Measures

Financial measures include comparing actual activity, such as revenues, to what was projected or budgeted. Many financial measures include targets for volume, such as the number of clients served in a month, patients seen, visits made, etc. When comparing actual costs and revenues to budgeted costs and revenues, it is most effective to focus on the variance, or difference, between the targeted goals and what actually occurred. Many organizations will track in both a raw number and percentage format. For example, if a target for 1 month was to serve 200 clients, and actual clients served was 100; then the variance would be 100, or 50% fewer clients were seen than projected. Many financial measures also employ the use of ratios because they are an indicator of how efficiently the program is operating. Common ratio measures may include the number of visits per occupational therapy practitioner; the number of staff hours or units of service generated in a given day, week, or month; or the cost of supplies per visit or unit of service. The value of measuring ratios lies in being able to monitor the proportion of resources used to deliver the intended service. Measuring gross variances alone can lead to a misinterpretation because they don't measure changes in volume against resources used. Often times, financial measures are not directly stated in the initial business plan goals or objectives, but are instead identified indirectly through operational, quality, or outcome measures.

Quality Measures—Structure, Process, and Outcome

Most non-financial measures fall into the broad categories of structure, process, outcomes, and consumer satisfaction,[24] and are considered to measure various aspects of quality. *Structural process* measures capture administrative issues or processes that direct and support the delivery of direct care. For example, in a school setting, a common measure may be the percent of students receiving occupational therapy services in a school-based program compared to the total number of students; or in some cases, the potential or anticipated number of students who have been identified in need of services. In a community setting, the percent of clients using the services as a proportion of the number of potential clients may be used as a measure. In the case of a wellness program that is designed to promote exercise opportunities to clients with physical limitations in a gym setting, a measure may be the percent of time specialized equipment is in use compared to the total time the wellness program is open. Most of these types of measures target the "volume" of activity or service being provided. Many target staffing efficiencies.

Process measures typically target clinical or service processes, meaning they measure whether or not you are actually doing what your policies or goals say you planned to do. The focus of these measures is typically on the use of specific evidence-based processes that occur during the delivery of care.[28] In the case of a free-standing private practice clinic, a measure could be the percent of clients who received a specific screening during the intake assessment when the target is to complete the screening on 100% of all clients. Another could be the percent who received targeted education during the initial visit. In the school setting, a process measure could be targeted at the rate of occupational therapy practitioner participation in the IEP process or the rate of occupational therapy practitioners who provide targeted education to parents or caretakers. In the previous wellness example, a process measure could be the rate of completion of a QOL questionnaire on the initial visit.

Outcome measures are often used to demonstrate accountability to external sources, such as funding sources, government agencies, or administrative bodies. The focus is to measure against the stated ultimate goal of the care or service delivered and to assess changes in health care status due to interventions. Examples could include the number of clients who achieved independence with cooking after participating in a meal preparation group, or the number of students who were able to successfully integrate into a class setting of peers after receiving targeted occupational therapy services. In the case of the wellness program, the proportion of clients reporting increased QOL measures after developing and participating in a regular exercise routine would be an outcome measure that is supported by a process measure.

SUMMARY

The AOTA Centennial Vision sees occupational therapy as a leading force in health care during the 21st century. This vision is driven by changing demographics, such as the growth of an aging population, obesity rates, changes in traditional family units, and increased cultural diversity stemming from immigration.[29] Coupled with pressures on reimbursement, new models of health care delivery are emerging and traditional models are shifting focus, exposing gaps in services and opening up new opportunities. The need for occupational therapy services is great at multiple levels, and the potential for delivering these needed services creates a global market of opportunity. The skills necessary to develop new programs at all levels are consistent with the skills, training, and education received by occupational therapy practitioners. Understanding changes in the environment, quickly identifying needs, and predicting trends are abilities that will ultimately lead to development of new and emerging practice areas (Table 30-4). Enhancing the person factors of occupational therapy practitioners through active engagement in the profession, applying knowledge and skills, and developing competencies continuously will lead directly to these new developments.

Table 30-4. *Evidence Table*

Ref	Key Idea and Purpose	Research Design and Methods; Level of Evidence	Results and Conclusions	Take Home Message
20	Importance of business planning	Descriptive Survey N=73	Effective planning is critical to long-range success	• Use experienced resources • Gather data/input from multiple sources • Base the plan on realistic assumptions • Use plans proactively for financial/budgeting purposes
12	Identify competencies and most effective model for leadership development	Quantitative Qualitative Survey N=883	Competency needs/skills vary with job roles	• Major competencies for leaders/business managers include: ◦ Advocacy ◦ Adaptation to change ◦ Verbal/written communication skills ◦ Development of partnerships ◦ Strategic planning ◦ Ethics knowledge ◦ Future focus thinking ◦ Ability to manage data/interpret ◦ Analytical thinking
24	Consumer perceptions of quality and service	Survey Quantitative Qualitative N=8000	Identified specific perceptions of health care consumers relating to what constitutes quality	• Client experience perceptions of quality include: ◦ Thorough assessment and explanation of results ◦ Involvement in decision making ◦ Active listening ◦ Communication in language understood ◦ Teamwork/courtesy/friendliness
			Identified facets of service quality	• Factors needed to provide and improve services include: ◦ Access to multiple data sources ◦ Accountability to standards ◦ Access to consultation to make improvements ◦ Identify/live service values/behaviors ◦ Monitor/control measures ◦ Reward/recognize

(continued)

Table 30-4 (continued).   *Evidence Table*

Ref	Key Idea and Purpose	Research Design and Methods; Level of Evidence	Results and Conclusions	Take Home Message
26	Identification of attributes geared at standardization of practices	Comprehensive literature review	Guidelines that were closest to existing norms requiring minimal change are more effective. Also, simple, concrete, and clearly defined guidelines were most effective.	• Keep standards simple, familiar, clear, concrete, and measurable
27	Identified characteristics of most effective clinical practice guidelines	Quantitative N = 86	Practice guidelines supported by evidence that do not require new skills and are not part of a complex decision-making matrix are effective.	• Guidelines, both operational and clinical, need to be kept simple and clear
23	To determine the types of strategies used in implementation	RCT N = 34	Strategies specifically tailored to individuals/interventions were most effective	• When developing business or marketing strategies, make sure they are matched with the specific intervention
28	To assess various strategies to use in evaluating processes	Qualitative Quantitative Descriptive N = 54	Audit/feedback; consensus building and development of a reminder system were most important	• When identifying and developing process measures, include the audit/feedback process details, agree on measures and definitions BEFORE the audit process begins, integrate "triggers" or reminders to help assure process steps are completed

REFERENCES

1. Jacobs K, McCormack GL. *The Occupational Therapy Manager.* 5th ed. Bethesda, MD: AOTA Press; 2011.
2. Centers for Medicare and Medicaid Services. History. CMS. gov: Centers for Medicare and Medicaid Services. http://www. cms.gov/About-CMS/Agency-Information/History/index. html?redirect=/History/. Updated June 13, 2013. Accessed October 7, 2013.
3. Centers for Medicare and Medicaid Services. Nursing Home Quality Initiative. CMS.gov: Centers for Medicare and Medicaid Services. http://www.cms.gov/Medicare/Quality-Initiatives-Patient-Assessment-Instruments/NursingHomeQualityInits/index.html. Updated September 20, 2013. Accessed October 27, 2013.
4. Bohmer RMJ. *Designing Care: Aligning the Nature and Management of Health Care.* Boston, MA: Harvard Business Press; 2009.
5. AOTA. AOTA: American Occupational Therapy Association. http://www.aota.org/. Updated 2013. Accessed October 27, 2013.
6. Sullivan A, Sheffrin SM. *Economics: Principles in Action.* Upper Saddle River, NJ: Pearson Prentice Hall; 2003.
7. *Business.* Merriam-Webster. http://www.merriam-webster. com/dictionary/business. Updated 2013. Accessed October 27, 2013.
8. Institute of Medicine: Committee on Quality of Health Care in America. *Crossing the Quality Chasm: A New Health System for the 21st Century.* Washington, DC: National Academy Press; 2013.
9. Brue G, Howes R. *Six Sigma.* New York, NY: McGraw-Hill; 2006.
10. Internet Center for Management and Business Administration, Inc. Quick MBA: Knowledge to Power Your Business. Quick MBA. http://www.quickmba.com. Updated 2010. Accessed October 7, 2013.
11. Baum CM. Centennial challenges, millennium opportunities. *Am J Occup Ther.* 2006;60(6):609-616.
12. Garman A, Scribner L. Leading for quality in healthcare: development and validation of a competency model. *J Healthc Manag.* 2011;56(6):373-382.
13. Medicare Program—General Information. Centers for Medicare and Medicaid Services. http://www.cms.gov/Medicare/Medicare-General-Information/MedicareGenInfo/index.html?redirect=/MedicareGenInfo/. Updated August 27, 2103. Accessed October 7, 2013.

14. Inpatient Rehabilitation Facility: Patient Assessment Instrument. Centers for Medicare and Medicaid Services. http://www.cms.gov/InpatientRehabFacPPS/downloads/CMS-10036.pdf. Updated January 2006. Accessed October 7, 2013.

15. CMS Manual System: Pub 100-02 Medicare Benefit Policy: Transmittal 144: Home Health Therapy Services. Centers for Medicare and Medicaid Services. http://www.cms.gov/transmittals/downloads/R144BP.pdf. Published May 6, 2011. Accessed October 7, 2013.

16. Braveman B. *Leading and Managing OT Services*. Philadelphia, PA: FA Davis; 2006.

17. Fazio LS. *Developing Occupation Centered Programs for the Community*. 2nd ed. Upper Saddle River, NJ: Pearson Prentice Hall; 2008.

18. Richmond T, Powers D. *Business Fundamentals for the Rehabilitation Professional*. 2nd ed. Thorofare, NJ: SLACK Incorporated; 2009.

19. Kansas State University. *Assessing the Feasibility of Business Propositions*. Kansas State University: Agricultural Economics. http://ageconomics.k-state.edu/. Accessed September 15, 2011.

20. Singhvi S. Business planning practices in small size companies: survey results. *Journal of Business Forecasting Methods and Systems*. 2008;19(2):3-8.

21. SBA.gov: US Small Business Administration. http://www.sba.gov. Accessed September 5, 2011.

22. Rathbone CLH. Turning on the cutting edge of reality. *Management Accounting*. 1999;77(11):16-20.

23. Baker R, Reddish S, Robertson N, Hearnshaw H, Jones B. Randomized controlled trial of tailored strategies to implement guidelines for the management of patients with depression in general practice. *Br J Gen Pract*. 2001;51:737-741.

24. Kennedy DM, Caselli RJ, Berry LL. A roadmap for improving healthcare service quality. *J Healthc Manag*. 2011;56(6):385-400.

25. Grol R, Wensing M, Eccles M. *Improving Patient Care—The Implementation of Change in Clinical Practice*. Edinburgh, Scotland: Elsevier; 2005.

26. Grol R, Eccles M, Maisonneuve H. Developing clinical practice guidelines: the European experience. *Dis Man Health Out*. 1998;4:255-266.

27. Burgers JS, Cluzeau FA, Hanna SE, Hunt SE, Grol R. Characteristics of high quality guidelines: evaluation of 86 clinical guidelines developed in ten European countries and Canada. *Int J Technol Asess Health Care*. 2003;19(1):148-157.

28. Baskerville NB, Hogg W, Lemelin J. Process evaluation of a tailored multifaceted approach to changing family physician practice patterns and improving preventive care. *J Fam Prac*. 2001;50:W242-W249.

29. Moyers P. A legacy of leadership: achieving our centennial vision. *Am J Occup Ther*. 2007;61(6):622-628.

KEY OCCUPATIONAL THERAPY CONCEPTS IN THE PERSON-OCCUPATION-ENVIRONMENT-PERFORMANCE MODEL

Their Origin and Historical Use in the Occupational Therapy Literature

Kathlyn L. Reed, PhD, OTR, FAOTA, MLIS

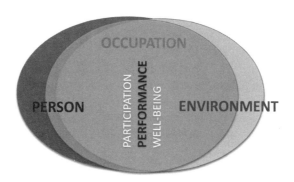

LEARNING OBJECTIVES

- Understand the purpose, functions, and value of concepts in evolving the knowledge base of a profession.
- Identify concepts associated with key periods in the history of the occupational therapy profession.
- Identify the key concepts underlying the PEOP Model.
- Review the historical use of key PEOP concepts within the occupational therapy literature.

- Identify types of conceptual practice models in occupational therapy.
- Appreciate the importance of carefully defining, using, documenting, and justifying terms when they are used in communicating the key ideas within a profession's body of knowledge.

KEY WORDS

- Achievement
- Adaptation

Christiansen CH, Baum CM, Bass J, eds.
Occupational Therapy: Performance, Participation, and Well-Being, Fourth Edition (pp 565-648).
© 2015 SLACK Incorporated.

- Autonomy
- Competence
- Coping
- Fitness
- Frameworks
- Function
- Health
- History
- Ideas
- Independence
- Interdependence
- Life balance
- Models
- Occupational balance
- Occupational justice
- Occupational performance
- Outcomes
- Prevention
- Quality of life
- Recovery
- Satisfaction
- Self-efficacy
- Self-management
- Theory
- Well-being

INTRODUCTION

As occupational therapy moves into relection and analysis around its second century of existence, what has gone before is one strategy for looking into the future. Occupational therapy was organized around ideas and applications that served the context of clients and practitioners at the time they were developed; however, changes in ideas and applications occur, as the context for practice has changed. Some of the original ideas and some of the changes may be useful in the future. The questions are: Which ideas? and How can they be evaluated? One approach is to examine the concepts. The history of the terms should help students, practitioners, and scientists in clearly defining and communicating key terms in interdisciplinary discourse. Specifically the concepts that are central to the PEOP Model will be discussed in this chapter.

(Editors' Note: This chapter uses APA style for citations and references because we believe this style more readily helps the reader associate the names of authors with the key concepts they originated or evolved in the occupational therapy literature.)

WHY CONCEPTS ARE IMPORTANT

In scientific theories, ideas are called *concepts* and occasionally *constructs* (Kerlinger, 1986, p. 26). Concepts are words or phrases used to label similarities between phenomena (Mosey, 1981, p. 32). Concepts are used to organize and synthesize thinking processes. Kim (1983) suggests concepts serve 6 functions, they are summarized in Table 31-1. The most important functions are the naming and framing of ideas and the definitions or descriptions which explain the parameters of the concept.

Organizing Concepts

The organization of concepts clarifies communication of thought by encouraging the sharing of ideas, which may facilitate elaboration and refinement (Rodgers & Knafl, 2000). Thus, concepts help to shape a profession's point of focus. Every profession needs to examine, clarify, and establish the boundaries of what constitutes its field of study and domain of concern. For occupational therapy, occupation is the field of study and occupational therapy is the application of that study. Concepts can also clarify the difference between the state of being (end result or product) and the state of action or becoming (process). Occupation may be described as a product (task, role, outcome), but occupational therapy is primarily concerned with the process of performing and participating in (doing) occupation(s). In addition, concepts can describe the thing pictured (entity) or a family of resemblances. In other words, a concept can apply to a single occupation, such as getting dressed; or to a group of occupations, such as ADL. Furthermore, concepts are a key element in constructing and understanding models and theories. Concepts act as the construction units or scaffolding of a model or theory.

Where Concepts Begin

Concepts derive from and are part of the language. Concepts developed within a specialized group are used to convey ideas needed to express the work of that group. For example, in trade groups, concepts often refer to particular equipment or materials, ie, to most people, a nail is a nail. However, to a carpenter a nail may be a common nail, a finishing nail, a brad nail, a roofing nail, a screw nail, a cut nail, or a boat nail. Each nail was designed for the particular purpose that it does best. Carpenters find the distinctions useful because they get better results by using the nail designed for the project at hand. Professionals also have developed specialized concepts to convey ideas useful to them. Occupational therapy has developed a number of concepts and has also borrowed many from both the common language and from specialized language of other

Table 31-1. *Functions of Concepts*

Functions

1. Facilitate the process of thinking about ideas by permitting the naming, labeling, and framing of things, events, events, and realities.

2. Are best explained as definitions or descriptions.

3. Can express symbolic constructs of real world phenomena (eg, spirituality expresses an idea that has no specific physical structure and may represent several cognitive meanings).

4. May refer to a single, unique case or entity or to a class of phenomena (eg, a person can speak about what is a purposeful activity to one individual or speak about purposeful activity as it relates to all media used in occupational therapy).

5. Can reference concrete or abstract phenomena using the same criteria (eg, the same rules can be applied to discussing a concrete concept such as eating or to an abstract concept such as wellness).

6. May be developed and used at either the specific or general level (eg, the concept of competence may be discussed as it is used in one model or as it is applied to all models).

professions; the source of the concepts may be lost or forgotten over the years. For example, the concept of activities of daily living (ADL) was not developed by occupational therapy practitioners, but came to the profession through physical medicine and rehabilitation, special education for orthopedically handicapped children, and physical therapy. This knowledge helps explains why there are many different definitions of ADL and why the emphasis varies from one profession to another. ADL in occupational therapy are usually described in terms of tasks, such as eating or dressing. ADL in physical therapy is more often described in terms of physical mobility, such as rolling over in bed or walking. Neither profession, however, owns the concept since it was developed from ideas synthesized from several different disciplines.

Another major influence on the development of concepts is philosophy. Models based on mechanistic philosophy, in which the person is viewed as passive, have one set of concepts and definitions for models based on organismic philosophy have another. Occupational therapy was organized primarily around the concepts from organismic philosophy, in which the individual is viewed as an active agent. However, during the middle part of the 20th century the profession was strongly urged to adopt mechanistic philosophy as an organizing base to appear more "scientific." In the latter half of the 20th century, the profession began to resist the pressure to use mechanistic philosophy and to return to the original organizing philosophic ideas. As a result, 5 periods of time can be used to roughly describe the development of concepts in the profession of occupational therapy. These are the preformative, formative, mechanistic, modern, and the post-modern periods. These time periods, major influences, and major contributions are detailed in Table 31-2.

What Concepts Are Needed?

While concepts are useful, too many concepts may clutter the information channels and confuse the intended audience. On the other hand, an insufficient number of concepts may lead to inadequate communication—causing gaps in understanding and possibly failures in application. Obviously, the right number of concepts is important, although the exact number may be difficult to determine. One way of determining how many concepts of what kind are needed or useful is to develop a working model of concept usage. The author has suggested that useful models in occupational therapy need to contain concepts in 3 areas: outcome, doing, and tools (Reed & Sanderson, 1999). *Outcome concepts* address the question "what are the goals, purposes, aims, objectives, or results of occupational therapy?" and explain why occupational therapy personnel should be allowed to intervene in a client's life situation and what change might result. An *outcome* is a statement that defines or describes what should have happened (changes occurred) by the end of occupational therapy intervention. *Doing concepts* address the question "what beliefs and assumptions underlie our views of humans as occupational beings" and explain how occupational therapy "works" as an applied profession to facilitate the change process. A doing concept describes a dynamic process designed to facilitate obtaining an outcome, but is not the outcome or end state itself. The doing process may involve changes designed to occur within the individual (internal

Table 31-2. *Periods and Influences in the Occupational Therapy Literature*

Name	Time Period	Major Influences and Contributions
Reformative period	1800 to 1899	*Major influence:* Moral Treatment and the Arts and Crafts Movement. *Major contribution:* Initial ideas which lead to the development and application of occupational therapy to clients in mental health institutions.
Formative period	1900 to 1929	*Major influence:* Philosophy of pragmatism and publications of early leaders and scholars. *Major contribution:* Many of the basic terms and concepts used today were developed during this period.
Mechanistic period	1930 to 1965	*Major influence:* Push by physicians to adopt the scientific (quantitative) method. *Major contribution:* Many of the formative concepts were forgotten and few new concepts were developed.
Modern period	1966 to 1995	*Major influence:* Return to ideas expressed in the publications of the formative period and acceptance of qualitative methods. *Major contribution:* Development of useful models of practice and expansion of the ideas about occupation and its contribution to performance of tasks and roles in everyday life. Also, research began to inform practice produced by evidence.
Post Modern period	1996 to present	*Major influence:* Organization of inter-related concepts of person, environment, and occupations as the 3 core concepts of occupational therapy, and development of models of practice based on the 3 core concepts.

environment), without the individual (external environment), or both at about the same time period. Tool concepts address the question "given those beliefs and assumptions, what concepts support where and how occupational therapy personnel choose to achieve their stated outcome(s) with individual or groups of clients?" *Tool concepts* explain the instruments of change or therapeutic interventions, what strategies are used and why the strategies are viewed as useful. Tools include media, modalities, methods, techniques, approaches, and contexts or environments. In occupational therapy, tools reflect the living conditions and situations of the clients being serviced, and thus the selection for a given individual or group is influenced by many factors. Examples from these 3 concept areas—outcomes, doing, and tools, along with definitions found in the occupational therapy literature—will be presented. Comments are provided for clarification.

OUTCOMES

Outcomes are the end point or terminal objective of an occupational therapy intervention. There are 2 forms of outcomes. An outcome may be "an agreed, clearly defined, expected or desired result of intervention (predetermined

outcome)" or an outcome may be "the result of therapeutic processes, which may be different from the initial objectives of therapy (actual outcome)" (Creek, 2003, p. 56). Samples of statements from early leaders show a variety of outcomes have been suggested. Examples of statements and the outcomes advanced are summarized in Table 31-3. The problem of discordance regarding outcome is also evident in the analysis of concepts related to outcome in the occupational therapy literature.

As an introduction to this next section on Outcomes, a short essay is presented to explain why clarity of language in necessary. Let's consider the word *function*. Clearly the profession of occupational therapy has incorporated the concept of function into the professional terminology. In the process, however, the concept has been overused to the point that clarity of communication is lost. Function has become a buzzword and a stand-in for more precise descriptors. Among the problems needed to be sorted out are the professional functions (role or purpose) of occupational therapy from the client functions (skills, training). In addition, the use of function as an outcome (person can function or person is functional), as doing (person is functioning, performing, or participating) or as a tool (use of a functional occupation, such as use of self-care, work, and play in intervention) is difficult to follow and probably

Table 31-3. *Early Outcomes in the Occupational Therapy Literature*

Outcomes

- The "aim of all curative work is to salvage the patient from a state of disability and unproductiveness and make him once more a useful unit of society" (Burnette, 1918, p. 20). *The outcome is focused on decreasing the effects of disability and increasing the productiveness and social contribution.*

- "A distinct advantage processed by the work-shop type of therapy consists in the fact that the patient here is a member of a social group and turns out a tangible product of economic value; he is thus brought to full realization of his social fitness and economic usefulness" (Baldwin, 1919, p. 7). *Thus, socialization and economic usefulness were again the desired outcomes.*

- "Occupational therapy at its best, first amuses, then actively interests the patient-the attitude of hopeless introspection is changed to one of positive...interest and progression" (Hall, 1921). *The outcomes focused on initiative and motivation to engage in occupation, as opposed to disinterest and idleness.*

- "The objects sought are to arouse interest, courage, and confidence to exercise mind and body in healthy activity: to overcome disability; and to re-establish capacity for industrial and social usefulness" (AOTA, 1923, p. 1). *The outcome focuses on health, work, and citizenship.*

- "The handicrafts are used... for the purpose of developing physical and mental effectiveness" (Hall, 1923). *Thus, fitness is stressed as an outcome.*

- "The present concept of therapy is that a person disabled by disease or injury... at the earliest possible moment shall be given active occupation that is graded, as rapidly as his strength permits, to normal levels of activity" (Willard & Spackman, 1947, p. vii). *The outcome is focused on normal activity and normalization.*

- "The task of occupational therapy is to prevent and reduce the incapacities resulting from illness" (Reilly, 1966, p. 300). *The outcome is reduction of incapacity.*

adds to the difficulty in communicating with other professions and the general public. Furthermore, function is used to refer to interventions based on remedial or restorative techniques, in which the parts are fixed in the hope that the whole will work to do whatever the person chooses to do. It also refers to intervention based on adaptation and coping, in which the focus is on what occupations the client needs to do and how such occupations can be done effectively and efficiently. Finally, there is a problem of clarifying the use of the concept of function within the profession without creating additional communication gaps with other groups who also use the term. For example the revised ICF defines functioning as "an umbrella term for body functions, body structures, activities, and participation. It denotes the positive aspects of the interaction between an individual (with a health condition) and that individual's contextual factors (environmental and personal factors)" (WHO, 2001). Such a broad use of the concept of function is even greater than used in occupational therapy, since discussion of function and structures within the body is usually not the primary focus of discussion by occupational therapy personnel, but rather function in relation to activities and participation. Another example of how a concept may be applied is mathematics,

in which the concept of function refers to a variable quantity which is expressed in relation to another quantity. Perhaps, the concept of function should be replaced with other concepts. As you read the other key concepts that are used in occupational therapy think about the need for clarity, or at least adopt the term that best means what you wish to communicate.

In contemporary literature, the following concepts related to outcome statements were identified by the author. They include achievement, adaptation (occupational adaptation), autonomy, competence (occupational competence), coping, fitness, function, health, identity (occupational identity, self-identity), independence, interdependence, life balance, mastery, occupational balance (imbalance), occupational justice, occupational performance, prevention, quality of life, recovery, satisfaction (life satisfaction), self-advocacy, self-efficacy, self-management, well-being, and wellness. The reader may quickly observe that there are more outcome concepts in the list than are included in the *Occupational Therapy Practice Framework* (AOTA, 2002c, 2008, 2014). The *Framework* needs expansion, or the concepts may need to reduced. These concepts and their definitions are summarized next.

Outcomes and Outcome Measures

- As defined in this section, outcomes are focused on measurable changes in the client as opposed to measurable changes in a therapy program (number of clients, cost per treatment unit, amount of personnel time).
- Outcomes refer to both the intended and unintended results of a therapy program (CAOT, 1991, p. 140).
- Outcomes are also viewed as the measured or observed consequence of an action. Outcomes may refer to a client's *desired outcome;* the *predetermined outcomes* that a service is expected to deliver, as described in a service level agreement or a commissioning contract; the *negotiated outcome* between a client and practitioner, as articulated in a goal; and the *actual outcome,* which is the measured effects of a specific intervention or the effects of a multidisciplinary or inter-agency management plan for the client (Cara & MacRae, 2013, p. 970).
- Outcome measurement involves the use of systematic or scientific methods to determine client outcome.
- Outcome measures are an aspect of program evaluation that evaluates the results of the intervention after the service has been provided (Hussey, Sabonis-Chafee, & O'Brien, 2007, p. 290)

Achievement

- Achievement is mentioned in Adolf Meyer's article: "to get the pleasure and pride of achievement ...is the basic remedy for the blasé tedium that characterizes the indifference or the hopeless depression" (Meyer, 1922, p. 7).
- Achievement means "getting some work or things done" (Meyer in Winter, 1952).
- Achievement is "competition with a standard of excellence" (McClelland, Atkinson, & Lowell, 1953; as stated in Reilly, 1974, p. 147).
- Parham and Fazio (1997) provided 2 definitions of achievement: "1) performance that is linked to public expectancies or standards of excellence, and 2) something accomplished, especially by ability or special effort; connotes final accomplishment of something noteworthy; an attainment" (p. 248).
- Jacobs and Jacobs (2009) defined *achievement behavior* as "guided by societal standards, the behavior facilitates risk-taking ability, and the development of a sense of competition" (p. 2).
- **Author's comment:** Other than Reilly's Occupational Behavior Model, the concept of achievement as an outcome criterion has received little attention in occupational therapy literature in recent years.

Adaptation, Occupational Adaptation

- Adaptation has been a concept since the beginning of the profession. In the early 1990s the focus was expanded to include the external factors in the environment that may affect or contribute to adaptation. Meyer (1922) said "no branch of medicine has learned as clearly as psychiatry that after all, many of these formidable diseases are largely problems of adaptation..." (p. 1). Meyer was referring to the idea that mental health problems were, in his opinion, more related to problems in adaptation or adjustment to contextual situations than to pathology of the brain, constitutional weakness, or poor upbringing. In this chapter, the focus is on the concept of individual or personal adaptation as a psychological concept, as opposed to species adaptation as a biological concept. The concept of adaptation can be viewed as an outcome (goal, objective, aim, purpose) as a doing process (adapting, changing, adjusting, performing, participating), and as a tool (method, technique, strategy). The distinction between the outcome and process are often fused together in definitions. However, when separated, the definitions of adaptation as doing appear under the section on Doing and as a tool under the section on Tools.
- King (1978) states that "individual adaptation refers to adjustments made by the individual that primarily enhance personal rather than species survival, and secondarily contribute to actualization of personal potential" (p. 431).
- Any change in structure, form, or habits of an organism to suit a new environment—in reflex action, decline in the frequency of impulses when the sensory nerve is stimulated repeatedly; in psychiatry, those changes experienced by an individual that lead to adjustment (Hopkins & Smith, 1978, p. 727; 1983, p. 915).
- Adaptation is "adjustment of an organism to its environment, or the process by which it enhances such fitness" (CAOT, 1991, p. 137).
- Schkade and Schultz (1992) defined adaptation as "a change in the functional state of the person as a result of movement toward relative mastery over occupational challenges" (p. 831). The term *movement* refers to a cognitive change, not a physical motion.
- Ryan (1993) said that adaptation is "satisfactory adjustment of individuals within their environment over time" (p. 357).
- Bonder and Wagner (1994) defined adaptation as adjustment to environmental conditions. When used to describe visual behavior, adaptation is the ability

of the eye to "adjust to increases and decreases in the amount of illumination in the environment" (p. 378). This is an example of physiological adaptation of the individual, not related to an occupational therapy outcome.

- Adaptation is viewed as an occupational engagement that leads to a "harmonious synergy between the person and the context, namely environment, culture, and time" (Fanchiang, 1996, p. 277).

- Christiansen and Baum (1997) defined adaptation as "a change a person makes in his or her response approach when that person encounters an occupational challenge. This change is implemented when the individual's customary response approaches are found inadequate for producing some degree of mastery over the challenge" (p. 591; used in AOTA, 2002c, p. 630).

- Parham and Fazio (1997) included both emphases in their definition of adaptation. The first is "a change or response to stress of any kind; many are normal, self-protective, and developmental" and the second is "a change in routine, materials, or equipment that enables a person with a disability to function independently or to participate more fully in an activity" (p. 248).

- Hagedorn (2000) described both internal and external adaptation in one definition by suggesting that adaptation is "any change in the occupational habits or organization of person which is made in order to meet environmental demands and restore fit or an alteration made by a practitioner or client to an object or environment in order to provide therapy or to improve the client's ability to perform" (p. 307).

- Stein and Roose (2000) also followed the attitude approach by defining adaptation as "the adjustment of a person to his or her environment as a reaction to a stressor or environmental demand" (p. 2).

- Stein and Cutler (2002) defined adaptation as "an adjustment of a person to his or her environment; a reaction to a stressor or environmental demand by an individual. Adaptation can also refer to the modification of an environment (eg, addition of more structure to the daily schedule), equipment, or materials (eg, providing cues in the work environment to enable the individual to function independently in work, leisure, or self-care)" (p. 613).

- A "change in function that promotes survival and self-actualization" (Hussey et al., 2007, p. 285)

- A change in response approach that the client makes when encountering an occupational challenge. "This change is implemented when the [client's] customary response approaches are found inadequate for producing some degree of mastery over the challenge"

(AOTA, 2008, p. 662, 669 [adapted from Schultz & Schkade, 1997, p. 474]).

- Brown and Stoffel (2011) defined adaptation as "adjustment of a person to fluctuating circumstances within or external to the individual" (p. 773) *(outcome)*.

- A change in response approach generated when encountering a challenge. It also refers to therapeutic intervention in which task demands are changed to be consistent with the individual's ability level; may involve modification by reducing demands, use of assistive devices, or changes in the physical or social environment (Schell, Gillen, & Scaffa, 2014, p. 1229)

- Occupational adaptation is the construction of a positive occupational identity and achieving occupational competence over time in the context of one's environment (Kielhofner, 2002, p. 122; 2008, p. 107).

- Occupational adaptation is the state of competency toward which human beings aspire. The existence and strength of this state in an individual is a function of the extent to which occupational responses have been effective and successfully generalized to a variety of occupational challenges (Schkade & Schultz, 1992, p. 831).

- Spatiotemporal adaptation is a continuous, ongoing state of the act of adjusting those bodily processes required to function within a given space at a given time (Hopkins & Smith, 1977, p. 728; 1983, p. 928).

- **Author's comment:** Adaptation, or its verb forms (to adapt, adapting, adapted), is the second most used word in the occupational therapy literature to be discussed in this chapter. The first is *occupation*, which is discussed under the section on Tools. *Adaptation* is used as an outcome (the goal is to have adapted, successfully, the self or group to perform under a given set of circumstance), a doing process (adapting self or making the necessary self-adjustments to do something in a given situation or condition), and as a tool (an adaptation to a method of performance, such as one-hand technique, or adaptation of an object or equipment in the external environment, such as elongating a handle to facilitate reaching). The multiple uses of the term *adaptation* within the occupational therapy literature are often not clearly articulated, making differentiating the usage difficult to follow. In this chapter, the uses of the word adaptation or verb forms related to the doing process are discussed under the section on Doing, and those related to tool use under the section on Tools.

Autonomy

- Autonomy appeared in Moorhead (1969), who speaks about the occupational role history and the critical variables to occupational function. The first listed variables are *autonomy* and *independence*, and are described as including "realistic perception of one's own assets and liabilities; ability to make stable decisions and implement them effectively; and competence in management of time, space, and personal needs" (p. 330). Use of the term *autonomy* has 2 meanings: outcome criterion and ethics principle. The 2 meanings are not clearly separated in the definitions.

- Hopkins and Smith (1979) defined autonomy as the "quality of being self-governing and self-determining" (p. 729).

- Erikson's concept of autonomy is discussed in Pratt and Allen (1985): "Erikson specified the relationship of autonomy to the child's increasing control over his body. This permits independent movement into the outer world" (p. 25). This description marks the change in definitions from being able to perform to being able to take control as well as perform.

- Reed and Sanderson (1983) defined autonomy as "the ability to act or perform according to one's own volition or direction" (p. 237).

- In 1995, Hagedorn defined autonomy as "capable of exercising choices and control over one's personal life" (p. 53).

- In 1997, Christiansen and Baum's definition of autonomy is similar, stating that autonomy is "reflected in the ability to make choices and have control over the environment" (p. 592).

- Cara and MacRae (1998) provided a more comprehensive definition by stating that autonomy means "self-determination and independence. The process of becoming autonomous is characterized by a gradual reduction in dependency and steady movement toward ever-greater independence. The process of and timing for becoming autonomous are largely determined by the cultural context of the family" (p. 666).

- Jacobs (1999) provided a succinct definition to autonomy as the "state of independence and self-control" (p. 13).

- Creek (2003) defined autonomy as "the capacity to make choices or to exercise freedom of the will. In order to choose to do something, the individual has to be aware of what options are available and how to access them. The ability to make choices depends on three types of autonomy: autonomy of thought, of will, and of action. Autonomy is not an all or nothing capacity but may vary at different times of life" (p. 34).

- The freedom to decide and the freedom to act (Hussey et al., 2007, p. 286).

- Creek (2008 [based on Gillon 1985; 1986]) defines autonomy as "the capacity to think, decide, and act on the basis of such thought and decision freely and independently and without... let or hindrance" (p. 60).

- In 2010, Creek, writing for the *European Network of Occupational Therapy in Higher Education*, defines autonomy as "the freedom to make choices based on consideration of internal and external circumstances and to act on those choices" (p. 25).

- Brown and Stoffel (2011) defined autonomy as "capacity of the client for self-direction and making his or her own choices, as opposed to authority, in which the therapist tells the client what to do" (p. 774).

- **Author's comment:** The definitions of autonomy stress the concepts of freedom of choice, independent action, and a sense of self-directedness. Autonomy is also a basic principle in professional ethics, so some definitions may directly or indirectly reflect an ethical value. In addition, autonomy and independence are related concepts, so some definitions may reflect the value of independence and independent action.

Competency, Competence, Occupational Competence, Role Competence

- The term *competency* related to clients first appears in occupational therapy literature in an article by Reilly (1966). She discussed the specifications for a psychiatric occupational therapy program and stated that "the fourth specification, therefore, speaks for the building of a milieu which acknowledges competency..." (p. 63). In the context of client outcomes, the concept of professional competence to practice occupational therapy is not discussed, nor is the legal definition of competence (knowing right from wrong). Robert White, a psychologist, originated the psychological concept in 1959. He stated that competence is "sufficient or adequate behavior to meet the demands of the situation or task" (1971, p. 273).

- The term *incompetence* appeared in 1930 in an article by Marjorie Taylor, but is not defined (p. 54).

- The first definition of competency appears in 1975 as the "ability to perform at a predetermined level" (AOTA, 1976, p. 262).

- Competency is the ability to perform skills to the level of efficiency required by physical, psychological and social health (CAOT, 1991, p. 137).

- The first definition of competence appears in Hopkins and Smith (1977), and is defined as the "quality of adequacy or possession of required skill, knowledge, or capacity" (p. 730; 1983, p. 918).

- Rogers (1982) described competence as "a transactional concept that involves effectiveness in interacting with the environment. It (competence) arises from an urge to learn about the environment by testing our actions upon it. Competence implies adaptability in organizing skills into integrated courses of action to serve innumerable purposes. Competence is an overall strategy of adaptation consisting of thinking, deciding, doing, and evaluating" (p. 709).

- Competence is defined by Allen (1985) as "an inference we make about the prerequisite ability required to do the task procedure" and "an estimate of the level of thought required to do a step in the task" (p. 73).

- Kielhofner (1985) stated that competence is "the quality of being able or having the capacity to respond effectively to the demands of one or a range of situations (p. 502).

- Competence, according to Mocellin (1988), "refers to the ability required to carry out a task, to the quality of being functionally adequate or having sufficient skill for a particular task, and to a potential which is realized at the moment of performance" (p. 5).

- Competence has also been defined as "the ability to answer all the requirements of an environment" (Polatajko, 1992, p. 196).

- Competence is the "achievement of skill equal to the demands of the environment" (Christiansen & Baum, 1997, p. 593).

- Creek (1997) added the idea of *life role* to her definition, which is that competence is "the ability to perform skills to a level that allows satisfactory performance of life roles" (p. 529).

- Parham and Fazio (1997) defined competence as "the state of being adequate to meet the demands of a task or situation" (p. 249).

- "Reilly's second hierarchical stage of play behavior, in which the play is driven by effectance motivation and practice tasks repeatedly in pursuit of competence and mastery of skills. In this stage, play builds on trust in the environment and generates self-confidence" (Parham & Fazio, 1997, p. 249).

- Punwar and Peloquin (2000) stated that competence is "the individual's adequacy or capacity in a given task" (p. 278).

- Hagedorn (2001) defined competence as "skilled and adequately successful completion of a piece of performance, task or activity. The performance should be effective within defined parameters, in specified contexts, and transferred adaptively to related settings" (p. 160).

- Christiansen and Townsend (2004) defined competence as "a match between the demands or challenges of a task or occupation and the knowledge and/or skills of an individual who has chosen to pursue that endeavor" (p. 276). The definition was modified in 2010 to read "a match between the environmental demands or challenges of an occupation and the knowledge and/or skills of persons" (p. 417).

- "The ability to interact effectively with the environment while maintaining individuality and growth, achievement of skill equal to the demands of the environment" (Christiansen & Baum, 2005, p. 544).

- Competence is analogous to self-efficacy, "a belief in an individual's own capability, which motivates him or her to act" (Brown & Stoffel, 2011, p. 776).

- Competence is an individual's capacity to perform his or her responsibilities, commonly used to reference demonstrated performance on a job or to professional practice (Schell et al., 2014, p. 1231). This is professional or job competence, not individual competence.

- Parham and Fazio (1997) defined competency behavior as "play that involves practice or repetition of fragments of activity sequences in pursuit of mastery of skills" (p. 249).

- Occupational competence by definition "is determined by the interaction of the individual and environment. (It) is the product of the dynamic interaction between the environment and the individual, each changing in response to the other" (Polatajko, 1992, pp. 196-197).

- "Occupational competence is the result of a goodness of fit between the person, the occupation, and the environment" (Polatajko, 1994, p. 592).

- "Occupational competence is the product of the dynamic interaction of the three dimensions of the individual, the environment, and occupation" (Martini et al., 1995, p. 16).

- "Occupational competence is adequacy or sufficiency in an occupational skill, meeting all requirements of an environment" (Law et al., 1997b, p. 40).

- Occupational competence seems to imply the ability to cope adequately with the 3 "duties of care" to self, neighbor, and state, while occupational dysfunction implies a breakdown in one or more of these areas (Hagedorn, 1995, p. 53).

- Occupational competence is the ability to perform needed occupations adequately, consistently, and effectively, to a required standard (Hagedorn, 2001, p. 166)

- Occupational competence is accomplished by minimizing the disabling effects of physical and mental impairments, and optimizing existing strengths (Rogers, 1984, p. 48).

- Occupational competence is the degree to which one sustains a pattern of occupational participation that reflects one's occupational identity. Occupational competence has to do with putting occupational identity into action in an ongoing way. Occupational competence includes the following (Kielhofner, 2008, p. 107):
  ◊ Fulfilling the expectations of one's roles and one's own values and standards for performance
  ◊ Maintaining a routine that allows one to discharge responsibilities
  ◊ Participating in a range of occupations that provide a sense of ability, control, satisfaction, and fulfillment
  ◊ Pursuing one's values and taking action to achieve desired life outcomes

- Occupational competence is "ability, skill, knowledge, and attitudes for engagement in occupations" (Christiansen & Townsend, 2010, p. 420).

- Occupational competence is the personal sense of achievement in one's performance of daily activities (Brown & Stoffel, 2011, p. 765).

- Occupational competence is the degree to which one is able to sustain a pattern of occupational participation that reflects one's occupational identity (Schell et al., 2014, p. 1357).

- Occupational competency is an individual's ability to perform in such a way as to fulfill his or her occupational identity (Duncan, 2006, p. 339).

- Role competence is the ability to effectively meet the demand of roles in which the client engages (AOTA, 2002c, p. 633; AOTA, 2008, p. 663).

- Role competence is the ability to meet the demands of roles (Hussey et al., 2007, p. 291).

- **Author's comment:** Competence is a complex concept. Occupational therapy practitioners must differentiate between competence to perform some daily occupations, but not necessarily all commonly performed occupations in a given society or role. For example, self-care competence but not work competence; competence to perform all role tasks identified by the individual and society (role competence); competence to perform work-related (job, vocation) tasks only; or other restricted area of competence (work competence or professional competence). As used in this chapter, the definitions refer to competence of the client, not competence of the practitioner as a professional person.

Coping

- Coping does not have as long a history with occupational therapy as adaptation. Yet they seem to be linked (Coelho, Hamburg, & Adams, 1974). The first definition was located in 1973 in a grant report on roles and functions. The definition of coping behavior "includes abilities and limitations in ability to sublimate drives, find sources of need gratification, tolerate frustration and anxiety, experience gratification and control impulses" (AOTA, 1973, p. 42).

- White (1974), a psychologist, suggested that adaptation is the master concept with 3 superordinate terms: *coping, mastery,* and *defense.* Coping is seen as "adaptation under relatively difficult conditions" (p. 49).

- Lazarus (1984), a psychologist, said that "coping has been widely and long regarded as having a central role in adaptation, yet it has defied universal agreement on definition" (p. 294).

- Lazarus and Folkman (1984) defined coping as *"constantly changing cognitive and behavioral efforts to manage specific external and/or internal demands that re appraised as taxing or exceeding the resources of the person"* (p. 141, italics in original).

- Kielhofner (1985) described coping as "the active psychosocial process through which persistent efforts are made to overcome and solve the problems and dilemmas of the person or those imposed by the environment" (p. 502).

- Zeitlin, Williamson, and Szczepanski (1988) defined coping as "a general term for the process of using learned adaptive behaviors to manage one's world. Coping is the process of making adaptation to meet personal needs and to respond to the demands of the environment" (pp. 1-2).

- Gage (1992) described coping as the process through which the individual manages to deal with the demands of stressful situations that tax or exceed the person's resources and the emotions generated by those situations in the person-environment relationship (pp. 353-354, based on Lazarus and Folkman, 1984).

- Stewart (1992) stated that "the mission of occupational therapy... is to enable people to cope with everyday activities" (p. 298).

- Williamson (1997) described coping as (a)n adaptation to environmental stress that is based on conscious or unconscious choice and that enhances control over behavior or gives psychological comfort" (p. 439).
- Brown and Stoffel (2011) defined coping as "adapting to and managing change, stress, or opportunity (e.g., acute or chronic illness, disability, pain, death, relocation, work, changes in family structure, new relationships, or new ideas) (p. 777)
- Coping is "conscious, volitional efforts to regulate emotion, cognition, behavior, physiology, and the environment in response to stressful events or circumstances" (Schell et al., 2014, p. 1232).
- Coping skills include the "ability to sublimate drives, find sources of need gratification, tolerate frustration and anxiety, experience gratification, and control impulses" (AOTA, 1978, p. 75).
- Punwar and Peloquin (2000) defined coping skills as "those abilities that enable an individual to identify and manage stress and related reactions" (p. 278, based on AOTA, 1989, p. 814).
- Coping skills includes identifying and managing stresses and related factors (AOTA, 1994, p. 1054).
- Coping skills include those abilities that enable an individual to identify and manage stress and related reactions (Punwar, 1994, p. 257).
- Stein and Roose (2000) defined coping skills as "an individual's ability to self-regulate stress and master the environment (p. 80).
- Cara and MacRae (2013) defined coping strategies as "strategies developed alone or through professional intervention that enable a disabled person to better cope with his or her circumstances" (p. 965).
- Situational coping refers to "skills and performance in handling stress and dealing with problems and changes in a manner that is functional for self and others" (*Uniform Terminology*, 1979, p. 901).
- **Author's comment:** Gage (1992) proposed a model of coping designed to help clients learn to cope with a disease process, but the model has not been widely quoted.

Fitness

- The term *fitness* has not been defined in occupational therapy literature, although the word has appeared since 1918. Three primary references to fitness in the current literature are to fitness to drive, general health and fitness, and physical fitness (organ system), such as cardiovascular fitness.

- Psychology dictionary definition is "generally, the extent to which an organism is prepared to succeed to some endeavor" (Reber & Reber, 2001, p. 277).
- The psychology dictionary definition is 1) in individual animals, their reproductive success, in consideration of competition for mates; 2) adaptation to the conditions of the environment—that is, capability of an organism, due to its structural organization, to meet the general conditions of life (Corsini, 2002, p. 379).
- The American Psychological Association definition is a set of attributes that people have or are able to achieve relating to their ability to perform physical work and to carry out daily tasks with vigor and alertness, without undue fatigue, and with ample energy to enjoy leisure pursuits. In biology, the extent to which an organism or population is able to produce viable off-spring in a given environment (VandenBos, 2007, p. 378).
- *Fitness for duty evaluation* is a psychological assessment of an employee's present mental state and functioning to estimate the employee's future functioning and determine whether that individual is able to safely and effectively perform his or her job duties (VandenBos, 2007, p. 378).
- Total fitness has 8 domains (Institute for Alternative Futures, 2009, p. 6):
  ◊ *Physical:* strength, endurance, flexibility, mobility
  ◊ *Environmental:* health/cold, altitude, depth
  ◊ *Medical:* immunization, screening
  ◊ *Spiritual:* expression, cognitive, behavioral, relational, family
  ◊ *Nutritional:* fuel, quality, prevent illness, behavioral
  ◊ *Psychological:* mental, emotional, behavior
  ◊ *Behavioral:* substance abuse, hygiene, risk mitigation
  ◊ *Social:* task cohesion, social cohesion, connectedness
- **Author's comment:** The concept of fitness is evolving in the occupational therapy literature, but does not have a working definition to date.

Function/Functionalism

- The concept of function as used in occupational therapy seems to be consistent with the idea of *functionalism* as expressed in functional psychology. Central figures in the founding of functionalism at the end of the 19th century were William James and John Dewey (Wolman, 1989).

- In functionalism, "the process of adjustment of the organism to the environment is central, as is a purposivistic interpretation of the process in which stimuli and responses are a chain of deeds and not separate entities" (Wolman, 1989, p. 141).

- Functionalism is the "philosophical doctrine of W. James, which considers mental phenomena their dynamic unity as a system of functions (geared to adapting the organism to its environment) for the satisfaction of needs that are biological in origin" (Eysenick et al., 1982, p. 395).

- Functionalism is a "theory claiming that the best, or only, way of defining something is in terms of what is does or the role it plays in the ongoing course of events" (Bothamley, 1993, p. 217).

- Functional psychology is the doctrine that "conscious processes or states such as those of willing (volition), thinking, emoting, perceiving, sensating are activities or operations of an organism in physical interrelationship with a physical environment and cannot be given hypostatized, substantive existence. These activities facilitate the organism's control, survival, adaptation, engagement or withdrawal, recognition, direction, etc." (Angeles, 1981, p. 107).

- Functional psychology considers "the mental process of sense perception, emotion, volition, and thought as functions of the biological organism in the adaptation to and control of its environment" (Runes, 1980).

- **Author's comment:** Functionalism arose as a protest against structural psychology, for which the task of psychology is the analysis and description of consciousness. The functional theory of the mind is characteristic of the pragmatism and instrumentalism of Pierce, James, Mead, and Dewey (Runes, 1962, p. 114). Many of the words used in these definitions and descriptions are familiar to occupational therapy personnel. Since none were written by occupational therapy practitioners, there appears to be an agreement of thought between the concept of functionalism and the use of function as a concept in occupational therapy.

Function/Functioning

- The word *function* appears in occupational therapy literature from the formative period. Meyer (1922) spoke of the "laws of function" as expansions of the laws of physics and chemistry (p. 9). Definitions, however, do not appear until 1981. Mosey (1981) stated that "function is the ability to engage comfortably at an age-appropriate level in performance components and the areas of occupational performance within the context of one's cultural, social, and nonhuman environment" (p. 82).

- Punwar (1994) defined function and functional performance as "a person's ability to perform those tasks necessary in their daily life" (p. 259; Punwar & Peloquin, 2000, p. 280).

- Baum and Edwards (1995) stated that practitioners focus "their efforts on function by using interventions to improve the occupational performance of persons who lack the ability to perform an action or activity considered necessary for their everyday lives" (p. 1019).

- Turner, Foster, and Johnson (1996) defined function as "an action performed to fulfill an allocated task" (p. 873).

- According to Christiansen and Baum (1997), function "as used by an occupational therapy practitioner, describes a behavior related to the performance of a task" (p. 596).

- Creek (1997) stated that function is the "possession of the skills necessary for successful participation in the range of roles expected of the individual" (p. 529).

- Hinojosa and Kramer (1997) stated that the term *function* is "viewed as the ability to perform activities required in one's occupations" (p. 866).

- Stein and Roose (2000) chose to define functional rather than function. Functional is "the degree of a client's independence in the performance areas of work/productivity and leisure" (p. 108).

- The WHO (2001) used the term *functioning* as "an umbrella term for body functions, body structures, activities, and participation. It denotes the positive aspects of the interaction between an individual (with a health condition) and that individual's contextual factors (environmental and personal factors)" (p. 212).

- Reflects an individual's performance of activities, tasks, and roles during daily occupations (Christiansen & Baum, 2005, p. 546).

- Function is defined as "action for which a person is fit; the ability to perform" (Hussey et al., 2007, p. 288).

- Creek (2010) writing for the European Network of Occupational Therapy in Higher Education (ENOTHE) defined function using 2 definitions. Function 1 is the underlying physical and psychological components that support occupational performance. Function 2 is the capacity to use occupational performance components to carry out a task, activity or occupation (p. 25). The difference between function as "underlying readiness at the organ level" as opposed to actual "doing or performing level" is an important distinction.

- Function (of an occupation) is what an occupation achieves, such as volunteering for a local service might achieve integration into the community (Schell, Gillen, & Schaffa, 2012, p. 1233).

Function as a Modifier

- Functional ability is "the skill to perform activities in a normal or accepted manner" (Reed & Sanderson, 1992, p. 339).
- Functional ability is having the ability to perform competently the roles, and occupations required in the course of daily life (Hagedorn, 2001, p. 166).
- Functional adaptation is the ability that when one cortical pathway is derailed, the possibility remains for another pathway in a non-traumatized area to carry the same information (Jacobs & Jacobs, 2009, p. 98).
- Kamenetz (1983) wrote that functional assessment includes ADL, but adds locomotion and communication.
- Functional assessment is the "observation of motor performance and behavior to determine if a person can adequately perform the required tasks of a particular role or setting" (Christiansen & Baum, 1991, p. 852).
- Functional assessment is the "observation of behavior in a natural context or one that closely simulates the natural context in order to understand how environmental factors affect performance or specific behaviors" (Schell et al., 2014, p. 1234).
- Functional capacity was originally evaluated on a functional evaluation from Bennett (1950, pp. 346-347).
- Functional capacity is the "capacity to perform aerobic work; maximal aerobic power defined by maximum oxygen consumption" (Bonder & Wagner, 1994, p. 382).
- Punwar (1994) defined functional communication as "the ability to utilize equipment or systems to enhance or provide basic communication with others" (p. 25; Punwar & Peloquin, 2000, p. 280).
- Functional dependence is the "inability to attend to one's own needs, including the basic activities of daily living" (Bonder & Wagner, 1994, p. 382).
- A functional group is a "group that includes the group leader's capitalizing on the use of group structure and therapeutic use of self to enhance the group process and individual function" (Unsworth, 1999, p. 477).
- Functional group is "designed to promote adaptation and health through group action and engagement in occupation" (Schell et al., 2014, p. 1234).

- Functional independence is the "ability to successfully perform the day-to-day activities expected of the person" (Christiansen & Baum, 1997, p. 596).
- Functional independence is the "ability to perform required activities and tasks of daily living without the assistance of another person (usually an undeclared combination of environment-free and environment-adjusted constructs)" (Christiansen, 2000, p. 402).
- Functional independence refers to the degree of a client's independence in the performance areas of work/productivity, self-care, and leisure (Stein & Cutler, 2002, p. 621).
- Functional limitations are the "restrictions or lack of ability to perform an action or activity in the manner or within the range considered normal that results from impairment or failure of an individual to return to the preexisting level or function" (Christiansen & Baum, 1997, p. 596).
- Punwar (1994) defined functional mobility as "the ability to move from one position or place to another" (p. 259; Punwar & Peloquin, 2000, p. 280).
- Functional mobility is the use of wheeled devices, such as strollers, transport chairs, or wheelchairs, to enable transportation if disability restricts it (Christiansen, 2000, p. 402; Christiansen & Matuska, 2004, p. 466; Christiansen & Matuska, 2011, p. 540).
- Functional performance is defined as the "ability to perform functional activities, ie, activities of daily living" (Bonder & Wagner, 1994, p. 382).
- Functional performance is defined as "having the ability to perform competently the roles, relationships, and occupations required in the course of daily life" (Hagedorn, 2000, p. 209).
- Functional position is a "position that allows a person to complete necessary functional activities, even if that position is fixed so that movement is limited to that single position" (Stein & Roose, 2000, p. 108).
- Functional skills are "skills that if not performed by the person in part or in full must be completed or performed by another; purposeful for a given person an valued by others" (Christiansen, 2000, p. 402).
- Psychosocial functions are "those mental functions that enable people to express their feelings, relate to others, and perceive themselves realistically" (Punwar, 1994, p. 264).
- Psychosocial functioning describes a person's ability to perform the tasks of daily life and to engage in mutual relationships with other people in ways that are gratifying to the individual and others, and that

meet the needs of the community in which the person lives (Murray et al., 2011).

- Sensory motor functions "a group of performance components that depend on the ability of the central nervous system to organize and use sensory stimuli for interactions with the external environment" (Punwar, 1994, p. 265).

Function as Term Used in Rehabilitation

- Pattee (1951) described functional occupational therapy as "for patients needing remedial exercise for the restoration of function of muscles or joints and for co-ordination" (p. 83).
- Coulter (1950) described functional therapy as "prescribed activities planned to assist in the restoration of articular and muscular function" (p. 452).
- Bennett (1950) defined functional training as "the specific use of physical, occupational and recreational therapy to assist the patient to "pass" the test items, representing the common obstacles encountered in daily living in a normal environment. Functional training is the attempt to teach a physically handicapped individual to safely and practically perform the basic physical activities that which is required of him when he returns home" (p. 351).
- Functional training involves the physical reconditioning of the patient through a carefully devised exercise and activity program in order to make him able to handle his body in the most efficient way so that he will be as independent as possible (Buchwald, 1952, p. 3).
- Kamenetz (1983) defined functional training or therapy is "therapeutic motions or exercises in the form of purposeful activities, such as balancing, walking, eating, dressing, in which a combination of motions is practiced rather than isolated motions of individual muscle groups or body parts" (p. 132).
- Functional training is "a remedial intervention system that uses cognitive or behavioral strategies to train and compensate for disabilities in the day-to-day activities expected of the person" (Christiansen, 2000, p. 402).
- Functional use training is the staged process of instructing a person with an upper-extremity amputation in how to use his or her prosthesis in the activities of daily living (Christiansen, 2000, p. 402).
- **Author's comment:** The use of the term *functional training* as described by Bennett and Buchwald morphed into what is now known as ADL. However, the term *functional* continues to be used in other contexts in the current literature.

Health

- First definition located in 1976, although the concept is mentioned in the formative period.
- Health "is an individual state of biological, social, and emotional well-being whereby an individual is capable and able to perform those tasks or activities which are important or necessary to him to promote and maintain a sense of well-being. The individual state of health is influenced by forces such as heredity, behavior, physical environment, and the economic and social system in which he lives" (Glossary to the Essentials for an Approved Program for the Occupational Therapy Assistant, 1976, p. 262).
- Other definitions of health have suggested that integrity of body, mind, spirit, and emotions create a condition of well-being or wholeness that permits the individual to function adequately or optimally in his or her environment in a balanced variety of roles and patterns of occupation; allows the person to contribute to the social and economic fabric of a community over the lifespan; is conducive to independent choice, opportunity, enjoyment of life, optimal function, life satisfaction; and is available even in the presence of illness, disease, or disability (Johnson, 1986, p vii; Spencer, 1989, p. 92; Christiansen & Baum, 1997, p. 597; Creek, 1997, p. 529; Townsend, 1997, p. 181).
- Rogers (1984) suggested that "health is manifested in the ability to carry out daily living tasks" (p. 47).
- Smith (1986) a nurse, suggested there are 4 models included in the concept of health. Occupational therapy has models of practice that address all 4 models of health:
  ◊ *Clinical model:* views health as the absence of disease
  ◊ *Role performance model:* considers health a state of optimum capacity of an individual for the effective performance of the roles and tasks for which one has been socialized
  ◊ *Adaptive model:* considers the environment as a central factor
  ◊ *Eudaemonistic model:* defines health as well-being and self-realization
- From an occupational perspective, health includes having choice, abilities, and opportunities for engagement in meaningful patterns of occupation for looking after self, enjoying life, and contributing to the social and economic fabric of a community over the lifespan to promote health, well-being, and justice through occupation (Townsend, 1997).
- A dynamic, functional state that enables the individual to undertake his normal occupational performance

satisfactorily. The state of complete physical, mental, and social well-being and not merely the absence of disease or infirmity (Creek, 2003, p. 54; Turner et al., 2002, 5th ed., p. 639).

- A complete state of physical, mental, and social well-being, and not just the absence of disease or infirmity (AOTA, OTTF-1, 2002; Sladyk, Jacobs, & MacRae, 2010, p. 616; Schell et al., 2014, p. 1234 [based on WHO, 1947, p. 29]).

- Health is a dynamic, functional state that enables the individual to perform her or his daily occupations to a satisfying and effective level and to respond positively to change by adapting activities to meet changing needs (Creek, 2003, p. 54).

- From an occupational perspective, health is a balance of physical, mental, and social well-being attained through socially valued and individually meaningful occupation, enhancement of capacities, and opportunity to strive for individual potential; community cohesion and opportunity; and social integration, support, and justice; all within and as part of a sustainable ecology, beyond the absence of illness, but not necessarily beyond disability (Christiansen & Baum, 2005, p. 546).

- Health is "the state of physical, mental, and social well-being" (Hussey et al., 2007, p. 288).

- Health is a resource for everyday life, not the objective of living. It is a state of complete physical, mental, and social well-being, as well as a positive concept emphasizing social and personal resources, and physical capacities (AOTA, 2008, p. 671 [adapted from the WHO, 1986]).

- **Author's comment:** In the occupational therapy literature, health is like the weather; everybody talks about it, but few do anything about it. Occupational therapy practitioners need to advance the understanding of the outcome of health and occupation. There is discussion about the relationship of occupation and health and an assumption that occupation contributes positively to health; but the profession continues to cite the WHO's definition of health instead of contributing to the definition by explaining how occupation can be used to change a person's health status, and thus the definition of health as a concept in occupational therapy.

Identity (Occupational Identity, Personal Identity, Individual Identity, Self-Identity)

- Identity is the individual's perception of self, and includes knowledge and judgments about and feelings toward the self (Mosey, 1986, p. 437).

- Identity is a "composite definition of the self and includes an interpersonal aspect…an aspect of possibility or potential (who we might become), and a values aspect (that suggests importance and provides a stable basis for choices and decision). Identity can be viewed as the superordinate view of ourselves that includes both self-esteem and self-concept, but also importantly reflects and is influenced by the larger social world in which we find ourselves" (Christiansen, 1999, pp. 548-549; AOTA, 2002, p. 631; Christiansen & Matuska, 2011, p. 541).

- Cumulative sense of who one is and wishes to become as an occupational being generated from one's occupational history (Crepeau, Cohn, & Schell, 2003, p. 1031).

- Composite sense of who one is and wishes to become as an occupational being generated from one's history of occupational participation (Kielhofner, 2002, p. 122).

- Hagedorn (2001) defined occupational identity as "The perceptions which an individual has of himself as an 'occupational being'; the names of occupations for which he feels ownership. Occupational identity contributes to a sense of personal identity and provides meaning to daily activities" (p. 166; Duncan, 2006, p. 339).

- Occupational identity is defined as "a composite sense of who one is and wishes to become as an occupational being generated from one's history of occupational participation. One's volition, habituation, and experience as a lived body are all integrated into occupational identity" (Kielhofner, 2008, p. 106).

- Occupational identity is "the socially constructed image of self as a participant in occupations" (Christiansen & Townsend, 2010, p. 421).

- Occupational identity is the composite sense of who one is and wishes to become as an occupational being, generated from one's history of occupational participation (Schell et al., 2014, p. 1238).

- Hagedorn (2001) defined role identity as "The roles which a person has which contribute to a sense of selfhood and place the individual in relationships with others" (p. 166).

- Self-identity and self-concept include the "ability to perceive self needs and expectations from those of others, identify areas of self-competency and limitations, accept responsibility for self, perceive sexuality of self; have self-respect, have appropriate body image, view self as being able to influence events" (AOTA, 1978, p. 74).

- Self-identity is the ability to perceive oneself as an autonomous, holistic, and acceptable person who has permanence and continuity over time (Mosey, 1986, p. 437).

- Self-identity is the composite, unique view of self that a person works at shaping to establish acceptance in the social community (Christiansen & Baum, 2005, p. 550).

- **Author's comment:** Identity or occupational identity seem to have 2 aspects that appear to be related, ie, the individual's sense of selfhood and the social identity in a social world including performance of occupation.

Independence

- Independence has been used since 1905, when Hall stated that "to encourage a feeling of independence it has been decided that when a patient can turn out work of value, this product may be sold..." (p. 31).

- Upham (1918b) stated that "the sooner he sees tangible evidence of his returning ability... the sooner he will believe [economic] independence possible" (p. 36).

- By the 1950s and 1960s, the definition of independence began to be related to self-care, ADL, and self-care devices. Zimmerman (1957) illustrates and discusses several self-help devices designed to increase independence.

- Hightower (1966) continued, "in achieving independence, training in the use of the residual ability is always necessary and training in the use of self-help devices or specialized equipment is often indicated" (p. 449).

- By the 1970s, the focus of independence has turned to independent living for the elderly in their own homes and communities, as evidenced by the articles written by Hasselkus and Kiernat (1973) and Warren (1974).

- Warren's statement (1974) seems typical: "while most older people prefer to live independently as long as they can manage for themselves, coping becomes increasingly strenuous with advanced age" (p. 439).

- In the first edition of the *Uniform Terminology* adopted in 1979, the 3 themes of economic, self-care, and living in community are integrated into one definition, which reads "independent living/daily living skills refer to the skill and performance of physical and psychological/emotional self-care; work, and play/leisure activities to a level of independence appropriate to age life-space, and disability" (AOTA, 2002a, p. 900).

- Rogers (1982) expanded the concept of independence by stating that "functional independence is not just a core concept of occupational therapy theory, it is the goal of the occupational therapy process" and that "independence connotes self-reliance, self-determination, self-directedness, and a perspective of personal control" (p. 709).

- Christiansen and Baum (1991) defined independence is "having adequate resources to accomplish everyday tasks" (p. 853).

- The profession views independence as the ability to self-determine activity performance, regardless of who actually performs the activity (AOTA, 1995, p. 1014).

- Hagedorn (1995) stated that independent means "able to do what is required to remain healthy, without needing someone else to help" (p. 53).

- Christiansen and Baum (1997) also used the phrase "functional independence," and defined it to mean "the ability to successfully perform the day-to-day activities expected of the person (depending on culture, age, and gender)" (p. 596).

- Jacobs (1999) defined independence as the "lack of requirement or reliance on another; adequate resources to accomplish everyday tasks" (p. 69).

- Cammack and Eisenberg (1995) defined independence as "the ability to perform a task without physical or cognitive assistance or supervision in a reasonable amount of time" (p. 70). They continued by stating that "this term is used in the rehabilitation taxonomy to reflect the highest level of functioning. It may be used to refer to independence with all activities of daily living (or) with one specific activity" (p. 70).

- Davis (1996) seems to agree with this description when she stated that to encourage independence the patient should begin with simple ADL tasks (p. 445).

- Rock (1996) also supported the independence in ADL view saying "the person is encouraged to analyze and perform the activities of personal hygiene and grooming, dressing, feeding, home management, communication, avocation, and vocation as independently as possible" (p. 584).

- Trombly (1995) suggested a goal be stated as "the patient will demonstrate independent sitting balance and trunk flexion and extension required for independently putting on and removing shoes and stocking" (p. 33).

- In the 1970s, the consumer-driven Independent Living Movement was underway, which was built on the concepts of freedom, dignity, self-determination, and choice; basically the civil right to live independent lives. This set up the divide between occupational therapy practitioners as those who treat to fix and those who enable people to live lives. Fortunately by the early 2000s, occupational therapy began to establish its role to enable the independence of individuals by removing barriers to active living and participation in the community.

- Brown and Gillespie (1992) have reminded occupational therapy personnel that "the concept of independence has permeated the cultural understanding of mental and physical health" (p. 1001).
- Jackson (1996) stated "the spirit of independence is a tenacious American value that permeates many social institutions in this country" (p. 351).
- Kielhofner (1997) encouraged occupational therapy personnel not to impose values derived from their own professional perspectives onto the client. He summarized the view of Hocking and Whiteford's (1995) article on values saying "the tradition occupational therapy values of independence and self-determination may conflict with cultural values of clients that emphasize interdependence" (p. 87). Not all clients want to be independent of others or living independent lives. Some clients value interdependence or prefer to be taken care of by family members.
- Whiteford and Wilcock (2000) suggested that occupational therapy personnel not view the concept of independence as a given in occupational therapy practice, but rather attempt to explore what independence may mean for the client.
- A self-directed state of being, characterized by an individual's ability to participate in necessary and preferred occupations in a satisfying manner irrespective of the amount or kind of external assistance desired or required.
  ◊ Self-determination is essential to achieving and maintaining independence.
  ◊ An individual's independence is unrelated to whether he or she performs the activities related to an occupation himself or herself, performs the activities in an adapted or modified environment, makes use of various devices or alternative strategies, or oversees activity completion by others.
  ◊ Independence is defined by the individual's culture and values, support systems, and ability to direct his or her life.
  ◊ An individual's independence should not be based on pre-established criteria, perception of outside observers, or how independence is accomplished (AOTA, 2002c, p. 660).
- Creek (2003) defined independence as "the position of not being dependent on authority; not relying on others for one's opinions or behaviors; being able

to do things for oneself; having choice, control and participation in society" (p. 54).
- Creek, writing for ENOTHE, defined independence as the "condition of being able to perform everyday activities to a satisfactory level" (2010, p. 25).
- **Author's comment:** The concept of independence is well-established in the occupational therapy literature, but has been criticized as based on Western values of self-reliance that may be in contrast to societies and cultures in which interdependence is acceptable viewed as a cultural norm. Understanding how to best use both concepts successfully may be a current challenge to occupational therapy practitioners.

Interdependence

- There are multiple meanings for the term *interdependence*. The primary meaning for this chapter is an interpersonal relationship between 2 or more people that is mutually beneficial or satisfying to both or all persons. Persons may share the performance and participation in several occupations. Often, interdependence occurs between family members or relatives, but may occur between friends, neighbors, or co-workers. Another meaning refers to cooperation between professional and professional disciplines. Inter-professional interdependence will not be discussed in this chapter.
- The term *interdependence* communicates that those in societies depend on collaboration and cooperation, and that no community-dwelling individual is truly independent (Baum & Christiansen, 1997, p. 35).
- The mutual dependence of 2 or more persons on one another (Punwar & Peloquin, 2000, p. 281).
- Reliance that people have on each other as a natural consequence of group living (Christiansen & Townsend, 2004, p. 277; Christiansen & Townsend, 2010, p. 419).
- Interdependence is a fundamental experience in shared occupations (Christiansen & Townsend, 2004, p. 145).
- Interdependence is the expression and satisfaction of being and doing with others (based on Condeluci, in Christiansen & Townsend, 2004, p. 145).
- Interdependence is founded on mutual respect, acknowledgement, accommodation, and cooperation that both connects people and provides them with the independence to develop their communities (Christiansen & Townsend, 2004, pp. 145-146).
- Positive interdependence generates mutual aid and reciprocal giving (Christiansen & Townsend, 2004, p. 145).

- Interdependence "engenders a spirit of social inclusion, mutual aid, and a moral commitment and responsibility to recognize and support difference" (Christiansen & Townsend, 2004, p. 146).

- *State,* or condition of being independent (self-reliant) (Hussey et al., 2007, p. 288).

- Creek, writing for ENOTHE, defined interdependence as "the condition of mutual dependence and influence between members of a social group" (Creek, 2010, p. 25).

- Interdependence is a "relationship between 2 people or things. [There is] interdependence between people, and between people and the natural world" (Creek, 2010, p. 127).

- Interdependence is reliance on others (Sladyk, Jacobs, & MacRae, 2010, p. 617).

- Brown and Stoffel (2011) defined interdependence as "a dynamic of being mutually and physically responsible to and sharing a common set of principles with others. It is the result of an individually chosen balance between personal abilities and aspiration and environmental resources that support occupational functioning" (p. 782).

- **Author's comment:** As noted under the concept of independence, occupational therapy practitioners, educators, and researchers need to be aware that societies and cultures differ in the view of how much the individual should rely on others while performing daily life activities. Self-reliance vs mutual reliance is important to consider when addressing the concepts of independence vs interdependence. The acceptability depends on the social and cultural norms.

Life Balance

- The term *life balance* first appeared in the occupational therapy literature in the glossary of a draft document for the *Occupational Therapy Practice Framework,* and is defined as "the dynamic balance of occupations among areas of self-care, work and productive activities, play and leisure activities, and rest and sleep that support health and satisfaction" (AOTA, 2002b, p. 56). The term was not included in the published version.

- Lifestyle balance implies a "satisfactory congruence between an array of actual and desired occupational patterns; what people want to spend their time doing and what they actually do" (Matuska & Christiansen, 2008, p. 11).

- A consistent and desired pattern of occupations that enables people to manage stress and promote health and well-being. Patterns may be viewed on several

dimensions, including time allocation, fulfillment of social roles, and meeting psychological needs. (Synonyms or closely related terms include role balance, work-related balance, work family balance, lifestyle balance, work-life balance, and occupational balance) (Christiansen & Townsend, 2010, p. 419).

- An emerging interdisciplinary concept related to the identification of lifestyle characteristics that engender health and well-being (related to the historical but unsubstantiated concept known in occupational therapy as occupational balance) (Christiansen & Matuska, 2011, p. 542).

- A satisfying pattern of daily activity that is healthful, meaningful, and sustainable to an individual within the context of his or her current life circumstances (Schell et al., 2014, p. 1235).

- Life imbalance is a state in which one's activity configurations limit or compromise participation in valued relationships; are incongruent for establishing or maintaining psychological health and a satisfactory identity; or are mundane, uninteresting, or unchallenging (Schell et al., 2014, p. 1235).

- Balanced lifestyle is *"a satisfying pattern of daily occupation that is healthful, meaningful, and sustainable to an individual with the context of his or her current life circumstances"* (italics in original citation, Matuska & Christiansen, 2008, p. 11).

- **Author's comment:** Life balance appears to be a broader, more inclusive concept than occupational balance, and may be a better choice for some clients. However, occupational therapy practitioners need to consider that achieving the goal of life balance may be unrealistic in short-term treatment situations where occupational balance may be a more achievable goal.

Mastery

- The term *mastery* appeared in a proposed theory of occupational therapy in 1968, but the term is not defined or described (Mazer, 1968, pp. 453-454 in Diagram II).

- Wantanabe (1968) defined mastery as the "ability and skill in recognizing and comprehending the options that society offers and making choices appropriately using one's human and nonhuman environment to meet one's own needs and abilities" (p. 440).

- Hopkins and Smith (1979) defined mastery as "command or grasp of a subject" (p. 734).

- Llorens (1976) used the term *mastery* but did not define it. Phrases included "mastery of the developmental tasks and adaptive skills according to the age" and "developmental mastery for successful adaptation" (p. 1). In 1991, she stated that "accomplishment of tasks is prefaced on the ability to achieve mastery of skills" and describes "levels of mastery for successful adaptation" (pp. 46-47). Level 1 is called "occupational performance enablers," which includes the sub-skills of sensory perception, sensory integration, motor coordination, psychosocial and psychodynamic responses, sociocultural development, and social language responses. Level 2 is called "activities and task of occupational performance," which includes the skill areas of self-care/self-maintenance, play/leisure, work/education, and rest/relaxation. Level 3 is called "occupational roles," which includes worker, student, volunteer, homemaker, parent, child, sibling, peer, and best friend or chum.

- Fidler and Fidler (1978) described mastery, but did not define the term. They said "the meaning and worth of one's doing or mastery is appreciably determined by the views and values of significant others" (p. 307).

- Christiansen and Baum (1991) defined mastery as "the achievement of skill to a criterion level of success" (p. 854).

- Schkade and Schultz (1992) used the term *relative mastery*, which is defined as "the extent to which the person experiences the occupational response as efficient (use of time and energy), effective (production of the desired result), and satisfying to self and society; that is, it is pleasing not only to the self but also to relevant others as agents of the occupational environment" (p. 835).

- Ryan (1993) defined mastery as "the desire to explore, understand, and to some extent, control oneself and an environment" (p. 362).

- Muñoz and Kielhofner (1995) also used the term *mastery*, stating that the achievement level "represents the fullest mastery over one's self and the environment" (p. 346).

- Parham and Fazio (1997) defined mastery as "the state of being competent" or of "having adequate skills to exert some degree of control over one's environment and situation" (p. 250).

- Christiansen and Townsend (2004) defined mastery as "proficiency in dealing successfully with the challenges of living that occur at any point in time" (p. 277).

- Brown and Stoffel (2011) defined mastery as "success; possession of consummate skills" (p. 783).

- Relative mastery is a person's phenomenological evaluation of the quality of his or her occupational response. This evaluation has 4 aspects: efficiency (use of time, energy, resources), effectiveness (the extent to which the desired goals was achieved), of satisfaction to self, and satisfaction to society (Schell et al., 2014, p. 1240).

- **Author's comment:** The *APA Dictionary of Psychology* (VanderBos, 2007) listed the term *mastery training*, which appears to summarize the intent of the definitions of mastery above. Mastery training is defined as "experimental or real-world training that prepares individuals for aversive situations or conflict by teaching them methods of assertion and constructive control over environmental conditions" (p. 557).

Occupational Balance (Occupational Imbalance)

- Balance as related to occupation has been a concept in the occupational therapy literature from the formative years. Meyer (1922) said "the big four—work and play and rest and sleep, which our organism must be able to balance even under difficulty."

- Dewey wrote in 1900 that "the fundamental point in the psychology of an occupation is that it maintain a balance between the intellectual and the practical phases of experience" (1990, p. 133 [reprint]).

- Reilly reestablished balance as an important concept in occupational therapy. She stated that "the concept of balanced daily living" should become "highly valued by us and that skills pertaining to planning and implementing daily living schedules" should be acquired (1966, p. 64).

- Mosey interpreted the temporal aspect of balance to mean equal amounts when she stated "temporal adaptation refers to one's ability to satisfy these needs (work, play and rest) in a relatively equal manner" (1981, p. 78).

- Llorens suggested another interpretation for the concept of balance. She said that "balance in the individual environment supports functional performance in activities of daily living, and independent living skills, in work and play, and learning and leisure" (1984, p. 30).

- Reed (1984) defined occupational balance as "a state in which a person's needs and demands are met through the performance of occupations in all three areas—self-maintenance, productivity, and leisure. Occupational balance requires an understanding of the person's needs and demands and an analysis of the types of tasks being done, their effectiveness in meeting needs and demands and the amount of time being spent or not spent to perform them. Balance is influenced by individual situations, performances (values), and age. Balance should be a dynamic process which can change as needs and demands change" (p. 501).

- Kielhofner (1985) spoke of role balance as "integration of an optimal number of appropriate roles into one's life" (p. 508).

- Mocellin (1995) returned to the theme of equal time speaking of "activity balance," and reports that in Australia the 8-hour working day was established in the skilled trades in the 1850s when the idea of 8 hours of work, 8 hours of play, and 8 hours of sleep was established (p. 505).

- Christiansen (1994) reviewed several categorization systems in his article on classification. The division into 3 groups is the most common and may have been an unintended consequence of the term *occupational performance*, as it was first defined in 1973, which stated that "occupational performance includes self-care, work, and play/leisure time performance" (AOTA, 1973, p. 41).

- Christiansen (1996) suggested the profession actually incorporates 3 different ideas within the concept of balance: (1) time budget approach, based on the assumption that daily activities can be classified according to intrinsic characteristics; (2) equivalent time spent among these categories will result in improved well-being; and (3) chronobiology, suggesting that well-being results when internal clocks and external behaviors (and occupations) are synchronized.

- Christiansen and Baum (1997) do not define balance as a single word, but rather define the phrase balance of occupations as "a belief, not substantiated by research, that a general configuration of daily occupation can contribute to health and well-being" (p. 592).

- Simpson (1997) defines occupational balance "as the state of balance among the performance areas of work, self-care, and leisure" (p. 7).

- Wilcock (1998) may have had a similar idea in mind when she defined occupational balance as "a balance of engagement in occupation that leads to well-being. For example, the balance may be among physical, mental, and social occupations; between chosen and obligatory occupations; between strenuous and restful occupations; or between doing and being" (p. 257; Wilcock, 2006, p. 343). The issues of choice and diversity are further supported by her definition of occupational imbalance as "a lack of balance or disproportion of occupation resulting in decreased well-being" (Wilcock, 1998, p. 257).

- "Managing [occupation] in a way that is personally fulfilling... and meets role demands... Each person has an individual balance schema that suits his or her health" (Reed & Sanderson, 1999, p. 99).

- A sense of balance is a perceived state, involving attitudes, goals, and perspective, interacting with time and expectations of sociocultural environment. Occupational balance is internally defined (Backman, 2004, p. 202).

- A regular mix of physical, mental, social, spiritual, and rest occupations that provide an overall feeling of well-being (Christiansen & Baum, 2005, p. 134).

- A concept referring to the distribution of time for engagement in the habits and routines of everyday occupations; an interpretive concept for assessing time use with reference to health, well-being, and quality of life when the patterns of occupation are taken into account for individuals, groups, and communities; perceived state of satisfactory participation in valued, obligatory, and discretionary activities; occurs when the impact of occupations on one another is harmonious, cohesive, and under control (Christiansen & Townsend, 2010, p. 420).

- Balance in one's daily routines, appreciating that balance is influenced by cultural beliefs and context (Brown & Stoffel, 2011, p. 785).

- Individual's perception of having the right amount of occupations and the right variation between occupations. Three perspectives of occupational balance are in relation to occupational areas, in relation to occupations with different characteristics, and in relation to time use (Wagman, Håkansson, & Bjöklund, 2012, p. 322).

- Christiansen and Townsend (2010) defined role balance as "satisfactory fulfillment of all valued roles" (p. 422).

- Often the opposite concept assists in clarifying the original concept. The following are some definitions of occupational imbalance. Although the temporal aspect dominates the definitions, the right (occupation right) to occupation that is neither under-occupied or over-occupied and the idea that lack of occupation can decrease health status, sense of well-being, and quality of life are evident.

  ◊ A lack of balance or disproportion of occupation resulting in decreased well-being (Wilcock, 1998, p. 257)

  ◊ A lack of variety in occupation, an undue focus on one occupation to the exclusion of others (Hagedorn, 2001, p. 166)

  ◊ A lack of balance between self-care, work, rest, and play/leisure that fails to meet an individuals' physical or psychosocial needs, thereby resulting in decreased health and well-being (Scaffa, Desmond, & Brownson, 2001, p. 44)

◊ Excessive time spent in one area, usually work, at the expense of another, usually leisure. May aggravate health and quality of life (Trombly & Radomski, 2002, pp. 746-747, attributed to Wilcock, 1998)

◊ Refers to a loss of balance between work, rest, and play (Creek, 2003, p. 28)

◊ Refers to states in which people are unable to participate in occupations that allow them to exercise their physical, social, and mental capacities (Larson, Wood, & Clark, 2003, p. 20)

◊ A temporal concept referring to the allocation of time for particular purposes; may be experimental at both individual and societal levels when people are over-occupied or under-occupied (Christiansen & Townsend, 2004, p. 253)

◊ An individual or group experience in which health and QOL are compromised because of being over-occupied or under-occupied (Christiansen & Townsend, 2004, p. 278; 2010, p. 421)

◊ Patterns of occupations that do not meet unique needs, interests, and commitments (Christiansen & Baum, 2005, p. 548)

◊ The social condition of being occupied too little or too much of the time to engage in meaningful and necessary occupations (Cara & MacRae, 2013, p. 970)

- **Author's comment:** The concept of occupational balance remains popular, and has become a complex concept with at least 3 dimensions: balance between occupations selected from different occupational areas, balance of characteristics between different occupations, and balance of time use between different occupations.

Occupational Justice (Occupational Injustice)

- Wilcock (1998) defined occupational justice as "the promotion of social and economic change to increase individual, community, and political awareness, resources, and equitable opportunities for diverse occupational opportunities, which enable people to meet their potential and experience well-being" (p. 257; 2006, p. 343).

- The concept of occupational justice is about "recognizing and providing for the occupational needs of individuals and communities as part [of] a fair and empowering society" (Wilcock & Townsend, 2000, p. 84).

- A critical perspective of social structures that promotes social, political, and economic changes to enable people to meet their occupational potential and experience well-being (Crepeau, Cohn, & Schell, 2003, p. 1031).

- The just and equitable distribution of power, resources, and opportunity so that all people are able to meet the needs of their occupational natures without compromising the common good (Christiansen & Baum, 2005, p. 548).

- Access to and participation in the full range of meaningful and enriching occupations afforded to others, includes opportunities for social inclusion and the resources to participate in occupations to satisfy personal, health, and societal needs (AOTA, 2008, p. 663, 672; adapted from Townsend & Wilcock, 2004b).

- Brown and Stoffel (2011) defined occupational justice as "the equitable opportunity and resources to enable people's engagement in meaningful occupations" (p. 765).

- The right of an individual or group to engage in occupations that are meaningful and enriching. Occupational justice describes the rights of individuals or groups to exert autonomy through choice in participation, and engagement in occupations that are in the typical range of occupations within the community and of significant value to the group or individual (Cara & MacRae, 2013, p. 970).

- Occupational injustice is an outcome of social policies and other forms of governance that structure how power is exerted to restrict participation in the everyday occupations of populations and individuals (Nilsson & Townsend, 2010, p. 58).

- **Author's comment:** The term *occupational justice* is credited to Wilcock in 1998 and is based on the concept of social justice. The concept of occupational justice as an outcome was accepted in the *Occupational Therapy Practice Framework*, second edition (AOTA, 2008) and is included in the third edition (AOTA, 2014). The concept has ethical as well as outcome considerations, since justice is a major concept in professional ethics.

Occupational Performance

- The term *occupational performance* first appeared in the occupational therapy literature in 1973 and was described as follows: "occupational performance includes self-care, work, and play/leisure time performance. Occupational performance requires learning and practice experiences with the role and developmental stage-specific tasks, and the utilization of all performance components. Deficits in task learning experiences, performance components, and/or life space, any result in limitations in occupational performance" (AOTA, 1973, p. 41).

- In 1974, the Task Force on Target Populations defined occupational performance as "the ability to accomplish the tasks related to a development stage; it includes the ability to develop and sustain a life style that is equally balanced among goal-directed activities—toward self-care, independence, contributions to others and gratification of personal needs" (AOTA, 1974, pp. 231-232). This definitions primarily addresses outcome.

- Occupational therapy practitioners treat problems and potential problems of occupational performance. The identified areas of occupational performance of concern to the practicing occupational therapy practitioner are work, education, play, self-care, and leisure (Llorens, 1976, pp. 1-2).

- In 1978 occupational performance was defined as "the performance of self-care, work, and play/leisure activities, the activities of daily living. The performance of these activities requires self-care, work, and play/leisure skills" (AOTA, 1978, p. 74).

- "The occupational performance [frame] of reference operationalizes occupational performance components of sensory, motor, psychological, social, and cognitive functions and the areas of self-care, work, play, learning, and leisure" (Llorens, 1984, p. 30).

- Nelson (1988) defined occupational performance as "the doing, the action, the active behavior, or the active responses exhibited within the context of an occupational perform" (p. 634). Clearly Nelson described a doing process.

- Punwar (1994) defined occupational performance as "an individual's total pattern of activities, ie, self-care, work, leisure, and organization of time" (p. 262).

- Law et al. (1996) defined occupational performance as "the outcome of the transaction of the person, environment, and occupation. It is defined as the dynamic experience of a person engaged in purposeful activities and tasks within an environment" (p. 16). Occupational performance is viewed as a complex, dynamic phenomenon that has both spatial and temporal considerations and is shaped by the transaction that occurs among the person, environment, and occupation in which the person engages. Occupational performance requires the ability to balance occupation and views of self and environment

that sometimes conflict, and to encompass changing priorities (p. 17). This definition and description outline both the outcome and doing process.

- Baum and Law (1997) stated that occupational performance is "the point when the person, the environment, and the person's occupation intersect to support the tasks, activities, and roles that define the person as an individual" (p. 281). This is a theoretical definition.

- Christiansen and Baum (1997) described occupational performance as the "accomplishment of tasks related to self-care/self-maintenance, work/education, play/leisure, and rest/relaxation; the unique term used by occupational therapy to express function as it reflects the individual's dynamic experience of engaging in daily occupations within the environment" (p. 600). This is an outcome definition.

- Creek (1997) defined occupational performance as "the actions of the individual elicited and guided by the occupational form" (p. 529). This is a doing process definition.

- Hagedorn (1997) described occupational performance as "human behavior having three areas: self-care, productivity, and leisure, which are based on the interaction of the individual's mental, physical, sociocultural, and spiritual performance components" (p. 145). This definition suggests criteria for an outcome statement.

- Jackson and Banks (1997) defined occupational performance as "task accomplishment in everyday living with a desirable role" (p. 460). Their definition is more consistent with the concept of tool. Townsend (1997) stated that occupational performance is the "ability to choose, organize, and satisfactorily perform meaningful occupations that are culturally defined and age-appropriate for looking after oneself, enjoying life, and contributing to the social and economic fabric of one's community" (p. 181; Hagedorn, 2001, p. 166). Again, criteria for an outcome statement are described.

- Gillen and Burkhardt (1998) explained that occupational performance is the ability to accomplish the tasks required by a certain role (p. 540). This definition suggests the doing application of the concept.

- Punwar and Peloquin (2000) defined occupational performance as "an individual's total pattern of activities, ie, self-care, work, leisure, and organization of time" (p. 282). This is yet another description of possible criteria for outcome.

- The ability to carry out activities of daily life (areas of occupation). Occupational performance can be addressed in 2 different ways:

◊ *Improvement:* used when a performance deficit is present, often as a result of an injury or disease process. This approach results in increased independence and function in ADL, IADL, education, work, play, leisure, or social participation.

◊ *Enhancement:* used when a performance deficit is not currently present. This approach results in the development of performance skills and performance patterns that augment performance or prevent potential problems from developing in daily life occupations (AOTA, 2002c, p. 632).

• The ability to carry out activities in the areas of occupation (Hussey et al., 2007, p. 289).

• Christiansen and Townsend (2004) defined occupational performance as "the task-oriented, completion, or doing aspect of occupations; often, but not exclusively, involving observable movement (p 278; 2010, p. 421).

• The act of doing and accomplishing a selected activity or occupation that results from the dynamic transaction among the client, the context, and the activity. Improving or enabling skills and patterns in occupational performance leads to engagement in occupations or activities (AOTA, 2008, pp. 672-673 [adapted in part from Law et al., 1996, p. 16]).

◊ *Improvement:* used when a performance limitation is present. These outcomes document increased occupational performance for the person, organization, or population.

◊ *Enhancement:* used when a performance limitation is not currently present. These outcomes document the development of performance skills and performance patterns that augment existing performance or prevent potential problems for developing in life occupations (AOTA, 2008, p. 662).

• Doing a task related to participation in a major life area; the accomplishment of the selected occupation resulting from the dynamic transaction among the client, the context and environment, and the activity (Schell et al., 2014, p. 1238).

• Occupational performance skills are those skills required for successful performance of the roles that are assumed by individuals in their lives. Most human roles fall into the categories of play, self-care, and work. (Hopkins & Smith, 1977, p. 735; 1983, p. 924)

• **Author's comment:** Performance appears to be used more frequently in the occupational therapy literature to describe a doing process, in which the verbs "to perform" and "performing" may appear. Occupational performance appears to be defined more in relation to a desired outcome. Perform,

performing, and performance are common English words. The profession of occupational therapy can only clarify their use within the profession. The concept of occupational performance is more unique to the profession and, thus, the profession can more easily direct its use. The same can be said for the concepts of performance areas, performance components, and performance contexts. These concepts developed primarily within the profession and their usage can be controlled by the profession. However, there may be some help from the new ICF document (WHO, 2001) where performance is defined as "a construct that describes, as a qualifier, what individuals do in their current environment, and in this way, brings in the aspect of a person's involvement in life situations" (p. 166).

Prevention

• Prevention became a concept in the occupational therapy literature in the late 1960s. West (1969), Wiemer (1972), and Finn (1972) discussed prevention as an aspect of community health and suggested several roles that occupational therapy personnel could fill.

• The 1979 *Uniform Reporting System* describes prevention as referring "to skills and performance in minimizing debilitation. It may include programs for persons where predisposition to disability exists, as well as for those who have already incurred a disability" (Hopkins & Smith, 1983, p. 905). Examples provided include energy conservation, joint protection and body mechanics, positioning, and coordination of daily living activities.

• In 1988, Levy discussed the health promotion and disease prevention programs as including "one or more elements of primary prevention (the prevention of disease before any symptoms are present), secondary prevention (screening, early detection, and early treatment of apparent disease in a person who has been defined as at risk), and tertiary prevention (the treatment of acquired disease in a manner designed to minimize the development of complications)" (p. 164).

• Promoting a healthy lifestyle at the individual, group, organizational, community (societal), and government or policy level (AOTA, 2002c, p. 633).

• The *Occupational Therapy Practice Framework,* 2nd edition (AOTA, 2008) described prevention as follows, "health promotion is equally and essentially concerned with creating the conditions necessary for health at individual, structural, social, and environmental levels through an understanding of the determinants of health, peace, shelter, education, food, income, a stable ecosystem, sustainable resources, social justice, and equity" (Kronenberg, Algado, & Pollard, 2001, p. 441).

- Occupational therapy promotes healthy lifestyle at the individual, group, organizational, community (societal), and governmental or policy level (adapted from Brownson & Scaffa, 2011, p. 663, 674).

- Promoting a healthy lifestyle and creating the conditions necessary for health (Christiansen & Matuska, 2011, p. 543).

- **Author's comment:** As used in occupational therapy practice, prevention does not seem to be a unique concept, but rather a part of the continuum of obtaining another objective. Working toward occupational balance for example automatically includes preventing occupational imbalance; the prevention is "built into" the desired concept. As written descriptions of prevention seem to be more focused on health promotion, perhaps the outcome should be health promotion, not prevention.

Quality of Life

- Concept first appears in the modern period in 1985. Kielhofner (1985) defines quality of life (QOL) as "positive feeling states captured by concepts like happiness, well-being, and hope" (p. 507).

- Punwar (1994) defines QOL as "considering a patients' satisfaction with life as well as his or her physical needs" (p. 264; Punwar & Peloquin, 2000, pp. 183-183).

- Eisenberg (1995) suggests that in the field of rehabilitation there are 3 meanings for the term *QOL:* (1) aspects of daily life that collectively are construed as positive and render a feeling that life is worth living, (2) aspects of a person's ability to perform ordinary ADL, and (3) the ability to realize life plans (p. 202). The first is based on affect, the second on performance, and the third on cognition.

- Christiansen and Baum (1997) define QOL as a "concept defined by an individual's perceptions of over-all life satisfaction and happiness with his or her living circumstances, including physical status and abilities, psychological well-being, social interactions, and economic conditions" (p. 602).

- Townsend (1997) defines QOL as "choosing and participating in occupations that foster hope, generate motivation, offer meaning and satisfaction, create a driving vision of life, promote health, enable empowerment, and otherwise address the quality of life" (p. 182).

- Individual level of "satisfaction with various aspects of life, including daily living, degree of choice, feelings of being in control, feeling able to succeed, ability to accomplish tasks and number and quality of relationships" (Creek, 2003, p. 58).

- Incorporates health, psychological state, level of independence, social relationships, and relationships with the environment (Christiansen & Baum, 2005, p. 549).

- A relative measurement of what is meaningful and what provides satisfaction to an individual (Hussey et al., 2007, p. 291).

- A client's dynamic appraisal of life satisfaction (perceptions of progress toward identified goals), self-concept (the composite of beliefs and feelings about themselves), health and functioning (including health status, self-care, capabilities), and socioeconomic factors (eg, vocation, education, income) (AOTA, 2008, pp. 663, 674; Christiansen & Matuska, 2011, p. 544).

- A term difficult to define in the medical literature, but generally meaning a concept broader than health or disease and consisting of such characteristics as good mobility, social relations, self-esteem, independent living, and other daily living factors (Cara & MacRae, 2013, p. 971).

- A measure of well-being; encompasses individual's perceptions of their position in life in the context of culture and value systems in which they live, and in relation to their goals, expectations, standards, and concerns (Schell et al., 2014, p. 1240).

- **Author's comment:** QOL is a complex concept that requires clarification to be useful as an outcome measure, because the term has both subjective and objective components that must be addressed in determining whether a person has a quality of life that is acceptable, good, or better from the viewpoint of the client.

Recovery (in Mental Health)

- Term as defined here is credited to William A. Anthony, a psychologist, in 1993.

- Recovery is "the processes by which people with mental illnesses come to be actively engaged in creating meaningful community lives in spite of the presence of intermittent or even pervasive and continuous mental illness" (Krupa & Clark, 2004 p. 69).

- Recovery is a "journey of healing and transformation enabling a person with a mental health problem to live a meaningful life in a community of his or her choice while striving to achieve his or her full potential" (Brown & Stoffel, 2011, p. 787).

- Recovery is a personal process of actively engaging in community life despite the ongoing presence of mental illness (Eisfelder & Gewurtz, 2012, p. 219; based on Krupa & Clark, 2004).
- A process of change through which individuals with mental disorders and substance abuse disorders improve their health and wellness, live a self-directed life, and strive to reach their full potential (Schell, Gillen, & Scaffa, 2014 [based on Substance Abuse and Mental Health Services Administration, 2011, SAMHSA's working definition of recovery, pamphlet]).
- **Author's comment:** Recovery is a new concept as an outcome measurement for occupational therapy. The role of occupational therapy remains fluid, which limits the outcome criteria available to measure the effectiveness or efficiency of occupational therapy services in attaining the goal of recovery.

Satisfaction (Client Satisfaction)

- Client satisfaction is the client's affective response to his or her perception of the process and benefits of receiving occupational therapy services (AOTA, 2002c, p. 630).
- Client satisfaction is a measure of the client's perception of the process and the benefits received from occupational therapy services (Hussey et al., 2007, p. 286).
- **Author's comment:** The concept of client satisfaction with the outcome of occupational therapy services has received limited attention in the occupational therapy literature, as evidenced by the lack of definitions. Although defined in the first edition of the *Occupational Therapy Practice Framework*, the term is not included in the glossary of terms for the second edition published in 2008, nor in the third edition published in 2014. In other words, occupational therapy practitioners and assistants state that a major tool of occupational therapy is a client-centered approach (see definitions under section on Tools), but little research is performed to determine if, in fact, client-centered care is in reality being delivered as determined by clients actually receiving occupational therapy services. McKinnon (2000) suggests 3 domains of client satisfaction be explored: satisfaction with accessibility to occupational therapy services, health outcomes attributed to occupational therapy services, and global satisfaction with occupational therapy services.

Satisfaction (Life Satisfaction)

- Hall (1905) described satisfaction saying that "the one great end to be obtained is self-forgetfulness and a pride and satisfaction in work and in life" (p. 32) and Meyer (1922) uses satisfaction several times in his article (p. 8).
- Dunton (1928) suggested that "stimulating heart action, respiration and blood circulation...yield some of the joy and satisfaction that wisely selected wholesome occupation provides in normal life" (p. 4).
- Satisfaction is the experience of pleasure and contentment with one's performance (Crepeau, Cohn, & Schell, 2003, p. 1033).
- Hopkins and Smith stated simply that life satisfaction is a "subjective sense of well-being" (1983, p. 923).
- Maguire (1983) described a model of life satisfaction in which "satisfaction depends on the degree of congruence between an individual's perceived resources and his or her expectations for participation in valued activities" (p. 167). Four assumptions were proposed: 1) a person's individual activity resources either enhance or constrain his or her ability to act, 2) activity expectations vary with each individual and particular social situation, 3) activity expectation may prescribe relative activity levels, and 4) a person's individual expectations may vary from the social norms of a particular situation.
- Life satisfaction is being able to do what the person wants and needs to do. The central concepts are pursuing valued interests, meaningful experiences, and relationships consistent with one's life plan (Christiansen & Baum, 2005, p. 547).
- Life satisfaction is one's overall satisfaction with the experiences of life (Christiansen & Townsend, 2010, p. 419).
- Life satisfaction is a person's satisfaction with the circumstances of her or his life. Life satisfaction is not necessarily correlated with the severity of a disability (Cara & MacRae, 2013, p. 968).
- Satisfaction with experience includes overall feelings and perceptions related to experiences (Schell et al., 2014, p. 1241).
- **Author's comment:** To assess life satisfaction, the client must have the cognitive capacity to evaluate the availability of one or more resources (time, place, object, event) in relation to some level or type of doing (more, less, different from, same as). Life satisfaction is a dynamic concept and changes, sometimes frequently, over a lifetime as conditions and situations change.

Self-Efficacy

- The concept of self-efficacy or *efficacy expectation* was originated in 1977 by Bandura, a psychologist, and was originally defined as "the conviction that one can successfully execute the behavior required to produce the outcome" (p. 193). In 1986, Bandura further defined perceived self-efficacy as "people's judgments of their capabilities to organize and execute a course of action required to attain designated types of performances" (p. 391). He continued by stating that judgment or perception of what a person can do is more critical than the skills or skill level, per se. In 1988 he wrote "concerned with beliefs in one's capabilities to mobilize the motivation, cognitive resources and courses of action need to meet given situational demands" (Bandura et al., 1988, p. 479).

- Self-efficacy first appeared in the occupational therapy literature when Crist and Stoffel (1992) referred to Bandura's (1977) 4 sources of judgments about one's self-efficacy that affect performance: emotional arousal, verbal and social persuasion, vicarious experience, and performance accomplishment (p. 436).

- Gage and Polatajko (1994) suggested there are 3 parameters of perceived self-efficacy, which are magnitude, strength, and generality.

- Self-efficacy is the feeling or perception that a person has about himself or herself as able to be successful in using a particular coping strategy or problem-solving approach, and the person's belief or self confidence in his or her performance capabilities with respect to the effectiveness or power to produce effects or intended results on a specific functional task or occupation. The feeling or belief is assumed to be an important determinant of actual performance, and predicts the likelihood that one will attempt a given behavior and continue working at it, despite possible difficulties, in new situations (Gage et al., 1994, p. 783; Christiansen & Baum, 1997, p. 433; Cara & MacRae, 1998, p. 688; Jacobs, 1999, p. 132; Hagedorn, 2000, p. 311; Stein & Roose, 2000, p. 284).

- "People's beliefs in their capabilities to organize and execute the courses of action required to deal with prospective situations" (AOTA, 2002c, p. 633 [based on Bandura, 1995]).

- An estimate by an individual as to his or her ability to manage a situation; the likelihood of something occurring (Christiansen & Baum, 2005, p. 550).

- Belief that oneself can overcome barriers or problems in spite of obstacles (Cara & MacRae, 2013, p. 972).

- Confidence in one's ability to take action (Schell et al., 2014, p. 1241).

- **Author's comment:** The definition of self-efficacy appears to be congruent with the Bandura's original definitions, which is important because when concepts enter the occupational therapy literature, changes in the limitations on meaning or descriptors may occur that are different from the original source or usage.

Self-Management (Chronic Disease Self-Management)

- The concept of self-management became popular in the medical literature around 1988. Most definitions of self-management describe a program that is a tool. Therefore, the concept of self-management as an outcome is still evolving. As an outcome, self-management would require the individual to take charge of (with appropriate supports) managing the chronic elements of his or her condition while participating in daily activities and meeting performance obligations to an acceptable level of personal satisfaction and QOL. Self-management thus requires combining several outcomes into a larger or mega-concept.

- Four categories are listed: coping skills, time, management, and self-control (AOTA, 1994, p. 1054), but no definition of self-management is stated.

- Active self-management includes (for arthritis): low impact exercise (eg, walking, swimming); range of motion exercises for specific joint; applying heat or cold to painful joints; relaxation; joint protection; massaging painful joints; a balance of rest, exercise and meaningful activities compatible with level of disability; use of cognitive coping methods such as distraction, imagery, and self-statements; and appropriate use of painkillers (Jefferson & Hammond, 2002, p. 625).

- Self-management approach assumes that people understand their own life circumstances and take action based on internal motivation and a sense of confidence in their ability to succeed. Knowledge alone does not result in self-management: knowledge accompanied by information, confidence, and support does (Packer, 2011, p. 3).

- Self-management programs teach the skills needed to carry out medical regimes specific to the disease, guide health behavior change, and provide emotional support for patients to control their disease and live functional lives (Augustine, Roberts, & Packer, 2011, p. 9).

- Self-management addresses not only the ongoing medical management of the condition, but also acknowledges the emotional impact and the need for the individual to engage in meaningful roles and activities. The emphasis is on self-efficacy, or increasing confidence in problem solving and decision making (White & Buyting, 2011, p. 11).

- "Self-management is a patient-focused approach to managing chronic conditions... by encouraging people to be actively involved in their own health care" (Gilbert et al., 2012, p. 1). Common elements include active participation of the individual in his or her treatment to minimize the effect of the condition, goal setting, problem solving, and self-management support.

- Self-management relates to the tasks that an individual does to live well with one or more chronic conditions. These tasks include gaining confidence to deal with medical management, role management, and emotional management (Packer, 2013, p. 1).

- Self-management principles include knowledge related to reducing the adverse consequences of disease on lifestyle, ie, understanding the disease and its causes, awareness of medications and their side effects, and recognition of practical techniques and devices that can prevent or reduce disease progression and improve function and quality of life (Christiansen & Matuska, 2004, p. 469; 2011, p. 544).

- **Author's comment:** Packer et al. (2012) stated that the aim of self-management programs is "to provide people with knowledge and skills needed to manage their risk factors, monitor their disease(s), make effective use of services, and/or manage the impact of disease on their lives" (p. 93). These aims should form the basis for evaluating self-management as an outcome, but instead the studies involving occupational therapy tend to use other outcome criteria, such as self-efficacy or quality of life. If self-management is to be a useful outcome for occupational therapy, then the concept of self-management needs to be measured directly, not indirectly.

- *Social Participation:* See *Doing* concepts.

Well-Being (Wellbeing)

- Well-being became a concept in the occupational therapy literature in the 1980s. Two themes have emerged: emotional/psychological end state (pleasure, happiness, satisfaction, comfort) and cognitive process of evaluating (perceiving, experiencing) life situation.

- Johnson (1986) defined well-being as "a state that transcends the limitations of body, space, time, and circumstances, and in which one is at peace with one's self and with others" (p. vii).

- Christiansen and Baum (1997) stated that well-being is "a subjective sense of overall contentment, thought to be defined by affective state and life satisfaction" (p. 606).

- Law, Steinwender, and Leclair (1998) stated that well-being refers to "the integration of a person's physical, mental, emotional, spiritual, and social characteristics" (p. 83).

- Wilcock (1998) suggested the concept of well-being should be explored from 3 individual aspects: physical, mental, and social; and 2 contexts: community and ecology. In other words, well-being is an interactive process between the individual and the surrounding in which the person lives.

- The ICF (WHO, 2001) defined well-being as "a general term encompassing the total universe of human life domains including physical, mental, and social aspects, that make up what can be called a 'good life.' Health domains are a subset of domains that make up the total universe of human life" (p. 211). The universe of well-being includes education, employment, environment, etc, as well as the health domains of seeing, speaking, remembering, etc (p. 212).

- A subjective experience consisting of feelings of pleasure or various feelings of happiness, health, and comfort, which can differ from person to person (Creek & Lougher, 2008, p. 583).

- Is experienced when people engage in occupations that they perceive (a) are consistent with their values and preferences, (b) support their abilities to competently perform valued roles, (c) support their occupational identities, and (d) support their plans and goals (Townsend & Polatajko, 2007, p. 374).

- Extent to which individuals experience a sense of vitality and satisfaction with their life and circumstances, as well as subjective perceptions of occupational performance, rather than objective measurements of the frequency or extent of participation in valued occupations (Crepeau, Cohn, & Schell, 2009, p. 1160).

- The affect or emotion about one's psychological, emotional, or physical state as perceived at a given moment (Christiansen & Townsend, 2010, p. 423).

- The state of being content, comfortable, and satisfied with one's self, relationships, and QOL (Sladyk, Jacobs, & MacRae, 2010, p. 624).

- The term *well-being* describes basic material satisfaction; freedom of choice; and action, health, security, and good social relations (Whittaker, 2012, p.437).

- Implies that basic survival needs are met and encompasses ideas such as health, happiness, and prosperity (Schell et al., 2014, p. 1243).

- Mental well-being is a feeling of contentment associated with emotional, intellectual, and spiritual satisfaction, enabling effective interaction with others and peace with self (Christiansen & Baum, 2005, p. 547).

- Christiansen and Townsend (2010) defined occupational well-being as "experiences of satisfaction and meaning derived from participation in occupations" (p. 421).

- **Author's comment:** The concept of well-being has several meanings. Aldrich (2011) identifies 5: eudaemonia (well-being equals happiness from "rational" activity carried out in a "virtuous" way), hedonism (well-being equals having more pleasure than pain), desire fulfillment (well-being equals having desires fulfilled), objective list (well-being equals checking off a list of recognizable qualities determined in advance), and prudential value list (well-being equals having the qualities inherent in the "characteristic human life"). These definitions seem to touch on all 5 meanings, with a focus on hedonism and desire fulfillment.

Wellness

- According to Johnson (1986) the concept of wellness began in the 1960s.

- Earliest reference in the occupational therapy literature is Reed and Sanderson (1980), in which wellness is described as "an optimal or ideal condition toward which to strive" (p. 92).

- In 1985, Johnson described wellness "as a context for living" (p. 129). In 1986, White defined wellness as "a lifestyle for well-being that a person chooses, regardless of the presence or absence of disabling conditions, to reach optimum potential" (p. 745).

- Reed and Sanderson (1992) suggested there are 3 uses of the term *wellness* that include (1) wellness as the polar opposite of illness, (2) wellness as a graduated scale with illness, and (3) wellness as a separate or nearly separate dimension from illness (p. 48). None of the 3 has been developed adequately in occupational therapy to be used as a consistent indicator of outcome. In addition, wellness is often associated with health promotion.

- Dunn (1977), one of the early advocates of wellness, defined wellness as an "integrated method of functioning which is oriented toward maximizing the potential of which the individual is capable; it requires that the individual maintain a continuum of balance of purpose and direction within the environment where he or she is functioning" (p. 4).

- Corsini (1999) said that wellness is "the emphasis in health and medical counseling toward healthy lifestyles, preventive measures, and self-treatment" (p. 1068).

- An active process through which individuals become aware of and make choices towards a more successful existence (AOTA, 2008, p. 676 [based on Hettler, 1984, p. 1117]).

- Wellness is more than a lack of disease symptoms; it is a state of mental and physical balance and fitness (AOTA, 2008, p. 676 [adapted from *Taber's Cyclopedic Medical Dictionary*, 1997, p. 2110]).

- The condition of being in good health (Hussey et al., 2007, p. 292).

- The individual's perception of a responsibility for psychological and physical well-being, as these contribute to overall satisfaction with one's life situation. It is also the outcome of health promotion (Schell et al., 2014, p. 1243).

- **Author's comment:** Wellness is another example of a concept that appears in the occupational therapy literature without adequate development and refinement to make it useful as an outcome criterion for occupational therapy services. In particular, a distinction between wellness and health promotion is needed. Is wellness the outcome and health promotion the tool, or is wellness the tool and health promotion the outcome?

Summary of Outcome Concepts

The choice of outcome criteria in occupational therapy includes a wide variety of concepts. The variety suggests several issues and possibilities that can be summarized as follows. There are many factors affecting outcome, both positive and negative, that may be internal to the person or external in the environment. Some concepts related to outcome are unclear and need further development and refinement to be useful as objectives and goals for establishing outcome criteria that can be measured. There continues to be a need for clearly articulated outcomes to occupational therapy services that can facilitate communication and interaction with consumers, other health care and education providers, and reimbursement sources. To be most useful to the profession, each outcome must be translated into an outcome assessment instrument with sound psychometric properties that can be used to measure change in individuals, groups, or communities in practice and research.

Doing

Doing has always been a central concept in occupational therapy. However, the meaning of doing, the rationale for doing, and the organization of the doing process have been explained in many ways over the years. The verb "to do" has numerous meanings, all of which can become part of doing. Examples include act, accomplish, achieve, approve, arrange, cause, change, clean, complete, conduct, condone, create, effect, execute, exert, explore, finish, fit, form, give, make, manage, move, pay, perform, prepare, proceed, render, serve, study, translate, travel, traverse, and work (Barnes & Noble, 1995, p. 576). The mere lack of specificity creates its own problem in explaining the role of doing in occupational therapy.

The meaning of "to do" is sometimes compared to the meaning of the verb "to occupy." Meanings provided for the word "occupy" include to take up, to fill up, to engage, to employ, to hold, to take, to control, to be a resident of, or to be a tenant of. Synonyms include use, busy, capture, and seize (Barnes & Noble, 1995, p. 1340). In essence, the meanings of the 2 words do not overlap. The verb "to occupy," thus, is not a synonym for the concept of doing. Rather, it relates to the rationale or purpose for selecting an occupation "to do," but not the process of actually doing or performing that occupation.

The rationale, explanation, or justification for "doing" in occupational therapy has been explained in several ways. Nine major rationales have been discussed in the literature, beginning with the formative ideas of occupational therapy that can be traced to the concept of moral treatment (Bockoven, 1971). Because of the influence of moral treatment and the arts and crafts movement on the early development of occupational therapy, some pertinent thoughts about moral behavior and treatment have been summarized in Table 31-4, while thoughts about the arts and crafts movement are summarized in Table 31-5. The rationales can be labeled moral (role modeling) behavior, habit and time organization, practice and experience, mechanotherapy, thought substitution, emotional release and gratification, functional training, skill and role building, and environmental interaction. Each rationale, an approximate time period, and corresponding goal(s) related to doing in occupational therapy practice has been summarized in Table 31-6. Some of the rationales remain in practice today, while others have been discarded, reorganized, or are in limited use.

Definitions of Doing in Occupational Therapy Literature

- Fidler and Fidler (1978) state that the word *doing* is selected to convey the sense of performing, producing, or causing. It is purposeful action in contrast to random activity, in that the action is directed toward the intrapersonal (testing a skill), the interpersonal (clarifying a relationship), or the nonhuman (creating an end product) (p. 305). A similar definition appears in Fidler and Fidler (1983, p. 268).
- Doing can mediate between one's inner and outer world, nurture the capacity to invest, teach realistic responses to success and failure, provide concrete evidence of one's capacities and limitations, test the reality base of fantasy and perceptions, and validate the ability to achieve and influence one's environment (Fidler & Fidler, 1978, p. 306).
- Brown and Stoffel (2011) define doing as "acting on the environment and interacting with other people" (p. 770).

Values and Beliefs About Doing

The rationales described in Table 31-5 provide some explanations of why doing is viewed as an important process, but do not explain why a given individual engages in doing. Polatajko (1992) and Mayer (2000) suggested there are several values or beliefs about occupation from an individual's perspective. Six of the values and beliefs can be related to doing: 1) doing occupation is a basic human need, 2) doing occupation is an essential component of life, 3) doing occupation organizes behavior, 4) doing occupation gives meaning to life, 5) doing occupation improves an individual's QOL, and 6) doing occupation enables a healthy lifestyle. These values and beliefs provide some of the rationale for why humans do occupations based on current models of practice. The same values and beliefs support the use of occupation as a therapeutic tool, that is discussed in the next section. The values and beliefs regarding doing require special consideration because of the literature written about them.

The *Uniform Terminology III* (Dunn, Foto et al., 1994) defined values as "identifying ideas or beliefs that are important to self and others" (p. 1054). Jacobs (1999) added that values are "operational beliefs that one accepts as one's own and determines behavior" (p. 154). Punwar and Peloquin (2000) defined values as "those ideas or beliefs that are intrinsically important to an individual" (p. 285). According to *Webster's New Universal Unabridged Dictionary* (Barnes & Noble, 1995) a belief involves "confidence in the truth or existence of something not immediately susceptible to rigorous proof" (p. 190). The following concepts relative to doing were identified as effectiveness, efficiency, indirect and direct focus on the disability, learning by doing, meaning or meaningfulness, moral rules practical doing, purposeful activity, and sociocultural relevance. All are summarized next.

Table 31-4. *Historical Context of Moral Treatment*

- Formative ideas of occupational therapy can be traced to the concept of moral treatment (Bockoven, 1971).

- Moral treatment was used to treat insanity of the moral senses in the 18th and 19th centuries.

- The rationale was based on the belief that "the brain could be damaged by 'moral' agencies such as emotional stress, overwork, religious fanaticism, and self-abuse" (Barton, 1987, p. 58).

- "Any stressor of a psychological nature was referred to as a 'moral' cause of damage to the brain" (Barton, 1987, p. 58).

- There were several moral sense theories, but basically they proposed that there was a special moral sense that either enabled a person to perceive special moral qualities of virtue and vice, or would arouse feelings of approval or disapproval of the ordinary human actions (Bothamley, 1993).

- The philosophy of moral treatment was based on the belief that a "mentally deranged person would recover moral reason in the company of persons of sound mind and kindly nature who helped the individual with the regimen of daily life" (Bockoven, 1971, p. 223).

- Caregivers (staff) lived with the clients in small units or houses and were with the clients at all times to provide role models and maintain the daily routine.

- Essential attitudes of the caregivers were respect for human beings as individual persons, respect for the rights of individuals under the law, and respect for the need of every individual to be engaged in creative and recreational activity with others (Bockoven, 1971).

- The ideas and ideals of moral philosophy and treatment set the stage for occupational therapy personnel to view clients from a humanitarian (kind care), humanistic (person is source of action and change), and holistic (person is an indivisible whole) perspective (Bockoven, 1971).

- Moral treatment broke down for 3 major reasons: (1) a rapid increase in the number of clients admitted to the psychiatric hospitals overwhelmed staff; (2) ethnic prejudice against new and different immigrant populations who had different cultures, attitudes, and beliefs; and (3) a shift in medical view from regarding mental illness as a moral-emotional problem to belief in incurable cellular damage in the brain (Bockoven, 1971, p. 2).

- Punwar (1994) defines moral treatment as "an 18th century approach to the treatment of mental illness that included the use of planned activities to help in normalizing patients' behavior" (p. 261).

- Wilcock (1998) defines moral treatment as "the first systematic treatment which commenced in the last decade of the 18th century providing responsible care for an appreciable number of people with mental illness; 'moral' was used in the early context as the equivalent of 'emotional' or 'psychological' (from the same root as morale) and also has to do with custom, conduct, way of life, and inner meaning" (pp. 256-257).

- Moral treatment was a movement during the 19th century that developed as a reaction to the inhumane care of the mentally ill who, up until that time, were abused and poorly treated. Arts and crafts, farming, and creative activities were emphasized in moral treatment (Stein & Cutler, 2002, p. 625).

- A movement grounded in the philosophy that all people, even the most challenged, are entitled to consideration and human compassion (Hussey, Sabonis-Chafee, & O'Brien, 2007, p. 289).

- An approach to mental disorders based on humane psychosocial care or moral discipline that emerged in the 18th century and came to the forefront for much of the 19th century, derived partly from psychiatry or psychology and partly from religious or moral concerns. The movement is particularly associated with reform and development of the asylum system in Western Europe at that time. It fell into decline as a distinct method by the 20th century due to overcrowding and misuse of asylums and the predominance of biomedical methods. The movement is widely seen as influencing certain areas of psychiatric practice up to the present day (Brown & Stoffel, 2011, p. 784).

- Term given for a movement characterized by the provision of humane conditions of care for person with mental illness, influenced by the ideas emanating from the age of enlightenment (Schell et al., 2014, p. 1236).

Table 31-5. *Arts and Crafts Movement*

- A social and artistic movement of the second half of the 19th century, emphasizing a return to handwork, skilled craftsmanship, and attention to design in the decorative arts, away from the mechanization and mass production of the Industrial Revolution ("Arts and crafts," 2001, p. 81).

- Social reform movement of the late 19th and early 20th centuries that promoted the use of fine arts and crafts to counter the alienation of industrialism (Crepeau et al., 2002, p. 1026).

- A late 19th-century movement born in reaction to the Industrial Revolution, emphasized craftsmanship and design (Hussey et al., 2007, p. 285).

- A movement originating in England that championed design and manual craftsmanship as a form of cultural resistance to the mechanization and impersonal production of industrialism (Schell et al., 2014, p. 1230).

- **Author's comment:** Schwartz (1998) states that whereas moral treatment provided the idea of using occupation involving labor and manual tasks, such as gardening or carpentry, the arts and crafts movement suggested the potential of crafts for both their curative process and satisfying outcome (p. 855). In other words, moral treatment provided the justification (why), but the arts and crafts movement provided the process (what) and tools with which to *do* (apply) the process.

Table 31-6. *Changes in Rationale for Interventions Using Occupational Therapy*

Intervention Rationale	Time Period	Primary Goal of "Doing" Occupational Therapy
Moral behavior (Bockoven, 1971; Barton, 1987)	1800-1899	Provide consistent role model for performing daily routines. (Helped shape development of occupational therapy when it was formally recognized as a discipline).
Habit and time organization (Hall, 1905, 1910; Meyer, 1951; Slagle, 1922)	1900-1939 Mental health 1966-Present All practice areas	Reestablish or reinforce personal habits and structure the daily routine into specific units of clock time. (Mental illness is viewed as the result of "habit disorder and faulty living" and, thus, habits must be corrected or reinstated and organized into a daily living routine called habit training.)
Pragmatism (James, 1898; Dewey, 1902; Tracy, 1910)	1900-1939 Mental health 1966-Present All practice areas	Provide opportunity for experience and practice in real occupation(s). (Experience and practice shape the interpretation of ideas, the meaning of concepts, and the understanding of reality.)
Curative work (Mock, 1918; Baldwin, 1919)	1918-1946 Physical disabilities	Provide functional re-education and functional restoration to persons with orthopedic conditions. (Restore person to usefulness, overcome deformities, or teach new functions through use of specific voluntary movements involved in occupations.)
Thought substitution (Dunton, 1915, p. 27; Farrar, 1906)	1915-Present	Focus attention on a desired (reality based) actions. *Mental:* Will prevent the person from focusing on undesired health (hallucination, depressive thought, non-reality) thinking, because brain can only focus on one thought at a time.

(continued)

Table 31-6 (continued).   *Changes in Rationale for Interventions Using Occupational Therapy*

Intervention Rationale	Time Period	Primary Goal of "Doing" Occupational Therapy
Emotional release and gratification (AOTA, 1958; Fidler & Fidler, 1958; Azima & Azima, 1959)	1940-1965 Mental health	Provide constructive outlets in a controlled setting to meet and satisfy emotional needs. (The id, ego, and superego and or psychosexual stages of development must be satisfied to permit the person to function normally in everyday life.)
Kinetic and metric occupational therapy (Licht, 1947; Spackman, 1947)	1947-Present Physical disabilities	Restore or improve muscle strength, joint mobilization, and coordination. Improve work tolerance (now called the biomechanical model).
Functional Training (Deaver & Brown 1945)	1945-Present Physical disabilities	Teach persons with long-term disabilities how to perform the physical demands of daily life using adapted or compensatory techniques and altered equipment as needed. (Persons who cannot have "normal" function rehabilitation restored should be taught alternate methods of performing the functional tasks of daily living.)
Skill and role building (Reilly, 1966; Muñoz & Kielhofner, 1995; Robertson, 1998)	1966-Present All practice areas	Gain or regain the skills which support task, role, and occupational performance in daily life. (Occupational performance requires competence in performing skills and tasks necessary to carry out each occupational role; as expected by the situation/context in which the person lives and to the level of satisfaction, purpose, and meaning desired by the individual.)
Environmental interaction (Dunning, 1972; Howe & Briggs, 1982)	1972-Present All practice areas	Changing the context or ecological system can facilitate or hinder an occupational performance as much as changing the individual's functional skills. (The external environment should be viewed as having potential to adapt to the individual's needs and to change to promote the individual's participation.)
Self-Management recovery (Melvin, 1998; Brown, 2001)	1998-Present All practice areas	The service use decides what changes are needed in attitudes, values, feelings, goals, skills, and/or roles to enable recovery. The therapist's role is to help the service user learn new approaches and organize new and existing resources so the individual regains control of his or her life.

Describing the Doing Process

Effectiveness (of Doing)

- Schkade and Schultz (1992) discussed effectiveness as one measure of evaluating relative mastery. They state that "relative mastery is the extent to which the person experiences the occupational response as... effective (production of the desired result)" (p. 835).

- Jacobs (1999) defined effectiveness as the "degree to which the desired result is produced" (p. 47).
- Hagedorn (2000) suggested that "the effective level is the level of occupation at which productive, meaningful activities are performed in order to enable the individual to achieve an adaptive fit with the individual's environment, which enhances and maintains survival, health, and well-being" (p. 308).
- *Webster's New Universal Unabridged Dictionary* (Barnes & Noble, 1995) defined *effective* as "adequate

to accomplish a purpose; producing the intended or expected result" (p. 622). Synonyms include capable or competent, and closely related concepts are effectual, efficacious, and efficiency.

- **Author's comment:** The concept of effective doing or doing that is effective is probably part of the subculture or "underground practice" of occupational therapy. The idea is so ingrained it has only recently surfaced for careful analysis. The knowledge of occupational therapy practice could be further enhanced by studying what constitutes "effective doing" and how occupational therapy personnel can promote in the client "doing which is effective." This can be translated today in the context of evidence that "doing" is effective.

Efficiency (of Doing)

- Hall (1905) stated that "it is hoped that the treatment of work will... substitute a simple but positive efficiency which will reorganize the life of the individual on better lines" (p. 32).
- Schkade and Schultz (1992) used efficiency in relation to relative mastery. "Relative mastery is the extent to which the person experiences the occupational response as efficient (use of time and energy)" (p. 835).
- *Webster's New Universal Unabridged Dictionary* (Barnes & Noble, 1995) defined efficient as "performing or functioning in the best possible manner with the least waste of time and effort" and "having and using requisite knowledge, skills, and industry" (p. 622). Synonyms include competent, capable, and reliable.
- **Author's comment:** Efficiency appears to be a type or quality of doing valued in occupational therapy practice. Additional clarification may enhance the understanding of how efficiency or efficient doing can benefit clients in their daily lives. On the other hand, some rituals or ceremonies are probably not efficient in terms of time, effort, knowledge, or skills. In what situations is non-efficiency acceptable or even desirable in human occupation?

Indirect and Direct Focus of Doing in Relation to Disability

- Doing can be focused indirectly or directly on the person's problems, and was the subject of an ongoing debate in the formative years of the profession.
- Upham (1918b) summarized the debate: the concrete value of occupation is its power to turn the patient's attention away from his disability into healthy channels of interest and effort. This is especially necessary for patients inclined to self-analysis and morbid

introspection. "There is a group of occupational therapeutists who believe the patient's disability should be uppermost in his mind. They related the occupation so closely to his disability that he is keenly conscious that occupation is a fundamental part of his cure. He is taught to be as faithful in that occupation as he would be in taking a drug" (p. 18). The side of the debate the practitioner took frequently depended on whether mental or physical disabilities were being addressed. In mental disability, the approach to health and living often includes redirecting attention away from the symptoms and behaviors that lead to dysfunctional living. In place of the dysfunctional behavior, attempts are made to attract the person's attention to more healthy and useful behaviors. Therefore, the person was asked to do occupations that redirected attention from immediate problems. In contrast, frequently the focus of attention in physical disabilities was directed to the dysfunction so that weakened muscles can be strengthened, range of motion can be increased, and endurance improved, for example. Specific occupations directed at the dysfunction were assumed necessary for the objectives to be obtained.

- **Author's comment:** Both approaches are valued today. In many cases, occupations are selected that address directly the nature of the person's problems. On the other hand, a person in pain may need occupations that focus awareness away from the particular location of that pain toward some other situation or object that can command attention. As attention is refocused, awareness and response to pain may decrease. Perhaps the real issue is to understand when to select occupations that will most benefit the client at a particular point in the therapeutic process. More study is needed to clarify whether to focus doing and attention indirectly or directly on the identified client problems.

Learning by Doing

- Learning by doing is a basic principle of the pragmatic philosophy. Although learning is a central part of the doing process, the value of learning was discussed only in the terms of learning academic subjects in the early literature; it has now become central to recovery.
- In 1977, Hopkins and Smith defined learning as the "relatively permanent change in behavior or in the capacity for behavior resulting from either experience or practice" (p. 734). Both experience and practice require doing an occupation.
- Christiansen and Baum (1991) stated that learning is "the enduring ability of an individual to comprehend

and/or competently respond to changes in information from the environment and/or from within the self. As one learns about the environment, alterations occur in the definition of the self and possible behaviors; as one learns about the self, alterations occur in the definition of the environment and possible behaviors" (p. 855). The focus of this definition is the contribution of learning through doing on the development of the self.

- Mosey (1994) stated that learning is "a process wherein there is a change in an individual's behavior in a given situation brought about by repeated experience in the situation, providing that the behavior cannot be explained on the basis of native response tendencies, maturation, or temporary states of the organism, such as fatigue or drugs" (p. 26). In other words, learning through doing changes a person's behavior.

- Learning is a permanent change in behavior as a result of experience and practice according to Schmidt (1988), as stated in Poole (1995, p. 265).

- Pedretti and Umphred (1996) used another definition of Schmidt's (1991) for motor learning which was "a set of processes associated with practice or experience leading to relatively permanent changes in the capability for responding" (p. 65).

- Kielhofner (1985) defined formal learning as "the transmission of cultural norms in situations where right and wrong ways of doing something are so taken for granted that explanations are not given" (p. 504). He also defined informal learning as "the transmission of cultural norms through imitation of role models, trial and error, and other intuitive processes that tend to be difficult to describe or pin down" (p. 504).

- The enduring ability of an individual to comprehend and/or competently respond to changes in information from the environment and/or from within the self. As one learns about the environment, alterations occur in the definition of the self and possible behaviors; as one learns about the self, alterations occur in the definition of the environment and possible behaviors (Christiansen & Baum, 2005, p. 547).

- Cara and MacRae (2013) defined learning as acquisition of new or adaptation of existing knowledge, which is the foundation for reflecting on facts, behaviors, and skills, or synthesizing information for multiple sources (p. 968).

- Stages of learning include 4 specific phases in which skills are learned during intervention from acquisition, through fluency, maintenance, and generalization (Christiansen, 2000, p. 405; Christiansen & Matuska, 2011, p. 538).

- Specificity of learning includes the condition of learning exactly what is taught, including environmental variables (Christiansen & Baum, 2005, p. 550).

Meaning and Meaningfulness of Doing

- The concepts of meaning or meaningfulness and their opposites, meaningless or meaninglessness, do not appear as issues in the early literature on occupational therapy. The first definitions appeared in 1985. Kielhofner spoke of the meaningfulness of activities as "an individual's disposition to find importance, security, worthiness, and purpose in particular occupations" (p. 505).

- Nelson (1988) said that "meaning or meaningfulness is the term to be used in labeling the individual's interpretation of the occupational form" and that "meaningfulness refers both to the perceptual sense it makes to the individual, as well as to the cognitive associations elicited in the individual" (p. 635). In 1994, he defined meaning as "the entire interpretive process in which an individual engages when encountering an occupational form" (p. 21).

- Christiansen and Baum (1997) explained that "meanings reflect our overall interpretations of life events. Most of our intentions and actions are filled with meaning. This meaning comes from the nature of a situation and how we interpret its significance based on our current goals, values, and past experiences. There are individual meanings and collective or shared meanings" (p. 53). They defined the word *meaning* as "the personal significance of an event as interpreted by an individual" (p. 599).

- Meaningful lives have an active life with opportunities for creative work and enjoyment, with the experience of beauty, art and nature, and meaning. People are able to adapt when they perceive their world as comprehensible, manageable, and meaningful. The concept of meaningful occupation or meaningfulness came into the occupational therapy literature in the modern period. The early literature contains the concept of interest and focuses on productivity and social usefulness. The term appears to be closely related to the concept of purpose (Christiansen & Baum, 2005, p. 547).

- Meaninglessness is lack of belief in the value, usefulness, or importance of daily occupations or lives (Christiansen & Baum, 1997, p. 599).

- Hagedorn (2000) suggested there is a problem with therapeutic meaningful doing, because it is often simulated doing and performed in a protected and artificial environment.

- Meaningful occupations are those occupations which have meaning or significance to the individual in terms of personal needs and environmental demands. The activity may be seen as a part of a goal to be reached or accomplished, or the activity may be done deliberately because the person wants to be able to do it (Reed, 1984, p. 502).
- Personal meaning includes satisfaction of conscious or unconscious needs and/or attribution of benefits derived from activities (Schell et al., 2014, p. 1238).
- **Author's comment:** The concept of meaningful occupation or meaningfulness came into the occupational therapy literature in the modern period. The early literature contains the concept of interest and focuses on productivity and social usefulness. The term appears to be closely related to the concept of purpose. In *Webster's New Universal Unabridged Dictionary* (Barnes & Noble, 1995), the words meaning and meaningful both list the word purpose as a synonym. Perhaps the intent of using the terms meaningful or meaningfulness is an attempt to expand the idea of practical or purposeful doing.

Occupational Behavior and Doing

- Behavior as a means of doing has been accepted in the occupational therapy literature for many years. The term *occupational behavior*, however, was introduced by Reilly in 1966 when she stated that "society programs its members for occupational behavior through sequential experience in play, family living, school, and recreation" and that "occupational behavior is developmentally acquired and is capable of being divided into various substrates for corrective purposes" (p. 64). In 1969, Reilly provided a definition of the concept stating that occupational behavior is the "entire developmental continuum of work and play" (p. 302).
- Matsutsuyu (1971) expanded Reilly's idea of occupational behavior by suggesting the "adult occupational behavior reflects an attempt to assimilate oneself into some identified group that meets one's own need for productivity, belonging, and life structuring activities" (p. 292).
- In 1973 occupational behavior was defined as "the person's use of time, energy, and attention to rest, play, and work" (Johnson, 1973, pp. 160-161).
- A more comprehensive definition was provided by Woodside, a student of Reilly's, in 1976 as "occupational behavior is that aspect of growth and development represented by the developmental continuum of play and work as they support competency, achievement, and occupational role" (p. 11).

- In 1977 occupational behavior was defined as "organization and action based on skills, knowledge, and attitudes to make functioning possible in life roles" (Hopkins & Smith, p. 735; 1983, p. 924).
- Punwar (1994) defined occupational behavior as "those behaviors or activities that an individual engages in, in order to fulfill his or her occupational roles" (p. 262).
- In 1997, Christiansen and Baum stated that occupational behavior is "the set of responses which allow the individual to maintain role competence" (p. 433).
- In 1997, Law et al. stated occupational behavior "is that aspect or class of human action that encompasses mental and physical doing" (1997b, p. 40).
- Creek, also in 1997, said that occupational behavior is the "active engagement in occupation" (p. 529).
- Jacobs (1999) stated that occupational behavior is a "set of responses which allow the individual to maintain role competence" (p. 97).
- Punwar and Peloquin (2000) defined occupational behavior as "those behaviors or activities that an individual engages in to fulfill his or her occupational roles" (p. 282).
- Christiansen and Townsend (2010) defined occupational behavior as "human action produced by the combined efforts and expressions of mind, body, and spirit" (p. 420).
- **Author's comment:** This is a good example of how terms evolve in a profession beyond the original parameters. Reilly did not include phrases such as skills, knowledge, and attitudes; make functioning possible; maintain role competence; encompasses mental and physical doing; or active engagement in occupation. She did, however, stress that occupational behavior was a developmental continuum involving work and play. Her student, Woodside, added "support competency, achievement, and occupational role," which may be assumed to be acceptable to Reilly. Concepts that take on a life of their own may stray considerably from the original meaning. Redefinition is not necessarily undesirable, but failure to acknowledge that new definitions have been written does create a discontinuity of thought about the concept, and confusion in the minds of the readers.

Practical Doing

- The concept of practical doing, or doing what is practical, dates to the formative years. Upham (1918b) stated that "an occupation may be said to be practical, which in some way trains or prepares the patient for his future vocation or employment.

An occupation which is merely time-wasting and which contributes no improved knowledge or skill or awakened interest and which possesses no special therapeutic advantages may be said to be trivial and useless. That occupation is most practical which best restores the patient's mental and physical vigor. After this first consideration that occupation is most useful which is most closely related to his economic future" (p. 36).

- Practicality is a cornerstone to the pragmatic philosophy. *Webster's New Universal Unabridged Dictionary* (Barnes & Noble, 1995) defined pragmatism as "a philosophical movement or system having various forms, but generally stressing practical consequences as constituting the essential criterion in determining meaning, truth, or value" (p. 1518).

- The *Concise Oxford Dictionary* (Thompson, 1995) made a similar statement. Pragmatism is "a philosophy that evaluates assertions solely by their practical consequences and bearing on human interests" (p. 1073).

- **Author's comment:** Current occupational therapy literature does not seem to reflect the idea of doing what is practical. Instead, the current term seems to be doing what is meaningful or purposeful. Is the concept of practical doing a sub-concept within the ideas of meaningfulness or purposefulness, or is it an overlooked concept which should be reinstated in current models of practice?

Socially and Culturally Relevant Issue of Doing

- The issue of socially and culturally relevant doing began to surface in the 1970s. Klavins (1972) was one of the first persons to point out that work and play had different values and beliefs in different cultures and subcultures.

- The *Uniform Terminology III* (Dunn, Foto et al., 1994) defined social as "availability and expectations of significant individuals, such as spouse, friends, and caregivers. Also includes larger social groups which are influential in establishing norms, role expectations, and social routines" (p. 1054). The same document defines cultural as "customs, beliefs, activity patterns, behavior standards, and expectations accepted by the society of which the individual is a member. Includes political aspects, such as laws that affect access to resources and affirm personal rights. Also includes opportunities for education, employment and economic support" (p. 1054).

- Kielhofner (1985) defined culture as "the beliefs and perception, values and norms, and customs and behaviors that are shared by a group or society and passed from one generation to the next through both formal and informal education" (p. 503).

- Christiansen and Baum (1991) stated that culture is "patterns of behavior learned through the socialization process, including anything acquired by humans as members of society: knowledge, values, beliefs, laws, morals, customs, speech patterns, economic production patterns, etc" (p. 850).

- Cara and MacRae (1998) stated that culture is "a conscious and unconscious internal process of identification with overt manifestations of traditions, beliefs and values, often involving the use of objects, which guide human beings in organizing their lives" (p. 667).

- Ryan (1992) defined cultural shift as "movement in response to societal forces that results in a dynamic change" (p. 359).

- Clark, Ennevor, and Richardson (1996) defined cultural place as "the place in which development occurs, the ecology and locally adapted environment which includes meanings, beliefs, values and conventional practice learned and shared by members of a community" (p. 390).

- Christiansen and Townsend (2010) defined culture as "shared experiences of meaning and social processes that create meanings (p. 418).

- Brown and Stoffel (2011) defined culture as "something that is learned and shared among members of a group and that is cumulative and dynamic, including a system of shared meaning through language and nonverbal communication. It is value laden and defines norms for roles, relationships, obligations, beliefs, health practices, and behavior" (p. 777).

- **Author's comment:** The relationship of doing and sociocultural issues has always been recognized to some degree as a significant issue in occupational therapy evaluation and intervention strategies. However, the full impact is beginning to be understood as multiculturalism becomes a larger factor in the delivery of occupational therapy services. Doing is a multi-faceted concept that will require addition study to understand and use as a therapeutic process.

Concepts Related to the Doing Process

There are several synonyms or closely related concepts expressed in the occupational therapy literature that are defined in the following sections. These concepts include activity, adapting, engaging, flow, performing, participating, and purposeful activity.

Activity, Activities

The term *activity* or *activities* is seen frequently in occupational therapy literature and has been part of the professional lexicon since the formative years. Perhaps the best known use of the term is in Patterson's (1922) definition of occupational therapy, which is "any activity, mental or physical, definitely prescribed and guided for the distinct purpose of contributing to, and hastening recovery from, disease or injury" (p. 21). This definition is more consistent with the concept of a tool or therapeutic use of activity. Thus, the earliest use of the term *activity* is as a synonym for *therapeutic occupation*. Clearly activity or activities can be used as therapeutic tools. However, current definitions are more consistent with the concept that activity is a behavioral unit or action, and are thus listed under the section on Doing. That stated, the relationship of the concepts of activity and occupation (and task) remain to be resolved. Is there a relationship and if so, what is the relationship?

The answer probably lies in the dictionary uses of the concepts themselves. Synonyms for the concept of activity include action, active, animation, deed, energy, exercise, exertion, function, liveliness, power, process, and work while synonyms for occupation include action, activity, art, business, calling, career, control, craft, employment, incumbency, job, line, occupancy, position, possession, profession, pursuit, seizure, settlement, tenure, trade, vocation, and work. Clearly the terms overlap, but activity is primarily described in terms of *doing* or *action terms*, while occupation includes both *outcomes* and *doing terms* that can be ultimately used as tools. Therefore, within the context of usage for occupational therapy, the concept of occupation is broader than the concept of activity, which is confirmed by the definitions of occupation listed as tools. On a historical note, both words and concepts appeared in dictionaries available to the founders of occupational therapy in 1917. The concept of occupation was chosen. Activity, as used most often in occupational therapy, seems to be related more to doing.

- Activity is a specific action, function or sphere of action that involves learning or doing by direct experience (Reed & Sanderson, 1992, p 330) *(doing)*.
- Activities are smaller units of behavior that comprise tasks (Trombly, 1995, p. 19) *(doing)*.
- Activity is considered to be the basic unit of a task. It is designed as a singular pursuit in which a person engages as part of his or her daily occupational experience (Law et al., 1996, p. 16) *(doing)*.
- Activity is being active in mind and/or body. Doing something, usually for a particular purpose (Turner, Foster, & Johnson, 1996, p. 873) *(doing)*.
- Activity is "productive action required for development, maturation, and use of sensory, motor, social,

psychological, and cognitive functions. Activity may be productive without yielding an object. It is also a valuable vehicle to acquire, maintain, or redevelop skills necessary to fulfill occupational roles and provide satisfaction" (Christiansen & Baum, 1997, p. 591; 2005, p. 543).

- An activity is performed by an individual for a specific purpose on a particular occasion (Creek, 1997, p. 529) *(doing)*.
- Activity is an integrated sequence of tasks that takes place on a specific occasion, during a finite period, for a particular purpose (Hagedorn, 1997, p. 142) *(pattern of doing, tools, outcome)*.
- Activities are the basic units of occupational performance and consist of specific behaviors directed toward the completion of a task, whereas tasks are a set of activities that share some purpose (Watson, 1997, p. 32) *(pattern of doing)*.
- Activity is a series of linked episodes of task performance that takes place on a specific occasion during a finite period for a particular reason. An activity is composed of an integrated sequence of chained tasks. A completed activity results in a change in the previous state of objective reality or subjective experience (Hagedorn, 2000, p. 307) *(pattern of doing)*.
- A term that describes a class of human actions that are goal directed (AOTA, 2002, p. 630) *(doing, outcome)*.
- State or condition of being involved (participant) in a general class of human actions that is goal-directed (Hussey et al., 2007, p. 285).
- Activity(ies) are an observable unit of behavior and recognizable sequence of actions taken together in a particular context; beyond tasks, yet without the complexity of occupations in the simple to complex hierarchy of task activities and occupations (Christiansen & Townsend, 2010, p. 417) *(doing)*.
- Activity choices are activities that are engaged in during play and leisure (Schell, Gillen, & Scaffa, 2014, p. 1229) *(doing)*.
- Activity restriction is the exclusion of certain activities, or restrictions in method or duration of performance (AOTA, 1978, p. 73).
- Occupational activities are those that are part of, or concerned with, the performance of an occupation. Thus, activities which lead to or facilitate the performance of occupation in self-maintenance, productivity, or leisure by an individual are occupational activities (Reed, 1984, p. 501).
- Occupational activities are tasks that are directly related to the individual's preferred occupational role. Such tasks must have person meaning and

occupational relevance; the individual must be the primary actor in the activity (Schell et al., 2014, p. 1237).

- Productive activities are those that provide a service or commodity needed by another, or that add new abilities, ideas, knowledge, artistic objects, or performances to the cultural tradition (Kielhofner, 1983, p. 32).

Adapting/Adaptation (Client)

- Punwar (1988) defined adaptation as "the act or process of adapting to changes in the external or internal environments (p. 255; Punwar & Peloquin, 2000, p. 277). *Note:* Reference to the process of doing.

- Gillen and Burkhardt (1998) defined adaptation as "coping with the changing characteristics of a task, the environment, or the method of carrying out a task so that an activity can be completed" (p. 536).

- Adaptation refers to the ability to anticipate, correct for, and benefit by learning from the consequences of errors that arise in the course of action (Kielhofner, 1995, p. 135). The word *action* was changed to "task performance" in AOTA, 2002c (p. 630).

- Occupational adaptation is the process. Refers specifically to how occupation and adaptation become integrated into a single internal phenomenon within the patient. A process-based, non-hierarchical, and non-stage specific explanation of the phenomenon is provided by Schkade and Schultz (1992, p. 830). They describe it further as the process through which the person and the occupational environment interact when the person is faced with an occupational challenge called for an occupational response reflecting an experience of relative mastery (Schkade & Schultz, 1992, p. 831).

- Occupational adaptation is a normative internal process that is activated by the individual when approaching and adapting to challenges to life; constructing a positive occupational identity and achieving occupational competence over time in the control of one's environment (Schell, Gillen, & Scalffa, 2012, p. 1237).

- Temporal adaptation is the influence of life space and role demands on the individual's orientation and allocation of time to the various areas of occupational performance (CAOT, 1991 p. 142).

- Temporal adaptation is the ability to organize one's time in order to fulfill occupational roles and personal responsibilities (Punwar, 1994, p. 266).

Engaging, Engagement in Occupation (Occupational Engagement)

- The term *engagement in occupation* recognizes the commitment made to performance in occupations or activities as the result of self-choice, motivation, and meaning, and alludes to the objective and subjective aspects of being involved in and carrying out occupations and activities that are meaningful and purposeful to the person (AOTA, 2002c, p. 631).

- Engagement is the state of being involved with occupations that are meaningful to the person (Christiansen & Matuska, 2004, p. 465; Christiansen & Matuska, 2011, p. 540).

- Engaging occupations are done with great commitment, enthusiasm, perseverance, and passion (Jonsson, Josephsson, & Kielhofner, 2001, p. 428).

- Basic to occupational engagement is a person's personal power to author choices (Polkinghorne, 1996, p. 299).

- Occupational engagement is the ability of a client to interact physically with the surrounding environment. Can be associated with leisure activities, but also with self-care and work activities as well (Pellerito, 2006, p. 543).

- Kielhofner (2008) defined occupational engagement as "clients' doing, thinking, and feeling under certain environmental conditions in the midst of therapy or as a planned consequence of therapy" (p. 171).

- Occupational engagement is one's doing, thinking, and feeling under certain environmental conditions in the midst of or as a planned consequence of therapy (Schell et al., 2014, p. 1237).

- **Author's comment:** The term *occupational engagement* began appearing in the occupational therapy literature in the 1990s, but is not unique to occupational therapy literature. The term also appears in the literature on mental retardation and development disabilities beginning in 1988 (Lancioni, Smeets, & Oliva).

Flow

- Flow is a concept developed and defined by Mihalyi Csikszentmihalyi, a psychologist, over several years of work that culminated in books published in 1975, 1988, and 1990. Flow began appearing in occupational therapy literature in the 1990s.

- Jacobs (1994) describes flow as "a positive feeling that occurs when there is a balance between perceived challenges and one's skills, and may include enjoyment, intense or total involvement, deep concentration, or the loss of one's sense of time" (p. 989).

- Christiansen and Baum (1997) defined flow as a "term describing the subjective quality of an experience" (p. 596).
- Neistadt and Crepeau (1998) expanded the explanation as a "state of deep concentration in which consciousness is well ordered; elements present are a feeling of control, loss of self-consciousness, transformation of time, and concentration on the task at hand" (p. 868).
- Wilcock (1998) defined flow as "a state of consciousness when people are so involved in an activity that nothing else seems to matter; of optimal experience, transcendence, and enjoyment when individuals are challenged but engaged within the scope of their abilities" (p. 255).
- Rebeiro and Polgar (1999) suggested that "flow may be useful in understanding those aspects of the occupation, environment, and person that contribute to a 'just right' challenge and to enabling occupational performance through enjoyable, structured, and purposeful activity" (p. 14).
- Christiansen and Townsend (2010) defined flow as a "term given by United States psychologist Mihalyi Csikzentmihalyi to the experience of engagement that occurs when an individual is deeply interested in a task or occupation and his or her skills are at a level that matches or exceeds the challenges of the task" (p. 418).
- Brown and Stoffel (2011) defined flow as "a timeless experience in an inherently satisfying activity wherein a person's skill just meets the challenge of the situation" (p. 780).

Participating, Participation

General Definitions of Participation

- Participation is a person's involvement in a life situation. It represents the societal perspective of functioning (WHO, 2001, p. 213).
- Involvement in a life situation; the action of taking part with others (Creek, 2003, p. 56).
- Participation refers to engagement in work, play, or ADL that are part of one's sociocultural context and that are desired and/or necessary to one's well-being (Forsyth & Kielhofner, 2006, p. 77).
- Participation is "the act of doing the occupation, planning for the occupation, maintaining a balance with other areas of occupation, and obtaining and appropriately using related tools and supplies" (Brown & Stoffel, 2011, p. 785).
- Participation is "involvement in a life situation" (Christiansen & Matuska, 2011, p. 543).

- Engaging in everyday activities and occupations that individuals want and need to do (Cara & MacRae, 2013, p. 971).
- Participation is involvement in life situations (eg, self-care tasks, domestic life, education, employment, social, and civic life). Participation encompasses positive participation (eg, observing others or listening). Occupational therapy practitioners generally include additional elements, such as the meaning of participation and peoples' subjective experience of participation (Schell, Gellen, & Scaffa, 2014, p. 1238).

Active Participation

- Concept that views humans as active agents in their own development (Christiansen & Townsend, 2010, p. 417).

Partial Participation

- Performance of a task or activity in part or in full that is made possible through one or more adaptations (eg, personal assistance on difficult steps, changes in the sequence or rules, modification of task materials, the addition of adaptive devices) (Christiansen, 2000, p. 403).
- Ability to perform part of an activity or a somehow modified activity rather than carrying out the entire task in a typical way (Christiansen & Matuska, 2011, p. 538).

Client Participation

- An active concept characterized by involvement and engagement and is driven in part by biological needs to act, find meaning, and connect with others through doing (Townsend & Polatajko, 2007, p. 365).
- Active participation by the individual in the process of therapy, as opposed to passive compliance, increases his choice, autonomy, responsibility for outcomes, and control over his care (Creek, 2007, p. 127). Client may participate in an activity without being fully engaged; that is, without feeling fully involved and committed. However, engagement in activity is not possible without participation (Creek, 2010, p. 179).

Occupational Participation

- Taking part in or sharing in valued occupation (Mackenzie & O'Toole, 2011, p. 383).
- The engagement of the individual's mind, body, and soul in goal-directed pursuits (Christiansen & Townsend, 2004, p. 276).
- Taking part in any occupation, whether by oneself or as part of a group (regardless of the reason for taking part); involvement in life situations, which encompasses all aspects of human functioning that involve learning; and applying knowledge, completing tasks,

communication, mobility, self-care, domestic life, interpersonal relationships, major life areas (such as education and employment) in community, social, and civic life (Crepeau et al., 2009, p. 1164).

- The act of doing the occupation, planning for the occupation, maintaining a balance with other areas of occupation, and obtaining and appropriately using related tools and supplies (Brown & Stoffel, 2011, p. 785).

- Refers to involvement in a life situation through occupation (Townsend & Polatajko, 2007, p. 371).

- Engagement in work, play, or ADL that are part of one's sociocultural context and that are desired and/or necessary to one's well-being (Schell et al., 2014, p. 1238).

Social Participation
- Concept dates back to Parton in 1932.

- Organized patterns of behavior that are characteristic and expected of an individual in a given position within a social system (Mosey, 1996, p. 340; AOTA, 2002c, p. 633).

- Involvement in situations through activity within a social context (Creek, 2010, p. 25).

- Participation is involvement in a life situation (WHO, 2001, p. 10).

- Involvement in a life situation; the action of taking part with others (Creek, 2003, p. 56).

- A person's performance of meaningful roles and occupations within preferred social groups, such as families, classrooms, work teams, organization, and communities (Cole & Donohue, 2011). Consists of verbal and interpersonal activity interactions among people (Sladyk, Jacobs, & MacRae, 2010, p. 623).

- Interpersonal interaction with others in a verbal or nonverbal mode, with or without involvement in an activity (Cole & Donohue, 2011, p. 29).

- The nature and extent of a person's involvement in life situations in relation to impairments, activities, health conditions, and contextual factors. A fundamental property of participation is the complex interaction between a person with impairment and/or disability and the context. Participation consists of all areas or aspects of human life, including the full experience of being involved in a practice, custom, or social behavior (based on WHO, 2001; Radowski & Latham, 2008, p. 2).

- Involvement in life situations and activities that include the capacity to execute and perform tasks (WHO, 2001; Sladyk, Jacobs, MacRae, 2010, p. 620).

- Involvement in a subset of activities that involves social interactions with others and that support social interdependence; organized patterns of behavior that are characteristic and expected of an individual; or a given position within a social system and encompasses that individual's engagement with family, peers, friends, and community members (Schell et al., 2014, p 1241).

Performing, Performance

- The concept of performance has appeared in the occupational therapy literature since the formative years. Meyer (1922) used the term *performance* 9 times. A typical comment is "we all know how fancy and abstract thought can go far afield...while *performance* is its own judge and regular and therefore the most dependable and influential part of life" (p. 5, italics in original article). Performance is discussed as reality, while thinking is sometime subject to "flights of fancy." Therefore, performance is more desirable in the real world.

- Although the term *performance* appears in Meyer's article (1922), the term *occupational performance* did not appear in the occupational therapy literature until 1973 in a grant report in which occupational performance is described as "the individual's ability to accomplish the tasks required by his role and related to his developmental stage. Roles include those of a preschooler, student, homemaker, employee, and retired work" (AOTA, 1973, p. 41).

- Fidler and Fidler (1978) described performance "as the ability, throughout the life cycle, to care for and maintain the self in a more independent manner, satisfy one's personal needs for intrinsic gratification, and contribute to the needs and welfare of others" (p. 310).

- Allen (1985) stated that "performance is the task behavior we see the patient do" (p. 73).

- Jackson and Banks (1997) suggested that performance is "routine task behavior" (p. 460).

- Law et al. (1997b) defined performance as "the actual execution or carrying out of an occupation" (p. 40).

Performance as a Modifier
- Performance has also been used in combination with other words, such as "performance areas," "performance components," and "performance contexts." In the *Uniform Terminology III* (Dunn, Foto et al., 1994), performance areas are defined as the "activities that the occupational therapy practitioner emphasizes when determining functional abilities" (p. 1047). They include ADL, work, productive activities, and play or leisure. Performance areas are tools.

- Performance capacity includes the mental and physical abilities that underlie skilled performance (Brown & Stoffel, 2011, p. 786).
- Performance capacity includes the ability to do things provided by the status of underlying objective, physical mental components, and corresponding subjective experience (Schell, Gillen, & Scaffa, 2014, p. 1238).
- Performance components "are the elements of performance that practitioners assess and, when needed, in which they intervene for improved performance" (Dunn, Brown, & McGuigan, 1994, p. 1047). They include sensorimotor, cognitive, psychosocial, and psychological aspects.
- Performance context are "situations or factors that influence an individual's engagement in desired and/or required performance areas" (Dunn, Brown, & McGuigan, 1994, p. 1047). Performance context consists of temporal aspects, and environmental aspects; as such they are examples of tools.
- Performance patterns are "patterns of behavior related to daily life activities that are habitual or routine. Performance patterns include habits and routines (AOTA, 2002c, p. 632).
- Performance skills are "features of what one does, not of what one has, related to observable elements of action that have implicit functional purposes" (AOTA, 2002c, p. 632 [adapted from Fisher & Kielhofner, 1995, p. 113]).
- Performance skills include motor skills, process skills, and communication/interaction skills (AOTA, 2002c, p. 632).
- Performance skills are small units of observable action that are linked together in the process of executing a daily life task performance (Hussey et al., 2007, p. 290).
- Performance skills are the smallest observable units of occupational performance; goal-directed actions a person carries out one by one when engaged in naturalistic and relevant daily life task performances (Schell et al., 2014, p. 1238).
- **Author's comment:** Performance appears to be used more frequently in the occupational therapy literature to describe a doing process, in which perform and performing may appear. Occupational performance appears to be defined more in relation to a desired outcome. Perform, performing, and performance are common English words. The profession of occupational therapy can only clarify their use within the profession. The concept of occupational performance is more unique to the profession and, thus, the profession can more easily direct its use. The

same can be said for the concepts of performance areas, performance components, and performance contexts. These concepts developed primarily within the profession and their usage can be controlled by the profession. However, there may be some help from the new ICF document (WHO, 2001) where performance is defined as "a construct that describes, as a qualifier, what individuals do in their current environment, and in this way, brings in the aspect of a person's involvement in life situations" (p. 166).

Purposeful Activity/Purposeful Doing/ Purposeful Action/Purposeful Occupation

- Purposeful doing has been widely used as a concept in occupational therapy literature. The most common phrase is purposeful activity. The phrase may have been adopted from the literature of the early 20th century. Dewey (1916) used the phrase in talking about work. "Like play, it (work) signifies purposeful activity and differs not in that activity is subordinated to an external result, but in the fact that a longer course of activity is occasioned by the idea of a result" (p. 204). Earlier in the same text he stated that "to do these things [acts] means to have a mind-for mind is precisely intentional purposeful activity controlled by perception of facts and their relationships to one another" (p. 103).
- Burnette (1918) stated "this improved state is our chance to turn the awakened activities towards more purposeful and dignified occupation" (p. 11).
- Upham (1919) stated "in all countries, purposeful exercise has been found the expedient way to cure weakened muscles and stiffened joints" (p. 211). Purposeful exercise is related to active doing, as opposed to passive.
- Perhaps the best explanation for purposeful activity comes from Bowman (1922) when she explained that "the fundamental principle of occupational therapy is a psychological principle: the substitution of a coordinated, purposeful activity, mental or physical, for scattered activities or the idleness which comes with weakened body or mind" (p. 172).
- Hopkins and Smith (1977) defined purposeful activity as "treatment when directed to a response that enhances neural integration" (p. 737; 1983, p. 926). In the context of this definition, purposeful activity is a tool.
- Mosey (1981) provided a current definition, stating that "purposeful activities are doing processes directed toward a planned or hypothesized end result. They provide an opportunity for investigating, trying out, and gaining evidence of one's capacities for

experiencing, responding managing, creating, and controlling" (p. 62).

- The CAOT (1991) defined purposeful activity as the "therapeutic application of tasks or actions that are goal-directed; valuable and useful to the client, and relevant to the client's life stage" (p. 141).

- Hinojosa, Sabari, and Pedretti (1993) stated that "an activity is purposeful if the individual is an active, voluntary participant, and if the activity is directed toward a goal that the individual considers meaning-ful... Purposeful activity is goal-directed behaviors or tasks that comprise occupations" (p. 1081).

- Christiansen and Baum (1997) provided a short-hand definition, stating that purposeful activities are "actions which are goal directed" (p. 602).

- Punwar and Peloquin (2000) defined purposeful activity as "meaningful occupation; an occupation with a goal" (p. 283).

- Hussey et al. (2007) defined purposeful activity as an activity used in treatment that is goal directed, individual is an active voluntary participant, and has both inherent and therapeutic goals (p. 291).

- In 2008, AOTA defined purposeful activity as goal-directed behavior or activity within a therapeutically designed context that leads to an occupation or occu-pations. Specifically, selected activity that allows the client to develop skills that enhance occupational engagement (p. 674).

- The idea of purpose and doing in occupational therapy probably began with the philosophy of prag-matism, as the statement by Dewey (1916) suggested. However, there were psychologists whose primary interest was purposive psychology; of these, William M. McDougall (1922) and Edward C. Tolman (1932) are best known. Peters (1953) summarized the assumptions of purposive psychology as 1) all behav-ior is purposive and 2) there are certain innate goal-seeking tendencies (p. 669). The development of pur-posive psychology parallels the early years of occupa-tional therapy. Basically, purposive psychology is "the doctrine that behavior is distinguished from purely mechanical change or from physiological activity" (English & English, 1958, p. 432). Purposiveness has a history of controversy, according to English and English (1958). "Some theorists regard purposiveness as an inadmissable concept in science because it can-not be directly observed. Others use purposiveness as the defining characteristic of human behavior. A third group distinguishes between purposive behav-ior, in which persistent striving is clearly evident, and nonpurposive behavior, in which striving, if present, is not so evident" (p. 432).

- If occupational therapy model builders and theorists are using purpose as one type of behavior in which an aim, end, plan, result, or goal is established to be attained by the person; the study of pragmatic philosophy should be the focus for clarification of the concept. If, on the other hand, model builders view purpose as purposiveness, in which all behavior is viewed as having a purpose, then the works of McDougall and Tolman should be studied further. The statement of *The Philosophic Base of Occupational Therapy* (AOTA, 1979a) appeared to use purposeful activity as the primary or central means of facilitat-ing adaptation. If this interpretation is correct, occu-pational therapy is using purposive psychology as an important source of its philosophical base.

- The use of the concept of purpose or purposiveness is not simple or straight forward. Occupational therapy model builders and theorists need to clarify the con-cept of purpose as a means of explaining human behavior within and outside the profession.

- Purposeful actions are activities that have meaning for individuals and/or groups as a whole (Schell et al., 2014, p. 1240).

- Purposeful activities are specifically selected activi-ties that allow the client to develop skills that enhance occupational engagement (Schell et al., 2014, p. 1240).

- Purposeful occupations are those occupations that are valued and sanctified by society and culture as completed tasks. Although the person performs the task, the individual may not understand the meaning or significance of the task, except to know that the sociocultural environment values the outcome that task completion brings about. Purposeful occupa-tions are most common in self-maintenance and productivity occupations. They are measured by sociocultural standards based on the values and norms adopted by a group of citizens. Such factors as socioeconomic status, educational level, and aptitude may be considered in establishing or applying criteria (Reed, 1984, pp. 502-503).

Self-Advocacy

- The term *self-advocacy* appeared in the title of an article published in 1993 (Schlaff, p. 943), but is not defined. Working definitions do not appear until the year 2000.

- The ability to express personal needs and work with-in a larger social or legal system to get those needs met (Christiansen, 2000, p. 404).

- Actively promoting or supporting oneself or oth-ers (individuals, organizations, or populations) requires an understanding of strengths and needs, identification of goals, knowledge of legal rights and responsibilities, and communicating these aspects to others (AOTA, 2008, p. 663, 675).

- Brown and Stoffel (2012) defined self-advocacy as "speaking up for oneself; it means that although a person with a disability may call upon the support of others, the individual is entitled to be in control of his or her own resources and how they are directed. It is about having the right to make life decisions without undue influence or control by others" (p. 788).

- **Author's comment:** The concept of self-advocacy must be separated from professional advocacy on the client's behalf, or professional advocacy to promote occupational therapy services in general. Self-advocacy requires that the client be learning to promote himself or herself in situations where self-interest is involved.

Patterns of Doing

The process of doing may be described in terms that gather together the doing into more identifiable patterns. These patterns include habit, rituals, roles, and routines.

Habit/Habits

- The concept of habit has been discussed in the occupational therapy literature since the early years. Hall, in 1905, talked about the potential of systematic work for a patient to "change his occupation and habits of life" (p. 30).

- Upham (1918a) stated that the instructors in occupational therapy should be able "to develop in them (war invalids) regular habits of work, habits which are self-disciplinary and will render the men valuable members of civil communities" (p. 18). Slagle (1922) continued the dialogue about habits by saying "occupation used remedially serves to overcome some habits, to modify others and construct new ones, to the end that habit reaction will be favorable to the restoration and maintenance of health" (p. 14).

- Meyer (1957) summarized the view of habits common to the formative years of occupational therapy by stating that habits are the essential fabric of the reactive resources of the organism. The doing of things forms the basic structure of the mental life, and habit formation is a process that applies to every item of human behavior. Habits of action and bringing things to completion are the basic conative resources of the organism. Disorganization of habits is the deterioration of the learned but fundamental ways of meeting life (p. 201).

- Habit continued to be an important concept into the 1930s, as evidenced by Pollack (1938) who said that "habit, as is well known, is responsible for practically all the daily activities of an individual, comprising as they do the habits of dressing, eating, drinking, speech, thought, play, or work" (p. 292).

- The current view of habits was expressed by Kielhofner (1985) as "images guiding the routine and typical ways in which a person performs" (p. 504). In 1995, Kielhofner added that habits are defined as "latent tendencies acquired from previous repetitions, mainly operating at a preconscious level and influencing a wide range of behavioral patterns that correspond to familiar habitats" (p. 65).

- Trombly (1995) defined habits as "chains of subroutines that are so well learned that the person does not have to pay attention to do them under ordinary circumstances" (p. 19).

- Parham and Fazio (1997) stated that habits are "skills that are performed so routinely that they have become automatic" and they "allow for efficiency in daily occupations" (p. 250).

- Neistadt and Crepeau (1998) explained that habits are "automatic behavior that is integrated into more complex patterns that enable people to function on a day-to-day basis; skills that are habituated are typically performed easily and with little effort" (p. 869; AOTA, 2002c, p. 631).

- Dunn (2000) took the concept of habit one step further and suggested that there is a continuum of habit beginning with habit impoverishment, followed by habit utility and habit domination. Habit impoverishment occurs when "habits are not established and cannot support daily life" (p. 8S). Habit utility occurs when "habits support performance in daily life and contribute to life satisfaction" and there is the "ability to follow rhythms of daily life" (p. 8S). Habit domination is a situation in which "habits are so inherent that they interfere with daily life" (p. 8S).

- Kielhofner (1985) may have had a similar idea in mind when he defined degree of organization in habits as "the degree to which one has a typical use of time which supports competent performance in a variety of environments and roles and provides a balance of activity" (p. 503) and rigidity/flexibility of habits as "the degree to which a person is able to change routines of behavior to accommodate periodic contingencies" (p. 508). Yet another aspect of habit is added by Kielhofner (1985) when he defined the social appropriateness of habits as "the degree to which one's typical behaviors are those expected and valued by the environments in which one performs" (p. 508).

- Habit is a recurring, largely automatic, pattern of time use within the context of daily occupation (Christiansen & Baum, 2005, p. 546; 2010, p. 420).

- Habits influence behavior in a semiautomatic way without need for conscious, deliberate action (Christiansen & Baum, 2005, p. 546).

- Christiansen and Townsend (2010) defined habit as "a repetitive pattern of occupation or time use; a disposition to act in a certain way, without conscious attention" (p. 419).

- Acquired tendencies to respond and perform in certain consistent ways in familiar environments or situations; specific, automatic behaviors performed repeatedly, relatively automatically, and with little variation (Schell et al., 2014, p. 1234).

Ritual or Rituals

- The concept of ritual did not appear in the literature with any frequency until 1987.

- Law (1987) wrote about ritual time "as the texture of experience, with patterns overlapping, interwoven, leading in all directions through all dimensions, like movement in dance" (p. 19).

- The first definition of rituals located is by do Rozario (1994), who defined rituals as "mythological activities and symbolic expression" (p. 48).

- Christiansen and Baum (1997) suggested that rituals are "patterns of behavior that have strong elements of symbolism attached to them" (p. 603).

- Crepeau (1994) stated that "ritual is distinguished from day-to-day routine by its connection to the symbols, beliefs, and values of the social group" (p. 6). She continued by stating that "ritualization structures social life and imbues it with meaning... Rituals have two major characteristics: repetition and dramatic presentation. Rituals involve repetition of occasion, content, or form. Occasion such as weddings, funerals, holiday celebrations, family dinners, and work-related meetings. Content refers to the particular words or actions of a ritual. Form refers to the sequence of actions" (p. 9).

- According to Reber and Reber (2001), there are 5 meanings for the term *ritual:* 1) any sequence of actions or behaviors that is highly stylized, relatively rigid, and stereotyped; 2) a culturally or socially standardized set of actions dictated by tradition; 3) an oft-repeated pattern of behavior which tends to occur at appropriate times, eg, the morning ritual of washing, grooming, and dressing; 4) a fairly elaborate, stereotyped set of behaviors that perhaps had functional origins that are no longer apparent; and

5) irrational, repetitive behaviors often observed in obsessive compulsive disorder (p. 634).

- Family rituals are a form of symbolic communication that conveys the family identity ("who we are"), imparts to the participant individuals a sense of belong to the family, and provides continuity of meaning across generations (Segal, 2004, p. 499).

- Ritual is a prescribed occupation that is intentional in nature and that typically holds special significance and meaning for those performing them (Christiansen & Baum, 2005, p. 550).

- Rituals are symbolic actions with spiritual, cultural, or social meaning; contributing to the client's identity; and reinforcing the client's values and beliefs. Rituals are highly symbolic, with a strong affective component and representative of a collection of events (AOTA, 2008, p. 674).

- Christiansen and Townsend (2010) defined ritual as "an established pattern of actions in a prescribed or ordered manner often performed as part of a ceremony or observance and typically having an associated meaning beyond the action itself" (p. 422).

Role, Roles, and Occupational Role

- The concept of role entered the occupational therapy through the work of Reilly (1966), who talked about *role* and *roles* but did not define the term. Actually, there are 2 separate but overlapping concepts. One concerns roles in general and their relationship to human doing. The other concerns the specific occupational roles that humans do to fulfill the productivity aspects of social participation and responsibility. Reilly apparently felt that a specific concept of occupational role was the most appropriate concern for occupational therapy (Moorhead, 1969). Moorhead (1969), a student of Reilly's, stated that the role concept "has been constructed as a frame of reference for conceptualizing man's interaction with his human and task-oriented environment. Social roles are viewed as institutionally prescribed and proper ways for an individual to participate in society and thus satisfy his needs and wants" (p. 329). She continued her discussion by stating that occupational role is one of 3 types of roles used in sociology. The other 2 are family roles and personal-sexual roles. Occupational role can be identified by social position and by the tasks performed. See Table 31-7 for definitions of occupational role.

- The term *role* is traced to French theater, where a role was the roll of paper upon which an actor's part was written (Reber & Reber, 2001, p. 635). Both sociology and psychology have adopted and adapted the term.

Table 31-7. *Definitions of Role or Roles*

- Roles identify functions one assumes or acquires in society (eg, worker, student, parent, church members) (AOTA, 1989, p. 814).
- Role is a set of behaviors that have some socially agreed upon functions, and for which there is an accepted code of norms. (Christiansen & Baum, 1991, p. 857; 1997, p. 603).
- Ryan (1993) stated that roles are "functions of the individual in society that may be assumed or acquired (homemaker, student, caregiver, etc)" (p. 364).
- Punwar (1994) defined roles as "those functions that one assumes or acquires in society, ie, the roles of worker, parent, student, etc." (p. 265).
- Creek (1997) stated that role is "the set of expectations placed on an individual in a particular social context that become part of his identity and influence his behavior. Each person plays a large number of roles, such as worker, parent, friend" (p. 530).
- Hagedorn (1997) defined role as "a social or occupational identity which directs the individual's social, cultural and occupational behavior and relationships" (p. 145).
- Kielhofner (1997) defined an internalized role "as a broad awareness of a particular social identify and related obligations that together provide a framework for appreciating relevant situations and constructing appropriate behavior" (p. 193).
- Jackson and Banks (1997) suggested that roles are a "set of expectations governing the behavior of persons holding a particular position in society" (p. 460).
- Parham and Fazio (1997) stated that a role is "the expected pattern of behavior associated with occupancy of a distinctive position in society" (p. 252).
- Townsend (1997) defined role as "a culturally defined pattern of occupation that reflects particular routines and habits; stereotypical role expectations may enhance or limit persons' potential occupational performance" (p. 182).
- Neistadt and Crepeau (1998) stated that "roles give people scripts to behave in ways consistent with their social roles, such as student, worker, or parent" (p. 872).
- Jacobs (1999) stated that a role is a "set of behaviors that have some socially agreed-upon functions and for which there is an accepted code of norms" (p. 127).
- Punwar & Peloquin (2000) defined role as "those functions that one assumes or acquires in society, ie, the roles of worker, parent, student, etc" (p. 284).
- Roles are behavioral expectations that accompany a person's occupied position or status in a social system (Crepeau et al., 2003, p. 1033).
- Hussey et al. (2007) defined role as a pattern of behavior that includes certain rights and duties that an individual is expected, trained, and encouraged to perform in a particular social situation (p. 291).
- AOTA (2008) defined roles as sets of behaviors expected by society, shaped by culture, and may be further conceptualized and defined by the client (p. 674).
- Role includes social constructs that carry behavioral expectations and contribute to a person's self-image and sense of identity (Creek, 2008, p. 583).
- Roles are normative models shaped by the culture (Crepeau et al., 2009, p. 1066)
- Roles are a set of socially agreed-upon behavioral expectations, rights, and responsibilities for a specific position or status in a group or in society. These may be further conceptualized and defined by individuals enacting the role(s) (Schell et al., 2014, p. 1240).
- Role performance includes identifying, maintaining, and balancing functions one assumes or acquires in society, eg, worker, student, parent, friend, religious participant (AOTA, 1994, p. 1054).

Occupational Role

- The concept of occupation role entered the occupational therapy literature as an important concept in 1966, when Reilly stated in a question and answer session that "occupational [role] acknowledges that man, in addition to having a social and sexual nature, has an economic nature as well" (p. 66). Oakley, Kiehofner, Barris, and Reichler (1986) credited the term *occupational role* to Edwin Thomas, a sociologist, who stated that "for all adults there are at least three key roles or role clusters; one is the individual's sex role... another is one's occupational role; and third the individual's family roles" (1966, p. 5).

- Moorhead (1969) suggested that people identify each other by the occupational roles they perform, and that the roles become incorporated into a personal identification system.

- Matsutsuyu (1971), another student of Reilly's, added that the concept of occupational role includes "housewife, student, retiree, and preschooler, as well as worker" (p. 292).

- Reed (1984) defined occupational roles as "collections of specific subcategories of occupational areas. Roles depend on age, ability, and circumstances. Roles have occupational standards. Generally, roles become more complex with age until retirement, at which time roles may be simplified. Roles depend on occupational performance of selected skills in various combinations and patterns" (p. 502).

- Occupational roles were defined as roles that had attributes that defined a person's position in society, as well as the tasks he or she must do (Iannone, 1987, p. 94).

- Creek (1990) stated that an occupational role is "the main social position held by an individual and the tasks performed in that position, for example, student, worker, or volunteer" (p. 547; 1997, p. 529; 2002, p. 587).

- Occupational role refers to the performance of behavior components on a continuum from productive activities (eg, homemaking, working, studying) to playful activities (eg, hobbies, sports, social recreation) (Vause-Earland, 1991, p. 27).

- Occupational roles are patterns of self-maintenance, work, leisure, and rest activities that are done on a regular basis and are strongly associated with social cultural roles (Hillman & Chaparro, 1995, p. 88).

- Parham and Fazio (1997) defined occupational role as "the expected pattern of behavior associated with occupancy of a distinctive position in society and that contributes to society in an economic sense.

Examples of occupational roles include player, preschooler, student, worker, homemaker, retiree" (p. 251).

- Stein and Roose (2000) defined role performance. The definition is a social component that includes the individual's position in a family, job, culture, nation, or religion. The role functions include husband/wife, occupational title, political leader, spiritual, counselor, parent/homemaker, and professional soldier. These role functions are gained through education and social and family expectations. Throughout one's life, role functions are assumed and changed (p. 265).

- Occupational role includes the social expectations and behavioral enactment of activities and routines by individuals (Crepeau, Cohn, & Schell, 2003, p. 1031).

- Occupational role is defined as being able to carry out the occupations that are central to the person's role; satisfaction with role performance (Christianen & Baum, 2005, p. 548).

- **Author's comment:** Occupational therapy authors have not maintained the distinction between the 3 types of roles suggested by Thomas (1966) and Reilly (1966). Occupational roles were described as economic or productive roles, as opposed to gender and family roles. Instead the term *occupational role* is being used to explain the designation and performance of all 3 types of roles. When terms and concepts are borrowed from other disciplines, the definition and meaning must be kept clearly in mind. At this time, there is no clear definition of the concept of occupational role.

Routine and Routines (Occupational Routines)

- The term *routine* comes from the French word for route.

- The concept of routine in relation to clients was discussed by Allen (1985), and was used as the basis for the development of the Routine Task Inventory. However, the concept is not defined. The focus is on routine task behavior which "is observed during the process of completing a routine task" (Allen, 1985, p. 11).

- Hagedorn (1995) defined routine as "an automated and habitual chain of tasks with a fixed sequence" (p. 301).

- Reber (1995) suggested that some rituals become routines whenever the symbolic elements of the behaviors are lost. He stated that there are connotations "that somehow a routine is a more mundane, stereotyped behavior pattern than a ritual" (p. 676).

- Christiansen and Baum (1997) stated that routines are "occupations with established sequences, such as the related sequence of tasks that characterizes personal care (bathing, dressing, grooming) at the start of the day" (p. 603).
- Corsini (1999) defined routine as "a set of coordinated behaviors usually conducted without conscious intention, such as always putting shoes first on the left rather than on the right foot" (p. 865).
- Christiansen (2000) defined routines as "behaviors that are repeated over time and organized into patterns and habits" (p. 404; Christiansen & Matuska, 2011, p. 544).
- Routine is habitual, repeatable, and predictable ways of acting (Christiansen & Baum, 2005, p. 550).
- Routines are patterned behaviors that have instrumental goals. Routines give life order, whereas rituals give it meaning (Segal, 2004, p. 499).
- Routines provide an orderly structure for daily living that extends over time and pertain to a particular set of activities within a defined situation (Christiansen & Baum, 2005, p. 550).
- Routines are "patterns of behavior that are observable, regular, repetitive, and that provide structure for daily life. They can be satisfying, promoting, or damaging. Routines require momentary time commitment and are embedded in cultural and ecological contexts" (AOTA, 2008, pp. 674-675).
- Christiansen and Townsend (2010) defined routine as "a regular or customary pattern of time use through activity and occupation" (p. 422).
- A type of higher order habits that involves sequencing and combining process, procedures, steps, or occupations and provide a structure for daily live (Schell et al., 2014, p. 1241).
- Body routines are sets of coordinated, habitual bodily actions sustaining a specific task or aim; for example, driving, cooking, or lawn mowing (Schell et al., 2014, p. 1230).
- Christiansen and Townsend (2004) defined occupational routines as recurring sequences of time use, such as the regimen repeated upon waking each day (p. 278).
- Time-space routines are sets of more or less habitual bodily actions extending through a considerable portion of time; for example, a getting-up routine, a going-to the-gym routine, or a going-to-church and lunch routine (Schell, Gillen, & Scaffa, 2014, p. 1243).

Task or Tasks

Task has been discussed under the section on Doing because most, but not all, definitions imply that task or tasks are performances required or expected of the individual. The relation of task to activity or occupation is being explored, but has not achieved consensus. For example, is a task a unit of activity or is a task composed of units of activity?

- Tasks are the sequence of actions engaged in to satisfy either societal requirements or internal motivations to explore and be competent (Kielhofner, 1985, p. 509) *(doing)*.
- Task is a stage in or component of an activity (Hagedorn, 1992, p. 92) *(doing)*.
- Tasks are objective set of behaviors necessary to accomplish a goal (Dunn, Brown, & McGuigan, 1994, p. 599) *(doing)*.
- A task is a self-contained stage in an activity. Tasks chain to form an activity (Hagedorn, 1995, p. 301) *(doing)*.
- Tasks are composed of activities which are smaller units of behavior (Trombly, 1995, p. 17) *(doing)*.
- Task is defined as a set of purposeful activities in which a person engages (Law et al., 1996, p. 16) *(doing)*.
- A task is the constituent parts of an activity (Turner, Foster, & Johnson, 1996, p. 873) *(doing)*.
- Tasks are viewed as combinations of action sharing some purpose recognized by the task performer (Christiansen & Baum, 1997, p. 56; 2005, p. 551) *(doing)*.
- Tasks are work assigned to, selected by, or required of a person related to a skill. A collection of activities related to accomplishment of a goal (Jackson & Banks, 1997, p. 460) *(doing)*.
- Tasks are a set of activities that share some purpose (Watson, 1997, p. 32) *(doing)*.
- Task-involved activity is activity characterized by engagement because a task is interesting, challenging, or has other inherent qualities (Christiansen & Baum, 2005, p. 551).

Person/Personal Characteristics

Recently, additional concepts related to doing have begun to appear. These concepts can be grouped as person or personal characteristics of the doer. Punwar (1994) refers to the range of skills, aptitudes, or abilities that an individual possesses as a person's repertoire (p. 265). The specific concepts are ability, action, capacity, interests, motivation, skill, and volition. One important problem to solve is the relation of ability to skill and capacity. Although there is a trend toward considering ability as more associated with in-born or genetic characteristics and skill with learning, the trend is not universally accepted. The difference between ability and capacity is less defined.

Ability and Abilities

- Ability is defined by Polatajko (1992) as "the power to do something, whether physical or mental" (p. 196 [based on *Webster Dictionary*, 1972]).

- Ability is defined by Trombly (1995) as referring to a "general trait that an individual brings with him when he begins to learn a new task" (p. 19).

- Christiansen and Baum (1997) provided a similar definition, by suggesting the ability refers to "general traits which are a product of genetic make-up and learning much of which occurs during childhood and adolescence" (p. 56). Both of the definitions are based on the work of Fleishman (1975), a human factors scientist.

- Corsini (1999) suggested well-learned behaviors in his definitions, which are "1) the physical, mental or legal competence to function; and 2) a present skill, such as being able to spell a certain word, perform arithmetic, ride a bicycle, or recite a poem" (p. 2).

- In 2005 Christiansen and Baum defined ability as "supports performance and engagement in activity and tasks, makes it possible to complete the tasks within time frame or to meet standards of performance" (p. 543).

- Problem-solving ability is the ability to recognize and define a problem, identify alternative plans, select a plan, implement, and evaluate the outcome (Punwar & Peloquin, 2000, p. 283).

Action and Actions

- Christiansen and Baum (1997) defined actions as "any observable behavior that is recognizable can be described as an 'action,' the basic building block of occupation" (p. 56). Actions taken during a task may be a reflection of the individual's capabilities, skills, and experiences (Christiansen & Baum, 2005, p. 543).

- Unsworth (1999) defined purposive action as the "capacities for productivity and self-regulation (including the capacity to structure an effective and fluent course of action by initiating, maintaining, switching, and stopping complex action sequences in an orderly manner) to realize a goal" (pp. 481-482).

Capacity and Capacities

- Bonder and Wagner (1994) defined capacity as "the ability to perform a task, in contrast to the performance of a task" (p. 379). *Note:* Focus is on the doing of the task rather than quality of the result.

- Christiansen and Baum (1997) defined capacity as "the immediate potential of the individual to perform tasks which support occupational performance" (p. 592).

- Jackson and Banks (1997) suggested that capacity "is the ability to perform a task" (p. 460).

- Wilcock (1998) said that capacity means "the innate and perhaps undeveloped potential, aptitude, ability, talent, trait, or power with which each individual is endowed" (p. 42).

- Jacobs (1999) stated that capacity is "one's best, includes present abilities as well as potential to develop new abilities" (p. 21).

- Unsworth (1999) described capacity as "possessing normal psychological, physiological, or anatomical structure or function" (p. 474).

- Corsini (1999) stated that capacity "refers to potential ability" (p. 2).

- WHO (2001) stated that capacity is a "construct that indicates... the highest probable level of functioning that a person may reach... Capacity is measured in a uniform or standard environment and, thus, reflects the environmentally adjusted ability of the individual" (p. 166).

- Refers to a person's potential for occupation and includes aspects of human anatomy (eg, bipedal location, opposable thumbs, binocular vision), cognitive functions (eg, consciousness, attention), and the abilities developed through maturational processes (eg, strength, coordination, language, problem solving). Capacities are age and gender specific; may not yet be developed; and are shaped by a person's genetic heritage, aptitudes, traits, context, and occupational history (Schell et al., 2014, p. 1230).

Interests

- *Interest* or *interests* is another term that appeared in the early literature of occupational therapy. The major supporter of the concept of interest was Dr. Dunton. In 1918, he said that "any form of work to be curative must be able to create some interest for the patient (p. 318). In 1928, he defined interest as "by interest is meant the state of consciousness in which the attention is attracted to a task, companies by a more or less pleasurable emotional state" (p. 6).

- The pragmatist philosopher William James is probably one source of influence. In his famous text (1890, reprinted 1950) he stated "only those items which I notice shape my mind—without selective interest, experience is an utter chaos. Interest alone gives accent and emphasis, light and shade, background and foreground—intelligible perspective, in a word" (James, 1950, p. 402).

- Matsutsuyu (1969) suggested that "interests are described as feelings, drives or reactions which are interest states and related to attitudes, values and other motivation indices such as attention, direction and sentiments" (p. 324). In her study of interests she suggested there are 6 assumptions about interests, which are: 1) interests are family influenced, 2) interests evoke affective response, 3) interests are choice states, 4) interests can be manifest in effective action, 5) interests can sustain action, and 6) interests reflect self-perception.

- Borys (1974) suggested that interests are "developmentally permanent, learned and related to achievement" (p. 36). She summarized the major issues and influences in interest theories as developmental learning, motivational learning, choice, and personality development and self-concept.

- Ryan (1993) stated that interests are "activity that the individual finds pleasurable... and... are those that maintain one's attention" (p. 361).

- Punwar (1994) defined interests as "those mental or physical activities that create pleasure and maintain attention" (p. 261).

- The *Uniform Terminology III* (Dunn, Foto et al., 1994) defined interests as "identifying mental or physical activities that create pleasure and maintain attention" (p. 1054).

- Kielhofner (1997) defined interests as "dispositions to find pleasure and satisfaction in occupations, and the self-knowledge of our enjoyment of occupations; encompasses attraction and preference" (p. 207).

- Punwar and Peloquin (2000) stated that interests are "those mental or physical activities that create pleasure and maintain attention" (p. 281).

- Stein and Roose (2000) provided an extensive definition. Psychological components that include an individual's choice in engaging in activities such as sports, reading, music, films, theater, arts and crafts, cuisine, and table games. The motivation to engage in activities depends upon the opportunities available to the individual, ability to do the activity, and the pleasure related to the activity (p. 131).

- Brown and Stoffel (2011) stated that interests are "one of the components of a volitional system, or things that give pleasure and satisfaction" (p. 782).

- Activity interests and preferences include affective responses to play and leisure activities, perceptions and awareness of self and environments in relation to play and leisure activities, and motivation to participate in specific play and leisure activities (Schell et al., 2014, p. 1229).

Intrinsic Motivation, Motivating, Motivation

- Although the term *intrinsic motivation* is fairly new in the occupational therapy literature, the concept itself is probably very old. Dunton (1925) discussed the use of upholstery as a therapeutic medium. He says "there are numerous small problems constantly arising which must be solved... Their solutions may demonstrate a variety of mental mechanisms. It is believed that this has much to with creating enjoyment in the task, but there also seems to be a marked satisfaction when the work has been completed" (p. 221).

- The concept of motivation, especially intrinsic motivation or effectance motivation, appeared in 1969. Florey (1969) said that there is general agreement that the "motivational construct refers to a mediating system, process, or mechanisms that attempts to account for the purposive aspects of behavior" (p. 319). She suggested that "intrinsic motivation builds toward self-reward in independent action that underlies competent behavior" (p. 320).

- Deci (1975), a psychologist, defined intrinsic motivations as "behaviors which a person engages in to feel competent and self-determining" (p. 61). He continued by saying that the primary effects of intrinsic motivation are on the tissues of the central nervous system, not on non-nervous system tissues. He stated there are 2 types of intrinsic motivation. One occurs where there is not stimulation and the person seeks it out. A person who does not get stimulation will not feel competent and self-determining. The other kind of intrinsic motivation occurs when a person attempts to conquer challenges or reduce incongruity that reduces dissonance. In conquering the challenges, the person feels competent and self-determining. An individual seeks out pleasurable stimulation and deals with any over-stimulation effectively. Therefore, the individual is able to engage in seeking and conquering challenges, which is optimal for that person.

- In 1977, Hopkins and Smith defined intrinsic motivation as the "will to act based on personal internal standards incentives, desires, and needs" (p. 734; 1983, p. 922).

- Sharrott and Cooper-Fraps (1986) defined intrinsic motivation as "a biologically inherent or innate urge to explore and master the environment," which is characterized by the desire to be a causative agent, resulting in behavior that is self-satisfying.

- Doble (1988) has suggested there are 4 determinants of intrinsic motivation which influence the amount and use of the concept within an individual. The determinants are identified as (1) orientation of the person to the task environment, (2) meaningfulness of the activity to the person, (3) provision of opportunities for personal control, and (4) generation of feelings of competence. Consideration of the 4 determinants suggests a variety of possible responses on the part of the person which affect the doing process.

- Punwar (1994) defined intrinsic motivation as "motivation that comes from within the individual; self-motivation" (p. 261; Punwar & Peloquin, 2000, p. 281).

- Reber (1995) defined intrinsic motivation as "any behavior that is dependent on factors that are internal in origin" and is derived from feelings of satisfaction and fulfillment" (p. 387).

- Corsini (1999) defined intrinsic motivation with 2 definitions. The first is "behavior done for its own sake rather than for some kind of reward or payoff, for example, fishing for the pleasure of doing so versus fishing to make a living", and the second is "the intellectual satisfaction derived from the understanding of a meaningful solution: engaging in an activity for its own sake" (p. 505).

- Creek (1997) defined intrinsic motivation as "an innate drive to use one's capacity for action (p. 529).

- Parham and Fazio (1997) stated that intrinsic motivation is "a prompt to action that comes from within the individual and is not prompted by outside influence" and a "drive to action that is rewarded by the doing of the activity itself rather than some external reward. Intrinsic motivation is widely accepted as an essential ingredient of play" (p. 250).

- Jacobs (1999) stated that intrinsic motivation is a "concept in human development that proposes that people develop in response to an inherent need for exploration and activity" (p. 72).

- Punwar and Peloquin (2000) suggested that intrinsic motivation is "motivation that comes from within the individual; self-motivation" (p. 281).

- Stein and Roose (2000) defined intrinsic motivation as "the internal motivation to achieve or perform an activity without external rewards. For example, an artist will continue painting without expecting any reward or praise. Individuals with intrinsic motivation have an internal locus of control" (p. 132).

- Christiansen and Townsend (2010) defined the purposive view of motivation as an "emphasis on goal-directed or intentional action caused by anticipated benefit or a desire to avoid harm" (p. 422).

- Christiansen and Townsend (2010) defined achievement motivation as a "psychological need to succeed or attain mastery" (p. 417).

Skill or Skills

- The word skill has become a popular concept in occupational therapy literature, especially in the modern period of occupational therapy literature. Kielhofner (1985) defined skills as "the abilities that a person has for the performance of various forms of purposeful behavior" (p. 508).

- Hagedorn (1992) described skill as "a specific ability or integrated set of abilities such as motor, sensory, cognitive or perceptual, learnt, and practiced to a standard required for the effective performance of a task or subtask" (p. 92). In 1995, she rephrased the description and stated skill is "the ability to put skill components together in smoothly integrated and sequenced, competent, performance" (Hagedorn, p. 301).

- Polatajko (1992) defined skill as "a developed proficiency or dexterity in some art, craft, or the like" (p. 196).

- Trombly (1995) defined skill as "an individual's ability to achieve goals under a wide variety of conditions with a degree of consistency and economy" (p. 19).

- Turner, Foster, and Johnson (1996) stated skill is "a performance component which evolves with practice" (p. 873).

- Christiansen and Baum (1997) defined skill as "pertains to the level of proficiency in a specific task" (p. 57).

- Parham and Fazio (1997) stated that skills are "consolidations of rule-based subroutines of behavior that produce goal-directed behavior; for example, the subroutines of grasping the handle of a pitcher, pouring, and holding a glass are combined in the skill of pouring a drink. Skills, when practiced repeatedly until automatic, become habits" (p. 253).

- Corsini (1999) defined skill as "an acquired high-order ability to perform complex motor acts smoothly and precisely" (p. 906). However, he also added that the term "sometimes includes knowledge or keen cognition" in some definitions outside psychology (p. 906).

- Observable, goal-directed actions that a person uses while performing (Schell et al., 2014, p. 1241).

- Daily living skills are those abilities needed to function in daily life, ie, grooming, dressing eating, etc (Punwar, 1994, p. 257; Punwar & Peloquin, 2000, p. 279).

- Developmental skills are those abilities that children develop as they go through normal developmental stages, ie, language, motor skills, etc (Punwar & Peloquin, 2000, p. 279).

- Occupational skills and capacities include an individual's ability to perform his or her occupation, including ADLs, work, and leisure activities that are important, meaningful, and purposeful to the individual (Brown & Stoffel, 2011, p. 785).

- Occupational performance skills observed as a person selects, interacts with, and uses task tools and materials; carries out individual actions and steps; and modifies performance when problems are encountered (Schell et al., 2014, p. 1239).

Volition (Will)

- The concept of volition appears in the early occupational therapy literature. Upham (1919) said that "in healthy minds, volition precedes action, and disordered minds may be normalized if volition can be born, and action and decision made clear and enforced. Volition may be helped by the selection of the right occupation" (p. 211).

- The concept seems to have come from J. Madison Taylor, a physician, who wrote at the beginning of the 20th century. It was reintroduced by Kielhofner in the 1980s. He used the concept as a volition subsystem, which is "an interrelated set of energizing and symbolic components which together determine conscious choices for occupational behavior" (Kielhofner, 1985, p. 509).

- In 1997, Kielhofner defined the term *volition* as "a system of dispositions and self-knowledge that predisposes and enables a person to anticipate, choose, experience, and interpret occupational behavior" (p. 208).

- Creek (1997) defined volition as "the ability to choose between alternative actions; exercise of the will, or the inner condition of the organism that initiates or directs its behavior toward a goal" (p. 530).

- Unsworth (1999) stated that volition is "the capacity to determine what one needs and wants to do and the capacity to conceptualize a future realization of one's needs and wants. Volition requires the capacity to formulate a goal or an intention and then to initiate task performance" (p. 484).

- Reber (1995) defined volition as "conscious, voluntary selection of particular action or choice from many potential actions or choices" (p. 848).

- Christiansen and Townsend (2010) defined volition as "choice or will, intentionality" (p. 423).

- Brown and Stoffel (2011) defined volition as "a person's motivation for action and different occupations... It influences both the individual's choice of occupation and his or her persistence when engaging in that occupation" (p. 792).

- Patterns of thoughts and feelings about oneself as an actor in one's world that occur as one anticipates, chooses, experiences, and interprets what one does (Schell et al., 2014, p. 1243).

- Volitional processes control intentions and impulses so that an action is carried out; mediate the enactment of decisions to act and protect them (Christiansen & Baum, 2005, p. 551).

- Volitional structures include a stable pattern of dispositions and self-knowledge generated from and sustained by experience (Kielhofner, Borell, Helrich, & Nygard, 1995, p. 41).

- Volitional subsystem is a system of dispositions and self-knowledge that predisposes and enables people to anticipate, choose, experience, and interpret occupational behavior (Kielhofner, 1995, p. 30).

Summary of Doing Concepts

Doing has both an internally and externally directed process. Internally, the person must be able to initiate some action through the sensorimotor or cognitive system and must have some direction toward interest, meaning, and purpose from the cognitive system. Externally, the context, especially the sociocultural environment, moderate and influence the doing process. In the past, occupational therapy literature has contained many articles concerning the internal processes, but more recently attention has also focused on the external process.

There are many concepts associated with the doing process. As occupational therapy practitioners have experienced, doing is not a simple concept; any single act of doing has many factors contributing to the action. As occupational therapy continues to develop its own philosophy and rationale for practice, understanding the doing process becomes more important to the explanation of why occupational therapy is useful in developing, maintaining, and restoring health and well-being. Table 31-8 lists the concepts that can influence the doing process.

TOOLS

Tools are the instruments of change, the change agents, used in intervention. Common descriptors have included media, modalities, methods, techniques, strategies, and

Table 31-8. *Factors That Can Influence Doing*

Physical (Location) Factors	Temporal (Time) Factors	Sociocultural Factors
• Place: home or institution	• Age/life span	• Gender
• Built or nature environment	• Time of day	• Race
• Terrain	• Sequence: 1st, 2nd, 3rd	• Ethnicity
• Climate	• Season of the year	• Socioeconomic status
• Temperature	• Speed and accuracy	• Role: Parent/child
• Altitude	• Taking turns	• Role: Supervisor/worker
• Weather	• Waiting in line	• Role: Staff/patient
• Location (inside or outdoors)	• Being on time	• Crowds
• Location (clinic or ward)	• Following directions	• Consumer
• Location (community)	• Stage/course of illness	• Customer
• Light and color	• Expectation for recovery	• Citizenship
• Sound or noise	• Start/stop a movement	• Laws/rules and regulations
• Odors/smells	• Start/stop an activity	• Values, beliefs, and attitudes
• Safety or fire hazard	• Repetitive motion	• Economics
• Indoor climate control	• Amount of time needed to perform a task	• Politics
• Furniture	• Number of steps to finish	• Customs, mores, social norms
• Room arrangement	• Short-term memory	• Personal habits, preferences
• Supplies/materials available	• Long-term memory	• Country of origin/birth
• Equipment available		• Relationships
• Steps/stairs/ramps		
• Doors		
• Windows		
• Tastes/texture		
• Tactile sensations		
• Gravity		
• Humidity		
• Soil		
• Water		
• Chemicals		
• Architecture		
• Technology		

approaches. At issue is what tools occupational therapy practitioners select when working with clients. The particular tool is not as important as the process of selection, as Upham (1918a) stated: "the success of occupational therapy does not lie in any particular craft or trade, but rather in the skill with which it is selected for a particular disability of the patient and the technique of allowing the patient's reaction, temperament, and fatigue to form the basic teaching" (p. 51). Although the exact tool may not be important, the use of tools is very important, since they are the means of initiating and maintaining the doing process. The discussion of tools begins with a naming problem and continues with discussions of assumptions about purposes and classification systems. The specific tools to address the person and environment concepts are found in Sections II and III of this text. This section contains the history of the occupation and activities tools used by occupational therapy personnel.

Notes: When used in occupational therapy, the word *occupation* tends to be used as the noun form of the verb "to occupy" and describes the process of doing, engaging, performing, acting, and participating in a therapeutically constructed use of time and space. On the other hand, the term *occupations* tends to be used as the plural form of the noun "occupation" and refers to the roles, activities, vocations, or functions that can be "named and framed" and organize the time and space of people's lifetimes. Furthermore, occupations can be classified or grouped into potential tools for therapeutic intervention. Once selected as part of a client's intervention plan, the selected occupations occupy the client's therapeutically constructed time and space. Perhaps the discussion is simply word play, but the difference between describing what a client is doing in a therapeutic context (occupying time and space) vs describing the occupations of a population (group of persons) seems important to understanding how occupation "works" in occupational therapy as an applied discipline.

Occupation

Occupation is the major tool used in occupational therapy. The concept of occupation appears to have been based at least in part on the work of John Dewey. Dewey stated in his book *School and Society* in 1900 that "by occupation I mean a mode of activity on the part of the child which reproduces, or runs parallel to, some form of work carried on in social life" (Dewey, 1990, p. 132 [reprint]). He continued by stating that "in a rough way, all occupations may be classified as gathering about man's fundamental relations to the world in which he lives through getting food to maintain life, securing clothing and shelter to protect and ornament it, and thus, finally, to provide a permanent home in which all the higher and more spiritual interests may center" (Dewey, 1990, p. 137 [reprint]).

In 1916, he stated simply that "an occupation is a continuous activity having a purpose" (p. 309). However, as the concept has evolved in the occupational therapy literature, occupation has been used to describe the outcome, the doing process, and the major tool. Therefore, each definition following has been analyzed to determine whether it addresses the outcome, doing, or tool aspect of occupational therapy most directly, because the term *occupation* is used in all 3 contexts. The appropriate term is identified at the end of the definition.

Definitions of Occupation as Doing (Process, Means)

- Chunks of culturally and personally meaningful activity in which humans engage that can be named in the lexicon of the culture (Clark et al., 1991, p. 301).

- Occupation is used as a general term that refers to engagement in activities, tasks, and roles for the purposes of meeting the requirement of living (Levine & Bradley in Christiansen & Baum, 1991) *(doing, outcome)*.

- Activity or task that engages a person's resources of time and energy; specially, self-maintenance, productivity, and leisure (Reed & Sanderson, 1992, p. 345).

- Human occupation is "doing culturally meaningful work, play, or daily living tasks in the stream of time and in the contexts of one's physical and social world" (Kielhofner, 1995, p. 30).

- Occupation is the relationship between an occupation form and an occupational performance. *Occupational form* is the objective set of circumstances, external to the person, which elicits, guides, or structures the person's occupational performance. *Occupational performance* is the voluntary doing of the person in the context of the occupational form (Nelson, 1994, pp. 10-11).

- Occupations are defined as "chunks" of activity within the stream of human behavior that are names in the lexicon of the culture (Zemke & Clark, 1996, p. 48).

- Occupation is defined as groups of self-directed, functional tasks and activities in which a person engages over the lifespan (Law et al., 1996, p. 16).

- Occupations are the ordinary and familiar things that people do every day (Christiansen & Baum, 1997, p. 600).

- Occupations are groups of activities and tasks of everyday life, named, organized, and given value and meaning by individuals and a culture. Occupation is everything people do to occupy themselves, including looking after themselves (self-care, enjoying life, leisure) and contributing to the social and economic fabric of their communities (productivity); the domain of concern and the therapeutic medium of occupational therapy (Townsend, 1997, p. 181) *(doing, outcome)*.

- Occupation is all the "doing" that has intrinsic or extrinsic meaning (Wilcock, 1998, p. 257).

- Occupation is the engagement in daily life activities that are meaningful and purposeful, including self-care, instrumental, vocation, educational, play and leisure, and rest and relaxation ADL (Gillen & Burkhardt, 1998, p. 540).

- Occupation is a form of human endeavor that provides longitudinal organization of time and effort in a person's life (Hagedorn, 2000, p. 309).

- Occupation is the active or "doing" process when one is engaged in goal-directed activity (Punwar & Peloquin, 2000, p. 282).

- Occupation is the culturally and personally meaningful and purposeful activities that humans engage in during their everyday lives. These occupations include the major functions of life, such as work, leisure, play, self-care, rest, sleep, and social interactions (Stein & Roose, 2000, p. 201).

- Occupation is "a person's personally constructed, one-time experience within a unique context" (Pierce, 2001, p. 138).

- Velde and Fidler (2002) defined occupation as "a dynamic, complex process of being engaged in 'doing'; the phenomenon of mind and body being occupied" (p. 5); the "dynamic process of being engaged in doing an activity" (p. 6); and the "process of being occupied, being engaged in a doing experience" (p. 7).

- Engagement or participation in a recognizable life endeavor (Christiansen & Townsend, 2004, p. 278).

- Occupation is engagement in activities, tasks, and roles for the purpose of productive pursuit; maintaining one's self in the environment; and for purpose of relaxation, entertainment, creativity, and celebration—activities in which people are engaged to support their roles (Christiansen & Baum, 2005, p. 600).

- Occupations are "things that people do to occupy life for intended purposes such as paid work, unpaid work, personal-care, care of others, leisure, recreation, or subsistence. Includes groups of activities and tasks of everyday life, named, organized, and given value and meaning by individuals and a culture. Categories used by researchers and governments to track human participation in the labor market and society" (Christiansen & Townsend, 2010, p. 421).

- Occupation is "everything people do to occupy themselves throughout a 24-hour day, including taking care of one-self (self-care), enjoying life (leisure), and contributing to social and economic everyday life in one's community (productivity)" (Brown & Stoffel, 2012, p. 785).

- In occupational therapy, occupations refer to the everyday activities that people do as individuals, in families, and with communities to occupy time and bring meaning and purpose to life. Occupations include things people need to, want to, and are expected to do (WFOT, 2012).

- Occupation is the things that people do that occupy their time and attention; meaningful, purposeful activity, the personal activities that individuals choose or need to engage in, and the ways in which each individual actually experience them (Schell et al., 2014, p. 1237).

- "Occupation is used to mean all the things people want, need, or have to do, whether of physical, mental, social, sexual, political, or spiritual nature, and is inclusive of sleep and rest. It refers to all aspects of actual human doing, being, becoming, and belonging" (Townsend & Wilcock, 2004a, p. 542).

Occupation as Potential Outcome Measures (Purpose, Goal, or End)

- All goal-directed use of time, energy, interest and attention in work, leisure, family, cultural, self-care, and rest activities (AOTA, 1972, p. 204).

- Occupation is the dominant activity of human beings, which includes serious, productive pursuits and playful, creative, and festive behaviors. It is the result of evolutionary processes culminating in a biological, psychological, and social need for ludic and productive activity (Kielhofner, 1983) *(occupational performance)*.

- Occupation is a person's actual practice that reflects his or her own beingness within the environmental context. The framework of a life is planned, drafted, and endlessly refined through active participation in daily occupation (Fanchiang, 1996, p. 277) *(participation)*.

- Occupation is that which defines and organizes a sphere of action over a period of time and is perceived by the individual as part of his personal and social identity (Turner, Foster, & Johnson, 1996, p. 873) *(occupational identity)*.

- Occupation is the engagement in activities, tasks, and roles for the purpose of productive pursuit; maintaining oneself in the environment; and for purposes of relaxation, entertainment, creativity, and celebration—activities in which people are engaged to support their roles (Christiansen & Baum, 1997, p. 600) *(social productivity, survival, play/leisure, occupational performance)*.

- Occupation defines and organizes a sphere of action over a period of time and is perceived by the individual as part of his or her social identity (Creek, 1997, p. 529) *(occupational identity)*.

- Occupation includes the ordinary tasks of human existence in which people create their self-image and identify and organize their lives (Cara & MacRae, 1998, p. 669) *(occupational identity)*.

- Occupation includes the daily activities typical for a culture that form a pattern of activity (Neistadt & Crepeau, 1998, p. 870) *(occupational performance)*.

- Human occupation is the total range of productive, purposeful and meaningful occupations in which people participate and is the area of human life with which occupational therapy practitioners are concerned (Hagedorn, 2000, p. 309) *(participation and tool)*.

- Occupation is a synthesis of doing, being, and becoming that is central to the everyday life of every person and that provides longitudinal organization of time and effort. Occupation is a basic need for people of all ages and is necessary for adaptation and survival (Creek, 2003, p. 32).

- Occupation is "activity in which one engages that is meaningful and central to one's identity" (Hussey et al., 2007, p. 289) *(occupation identity)*.

- Occupations are activities that bring meaning to the daily lives of individuals, families, and communities and enable them to participate in society (AOTA, 2011) *(quality of life, life satisfaction)*.

Occupation as Tool (Therapeutic Change Agent, Natural Change Agent)

- Therapeutic occupations are those occupations or activities that are used as part of an intervention program. To qualify as a therapeutic occupation there must be a purpose or goal toward which the occupation is being directed. Although most occupations can be used for therapeutic purposes, the most common ones are those that fall into the categories of self-maintenance, productive, or leisure time activities (Reed, 1984, p. 501).

- Occupation is appropriate to use when the person's abilities, motivations, and goals come together to enable role performance (Trombly, 1995, p. 237).

- Therapeutic occupation includes any purposeful activity used to prevent physical or mental dysfunction or to restore or improve function to a normal level (Punwar, 1994, p. 262; Punwar & Peloquin, 2000, p. 282).

- Therapeutic use of occupations and activity includes the selection of activities and occupations that will meet the therapeutic goals (Hussey et al., 2007, p. 292).

Reading the definitions of occupation leads to 3 conclusions. First, more than 1 idea is being conveyed in the use of the term *occupation*. Since these definitions were all written by authors in the profession, a second conclusion is evident. Occupational therapy personnel use the term *occupation* to convey the essential reality of the profession—occupation is both process and product. As Trombly (1995) has said, occupation is both means and ends. Occupation is both the means by which occupational therapy is delivered and the results of having engaged in or received occupational therapy services. Practitioners guide clients to engage in occupation to learn or relearn how to engage in occupation in the future, thus there is both a present and future time reference. The process takes time and energy and is composed of actions, tasks, and roles with labels such as washing clothes (activity) to provide clean clothing (task) as a homemaker (role). The product is influenced by factors such as health or disability status, sociocultural customs, economic means, geography, political situation, religious rituals, and personal preferences. All of the factors that affect the use of the term *occupation* used in occupational therapy should appear in the description of the term as used by occupational therapy personnel. A third conclusion is that the term *occupation* is not often used to describe occupation as the tool used in occupational therapy.

Occupation is the primary, most important therapeutic tool used in occupational therapy practice. Clarification is clearly in order. The profession must come to some agreement about the central term and concept in the field. Based on a word analysis of the definitions above, 9 assumptions are proposed that should be considered in a comprehensive definition of occupation as it is used in occupational therapy today. These are listed in Table 31-9. Table 31-10 reviews how the term *occupation* is used in the literature.

Occupational Dysfunction

- Problems with performing occupations have also been defined using the term *occupational dysfunction*.

- Occupational dysfunction includes problems of planning for occupations to be done, actually performing the occupations, and evaluating the effectiveness (feedback) of such performance. Dysfunction may be observed in the failure to perform an occupation in which the skills are available, inability to perform an occupation because the skills cannot be done, and nonperformance of an occupation because the opportunity has not arisen or has not been taught (Reed, 1984, p. 501).

- Occupational dysfunction includes "losses in any of the aspects of human functioning, loss of motivation, drastic changes in environment, or cultural inaccessibility results in disability or handicap" (Trombly, 1995, p. 23).

Table 31-9. *Assumptions About Occupation*

- Occupation(s) can be named, defined, described, and framed.
- Occupation is composed of activities, tasks, components, and roles.
- Occupation has an organizing, organizational, pattern, or sequencing effect on people.
- Occupation occurs in a physical dimension of time (temporal) and space (spatial).
- Occupation occurs in a personal, social and cultural dimension, environment, context or situation.
- Occupation involves a doing process that requires internal and external resources, such as effort, energy, abilities, capacities, motivation, supplies, tools, and equipment.
- Occupation may be done or performed for a variety of reasons, functions, interests, meanings, purposes, values, or beliefs.
- Occupation can meet a variety of personal or individual goals or outcomes, such as increased or improved self-image, self-identity, occupational identity, or self-efficacy.
- Occupation can meet a variety of sociocultural goals or outcomes, such as economic, political, and institutional.
- Occupation can be subdivided into a number of categories for convenience, clarification, classification, or taxonomy.

Table 31-10. *Use of Term* Occupation *in Occupational Therapy Literature*

- Occupation involves the engagement of the whole person in the performance of occupational activities or tasks.
- Occupation can contribute to a person's sense of well-being and state of health.
- Occupation can enable a person to meet individual needs and societal demands.
- Occupation can facilitate the attainment of adaptive behavior, mastery, autonomy, efficacy, control, or sense of competence within the environment, context, or situation because the person is able to produce an effect.
- Occupation can be used to attain, maintain, or regain skills necessary to fulfill social roles.
- Occupation can be used to maintain, prevent, or slow the loss of skills
- Occupation can be used to help a person learn to organize his or her life and use resources to reduce the impact of disability.
- Occupation can facilitate normal development throughout the lifespan.
- Occupation can be graded to accommodate different learning abilities.
- Occupation can be used to enhance skills in a variety of performance components, areas, or contexts.
- Occupation can be used in changing (increase or decrease) the level of participation, performance, and responsibility assumed by a person.

Based on Reed, K. L., & Sanderson, S. N. (1999). *Concepts of occupational therapy* (4th ed.). Philadelphia, PA: Lippincott Williams & Wilkins; and Yerxa, E. J. (1996). The social and psychological experience of having a disability: implications for occupational therapists. In L. W. Pedretti (Ed.), *Occupational therapy: practice skills for physical dysfunction* (pp. 253-274). St. Louis, MO: Mosby.

- Kielhofner (1995) stated that "we recognize occupational dysfunction when an individual has difficulty performing, organizing, or choosing occupations. We also recognize it when the pattern of occupational behavior exhibited by a person fails to provide a basic quality of life to the individual and/or meet reasonable expectations of the environment… Occupational dysfunction is multifaceted" (p. 155).
- Occupational dysfunction "is a phenomenon that is 'nested' in a complex of factors, all of which reflect

and contribute to the sustaining the performance, patterns of behavior, identities, choices, and so on, that reflect a life in trouble" (Whiteford, 2000, p. 201).

- Inability to maintain one's self; that is, care for self, dependents, and home; to advance oneself through work, learning, and financial management; or to enhance the self by engaging in self-actualizing activities that add enjoyment of life (Trombly & Radomski, 2002, p. 2).
- Inability to engage in one or more of the roles that are important to the client in the manner in which he or she wants to engage in them (Trombly & Radomski, 2002, p. 31).
- Scaffa stated that "occupational dysfunction is multidimensional, resulting from the interplay of biological, psychological, and ecological factors" (Scaffa, 2001, p. 141).

Types of Occupation

ADL, self-maintenance, IADL, self-care, work, leisure, play, and task are terms to describe types or categories of occupation. Some of the terms have a long history in occupational therapy literature, while others were created more recently. These are discussed below.

Activities of Daily Living

The term *activities of daily living* first appears in the occupational therapy literature in the second edition of Willard and Spackman (Holdeman, 1954) in the chapter on the treatment of polio. Holdeman, the chapter author, stated that "the function, or activities of daily living (A.D.L.), test is a guide in evaluating his (the client's) process" (p. 262).

Activities of daily living, however, was not the original name for what is now called ADL. The original name for the assessment of daily living skills was the "achievement record" (Sheldon, 1935). An example of an achievement record appeared in Livingstone (1950). A second name was "physical demands of daily life" (Deaver & Brown, 1945). Deaver, a physician, and Brown, a physical therapy practitioner, developed a scale with 3 headings: location, self-care activities, and hand activities. An assessment protocol based on Deaver and Brown appears in MacLean's (1949) article on the management of polio. Smith (1945) credited Deaver with initiating the program of training in daily life tasks. Smith said that Deaver became concerned with the number of clients who, in spite of many months of treatment, "could not perform the ordinary routine tasks required in daily life although they were capable of being taught to do so" (Deaver & Brown, 1945, p. I). Between the years 1945 and 1949, the name changed from "physical

activities of daily life" to "functional activities" to "activities of daily living" (Buchwald, 1949, p. 491). Since then, the phrase *activities of daily living* has been defined in numerous ways in the occupational therapy literature, such as "independent living/daily living skills" in the 1979 *Uniform Terminology for Reporting Occupational Therapy Services* (AOTA, 1979b) and 1981 *Entry-Level Role Delineation for OTRs and COTAs* (AOTA, 1981).

- AOTA (1978) first defined ADL as "the components of everyday activities including self-care, work and play/leisure activities" (p. 73).
- Mosey (1986) said that ADL are "all those activities that one must engage in or accomplish in order to participate with comfort in other facets of life. These activities may be subdivided into self-care, communication and travel... and... responsibilities of being a homemaker or home manager" (p. 8).
- Reed and Sanderson (1992) defined ADL as "the tasks that a person must be able to perform in order to care for the self independently, including self-care, communication, and travel" (p. 330).
- Ryan's (1993) definition was an "area of occupational performance that refers to grooming, oral hygiene, dressing, feeding and eating, medication routine, socialization, functional communication, functional mobility, and sexual expression activities" (p. 357).
- Bonder and Wagner (1994) defined ADL as "basic activities that support survival, including eating, bathing, toileting, and hygiene and grooming" (p. 378).
- Trombly (1995) said that ADL "includes those tasks that a person regularly does to prepare for, or as an adjunct to, participating in his or her social and work roles" (p. 289).
- Pedretti (1996) stated that "ADL require basic skills and include task of mobility, self-care, communication, management of environmental hardware and devices, and sexual expression" (p. 463).
- Christiansen and Baum (1997) defined ADL as "typical life tasks required for self-care and self-maintenance, such as grooming, bathing, eating, cleaning the house, and doing laundry" (p. 591).
- Gillen and Burkhardt (1998) stated that ADL are "the activities usually performed in the course of a normal day, such as eating, toileting, dressing, washing, and grooming" (p. 536).
- Neistadt and Crepeau (1998) suggested ADL are "self-maintenance tasks considered necessary for meeting the demands of daily living, including such as activities as bathing, dressing, grooming, oral hygiene, eating, taking medication, and communication" (p. 866).

- Christiansen (2000) said that ADL are "activities or tasks that a person does every day to maintain personal independence" (p. 399).

- Stein and Roose (2000) defined ADL as "tasks that are essential for self-care, including dressing, grooming, feeding, mobility/transferring, bathing, and toileting" (p. 1).

- Activities that are oriented toward taking care of one's own body (AOTA, 2002c, p. 630 [adapted from Rogers & Holm, 1999]). Includes bathing, showering, bowel and bladder management, dressing, eating, feeding, functional mobility, personal device care, personal hygiene and grooming, sexual activity, sleep, rest, and toilet hygiene.

- An area of occupation that includes activities oriented toward taking care of one's own body. Also referred to as basic activities of daily living (BADL) and personal activities of daily living (PADL) (Christiansen & Matuska, 2004, p. 463; 2011, p. 537).

- Activities involved in taking care of one's own body, including such things as dressing, bathing, grooming, eating, feeding, person device care, toileting, sexual activity, and sleep/rest (Hussey et al., 2007, p. 285).

- Tasks that are typically performed in a habitual manner; every day; and across all age groups, genders, and cultures (Brown & Stoffel, 2011, p. 773).

- Activities are oriented toward taking care of one's own body, such as bathing/showering, bowel and bladder management, dressing, feeding, functional mobility, person device care, personal hygiene and grooming, sexual activity, and toilet hygiene (Schell, Gillen, & Scaffa, 2014, p. 1229).

Some substitute the concept self-care or self-maintenance for ADL. Of interest may be definitions used in the MEDLINE database, in which self-care is the individual's ability to perform the tasks for him- or herself, whereas ADL require the help or supervision of another person to perform. Self-maintenance is emerging and is included as a new intervention. Which idea is being conveyed in the occupational therapy literature?

Self-Care

- AOTA (1978) defined self-care skills as "skills such as dressing, feeding, hygiene/grooming, mobility, and object manipulation" (p. 75). The definition includes 2 subcategories: mobility and object manipulation.

- Letts, Fraser, Finlayson, and Walls (1993) defined self-care as "the decisions and actions individuals take in the interest of their own health and for the health of family members, eg, eating a balanced diet, choosing to exercise regularly, pre-natal care" (p. 8).

- Trombly (1995) suggested self-care involved "activities or tasks done routinely to maintain the client's health and well-being, considering the environment and social factors" (p. 352).

- Jacobs (1999) said that self-care are the "personal activities an individual performs to prepare for and maintain a daily routine" (p. 131).

- Christiansen (2000) used the term *self-care occupations*, which was defined as "those basic personal care activities such as eating, grooming, dressing, mobility, and personal hygiene" (p. 404).

- Stein and Roose stated that self-care includes "activities that are completed daily to maintain good hygiene and good appearance, meet basic needs such as eating and voiding, and move from one necessary area (such as the kitchen) to another (the bathroom)" (p. 273).

- Basic self-care includes personal activities, such as eating, grooming, hygiene, and mobility, that are necessary for maintenance of the self within the environment (Christiansen & Baum, 2005, p. 543).

- **Author's comment:** Medical Subject Headings (MESH) defines self-care as taking care of one's own needs (Wos, 1984). ADL refer to personal needs performed by others. Is there an advantage to using self-care over ADL or vice versa?

Self-Maintenance

- Reed and Sanderson (1992) defined self-maintenance occupations as "those activities or tasks that are done routinely to maintain the person's health and well-being in the environment, ie, dressing, feeding" (p. 352).

- Christiansen (2000) also suggested that self-maintenance could be used as a synonym for ADL. He defined self-maintenance as "the ability to handle tasks ranging from basic personal care, including dressing, eating, grooming, toileting, and getting around (mobility), to doing laundry, using the telephone, shopping, banking, and managing medications" (p. 404).

- Occupations pursued to enable participation in the social world, related to personal care and existence in the community (Christiansen & Baum, 2005, p. 550).

Education

- Although the term used today is *education*, the early literature used the term *re-education*. Barton (1917) wrote a book entitled *Re-education: An Analysis of the Institutional System of the United States* about the need and value of work activities in social institutions.

- Education in the form of patient or client education has been a part of occupational therapy intervention for many years. The concept of helping clients to seek, obtain, and participate in educational activities outside of the therapy session is most associated with school-based settings.

- Education includes activities needed for learning and participating in the environment (AOTA, 2008, p. 632).

- Format educational participation includes the categories of academic (eg, math, reading working on a degree), nonacademic (eg, recess, lunchroom, hallway), extracurricular (eg, sports, band, cheerleading, dances), and vocation (pre-vocational and vocational) participation (AOTA, 2008, p. 632).

- Internal personnel educational needs or interests exploration. Identifying topics and methods for obtaining topic-related information or skills (AOTA, 2008, p. 632).

- Informal personal education participation is participating in classes, programs, and activities that provide instruction/training in identified areas of interest (AOTA, 2008, p. 632).

Instrumental Activities of Daily Living

- IADL became a phrase in 1969 when Lawton and Brody published an article on the subject and become popular with the publication of the assessment by Lawton in 1971. The concept did not start appearing in occupational therapy literature until the 1990s.

- IADL included what were considered hierarchically more complex tasks, such as using the telephone, making meals, and managing medications (Hasselkus, 1993, p. 745).

- Bonder and Wagner (1994) defined IADL as "higher order activities which support independence, including housekeeping, shopping, and budgeting and money management" (p. 383).

- According to Pedretti (1996) IADLs involved "more advanced problem-solving skills, social skills, and complex environment interaction, such as home management and community living skills, health management, and safety preparedness" (p. 463).

- Jackson and Banks (1997) defined IADLs as "higher-order activities that support independence, including housekeeping duties, shopping, budgeting, and money management" (p. 460).

- Unsworth (1999) stated that IADL are "domestic and community activities of daily living, such as cleaning, shopping, and driving (p. 478).

- Christiansen (2000) defined IADL as "more complex activities or tasks that a person does to maintain independence in the home and community" (p. 402).

- Piersol and Ehrlich (2000) said that IADL are "activities other than BADL that related to the ability to manage independently at home, eg, laundry, shopping, and money management" (p. 200).

- Stein and Roose (2000) define IADL as "tasks that involve participation of a client with the physical and/or social environment, including home management, money management, communication, safety, community living skills, work, and leisure activities" (p. 130).

- Includes telephone, food preparation, housekeeping, laundry, shopping, money management, use of transportation, and medication management as important occupations necessary for living independently in the community (Christiansen & Baum, 2005, p. 546).

- Activities, such as meal preparation, money management, and care of others, that involve interacting with the environment, often complex, and may be considered optional (Hussey et al., 2007, p. 288).

- More complex activities than BADL that require interaction with the environment and/or others, such as grocery shopping, using public transportation, and money management (Brown & Stoffel, 2011, p. 782).

- Activities to support daily life within the home and community that often require more complex interactions than self-care used in ADLs (Christiansen & Matuska, 2011, p. 541).

- IADL include 12 activity categories: care of others, care of pets, child rearing, communication management, community mobility, financial management, health management and maintenance, home establishment and management, meal preparation and clean up, religious observance, safety and emergency precautions, maintenance, and shopping (Schell, Gillen, & Scaffa, 2014, p. 1235).

- **Author's comment:** Generally, IADL are assumed to require additional cognitive skills (less dependent on rote or procedural memory, more flexibility required). The exact number and type depends on occupational roles performed by the person.

Leisure

The term *leisure* comes from the Latin verb "licere" that means "to be permitted." Leisure is not as widely defined as work. Early definitions of leisure did not always differentiate leisure from play. The diversity of opinion as to what constitutes leisure is evident in the definitions following.

- Play/leisure refers to skill and performance in choosing, performing, and engaging in activities for amusement, relaxation, spontaneous enjoyment, and/or self-expression (AOTA, 1979b, p. 902).

- Leisure is time when one is free from family and other social responsibilities, ADL, and work (Mosey, 1986, p. 85).

- Leisure includes those activities or tasks done for the enjoyment and renewal that the activity or task brings to the person, which may contribute to the promotion of health and well-being, ie, bowling, collecting antiques (Reed & Sanderson, 1992, p. 343).

- Leisure is non-work or free time spent in adult play activities that have an influence on the quality of life (Ryan, 1993, p. 361).

- Leisure is defined as "experiences characterized by choice on the part of the individual, personal control, internal motivation, disengagement from the stresses of everyday life, and total absorption" (Bonder & Wagner, 1994, p. 383).

- Leisure includes activities or tasks that are not obligatory and that are done for enjoyment (Trombly, 1995, p. 44), or components of life free from work and self-care activities (Trombly, 1995, p. 352).

- Leisure is that category of occupations for which freedom of choice and enjoyment seem to be the primary motives. (Christiansen & Baum, 1997, p. 598; 2005, p. 547).

- Leisure is:
  ◊ Freedom from the demands of work or duty
  ◊ Free or unoccupied time; a block of time in which there is no external pressure to generate a product
  ◊ Unhurried ease
  ◊ Play, particularly play in adulthood; leisure in this sense is usually associated with a conviction that is necessary for individual life satisfaction and maintenance of social order and legitimate times, spaces, and practices associated with leisure
  ◊ A non-obligatory activity that is intrinsically motivated and engaged in during discretionary time; that is, time not committed to obligatory occupations such as work, self-care, or sleep (Parham & Fazio, 1997, p. 250; AOTA, 2002c, p. 632)

- Leisure includes activities driven by internal motivation, implies freedom of choice, and is not usually done within time constraints (Neistadt & Crepeau, 1998, p. 870).

- Leisure is a major occupation and performance area that relates to the individual's use of free time. It is related to intrinsic motivation, QOL, personal freedom, life satisfaction, relaxation, health, lifestyle, amusement, self-actualization, and pleasure. Leisure occupations include a wide range of activities, such as gardening, sports, hobbies, social clubs, music, and traveling, that are related to the specific interests of an individual. Cultural, psychological, social, developmental, family, and educational factors may influence leisure choices (Stein & Roose, 2000, p. 142).

- Activities that are freely selected by an individual that he or she participates in during self-allocated time. Leisure activities are varied and selected on the basis of meaning, pleasure, personal fulfillment, relaxation, and other attributes of significance to the individual (Duncan, 2006, p. 339).

- Leisure is "free or uncommitted time or opportunity to do something" (Christiansen & Townsend, 2010, p. 419).

- A non-obligatory activity that is intrinsically motivated and engaged in during discretionary time; that is, time not committed to obligatory occupations such as work, self-care, or sleep (Christiansen & Matuska, 2011, p. 542).

- A non-obligatory activity that is intrinsically motivated and engaged in during discretionary time; that is, time not committed to obligatory occupations such as work, self-care, or sleep (Brown & Stoffel, 2011, p. 783).

- Leisure exploration is identifying interests, skills, opportunities, and appropriate leisure activities (AOTA, 2008, p. 632).

- Leisure participation is planning and participating in appropriate leisure activities; maintaining a balance of leisure activities with other areas of occupation; and obtaining, using, and maintaining equipment and supplies as appropriate (AOTA, 2008, p. 632).

Themes include a temporal relationship to other occupations (done in free time or non-work time), control of choice (freedom to choose, not obligatory), related to health and well-being (promote health, enjoyment, quality of life), may be considered an adult form of play, and variety of activities from which to choose. The lack of consensus on what constitutes leisure may be one factor in the lack of development of leisure in many practice settings.

Play

The concept of play became popular in the models of occupational therapy due to Reilly's (1966) interest. Thereafter, most discussions of occupational therapy media include play. Based on these definitions, play is a complex term that has only received serious study in occupational therapy in the modern period. The role of play in child development and the relation of play to adult work skills have been discussed, but consensus has not been achieved.

- Play is a departure from reality, from the social prescriptions of everyday living (Shannon, 1970, p. 113).
- Play is activity voluntarily engaged in for pleasure (Hopkins & Smith, 1983, p. 925).
- Play is spontaneous behavior initiated for pleasure, fun, or experimentation; a motive or activity characterized by freedom to explore, unrestricted by a utilitarian goal or expected result (Spencer, 1989, p. 92).
- Play includes activities carried on as part of one's leisure occupation that develop skills in and permits self-expression, competition, exploration, and make believe. Most play has rules that govern the conduct of the specific play activity. Skills learned in play may be applied to work and productive occupations (Reed & Sanderson, 1992, p. 347).
- Play is an intrinsic activity that involves enjoyment and leads to fun; spontaneous, voluntary, and engaged in by choice (Ryan, 1993, p. 363).
- Play includes a variety of occupations that constitute a pleasurable way of passing time and are also the medium through which a wide range of skills can be learned and rehearsed (Creek, 1997, p. 529).
- Play is a category of occupations characterized by choice, expression, and development (Christiansen & Baum, 1997, p. 601).
- Play is:
  ◊ An attitude or mode of experience that involves intrinsic motivation; emphasis on process rather than product and internal rather than external control; and an "as-if" or pretend element; takes place in a safe, unthreatening environment with social sanctions.
  ◊ Also any spontaneous or organized activity that provides enjoyment, entertainment, amusement, or diversion (Parham & Fazio, 1997, pp. 251-252).
- Play involves choosing, performing, and engaging in an intrinsically motivated activity (attitude or process) that is experienced as pleasurable (Jacobs, 1999, p. 112).
- Play and leisure activities are intrinsically motivating activities that provide pleasure, relaxation, and expression of creativity (Neistadt & Crepeau, 1998, p. 871).
- Play is "the primary occupation of childhood; also a term often used interchangeably with leisure to describe the non-work activities of adults" (Christiansen & Baum, 2005, p. 549).
- Play is "the spontaneous, enjoyable, free from rules, internally motivated activity in which there is no goal or purpose" (Hussey et al., 2007, p. 289). (*Note:* Probably not the best definition. Play often has rules and is one of main ways people learn to understand and follow rule-based behavior. Play often has a goal or purpose; to explore different ways of doing things or imitating behavior [playing house or playing fireman] or trying out new skills [riding a bicycle].)
- Play is "any spontaneous or organized activity that provides enjoyment, entertainment, amusement, or diversion" (Brown & Stoffel, 2011, p. 786).
- Play is "an area of occupation that provides enjoyment, entertainment, amusement or diversion" (Christiansen & Matuska, 2011, p. 543).
- Play or leisure activities includes intrinsically motivating activities for amusement, relaxation, spontaneous enjoyment, or self-expression (Dunn, Foto et al., 1994).
- Play and leisure activity interest/preferences, and activity choices related to play and leisure performance (Schell et al., 2014, p. 1239).
- Play exploration includes identifying appropriate play activities, which can include exploration play, practice play, pretend play, games with rules, constructive play, and symbolic play (AOTA, 2008, p. 632).
- Play participation includes participating in play; maintaining a balance of play with other areas of occupation; and obtaining, using and maintaining toys, equipment, and supplies appropriately (AOTA, 2008, p. 632).

A summary of these ideas is that play is characterized by pleasure, fun, experimentation, exploration, self-expression, competition, and make believe; that play does not have a utilitarian goal, but does contribute to learning or rehearsing a wide range of skills that can be applied to productive occupations and permits self-expression; that play involves intrinsic motivation, choice, and voluntary participation that may be spontaneous or organized, and is process rather than product or goal oriented; that play does have rules that govern the conduct of the specific play activity; and that play may result in entertainment, amusement, diversion, passing time, and/or relaxation.

Productivity, Productive

- Productivity includes activities that are recognized by society as making an economic contribution. May include paid employment, volunteer work, homemaking, or caregiving activities to which a monetary value can be fixed (Bonder & Wagner, 1994, p. 386).
- Productivity includes activities and tasks that are done to enable the person to provide support to the

self, family, and society through the production of goods and services (CAOT, 1995, p. 141).

- Productivity occupations are those activities or tasks that are done to enable the person to provide support to the self, family, and society through the production of goods and services to promote health and well-being, ie, secretary, mechanic, homemaker (Reed & Sanderson, 1992, p. 348).

- **Author's comment:** Productivity can also be viewed as a management tool to measure the ratio between output and the resources expended to obtain that output. This definition is not generally what occupational therapy practitioners are describing when they use the term *productivity*.

The consensus in occupational therapy seems to be that there are several categories of work or productive activity, and that the work occurs in a variety of settings. A summary of ideas expressed in the definitions is that work involves participating in socially purposeful, meaningful, and productive activities that includes services or commodities to maintain or advance society and individuals (with labels such as remunerative employment, subsistence, home management, care of others, education, avocation, or vocation), and is characterized as having a predetermined manner or standard of performance.

Rest and Sleep

- The terms *rest* and *sleep* are part of the "big four" discussed by Meyer (1922) that included work, play, rest, and sleep (p. 6). Although work and play received much attention in the intervening years, rest and sleep received very little. In addition, sleep itself may be more correctly considered a physiological state or process, and not an occupation that can be used as a therapeutic tool. However, participation in sleep-related activities and preparation for sleep can be considered as tools.

- Rest includes quiet and effortless actions that interrupt physical and mental activity, resulting in a relaxed state (Nurit & Michel, 2003, p. 227).

- Rest "includes identifying the need to relax; reducing involvement in taxing physical, mental or social activities; and engaging in relaxation or other endeavors that restore energy, calm, and renewed interest in engagement" (AOTA, 2008, p. 632).

- Rest is a period of relaxing or ceasing to engage in strenuous or stressful activity (Schell et al., 2014, p. 1240).

- Sleep includes a series of activities resulting in going to sleep, staying asleep, and ensuring health and safety through participation in sleep, involving engagement with the physical and social environments (AOTA, 2008, p. 632).

- Sleep hygiene includes habits, environmental factors, and practices that may influence the length and quality of one's sleep (Schell et al., 2014, p. 1241).

- Sleep participation includes taking care of the personal need for sleep, such as cessation of activities to ensure onset of sleep, napping, dreaming, sustaining a sleep state without disruption, and night-time care of toileting needs or hydration; negotiating the needs and requirements of others within the social environment; interacting with those sharing the sleeping space (such as children or partners), providing night-time caregiving (such as breastfeeding), and monitoring the comfort and safety of others (such as the family while sleeping) (AOTA, 2008, p. 632).

- Sleep preparation includes engaging in routines that prepare the self for a comfortable rest, such as grooming and undressing, reading or listening to music to fall asleep, saying goodnight to others, and meditation or prayers; determining the time of day and length of time desired for sleep or the time needed to wake; and establishing sleep patterns that support growth and health (patterns are often personally and culturally determined) (AOTA, 2008, p. 632).

- Sleep preparation includes preparing the physical environment for periods of unconsciousness, such as making the bed or space on which to sleep, ensuring warmth/coolness and protection, setting an alarm clock and securing the home, such as locking doors or closing windows or curtains, and turning off electronics or lights (AOTA, 2008, p. 632) *(social participation, see under Doing).*

Work

The term *work* has appeared in the occupational therapy literature since the earliest articles were published, and descriptions of work appear frequently. Values, beliefs, and social customs regarding work also appear. The first documented definition written for the profession of occupational therapy was published in 1979.

- Work refers to skill and performance in participating in socially purposeful and productive activities. These activities may take place in the home, employment setting, school, or community (AOTA, 1979b, p. 901).

- Work includes all forms of productive activity, regardless of whether they are reimbursed (Jacobs, 1985, p. 11).

- Work is any formal activity that prepares one for (or involves) earning a living, being a student, or remunerative employment (Mosey, 1986, p. 71).

- Work activities include home management, care of others, educational activities, and vocational activities (AOTA, 1989, p. 812).
- Work involves serious mental and/or physical effort directed toward purposeful production of something, a known objective or outcome, a self-imposed or other-imposed utilitarian activity to be performed in a predetermined manner and standard of performance (Spencer, 1989, p. 92).
- Work and productive activities include purposeful activities for self-development, social contribution, and livelihood. Includes home management, care of others, educational activities, and vocational activities (AOTA, 1994, p. 1052).
- Refers to activities both paid and unpaid, which provide services or commodities to others (eg, ideas, knowledge, help, information-sharing, utilitarian or artistic objects, and protection) (Kielhofner, 1995, p. 3).
- Work involves activities or tasks done to provide support to the self, family, and society (Trombly, 1995, p. 352).
- Work is any activity, physical or mental, undertaken to achieve a desired outcome (Turner, Foster, & Johnson, 1996, p. 873).
- Work is a category of occupation in which an individual engages for the primary purpose of subsistence (Christiansen & Baum, 1997, p. 606).
- Work is any productive activity, whether paid or unpaid, that contributes to the maintenance or advancement of society as well as the individual. The work in which an individual spends the most time usually becomes both an occupation and a major social role (Creek, 1997, p. 530).
- Work and productive activities are activities that enable people to contribute to society, to support themselves and others dependent on them through work-related activities, and to manage day-to-day activities such as shopping and cleaning (Neistadt & Crepeau, 1998, p. 873).
- Work includes paid or unpaid activity that contributes to subsistence, produces a service or product, and is culturally meaningful to the worker (Stein & Roose, 2000, p. 327).
- Work includes activities needed for engaging in remunerative employment or volunteer activities (AOTA, 2002c, p. 633; based on Mosey, 1996, p. 341).
- Work has a product or result of value to society or an individual, but typically is an aspect of a division of labor that enables the individual to survive as a member of society and promotes the survival of the

society as a whole. In occupational therapy, work means the range of productive activities and tasks which the individual feels obligated to perform and to which time is allocated as a priority, because it is necessary for his or her own benefit or that of others (Duncan, 2006, p. 341).
- Work is "an activity required for subsistence" (Christiansen & Baum, 2005, p. 551).
- An area of occupation that includes activities related to remunerative employment or volunteerism (Christiansen & Matuska, 2011, p. 546).
- Work is a "means of providing a financial or other source of reward to support our daily existence and to help us to meet our need for food and shelter... working holds some meaning for the individual and is tied in some way to his or her identity as a worker and a person" (Braveman, 2012, p. 3).
- Work is exertion or effort directed to accomplish something (Schell et al., 2014, p. 1243).
- Work skills are skills, such as work habits, workmanship, and actual skills related to specific job tasks. The skills may refer to the work of the student, home manager, or paid employee. Home manager skills include as cooking, budgeting, shopping, clothing maintenance, house cleaning, and maintenance (AOTA, 1978, p. 75).

Successful Application of Tools

Tools can be conceptualized based on their success as therapeutic agents. Turner and MacCaul (1996) suggest there are 8 factors that determine the success of a tool for use within occupational therapy practice. These are flexibility, adaptability, relevance, therapeutic richness, usability, defensible and justifiable, robust and replaceable, and finally appropriateness and acceptability. These characteristics are presented in Table 31-11.

Influential Factors, Conditions, or Situations

In occupational therapy practice, tools include factors, conditions, or situations that can influence or change how, why, or where a tool is used. Sometimes the factors, conditions, or situations themselves become tools that can be manipulated or modified to change how an occupation is done. These factors include context, environment, and ecology. Following are some definitions.

Context

- The concept of context is a recent addition to the occupational therapy literature.

Table 31-11. *Tool Use in Occupational Therapy*

- Tools should be flexible, so they can be used in a variety of ways for long and short periods of time and offer a wide variety of therapeutic components.
- Tools should be adaptable, so they can be used within and without the normal domain of expected use. Tools should be relevant to the therapeutic needs, culture, age, and gender requirements of the people who use them.
- Tools should be rich in therapeutic components, so that the occupation offers sufficient therapeutic value, as opposed to non-therapeutic elements.
- Tools should be used by a variety of therapy staff and not be dependent on the skills of 1 or 2 people with specialized training.
- Tools should be therapeutically and professionally justifiable and defended within the scope of occupational therapy practice.
- Tools should be useable within existing resources including staff, time, environment, and cost.
- Tools should be robust and replaceable and conform to health and safety regulations.
- Tools should be aesthetically pleasing and culturally, gender, and age appropriate and acceptable to the clients who will use them.

Adapted from Turner, A., & MacCaul, C. (1996). The therapeutic use of activity. In A. Turner, M. Foster, & S. E. Johnson (Eds.), *Occupational therapy and physical dysfunction: principles, skills, and practices* (4th ed., pp. 125-157). New York, NY: Churchill Livingstone.

- Ryan (1993) stated that context "refers to the social, physical and psychological milieu of the situation" (p. 358).
- Gillen and Burkhardt (1997) defined context as the "circumstances associated with a particular environment or setting" (p. 537).
- Parham and Fazio (1997) suggested that context is "the situation in which an event occurs; includes physical, symbolic, social, cultural, and historical dimensions" (p. 249).
- Neistadt and Crepeau (1998) divided context into 2 aspects: temporal and environmental. "Temporal aspects [include] chronological, culture, developmental, life cycle, disability status; environmental aspects [include] physical, social, cultural" (p. 868).
- Unsworth (1999) did not define context, but did define 2 concepts based on context. Contextual congruence is "a simple environment that requires minimal processing demands...a congruent environment is designed to match the task with the goal" (p. 476). Contextual interference was described as "potential destructors that are normally found in an environment. An environment with contextual interference is complex, requires higher processing demands, and is usually designed to make a goal more difficult to achieve in order to strengthen a learning pattern" (p. 476).

- The setting in which the occupation occurs includes cultural, physical, social, personal, spiritual, temporal, and virtual conditions within and surrounding the client that influence performance (Hussey et al., 2007, p. 287).
- Context includes a variety of inter-related conditions (cultural, physical, social, spiritual, temporal, and virtual) within the surrounding individuals that influence performance; includes the external physical, social, economic, political, and cultural environments in which people function and is sometimes referred to as contextual or environment features or influences (Schell et al., 2014, p. 1231).
- Cultural context includes customs, beliefs, activity patterns, behavior standards, and expectations accepted by the society of which the individual is a member. It includes political aspects, such as laws that affect access to resources and affirm personal rights. Opportunities for education, employment, and economic support are also included (Brown & Stoffel, 2011, p. 777).

Environment

Slagle, in 1923, speaks to the importance of the environment in her article about developing occupational therapy programs in the state of New York. She states that a "complete change of environment" is important in deciding where to locate "the occupational center" and that the location should be away from the ward (p. 597). Thus, concern about environmental issues, such as the arrangement and organization of space, have been discussed in the occupational therapy literature for many years, but the formal interest in environment seems to have started with Dunning's article (1972). Dunning summarized 5 environmental issues: 1) the function and meaning of space; 2) the satisfaction of need through spatial organization; 3) the effect of the environment on social interaction and role performance; 4) environmental influences as these shape psychological processes of learning, perception, cognition, and emotion; and 5) the importance of environmental design and urban planning on human behavior and the quality of life (p. 292). Thereafter, definitions of environment began to appear.

- Hopkins and Smith (1977) defined environment as "a composite of all external forces and influences affecting the development and maintenance of an individual" (p. 731).
- Kielhofner (1985) defined environment as "the objects, persons, and events with which a system interacts" (p. 503).
- Christiansen and Baum (1997) defined environment as "the external social and physical conditions or factors which have the potential to influence an individual" (p. 595).
- Creek (1997) defined environment as "the human and nonhuman surroundings of the individual, including objects, people, events, cultural influences, social norms, and expectations" (p. 529).
- Neistadt and Crepeau (1998) described environment as including "physical (geography, buildings, objects) and social (people, culture, surroundings)" (p. 868).
- Environment is "the external social and physical conditions or factors that have the potential to influence an individual" (Christiansen & Baum 2005, p. 545).
- Brown and Stoffel (2011) defined environment as "the milieu, the aggregate of all of the external conditions and influences affecting the life and development of an individual" (p. 379).
- Environment(s) include particular physical, social, cultural, economic, and political features within a person's everyday life that affects motivation, organization, and performance (Schell et al., 2014, p. 1233).
- Cultural environment ethos and value system of a particular people or group (CAOT, 1991, p. 138).
- Cultural environment includes culture references to values, beliefs, customs, and behaviors that are transmitted from one generation to the next. Culture affects performance by prescribing norms for the use of time and space, and influencing beliefs regarding the importance of activities, work, and play. It also

influences choices in what people do, how they do it, and how important it is to them (Christiansen & Baum, 2005, p. 545 [based on Alman & Chelmens, 1984]; Hall, 1973).
- The natural environment includes geographical features such as terrain, hours of sunlight, climate, and air quality. The natural environment can be a significant factor in determining whether or not an individual's physical limitations are disabling (Christiansen & Baum, 2005, p. 547).
- Physical environment includes natural and manmade surroundings of an individual, and structural living space boundaries (CAOT, 1991, p. 138).
- Physical environment includes the natural and built nonhuman environment, and objects in them (AOTA, 2008, p. 673).
- Environmental attributes include aspects of the environment that can influence an individual's occupational performance in either a negative or positive way (Christiansen & Baum, 2005, p. 545).
- Social environment includes patterns of relationships of people living in an organized community (CAOT, 1991, p. 138).
- The social environment includes the standing of an individual within the group that shapes behavior and attitudes toward self. Social rejection and isolation can have devastating psychological consequences. Social policies govern the availability of resources that control access to services and work (Christiansen & Baum, 2005, p. 550).

A summary of the ideas includes the environment is a composite of all external forces; influences; surroundings, such as physical factors or conditions (geography, building, objects); and social factors or conditions (people, events, culture, social norms and expectation) that have the potential to influence or affect the development and maintenance of an individual. Some writers have subdivided environment in additional categories, which are described in the following definitions.

- Hagedorn (1995) made a distinction between the external environment, which is "the physical and psychosocial environment; the world and universe" (p. 298) and the internal environment, which is "the abstract area in which the individual experiences his inner personal existence and actions" (p. 299).
- Gillen and Burkhardt (1997) also defined environment as including both "the external and internal surroundings that influence a person's development (including the person's own psyche)" (p. 538).
- In 1978, AOTA defined environmental adaptations and structuring environment. Environmental adaptation is defined as "structural or positional

changes designed to facilitate independent living and/or increase safety in the home, work or treatment settings, ie, the installation of ramps, bar; change in furniture heights; adjustment of traffic patterns" (p. 74). Structuring environment is defined as "the organization of the client's time, activities, and/or physical environment in order to enhance performance" (p. 75).

- Hagedorn (1997) also defined environmental adaptation, environmental analysis, and environmental demand. *Environmental adaptation* includes "changing the physical or social features of an environment to enhance performance, promote or restrict a behavior, or provide therapy" (p. 144). *Environmental analysis* is the "observation of features in the physical or social environment and interpretation of their significance or patient performance or therapy" (p. 144). *Environmental demand* is "the combined effect of elements in the environment to produce expectations for certain human actions and reactions" (p. 144). She also defined environmental demand as "the challenges presented by an environment which press the individual to respond by appropriate occupational performance" (2000, p. 308).

- Parham and Fazio (1997) defined environmental negotiation as "those transactions required to succeed in moving through, over, or around obstacles in the physical surroundings; involves the organization of space, time, and social interactions." They defined environmental control system as "any structure, design, instrument, contrivance or device that enables a person with a disability to effect changes in the surroundings in which daily routines take place and thereby gain more functional independence" (p. 249).

Ecology

There are relatively few definitions of ecology in the current occupational therapy literature.

- The first appears in Howe and Briggs (1982), who defined ecology as "the study of the relationship between organisms and their environments" (p. 322).

- Dunn, Brown, and McGuigan (1994) stated that ecology "is concerned with the interrelationships of organisms and their environments" (p. 595).

- Wilcock (1998) defined ecology as "the scientific study of organisms in their natural environment, including the relationships of different species with each other and the environment" (p. 254).

- Ecological sustainability is defined as "to uphold and support the ecology and ecosystems by practices which maintain, and continue to maintain, the

natural environment and relationships of different species" (Wilcock, 1998, p. 254).

- Ecological systems analysis is described as "a model that presents behavior as the result of interaction between an individual with an inherent biopsycholosocial makeup and a given environmental system" (Neistadt & Crepeau, 1998, p. 868).

- Ecology of human performance is described as "a framework for considering the transaction among persons, tasks, and the contexts (ie, temporal, cultural, social, and physical environments) for daily life" (Christiansen & Baum, 1997, p. 595).

- "A framework that emphasizes that the ecology, or the interaction between a person and the context, affects human behavior and task performance" (Neistadt & Crepeau, 1998, p. 868).

Clearly, the interest in occupational therapy for considering contextual issues is expanding. As more occupational therapy practice moves further away from controlled environments, such as a hospital or clinic, the need to understand the context becomes more important. This is because the practitioner enters the client's or consumer's world, where the rules are not determined by the practitioner. Concepts of practice must describe these tools as well as more tradition tools.

Types of Practice Models

Practice models are the composite tools of the profession. They organize ideas and strategies together into a "blueprint" for practitioners to follow. Basically, there are 2 major types of practice models: *body-centered* and *person-centered*. Body-centered models organize the structure (anatomy) and function (physiology) into identifiable "packages." Examples in occupational therapy are the biomechanical model, which stresses the relationship of muscle, bone, nerve, tendon and related soft tissues to each other to produce motor actions and skills. Facilitation techniques (neurodevelopmental therapy, sensory integration, proprioceptive neuromuscular facilitation) stresses the relationship of the nervous system to sensory input and motor output. Cognitive rehabilitation models stress approaches to perception, learning, and memory. The goal is to remediate, restore, or repair any damage or disruption (impairment and activity limitations) to the "normal" structural and functional integrity of the body parts and relationships so the body can return to as normal a pattern of performance as possible, depending on the nature of the disease, disorder, injury, or condition. In contrast, person-centered models assume there is an interaction or transaction between the person (client, patient, student, resident), the environment (context, situation), and the occupations (activities, tasks, roles) to be performed, which can be disrupted leading to participation restrictions. "Normal" is not prescribed in advance, based on average performance of various collated data, but is instead negotiated between the person, the practitioner, and significant others in the person's living situation, based on factors such as values, preferences, and available resources. The goal is to encourage (enable, empower) participation in occupation(s) by facilitating performance through whatever means are effective, efficient, and satisfying for the person (client). Following are some definitions found in the occupational therapy literature.

Body Factor-Centered Models

- Biomechanical frame of reference is used to treat individuals with activity limitations due to impairment in biomechanical body structures and functions (James in Crepeau et al., 2002, p. 240).

- Biomechanical frame of reference is derived from theories in kinetics and kinematics used with individuals who have deficits in the peripheral nervous, musculoskeletal, integumentary (eg, skin), or cardiopulmonary system (Hussey et al., 2007, p. 286).

- Biomechanical approach is a therapeutic intervention focused on improving body movement and strength; typically identified with remediation or improvements in strength, range of motion, or endurance (Schell et al., 2014, p. 1230).

- Cognitive disability frame of reference is based on the premise that cognitive disorders in those with mental health disabilities are caused by neurobiologic deficits or deficits related to the biologic functioning of the brain (Hussey et al., 2007, p. 286).

- Cognitive rehabilitation is a systematic intervention, based on assessment, that may use the range of approaches from remedial to compensation to address the variety of cognitive limitations experienced by a client (Christiansen & Baum, 2005, p. 544).

- Developmental frame of reference postulates that practice in a skill set will enhance brain development and help the child progress through the stages (Hussey et al., 2007, p. 287).

- Facilitation techniques include selection, grading, and modification of sensory input that attempts to encourage motion in a non-functioning muscle or muscle group (AOTA, 1978, p. 74).

- Inhibition techniques include selection, grading, and modification of sensory input that attempts to decrease muscle tone, or excess motion that interferes with function (AOTA, 1978, p. 74).

- Rehabilitation is the restoration to a disabled individual of maximum independence, commensurate with his limitations, by developing his residual capacities (Hopkins & Smith, 1977, p. 737; 1983, p. 926).

- Rehabilitation is a process of intervening to assist an individual to regain previous function loss as a result of an illness or injury (Bonder & Wagner, 1994, p. 386). *Note:* The definition does not specify what type of function (physiological or participation).

- Sensory integration is the organization of sensory input for practical use; the ability to respond to sensory stimuli in a purposeful way (Punwar & Peloquin, 2000, p. 284).

- Sensory integration is the organization of sensations to form perceptions, behaviors, and to learn; a neurological process and theory of the relationship between the neural organization of sensory processing and behavior (Crepeau et al., 2002, p. 1034).

- Task-oriented training includes a wide range of interventions, such as treadmill training, walking training on the ground, bicycling programs, endurance training and circuit training, sit-to-stand exercises, and reaching tasks for improving balance. In addition, use is made of arm training using functional tasks, such as grasping objects, constraint-induced therapy, and mental imagery. Such training is task and patient focused and not occupational therapy practitioner focused (Schell et al., 2014, p. 1242).

Person/Environment (Client)-Centered Models

- Client-centered approach to practice began with Carl Rogers. In his book, *The Clinical Treatment of the Problem Child* (Rogers, 1939) he described a practice that was non-directive and focused on concerns as expressed by the client receiving the service—and recognized the person's unique cultural values. The role of the occupational therapy practitioner, according to Rogers, is to facilitate problem solving through stimulating the person's desire and ability to understand problems and propose solutions that are appropriate for his or her life. Constructs include learning theory, non-directiveness, and non-judgmental approach (Law & Mills, 1998, p. 4).

- Client-centered approach:
  ◊ Philosophy of service committed to respect for and partnership with people receiving services. Emphasizes the individual recipient of service with a focus on developing, restoring, or adapting the individual's skills, and organizing and using assistance available in natural supports from family and friends (Crepeau et al., 2009, p. 1155).

  ◊ Embraces the possibility that the client's beliefs and attitudes may be different from those of the practitioner (Creek & Lougher, 2008, p. 579).

◊ An approach to providing occupational therapy that recognizes the autonomy of the person receiving services, as well as the need for client choice in making decisions regarding occupational needs. This approach emphasizes respect for the client and builds on the strengths that clients bring to the occupational therapy encounter (Cara & MacRae, 2013, p. 964).

- Client-centered practice:
  ◊ Is an approach to service that embraces a philosophy of respect for, and partnership with, people receiving services (Law, Baptiste, & Mills, 1995, p. 253).
  ◊ Is a therapeutic orientation whereby disabled clients engage the assistance and support of a practitioner to facilitate their problem solving and the achievement of their goals. The origins of client-centered practice come from the work of Carl Rogers (1942). Rogers described client-centered therapy as a non-directive approach where the practitioner's role is to create an environment of trust and support, furnishing clients with the opportunity to utilize their own problem-solving capacities to realize their therapeutic goals (McColl & Bickenbach, 1998, pp. 184-185).
  ◊ Is a therapeutic orientation whereby disabled clients engage the assistance and support of a practitioner to facilitate their problem solving and the achievement of their goals (McColl & Bickenbach, 1998, p. 184).
  ◊ An approach in which the client, family, and significant others are active participants throughout the therapeutic process (Hussey et al., 2007 p. 286).
  ◊ Is an orientation that honors the desires and priorities of clients in designing and implementing interventions (AOTA, 2008, p. 670).
  ◊ An approach to providing occupational therapy that recognizes the autonomy of the person receiving services, as well as the need for client choice in making decisions regarding occupational needs. This approach emphasizes respect for the client and builds on the strengths clients bring to the occupational therapy encounter (Cara & MacRae, 2013, p. 964).
  ◊ An orientation that honors the desires and priorities of clients in designing and implementing interventions (Adapted from Dunn, 2000, p. 4; AOTA, 2008, p. 670; Sladyk et al., 2010, p. 613).
- Client-centered care:
  ◊ Therapeutic interventions where the person who is receiving services has a major role in the decision making regarding his or her care. The practitioner

takes a collaborative rather than authoritarian role (Sladyk, Jacobs, & MacRae, 2010, p. 613).
  ◊ An approach to service that incorporates respect for and partnership with clients as active participants in the therapy process. This approach emphasizes client's knowledge and experience, strengths, capacity for choice, and overall autonomy (Schell, Gillen, & Scaffa, 2012, p. 1230).

- Client-centered enablement is based on enablement foundations and employs enablement skills in a collaborative relationship with clients who may be individuals, families, groups, communities, organizations, or populations, to advance a vision of health, well-being, and justice through occupation (Townsend & Polatajko, 2007, p. 365).
- Client-centered occupation-based approaches include occupational therapy interventions and models that emphasize participation in roles and activities as the primary goal of care and engender the active participation of clients in the goal-setting process (Christiansen & Matuska, 2011, p. 538).
- Client-centered practice:
  ◊ A partnership between a client and practitioner that serves to empower a client toward reaching goals of his or her own choosing "An approach to therapy that supports a respectful partnership between therapists and clients" (Law, Baptiste, & Mills, 1995, p. 256).
  ◊ Collaborative and partnership approaches used in enabling occupation with clients who may be individuals, groups, agencies, governments, corporations, or others. Client-centered occupational therapy practitioners demonstrate respect for clients, involve clients in decision making, advocate with and for clients' needs, and otherwise recognize clients' experience and knowledge (Townsend, 2002, p. 180).
  ◊ A partnership between the practitioner and client in which the client's occupational goals are given priority during assessment and treatment. The practitioner listens to and respects the client's standards, and adapts the intervention to meet the client's needs. The client actively participates in negotiating goals for intervention and making decisions (Creek, 2003, p. 50).
  ◊ A collaborative process in which the practitioner, client, and other interested parties negotiate and share choice and control (Creek & Lougher, 2008, p. 579).
  ◊ Emphasis on a client's autonomy and right to choose goals and/or interventions based on his or her identified needs for services (Brown & Stoffel, 2011, p. 775).

◊ A partnership between a practitioner and a client that empowers the client to reach fulfillment in his or her everyday life (Duncan, 2006, p. 337). *Note:* Concept of shared responsibility.

◊ Client-centered practice includes the following concepts: a) a recognition of each clients' unique perspectives; b) a shift in power toward the client having more say in defining and directing intervention; c) a shift to an enablement intervention model; d) an understanding of the importance of the influence on intervention of the client's culture, preferences, interests, roles, and environments; 3) an understanding of the importance of flexible and dynamic intervention that emphasizes learning and problem solving; and f) respect for the client's values, regardless of whether they are shared by the practitioner (Sladyk et al., 2010, p. 613).

• Client-centered therapy is a type of psychotherapy developed by Rogers (1951) that emphasizes the relationship between the client and practitioner, and empowers the client to facilitate psychological growth (Stein & Cutler, 2002, p. 617).

• Client collaboration/client-centered approach to treatment that demonstrates respect for and partnership with the individual or group receiving the service (Crepeau et al., 2003, p. 1027).

• Context-focused therapy is occupational therapy in which the environment and environmentally situated occupations are modified as the mode of intervention (Schell et al., 2014, p. 1231).

• Empowerment models are also referred to as consumer/supervisor models, in which consumers have much greater control over services and may actually provide them (Christiansen & Matuska, 2004, p. 465).

• Environment-focused intervention includes environmental solutions that have the potential to indirectly influence a person's thoughts and beliefs. Educating family, friends, caregivers, and health care professions using the same teaching/learning and cognitive behavior treatment strategies and techniques used with clients is an environmentally focused intervention that can indirectly have a profound impact on modifying a person's dysfunctional beliefs (Brown & Stoffel, 2011, p. 777).

• Habit training:

◊ A re-education program dedicated to restoring and maintaining health by directing activity to construct new habits and discard ineffective ones (Hussey et al., 2007, p. 288).

◊ The development of cultural, personal, and occupational habits in the client with mental illness (Cara & MacRae, 2013, p. 967).

• Health promotion:

◊ A set of activities designed to maximize wellness or function (Bonder & Wagner, 1994, p. 382).

◊ Any planned intervention or services designed to provide individuals and communities with resistance to health threats, often by modifying policy or the environment to decrease potentially harmful interactions (Christiansen & Baum, 2005 [based on the Joint Committee on Health Education and Promotion Terminology, 2001, p. 101]).

• Life redesign is an approach utilized in occupational therapy to help clients make life changes that are healthy, meaningful, and satisfying. It was originally designed specifically for the well elderly, but the approach is now used with a variety of populations (Cara & MacRae, 2013, p. 968).

• Milieu therapy includes treatment using the manipulation of the socioenvironmental setting to benefit the patient (Hopkins & Smith, 1977, p. 734).

• Milieu treatment is a treatment approach that sets rules and expectations for the entire community as they interact together, and originally all staff, whether health professions or maintenance people, were trained in how to respond in a similar manner to the community (Cara & MacRae, 2013, p. 969).

• Occupational adaptation is a model of practice that proposes that occupational therapy practitioners examine how they may change the person, environment, or task so the client may engage in occupations (Hussey et al., 2007, p. 289).

• Person-centered occupational therapy is a partnership between the practitioner and the individual receiving intervention (Sumsion, 1999, p. 56). "The client's occupational goals are given priority and are at the center of assessment and treatment. The practitioner listens to and respects the client's standards and adopts the intervention to meet the client's needs. The client participates actively in negotiating goals for intervention and is empowered to make decisions. The practitioner and the client work together to address the issues presented by a variety of environments to enable the client to fulfill his or her role expectations" (Turner, Foster, & Johnson, 2002, p. 32).

• PEOP Model is a conceptual model used by occupational therapy practitioners to guide clinical reasoning and plan interventions. It emphasizes that occupational performance is influenced by the capacities of the individual, the characteristics of the occupation, and the resources and task demands of the environment (Brown & Stoffel, 2011, p. 786).

Intervention Programs

- PEOP Model is a model of practice that provides definitions and describes the interactive nature of human beings (Hussey et al., 2007, p. 289).

Intervention Programs

- Accommodation approach includes the use of compensatory strategies to help older persons live with a disability (Hasselkus, 1993, p. 748).

- When practitioners adapt, they "design a more supportive context for the person's performance... might enhance some contextual features to provide cues and reduce other features to minimize distractibility" (Dunn, Brown, & McGuigan, 1994, p. 604).

- Neistadt and Crepeau (1998) also followed the idea of changes generated external to the individual in their definition of adaptation: "making the task simpler or less physically demanding to promote independent function" before proceeding to the second part; "changing in response to new demands or expectations" (p. 866). The first part of definition appears to be directed at the practitioner, while the second part appears directed as the client.

- Unsworth (1999) said that adaptation involved "promoting quality of occupational performance by modifying the method used to accomplish a task, modifying the task itself, or changing the environment" (p. 473).

- Adaptation/modification includes reducing environmental barriers by changing the existing environment or the features of the task in which the client will engage (Christiansen & Baum, 2005, p. 544).

- Adaptive includes emphasizing changing the task or aspects of the environment to minimize the effect of underlying deficits, and/or related behaviors in areas of functional performance, eg, reducing the amount of written work (Chu, 2002, p. 378).

- The alter intervention emphasizes selecting a context that enables the person to perform with current skills and abilities, "the occupational therapist would consider the person's skills, abilities, and difficulties and find a context that was compatible with this performance profile" (Dunn, Brown, & McGuigan, 1994, p. 603).

- Compensation includes the use of environmental supports to avert occupational performance problems associated with a personal performance constraint (Christiansen & Baum, 2005, p. 544).

- Compensatory includes emphasizing and minimizing the effect of underlying deficits in areas of function performance, eg, using different color codes to classify lesion files and using a checklist to help the person follow each step of a task (Chu, 2002, p. 379).

- Compensatory includes finding a new way to accomplish a task when performance capacities are limited; occurs through modifying the task or environment (Christiansen & Matuska, 2004, p. 464; 2011, p. 538).

- The compensatory approach is an intervention approach whereby the occupational therapy practitioner adapts the environment, tasks, or teaching method to compensate for the cognitive impairment (Brown & Stoffel, 2011, p. 776).

- Compensatory techniques are used by clients to aid in daily activities. These devices (physical or not) help the client compensate for disabilities, aging-related challenges, or both (Pellerito, 2006, p. 540).

- Therapeutic intervention includes creating circumstances that promote more adaptable or complex performance in context (Dunn, Brown, & McGuigan, 1994, p. 604).

- Create, Promote (as health promotion) includes an intervention approach that does not assume a disability is present or that any factors would interfere with performance. This approach is designed to provide enriched contextual and activity experiences that will enhance performance for all persons in the natural contexts of life (AOTA, 2002c, p. 627 [based on Dunn, McGlain, Brown, & Youngstrom, 1998]).

- A developmental program is designed for an individual who has not developed or learned the skills and tasks appropriate to chronological age (Reed & Sanderson, 1980, p. 80).

- Empowerment:
  ◊ Is a social action process that promotes participation of people, organizations, and community in gaining control over their lives in their community and the larger society (CAOT, 1993, p. 80 [based on Wallerstein & Bernstein, 1988, p. 380]).

  ◊ Means the process of supporting individuals and providing them with opportunities to take control for themselves. It means devolving decision making to local levels and encouraging individual responsibility. Empowerment is about giving control and choice; about participation and consultation. It requires having information to work on and the ability to respond (Stewart, 1994, p. 248).

  ◊ Is personal and social processes that transform visible and invisible relationships so that power is shared more equally (Townsend, 1997, p. 180).

  ◊ Is "a complex participatory process aimed at achieving greater social justice and equity through enabling groups with disadvantages to exercise power and influence" (Christiansen & Townsend, 2004, p. 276). The definition was modified in 2010 to "a complex, participatory process of individual, group, and social change aimed at achieving greater societal justice and equity through enabling groups who are disempowered or otherwise disadvantaged or oppressed to exercise greater power, entitlement, privilege and overall influence as citizens" (Christiansen & Townsend, 2010, p. 418).

◊ The sense of acquiring personal strength through knowledge and skills (Duncan, 2006, p. 338).

◊ Brown and Stoffel (2011) defined empowerment as "increasing the spiritual, political, social, or economic strength of individuals and communities. It often involves developing confidence in one's own capacities" (p. 778).

• Enablement:

◊ Polatajko (1992) described enablement as "the positive form of the term disablement." Enablement incorporated "the concepts of skills, ability and competence as they relate to occupation. Enablement is rooted in a belief in the rights of the individual to autonomy" (p. 196) *(tool, outcome of competence or autonomy)*.

◊ An educational process that occurs within the client-occupational therapy practitioner relationship. Enablement helps people to learn about themselves and their situation, and about their ability to make decisions which fulfill their sense of purpose of in life (CAOT, 1993, p. 80) *(tool, service delivery)*.

◊ Stewart (1994) described enablement as "helping the individual to achieve what is important to that person, and not necessarily about seeking normality or conformity. It is about helping people to respond to their circumstances; to assert their individuality and establish their goals. It is about establishing cooperative relations. It is about removing barriers and creating opportunities which will help individuals to explore new areas, develop skills, and gain mastery over their environment in keeping with their own aspirations" (p. 248) *(tool, outcome of achievement or mastery)*.

◊ The process of helping the individual to achieve what is important to her or him, to respond to her or his circumstances, to assert her or his individuality, and establish her or his goals (Creek, 2003, p. 52 [based on Steward, 1992]) *(tool, outcome of achievement)*.

◊ Is providing a person with the means to develop and maintain an occupational life trajectory premised on attaining a state of well-being (Urbanowski, 2005, p. 303) *(tool)*.

◊ The active involvement of clients in therapy (Duncan, 2006, p. 338).

◊ Processes of facilitating, guiding, coaching, educating, prompting, listening, reflecting, encouraging, or otherwise collaborating with people so that individuals, groups, agencies, or organizations have the means and opportunity to be involved in solving their own problems; enabling is the basis of occupational therapy's client-centered practice and a foundation for client empowerment and justice; enabling is the most appropriate form of helping when the goal is occupational performance (Townsend, 1997, p. 180).

◊ Focus on occupation, is the core competency of occupational therapy—what occupational therapy practitioners actually do—and draws on an interwoven spectrum of key and related enablement skills, which are value-based, collaborative, attentive to power inequities and diversity, and charged with visions of possibility for individual and/or social change (Townsend, 2007, p. 367).

◊ The positive form of the term *disablement*; creation of the opportunity to participate in life's tasks and occupations irrespective of physical or mental impairment or environmental challenges (Christiansen & Townsend, 2004, p. 276). Use of processes such as adaptation, advocacy, collaboration, coordination, education, and design in mutual, reciprocal relationships with others to create opportunities, policies, legislation, and economic conditions, while also prompting others to develop the personal factors to participate to their highest potential in the occupations that they need and want to do as citizens; to promote health, well-being, and social inclusion, irrespective of physical or mental impairment or environmental challenges (Christiansen & Townsend, 2010, p. 418).

◊ The process of creating opportunities to participate in life's tasks and occupations irrespective of physical or mental impairment or environmental challenges (Creek, 2010; adapted from Christiansen & Townsend, 2004, p. 278).

• Enabling occupation includes enabling people to "choose, organize, and perform those occupations they find useful and meaningful in their environment" (Townsend, 1997, 2002, p. 180) *(tool)*.

• Environmental adjustment is an "alternative to the remediation... when change and recovery within the individual have achieved a level of function that can be expected [but] further improvement... can be expected if the external environment is changed to reduce barriers to performance" (Reed & Sanderson, 1980, p. 80).

- Establish or restore (remediate) includes the occupational therapy practitioner identifying the person's skills and barriers to performance, and designing interventions that improve the person's skills and abilities (Dunn, Brown, & McGuigan, 1994, p. 603).

- Establish, restore (remediation, restoration) is an intervention approach designed to change client variables to establish a skill or ability that has not yet developed or to restore a skill or ability that has been impaired (AOTA, 2002c, p. 627 [adapted from Dunn, McClain, Brown, & Youngstrom, 1998]).

- Establishment includes attaining a new skill (Christiansen & Baum, 2005, p. 549).

- Functional approach includes emphasizing and facilitating mastery of tasks, eg, specific motor skills training, practice of handwriting skills, etc. It is important to equip the person with adequate skills to cope with the demands of different learning and daily activities (Chu, 2002, p. 377).

- Grading is an activity chosen that matches the capabilities of the individual. As the individual masters an activity, then a slightly more difficult activity is introduced (Bonder & Wagner, 1994, p. 382).

- Measurable increase or decrease in activity, graded by length of time, size, degree of strength required or amount of energy expended (Duncan, 2006, p. 338).

- Habilitate is to educate or train (the mentally or physically handicapped, the disadvantaged) to function better in society (Hopkins & Smith, 1977, p. 733).

- Client is able to perform many skills independently, but must continue to perform these skills in order to maintain health (Reed & Sanderson, 1980, p. 81).

- Management includes emphasizing and minimizing distressing or disruptive feelings and behavior so that the dyspraxic child is able to deal more directly with primary problems, eg, psychological support, praise/reward, social skill training, etc (Chu, 2002, p. 379).

- Maintain is an intervention approach designed to provide the supports that will allow clients to preserve the performance capabilities they have regained, that continue to meet their occupational needs, or both. The assumption is that, without continued maintenance intervention, performance would decrease, occupational needs would not be met, or both; thereby affecting health and quality of life (AOTA, 2002c, p. 627; Christiansen & Matuska, 2011, p. 542).

- Maintenance is an approach that emphasizes preserving and supporting the child's current level of function in a protected environment, eg, use of high-power IT equipment for a dyspraxic child who

has extreme difficulty in manual handwriting skills (Chu, 2002, p. 379).

- Modification is an intervention approach directed at finding ways to revise the current context or activity demands to support performance in the natural setting, including compensatory techniques such as enhancing some features to provide cues or reducing other features to reduce distractibility (Christiansen & Matuska, 2011, p. 542).

- Modify (compensation, adaptation) is an intervention approach directed at "finding ways to revise the current context or activity demands to support performance in the natural setting... [includes] compensatory techniques, including enhancing some features to provide cues, or reducing other features to reduce distractibility" (AOTA, 2002c, p. 627 [based on Dunn, McClain, Brown, & Youngstrom, 1998]).

- Occupation-based intervention refers to the use of occupation as a treatment modality, and emphases occupations that are meaningful and pertinent to the client's daily life and goals for living (Cara & MacRae, 2013, p. 970).

- Prevent (disability prevention) is an intervention approach designed to address clients with or without a disability who are at risk for occupational performance problems. This approach is designed to prevent the occurrence or evolution of barriers to performance in context; interventions may be directed at client, context, or activity variables (AOTA, 2002c, p. 627 [adapted from Dunn, McClain, Brown, & Youngstrom, 1998]).

- Prevent:
  ◊ Occupational therapy practitioners can create interventions to change the course of events by addressing person, context, and task variables to enable functional performance to emerge (Dunn, Brown, & McGuigan, 1994, p. 604).
  ◊ Supporting occupational performance by anticipating problems and taking actions to avert problems that will impact occupational performance (Christiansen & Baum, 2005, p. 549).

- Prevention:
  ◊ A prevention program is focused on keeping problems from happening (primary prevention) or, if a problem has developed, to keep it from getting worse (secondary prevention) (Reed & Sanderson, 1980, p. 79).
  ◊ Refers to skill and performance in minimizing debilitation. It may include programs for persons where predisposition to disability exists, as well as for those who have already incurred a disability. This includes, but is not limited to, energy conservation,

joint protection/body mechanics, positioning, and coordination of daily living activities (AOTA, 1981, 827).

- Prevention approach includes the maintenance of current health status and the prevention of decline or injury (Hasselkus, 1993, p. 748).

- Remedial:
  ◊ Emphasizes "facilitating the improvement of underlying process, eg, improving practice function in a [person] with dyspraxia. It is diagnostic-prescriptive in nature... approach assumes that adequate skill performance depends on the integrity and integration of the [person's] sensory, perceptual, cognitive, and motor performance components" (Chu, 2002, p. 377).

  ◊ An intervention that is designed to improve or establish a skill or ability that has not yet been developed in order to meet the requirements of task demands (Christiansen & Matuska, 2011, p. 544).

- Remediation:
  ◊ Strategies that focus on restoring or improving function within performance components, such as in sensation, cognition, or voluntary movement, and includes training. (Christiansen, 2000, p. 404).

  ◊ Correct the problem (Christiansen & Baum, 2005, p. 549).

  ◊ Intervention designed to change a client's body functions, structures, values, skills, beliefs, performance skills, performance patterns, and overall occupational performance (Christiansen & Matuska, 2011, p. 544).

  ◊ An intervention approach designed to change client variables to establish a skill or ability that has not yet developed or to restore a skill or ability that has been impaired (Schell et al., 2014, p. 1240).

- Remediation program:
  ◊ Accepts individuals who have lost skills to illness or trauma, but can be expected to regain some skills or relearn some activities through a "specialized intervention" program (Reed & Sanderson, 1980, p. 80).

  ◊ A course of action determine by the DRS (driver rehabilitation specialist) to help the client develop the necessary client factors, such as strength or cognitive skills, to meet predetermined goals, such as passing a standard license test (Pellerito, 2006, p. 544).

- Resolve includes supporting occupational performance by identifying performance problems and taking action to correct them (Christiansen & Baum, 2005, p. 549).

- Restoration includes recovering a skill that was lost (Christiansen & Baum, 2005, p. 549).

- Restoration approach includes the use of rehabilitative techniques to help an older person regain maximum function (Hasselkus, 1993, p. 748).

- Restorative occupation includes using occupations to facilitate restoring person factors and/or body function (Schell et al., 2014, p. 1240).

- Therapeutic adaptations refers to the "design and/or restructuring of the physical environment to assist self-care, work, and play/leisure performance. [Includes] orthotics, prosthetics, [and] assistive/adaptive equipment" (AOTA, 1981, p. 837).

SUMMARY

This review of the history and use of selected occupational therapy concepts points out the importance of and need for a better understanding and use for the concepts within the field of occupational therapy. Many of the concepts used in occupational therapy models, theories, frameworks, and position papers originated outside the field of occupational therapy. Some concepts have been adopted without modification; other concepts have been modified to suit the intent of occupational therapy writers, leaders, practitioners, and researchers. A frequent modification is the addition of the word "occupational" in front of a common English word (ie, occupational balance, occupational competence, occupational identity, occupational justice, occupational performance, occupational readiness, etc). While creating a vocabulary is inherent in the development of a profession's unique knowledge base, adding an adjective (occupational) to any noun does not automatically make the resulting phrase a useful part of the professional vocabulary. To be useful, the phrase must be carefully defined to describe phenomena that are unique to the knowledge base of occupational therapy. Simply adding words and phrases does not necessarily advance the profession's body of knowledge, but instead may add to the vagueness and lack of clarity—neither of which is needed. As occupational therapy practitioners communicate with other professions, occupational therapy writers and leaders must identify and understand the source of the concept or concepts being discussed and indicate what, if any, modifications have been made to the formative ideas about that concept from the original discipline's literature. Doing one's professional "homework" is part of the scholarly advancement of knowledge and professional literature. There is work yet to be done. The concepts of occupational therapy must be better integrated within the knowledge base. Hierarchies and taxonomies are examples of classification systems, but models and theories can perform a similar purpose of structuring and organizing the concepts into logical groups and sequences. Currently, the number of concepts and the lack of organization are barriers to effective student learning and to sharing ideas within and without the profession. Terms and concepts translate into learning definitions and understanding where and when to apply the information. Occupational therapy does encompass a wide range of ideas, so the number of terms and concepts is likely to be large. This chapter has been my attempt to begin the work to organize the professions concepts.

Techniques Used in This Chapter to Study Concepts

Several techniques have been used to study the concepts in this chapter. All of these techniques can be used to better organize and refine concepts in occupational therapy. The specific techniques have included the following:

- Use in context as the term or concept appeared in the original text of an article written by a prominent writer in the occupational therapy literature.

- Definitions of terms and concepts as they appear in glossaries of textbooks of occupational therapy, including multiple meanings of the same term.

- Definitions appearing in standard dictionaries of the English language, especially unabridged dictionaries that list multiple meanings of the same term. Also definitions appearing in specialized dictionaries, such as psychology and rehabilitation. Specifically addressed was the origin of a term as stated in a dictionary, comparison of terms and concepts using synonyms and antonyms, and word/phrase themes from published articles or books.

- Explanation of concepts that have developed from philosophy and different philosophical views of the world.

- Explanation of the use of concepts from another discipline, especially when the concept is used as described in the originating discipline or if the concept has been changed in the occupational therapy literature.

- Comparison of definitions of a term or concept over a time period by examining definitions from dictionaries published several years apart.

- Comparison of usage of a term or concept over a time period by examining use from articles or books published several years apart.

- Examination of the assumptions stated in the development of a concept or associated with an existing conceptual model.

- Examination of how concepts have appeared and been organized in various models of practice in occupational therapy.

A technique not used in this chapter, but used in nursing literature (Walker & Avant, 1995; Rodgers & Knafl, 2000) is the case method, in which the term or concept is developed in a short case study that is designed to convey the current usage in context so that other usages can be compared and contrasted against the case. The case method approach is useful for examining one concept, but would have been too lengthy to use in this chapter.

Finally, words, terminology, and concepts are most useful when they convey ideas or notions that are important to the communication system in which they are used. Concepts should be developed and nurtured carefully to ensure that their meaning and intent is clear and articulated with other concepts in a relationship that conveys the relationship of one concept to another. Fuzzy logic (a computer term) is not needed when communicating the profession's body of knowledge, and word salad (a jumble of incoherent words or neologisms) is not helpful in professional communication. There should be rules in professional communication such as (1) do not create new words or phrases if an existing word or phrase will do, (2) clearly define any new word or phrase, (3) justify why the new word or phrase is needed, and (4) carefully explain where the new word or phrase "fits" into the professional vocabulary and relates to other existing concepts. When in doubt, keep it simple.

Note From the Author and Editors

As this chapter was being prepared for publication, a 3rd edition of the AOTA *Occupational Therapy Practice Framework* was published (AOTA, 2014). The key revisions include a change in the definition of client to include individuals, groups, and populations; a modification to the description of occupational therapy's domain and process, described as "achieving health, well-being, and participation in life through engagement in occupation"; and some modifications in how interventions and types of service delivery are organized and defined (AOTA, 2014, p. S4). For example, self-advocacy and group interventions have been added as intervention types, while consultation is described as a type of service delivery, and therapeutic use of self is recognized not as a type of intervention, as it had previously been viewed, but a characteristic that is now seen as integral to all types of interventions (AOTA, 2014, p. S2).

No doubt, this document, which influences how terms are defined and used by occupational therapists in the United States, will continue to evolve. The reader should view these changes as emblematic of the ongoing manner in which concepts and terms evolve and change over time. By observing these changes in the newest version of the AOTA *Framework*, one can clearly see that refinements in how groups use terms and concepts continue to alter the language of the profession.

Selected terms relevant to this chapter and their definitions and uses as contained in the 2014 AOTA *Practice Framework* are as follows:

- *Autonomy*: Not defined individually, but mentioned as an aspect of client-centered practice: "The intervention process consists of the skilled services provided by occupational therapy practitioners in collaboration with clients to facilitate engagement in occupation related to health, well-being, and participation" (AOTA, 2014, p. S41).

- *Areas of occupation*: Redefined as simply "occupations" (AOTA, 2014, p. S2).

- *Clients*: Redefined as "persons, groups, and populations" (AOTA, 2014, p. S2).

- *Competence*: Reference is made only to occupational therapists' professional competence (AOTA, 2014, p. S47).

- *Coping*: Not redefined; mentioned in relation to mental health: "Similarly, services addressing independent living skills for adults coping with serious and persistent mental illness may also address the needs and expectations of state and local services agencies and of potential employers" (AOTA, 2014, p. S11).

- *Context*: Defined as a "variety of interrelated conditions within and surrounding the client that influence performance, including cultural, personal, temporal, and virtual contexts" (AOTA, 2014, p. S42).

- *Engagement in occupation*: No change from 2008 Framework.

- *Fitness*: Listed under Health Management and Maintenance with IADL. Defined as "developing, managing, and maintaining routines for health and wellness promotion, such as physical fitness, nutrition, decreased health risk behaviors, and medication routines" (AOTA, 2014, p. S19).

- *Framework*: No addition or change found for this term.

- *Function*: Term used only to describe body functions in the context of practitioners having knowledge of them and understanding their impact on engagement in occupation (AOTA, 2008; 2014, p. S23).

- *Health*: Defined as "a state of complete physical, mental, and social well-being, and not merely the absence of disease or infirmity" (WHO, 2006, p. 1; 2014, p. S42).

- *Independence*: No change.

- *Interdependence*: Defined in glossary as the "reliance that people have on one another as a natural consequence of group living" (Christiansen & Townsend, 2010, p. 419). "Interdependence engenders a spirit of social inclusion, mutual aid, and a moral commitment and responsibility to recognize and support difference" (Christiansen & Townsend, 2010, p. 187; AOTA, 2014, p. S43).

- *Life balance*: Not mentioned.

- *Models*: Occupational therapy practitioners use theoretical principles and models, knowledge about the effects of conditions on participation, and available evidence of the effectiveness of intervention to guide their reasoning (AOTA, 2014, p. S12).

- *Occupation*: Defined as "the daily life activities in which people engage" (AOTA, 2014, p. S6) and elaborated to identify aspects of its complexity, including context, client characteristics, performance dimensions, temporal aspects, perceived meaning, and major categories.

- *Occupational Therapy*: Comprehensively defined as "the therapeutic use of everyday life activities (occupations) with individuals or groups for the purpose of enhancing or enabling participation in roles, habits, and routines in home, school, workplace, community, and other settings. Occupational therapy practitioners use their knowledge of the transactional relationship among the person, his or her engagement in valuable occupations, and the context to design occupation-based intervention plans that facilitate change or growth in client factors (body functions, body structures, values, beliefs, and spirituality) and skills (motor, process, and social interaction) needed for successful participation. Occupational therapy practitioners are concerned with the end result of participation and thus enable engagement through adaptation and modifications to the environment or objects within the environment when needed. Occupational therapy services are provided for habilitation, rehabilitation, and promotion of health and wellness for clients with disability- and non–disability-related needs. These services include acquisition and preservation of occupational identity for those who have or are at risk for developing an illness, injury, disease, disorder, condition, impairment, disability, activity limitation, or participation restriction" (AOTA, 2014, p. S1).

- *Occupational balance*: Not mentioned explicitly. However, the document does state that "the extent to which a person is involved in a particular occupational engagement is also important. Occupations can contribute to a well-balanced and fully functional lifestyle or to a lifestyle that is out of balance and characterized by occupational dysfunction" (AOTA, 2014, p. S6).

- *Outcomes*: Determinants of success in reaching the desired end result of the occupational therapy process. Outcome assessment information is used to plan future actions with the client and to evaluate the service program (i.e., program evaluation) (AOTA, 2014, p. S10).

- *Performance skills*: Redefined as "observable elements of action that have an implicit functional purpose; skills are considered a classification of actions, encompassing multiple capacities (body functions and body structures) and, when combined, underlie the ability to participate in desired occupations and activities" (AOTA, 2014, p. S25).

- *Prevention*: One of five approaches to intervention identified in the 2014 Framework. Defined as an intervention approach designed to address the needs of clients with or without a disability who are at risk for occupational performance problems (AOTA, 2014, p. S33).

- *Quality of life*: Dynamic appraisal of the client's life satisfaction (perceptions of progress toward goals), hope (real or perceived belief that one can move toward a goal through selected pathways), self-concept (the composite of beliefs and feelings about oneself), health and functioning (e.g., health status, self-care capabilities), and socioeconomic factors (e.g., vocation, education, income) (AOTA, 2014, p. S35).

- *Recovery*: Not referenced in the 2014 Framework.

- *Satisfaction*: Not mentioned or defined as an individual term in the 2014 Framework. Contained in other descriptions regarding the client, including quality of life.

- *Self-efficacy*: Not mentioned as a stand-alone term but as a type of client outcome.

- *Self-management*: Not identified as a stand-alone term. However, it is mentioned as a focus of intervention in services to groups and populations (e.g., "The intervention focus often is on health promotion activities, self-management, educational services, and environmental modification") (AOTA, 2014, p. S15).

- *Theory*: Not defined as a stand-alone term but used as a synonym for framework or model.

- *Well-being*: Not used as a stand-alone term, but the following sentence shows that it is viewed as a type of intervention outcome: "The intervention process consists of the skilled services provided by occupational therapy practitioners in collaboration with clients to facilitate engagement in occupation related to health, well-being, and participation" (AOTA, 2014, p. S14).

REFERENCES

Aldrich, R. M. (2011). A review and critique of well-being in occupational therapy and occupational science. *Scandinavian Journal of Occupational Therapy, 18,* 93-100.

Allen, C. A. (1985). *Occupational therapy for psychiatric diseases: Measurement and management of cognitive disabilities.* Boston, MA: Little, Brown, and Company.

Angeles, P. W. (1981). *Dictionary of philosophy.* New York, NY: Barnes & Noble.

Anthony, W. A. (1993). Recovery from mental illness: The guiding vision of the mental health service system in the 1990s. *Psychosocial Rehabilitation Journal, 16,* 11-23.

AOTA. (1923). *Principles of occupational therapy, Bulletin No. 4.* New York, NY: The Association.

AOTA. (1958). *Objectives and functions of occupational therapy.* Dubuque, IA: William C. Brown Book Co.

AOTA. (1972). Occupational therapy: Its definition and functions. *American Journal of Occupational Therapy, 26,* 204-205.

AOTA. (1973). *The roles and functions of occupational therapy personnel* (Grant Contract No. N01-AH-24172). Rockville, MD: The Association.

AOTA. (1974). Task force on target populations, Report II. *American Journal of Occupational Therapy, 28*(4), 231-236.

AOTA. (1976). Essentials of an approved education program for the Occupational Therapy Assistant. *American Journal of Occupational Therapy, 30*(4), 245-263.

AOTA. (1978). Uniform terminology for reporting occupational therapy services. In *Manual on Administration* (pp. 73-75). Dubuque, IA: Kendall/Hunt Publishing Co.

AOTA. (1979a). The philosophical base of occupational therapy. *American Journal of Occupational Therapy, 33,* 785.

AOTA. (1979b). Uniform terminology for reporting occupational therapy services. In H. L. Hopkins & H. D. Smith (Eds.), (1983). *Willard and Spackman's occupational therapy,* (6th ed., pp. 899-907). Philadelphia, PA: J. B. Lippincott.

AOTA. (1981). Entry-level role delineation for OTRs and COTAs. In H. L. Hopkins & H. D. Smith (Eds.), (1988). *Willard and Spackman's occupational therapy* (7th ed., pp. 814-828). Philadelphia, PA: J. B. Lippincott.

AOTA. (1989). Uniform terminology for occupational therapy (2nd ed.). *American Journal of Occupational Therapy, 43*(12), 808-815.

AOTA. (1994). Uniform terminology for occupational therapy (3rd ed.). *American Journal of Occupational Therapy, 48,* 1047-1054.

AOTA. (1995). Position paper: Broadening the construct of independence. *American Journal of Occupational Therapy, 49*(10), 1014.

AOTA. (2002a). Broadening the construct of independence (position paper). *American Journal of Occupational Therapy, 56,* 660.

AOTA. (2002b). Glossary. In *Occupational therapy practice framework: domain and process.* Draft XVIII Final—January, Commission on Practice. Unpublished.

AOTA. (2002c). Occupational therapy practice framework: domain and process. *American Journal of Occupational Therapy, 56*(6), 609-639.

AOTA. (2008). Glossary. In Occupational therapy practice framework: domain and process (2nd ed.). *American Journal of Occupational Therapy, 62*(6), 625-683.

AOTA. (2011). The philosophical base of occupational therapy. *American Journal of Occupational Therapy, 65*(6 Suppl.), S65.

AOTA. (2014). Occupational therapy practice framework: Domain and process. *American Journal of Occupational Therapy, 68*(Supplement 1), S1-S51.

Arts and crafts movement. (2001). In M. Agnes & D. B. Guralnik (Eds.). Webster's New World College Dictionary (4th ed., p. 81). Foster City, CA: IDG Books Worldwide Inc.

Augustine, H., Roberts, J., & Packer, T. (2011). Everyday participation: important outcomes for people with chronic conditions. *Occupational Therapy Now, 13*(4), 8-10.

Azima, H., & Azima, F. (1959). Outline of a dynamic theory of occupational therapy. *American Journal of Occupational Therapy, 13*(5), 215-221.

Backman, C. L. (2004) Occupational balance: exploring the relationship among daily occupations and their influence on well-being. *Canadian Journal of Occupational Therapy, 71*(4), 202-209.

Baldwin, B. T. (1919). *Occupational therapy applied to restoration of function of disabled joints. (Walter Reed Monograph).* Washington, DC: Walter Reed General Hospital.

Bandura, A. (1977). Self-efficacy: toward a unifying theory of behavioral change. *Psychological Review, 84,* 191-215.

Bandura, A. (1986). *Social foundations of thought.* Englewood Cliffs, NJ: Prentice Hall.

Bandura, A., Cioffi, D., Taylor, C. B., & Brouillard, M. E. (1988). Perceived self-efficacy in coping with cognitive stressors and opiate activation. *Journal of Personality and Social Psychology, 55,* 479-488.

Barnes & Noble. (1995). *Webster's new universal unabridged dictionary.* New York, NY: Barnes & Noble.

Barton, G. E. (1917). *Re-education: an analysis of the institutional system of the United States.* Boston, MA: Houghton Mifflin.

Barton, W. E., (1987). *The history and influence of the American Psychiatric Association.* Washington, DC: The Association.

Baum, C., & Christiansen, C. (1997). The occupational therapy context: philosophy-principles-practice. In C. Christensen & C. Baum (Eds.), *Occupational therapy: enabling function and well-being* (pp. 27-45). Thorofare, NJ: SLACK Incorporated.

Baum, C., & Edwards, D. (1995). Occupational performance: occupational therapy's definition of function. *American Journal of Occupational Therapy, 49*(10), 1019-1020.

Baum, C. M., & Law, M. (1997). Occupational therapy practice: focusing on occupational performance. *American Journal of Occupational Therapy, 51*(4), 277-288.

Bennett, R. L. (1950). Rehabilitation in poliomyelitis. In H. H. Kessler (Ed.), *The principles and practice of rehabilitation* (324-360). Philadelphia, PA: Lea & Febiger.

Bockoven, J. S. (1971). Occupational therapy—a historical perspective, legacy of moral treatment—1800s to 1910. *American Journal of Occupational Therapy, 25*(5), 223-225.

Bonder, B. B., & Wagner, M. B. (1994). Glossary. In B. B. Bonder & M. B. Wagner (Eds.), *Functional performance in older adults* (pp. 378-387). Philadelphia, PA: F. A. Davis.

Borys, S. S. (1974). Implications of interest theory for occupational therapy. *American Journal of Occupational Therapy, 28*(1), 35-38.

Bothamley, J. (1993). *Dictionary of theories.* London, England: Gale Research International Ltd.

Bowman, E. (1922). Psychology of occupational therapy. *Archives of Occupational Therapy, 1*(3), 171-178.

Braveman, B. (2012). Work in the modern world. In B. Braveman & J. J. Page (Eds.), *Work: Promoting participation & productivity through occupational therapy* (pp. 2-27). Philadelphia, PA: F. A. Davis.

Brown, C. (Ed). (2001). *Recovery and wellness: models of hope and empowerment for people with mental illness.* New York, NY: Haworth Press.

Brown, C., & Stoffel, V. C. (2011). Glossary. In C. Brown & V. C. Stoffel (Eds.), *Occupational therapy in mental health: a vision for participation* (pp. 773-792). Philadelphia, PA: F. A. Davis.

Brown, C., & Stoffel, V. C. (2012). *Occupational therapy in mental health: A vision for participation.* Philadelphia, PA: F. A. Davis.

Brown, K., & Gillespie, D. (1992). Recovering relationships: a feminist analysis of recovery models. *American Journal of Occupational Therapy, 46*(11), 1001-1005.

Buchwald, E. (1949). Functional training. *Physical Therapy Review, 29*(11), 491-496.

Buchwald, E. (1952). *Physical rehabilitation for daily living.* New York, NY: McGraw-Hill.

Burnette, N. (1918). *Invalid occupation in war hospitals (Manual No. 1).* Ontario, Canada: Department of Soldiers Civil Re-Establishment, Invalided Soldiers' Commission, Vocational Branch.

Cammack, S., & Eisenberg, M. G. (Eds.). (1995). *Key words in physical rehabilitation: A guide to contemporary usage.* New York, NY: Springer Publishing Co.

CAOTA. (1991). *Occupational therapy guidelines for client-centred practice.* Toronto, ON: CAOTA.

CAOTA. (1993). *Occupational therapy guidelines for client-centred mental health practice.* Toronto, ON: CAOTA.

Cara, E., & MacRae, A. (1998). Glossary. In E. Cara & A. MacRae (Eds.). *Psychosocial occupational therapy: a clinical practice.* New York, NY: Delmar Publishers.

Cara, E., & MacRae, A. (2013). *Psychosocial occupational therapy: An evolving practice* (3rd ed.). Independence, KY: Delmar Cengage Learning.

Christiansen, C. (1994). Classification and study in occupation: a review and discussion of taxonomies. *Journal of Occupational Science: Australia, 1*(3), 3-21.

Christiansen, C. (1996). Three perspectives on balance in occupation. In R. Zemke & F. Clark (Eds.). *Occupational science: the evolving discipline* (pp. 431-451). Philadelphia, PA: F. A. Davis.

Christiansen, C. (1999). Defining lives, occupation as identify, *American Journal of Occupational Therapy, 53,* 548-549.

Christiansen, C. H. (2000). *Ways of living* (2nd ed.). Bethesda, MD: American Occupational Therapy Association.

Christiansen, C., & Baum, C. (1991). Glossary. In C. Christiansen & C. Baum (Eds.), *Occupational therapy: overcoming human performance deficits* (pp. 847-860). Thorofare, NJ: SLACK Incorporated.

Christiansen, C., & Baum, C. (1997). Glossary. In C. Christiansen & C. Baum (Eds.), *Occupational therapy: enabling function and well-being* (2nd ed., pp. 591-606). Thorofare, NJ: SLACK Incorporated.

Christiansen, C., & Baum, C. (2005). Glossary. In C. Christiansen & C. Baum (Eds.). *Occupational therapy: performance, participation, and well-being* (pp. 543-554). Thorofare, NJ: SLACK Incorporated.

Christiansen, C. H., & Matuska, K. M. (2004). *Ways of living: Intervention strategies to enable participation* (3rd ed.). Bethesda, MD: AOTA Press.

Christiansen, C. H., & Matuska, K. M. (2011). *Ways of living: Intervention strategies to enable participation* (4th ed.). Bethesda, MD: AOTA Press.

Christiansen, C., & Townsend, E. A. (2004). *Introduction to occupation: the art and science of living.* Upper Saddle River, NJ: Prentice-Hall.

Christiansen, C.H., & Townsend, E.A. (2010). *Introduction to occupation: The art and science of living* (2nd ed). Upper Saddle River, NJ: Pearson.

Chu, S. (2002). Children with developmental dyspraxia. In C. S. Hong & L. Howard (Eds.), *Occupational therapy in childhood* (pp. 365-383). London, England: Whurr.

Clark, F. A., Parham, D., Carlson, M. E., Frank, G., Jackson, J., Peirce, D., Wolfe, R. J., & Zemke, R. (1991). Occupational science: Academic innovation in the service of occupational therapy's future. *American Journal of Occupational Therapy, 45*(4), 300-310.

Clark, F., Ennevor, B. L., & Richardson, P. L. (1996). A grounded theory of techniques for occupational storytelling and occupational story making. In R. Zemke & F. Clark (Eds.), *Occupational science: the evolving discipline* (pp. 373-392). Philadelphia, PA: F. A. Davis.

Coelho, G. V., Hamburg, D. A., & Adams, J. E. (Eds.). (1974). *Coping and adaptation*. New York, NY: Basic Books.

Cole, M. B., & Donohue. M. V. (2011). *Social participation in occupational contexts in schools, clinics, and communities*. Thorofare, NJ: SLACK Incorporated.

Corsini, R. (1999). *The dictionary of psychology*. New York, NY: Brunner/Routledge.

Corsini, R. (2002). *The dictionary of psychology*. Philadelphia, PA: Brunner/Mazel.

Coulter, J. S. (1950). Occupational therapy in a private general hospital. In *American Medical Association handbook of physical medicine and rehabilitation* (pp. 452-483). Philadelphia, PA: Blackiston Co.

Crepeau, E. B. (1994). Rituals. In C. B. Royeen (Ed.), *The practice of the future: putting occupation back into therapy. AOTA self-study series #6* (pp. 1-32). Bethesda, MD: AOTA.

Crepeau, E. B., Cohn, E. B., & Schell, B. A. B. (2003). *Willard & Spackman's occupational therapy* (10th ed.). Philadelphia, PA: Lippincott Williams & Wilkins.

Crepeau, E. B., Cohn, E. B., & Schell, B. A. B. (2009). *Willard & Spackman's occupational therapy* (11th ed.). Philadelphia, PA: Lippincott Williams & Wilkins.

Creek, J. (1997). Glossaries—occupational therapy terms. In J. Creek (Ed.), *Occupational therapy and mental health* (2nd ed., pp. 529-530). New York, NY: Churchill Livingstone.

Creek, J. (2003). *Occupational therapy defined as a complex intervention*. London, England: College of Occupational Therapist.

Creek, J. (1990). *Occupational therapy and mental health*. Edinburgh, Scotland: Churchill Livingstone.

Creek, J. (2002). Occupational therapy and mental health (3rd ed.). Edinburgh, Scotland: Churchill Livingstone.

Creek, J. (2007). Engaging the reluctant client. In J. Creek & A. Lawson-Porter (Eds.). *Contemporary issues in occupational therapy: Reasoning and reflection* (pp. 127-142). West Sussex, England: John Wiley & Sons.

Creek, J. (2008). Glossary. In Creek, J. *Occupational therapy in mental health* (4th ed., pp. 579-583). Edinburgh, Scotland: Churchill Livingstone Elsevier.

Creek, J. (2010). *The core concepts of occupational therapy: a dynamic framework for practice*. London, England: Jessica Kingsley Publishers.

Creek, J., & Lougher, L. (2008). *Occupational therapy and mental health* (4th ed.). Edinburgh, Scotland: Churchill Livingstone Elsevier.

Crist, P. A. H., & Stoffel, V. C. (1992). The Americans with Disabilities Act of 1990 and employees with mental impairments: personal efficacy and the environment. *American Journal of Occupational Therapy, 46*(5), 434-443.

Csikszentmihalyi, M. (1975). *Beyond boredom and anxiety*. San Francisco, CA: Jossey-Bass.

Csikszentmihalyi, M. (1990). *Flow: the psychology of optimal experience*. New York, NY: Harper & Row.

Csikszentmihalyi, M., & Csikszentmihalyi, I. S. (1988). *Optimal experience: psychological studies of flow in consciousness*. Cambridge, England: Cambridge University Press.

Davis, J. Z. (1996). Neurodevelopmental treatment of adult hemiplegia: the Bobath approach. In L. W. Pedretti (Ed.), *Occupational therapy: practice skills for physical dysfunction* (4th ed., pp. 435-461). St. Louis, MO: Mosby.

Deaver, G. G., & Brown, M. E. (1945). *Physical demands of daily life: an objective scale for rating the orthopedically exceptional. (Studies in rehabilitation I)*. New York, NY: Institute for Crippled and Disabled.

Deci, E. L. (1975). *Intrinsic motivation*. New York, NY: Plenum Press.

Dewey, J. (1916). *Democracy and education: an introduction to the philosophy of education*. New York, NY: Macmillian. Reprinted edition by Simon & Schuster Inc., New York.

Dewey, J. (1990). *The school and society and the child and the curriculum: a centennial edition*. Chicago, IL: University of Chicago Press (reprint of *The child and curriculum*, 1902; and *The school and society*, 1900, 1915 [Rev. ed.], and 1943).

Doble, S. (1988). Intrinsic motivation and clinical practice: the key to understanding the unmotivated client. *Canadian Journal of Occupational Therapy, 55*(2), 75-81.

do Rozario, L. (1994). Ritual, meaning, and transcendence: the role of occupation in modern life. *Journal of Occupational Science: Australia, 1*(3), 46-53.

Duncan, E. A. S. (2006). Glossary. In E. A. S. Duncan (Ed.), *Foundations for practice in occupational therapy* (4th ed., pp. 337-341). Edinburgh, Scotland: Elsevier, Churchill Livingstone.

Dunn, H. L. (1977). *High level wellness*. Thorofare, NJ: Charles B. Slack.

Dunn, W. W. (2000). Habit: what's the brain got to do with it? *Occupational Therapy Journal of Research, 20*(Suppl.), 6S-20S.

Dunn, W., Brown, C., & McGuigan, A. (1994). The ecology of human performance: a framework for considering the effect of context. *American Journal of Occupational Therapy, 48*(7), 595-607.

Dunn, W., Foto, M., Hinojosa, J., Schell, B., Thomson, L. K., & Hertfelder, S. D. (1994). Uniform terminology (3rd ed.). *American Journal of Occupational Therapy, 48*(11), 1047-1054.

Dunning, H. (1972). Environmental occupational therapy. *American Journal of Occupational Therapy, 26*(6), 292-298.

Dunton, W. R. (1915). *Occupation therapy*. Philadelphia, PA: Saunders.

Dunton, W. R. (1918). The principles of occupational therapy. *Public Health Nurse, 18*, 316-321.

Dunton, W. R. (1925). Economic studies of crafts: 1. Upholstery. *Occupational Therapy and Rehabilitation, 4*(2), 219-222.

Dunton, W. R. (1928). *Prescribing occupational therapy*. Springfield, IL: Charles C. Thomas.

Eisenberg, M. G. (1995). *Dictionary of rehabilitation*. New York, NY: Springer Publishing Co.

Eisfelder, R., & Gewurtz, R. (2012). Mental health and work. In B. Braveman & J. J. Page (Eds.), *Work: promoting participation & productivity through occupational therapy* (pp. 198-220). Philadelphia, PA: F. A. Davis.

English, H. B., & English, A. C. (1958). *A comprehensive dictionary of psychological and psychoanalytical terms: a guide to usage*. New York, NY: David McKay Company, Inc.

Eysenick, H. J., Arnold, W., & Meili, R. (1982). *Encyclopedia of psychology*. New York, NY: Continuum Publishing Co.

Fanchiang, S. C. (1996). The other side of the coin: growing up with a learning disability. *American Journal of Occupational Therapy, 50*(4), 277-285.

Farrar, C. B. (1906). The making of psychiatric records. *American Journal of Insanity, LXII*, 479-485.

Fidler, G. S., & Fidler, J. W. (1958). *Introduction to psychiatric occupational therapy*. New York, NY: Macmillian Co.

Fidler, G. S., & Fidler, J. W. (1978). Doing and becoming: purposeful action and self-actualization. *American Journal of Occupational Therapy, 32*(5), 305-310.

Fidler, G. S., & Fidler, J. W. (1983). Doing and becoming: the occupational therapy experience. In G. Kielhofner (Ed.), *Health through occupation*. Philadelphia, PA: F. A. Davis.

Finn, G. L. (1972). The occupational therapist in prevention programs. *American Journal of Occupational Therapy, 26*(2), 59-66.

Fleischman, E. A. (1975). Toward a taxonomy of human performance. *American Psychologist, 30*(12), 1127-1149.

Florey, L. (1969). Intrinsic motivation: the dynamics of occupational therapy theory. *American Journal of Occupational Therapy, 23*(4), 319-322.

Forsyth, K., & Kielhofner, G. (2006). Model of human occupation: Integrating theory into practice and practice into theory. In E. A. S. Duncan (Ed.). *Foundations for practice in occupational therapy* (pp. 69-107). Edinburgh, Scotland: Churchill Livingstone.

Gage, M. (1992). The appraisal model of coping: an assessment and intervention model for occupational therapy. *American Journal of Occupational Therapy, 46*(4), 353-362.

Gage, M., Noh, S., Polatajko, H. J., & Kaspar, V. (1994). Measuring perceived self-efficacy in occupational therapy. *American Journal of Occupational Therapy, 48*(9), 783-790.

Gage, M., & Polatajko, H. J. (1994). Enhancing occupational performance through an understanding of perceived self-efficacy. *American Journal of Occupational Therapy, 48*(5), 452-461.

Gilbert, M. M., Chamberlain, J. A., White, C. R., Mayers, P. W., Pawsy, B., Liew, D. … Castle, D. J. (2012). Controlled clinical trial of a self-management program for people with mental illness in an adult mental health service—the Optimal Health Program (OHP). *Australian Health Review, 36*, 1-7.

Gillen, G., & Burkhardt, A. (1998). Glossary. In G. Gillen & A. Burkhardt (Eds.), *Stroke rehabilitation: a function-based approach* (536-541). St. Louis, MO: Mosby.

Hagedorn, R. (1992). *Foundations for practice in occupational therapy*. Edinburgh, Scotland: Churchill Livingstone.

Hagedorn, R. (1995). Glossary. In R. Hagedorn, *Occupational therapy: perspectives and processes* (pp. 297-302). Edinburgh, Scotland: Churchill Livingstone.

Hagedorn, R. (1997). Glossary. In R. Hagedorn, *Foundations for practice in occupational therapy* (2nd ed., pp. 141-147). New York, NY: Churchill Livingstone.

Hagedorn, R. (2000). Glossary. In R. Hagedorn, *Tools for practice in occupational therapy: a structured approach to core skills and processes* (pp. 307-312). Edinburgh, Scotland: Churchill Livingstone.

Hagedorn, R. (2001). Glossary. In R. Hagedorn, *Foundations for practice in occupational therapy* (3rd ed., pp. 157-167). Edinburgh, Scotland: Churchill Livingstone.

Hall, H. J. (1905). The systematic use of work as a remedy in neurasthenia and allied conditions. *Boston Medical and Surgical Journal, CLII*(2), 29-32.

Hall, H. J. (1910). The work-cure. *Boston Medical and Surgical Journal, LIV*(1), 13-15.

Hall, H. J. (1921). Forward steps in occupational therapy during 1920. *Modern Hospital, 16*, 245-247.

Hall, H. J. (1923). *OT: A new profession*. Concord, NH: Rumford Press.

Hall, H. J. (1973). *O.T.: A new profession*. Concord, NH: Rumford Press.

Hasselkus, B. R. (1993). Functional disability and older adults. In H. L. Hopkins & H. D. Smith (Eds.), *Willard and Spackman's occupational therapy* (8th ed., pp. 742-752). Philadelphia, PA: J. B. Lippincott.

Hasselkus, B. R., & Kiernat, J. M. (1973). Independent living for the elderly. *American Journal of Occupational Therapy, 27*(4), 181-190.

Hightower, M. D. (1966). Independence through activities of daily living. *Delaware Medical Journal, 38*(8), 449-455.

Hillman, A. M., & Chapparo, C. J. (1995). Occupational role performance in men following a stroke. *Journal of Occupational Science: Australia, 2*(3), 88-99.

Hinojosa, J., & Kramer, P. (1997). Fundamental concepts of occupational therapy: occupation, purposeful activity, and function. *American Journal of Occupational Therapy, 51*(10), 864-866.

Hinojosa, J., Sabari, J., & Pedretti, L. (1993). Position paper: purposeful activities. *American Journal of Occupational Therapy, 47*(12), 1081-1082.

Hocking, C., & Whiteford, G. (1995). Multiculturalism in occupational therapy: a time for reflection on core values. *Australian Occupational Therapy Journal, 42*(4), 172-175.

Holdeman, E. E. (1954). Occupational therapy for patients with anterior poliomyelitis. In H. S. Willard & C. S. Spackman (Eds.), *Principles of occupational therapy* (pp. 256-273). Philadelphia, PA: J. B. Lippincott.

Hopkins, H. L., & Smith, H. D. (1977). Glossary. In H. L. Hopkins & H. D. Smith (Eds.), *Willard and Spackman's occupational therapy* (5th ed., pp. 727-740). Philadelphia, PA: J. B. Lippincott.

Hopkins, H., & Smith, H. (1978). *Willard & Spackman's occupational therapy* (5th ed.). Philadelphia, PA: Lippincott.

Hopkins, H. L., & Smith, H. D. (1983). Glossary. In H. L. Hopkins & H. D. Smith (Eds.), *Willard and Spackman's occupational therapy* (6th ed., pp. 915-930). Philadelphia, PA: J. B. Lippincott.

Howe, M. C., & Briggs, A. K. (1982). Ecological systems model for occupational therapy. *American Journal of Occupational Therapy, 36*, 322-327.

Hussey, S. M., Sabonis-Chafee, B., & O'Brien, J. C. (2007). Glossary. In S. M. Hussey, B. Sabonis-Chafee, & J. C. O'Brien (Eds.), *Introduction to occupational therapy* (3rd ed., pp. 285-293). St. Louis, MO: Mosby Elsevier.

Iannone, M. (1987). A cross-cultural investigation of occupational role. *Occupational Therapy in Health Care, 4*(1), 93-101.

Institute for Alternative Futures. (2009). *Conference report: Total fitness for the 21st century*. Alexandria, VA: Uniformed Services University, Consortium for Health and Military Performance.

Jackson, J. (1996). Living a meaningful existence in old age. In R. Zemke & F. Clarke (Eds.), *Occupational science: the evolving discipline* (339-362). Philadelphia, PA: F. A. Davis.

Jackson, S. J., & Banks, R. M. (1997). Home management—glossary. In J. Van Deusen & D. Brunt (Eds.), *Assessment in occupational therapy and physical therapy* (pp. 459-460). Philadelphia, PA: W. B. Saunders.

Jacobs, K. (1985). *Occupational therapy. Work-related programs and assessments*. Boston, MA: Little, Brown, & Co.

Jacobs, K. (1994). Flow and the occupational therapy practitioner. *American Journal of Occupational Therapy, 48*(10), 989-996.

Jacobs, K. (1999). *Quick reference dictionary for occupational therapy*, 2nd ed. Thorofare, NJ: SLACK Incorporated.

Jacobs, K., & Jacobs, L. (2009). *Quick reference dictionary for occupational therapy* (5th ed.). Thorofare, NJ: SLACK Incorporated.

James, W. (1890). *The principles of psychology*. New York, NY: Henry Holt & Co. Reprint 1950, New York, NY: Dover Press.

James, W. (1950). *The principles of psychology* (Vol. 1, p. 402). New York, NY: Dover. Reprint originally published by Henry Holt and Company in 1890.

Jefferson, P., & Hammond, A. (2002). Osteoarthritis. In A. Turner, M. Foster, & S. E. Johnson (Eds.), *Occupational therapy and physical dysfunction* (5th ed., pp. 617-636). Edinburgh, Scotland: Churchill Livingstone.

Johnson, J. (1973). Task force on target populations, part 1. *American Journal of Occupational Therapy, 28*(3), 158-163.

Johnson, J. A. (1985). Wellness: its myths, realities, and potential for occupational therapy. *Occupational Therapy in Health Care, 2*(2), 117-138.

Johnson, J. A. (1986). New dimensions in wellness: a context for living. Thorofare, NJ: SLACK Incorporated. *Current Practice Series in Occupational Therapy, 1*(4), 1-134.

Jonsson, H., Josephsson, S. & Kielhofner, G. (2001). Narratives and experience in an occupational transition: a longitudinal study of the retirement process. *American Journal of Occupational Therapy, 55*(1), 424-432.

Kamenetz, H. L. (1983). *Dictionary of rehabilitation medicine.* New York, NY: Springer Publishing Co.

Klavins, R. (1972). Work-play behaviors: cultural influences. *American Journal of Occupational Therapy, 26*(4), 176-179.

Kerlinger, F. N. (1986). *Foundations of behavioral research* (3rd ed.). San Diego, CA: Academic Press.

Kielhofner, G. (1983). Occupation. In H. L. Hopkins & H. D. Smith (Eds.), *Willard and Spackman's occupational therapy* (6th ed., pp. 31-41). Philadelphia, PA: J. B. Lippincott.

Kielhofner, G. (1985). Glossary. In G. Kielhofner (Ed.), *A model of human occupation: theory and application* (pp. 501-509). Baltimore, MD: Williams & Wilkins.

Kielhofner, G. (1995). *A model of human occupation: therapy and application* (2nd ed.) Baltimore, MD: Williams & Wilkins.

Kielhofner, G. (1997). *Conceptual foundations of occupational therapy* (2nd ed.). Philadelphia, MD: F. A. Davis.

Kielhofner, G. (2002). *A model of human occupation: theory and application* (3rd ed.). Philadelphia, PA: Lippincott Williams & Wilkins.

Kielhofner, G. (2008), *A model of human occupation: theory and application* (4th ed.). Philadelphia, PA: Wolters Kluwer, Lippincott Williams & Wilkins.

Kielhofner, G., Borell, L., Helfrich, C., & Nygard, L. (1995). Volitional subsystem. In G. Kielhofner (Ed.), *A model of human occupation: theory and application* (2nd ed., pp. 39-62). Baltimore, MD: Williams & Wilkins.

Kim, H. S. (1983). *The nature of theoretical thinking in nursing.* Norwalk, CT: Appleton-Century-Crofts.

King, L. J. (1978). Toward a science of adaptive responses. *American Journal of Occupational Therapy, 32*(7), 429-437.

Kronenberg, F., Algado, S. E., & Pollard, N. (2001). *Occupational therapy without borders–Volume 1: Learning from the spirt of survivors.* Edinburgh, Scotland: Churchill Livingstone.

Krupa, T., & Clark, C. (2004). Occupational therapy in the field of mental health: promoting occupational perspectives on health and well-being. *Canadian Journal of Occupational Therapy, 71*(2), 69-74.

Lancioni, G. E., Smeets, P. M., & Oliva, D. (1988). A computer-aided program to supervise occupational engagement of severely mentally retarded persons. *Behavioral Residential Treatment, 3*(1), 1-17.

Larson, B., Wood, W., & Clark, F. (2003). Occupation science: Building the science and practice of occupation through an academic discipline. In E. B. Creapeu, E. S. Cohn, & B. A. B. Schell (Eds.), *Willard and Spackman's occupational therapy* (10th ed., pp. 15-26). Philadelphia, PA: Lippincott Williams & Wilkins.

Law, J. F. (1987). Time perception and rehabilitation of the elderly. *Physical and Occupational Therapy in Geriatrics, 5*(4), 17-30.

Law, M., & Mills, J. (1998). Client-centered occupational therapy. In M. Law (Ed.). *Client-centered occupational therapy* (pp. 1-8). Thorofare, NJ: SLACK Incorporated.

Law, M., Baptiste, S., & Mills, J. (1995). Client-centred practice: What does it mean and does it make a difference? *Canadian Journal of Occupational Therapy, 62*(5), 250-257.

Law, M., Cooper, B., Strong, S., Steward, D., Rigby, P., Letts, L. (1996). The person-environment-occupation model: a transactive approach to occupational performance. *Canadian Journal of Occupational Therapy, 63*(1), 9-23.

Law, M., Cooper, B., Strong, S., Steward, D., Rigby, P., Letts, L. (1997a). Theoretical contexts for the practice of occupational therapy. In C. Christiansen & C. Baum (Eds.), *Occupational therapy: enabling function and well-being* (2nd ed., pp. 73-102). Thorofare, NJ: SLACK Incorporated.

Law, M., Polatajko, H., Baptiste, S., & Townsend, E. (1997b). Core concepts of occupational therapy (pp. 29-56). In E. Townsend (Ed.), *Enabling occupation: an occupational therapy perspective.* Ottawa, ON: CAOT.

Law, M., Steinwender, A., & Leclair, L. (1998). Occupation, health, and well-being. *Canadian Journal of Occupational Therapy, 65*(2), 81-91.

Lawton, M. P. (1971). The functional assessment of elderly people. *Journal of the American Geriatric Society, 19*(6), 465-481.

Lawton, M. P., & Brody, E. M. (1969). Assessment of older people self-maintaining and instrumental activities of daily living. *Gerontologist, 9*(3), 179-186.

Lazarus, R. S. (1984). Coping. In R. J. Corsini (Ed), *Encyclopedia of psychology* (Vol. 1, pp. 294-296). New York, NY: John Wiley & Sons.

Lazarus, R. S., & Folkman, S. (1984). *Stress, appraisal, and coping.* New York, NY: Springer Publishing Co.

Letts, L., Fraser, B., Finlayson, M., & Walls, J. (1993). *For the health of it! Occupational therapy within a health promotion framework.* Ottawa, ON: CAOT.

Levy, L. (1988). The health care delivery system today. In H. L. Hopkins & H. D. Smith (Eds.), *Willard and Spackman's occupational therapy* (7th ed., pp. 153-164). Philadelphia, PA: Lippincott.

Licht, S. (1947). Kinetic analysis of crafts and occupations. *Occupational Therapy and Rehabilitation, 26,* 75-78.

Livingstone, D. M. (1950). Achievement recording for the cerebral palsied. *American Journal of Occupational Therapy, 4*(2), 66-67, 74.

Llorens, L. A. (1976). *Application of a developmental theory for health and rehabilitation.* Rockville, MD: AOTA.

Llorens, L. A. (1984). Changing balance: environment and individual. *American Journal of Occupational Therapy, 38*(1), 29-34.

Mackenzie, L., & O'Toole, G. (2011). *Occupation analysis in practice.* West Sussex, England: Wiley-Blackwell.

MacLean, F. M. (1949). Occupational therapy in the management of poliomyelitis. *American Journal of Occupational Therapy, 3*(1), 20-27.

Maguire, G. H. (1983). An exploratory study of the relationship of valued activities to the life satisfaction of elderly persons. *Occupational Therapy Journal of Research, 3*(3), 164-172.

Martini, R., Polatajko, H. J., Wilcock, A. (1995). ICIDH-PR: A potential model for occupational therapy. *Occupational Therapy International, 2*(1), 1-21.

Matsutsuyu, J. S. (1969). The Interest Check List. *American Journal of Occupational Therapy, 34*(4), 323-328.

Matsutsuyu, J. (1971). Occupational behavior: A perspective on work and play. *American Journal of Occupational Therapy, 25*(6), 291-294.

Matuska, K., & Christiansen, C. (2008). *Life balance: Multidisciplinary theories and research*. Bethesda, MD: AOTA Press.

Mayer, C. A. (2000). The Casson Memorial Lecture 2000: reflect on the past to shape the future. *British Journal of Occupational Therapy, 63*(8), 358-366.

Mazer, J. (1968). Toward an integrated theory of occupational therapy. *American Journal of Occupational Therapy, 22*(5), 452-456.

McClelland, D. C., Atkinson, J. W., & Lowell, E. L. (1953). *The achievement motive*. New York, NY: Appleton-Century-Crofts.

McColl, M. A., & Bickenbach, J. E. (1998). *Introduction to disability*. London, England: W. B. Saunders.

McDougell, W. (1923). Purposive or mechanical psychology. *Psychological Review, 30*, 273-289.

McKinnon, A. L. (2000). Client values and satisfaction with occupational therapy. *Scandinavian Journal of Occupational Therapy, 7*, 99-106.

Melvin, J. L. (1998). Self-management for fibromyalgia. *OT Practice, 3*(4), 39-43.

Meyer, A. (1922). The philosophy of occupation therapy. *Archives of Occupational Therapy, 1*(1), 1-10.

Meyer, A. (1951). Remarks on habit disorganization in the essential deteriorations, and the relation of deterioration to the psychasthenic, neurasthenic, hysterical and other constitutions. In E. Winters (Ed.), *The collected papers of Adolf Meyer (Vol. II). Psychiatry*. Baltimore, MD: Johns Hopkins Press.

Meyer, A. (1952). What is the safest psychology for a nurse? In E. Winter (Ed.). *The collected papers of Adoph Meyer* (Vol. IV, p. 85). Baltimore, MD: Johns Hopkins Press.

Meyer, A. (1957). *Psychobiology*. Springfield, IL: Charles C. Thomas.

Mocellin, G. (1988). A perspective on the principles and practice of occupational therapy. *British Journal of Occupational Therapy, 51*(1), 4-7.

Mocellin, G. (1995). Occupational therapy: a critical overview, Part 1. *British Journal of Occupational Therapy, 58*(12), 502-506.

Mock, H.E. (1918). Curative work. *Carry On, 1*(9), 12-15.

Moorhead, L. (1969). The occupational history. *American Journal of Occupational Therapy, 23*(4), 329-334.

Mosey, A. C. (1981). *Occupational therapy: configuration of a profession*. New York, NY: Raven Press.

Mosey, A. C. (1986). *Psychosocial components of occupational therapy*. New York, NY: Raven Press.

Mosey, A. C. (1994). Working taxonomies. In C. B. Royeen (Ed.), *Introduction to cognitive rehabilitation. AOTA self-study series* (Vol. 1, pp. 23-34). Bethesda, MD: AOTA.

Mosey, A. C. (1996). *Applied scientific injury in the health professions: an epistemological orientation* (2nd ed). Bethesda, MD: AOTA.

Muñoz, J. P., & Kielhofner, G. (1995). Program development (pp. 343-370). In G. Kielhofner (Ed), *A model of human occupation: theory and application* (2nd ed.). Baltimore, MD: Williams & Wilkins.

Murray, G., Suto, M., Hole, R., Hale, S., Amari, E., & Michalak, E. E. (2011). Self-management strategies used by "high functioning" individuals with bipolar disorder: from research to clinical practice. *Clinical Psychology and Psychotherapy, 18*, 95-109.

Neistadt, M. E., & Crepeau, E. B. (1998). Glossary. In M. E. Neistadt & E. B. Crepeau (Eds.), *Willard and Spackman's occupational therapy* (9th ed., pp. 866-673). Philadelphia, PA: Lippincott.

Nelson, D. L. (1988). Occupation: form and performance. *American Journal of Occupational Therapy, 42*(10), 633-641.

Nelson, D. L. (1994). Occupational form, occupation performance, and therapeutic occupation. In L. C. B. Royeen (Ed.), *The practice of the future: putting occupation back into therapy* (Vol. 2, pp. 10-48). Rockville, MD: AOTA.

Nilsson, I., & Townsend, E. (2010). Occupation justice—bridging theory and practice. *Scandinavian Journal of Occupational Therapy, 17*(1), 57-63.

Nurit, W., & Michel, A. B. (2003). Rest: a qualitative exploration of the phenomenon. *Occupational Therapy International, 10*, 227-238.

Oakley, F., Kiehofner, G., Barris, R., & Reichler, R. (1986). The role checklist: Development and empirical assment of reliability. *Occupational Therapy Journal of Research, 6*, 157-170.

Packer, T. (2011) An occupation-focused approach to self-management. *Occupational Therapy Now, 13*(5), 3-4.

Packer, T. (2013). Editorial: self-management interventions: using an occupational lens to rethink and refocus. *Australian Occupational Therapy Journal, 60*, 1-2.

Packer, T. L., Boldy, D., Ghahari, S., Melling, L., Parsons, R., & Osborne, R. H. (2012). Self-management programs conducted within a practice setting: who participates, who benefits and what can be learned? *Patient Education and Counseling, 87*(1), 93-100.

Parham, L. D., & Fazio, L. S. (1997). Glossary. In L. D. Parham & L. S. Fazio (Eds.). *Play in occupational therapy for children* (pp. 248-254). St. Louis, MO: Mosby, Pratt & Allen. (1985).

Parham, L. D., & Fazio, L. S. (1997). Play in occupational therapy for children. St. Louis, MO: Mosby.

Parten, M. B. (1932). Social participation among pre-school children. *Journal of Abnormal and Social Psychology, 27*(3), 243-288

Pattee, G. (1951). Occupational therapy for the medical patient. In F. H. Krusen (Ed.), *Physical medicine and rehabilitation for the clinician* (pp. 83-94). Philadelphia, PA: W. B. Saunders Co.

Patterson, H. A. (1922). The trend of occupational therapy for the tuberculous. *Archives of Occupational Therapy, 1*(1), 1924.

Pedretti, L. W. (1996). *Occupational therapy: Practice skills for physical dysfunction* (4th ed.). St. Louis, MO: Mosby.

Pedretti, L. W., & Umphred, D. A. (1996). Motor leaning and teaching activities in occupational therapy. In L. W. Pedretti (Ed.), *Occupational therapy: practice skills for physical dysfunction* (4th ed., pp. 65-75). St. Louis, MO: Mosby.

Pellerito, J. M., Jr. (2005). *Driver rehabilitation and community mobility: Principles and practice*. St. Louis, MO: Elsevier Mosby.

Pellerito, J. M. (2006). Glossary. In J. M. Pellerito (Ed.), *Driver rehabilitation and community mobility*. St. Louis, MO: Elsevier Mosby.

Peters, R. S. (1953). *Brett's history of psychology*. London, England: Macmillian Company.

Pierce, D. (2001). Untangling occupation and activity. *American Journal of Occupational Therapy, 55*(2), 138-146.

Piersol, C. V., & Ehrlich, P. L. (2000). Glossary. In C. V. Piersol & P. L. Ehrlich (Eds.), *Home health practice: a guide for the occupational therapist* (pp. 99-202). Bisbee, AZ: Imaginart.

Polatajko, H. (1992). Naming and framing occupational therapy: a lecture dedicated to the life of Nancy B. *Canadian Journal of Occupational Therapy, 59*(4), 189-200.

Polatajko, H. (1994). Dreams, dilemmas, and decisions for occupational therapy practice in a new millennium: a Canadian perspective. *American Journal of Occupational Therapy, 48*(7), 590-594.

Polkinghorne, D. E. (1996). Transformative narratives: from victimic to agentic life plots. *American Journal of Occupational Therapy, 50*(4), 299-305.

Pollack, B. (1938). Aims and ideals of occupational therapy in state hospitals. *Occupational Therapy and Rehabilitation, 11*, 291-300.

Poole, J. L. (1995). Learning. In C. A. Trombly (Ed.), *Occupational therapy for physical dysfunction* (4th ed., pp. 265-276). Baltimore, MD: Williams & Wilkins.

Pratt, R. N., & Allen, A. S. (1985). *Occupational therapy for children* (2nd ed.). St. Louis, MO: Mosby.

Punwar, A. J. (1988). *Occupational therapy: Principles and practice.* Baltimore, MD: Williams & Wilkins.

Punwar, A. J. (1994). *Occupational therapy: Principles and practice* (2nd ed.). Baltimore, MD: Williams & Wilkins.

Punwar, A. J., & Peloquin, S. M (2000). Glossary. In A. J. Punwar & S. M. Peloquin. *Occupational therapy: principles and practice* (3rd ed., pp. 277-286). Philadelphia, PA: Lippincott Williams & Wilkins.

Radowski, M. V., & Trombly Latham, C. A. (2008). *Occupational therapy for physical dysfunction* (6th ed.). Philadelphia, PA: Wolters Kluwer.

Rebeiro, K. L., & Polgar, J. M. (1999). Enabling occupational performance: optimal experiences in therapy. *Canadian Journal of Occupational Therapy, 66*(1), 14-22.

Reber, A. S. (1995). *Dictionary of psychology* (2nd ed.). London, England: Penguin Books.

Reber, A. S., & Reber, E. (2001). *The Penguin dictionary of psychology* (3rd ed.). London, England: Penguin Books.

Reed, K. L. (1984). *Models of practice in occupational therapy.* Baltimore, MD: Williams & Wilkins.

Reed, K. L. (1986). Tools of practice: heritage or baggage. *American Journal of Occupational Therapy, 40*(9), 597-505.

Reed, K. L., & Sanderson, S. R. (1980). *Concepts of occupational therapy.* Baltimore, MD: Williams & Wilkins.

Reed, K. L., & Sanderson, S. R. (1983). Glossary. In K. L. Reed & S. R. Sanderson, *Concepts of occupational therapy* (2nd ed., pp. 329-357). Baltimore, MD: Williams & Wilkins.

Reed, K. L., & Sanderson, S. R. (1992). *Concepts of occupational therapy* (3rd ed.). Baltimore, MD: Williams & Wilkins.

Reed, K. L., & Sanderson, S. N. (1999). *Concepts of occupational therapy* (4th ed.). Philadelphia, PA: Lippincott Williams & Wilkins.

Reilly, M. (1966). A psychiatric occupational therapy program as a teaching model. *American Journal of Occupational Therapy, 20*(2), 61-67.

Reilly, M. (1969). The educational process. *American Journal of Occupational Therapy, 23*(4), 299-307.

Reilly, M. (1974). *Play as exploratory learning.* Beverly Hills, CA: Sage Publications.

Robertson, S. C. (1998). Treatment for psychosocial components: Intervention for mental health. In M. E. Neistadt & E. B. Crepeau (Eds.), *Willard and Spackman's occupational therapy* (9th ed., pp. 450-454). Philadelphia, PA: Lippincott.

Rock, L. M. (1996). Upper extremity amputations and prosthetics: section 1: amputations and body-powered prostheses. In L. W. Pedretti (Ed.), *Occupational therapy: practice skills for physical dysfunction* (4th ed., pp. 576-585). St. Louis, MO: Mosby.

Rodgers, B. L., & Knafl, K. A. (2000). *Concept development in nursing: foundations, techniques, and applications* (2nd ed.). Philadelphia, PA: W. B. Saunders Co.

Rogers, C. (1939). *Clinical treatment of the problem child.* Boston, MA: Houghton-Mifflin.

Rogers, C. (1942). *Counseling and psychotherapy: Newer concepts in practice.* Boston, MA: Houghton-Mifflin.

Rogers, C. (1951). *Client-centered therapy: Its current practice, implications and theory.* Boston, MA: Houghton-Mifflin.

Rogers, J. C. (1982). The spirit of independence: the evolution of a philosophy. *American Journal of Occupational Therapy, 36*(11), 709-715.

Rogers, J. C. (1984). Why study human occupation? *American Journal of Occupational Therapy, 38*(1), 47-49.

Ryan, S. (1992). *The combined volume: COTA, second edition and practice issues in occupational therapy.* Thorofare, NJ: SLACK Incorporated.

Ryan, S. (1993). Glossary. In S. Ryan (Ed.), *Practice issues in occupational therapy: intraprofessional team building.* Thorofare, NJ: SLACK Incorporated.

Runes, D. D. (1962). *Dictionary of philosophy.* Totowa, NJ: Littlefield, Adams, & Co.

Runes, D. D. (1980). *Dictionary of philosophy* (p. 114). Totowa, NJ: Littlefield, Adams, & Co.

Scaffa, M. (2001). *Occupational therapy in community-based practice settings.* Philadelphia, PA: F. A. Davis.

Scaffa, M. E., Desmond, S., & Brownson, C. A. (2001). Public health, community health, and occupational therapy. In *Occupational therapy in community-based practice settings* (pp. 35-50). Philadelphia, PA: F. A. Davis.

Schell, B. A. B., Gillen, G., & Scaffa, M. E. (2012). Glossary. In B. A. B. Schell, G. Gillen, & M. E. Scaffa (Eds.), *Willard and Spackman's occupational therapy* (12th ed., pp. 1129-1243). Philadelphia, PA: Wolters Kluwer.

Schell, B. A. B., Gillen, G., & Scaffa, M. (2014). *Willard & Spackman's occupational therapy* (12th ed.). Philadelphia, PA: Wolters Kuwer.

Schkade, J. K., & Schultz, S. (1992). Occupational adaptation: toward a holistic approach for contemporary practice, part 1. *American Journal of Occupational Therapy, 46*(9), 829-837.

Schlaff, C. (1993). From dependency to self-advocacy: redefining disability. *American Journal of Occupational Therapy, 47*(10), 943-948.

Schmidt, R. A. (1988). *Motor control and learning: a behavioral emphasis.* Champaign, IL: Human Kinetics Publishers.

Schmidt, R. A. (1991). Motor learning principles for physical therapy. In *Contemporary management of motor control problems: proceedings of the II-STEP conference.* Alexandria, VA: American Physical Therapy Foundation.

Schwartz, K. B. (1998). The history of occupational therapy. In M. E. Neistadt & E. B. Crepeau (Eds.), *Willard and Spackman's occupational therapy* (9th ed., pp. 854-860). Philadelphia, PA: Lippincott.

Segal, R. (2004). Family routines and rituals: a context for occupational therapy interventions. *American Journal of Occupational Therapy, 58*(5), 499-508

Shannon, P. D. (1970). Work adjustment and the adolescent soldier. *American Journal of Occupational Therapy, 24*(2), 111-115

Sharrott, G. W., & Cooper-Fraps, C. (1986). Theories of motivation in occupational therapy: an overview. *American Journal of Occupational Therapy, 40*(4), 249-257.

Sheldon, M. P. (1935). Physical achievement record for use with crippled children. *Journal of Health and Physical Education, 6*(5), 30-31, 60.

Simpson, P. L. (1997). Occupational balance: a holistic frame of reference of physical disability practice. *Journal of Occupational Therapy Students,* 7-18.

Sladyk, K., Jacobs, K., & MacRae, N. (2010). *Occupational therapy essentials for clinical competence.* Thorofare, NJ: SLACK Incorporated.

Slagle, E. C. (1922). Training aides for mental patients. *Archives of Occupational Therapy, 1*(1), 11-17.

Slagle, E. C. (1923). A year's development of occupational therapy in New York state hospitals. *State Hospital Quarterly, 8,* 590-603.

Smith, J. N., Jr. (1945). Preface. In G. G. Deaver & M. E. Brown (Eds.). *Physical demands of daily life: An objective scale for rating the orthopedically exceptional.* New York, NY: Institute for the Crippled and Disabled.

Smith, J. A. (1986). The idea of health: doing foundational inquiry. In P. L. Munhall & C. J. Oiler (Eds.), *Nursing research: a qualitative perspective* (pp. 251-262). Norwalk, CT: Appleton-Century-Crofts.

Spackman, C. S. (1947). Occupational therapy for patients with physical injuries. In H. S. Willard & C. S. Spackman (Eds.), *Principles of occupational therapy* (pp. 175-273). Philadelphia, PA: J. B. Lippincott.

Spencer, E. A. (1989). Toward a balance of work and play: promotion of health and wellness. *Occupational Therapy in Health Care, 5*(4), 87-99.

Stein, F., & Cutler, S. F. (2002). Glossary. In F. Stein & S. F. Cutler, *Psychosocial occupational therapy: a holistic approach* (2nd ed., pp. 613-637). New York, NY: Delmar/Thompson Learning.

Stein, F., & Roose, B. (2000). *Pocket guide to treatment in occupational therapy.* San Diego, CA: Singular Publishing Co.

Stewart, A. (1994). Empowerment and enablement: occupational therapy 2001. *British Journal of Occupational Therapy, 57*(7), 248-254

Stewart, A. M. (1992). The Cason Memorial Lecture 1992: always a little further. *British Journal of Occupational Therapy, 55*(8), 296-301.

Sumsion, T. (1999). *Client-centred practice in occupational therapy: A guide to implementation.* Edinburgh, Scotland: Churchill Livingstone.

Taylor, M. (1930). Rehabilitation of the disabled through occupational therapy. *Hospital Social Service, 23,* 54-56.

Thomas, E. J. (1966). Problems of disability from the perspective of role theory. *Journal of Health and Human Behavior, 7*(1), 2-11.

Thompson, E. (Ed.). (1995). *The concise oxford dictionary* (9th ed.). Oxford, England: Clarendon Press.

Tolman, E. C. (1932). *Purposive behavior in animals and men.* New York, NY: Century.

Townsend, E. (1996). Enabling empowerment: using simulation versus real occupations. *Canadian Journal of Occupational Therapy, 63*(2), 114-128.

Townsend, E. (1997). Key terms. In E. Townsend (Ed.), *Enabling occupations: an occupational therapy perspective* (pp. 179-182). Ottawa, ON: CAOT.

Townsend, E. (2002). *Enabling occupation: An occupational therapy perspective.* Ottawa, ON: Canadian Association of Occupational Therapists.

Townsend, E. (2007). *Enabling occupation II: Advancing an occupational therapy vision for health well-being & justice through occupation.* Ottawa, ON: Canadian Association of Occupational Therapists.

Townsend, E., & Polatajko, H. (2007). Enabling occupation II: Advancing an occupational therapy vision for health well-being & justice through occupation. Ottawa, ON: Canadian Association of Occupational Therapists.

Townsend, E., & Wilcock, A. A. (2004a). Occupational justice. In C. H. Christiansen & E. A. Townsend (Eds.), *Introduction to occupation: The art and science of living* (pp. 243-273). Upper Saddle River, NJ: Prentice Hall.

Townsend, E., & Wilcock, A. A. (2004b). Occupational justice and client-centred practice: A dialogue in progress. *Canadian Journal of Occupational Therapy, 71*(2), 75-87.

Tracy, S. E. (1910). *Studies in invalid occupations.* Boston, MA: Whitcomb & Barrows.

Trombly, C. A. (1995). Planning, guiding, and documenting therapy. In C. A. Trombly (Ed.), *Occupational therapy for physical dysfunction* (4th ed., pp. 29-40). Baltimore, MD: Williams & Wilkins.

Trombly, C. A., & Radomski, M. V. (2002). *Occupational therapy for physical dysfunction* (5th ed.). Philadelphia, PA: Lippincott Williams & Wilkins.

Turner, A., Foster, M., & Johnson, S. E. (1996). Glossary. In A. Turner, M. Foster, & D. E. Johnson (Eds.), *Occupational therapy and physical dysfunction: principles, skills, and practices* (4th ed., pp. 873). New York, NY: Churchill Livingstone.

Turner, A., Foster, M., & Johnson, S. E. (2002). Glossary. In A. Turner, M. Foster, & S. E. Johnson (Eds.), *Occupational therapy and physical dysfunction: principles, skills, and practices* (5th ed.). New York, NY: Churchill Livingstone.

Turner, A., & MacCaul, C. (1996). The therapeutic use of activity. In A. Turner, M. Foster, & S. E. Johnson (Eds.), *Occupational therapy and physical dysfunction: principles, skills, and practices* (4th ed., pp. 125-157). New York, NY: Churchill Livingstone.

Unsworth, C. (1999). Glossary of terms. In C. Unsworth (Ed.), *Cognitive and perceptual dysfunction: a clinical reasoning approach to evaluation and intervention* (pp. 473-484). Philadelphia, PA: F. A. Davis.

Upham, E. G. (1918a). *Training of teachers for occupational therapy for the rehabilitation of disabled soldiers and sailors (Federal Board for Vocational Education Bulletin, No. 6).* Washington, DC: Government Printing Office.

Upham, E. G. (1918b). *Ward occupations in hospitals (Federal Board for Vocational Education, Re-Education Series, No. 4).* Washington, DC: Government Printing Office.

Upham, E. G. (1919). Occupational therapy and the trained nurse. *Modern Hospital, 12,* 210-212.

Urbanowski, R. (2005). Transcending practice borders through perspective transformation. In F. Kronenberg, S. Simó Algado, & N. Pollard (Eds.), *Occupational therapy without borders* (pp. 302-312). Edinburgh, Scotland: Elsevier.

VandenBos G. R., & American Psychological Association (APA). (2007). *APA Dictionary of Psychology.* Washington, DC: APA.

Vause-Earland, T. (1991). Perception of role assessment tools in the physical disability setting. *American Journal of Occupational Therapy, 45*(1), 26-31.

Velde, B., & Fidler, G. (2002). *Lifestyle performance.* Thorofare, NJ: SLACK Incorporated.

Wagman, P., Håkansson, C., & Björklund, A. (2012). Occupational balance as used in occupational therapy: a concept analysis. *Scandinavian Journal of Occupational Therapy, 19*(4), 322-327.

Walker, L. O., & Avant, K. C. (1995). *Strategies for theory construction in nursing.* Upper Saddle River, NJ: Prentice Hall.

Wantanabe, S. (1968). Four concepts basic to the occupational therapy process. *American Journal of Occupational Therapy, 22,* 439-445.

Warren, H. H. (1974). Self-perception of independence among urban elderly. *American Journal of Occupational Therapy, 28*(6), 329-336.

Watson, D. (1997). *Task analysis: An occupational performance approach.* Bethesda, MD: American Occupational Therapy Association.

West, W. L. (1969). The growing importance of prevention. *American Journal of Occupational Therapy, 23*(3), 226-231.

WFOT. (2012). Definition "occupation." Retrieved August 12, 2013, from http://www.wfot.org/aboutus/aboutoccupationaltherapy/definitionofoccupationalttherapy.aspx.

White, C. M. (2011). Heart-happy occupations in a cardiac rehabilitation circuit. *Occupational Therapy Now, 13*(5), 11-13.

White, C. M., & Buyting, P. L. (2011). Sense of doing: Heart-happy occupations in a cardiac rehabilitation circuit. *Occupational Therapy Now, 13*(5), 11-12.

White, R. (1971). The urge toward competence. *American Journal of Occupational Therapy, 25*(6), 271-274.

White, R. (1974). Strategies of adaptation: an attempt at systematic description. In S. V. Coelho, D. A. Hamburg, & J. E. Adams (Eds.), *Coping and adaptation* (pp. 47-68). New York, NY: Basic Books.

White, V. K. (1986). Promoting health and wellness: a theme for the eighties. *American Journal of Occupational Therapy, 40*(11), 743-748.

Whiteford, G. (2000). Occupational deprivation: global challenge in the new millennium. *British Journal of Occupational Therapy, 63*(5), 200-204.

Whiteford, G. E., & Wilcock, A. A. (2000). Cultural relativism: occupation and independence reconsidered. *Canadian Journal of Occupational Therapy, 67*(5), 324-336.

Whittaker, B. (2012). Sustainable global wellbeing: a proposed expansion of the occupational therapy paradigm. *British Journal of Occupational Therapy, 75*(9), 436-439.

WHO. (2001). *International classification of functioning, disability, and health.* Geneva, Switzerland: Author.

Wiemer, R. B. (1972). Some concepts of prevention as an aspect of community health. *American Journal of Occupational Therapy, 26*(1), 1-9.

Wilcock, A. A. (1993). Keynote paper: biological and sociocultural aspects of occupation, health, and health promotion. *British Journal of Occupational Therapy, 56*(6), 200-203.

Wilcock, A. A. (1998). *An occupational perspective of health.* Thorofare, NJ: SLACK Incorporated.

Wilcock, A. A. (2006). *An occupational perspective of health.* Thorofare, NJ: SLACK Incorporated.

Wilcock, A. A., & Townsend, E. A. (2000). Occupational terminology interactive dialogue. *Journal of Occupational Science, 7*(2), 84-86.

Willard, H. S., & Spackman, C. S. (1947). *Principles of occupational therapy.* Philadelphia, PA: J. B. Lippincott.

Williamson, G. G. (1997). Coping and young children with motor deficits. In J. D. Noshpitz (Ed.), *Handbook of child and adolescent psychiatry, Vol. 1, infants and preschoolers: development and syndromes* (pp. 439-452). New York, NY: John Wiley & Sons.

Wolman, B. B. (1989). *Dictionary of behavioral science* (2nd ed.). San Diego, CA: Academic Press.

Woodside, H. (1976). Dimensions of the occupational behaviour model. *Canadian Journal of Occupational Therapy, 43*(1), 11-14.

Wos, M. (1984). *MESHin' around.* Milwaukee, WI: Author.

Wrobel, S. (1994). *Concept formation and knowledge revision.* Dordrecht, Netherlands: Kluwer Academic Publishers.

Yerxa, E. J. (1996). The social and psychological experience of having a disability: implications for occupational therapists. In L. W. Pedretti (Ed.), *Occupational therapy: practice skills for physical dysfunction* (pp. 253-274). St. Louis, MO: Mosby.

Zeitlin, S., Williamson, G. G., & Szczepanski, M. (1988). *Early coping inventory: a measure of adaptive behavior (manual).* Bensenville, IL: Scholastic Testing Service.

Zemke, R., & Clark, F. (1996). *Occupational science: The evolving discipline.* Philadelphia, PA: F. A. Davis.

Zimmerman, M. E. (1957). Ideas for independence. *Crippled Child, 34*(5), 7-8.

Financial Disclosures

Dr. Kate Barrett has no financial or proprietary interest in the materials presented herein.

Dr. Julie D. Bass has no financial or proprietary interest in the materials presented herein.

Dr. Carolyn M. Baum has no financial or proprietary interest in the materials presented herein.

Dr. Sally Bennett has no financial or proprietary interest in the materials presented herein.

Dr. Catana Brown has no financial or proprietary interest in the materials presented herein.

Dr. Leeanne M. Carey has no financial or proprietary interest in the materials presented herein.

Dr. Charles H. Christiansen has no financial or proprietary interest in the materials presented herein.

Dr. Penelope A. Moyers Cleveland has no financial or proprietary interest in the materials presented herein.

Ms. Jane A. Davis has no financial or proprietary interest in the materials presented herein.

Dr. Lisa L. Dutton has no financial or proprietary interest in the materials presented herein.

Dr. Aaron M. Eakman has no financial or proprietary interest in the materials presented herein.

Dr. Gunilla Eriksson has no financial or proprietary interest in the materials presented herein.

Dr. Lena-Karin Erlandsson has no financial or proprietary interest in the materials presented herein.

Dr. Marcia Finlayson has no financial or proprietary interest in the materials presented herein.

Dr. John D. Fleming has no financial or proprietary interest in the materials presented herein.

Mr. Alec I. Hamilton has no financial or proprietary interest in the materials presented herein.

Ms. Anita L. Hamilton has no financial or proprietary interest in the materials presented herein.

Dr. Joy Hammel has no financial or proprietary interest in the materials presented herein.

Ms. Kathryn Haugen has no financial or proprietary interest in the materials presented herein.

Mr. Stan A. Hudson has no financial or proprietary interest in the materials presented herein.

Dr. Hans Jonsson has no financial or proprietary interest in the materials presented herein.

Dr. Naomi Josman has no financial or proprietary interest in the materials presented herein.

Ms. Marian Keglovits has no financial or proprietary interest in the materials presented herein.

Dr. Danbi Lee has no financial or proprietary interest in the materials presented herein.

Dr. Margareta Lilja has no financial or proprietary interest in the materials presented herein.

Dr. Sok Mui Lim has no financial or proprietary interest in the materials presented herein.

Dr. Adina Maeir has no financial or proprietary interest in the materials presented herein.

Dr. Kathleen Matuska has no financial or proprietary interest in the materials presented herein.

Dr. Sara E. McEwen has no financial or proprietary interest in the materials presented herein.

Ms. Patricia Nellis has no financial or proprietary interest in the materials presented herein.

Dr. René Padilla has no financial or proprietary interest in the materials presented herein.

Dr. Helene J. Polatajko has no financial or proprietary interest in the materials presented herein.

Dr. Jan Miller Polgar has no financial or proprietary interest in the materials presented herein.

Dr. Kathlyn L. Reed has no financial or proprietary interest in the materials presented herein.

Dr. Sylvia Rodger has no financial or proprietary interest in the materials presented herein.

Dr. Sandra L. Rogers has no financial or proprietary interest in the materials presented herein.

Ms. Shlomit Rotenberg-Shpigelman has no financial or proprietary interest in the materials presented herein.

Mr. Jon Sanford has no financial or proprietary interest in the materials presented herein.

Dr. Carol Haertlein Sells has no financial or proprietary interest in the materials presented herein.

Dr. Diane L. Smith has no financial or proprietary interest in the materials presented herein.

Dr. Susan Stark has no financial or proprietary interest in the materials presented herein.

Dr. Virginia C. Stoffel has no financial or proprietary interest in the materials presented herein.

Dr. Gretchen V. M. Stone has no financial or proprietary interest in the materials presented herein.

Ms. Verena C. Tatzer has no financial or proprietary interest in the materials presented herein.

Dr. Timothy J. Wolf has no financial or proprietary interest in the materials presented herein.

Dr. Jenny Ziviani has no financial or proprietary interest in the materials presented herein.

Index

ability/abilities, 393, 612
abnormal synergies, 273
Absolute Intensity testing, 292
Accessibility for Ontarians with Disabilities of 2005 (Canada), 449
accidents, in childhood occupation, 141
accommodation, 25, 634
achievement, 570
action
    concepts of, 612
    planning, 505–506
    purposeful, 605–606
Action Research Arm Test, 276
Active Lifestyle All Your Life Intervention Program, 179–180
active participation, 603
activities of daily living (ADL), 13, 14, 41, 621–622
Activities Scales for Kids, 139
activity/activities
    in daily occupation, 115–116
    definition of, 43
    doing and, 601–602
    health and, 9–10, 16–17
    internal clocks and, 17
    meaningfulness of, 314–315
    patterns of with aging, 177
    purposeful, 605–606
    sensory factors in, 250
    stress and, 16–17
Activity Card Sort, 237, 299, 323, 324, 351, 371
Activity in Context and Time (ACT), 125
adaptation, 144, 570–571, 602, 634
Adaptive Behavior Assessment System, 2nd ed (ABAS-II), 139
adolescence/adolescents, 130
    assessing occupations and performance of, 135
    development and occupation in, 134–135
    journals relevant to, 152
    mental health conditions in, 142
    organizations serving, 151
adult occupations, 157–166
adulthood
    demands of, 158
    occupational competence in, 159–160
    stages of, 158–159
advocacy, 431–434
    for assistive technology, 454
    dimensions of, 477–478
    structures supporting, 478
Advocacy-Clients, 433
Advocacy-Community, 433
Advocacy-Community Empowerment, 433
Advocacy-Education, 433
Advocacy-Political Competence, 433

Affordable Care Act, self-management services and, 509
age
    in cultural identity, 341
    in occupation patterns, 123
age coding, 170
ageism, 170
aging
    early theories of, 176–178
    occupational performance deficits with, 180
    occupational perspective on, 172–176
    positive aspects of, 176–177
aging society, 172–173
AgingCare.com, 166
Air Carrier Access Act, 403
alliance, client-practitioner, 85–86
altruism, evolutionary perspective on, 369
Alzheimer's disease, 236
American Academy of Sleep Medicine, 166
American Association of People with Disabilities, 352
American Community Survey, 374
American Medical Association Ethical Code, 474
American Occupational Therapy Association (AOTA)
    Blueprint for Entry-Level Education of, 84
    Centennial Vision of, 560
    Code of Ethics of, 469–473
    position of on public/community health interventions, 540–541
    Practice Framework, 3rd edition (*See Framework*)
Americans with Disabilities Act of 1990 (ADA), 402, 403, 425, 429, 449
    Accessibility Guidelines of, 408
    Checklist for Readily achievable Barrier Removal of, 410
    intention of, 423
Americans with Disabilities Amendments Act of 2008, 425, 429
amyotrophic lateral sclerosis, motor function impairment in, 269, 270
anosognosia, 237
apnea, sleep, 299
applied behavioral analysis (ABA), 261, 514
Architectural Barriers Act (ABA), 404, 425
areas of occupation, 639
Arm Motor Ability Test (AMAT), 276
arts and crafts movement, 595
Ask Dr. Wiki, 519
Assessment of Motor and Process Skills (AMPS), 139, 276, 351
    School Version of (School AMPS), 138
assessments
    in business planning, 555–556
    functional, 577
    in PEOP Model, 61–62
assimilation, 25
assistive devices, 399–400
    abandonment rates for, 84
    use and discontinuance of, 445

assistive technology
    acquisition of, 452
    advocacy for, 454
    categories of, 443–446
    definition of, 442–443
    as enabler, 442
    human activity model for, 447–448
    interventions with, 452–454
        assessment and evaluation of, 448–452
        evidence base of, 455–462
        outcomes of, 455
    legislation related to, 448
    matching children and, 450
    narrative perspective and background literature on, 442–448
    organizations and resources for, 445
    in PEOP Model, 442
    principles of selecting, 446–447
    selection process for, 452
    training/education in, 454
Assistive Technology Act of 1998/2004, 443, 449
assistive technology team members, 445
asTex test of touch sensibility, 259
asthma, 141
AT Device Predisposition Assessment, 450
AT Outcomes Profile-Mobility, 451
attachment theory, 131
attention, 149, 235
attention deficit hyperactivity disorder (ADHD), 140, 234, 235, 237
attitudes, in occupational change, 84–85
attitudinal barriers, 18
attribution theory, 84
audition, 251, 254
auditory learning, 150
auditory tests, 258–259
augmentative and alternative communication devices, 444
authenticity, 87, 88
autism spectrum disorder, 140, 257
autonomy, 471, 572
    definition of, 639
    need for, 317–318
awareness, 236–237
Awareness of Social Inference Test (TASIT), 240

Baddeley-Hitch model, 235
balance, 255, 582
    assessment of, 274
    conceptualizations of, 118–120
    interventions for, 281
    loss of, 255–256
    occupational, 583–585
balance tests, 275
balance training, 277
Baltes Selective Optimization with Compensation Theory, 26–27
Bandura social cognitive theory, 32, 85, 132–133
basic activities of daily living (BADL), 13
Basic Psychological Needs Scale, 327
bathing performance, environmental factors impacting, 398
Beck Depression Inventory, 222
Beecher, Henry Ward, 81–82
behavior
    definition of, 514–515
    learning and, 32
Behavior, Rating Inventory of Executive Function , 237
Behavior, Rating Inventory of Executive Function–Adult version (BRIEF-A), 238

Behavior Risk Factor Surveillance System (BRFSS), 202
behavioral, errorless learning techniques, 242
Behavioral Assessment of the Dysexecutive Syndrome (BADS), 240
Behavioral Inattention Test (BIT), 239
behavioral learning, 486–487, 491, 493
Behavioral Risk Factor Surveillance System, 374
behaviorism, 43
behaviorist education theories, 514–515
Belmont Report, 474
beneficence, 471
Berg Balance Scale (BBS), 274, 275
Berkman-Syme Social Network Index, 374
Better Life Index of Well-Being, 207
Bioecological or Ecological Systems Theory, 137–141
biological clock
    activities and, 17
    occupation patterns and, 122
biological rhythms, habits and routines in, 123
biomechanical frame of reference, 42, 631
biomedical-based models, 51
blindness, 253–254
Blogger, 519
blogs, 518, 519
body
    beliefs about, 343–345
    composition of, 291
    functions of, 43
body factor-centered models, 631
body mass index (BMI), 291
Body-Weight Percentage test, 291, 294
bond, in working alliance, 86
Bordin theory, 85–86
boredom, 322–323
Boredom Proneness Scale, 327
Borg Exertion Scale, 295, 296
Borg Rating of Perceived Exertion, 293, 295
Bowlby, John, 131
Box and Block Test, 276
Braden Scale, 303
brain injury, acquired, 235
Bronfenbrenner's ecological systems theory, 33–34, 137–141, 392–393
built environment, modifying, 399
bundling services, 550
burnout, 161
business
    definition of, 551
    forms of, 552
    fundamentals of, 550
    identifying and defining, 556
    structures of, 551–552
business plan, 557–559
    assessments and evaluations in, 555–556
    implementing, 559
business skills, 552–553
butterfly effect, 190

calibration, 132
calisthenics, 294
Canada Mortgage and Housing Corporation (CMHC), 409
Canadian Index of Well-Being, 206
Canadian Model of Occupational Performance (CMOP), 34, 38, 51, 390
    Enabling Occupation II (CMOP-E), 38–39
Canadian Occupational Performance Measure (COPM), 96, 258, 323, 324, 351
capacity, concepts of, 612

cardiorespiratory endurance, 296
cardiorespiratory function, 291–296
cardiovascular assessments, 292–294
Care for Chronic Conditions Model, 211
career responsibilities, 159
caregiver strain, 523
caregiving
    activities of, 161–163
    policies affecting, 402
Center for Epidemiological Studies-Depression Scale, 222
Centers for Disease Control and Prevention (CDC)
    calculating poor health costs, 532
    Health-Related Quality of Life-14 Healthy Days Measure of, 205–206
    Obesity Resource Center of, 166
central nervous system disorders, 269
cerebral palsy, 140
    interventions for, 146–148
    motor function impairment in, 270
    sensory impairment in, 256
    skill acquisition interventions for, 143–144
certification, ethical codes and, 472–473
chaining, 494
change, managing, 559
CHANGE (Community Health Assessment aND Group Evolution), 367, 374
Child-Initiated Pretend Play Assessment (ChiPPA), 136
childbearing decisions, 159
childhood
    acquired health conditions of, 141
    developmental conditions of, 140
    early, 130, 132–133
    journals relevant to, 152
    middle, 130, 133–134
    occupations of, 130–152
    play/leisure occupation measures for, 136–137
    stages of, 130
childhood cancers, 141
children
    assessing occupations and performance of, 135
    interventions supporting skill acquisition for, 143–144
    mental health conditions in, 142
    organizations serving, 151
Children Helping Out: Responsibilities, Expectations and Supports (CHORES), 139
Children's Assessment of Participation and Enjoyment, 323, 324
    Preferences for Activities of Children, 137, 351
chorea, 276–277
Chronic Care Model, 501–502, 509
chronic illness management, 507
chronic illness self-management, 590–591
chronobiology, 122
chronosystems, in children's occupation, 137–141
chronotherapeutics, 122
circadian desynchronosis, 122
Civil Rights of Institutionalized Persons Act, 403
classifications, 24
    in cognitive development, 133
    definition and purposes of, 43
    of ICF, 43–45
Clean Air Act, 425
client advocacy, 477–478
client-centered practice, 83, 631–634
    culturally sensitive, 350–353
    PEOP Model in, 52–53, 60
    self-management goals of, 508

Client-Centered Practice of Occupational Therapy, 390
clients
    adaptation of, 602
    definition of, 639
    participation of, 603
    preferences, values, and circumstances of, 102
    satisfaction of, 589
clinical expertise, 101–102
clinical reasoning, 103
clock drawing tests, 237, 240
clothing, in status, 344
Cochrane Collaboration, 94–95
cognition, 234
    assessments and evaluations of, 237–241
    background literature on, 235–237
    in Canadian model, 38
    interventions for, 241–244
    narratives for, 234–235
    organizations and journals focusing on, 245
    supporting and hindering learning, 489–490
Cognitive-Behavioral Intervention Framework, 42–43
cognitive-behavioral therapy, 223, 303
cognitive development stages, 131–135
cognitive development theory, 25–26
cognitive disabilities, 234, 631
cognitive-functional observations, 237–241
cognitive impairment, mild (MCI), 147, 234, 235
cognitive learning, 486
    assessment of, 492–493
    background literature on, 486–492
    versus behavioral learning, 487
    theories of, 487–488
Cognitive Orientation to Daily Occupational Performance (CO-OP), 143, 261, 494–495
Cognitive Performance Test (CPT), 239
cognitive rehabilitation, 631
    DIM strategy for, 495
cognitive technologies, 442, 444, 453
cognitive tests, 237–241
collaborative goal-setting principles, 53
collaborative purposeful work, 86
collaborative writing applications, 519
collective action, for public health, 529–531
collectivism, 342–343
Color Trails Test, 239
common good, 469
communication
    digital, 518, 519
    functional, 577
    in interprofessional teams, 473–476
communication devices, 442, 444, 453
communication skills, 236, 553
communities of practice concept, 103
community
    assessment of physical environment in, 410–411
    collapse of, 368
    disease impact on, 536
    environment of, 405, 406
    as exosystem, 393
    interdependent, 368–369
    modifications of, 407–408
    older adult activities in, 174
    in Public Health Assessments, 537
    social capital of, 369, 379
community-based programs, reimbursement in, 555

community-centered interventions, 70
community health
    assessments in, 529–532
    definition of, 528–529
    interventions in, 537–544
    narratives for, 529–532
    outcomes for, 541
Community Health Assessment Toolkit, 536–537
Community Health Environment Checklist (CHEC), 408, 409
COMPASS, 451
compensatory approach, 634
competence/competency, 572–574
    continuing, 478–482
    definition of, 639
    development of, 478–481
    need for, 317–318
Competent Occupational Performance in the Environment Model, 390
Comprehensive Assessment and Solution Process for Aging Residents (CASPAR), 409
Comprehensive Assessments of Reform Efforts, 432
computer access technology, 444
Computerized Cognitive Training (CCT), 241, 242
computers, 444, 518–522
concepts
    functions of, 567
    importance of, 566–568
    origin of, 566–567
    in PEOP Model, 568–639
concrete operational stage, 133
conditioning, 43
conduct disorder, 142
confidentiality, 471, 472
conservation, 133
constraint-induced movement therapy/training, 143, 277
constructivist learning theory, 515
consumer-driven health care, 95
Consumer Product Safety Act, 425
Contemporary Task-Oriented Approach Model, 390
content management systems, 518, 519
content publishing systems, 518, 519–520
context, 41, 627–628, 639
context-focused therapy, 633
Contextual Memory Test (CMT), 239
Continuity and Adaptation Theory, 176–178
continuity theory, 170
continuous quality improvement (CQI) projects, 476
control
    lifespan theory of, 316–317
    strategies for, 325
controls, design of, 398
co-occupation, 116
cooperation, evolutionary perspective on, 369
coordination disorders
    assessment of, 274–277
    interventions for, 143, 281
COPE, 327
coping, 574–575
    definition of, 639
    in personal narratives, 221
    through meaning, 320–321
core effect, concept of, 16–17
corporation, 551–552
Craig Hospital Inventory of Environmental Factors (CHIEF), 408, 411
critical thinking, 103–104
criticality, zone of, 190

crying, 131
cultural beliefs, in assistive technology assessment, 449–450
cultural competence assessment tools, 348–350
Cultural Competence Health Practitioner Assessment, 348
Cultural Competence Self-Assessment Questionnaire, 349
Cultural Fitness Survey, 348
cultural identity, sources of, 340–346
Cultural Onion Model, 339
Cultural Self-Efficacy Scale, 348
cultural structures, 123–124
cultural syndromes, 336
cultural validity, 351–352
culturally and linguistically appropriate service (CLAS), 346–347
culture, 41, 335–336, 354
    affecting occupational performance, 401
    assessments and evaluations of, 346–352
    boundaries of, 338–339
    conscious and unconscious, 338
    definition of, 335–336
    doing concept and, 600
    gender and, 144
    interventions for, 350–353
        outcomes of, 353–354
    levels of, 339–340
    narrative and background literature on, 337
    national and international efforts to address, 352–353
    shared, 337–338
curative services, 519
Current Procedure Technology codes, 554–555

daily occupation
    observing and measuring, 124–125
    patterns of
        defining, 115–118
        health and, 118–121
        integrating, 117–118
        occupations building, 116–117
Daily Stress Inventory, 301
Day Reconstruction Method, 222
decentering, 133
decision making
    context of, 102–103
    ethical, 468–469, 470
    process of, 93
decline, growth and, 26–27
Delicious, 519
deontologic approach, 469
depression, 490
deprivation, 209
Descartes, René, 8
development
    in adolescence, 134–135
    in early childhood, 132–133
    in infancy and toddlerhood, 130–132
    in middle childhood, 133–134
developmental conditions, 135–137, 140, 208
developmental coordination disorder, 140, 145, 256
developmental delay, 208–209
developmental frame of reference, 631
developmental learning theories, 515
dialectical behavior therapy, 223–224
Difficulties in Emotional Regulation Scale, 222
Diigo, 519
Direct Assessment of Functional Status-Revised, 351
Disabilities Discrimination Act (UK), 449

Disability Adjusted Life Year (DALY), 375, 532
Disability Assessment Schedule (WHO), 201
disability/disabilities
    definition of, 43
    developmental, 208
    doing and, 597
    excess, 26
    health and, 9–10
    intellectual, 140
    management of, 507
    as participation restriction, 18
    as person-environment misfit, 388
    social aspects of, 389
Disability Discrimination Act of 1992 (Australia), 449
disability-free life expectancy, 173–174
disability-related organizations, 438–439
Disability Rights International, 352
Disabled Parents Network, 352
Disabled People's International, 352
discrimination policies, 426
discriminatory practices, 345–346
discussion forums, online, 520
disease, impact on communities, 536
Disease Activity Score, 96
disease prevention programs, community, 531
disengagement, 107, 175
disorder, 10
disparities
    culture and, 345–346
    in health, 365
    in population health, 209
Do It Now Project, 179
documentation
    for Medicare reimbursement, 553–554
    oral, 477
    purposes of, 476
    technology in, 476–477
    written, 477
doing, 593
    concepts of, 567–568, 593, 600–607, 615–617
    disability and, 597
    effectiveness of, 596–597
    efficiency of, 597
    factors influencing, 616
    learning by, 597–598
    meaning and meaningfulness of, 598–599
    occupation as, 617–618
    occupational behavior and, 599
    patterns of, 607–611
    person/personal characteristics and, 611–615
    practical, 599–600
    process of, 598–600
    purposeful, 605–606
    socially and culturally relevant issue of, 600
    values and beliefs about, 593–596
doing the right things right, 94, 97
double effect, 469
Down syndrome, 140
Dunton's Credo, 83
duties, ethical decision making and, 469
Dynamic Interactional Model (DIM), 495
dynamic performance analysis, 261
dynamic systems theory, 29–30
dynamic teaming, 473
dynamometry, hand-held, 275

dysdiadochokinesis, 274
Dysexecutive Questionnaire (DEX), 238
dyslexia, 140

eating disorders, 142
ecological approach to perception and action theory, 29–30
Ecological Systems Model, 389
ecological systems theory, 33, 34
ecological theory of adaptation and aging, 32–33
ecology, 630
Ecology of Human Performance Model, 390
economic accountability, 97
economic environment, 425–426
education, 622–623
    activities of, 14, 15
    aligning with PEOP Model, 550–552
    digital technology in, 518–522
    as enablement tool, 514–515
    learning and, 515–517
    occupational therapy and, 513
education environment, 422–437
Education for All Handicapped Children Act of 1975, 402, 427
educational interventions
    in childhood occupation, 137
    life balance program in, 516
    outcomes for, 523
    using PEOP Occupational Therapy Process, 514, 522–523
Educational Technology Predisposition Assessment, 450
educator role, preparing for, 517–518
effectiveness
    of doing, 596–597
    in PEOP Model, 72–73
efficacy, 72–73
efficiency of doing, 597
effortful control, 149
elderhood, 170–176
elderly parents, caregiving of, 162–163
elderly persons
    multisensory processing problems in, 256
    occupational performance deficits and, 180, 181
    preventive occupation-based interventions for, 178–180
    sensory impairment in, 257
electronic health records, 476–477
elimination disorders, 142
Elluminate, 520
emergence, 190
emergent awareness, 237
emerging practice, 473
emotional intelligence, 517–518
emotional support, 400–401
emotions, 12
    management of, 503
    meaning and, 319–321
    regulation of, 220
empathy, 87, 88
employer-provided health benefits, 11
employment
    disparities in, 160–161
    in occupation patterns, 124
empowerment, 634–635
ENABLE-AGE Project, 180
enablement, 87, 89, 514–515, 635
Enabler Model, 396–397, 399, 409
Enabling-Disabling Process Model, 389
ENACT, THRIVE, 374

encopresis, 142
engagement, 176–178, 602
Engagement in Meaningful Activities Survey (EMAS), 322
engaging occupations, 176, 177
Englehardt, H. Tristram Jr, 9, 77
enuresis, 142
environment, 5, 41, 387–388
    adjustments of, 242–244, 630, 635–636
    analysis of, 630
    assessment of for business, 555
    in Canadian model, 38–39
    categories of, 399–400
    cultural, 335–354
    definition of, 43, 422
    health policies and, 423–426
    impairments and, 396–397
    international classification of, 392, 393, 394–395
    interventions addressing
        in community, 407–408
        at home, 405–407
    layers of, 402–405
    learning and, 491
    management of, 507–508
    in MOHO, 36
    occupational and rehabilitative models addressing, 388–390
    in occupational performance, 334, 399–405, 137–142
    in occupational therapy, 628–630
    in PEOP Model, 50, 54–55
    physical, psychobiological, and societal constructs of, 389
    physical and natural, 387–417
    public policy and, 422–439
    social, 359–383
    technological, 442–463
    theories supporting understanding of, 25
environment behavior studies (EBS), 389–399
environment-centered models, 631–634
environment level theories, 32–33
environmental adaptations, 242, 243–244, 630
environmental barriers, 180, 397
environmental boundaries, 337
environmental demand, 630
Environmental Press Model, 32–34, 393–396, 491, 492
environmental sensitivity, 124
Epworth Sleepiness Scale, 299
ethical codes, 469–473, 474–475
ethics
    in decision making, 468–469
    principles of, 469, 470–472
    supporting intervention, 468–473
ethnicity, 340–341
EuroQol Index, 96
eustress, 300
evaluation/assessment skills, business, 553, 555–556
Evaluation of Social Interaction (ESI), 240
everyday activities, 12, 13–16
Everyday Memory Questionnaire (EMQ), 237, 238
evidence, hierarchies of, 99
Evidence-Based Medicine Working Group, proposal of, 95
evidence-based policy making, 433–434
evidence-based practice, 4, 93–94, 95
    clients' preferences, values, and circumstances in, 102
    clinical and professional expertise in, 101–102
    in clinical context, 102–106
    context of, 95–98
    expectations for, 77

goal of, 95
    origins of, 94–95
    PEOP Model, 60–61
    research evidence in, 98–101
evolutionary biology, 369
excess disabilities, 26
Executive Function Performance Test (EFPT), 240, 241
executive functions, 236
exercise, 305–307
exosystems, 137–141, 393
Expanded Chronic Care Model, 500, 501–502
expectancy-value appraisal, 490
expertise, clinical and professional, 101–102
explanatory model, 345

Facebook, 518, 520
faculties, organizing framework for, 4
failure to thrive, 367–368
Fair Housing Act, Amendments to (1988), 402, 403
fall prevention, in home, 407
family
    in children's occupation, 137–141
    older adult activities in, 174
Family and Medical Leave Act (FMLA), 161
family-friendly policy, 191
Family Impact of Assistive Technology Scale (FIATS), 450
Farmville, 521
feasibility assessment, 556
feedback, in motor learning, 277–278
fetal alcohol syndrome, 140
fidelity, 471
figurative intelligence, 25
financial measures, 559–560
fine motor skills, 133
fitness, 296, 575, 639
5 A's, 504
flexibility, 291, 296
Flinder's Program, 503, 504, 508
flow, 149, 602–603
Fluidsurveys, 520
focus groups, 101–102
formal operations stage, 134–135
for-profit organizations, 187, 193
foundational knowledge, 112
Four-Quadrant Model of Facilitated Learning, 516
fourth age, theory of, 170, 176–178
fragile X syndrome, 140
frames of reference, 24, 40–42
Framework
    key definitions of, 639–640
    occupations defined in, 193
    on organizations' role, 186
    time use measures of, 202–205
Frankl, Victor, 76
freedom, retirement and, 175–176
Fugl-Meyer Assessment, 273, 275, 280
function, 575–576
    concept of, 568–569, 639
    as modifier, 577–578
functional approach, 636
functional electrical stimulation, 280
Functional Independence Measure for Children, 139
Functional Reach Test, 274, 275
functional skills, 577
Functional Tactile Object Recognition Test (fTORT), 259

functional training, 578
functionalism, 575–576
functioning, 43, 576–577
Functioning Everyday in a Wheelchair Seating-Mobility Outcomes Measure, 451
Future of Public Health Committee, Study of (IOM), 201

gaming, 521
gender
    in childhood occupation, 144
    in cultural identity, 341
    in occupation patterns, 123
gender roles, changing, 159
Geneva Convention, 474
Genttle's Taxonomy of Movement Tasks, 279, 280, 281
Gini Index, 375
Global Competencies Inventory, 348
goals
    setting, 505–506
    in working alliance, 86, 88
Google Drive, 518, 519
Google Hangout, 518
Google Scholar, 519
Gottlieb Visual Field Awareness System, 260
government organizations, 187
    occupational performance of, 193
    population health information of, 210–211
gratification, delayed, 132
Grating orientation discrimination test, 259
Groningen Fitness Test for the Elderly, 295–296, 297–298
groups
    health attitudes of, 8–9
    occupation of, 114
growth, decline and, 26–27
Guillain-Barré syndrome, 269, 270
gustatory function testing, 259
gustatory sense, 251, 256

habit training, 633
habits, 35–36, 41, 122–123, 607–608
habituation, 35–36
HALex, 375
Hand Active Sensation Test, 259
Hand Arm Bimanual Intensive Training (HABIT), 143
Hand Function Survey, 259
hand injury, 257
happiness, 76
hardware, adaptive, 399–400
Hassle Scale, 301
head injury, 257
healing, beliefs about, 345
health
    activities and, 16–17
    beliefs about, 343–345
    concepts of, 578–579
    daily occupation patterns and, 118–121
    definitions of, 8, 10–12, 639
    determinants of, 536
    disparities in, 365
    environment and policies of, 423–426
    holistic view of, 31
    for individuals, groups, and populations, 8–10
    inequalities of, 365, 375
    inequities of, 365
    in occupational performance, 12, 135–137

    as order, 10
    in PEOP Model, 422
    perceptions and understandings of, 8
    of populations, 17–18, 200–201
    social capital and, 369–370
    social determinants of, 361–367, 366, 371–378
    social model of, 30–31
    WHO definition of, 423–425
Health Assessment Questionnaire (HAQ), disability index of, 96
health behaviors, 201–202
health benefits programs, 11
Health Canada, 366
health care
    accessibility of, 95, 426
    affordability of, 426
    costs of, 426
    in industrial nations, 18–19
health care business
    evolution of, 550
    mission, vision, and value statements in, 556–559
    outcomes and, 559–560
    reimbursement in, 553–555
    research on, 561–562
health care environment, 422–437
health care organizations, 438–439
Health Care Technology Predisposition Assessment, 450
Health Coaching, 504
health equity, 364
Health Impact Assessment, 432
Health Information Technology for Economic and Clinical Health Act (HITECH), 476
Health Insurance Portability and Accountability Act (HIPAA), 473, 474, 476
health policies, international, 425
health promotion, 196, 531, 633
health-related quality of life (HRQOL), 76, 304
    in populations, 205–206, 208
Health Related Quality of Life–14 Healthy Days Measure, 205–206
health status, 342
Health Through Occupation, 314
healthy days, 375
Healthy People 2020, 366
    goals and measures of, 211
hearing, 254
hearing devices, 444, 453
hearing tests, 258–259
heart rate, target, 293
helping alliance, 85
helping encounter, 85
Helsinki Declaration, 474
Hierarchical Model of Motor Control, 268
Hippocrates, 8
Hippocratic Oath, 474
holistic view, 31
home
    modifications of, 397–398, 401–402, 405–407
    physical environment in, 409–410
Home and Community Environment Assessment (HACE), 408, 411
Home Environment Assessment Protocol (HEAP), 409
HOME-FAST, 407, 409
Home Health Agencies (HHA), 554
home meal service, 400–401
Home Observation for Measurement of the Environment (HOME), 410
Hope Scale, 222
household activities, 163

Housing Enabler, 407
Human Activity Assistive Technology Model (HAAT), 442, 447–448
human occupation, 82, 125–126
    change in, 83–85
    complexity of, 114–115
    essential aspects of, 83
    group level, 114
    individual level, 114
    patterns of, 126
human rights, 11
hypermetria, 274
hypersensitivity, 257
hypometria, 274

identity
    concepts of, 579–580
    occupation and, 224
    with PEOP occupational therapy, 75
    in personal narratives, 220
illness
    as disorder, 10
    as participation restriction, 18
    stigmatization of, 9
imbalance
    occupational, 583–585
    in population health, 209
immunizations, attitudes toward, 9
Impact of Vision Impairment Questionnaire, 258
impairments, 43
    environmental factors and, 396–397
implementation skills, 553
impulse control, 149
In-Home Occupational Performance Evaluation (I-HOPE), 410
inactivity, 164
incompetence, 572
independence/autonomy
    concepts of, 580–581
    development of, 132
    supporting, 84
individual
    definition of, 5
    health attitudes of, 8–9
individualism, 342–343
Individuals with Disabilities Education Act (IDEA), 402, 404
    Amendments of 2004, 429, 448
inequalities, health, 365
infancy, development and occupation in, 130–132
infectious disease, 8–9
information
    integrating sources of, 94, 103–104
    transfer and generalization of, 489
informational support, 400–401
informed consent, 471–472
informed risk management, 509
inhibition, 149
injustice, 209
    occupational, 585
inpatient rehabilitation facilities, 554
insight, 236–237
insomnia, 164, 166, 299
institutional environment, 450
Institutional Review Boards (IRBs), 472
instrumental activities of daily living (IADL), 13, 14, 41, 623
intentional relationship, 85

interactive encounter, 85
Intercultural Development Inventory, 348
Intercultural Effectiveness Scale, 348
interdependence, 581–582, 639
interdisciplinary teams, 473–476
interests, concepts of, 612–613
International Classification of Activities for Time-Use Statistics (ICATUS), 202
International Classification of Functioning, Disability and Health (ICF), 43, 45, 69, 350, 389, 392–395
    assistive technology definition of, 442–443
    principles of, 44
    related to policy, 422–425
Internet
    as education tool, 518–522
    health care information on, 95, 96–97
Interpersonal Support Evaluation List, 374
interprofessional teams, 473
interventions, 634–637
    emerging approaches to, 466
    principles of, 466
Inventory for Assessing the Process of Cultural Competence Among Health Care Professional, 349
Inventory of Socially Supportive Behaviors, 375
involuntary movement, 276–277
iTunes, 520

Jebsen Taylor Hand Function Test, 259
jet lag, 17, 122
Joomla, 518
justice. *See also* injustice; social justice
    distributive, 97–98, 469
    occupational, 209, 585
    procedural, 471
juvenile rheumatoid arthritis, 141

Kawa (River) Model, 34, 36–37, 222
Kettle Test, 239, 241
Kids Count Data Center, 374
Kinesthesia Test, 259
kinesthetic learning, 150
King's Model of Meaning of Life Experiences, 325
Klein, Bonnie Sherr, 82–83
knowledge
    clinical, 101
    declarative, 488–489
    foundational, 548
    procedural, 488
knowledge to action process, 104–106
knowledge translation, 104–106
knowledge workers, 195–196
Knox Pre-school Play Scales, Revised, 136

Labor, US Department of, 166
language
    in cultural identity, 341
    impairment of, 140
Language Activity Monitor, 451
laws
    related to assistive technology, 448
    related to occupational performance, 402, 403–404
    related to occupational therapy practices, 425–429
Lawton's environmental press theory, 13, 32–33, 34
Leading Health Indicators (LHIs), 532

learning, 515–516
    authentic, 516
    behavior and, 32
    behavioral approaches to, 493
    characteristics supporting and hindering, 489–492
    cognitive approaches to, 492–495
    core concepts of, 488
    definition of, 486
    by doing, 597–598
    errorless, 494
    factors affecting, 479–480
    generalization of, 489
    learner-centered, 516
    lifelong, 478–482
    memory and, 235–236
    mental states and, 31
    motor, 493
    neurofunctional approach to, 493–494
    observational, 31
    person-centered strategy for, 486–495
    task-specific, 242, 243
    transformative, 516–517
learning cultures, 478–479
learning disabilities, specific, 140
learning infrastructure, 480–481
learning-related skills, 132
learning styles, 149–150, 517
learning theories, 517
    constructivist, 515
    developmental, 515
    education and, 514
leisure, 15–16, 623–624
    activities of, 14
        adult, 163
        of older adults, 174
        in work-life balance, 118
    in Canadian model, 38
leukemia, 141
licensure, ethical codes and, 472
life balance, 119–120, 516, 582
    assessments for, 165
    factors affecting, 164
    in personal narratives, 221
Life Balance Inventory (LBI), 165
life coaching approach, 164
life energy, 37
life expectancy, 173–174
    disability-free, 173–174
life experience, 177, 316
life imbalance, 163–164
life partners, choosing, 159
life redesign, 633
Life Regard Index (LRI), 76
life roles, 250
life satisfaction, 75–76, 158, 589
lifespan human development principles, 26–27
lifespan theory of control, 316–317
Lifestyle Matter project, 179
Lifestyle Redesign program, 179
limitations, functional, 577
LinkedIn, 518, 520
Loewenstein Occupational Therapy Cognitive Assessment (LOTCA), 239
logical thought, 134–135

macrosystems, 103, 137–141, 393
manipulation technology, 444, 453
manual dexterity, 132
Manual Form Perception Test, 259
Manual Muscle Testing (MMT), 272–273, 275
marriage, 159
mass practice, in motor learning, 493
mastery, 84, 582–583
    occupations providing, 223, 224
MATCH Strategy, 143
maximum performance potential, zone of, 26
Mayo Clinic: Insomnia, 166
McGill Pain Questionnaire, 302
McMaster University Medical School
        Evidence-Based Medicine Working Group at, 98, 101
        problem-based learning approach at, 94–95
meaning, 313–314
    assessments and evaluations of, 322–323
    coping through, 320–321
    creation of, 76–77
    of doing, 598–599
    emotions and, 319–321
    global and situational, 318–319
    interventions related to, 323–325
    narrative perspective on, 315–316
    in occupational therapy, 314–315
    organizations and journals focusing on, 328
    outcomes related to, 326
    spirituality and, 321–322
Meaning in Life Questionnaire, 327
meaning-making model, 318–319
meaning of life experiences model, 316
Meaningful Activity Participation Assessment, 324
means, ordinary vs extraordinary, 469
Measure of Quality of the Environment (MQE), 411
Medicaid services, 9
medical body, 344
medical management, 503, 507
Medical Outcome Health Survey Short Form, Version 2, 327
Medicare
    documentation for reimbursement, 476
    Part A, 553–554
    Part B, 554–555
Medicare Therapy Cap, 422
Medicare—Support for Caregivers, 166
memory, 235–236
meningitis, 141
mental health
    in children and youth, 142
    in occupational performance, 135–137
    recovery in, 588–589
mental retardation, 140
mental states, in learning, 31–32
mesosystems, 103, 137–141, 392–393
metabolic equivalent (MET) levels, 291, 296
meta-cognition, 134–135
metacognitive treatment approach, 241–243
metamemory, 236
microsystems, 103, 137–141, 392
mid-life crisis, 159
mind, theory of, 236
Mini Mental Status Examination (MMSE), 237, 238
Minimum Data Set (MDS) assessment, 371
mission statements, 188, 189, 556

Moberg pick up test, modified, 259
MOBILATE project, 175
mobility
    functional, 577
    interventions for, 454
mobility devices, 442, 443–444
Mobility International USA, 352
Mobilizing Action toward Community Health (MATCH), 531
Mobilizing for Action through Planning and Partnerships (MAPP), 531
Model for the Practice of Occupational Therapy, 390
Model of Human Occupation (MOHO), 34–35, 84, 224, 390
    central focus of, 51
    environment of, 36
    occupational identity and competence in, 36
    occupational performance in, 36
    person components of, 35–36
    role performance in, 75
models, 24, 639
modification, 634
Modified Ashworth Scale (MAS), 272, 275
Modified Borg Perceived Exertion Scale, 295
Modified Caregiver Strain Index (MCSI), 523
Modified Tardieu Scale (MTS), 272, 275
Montreal Cognitive Assessment (MoCA), 237, 238
mood
    disorders of, 142
    occupations enhancing, 223, 224
    in personal narratives, 220
moral treatment, historical context of, 594
More Knowledgeable Other, 26
motivation
    in childhood occupation, 149
    concepts of, 613–614
    learning and, 490
    in personal narratives, 221
Motivational Interviewing, 223, 224, 504
Motivational Theory of Life Span Development, 325
Motor Activity Log, 276
Motor Assessment Scale (MAS), 275
motor behavior
    definition of, 27, 28
    models of, 27–30
    theories of, 27–30, 28
motor control
    in common health conditions, 269
    definition of, 28
    in PEOP Occupational performance model, 268, 269
    theories of, 268
motor development, 28
motor factors
    assessments and evaluations of, 269–277
    interventions for, 277–281
        outcomes of, 281–282
    organizations and journals focusing on, 282
motor function impairment, conditions associated with, 269, 270
motor learning, 29–30, 261, 277–279, 493
Multicontext Treatment Approach, 242
Multicultural Counseling Inventory, 349
multiculturalism, 345–346
Multidimensional Health Locus of Control Scale, 222
multidirectionality, 26–27
multidisciplinary teaming, 473–476
Multifactorial Memory Questionnaire (MMQ), 238
Multinational Time Use Study (MTUS), 202

Multiphasic Environmental Assessment Procedure (MEAP), 410
    Physical and Architectural Features Checklist of, 407
Multiple Errand Test (MET), 241
multiple sclerosis, 257, 270
multisensory impairments, 261
    assessments of, 251
    processing, 256, 259
    temporal processing, 257
muscle endurance
    assessments of, 292–294
    interventions for, 296
    in physical fitness, 290–291
muscle hypertonicity, 271–272
muscle rigidity, 270–271, 280
muscle strength, 290, 296
muscle tone, 270–272, 280
musculoskeletal injuries, 141
myasthenia gravis, 270
Myers-Briggs Type Indicator, 87–89

Nahemow theory, 34
narratives, 5
    in authentic learning, 516
    for communication health, 529–532
    in educational interventions, 522
    for health and public policies, 422–426, 529–532
    of organizational "story," 195
    in PEOP Model, 61
    in understanding meaning, 315–316
National Board for Certification of Occupational Therapy (NBCOT), 472–473
National Council on Disability, 353
National Dye Institute's Visual Function Questionnaire, 258
National Health and Nutrition Examination Survey (NHANES), 202
National Medical Rehabilitation Research Center Model, 391
National Organization of Disability, 353
National Survey on Drug Use and Health (NSDUH), 202
natural change agent, 619
natural environment, 400
Netvibes, 519
networking, 518, 519
Neurobehavioral Cognitive Status Examination, 239
neurodevelopmental approaches, 281
neurodevelopmental training, 281
neurofunctional learning, 493–494
Neurofunctional Treatment, 242
neuromuscular disorders, 269
neuropathic pain, 301
nociceptors, 301
nonmaleficence, 471
nonprofit organizations, 187, 193
Numeric Rating Scale, 302
Nuremburg Codes, 474
nutrition, 296–298

obesity, 164, 540
observational learning, 31
occupation. See also human occupation
    of adulthood, 157–166
    age coding, 170
    areas of, 13–16
    assumptions about, 620
    building daily occupation patterns, 116–117
    of childhood, 130–152

complexity of, 114–115
concepts of, 617
daily patterns of
    defining, 115–118
    health and, 118–121
definitions of, 4, 83, 130, 193, 639
as doing, 617–618
emotions and meaning in, 319–320
essential aspects of, 83
extrinsic factors impacting, 123–125
group level, 114
hidden, 117
hierarchies of, 115
holistic view of, 31
idiosyncratic nature of, 83
individual level, 114
intrinsic factors impacting, 121–123
lack of, 120–121
learning and, 491–492
main, 117
multiple dimensions of, 114
of organizations, 185–196
in PEOP Model, 50
of populations, 200–212
as potential outcome measures, 618–619
as predictor of survival in old age, 178
purposeful, 605–606
sequences building up, 115–116
as therapeutic change tool, 619
therapeutic potency of, 83
time and, 121
types of, 621–627
unexpected, 117
value and meaning in, 83
occupation-based models, 51, 59–60
occupation patterns, 120–122
Occupational Adaptation Model, 390, 570–571
occupational balance, 639–640
occupational behavior, 599
occupational change, 83–85
occupational community, 177
occupational competence, 36, 159–160, 390, 572–574
occupational deprivation, 160–161
occupational dysfunction, 619–621
occupational engagement, 602
Occupational Gap Questionnaire, 324
Occupational Health and Safety Act, 425
occupational identity, 36, 177
occupational imbalance, 160, 209
occupational outcomes, in historical context, 73–75
occupational participation, 603–604
occupational performance, 4, 8, 75
    assistive technology enabling, 442
    audition in, 254
    concepts of, 585–587
    developmental conditions and, 135–137
    environment factors affecting, 137–142, 334, 393
        in home, 397–398
        organizing continuum for understanding, 402–405
    everyday activities and, 13–16
    focus on, 52
    health and, 12, 135–137
    in MOHO, 36
    multisensory processing in, 256
    in older adults, 180, 181

olfactory and gustatory sensation in, 256
organization occupations and, 193–194
in PEOP Model, 40
person-centered model of, 36–37
person factors affecting, 142–150, 216
population health and, 17–18
promoting, 196
public policies influencing, 426–429
sensory factors in, 250
social supports affecting, 400–401
socioeconomic and political influences on, 401–402
somatosensation in, 255
strategies to improve, 399
vestibular sense in, 255
vision in, 253
Occupational Performance Coaching, 143
Occupational Performance History Interview-II, 222, 299, 352
Occupational Questionnaire, 237
occupational roles, 75, 610
occupational routine, 610–611
occupational task observation, 259
occupational therapy
    addressing environment, 388–389
    AOTA definition of, 82
    approaches in, 64
    biomechanical frame of reference in, 42
    CAOT definition of, 82
    central concepts of, 4–5
    changing rationale for, 595–596
    concepts of, 10, 112, 639
    domain of, 41
    for education, 515
    goals and outcomes of, 72
    in PEOP Model, 55, 62, 72–77, 566–640
    process of, 41–42
    tools for, 615–630
occupational therapy literature, periods and influences in, 568
Occupational Value Assessment with Predefined Items, 322, 324
odor detection evaluation, 259
old age, productive activity in, 178
older adults. *See also* aging; elderhood; elderly persons
    activity patterns of, 174–175
    as burden or resource, 172–173
    caring for grandchildren, 174
    definitions of, 170
    life expectancy and disability-free life expectancy of, 173–174
    stereotypes of, 170
olfactory sense, 251, 256
online trust, 521–522
ontogeny, 26
OPC Study, 145
operative intelligence, 25
oppositional defiant disorder, 142
oral reports, 477
order, 10
organization, 5
    activity demands of, 193–194
    assessment of, 555–556
    behavior of, 187
    complexity and change in, 190
    contexts and environments of, 194
    culture of, 188
    ethical codes related to, 473
    international perspective on social role of, 192–194
    needs assessment of, 195

occupational needs of, 193
occupational performance of, 196
occupations of, 185–196
PEOP process in, 194–196
principles of interventions for, 196
resources for, 192
roles of, 189–192
social roles of, 186
"story" of, 195
structure of, 187–188
SWOT analysis of, 194–195
types of, 187–190
vision and mission statements of, 188
organization-centered approach, 70–71
assessment and evaluation in, 71
outcomes of, 72
for self-management, 500–509
Organization for Economic Co-Operation and Development (OECD), mission of, 207
organizational behavior, 191
organizational effectiveness, fostering, 195–196
organizational evaluation, 195–196
organizational theory, 189
OTseeker database, 96
Ottawa Charter for Health Promotion, 11, 31, 201
Outcome and Assessment Information Set (OASIS), 554
outcomes, 568–569
concepts of, 567, 570–592
definition of, 640
ethical assessment of, 468–469
measures of, 77, 560, 570, 618–619
in occupational therapy literature, 569
Outcomes Assessment Information Set (OASIS), 550

Paediatric Activity Card Sort (PACS), 137, 324
pain, 301–303
Pain Intensity Scale, 302
PaperLi, 519
parallel play, 132
paralysis, 257
parenting, 162, 165
Parenting Daily Hassles (PDH), 165
Parkinson's disease, 270, 274
Parsons, Talcott, 9
participation, 5
assistive technology enabling, 442
attitudinal barriers to, 18
concepts of, 603–604
definition of, 43
with PEOP occupational therapy, 74–75
in population health, 17–18
public policies influencing, 426–429
restrictions on, 18
self-management and, 507
social factors and, 380–383
studies of, 16
Participation and Environment Measure for Children and Youth, 323, 324, 325
Partnering for Change, 145
partnership approaches, 632
partnerships, 83, 551, 552
Patient Activation Measure (PAM), 506
Patient Assessment Instrument (PAI), 550, 554
Patient Health Questionnaire-9, 222

Patient-Reported Outcome Measurement Information System (PROMIS), 208
patient-reported outcomes, 207–208
Patient's Bill of Rights, 475
Pediatric Evaluation of Disability Inventory (PEDI), 139, 352
Pediatric Interest Profiles (PIP), 137
peer groups, 134
peer review, 476
peer support services, 223, 225
perceived behavioral control, 85
Perceived Stress Scale, 301
perception, sensory factors in, 250
performance, 604. See also occupational performance
capacity for, 36
as modifier, 604–605
patterns of, 41
social factors and, 380–383
performance skills, 41, 640
peripheral nerve disorders, 261
person-centered interventions, 36–37, 63–67, 631–634
assessment and evaluation in, 66
PEOP Model in, 63–67
person-centered learning strategy, 486–495
person-centered narrative, 65–66
person-environment fit, 393–396
person-environment interaction, 395–396
person-environment misfit, 388
person-environment models, 389–399
Person-Environment-Occupation Model, 390
Person-Environment-Occupation-Performance (PEOP) Model, 1–2, 34, 39–40, 49–50, 189
aligning occupational training/education with, 550–552
central concepts of, 4–5
client-centered practice of, 52–53
concepts of, 566–640
description of, 53–55
domains of knowledge in, 50
efficacy and effectiveness in, 72–73
environment factors of, 50, 54–55, 334, 390
cultural, 335–354
health, education, social, and public policy, 422–439
physical and natural, 387–417
social, 359–383
technological, 442–463
environmental modification in, 408–413
ethical principles in, 468
framework in, 40–42
Healthy People 2020 Goals and Measures related to, 211
occupational performance focus of, 52
in occupational therapy services planning, 55
origins and aims of, 50–53
outcomes of, 73–74
person factors of, 50, 53–54, 216
cognitive, 234–245
meaning and spirituality in, 313–328
motor, 268–282
physiological, 290–309
psychological, 218–231
sensory, 250–262
population-centered approach in, 528–545
population occupations in, 200
self-management in, 500–509
systems perspective of, 52
values collaboration of, 51–52

Person-Environment-Occupation-Performance (PEOP) Occupational Therapy Process, 2, 58–59
   assessment and evaluation in, 61–62, 63
   client-centered, 60
   in cognitive learning, 486–493
   educational interventions using, 514, 522–523
   evidence-based, 60–61
   interventions in, 62
   narrative in, 61
   organization-centered, 59–60, 194–196, 373
   in organizations, 194–196
   outcomes of, 62–63, 72–77
   person-centered, 372
   in planning organization-centered interventions, 70–72
   in planning person-centered interventions, 63–67
   in planning population-centered interventions, 67–70
   population-centered, 373
   for sensory impairment assessment, 258
person factors, 5
   cognitive, 234–245
   concepts of, 611–615
   meaning and spirituality in, 313–328
   in MOHO, 35–36
   motor, 268–282
   in occupational performance, 142–150, 216
   in PEOP Model, 50, 53–54
   physiological, 290–309
   psychological, 218–231
   sensory, 250–262
   supporting and hindering learning, 489–491
   theories supporting, 25, 96–97
personal causation, 35
personal context, 41
personal environment, 402–404, 406
Personal Meaning Profile (PMP), 76–77
personal self, 87
personality characteristics, 87–89
personality typing tool, 87–89
Pew Health Professions Commission report, 468, 473
Physical Activity Readiness Questionnaire (PAR-Q), 293, 296
physical environment
   assessments of, 409–411
   interventions addressing, 414–417
   public policies affecting, 425
physical fitness
   intervention for, 296
   physiological factors in, 290–296
   quality of life and, 304
physical space, 388, 397
physiological factors, 290–304
   on occupation patterns, 122
   organizations and journals focusing on, 309
   resources for, 308
   studies related to, 305–307
   supporting and hindering learning, 490
Piaget, Jean, cognitive development theory of, 25, 131–135
Pilot RCT of CO-OP, 145
Pinterest, 519
Pittsburgh Sleep Quality Index (PSQI), 165, 299
Planned Approach to Community Health (PATCH), 531
planning skills, business, 553
plasticity, 26
play, 14–15, 132, 163, 624–625
Play History, 136

play/leisure occupation measures, 136–137
Playfulness, Test of, 136
playgroups, 132
podcasts/video casts, 520
policy environment, 137–141
Policy Implementation Assessment Tool, 432
political environment, 141
political factors, 401–402
population
   definition of, 5, 200
   ethical codes related to, 473
   health attitudes of, 9
   health of, 200–201, 208
      current priorities for, 209–210
      information sources for, 210–211
   occupation-based concepts of, 201–208
   occupational performance of, 17–18
   occupations of, 69, 200–212
   at risk, 209–210
population-centered approach, 67–70, 528–545
   AOTA position on, 540–541
   assessment and evaluation in, 69–70, 532–537
   characteristics of, 540
   interventions in, 537–544
   narrative for, 68, 529–532
   outcomes of, 70, 541
   purpose of, 537–540
Positive Affect–Negative Affect Schedule, 301, 327
Positive Behavioral Support (PBS), 514
post-traumatic stress disorders, 142
postural control, 274, 281
poverty, 164
power, divisions of, 343
practical support, 400–401
practice, law of, 278–279
practice evidence, 101–102
practice models, 630–637
practitioner-client trust, 86
Prader-Willi syndrome, 140
PRECEDE-PROCEED model, 531
Preferences for Activities for Children, 323, 324
Pregnancy Risk Assessment Monitoring System (PRAMS), 202
pre-operational stage, 132
preservation of life, 10
prevention, 636–637
   concepts of, 587–588
   definition of, 640
Prezi, 520
process measures, 560
productivity, 38, 625–626
products
   affecting performance, 399–400
   designing, 398
professional accountability, 95–97
professional advocacy, 477–478
professional associations, 478
   ethical codes and, 472–473
professional community of practice, 103
professional development, 97, 478–482
professional expertise, 101–102
professional identity, 466
professional interactions, 473
professionalism, principles supporting, 468–482
proprioception, 251

proprioceptive neuromuscular facilitation (PNF), 281
psychological factors
    assessments of, 219, 222
    interventions for, 219–226
    in learning, 490
    narratives and background literature on, 218–219
    organizations and journals focusing on, 231
    studies on, 227–230
    terms associated with, 220–221
psychoneuroimmunology, 17, 121, 320
psychosocial functioning, 577
Psychosocial Impact of Assistive Devices Scale (PIADS), 450
public access policies, 426
public environment, 405, 406
public health
    assessments in, 529–532
    current priorities for, 209–210
    definition of, 200, 528–529
    interventions for, 537–544
    narratives for, 529–532
    outcomes for, 541
    population health and, 200–201
Public Health Assessment, 537
public policies
    affecting environment, 422–437
    affecting occupational performance, 401–402
    assessments and evaluations of, 430–431, 432, 436–437
    evidence-based, 434
    ICF areas related to, 422–425
    influencing performance, participation, and well-being, 426–429
    interventions for, 431–434
    modification of, 434–436
    narrative perspective and background literature for, 422–426
    in PEOP Model, 422
    process of, 423
    resources for, 437–439
public self, 87
PubMed database, 96, 519
purpose, meaning and, 314–315
Purpose in Life Test, 327

quality measures, 560
quality of care, in population health, 18
quality of life (QOL), 10–11. *See also* health-related quality of life (HRQOL)
    concepts of, 588
    definition of, 640
    with motor control impairments, 281–282
    with PEOP occupational therapy outcome, 76–77
    of populations, 205–206
quality of life scales, vision-related, 258
Quebec User Evaluation of Satisfaction with Assistive Technology (QUEST 2.0), 450

RA Work Instability Scale, 96
race, 340
racism, 345–346
reactivity, 149
Reasoned Action and Planned Behavior Theory, 84–85
recovery, mental health, 588–589
Recreating Health Professional Practice for a New Century (Pew), 468
reflective practice, 101, 103
Reflex Model, 268

reflexes
    assessment of, 269–270
    infant, 130–131
    primitive, 269–270, 271
    testing, 275
reflexive exercises, 89–91
reflexivity, 87, 88
regulation, 149
rehabilitation
    function in, 578
    models for, 389, 631
Rehabilitation Act Amendments, 428
Rehabilitation Act of 1973, 404, 425, 427, 448
Rehabilitation International, 353
reimbursement, 553–555
reinforcement, positive and negative, 43
relatedness, need for, 317–318
Relative Intensity Test, 292
religion
    in cultural identity, 341
    health attitudes and, 9
remedial approach, 241, 242
remediation programs, 637
repetition, in motor learning, 493
Repetition Maximum test, 291, 293
research
    appropriateness of, 98–99
    in evidence-based practice, 98–101
    problems and opportunities in, 100–101
    qualitative, 100–101
    quantitative, 99
    rigorous, 99–100
    types of, 99
Resident Assessment Instrument (RAI), 550
resilience, 121, 149
Resilience Quotient, 222
resource availability, 103
resource utilization group (RUG), 554
respect, 346
respect for persons, 469
responsible collaboration, 87, 88
rest, 13, 14, 626
restorative approach, 241, 242
re-structuring, 399
retirement, 175–176
    transition to, 159
risk contracting, 509
ritual, 608
Rivermead Behavioral Memory Test, 3rd ed (RBMT-3), 240
Robert Wood Johnson Foundation, 366, 378, 380, 432, 531
Rogers, J.C., 10
role competence, 572–574
roles, 36, 41, 608–611
    expectations for, 159–160
    management of, 503, 507
    performance of, 75
Romberg test, 274
routine, 122–123, 610–611
Routine Task Inventory Expanded (RTI-E), 238
Ryff Scales of Psychological Well-Being, 327

Safe Drinking Water Act, 425
Safety Assessment of Function and the Environment for Rehabilitation (SAFER-Tool; SAFER-HOME), 410
safety awareness, 133
safety-related behavior, 191
salutogenesis, 17
sandwich generation, 162–163
SandwichGeneration.org, 166
satisfaction, 589
Satisfaction with Life Scale (SWLS), 76, 222, 327
SBAR method, 476
scaffolding, 26, 494
schizophrenia
    childhood, 142
    low occupational complexity in, 120–121
scholarly databases, 519
school-based services, reimbursement for, 555
school environment, 411–412
School Function Assessment, 138
School Outcomes Measure, 138
School Setting Interview (SSI), 138, 411
school work occupations, measures of, 138
Scoopit, 519
seating devices, 443–444
seating interventions, adaptive, 144
second career, 171
Second Life, 520
selective optimization with compensation theory, 26–27
self
    in client-therapist alliance, 87, 89
    knowledge of, 86–87
    personal/private, 87
    social/public, 87
    therapeutic use of, 82, 85–89
    tools for understanding, 87–89
self-advocacy, 606–607
Self-Awareness of Deficits Interview (SADI), 237, 238
self-care, 622
    in adolescence, 134
    in Canadian model, 38
    development of, 132
    in middle childhood, 133
self-care occupations measures, 139
self-concept, 87, 220
self-control, 572
self-determination theory, 317–318
self-efficacy, 32, 85
    in adulthood, 160
    concepts of, 590
    learning and, 490
    in personal narratives, 220
    social learning and, 31–32
    theory of, 224, 505
Self-Efficacy Gauge, 222
self-esteem, 220
self-feeding, 132
self-identity, 579–580
self-maintenance, 139, 622
self-management, 500, 507–508
    behaviors and skills of, 502
    broader context for, 500–502
    chronic illness, 590–591
    definition of, 502, 640
    interventions for, 500, 505–506, 508–509

outcomes for, 503–505
participation and, 507–508
population-centered interventions for, 540
principles of, 508
process of, 502–503
theoretical underpinnings of, 505–506
self-organization, 189, 190
self-realization, 75
Self-Regulation Skills Interview (SRSI), 238
semi-personal environment, 404–405
Semmes-Weinstein monofilaments test, 259
Sense of Coherence Scale, 327
sensemaking, 313–314, 328
    assessments and evaluations of, 322–323
    interventions for, 323–325
    outcomes related to, 326
sensory deficits/impairments, 257–259, 251–253
    interventions for, 259–261
    organizations and journals focusing on, 262
    outcomes of, 261–262
    populations and conditions affected by, 256–257
sensory factors, 253–256
    assessments and evaluations of, 251, 257–259
    definition, role, and impact of, 252–253
    major health conditions or disabilities influenced by, 250
    narrative and background literature on, 252
    understanding, 250–252
sensory gating impairment, 257
sensory integration, 261, 631
sensory motor functions, 578
sensory motor stage, 131–132
sensory perception, 252–253
sensory retraining, 261, 262
separation anxiety disorder, 142
seriation, 133
service quality, 191
shape/texture identification test, 259
shiftwork, 120
skill acquisition interventions, 143–144
skilled nursing facilities, reimbursement for, 554
skills, 36
    concepts of, 614–615
    environment interaction with, 393
skin
    integrity of, 303–304
    symbolic, 344
Skype, 518, 520
Slagle, Eleanor Clarke, 73
sleep, 13, 298
    assessments for, 165, 299
    concepts of, 626
    in daily occupation patterns, 117, 118
    duration of, 15
    health and, 299
    interventions for, 299
    pathologies of, 299
    patterns of throughout life, 299
    resources of, 166
    time spent in, 117
sleep deficits/disorders, 13–15, 164
SleepCenters.org, 166
Slideshare, 520
smell, sense of, 256
social awareness, 236

social bookmarking, 519
social capital, 368
    assessments addressing, 371, 375
    of communities, 369
    definition of, 364, 368–369
    health and, 369–370
    interventions addressing, 379
    PEOP Model and, 370
Social Capital Assessment Tool, 375
Social Capital Integrated Questionnaire (SOCAP IQ), 375
social class, 341–342
social cognitive theory, 85
social cohesion, 364
social connectedness, 364
social context, 103
social development, 25–26, 134
social emotional development, 135
social environment, 422–437
    in assistive technology assessment, 449
    in childhood occupation, 137–141
    health and, 9–10
    international perspective on, 192–194
    organizations' role in, 186, 192–194
    supporting and hindering learning, 491
social factors, 359–360
    assessments and evaluations of, 370–371
    in health, 361–367
    interventions addressing, 371–379
    narrative perspective on, 360–361
    organizations focusing on, 380
    PEOP Occupational Therapy Process and, 370
    resources for, 379–383
    studies of, 381–383
social groups, 600
social justice, 97–98, 471
social learning theory, 31–32, 132–133
social life, 123–124
social network sites, 520
social networks, 8–9, 223, 224, 225
social participation, 14, 16, 389, 604
social policies, 9
social problem solving, 505–506
Social Readjustment Rating Scale, 301
Social Relationship Scale, 374
Social Security Amendments of 1965, 9
social skills, 236
social support, 225–226, 367–368
    affecting performance, 400–401
    assessments addressing, 374–375
    definition of, 364
    interventions addressing, 378–379
    lack of, 367–368
Social Support Questionnaire, 374
sociocultural environment, public policies affecting, 425–426
socioeconomic factors, 401–402
socioemotional development, 133
somatic sensation, 254
somatosensation, 254–255
somatosensory function tests, 259
somatosensory impairments, 255, 257, 261
sound repetition screening tests, 259
SPARX, 521
spasticity, 270–271, 280
Spielberger State-Trait Anxiety Inventory for Adults, 222
spinal cord injury, 257, 270

spirituality, 313–314
    assessments and evaluations of, 322–323
    in Canadian model, 38
    interventions for, 323–325
    learning and, 490–491
    meaning and, 321–322
    organizations and journals focusing on, 328
    outcomes related to, 326
Stanford CDSM program, 504, 505, 508, 509
states, 25
stewardship, 469
Stimulus Generalization Training, 261
Stimulus Specific Training, 261
Storify, 519
strength
    interventions for, 280–281
    testing, 272–273
strength training, 277
stress, 299–300
    activity and, 16–17
    adaptation to, 17
    assessment and interventions for, 300
    categories of, 300
    in learning process, 490
    meaning and, 320–321
    measures of, 301
stretch reflexes, 269, 271
    hyperactive, 270
stretching, 277, 280
stroke survivors
    motor function impairment in, 270
    motor recovery measures for, 273
    sensory impairment in, 257
    sensory retraining programs for, 261
    somatosensory loss in, 255
structural process measures, 560
Study of the Effectiveness of Neurorehabilitation on Sensation (SENSe), 261, 262
subjective norms, 84–85
suicide, in children and youth, 142
support groups, 223, 225
Survey of Technology Use, 450
SurveyMonkey, 520
Swinburne University Emotional Intelligence Test, 327
SWOT (strengths, weaknesses, opportunities, and threats) analysis, 194–195, 555–556, 557
Symbolic and Imaginative Play Developmental Checklist (SIPDC), 136
Symbolic Play Test, 136
systems change framework, 500
Systems Model of Motor Control, 268, 269
systems theory, 52, 189

Tactile Discrimination Test, 259
Task/Context-Focused Approach, 144
task-oriented training, 277, 279–280, 631
task-specific learning, 242, 243
tasks, 611
    in daily occupation, 115–116
    in working alliance, 86
taste, sense of, 256
technology, 442. *See also* assistive technology; computers
    affecting performance, 399–400
    digital, in education, 518–522
    in documentation, 476–477
    evidence base of, 455–462

temperament, 149
temporal pattern, 121
theories, 24–25. *See also* specific theories
therapeutic alliance, 85–86
therapeutic change agent, 619
third age, 170, 175–178
time, experience of, 121–122
time budget methods, 124
time geography methodology, 124–125
time use, 118–119
    computer programs to analyze, 125
    in cultural context, 343
    measuring, 124–125
    occupation and, 121
    of older adults, 174–175
    patterns of, 120
    of populations, 202–205
    society and cultural structures influencing, 123–124
Timed Up and Go (TUG) test, 274, 275
toddlerhood, development and occupation in, 130–132
toileting, 132
tool concepts, 568
touch, 251
Tourette syndrome, 140
transformations, 25
transitions, 159
    to adolescence, 134
    to adulthood, 158–159
    in childhood development, 133
translational research, 104–106
traumatic brain injury, 141
    cognitive deficits with, 234
    motor function impairment in, 270
    participation and well-being with, 16
    sensory impairment with, 257
    spasticity in, 280
treadmill test, 292
tremors, 276
trust, in online environment, 521–522
truth, in cultural context, 342
Twitter, 518, 519
2-point Disk-Criminator, 259

underemployment, 161
unemployment, 121, 160–161
Unemployment Insurance, 166
United Nations High Commission for Refugees, 353
University of Kansas Community Tool Box, 378
University of Rhode Island Change Assessment, 222
utilitarian approach, 469

VA Caregiver Support Services, 166
VAK model, 150
Value and Meaning in Occupations (ValMO) model, 322
values, 35
    about doing, 593–596
    of client, 102
    in cultural identity, 342
values collaboration, 51–52
veracity, 471
vertigo, 255–256
vestibular function tests, 259
vestibular sense
    deficits in, 255–256, 261
    evidence-based assessments of, 251

    key knowledge about, 255
    in occupational performance, 255
vestibulo-ocular reflex, 255
Vineland Adaptive Behavior Scales, 2nd ed (Vineland-II), 139
virtual pinboard, 519
virtual presentation, 520
virtual worlds, multi-user, 520
vision, 253
    assessments of, 251
    impairments of, 256, 257, 260–261
    loss of, 253–254, 258
vision statements, 556
vision technologies, 444, 454
visual acuity testing, 258
visual analog scales (VAS), 96, 302
visual field tests, 258
visual learning, 150
VISUAL-TimePAcTS, 125
Vocational Rehabilitation Act of 1920, 402
voice over Internet protocol (VoIP), 518, 520
volition, 35, 149, 615
Volitional Questionnaire and Pediatric Volitional Questionnaire, 222
volume of oxygen measure, 292
Voting Accessibility for the Elderly and Handicapped Act, 423, 425, 428
Vygotsky, Lev, 25–26

water, as life energy, 37
Watson, John B., 43
Ways of Coping Questionnaire, 222, 327
Weinstein Enhanced Sensory Test (WEST), 259
well-being, 5, 76
    assessments of, 327
    assistive technology enabling, 442
    balance in, 119–120
    concepts of, 30, 207, 591–592, 640
    emotions and meaning in, 319–321
    factors in, 30
    health and, 12, 30–31
    holistic view of, 31
    measures of, 206–208
    participation and, 16
    in personal narratives, 221
    of populations, 206–207
    public policies influencing, 426–429
    social factors and, 380, 381–383
    subjective, 76
well elderly persons, 178–180
wellness, 592
Westmead Home Safety Assessment, 407, 410
Wheelchair Outcome Measures (WhOM), 451
Wheelchair Skills Test, 451
wheelchairs, 442, 444
Whiteford, Gail, 9–10
Wii, 521
Wikipedia, 519
wikis, 518, 519
will, 615
Wolf Motor Function Test (WMFT), 276
women
    changing roles of, 159
    leisure occupations of, 163
Wordpress, 519
Words With Friends, 521
work, 15, 160–161
    activities of, 14

analogues for, 177
concepts of, 626–627
resources of, 166
Work Addiction Risk Test (WART), 165
Work Environment Impact Scale (WEIS), 411
Work Experience Survey, 411
work-family balance, 191
work-leisure balance, 163
work-life balance, 118
workaholism, 161, 165
working alliance, 85–87
Working America AFL-CIO: Unemployment Lifeline, 166
workplace assessment, 411
Workplace Technology Predisposition Assessment, 450
World Federation of Occupational Therapists (WFOT), core competencies of, 192–193
World Health Organization (WHO)
    Commission on the Social Determinants of Health, 363–365, 367
    health definition of, 11–12
    Health Promotion Conference, 31
    holistic view of, 30
    International Classification of Functioning, Disability and Health, 43–45, 350
    Ottawa Charter for Health Promotion of, 11, 31, 201
    purpose of, 353
    quality of life measure of, 206
World of Warcraft, 521
wound care training, 303
Wrist Position Sense Test, 259

xenophobia, 345–346

Years Lived with Disability (YLD), 532
Years of Life Lost (YLL), 532
Youth Risk Behavior Surveillance System (YRBS), 202
YouTube, 520

zeitgebers, 122
ZohoWriter, 519
Zone of Proximal Development, 26

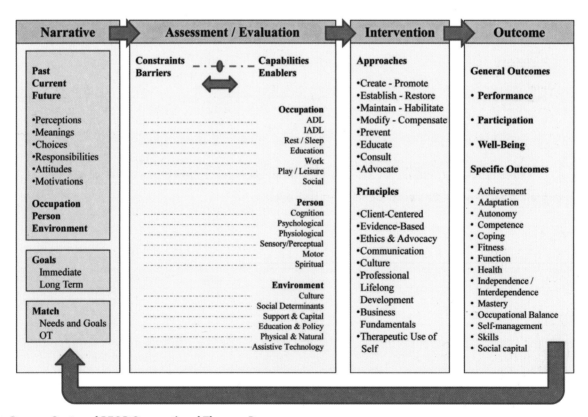

Narrative	Assessment / Evaluation	Intervention	Outcome

Narrative

Past
Current
Future

•Environments
•Behaviors
•Demographics
•Disparities
•Incidence
•Prevalence

Occupation
Person
Environment

Goals
General
Occupational

Match
Needs and Goals
OT

Assessment / Evaluation

Constraints   Capabilities
Barriers   Enablers

Occupation
Learning
General Tasks
Communication
Mobility
Domestic Life
Interpersonal
Major Life Areas
Community

Population
Cognition
Psychological
Physiological
Sensory/Perceptual
Motor
Spiritual

Environment
Culture
Social Determinants
Support & Capital
Education & Policy
Physical & Natural
Assistive Technology

Intervention

Approaches

•Create - Promote
•Establish- Restore
•Maintain - Habilitate
•Modify - Compensate
•Prevent
•Educate
•Consult
•Advocate

Principles

•Client-Centered
•Evidence-Based
•Ethics & Advocacy
•Communication
•Culture
•Professional
 Lifelong
 Development
•Business
 Fundamentals
•Therapeutic Use of
 Self

Outcome

General Outcomes

•**Performance**

•**Participation**

•**Well-Being**

Specific Outcomes

• Access: Health and
  Prevention Services
• Educational
  Achievement
• Employment
• Good Nutrition
  and Physical Activity
• Health: Indicators
  and Equality
• Injury and Violence
  Prevention
• Mental Health
• Home, Community and
  Workplace Safety
• Social Participation
• Fall Prevention

Population-Centered PEOP Occupational Therapy Process

Narrative	Assessment / Evaluation	Intervention	Outcome

Narrative

Past
Current
Future

•Perceptions
•Meanings
•Choices
•Responsibilities
•Attitudes
•Motivations

Occupation
Person
Environment

Goals
Immediate
Long Term

Match
Needs and Goals
OT

Assessment / Evaluation

Constraints   Capabilities
Barriers   Enablers

Occupation
ADL
IADL
Rest / Sleep
Education
Work
Play / Leisure
Social

Person
Cognition
Psychological
Physiological
Sensory/Perceptual
Motor
Spiritual

Environment
Culture
Social Determinants
Support & Capital
Education & Policy
Physical & Natural
Assistive Technology

Intervention

Approaches

•Create - Promote
•Establish - Restore
•Maintain - Habilitate
•Modify - Compensate
•Prevent
•Educate
•Consult
•Advocate

Principles

•Client-Centered
•Evidence-Based
•Ethics & Advocacy
•Communication
•Culture
•Professional
 Lifelong
 Development
•Business
 Fundamentals
•Therapeutic Use of
 Self

Outcome

General Outcomes

• **Performance**

• **Participation**

• **Well-Being**

Specific Outcomes

• Achievement
• Adaptation
• Autonomy
• Competence
• Coping
• Fitness
• Function
• Health
• Independence /
  Interdependence
• Mastery
• Occupational Balance
• Self-management
• Skills
• Social capital

Person-Centered PEOP Occupational Therapy Process